# Endocrinology in Clinical Practice

**Second Edition**

# Endocrinology in Clinical Practice

## Second Edition

**Edited by**

**Philip E. Harris**
Ipsen Biopharm Ltd.
and
Honorary Consultant Endocrinologist
University Hospital Lewisham
London, UK

**Pierre-Marc G. Bouloux**
Director of the Centre for Neuroendocrinology
Royal Free Campus, University College London Medical School
London, UK

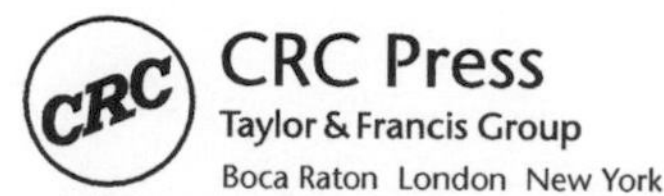


CRC Press is an imprint of the
Taylor & Francis Group, an **informa** business

CRC Press
Taylor & Francis Group
6000 Broken Sound Parkway NW, Suite 300
Boca Raton, FL 33487-2742

First issued in paperback 2020



ISBN-13: 978-1-138-03305-4 (pbk)



**Visit the Taylor & Francis Web site at**
**http://www.taylorandfrancis.com**

**and the CRC Press Web site at**
**http://www.crcpress.com**

# Contents

# Foreword by Dr. Ken Ho

Endocrinology is one of the most dynamic disciplines in biomedical science. It is among the most quantitative of the clinical specialties in which the marriage of basic and clinical sciences is very strong. The molecular revolution has led to an explosion of new information, bringing exciting insights and discoveries that have changed concepts of disease causation and treatment. How can all this information reach the practicing endocrinologist or trainee in a digestible form? What is required is a book that lays out the endocrine landscape, detailing where and how this is changing in ways that advance patient care.

It is this challenging confluence of research and patient care that has driven my work over 30 years as an endocrinologist and clinical scientist and now research director at a major teaching hospital in Australia, collaborating with likeminded colleagues internationally. My major area of interest is the neuroendocrine basis of metabolic disease with particular focus on the role of pituitary hormones.

I first met Philip and Pierre in London at the Clinical Endocrinology Trust Medallist of the British Endocrine Societies in 2000. We formed a strong bond through our shared fascination with, and commitment to, advancing the teaching, research, and management of endocrine disease. Philip and Pierre epitomize a rare breed: consultant endocrinologists with a passion to bring in advances to clinical practice. They are the beneficiaries of training at St. Bartholomew's Hospital, London, with Professor Michael Besser, and inspired by their mentor, they were drawn to neuroendocrinology, a field that demands a deep understanding of systems biology and its relevance to human disease. Together, they have made significant contributions: Philip in thyroid and pituitary disease, Pierre in reproductive endocrinology. Philip has carved a highly successful career for himself in the pharmaceutical industry while holding a consultant endocrinologist appointment at University Hospital Lewisham, London. As vice-president of Scientific Affairs at Ipsen, he provides strategic direction and opportunities in the development of new compounds, and he also takes collaborative opportunities to key opinion leaders at leading centers internationally. He brings an industry perspective to knowledge transfer in the advancement of patient care. Pierre, as Director of the Neuroendocrine Centre at the Royal Free Hospital, continues to advance research into the genetic basis of central hypogonadism. They both share a love of teaching and mentoring. Pierre brings in a particular brand of humor to teaching that is both memorable and highly engaging. Nothing stands clearer in my mind than the roars of laughter that interspersed a meet-the-professor delivery by Pierre at a 2007 meeting in Sao Paolo, Brazil. Together, they have assembled a distinguished authorship team from the United Kingdom, Europe, and the United States, the members of which, like themselves, are not only world leaders but also practicing endocrinologists.

In this second edition, Philip and Pierre have harnessed advances in clinical practice in a readable and succinct style by drawing on their considerable knowledge, experience, and network as leading consultant endocrinologists. This is a well-crafted compendium of practical information, invaluable for the clinical endocrine readership who will find relevant basic science covering the tenets of endocrine disease dovetailed to practical assessment, investigation, and management of the patient.

Buy it, read it, and keep it.

Ken Ho
*Professor of Medicine, University of Queensland*
*Chair, Centres for Health Research, Princess Alexandra Hospital*
*Translation Research Institute, Brisbane, Australia*
*Past President, Growth Hormone Research Society*
*President, Pituitary Society*

# Preface

The objective of the first edition was to provide cutting-edge information on clinical practice for practicing endocrinologists and doctors training in endocrinology. The second edition retains this ethos, but it has been extensively updated and modified. Endocrinology is moving toward an increasingly personalized approach to patient management. This is reflected by the increased focus on mechanisms of disease and biomarkers.

Certain subjects, such as neuroendocrine disease (Chapter 1), take a more generalized approach to the field, before focusing on specific diseases. The chapter is supported by protocols for pituitary function testing in the appendix. Separate chapters have been assigned to pituitary radiotherapy and surgery. Other chapters are more specifically focused from the outset. There is a dedicated chapter for imaging, which has changed considerably in the past few years, particularly with the increasing use of positron emission tomography.

A major stride forward has been achieved in the field of pituitary disease with the identification of aryl hydrocarbon receptor–interacting protein mutations in a proportion of patients with familial isolated pituitary adenomas. Accordingly, there is a new chapter dedicated to this topic. Neuroendocrine tumors are included for the first time as a separate chapter, because the incidence of this disease is increasing rapidly, and endocrinologists frequently take a leading role in their management. Closely linked to neuroendocrine tumors, there is a new chapter on hereditary primary hyperparathyroidism and multiple endocrine neoplasia. New chapters on disorders in calcium regulation and genetics of infertility reflect the mechanistic and genomic advances that have been made in recent times. Finally, there is a new chapter on the endocrinology of aging, focusing on the highly relevant endocrinological changes that occur in this group of individuals, who form an increasing part of the clinician's responsibilities.

A separate pharmacopeia has not been included in this edition, because details of pharmacological treatments are included in each chapter where relevant.

We are most grateful to our colleagues who have kindly found the time to contribute to this book. Finally, as ever, our thanks to our families for their patience and support during this endeavor.

Philip E. Harris
Pierre-Marc G. Bouloux

# Editor Biographies

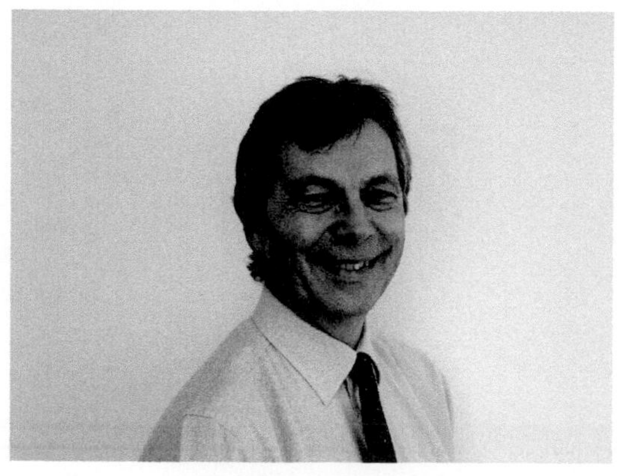

**Philip E. Harris** trained in endocrinology as an MRC Training Fellow at the University of Wales College of Medicine, at St. Bartholomew's Hospital, London, and The University of Newcastle upon Tyne. In 1990–1991, Dr. Harris worked as an MRC Travelling Fellow at the Endocrine and Reproductive Endocrine units, Massachusetts General Hospital, Boston, USA. In 1994, he was appointed senior lecturer and consultant endocrinologist at King's College Hospital, London. His main clinical and research interest is in the field of endocrine oncology, in particular, pituitary disease. Dr. Harris is currently vice president for Scientific Affairs, Ipsen Biopharm Ltd. He is also an Honorary Consultant in Endocrinology at University Hospital Lewisham, London.

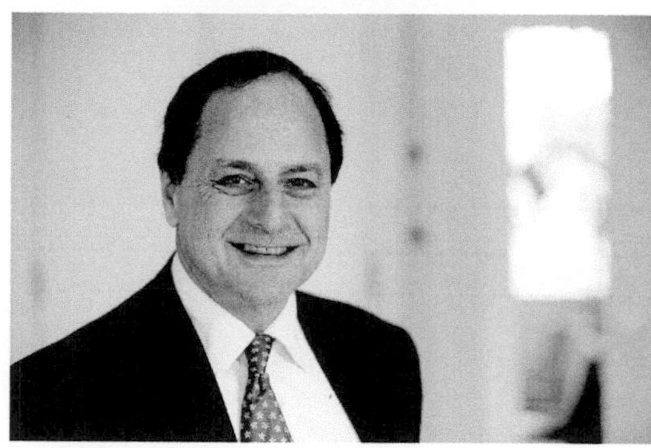

**Pierre-Marc G. Bouloux** is presently director of the Centre for Neuroendocrinology at the Royal Free and University College Medical School. He was an MRC Training Fellow under Michael Besser at St. Bartholomew's Hospital and was subsequently lecturer in medicine at the University Department of Medicine at St. Bartholomew's Hospital. He has held his present post since 1991. In addition to running a clinical service, he also has a special interest in neuroendocrinology. He has published more than 150 peer-reviewed publications.

# Contributors

**Thankamma Ajithkumar**
Department of Clinical Oncology
Norfolk and Norwich University Hospital
Norwich, UK

**Anjali Amin**
Endocrinology, Imperial AHSC
St Mary's Hospital
London, UK

**Renata S. Auriemma**
Department of Endocrinology
Centre Hospitalier Universitaire de Liège
University of Liège
Liège, Belgium

**Simon Aylwin**
Department of Endocrinology
King's College Hospital
London, UK

**Garni Barkhoudarian**
John Wayne Cancer Institute
Los Angeles, California

**Rachel L. Batterham**
Centre for Obesity Research
Department of Medicine
Rayne Institute
University College London
London, UK

**Albert Beckers**
Department of Endocrinology
Centre Hospitalier Universitaire de Liège
University of Liège
Liège, Belgium

**Arie Berghout**
Department of Internal Medicine
Diakonessenhuis Utrecht
Utrecht, the Netherlands

**Shalender Bhasin**
Centre for Neuroendocrinology
Royal Free Campus
University College Medical School
London, UK

**Jamshed Bomanji**
Institute of Nuclear Medicine
University College London
London, UK

**Pierre-Marc G. Bouloux**
Centre for Neuroendocrinology
Royal Free Campus
University College Medical School
London, UK

**Michael Brada**
Radiation Oncology
University of Liverpool Clatterbridge Cancer Centre NHS Foundation Trust
Wirral, UK

**David R. Clemmons**
Department of Medicine
University of North Carolina
Chapel Hill, North Carolina

**John M. Connell**
College of Medicine, Dentistry and Nursing
Ninewells Hospital and Medical School
Dundee, Scotland

**Adrian F. Daly**
Department of Endocrinology
Centre Hospitalier Universitaire de Liège
University of Liège
Domaine Universitaire du Sart-Tilman
Liège, Belgium

**William M. Drake**
Department of Endocrinology
St. Bartholomew's Hospital
London, UK

**Stephen Franks**
Reproductive Endocrinology
Institute of Reproductive and Developmental Biology
Imperial College London
Hammersmith Hospital
London, UK

**Marie Freel**
Institute of Cardiovascular and Medical Sciences
University of Glasgow
Glasgow, Scotland

**Philip E. Harris**
Ipsen Biopharm Ltd.
and
Honorary Consultant Endocrinologist
University Hospital Lewisham
London, UK

**Laszlo Hegedüs**
Endocrinology
University of Southern Denmark
and
Department of Endocrinology and Metabolism
Odense University Hospital
Odense, Denmark

**Gudmundur Johannsson**
Department of Endocrinology
Institute of Medicine
Sahlgrenska Academy
University of Gothenburg
Gothenburg, Sweden

**Efthimia Karra**
Centre for Obesity Research
Department of Medicine
Rayne Institute
University College London
London, UK

**Catharina Larsson**
Department of Oncology-Pathology
Karolinska Institutet
Karolinska University Hospital
Stockholm, Sweden

**Edward R. Laws, Jr.**
Pituitary/Neuroendocrine Program
Department of Neurosurgery
Brigham and Women's Hospital
Harvard Medical School
Boston, Massachusetts

**Yanhe Lue**
Division of Endocrinology
Department of Medicine
Harbor UCLA Medical Center and Los Angeles Biomedical Institute
Torrance, California

**Frances McManus**
Institute of Cardiovascular and Medical Sciences
University of Glasgow
Glasgow, Scotland

**Alex F. Muller**
Department of Internal Medicine
Internist and Endocrinologist
Diakonessenhuis Utrecht
Utrecht, the Netherlands

**Anna G. Nilsson**
Department of Endocrinology
Institute of Medicine
Sahlgrenska Academy
University of Gothenburg
Gothenburg, Sweden

**Dermot O'Toole**
Department of Clinical Medicine and Gastroenterology
St. James's Hospital and Trinity College
Dublin, Ireland

**Maxime Palazzo**
Department of Pancreatology and Neuroendocrine Tumours
Beaujon Hospital and University Paris 7
Paris, France

**Sofia Rahman**
Centre for Obesity Research
Department of Medicine
Rayne Institute
University College London
London, UK

**Stephen Robinson**
Consultant Endocrinologist Imperial AHSC
St Mary's Hospital
London, UK

**Philippe Ruszniewski**
Department of Pancreatology and Neuroendocrine Tumours
Beaujon Hospital and University Paris 7
Paris, France

**Rakesh Sajjan**
Institute of Nuclear Medicine
University College London
London, UK

**David Scott-Coombes**
Department of Endocrine Surgery
University Hospital of Wales
Cardiff, UK

**Dolores Shoback**
Endocrine Research Unit
Department of Veterans Affairs medical Center
University of California
San Francisco, California

**Terry J. Smith**
Frederick G.L. Huetwell
Ophthalmology and Visual Sciences and Internal Medicine
University of Michigan Medical School
Ann Arbor, Michigan

**Michael J. Stechman**
Department of Endocrine Surgery
University Hospital of Wales
Cardiff, UK

**Prasanth N. Surampudi**
Division of Endocrinology
Department of Medicine
Harbor UCLA Medical Center and Los Angeles Biomedical Institute
Torrance, California

**Ronald Swerdloff**
Division of Endocrinology
Department of Medicine
Harbor UCLA Medical Center and Los Angeles Biomedical Institute
Torrance, California

**Emma Tham**
Department of Clinical Genetics
Karolinska University Hospital
and
Department of Molecular Medicine and Surgery
Karolinska Institutet
Stockholm, Sweden

**Peter J. Trainer**
Department of Endocrinology
The Christie Foundation NHS Trust
Manchester Academic Health Science Centre
Manchester, UK

**Stylianos Tsagarakis**
Department of Endocrinology, Diabetes and Metabolism
Evangelismos Hospital
Athens, Greece

**Marinella Tzanela**
Department of Endocrinology, Diabetes and Metabolism
Evangelismos Hospital
Athens, Greece

**Ploutarchos Tzoulis**
Centre for Neuroendocrinology
Royal Free Campus
University College Medical School
London, UK

**Vladimir Vasilev**
Department of Endocrinology
Centre Hospitalier Universitaire de Liège
University of Liège
Liège, Belgium

**Dimitra Argyro Vassiliadi**
Department of Internal Medicine
Endocrine Unit
"Attikon" University Hospital
Athens, Greece

**Christina Wang**
Division of Endocrinology
Department of Medicine
Harbor UCLA Medical Center and Los Angeles Biomedical Institute
Torrance, California

**Ben Whitelaw**
Department of Endocrinology
King's College Hospital
London, UK

**Ahmed Yousseif**
Centre for Obesity Research
Department of Medicine
Rayne Institute
University College London
London, UK

# 1

# Neuroendocrine disease

*Philip E. Harris*

## *The normal hypothalamic–pituitary axis (see Chapter 5, Figure 5.1)*

Normal anterior pituitary function is under the central control of the hypothalamus and higher centers. Hypothalamic releasing and inhibitory factors are secreted into the capillaries of the hypophysial portal circulation at the median eminence. The neurohypophysis consists of neurons arising from the magnocellular and parvocellular neurons of the supraoptic and paraventricular nuclei. The anatomical relationships of the hypothalamus and surrounding brain structures can be clearly demonstrated on magnetic resonance imaging (MRI) scan. The posterior pituitary (neurohypophysis) characteristically has a high signal on T1-weighted images that is lost in cranial diabetes insipidus (Figure 1.1).

## *Classification of hypothalamic–pituitary disease*

Hypothalamic–pituitary disease is associated with increased mortality.[1] Endocrine dysfunction secondary to hypothalamic disease (Table 1.1) usually results in hypopituitarism. Rarely, activation of the hypothalamic–pituitary axis can occur. A well-recognized but rare example of this activation is precocious puberty, which may be associated with hypothalamic tumors such as neurofibromas, hamartomas, and pinealomas. Very rarely, hypothalamic tumors can produce releasing factors, resulting in pituitary hyperfunction. Acromegaly has been reported to occur as a result of the hypothalamic production of growth hormone–releasing hormone (GHRH) from hypothalamic tumors.[2] Similarly, Cushing's syndrome has been reported in association with the production of corticotropin-releasing hormone (CRH) by hypothalamic gangliocytomas.[3] Hyperprolactinemia is a frequent accompaniment of hypothalamic disease, secondary to damage of the dopaminergic (D2) neurons in the arcuate nucleus. Diabetes insipidus may complicate hypothalamic disease, in contrast to primary pituitary disease, where diabetes insipidus is almost never seen. There are certain clinical features that are indicative of hypothalamic disease rather than of pituitary disease. Obesity and hyperphagia pose major clinical problems for which there is, at present, no simple solution. Somnolence is also a characteristic feature that often occurs in conjunction with hyperphagia and obesity. Thermodysregulation and psychiatric disturbance can also occur[4] (Table 1.2).

Pituitary tumors are classified preoperatively in terms of function and size (Figures 1.2 through 1.5). There are several ways of classifying pituitary tumor size and invasion. In practice, most clinicians classify tumors on the basis of MRI or high-resolution computerized tomography (CT) imaging as grades 1–4 (Table 1.3). Postoperatively, tumors are routinely classified on the basis of histology and immunocytochemistry (Figure 1.6). The World Health Organization (WHO) 2004 classification of pituitary tumors describes typical adenoma; atypical adenoma with abnormal morphology: elevated proliferative indices (Ki-67 >3%, >2 mitoses/ 10 high power fields) and extensive nuclear p53 immunoreactivity; carcinoma. Functional classification is now well established but lacks predictive value[5] (Table 1.4). The identification and application of novel molecular markers is now being

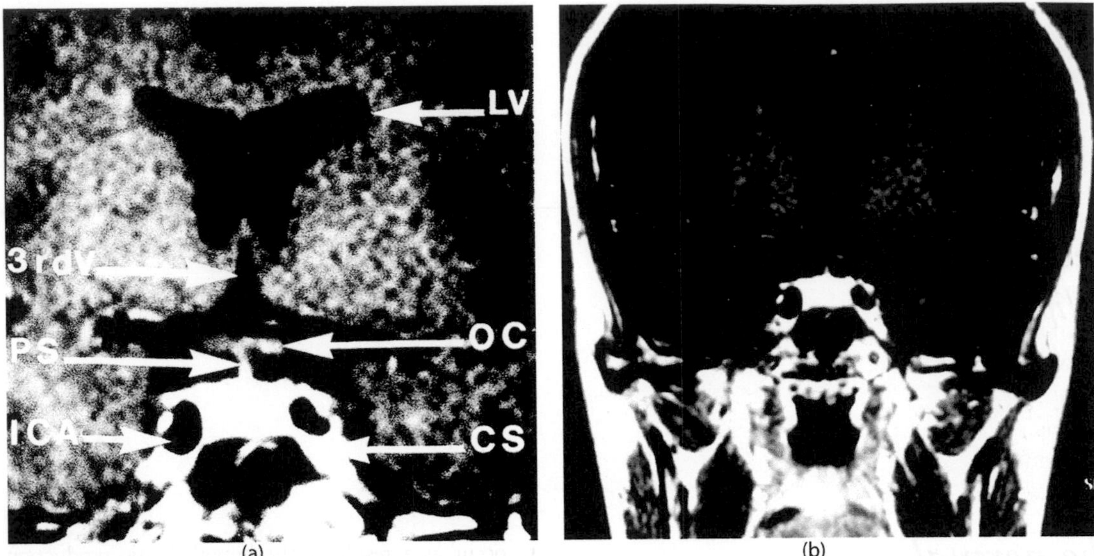


*Figure 1.1*
*Coronal MRI scan (T1-weighted) demonstrating the pituitary gland, hypothalamus, and surrounding structures; scan a is an enlargement of scan b. LV, lateral ventricle; 3rd V, third ventricle; OC, optic chiasm; PS, pituitary stalk; ICA, internal carotid artery; CS, cavernous sinus (includes third, fourth, first and second divisions of fifth and sixth cranial nerves).*

used to develop a more accurate prognostic classification of pituitary tumors, as clinical practice increasingly moves toward the personalized care of patients.[6] Pituitary carcinomas are very rare.[7]

Unlike hypothalamic disease that is usually manifested by hormone deficiency syndromes, pituitary tumors present with a wide variety of different features. In general, pituitary tumors can present with local pressure effects (Table 1.5), hypopituitarism, and/or syndromes of hormone excess.

An empty or partially empty sella on pituitary imaging (Figure 1.7) does not necessarily indicate an underlying pathology because this finding may represent a normal anatomical variant. Empty sella may also be seen in patients after pituitary surgery, radiotherapy, macroprolactinomas treated with dopamine (DA) agonists, and pituitary apoplexy.

Pituitary apoplexy usually occurs as a result of infarction of a pituitary tumor. It characteristically presents with a sudden onset of severe, debilitating headache that can last for several days, sometimes in association with cranial nerve lesions and acute onset of visual loss (Figure 1.8). Occasionally, patients may develop visual field defects, due to herniation of the optic chiasm into the fossa (see Chapter 24).

The optic chiasm is normally situated directly over the pituitary gland (80%), prefixed (15%), and postfixed (5%). The characteristic early field defect seen with a symmetrical suprasellar extension impinging on normally located chiasm is a bitemporal superior quadrantopia (Figure 1.9). This defect is due to the initial involvement of the decussating fibers originating from the inferior and nasal retinas. Further tumor growth involves the upper nasal fibers, with the development of the classical bitemporal hemianopia. Other patterns of visual disturbance are also frequently seen, depending upon the position of the chiasm and the site of suprasellar extension (Figure 1.10).

# Principles of treatment

## Pituitary surgery (see Chapter 3)

Neuroendocrine tumors should be managed in specialist centers. The management of these tumors requires a multidisciplinary approach involving specialists in endocrinology, neurosurgery, neuroradiology, radiotherapy, and neuropathology who have a particular interest in the subject. The cure of a pituitary tumor should aim for the complete removal of the tumor, with reversal of associated pressure effects such as visual field defects, the normalization of abnormal hormone secretion and

| |
|---|
| Congenital hypophysiotrophic hormone deficiencies |
| Isolated GnRH deficiency (olfactory–genital syndrome—Kallman's syndrome) |
| Isolated TRH deficiency |
| Isolated GHRH deficiency |
| Hypothalamic tumors |
| Craniopharyngioma |
| Arachnoid cyst |
| Hamartoma |
| Gangliocytoma |
| Glioma |
| Choristoma |
| Chordoma |
| Hypothalamic infiltration |
| Sarcoidosis |
| Histiocytosis X |
| Metastatic disease, e.g., breast |
| Infection |
| Tuberculosis |
| Meningitis |
| Viral encephalitis |
| Trauma |
| Stalk section, e.g., road traffic accident |
| Direct hypothalamic damage, e.g., surgery |
| Cranial irradiation |
| Vascular |
| Infarct |
| Aneurysm, subarachnoid hemorrhage |
| Arteriovenous malformation |

GnRH, gonadotrophin-releasing hormone; TRH, thyrotropin-releasing hormone; GHRH, growth hormone–releasing hormone.

***Table 1.1***
*Classification of hypothalamic diseases.*

associated metabolic abnormalities, the reversal of abnormal pituitary function, or the retention of normal pituitary function.

## *Perioperative medical management (see also Appendix)*

Patients undergoing pituitary surgery should be managed jointly by the neurosurgeon and the endocrinologist.

| |
|---|
| Disorders of food intake |
| Hyperphagia |
| Anorexia |
| Disorders of temperature regulation |
| Hyperthermia |
| Hypothermia |
| Poikilothermia |
| Disorders of drinking |
| Adipsia |
| Compulsive drinking |
| Disorders of sleep and consciousness |
| Somnolence |
| Altered sleeping patterns |
| Disorders of psychological functioning |
| Behavioral changes |
| Altered cognition |
| Disorders of neurological functioning |
| Raised intracranial pressure |
| Epilepsy |
| Impaired motor function |
| Impaired sensory function |
| Impaired autonomic function |

***Table 1.2***
*Non-endocrine manifestations of hypothalamic disease.*

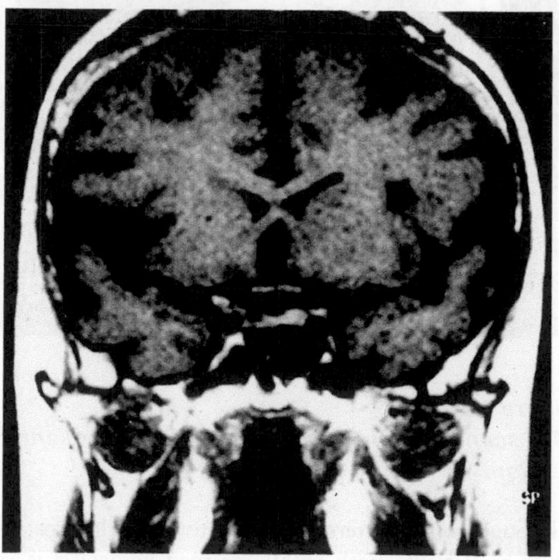

***Figure 1.2***
*Coronal MRI scan (T1-weighted) demonstrating a pituitary microadenoma (hypodense area on the right).*

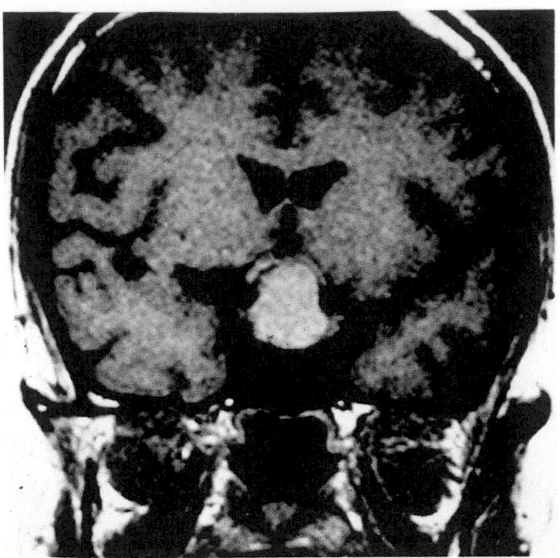

**Figure 1.3**
*Coronal MRI scan (T1-weighted) demonstrating a pituitary macroadenoma with suprasellar extension, compressing the optic chiasm.*

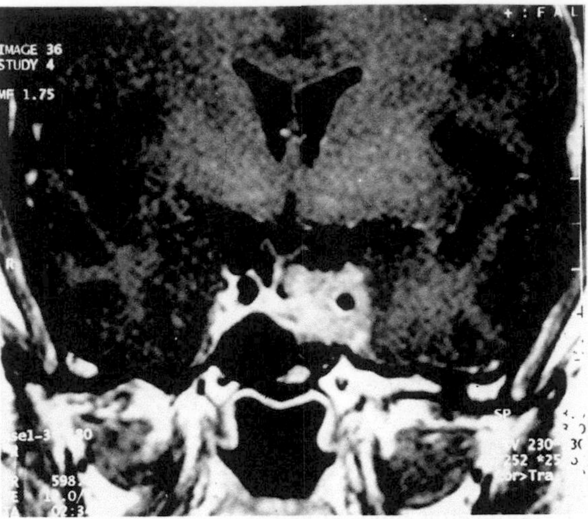


**Figure 1.4**
*Coronal MRI scan demonstrating an invasive pituitary macroadenoma, extending into the left cavernous sinus, with suprasellar extension.*

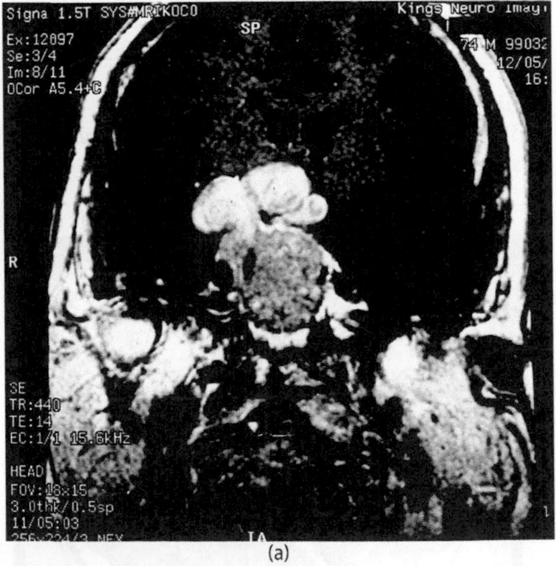


(a)

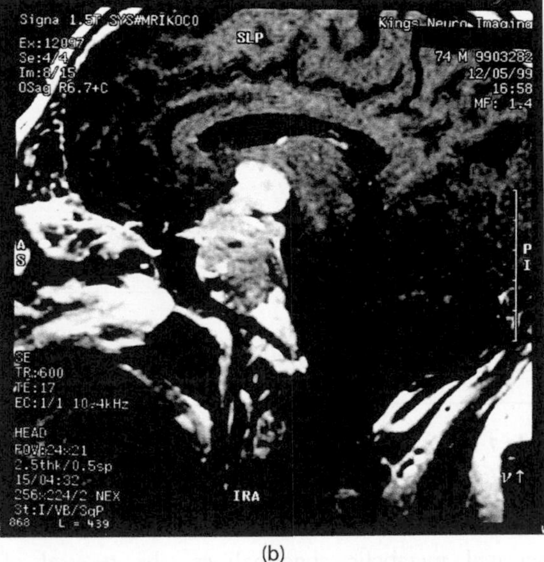


(b)

**Figure 1.5**
*MRI scan (T1-weighted) demonstrating a giant invasive macroadenoma. (a) Coronal section. (b) Sagittal section.*

Although some centers elect not to give glucocorticoid cover to patients with small microadenomas, it is certainly a safe policy to routinely provide all patients with perioperative glucocorticoid cover. Patients are frequently overtreated with glucocorticoids perioperatively, with consequent attendant risks of hypertension, glucose intolerance, poor wound healing, wound infections, and electrolyte disturbances. It is usually unnecessary to provide anything more than a modest increase in what would normally be replacement therapy. Patients with Cushing's

| Tumor grade | Tumor size |
|---|---|
| 1 | Microadenoma (<1 cm in diameter) |
| 2 | Macroadenoma (>1 cm in diameter); enclosed within sella, no erosion |
| 3 | Macroadenoma with enlarged sella |
| | Localized erosion/destruction |
| | Invasive macroadenoma |
| 4 | Giant macroadenoma (>4 cm in diameter) |

***Table 1.3***
*Imaging classification of pituitary tumor size (see Figures 1.2–1.5).*

syndrome should be treated with a higher dose of glucocorticoids than other patients. All patients should receive routine antibiotic prophylaxis as dictated by local neurosurgical preference.

Postoperative diabetes insipidus is not uncommon in the first 2–3 days in patients who have undergone surgery for macroadenomas, but in most cases it is transient. This may be masked if the patient is hypoadrenal. A detailed fluid balance chart is mandatory. The diagnosis is confirmed by the demonstration of polyuria (urine output >200 mL/h), plasma osmolality (>300 mOsmol/kg), and inappropriately dilute urine (<150 mOsmol/kg). There may be evidence of intravascular fluid depletion, with high-normal plasma sodium and high plasma urea and creatinine. If treatment is required, the patient should be given 1 μg of desmopressin acetate subcutaneous (s.c.). It is extremely dangerous for the patient to be given desmopressin without clear documentation of diabetes insipidus.

Ideally, patients should undergo a full endocrine assessment before discharge from the hospital, or failing this time frame, within 4–6 weeks of discharge. In the latter event, the patient should be discharged home on glucocorticoid replacement therapy.

# Medical treatment

## Dopaminergic agonists

Dopaminergic (D2) agonists are the first-line treatment of choice for prolactinomas.[8] They may also be used in acromegaly.[9] The first D2 agonist that became available was the ergot bromocriptine. A major side effect of bromocriptine is nausea and vomiting. Postural hypotension is a less frequent problem. Psychiatric complications occur very rarely, but they can be extremely serious[10] (Table 1.6).[12] Most patients can tolerate bromocriptine if it is commenced as a small dose (1–2.5 mg) last thing at night with a snack. To minimize the postural effect, the patient should be instructed not to get up out of bed on the first night. After three nights, the bedtime dose can be doubled; thereafter, the total dose can be slowly increased according to tolerance, by starting doses with breakfast and then later with lunch. If this approach is done slowly, the majority of patients will be able to tolerate bromocriptine given in split doses, three times daily. Some patients may be controlled on twice- or once-daily doses. Therapeutic dosages are usually in the region of 2.5–15 mg/day. There remains, however, a small group of approximately 10%–15% of patients who have genuine intolerance to oral bromocriptine.

Quinagolide is a nonergot that can be administered orally once or twice a week. The usual starting dose as provided in the manufacturer's "starting pack" is 25 μg/day for the first 3 days, 50 μg/day for the next 3 days, and then 75 μg/day. The usual maintenance dose is between 75 and 150 μg/day.

Cabergoline is a D2 agonist with a more prolonged duration of action. It has improved tolerability and efficacy compared with other D2 agonists, and it is the recommended D2 agonist of choice by the Endocrine Society.[11–13] It is usually administered as a once- or twice-weekly dose, although it can be given more frequently, up to daily, if necessary. The usual starting dose is 0.25 mg, with the dose being titrated as necessary. Most patients can be controlled on between 0.25 and 0.5 mg twice weekly. Some patients may require total doses of over 4.5 mg weekly.

The Endocrine Society recommends that women with prolactinomas discontinue D2 agonist therapy as soon as they discover that they are pregnant.[13] There may, however, be situations where treatment needs to be continued. There are currently no data available to suggest that D2 agonist therapy is teratogenic. The most extensive safety data available are for bromocriptine.[14,15] There are more limited safety data available for cabergoline.[16]

Treatment of patients with Parkinson's disease with high doses of cabergoline (≥3 mg daily) has been shown to be associated with an increased risk of valvular fibrosis and moderate-to-severe valvular regurgitation. This response is due to agonist activity at the 5-HT2b receptor. These doses are much higher than those routinely used in the management of prolactinomas or acromegaly. Current published data are largely from cross-sectional studies.[13,17] Presently, the consensus is that there is no increased risk of valvulopathy with the typical doses of 1–2 mg/week, but definitive risk assessment requires the results of long-term prospective follow-up with large cohorts of patients.

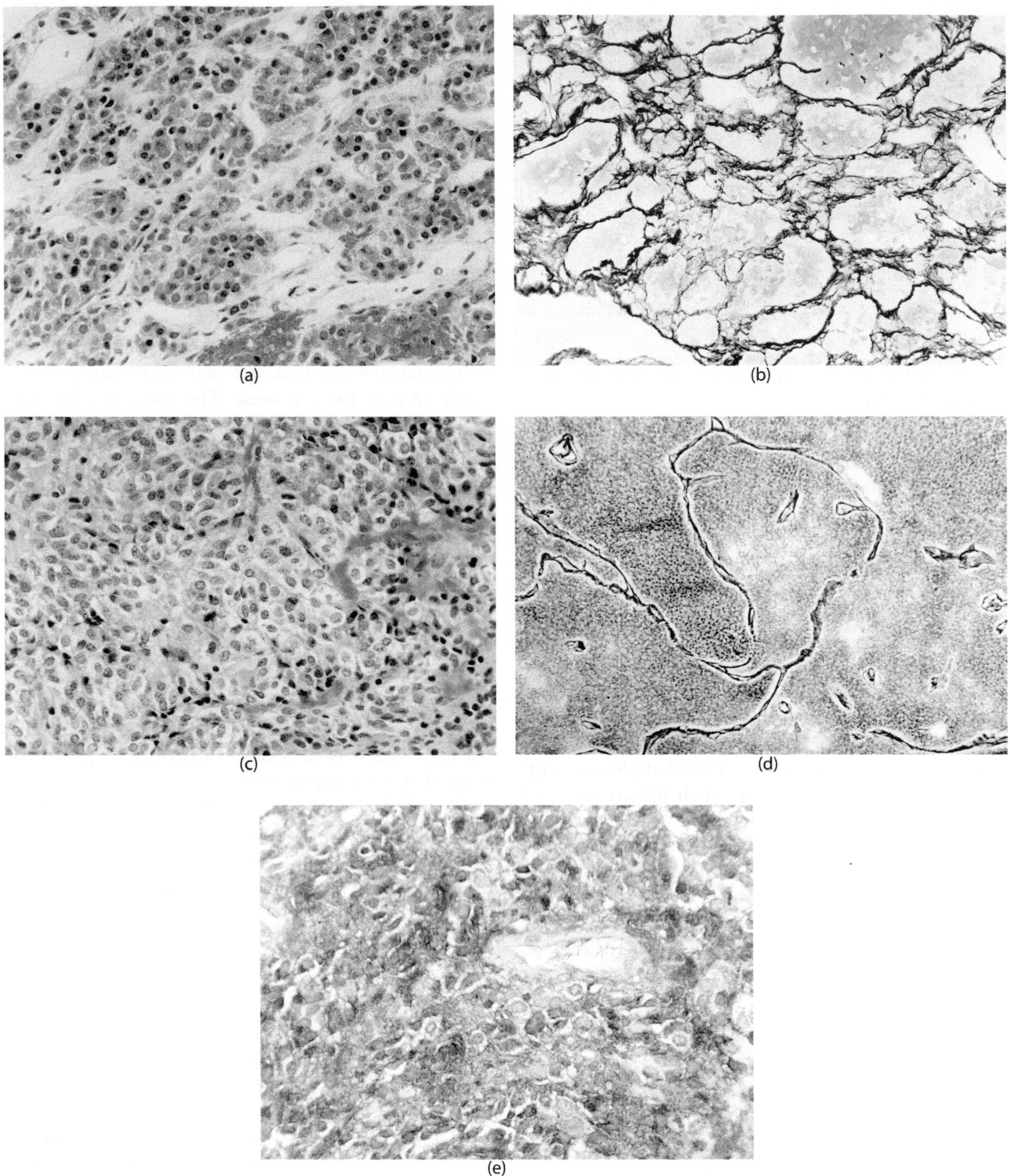

**Figure 1.6**
*(a) Normal adenohypophysis; hematoxylin and eosin stain. (b) Adenohypophysis demonstrating normal reticulin patterning. (c) Pituitary adenoma; hematoxylin and eosin stain. (d) Pituitary adenoma demonstrating disruption of reticulin patterning. (e) Prolactinoma demonstrating immunostaining for prolactin.*

| Tumor type | Transcription factors | Hormones, others |
|---|---|---|
| Somatotroph adenoma | | |
| • Densely granulated | Pit-1 | GH, α-subunit |
| • Sparsely granulated | Pit-1 | GH, keratin whorls (fibrous bodies) |
| • Mammosomatotroph/mixed adenoma | Pit-1, ER | GH, PRL, α-subunit |
| Lactotroph adenoma | | |
| • Sparsely granulated | Pit-1, ER | PRL, Golgi pattern |
| • Densely granulated | Pit-1, ER | PRL, diffuse cytoplasmic |
| • Acidophil stem cell | Pit-1 ER | PRL, GH, keratin whorls (fibrous bodies) |
| Thyrotroph | Pit-1, TEF, GATA-2 | β-TSH, α-subunit |
| Plurihormonal | Pit-1, ER, TEF, GATA-2 | GH, PRL, β-TSH, α-subunit |
| Corticotroph adenoma | Tpit | ACTH, keratins |
| Gonadotroph adenoma | SF-1, ER, GATA-2 | β-FSH, β-LH, α-subunit |
| Hormone-negative/null cell adenoma | None | None |
| Unusual plurihormonal adenoma | Multiple | Multiple |

*Source:* Al-Shraim M, Asa SL, *Acta Neuropathol*, 111, 1–7, 2006. With permission.
ER, estrogen receptor; GH, growth hormone; PRL, prolactin; TEF, thyrotroph embryonic factor; TSH, thyroid-stimulating hormone; ACTH, adrenocorticotropic hormone; FSH, follicle-stimulating hormone; LH, luteinizing hormone; SF, steroidogenic factor.

**Table 1.4**
*Classification of pituitary adenomas by cytodifferentiation.*

Headache—dural stretching, sudden bleed, or infarction
Visual field defect (see Figure 1.10)
CSF rhinorrhea
Cavernous sinus invasion—cranial nerve palsies: 3rd, 4th, 5th (ophthalmic and mandibular divisions), 6th
Hydrocephalus
Epilepsy—temporal lobe invasion
Facial pain—invasion of maxillary, sphenoid sinuses

**Table 1.5**
*Local complications of pituitary tumors.*

## *Somatostatin analogs*

Somatostatin (SS) analogs provide a means for the medical management of somatotroph adenomas. They are also efficacious in several other endocrine conditions[18] (Table 1.7). Five G-protein-linked human SS receptors (SST1–5) have been cloned. SS analogs bind to the SST2, 3, and 5.[19] SS receptors 2 and 5 are the principal mediators of the actions of SS analogs in the inhibition of growth hormone (GH) secretion in somatotroph adenomas. In addition to the inhibition of hormone release, SS analogs produce a variable degree of shrinkage of somatotroph adenomas.[20] They are also effective in thyrotropin-secreting pituitary adenomas (TSH-omas).

The presence of SST2 and 5 *in vivo* can be demonstrated using SST scintigraphy with $^{111}$In-labeled pentetreotide[21] (Figure 1.11). Positive SST scintigraphy, however, does not necessarily indicate sensitivity of pituitary tumors to SS analog therapy.[22]

Octreotide is a short-acting SS analog that needs to be given by s.c. injection three to four times daily.[18] A usual starting dose is 100 μg three times daily and can be titrated upward as necessary. Most acromegalic patients can be managed with total daily doses

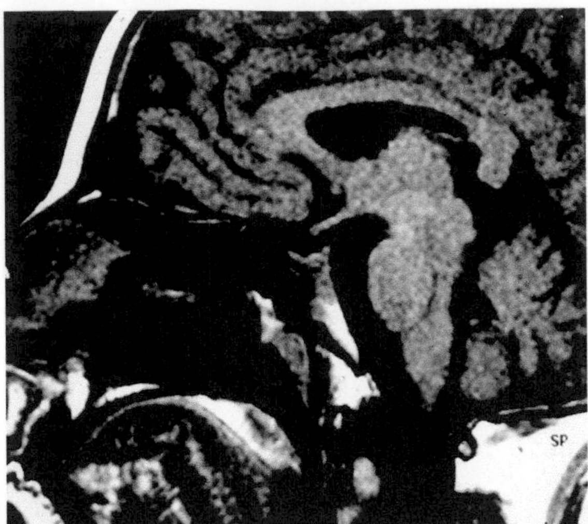


**Figure 1.7**
*Sagittal MRI scan (T1-weighted) demonstrating an empty sella. Note the herniation of cerebrospinal fluid (CSF) into the fossa.*

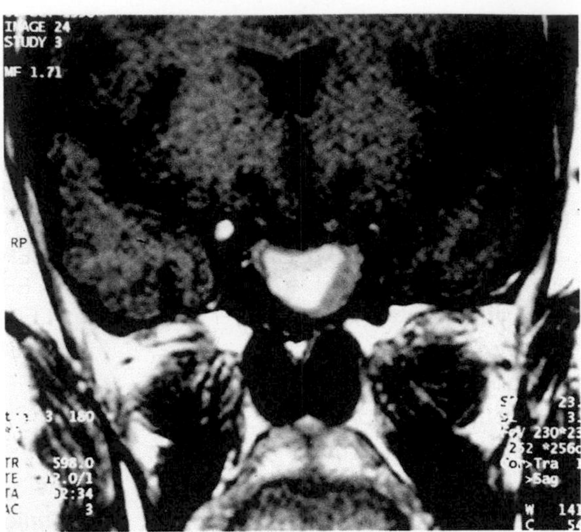


**Figure 1.8**
*Coronal MRI scan (T1-weighted) demonstrating pituitary apoplexy. Note the high signal, indicative of hemorrhage.*

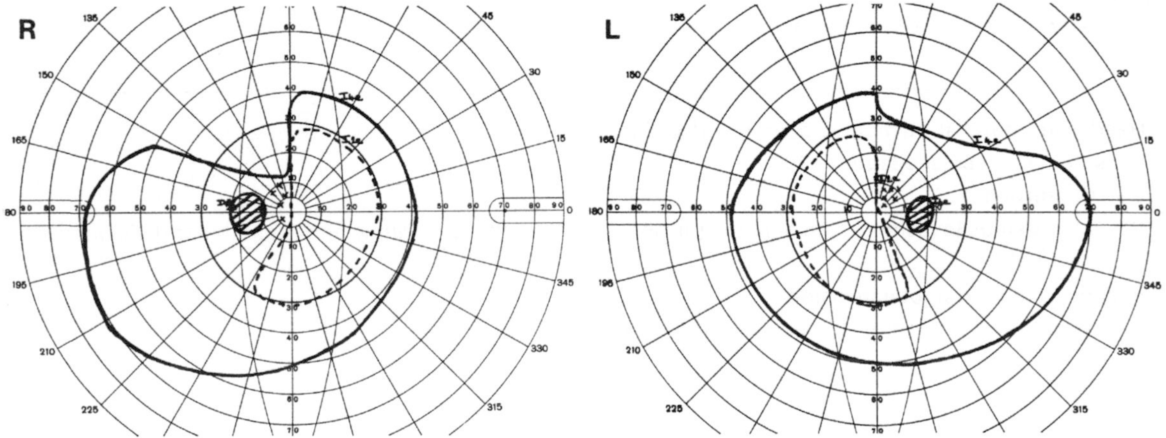


**Figure 1.9**
*Goldman perimetry demonstrating a bitemporal superior quadrantopia.*

of 600 µg or less. Unlike functioning neuroendocrine tumors, tachyphylaxis does not occur. The depot preparations of the SS analogs octreotide and lanreotide are now most widely used (Figure 1.12). Octreotide LAR (long-acting repeatable octreotide) consists of an octreotide-impregnated biodegradable polymer matrix, which is given by intramuscular (i.m.) injection monthly. The starting dose is 10 mg i.m. and may be increased to 20 and 30 mg i.m. or to 2 × 20 mg i.m. injections monthly.[23]

There are two lanreotide formulations. Lanreotide LA consists of copolymer microparticles in a 30 mg dose. It is initially given by i.m. injection every 14 days, with adjustment of dosage every 7–10 days, if necessary, to obtain therapeutic control. Lanreotide Autogel (lanreotide Depot in the USA) is an aqueous microparticle formulation in a prefilled syringe. It is available in three doses: 60, 90, and 120 mg. It is administered by deep s.c. injection.[24] An important advantage of lanreotide Autogel is the potential for the patient to self-inject.

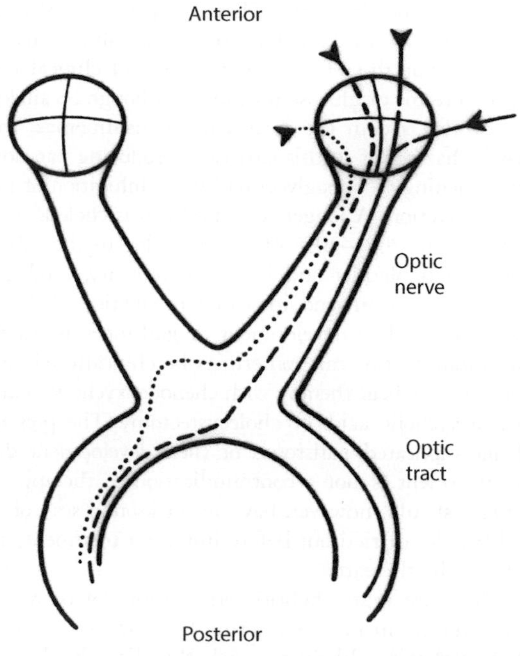


| Site of lesion | Visual field/acuity |
|---|---|
| 1. Optic nerve | Ipsilateral reduced acuity/blindness<br>Optic atrophy with long-standing lesion |
| 2. Optic nerve/chiasm (junctional syndrome) | Ipsilateral scotoma with reduced acuity<br>Contralateral temporal hemianopia |
| 3. Optic chiasm | Bitemporal hemianopia<br>Superior bitemporal quadrantopia |
| 4. Posterior chiasm | Bitemporal scotoma |
| 5. Optic tract | Homonymous hemianopia |

***Figure 1.10***
*Classical visual disturbances produced by pituitary tumors. Solid line, uncrossed temporal fibers; dashed line, superior nasal fibers; dotted line, inferior nasal fibers. The sites of the lesions are indicated by the numbers. (Modified from Melen O, Neuro-ophthalmic Features of Pituitary Tumors. In: Moiltch ME (ed),* Pituitary Tumors: Diagnosis and Management. Endocrinol Metab Clin North Am *1987; 16:585-608. With permission.)*

- Nausea and vomiting ~60%
- Postural hypotension ~25%
- Constipation ~10%
- Dry mouth
- Abdominal pain, dyspepsia
- Flushing
- Nasal congestion
- Headache
- Leg cramps
- Fatigue, weakness
- Psychiatric
- Pleuro-pulmonary
- Digital vasospasm
- Hypertension
- Thromboembolic events, particularly postpartum

*Source:* Verhelst J et al., *J Clin Endocrinol Metab* 84, 2518–22, 1999.

***Table 1.6***
*Side effects of DA agonists.*

- Somatotroph adenoma
- Thyrotroph adenoma
- Nonfunctioning pituitary adenoma (rarely)
- Medullary carcinoma of thyroid
- Neuroendocrine tumors
  - Functioning carcinoid
  - Nonfunctioning midgut (tumor stabilization)
  - Pancreatic
    - Gastrinoma
    - Insulinoma
    - Glucagonoma
    - Somatostatinoma
    - Vipoma
    - Polypeptidoma (PPoma)

***Table 1.7***
*Endocrine tumors responsive to somatostatin analogs.*

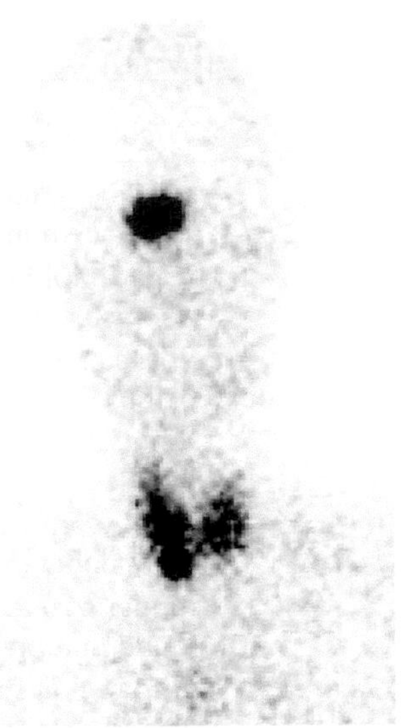

***Figure 1.11***
*Pituitary thyrotroph adenoma demonstrating binding of $^{111}$In pentetreotide. The patient has a goiter and is thyrotoxic, as evidenced by the binding of $^{111}$In pentetreotide by the thyroid.*

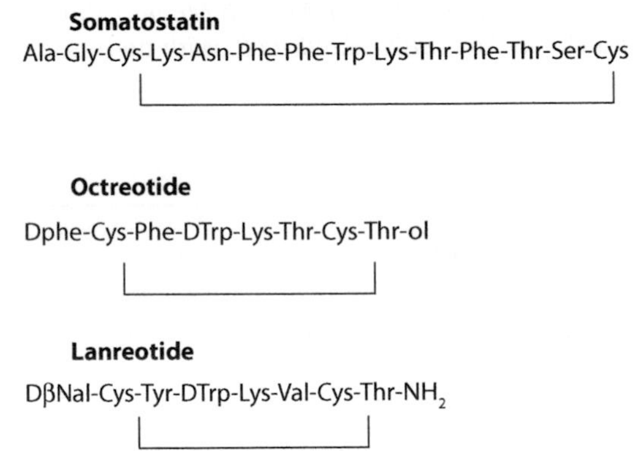


***Figure 1.12***
*Amino acid sequences of somatostatin-14, octreotide, and lanreotide.*

Most patients are treated by dose escalation to an optimized dose for therapeutic control. In addition, Autogel has extended injection interval on its label, enabling the injections to be spaced out up to 6–8 weeks in well-controlled patients.[25] A new injection pen is now available that incorporates a needle guard.

Side effects to SS analogs occur in about 30% of patients. The most frequent acute side effect is abdominal colic. This condition may be associated with diarrhea, steatorrhea, and flatulence. These symptoms usually disappear after 10–14 days of treatment. SS inhibits insulin secretion, but this effect is not usually of clinical relevance in terms of glucose tolerance. Although SS analogs can be effective in the treatment of insulinomas, they may be hazardous in this situation, producing paradoxical worsening of hypoglycemia by the inhibition of glucagon secretion. A longer term problem is cholelithiasis, occurring in 20%–30% of patients, due to the inhibition of gall bladder and intestinal motility, inhibition of cholecystokinin, and increased production of deoxycholic acid.[18] The development of gallstones is usually asymptomatic but can sometimes be clinically relevant, requiring medical therapy with chenodeoxycholic acid or ursodeoxycholic acid, or cholecystectomy. The presence of uncomplicated gallstones or their development during treatment is not a contraindication to therapy. All patients should, however, have an ultrasound scan of the gall bladder carried out before initiating treatment, and periodically thereafter.

There are many hybrid formulations of octreotide LAR and biosimilar long-acting formulations in development that are likely to reach the clinic in the near future. Over a longer time frame, oral and transdermal formulations may become available.

Pasireotide is a multi receptor-targeted agonist with high affinity for SST1–3 and, in particular, for SST5. Unlike conventional SS analogs, pasireotide does not induce internalization of SST2. Hyperglycemia is a frequent side effect with pasireotide, due to its high affinity for SST5.[26,27]

A novel concept is that of SS-DA chimeric molecules. Chimeric molecules have been shown to have markedly increased potency and efficacy compared with octreotide or octreotide combined with a DA analog in somatotroph adenoma cells *in vitro*.[28] The chimeric molecule BIM23A760 has been tested in normal human volunteers and in patients with acromegaly. It has been shown to be safe and to inhibit GH and insulin-like growth factor I (IGF-I) levels. New chimeric analogs are currently in development for clinical testing.

### *Pegvisomant*

Pegvisomant is a pegylated recombinant 191 amino acid analog of human GH. It has eight mutations at site 1 that increase binding to the GH receptor. It has a further mutation at site 2 that inhibits binding to the GH receptor. As a result, the molecule acts as a competitive GH receptor antagonist by inhibiting receptor dimerization.[29] Pegylation of four or five moieties results in an increased half-life of 72 h, with reduced immunogenicity. The drug is given by s.c. injection. It is indicated for the treatment of acromegaly. Treatment with 10–30 mg daily has resulted in the normalization of

IGF-I in >90% of patients in clinical trials.[30,31] The fall in IGF-I is mirrored by similar reductions in serum IGF-binding protein-3 (IGFBP-3) and acid-labile subunit (ALS). In contrast, however, serum GH levels more than double.[30] The drug is well tolerated, with dose-related improvements in symptomatic and metabolic parameters. In particular, in contrast to SS analogs, glucose homeostasis tends to improve. Unlike SS and DA analogs, the drug does not target the somatotroph adenoma. Although there have been concerns about the possibility of tumor growth with pegvisomant, there is no evidence of this response at present. Hepatotoxicity has been reported in patients treated with pegvisomant, usually in the form of elevated transaminases. These levels frequently return to normal, even if treatment is continued. A direct causal relationship has however been demonstrated in a few patients on rechallenging with pegvisomant. In the ACROSTUDY observational registry, the frequency of abnormal liver function tests ≥3 times the upper limit of normal was 2.5%. In consequence, all patients treated with pegvisomant should be regularly monitored. Local injection site reactions, including lipohypertrophy, are occasional complications.[32]

### *Temozolomide*

There have been recent reports of aggressive pituitary tumors and carcinomas that have been refractory to conventional therapies, demonstrating tumor shrinkage and reduced hormone secretion in response to treatment with temozolamide. Temozolamide is an alkylating chemotherapeutic agent used in the treatment of glioblastoma multiforme. It is administered orally in a cyclical regimen. Low expression of the DNA repair enzyme 06-methylguanine DNA methyltransferase (MGMT) has been shown to correlate with tumor response to treatment. The relationship of MGMT expression and promoter methylation in pituitary tumors to treatment response, however, is unclear.[33] Efficacy has been reported in 24/40 (60%) of the cases, although relapse usually occurs. It is generally well tolerated. Fatigue is common, and hemotological toxicity may occur, requiring dose reduction or drug withdrawal.

### *New targeted therapies*

Chemotherapy has been largely disappointing in the management of pituitary carcinomas. The identification of new molecular targets for the medical treatment of aggressive pituitary tumors is an area of interest for many research groups. The mammalian target of rapamycin (mTOR) signaling pathway has a central role in the control of cell proliferation. The mTOR inhibitor everolimus inhibits pituitary cell proliferation and is the subject of ongoing clinical trials in patients with aggressive pituitary tumors.

## *Radiotherapy (see Chapter 4)*

Conventional radiotherapy is now used much more sparingly than in the past. It is usually reserved for control of tumor growth rather than secretion. It has a slow onset of action and is associated with the development of hypopituitarism and other sequelae. In some centers, stereotaxic radiotherapy, delivering a single dose of irradiation (gamma knife, LINAC, proton beam), is being increasingly used.

# *Hypopituitarism (see Chapter 5)*

Hypopituitarism is one of the most frequent clinical problems in neuroendocrinology. It may occur *de novo*, or as a secondary event, most often as a result of surgery and/or radiotherapy (Table 1.8). Several relatively

| Causes |
|---|
| Hypothalamic |
| Craniopharyngioma |
| Sarcoidosis |
| Histiocytosis X |
| Glioma |
| Metastatic disease, e.g., breast cancer |
| Radiotherapy |
| Trauma |
| Infection, e.g., tuberculosis, mycoses, syphilis, toxoplasmosis, Whipple's disease |
| Genetic, e.g., septo-optic dysplasia |
| Infiltrative/invasive, e.g., meningioma, chordoma, dysgerminoma |
| Pituitary |
| Pituitary tumor |
| Pituitary apoplexy |
| Sheehan's syndrome |
| Empty sella syndrome |
| Lymphocytic hypophysitis |
| Surgery |
| Radiotherapy |
| Genetic, e.g., inactivating mutations of POU-1 and PROP-1 |

**Table 1.8**
*Causes of hypopituitarism.*

small, retrospective studies have demonstrated an association between hypopituitarism and reduced life expectancy.[34–37] There has been a particular association found with vascular disease in all but one of these studies. A large retrospective study of 2279 patients with presumed nonfunctioning pituitary adenomas included in the Swedish Cancer Registry (1958–1991) found an increased standardized mortality ratio (SMR) of 2.0. The SMR was higher in women. Cardiovascular and cerebrovascular diseases were the most common causes of mortality. Although endocrine data were not available, it was assumed that the majority of these patients were hypopituitary.[38] A prospective study of 1014 U.K. patients between 1992 and 2000 with a diagnosis of hypopituitarism (111 patients underwent dynamic testing) confirmed an increase in mortality (SMR 1.87), with an increased mortality in women (SMR 2.29) compared with men (SMR 1.57). Craniopharyngioma, in particular, was shown to have a relatively poor prognosis (SMR 9.28). The excess mortality was associated with vascular and respiratory causes.[39] The causes of increased mortality in hypopituitarism are likely to be multifactorial, in part dependent upon the underlying pathology, previous radiotherapy, and adequacy of pituitary hormone replacement therapy. Growth hormone deficiency (GHD), in particular, with its associated cardiovascular risk factors, has been considered to be relevant, but an unequivocal association has yet to be demonstrated.

Hypopituitarism classically develops in the sequential manner GH > luteinizing hormone (LH)/follicle-stimulating hormone (FSH) > adrenocorticotropic hormone (ACTH) >TSH.[40] Prolactin deficiency is usually a late event and does not appear to be of clinical significance, except in women who want to breastfeed. The developmental sequence of hormone deficiency can vary, although it is true to say that in pituitary adenomas, GH is almost invariably affected first. Diabetes insipidus is not associated with pituitary adenomas. It is a frequent transient phenomenon after pituitary surgery and may become permanent. *De novo* central diabetes insipidus is typically associated with hypothalamic disease or other pathologies, such as lymphocytic hypophysitis.

Hypopituitary patients who present *de novo* often give a preceding history of severe lethargy and weakness that may have been present over many years. Premenopausal women are more likely to present earlier than men due to the development of secondary amenorrhea. Male patients may or may not volunteer a history of erectile dysfunction and loss of libido, but these symptoms are usually described on direct questioning. Patients may describe a loss of axillary and pubic hair. Male patients also loose body hair, and facial hair growth diminishes. In severe cases, patients develop additional symptoms of hypothyroidism, such as cold intolerance. Osteoporosis may result in the development of fractures. Ischemic heart disease frequently develops. Often, patients are unable to participate in normal daily activities and work.

Clinical examination may appear to be unremarkable, particularly in women. On closer inspection, however, most patients will have a smooth, sallow facial appearance and thin skin. Male patients, in particular, develop the classical appearance with loss of facial hair. Most patients will have a diminution or loss of axillary and pubic hair (Figure 1.13). Profoundly hypopituitary patients may be hypotensive with cold skin and delayed tendon reflexes. Because of its insidious development, hypopituitarism is frequently missed and this oversight may have very serious consequences for the patient. Hypopituitarism is particularly likely to be missed in male patients with nonfunctioning pituitary tumors and prolactinomas. It is important to enquire about the sudden onset of what is often an extremely severe headache, suggesting pituitary apoplexy[41] (Figure 1.8) (see Chapter 24). In these circumstances, the patient will often describe the acute onset of symptoms after the event. Similarly, the onset of a severe headache in the peripartum period, followed by failure of lactation, should suggest the possibility of Sheehan's syndrome.[42]

The most frequent causes of hypopituitarism are pituitary surgery and hypothalamic–pituitary irradiation. These causes are predictable and should be detected early with specialist follow-up. It is uncommon for radiotherapy to result in the development of clinically significant hypopituitarism earlier than 1 year after treatment. All patients should have a full pituitary assessment immediately after pituitary surgery. Patients who receive radiotherapy should have baseline endocrinology checked at 6 months posttreatment, followed by a full pituitary assessment at 1 year, and regular periodic assessments thereafter.

## Differential diagnosis of suprasellar and sellar tumors

There is a large differential diagnosis for both suprasellar and sellar tumors[43] (Table 1.9). In practice, the majority of sellar tumors are pituitary adenomas. Probably the most important pathology to consider in the differential diagnosis of space-occupying lesions in this area is an aneurysm. Aneurysms can mimic large pituitary adenomas. If there is any doubt about the diagnosis, magnetic resonance (MR) angiography or conventional carotid angiography should

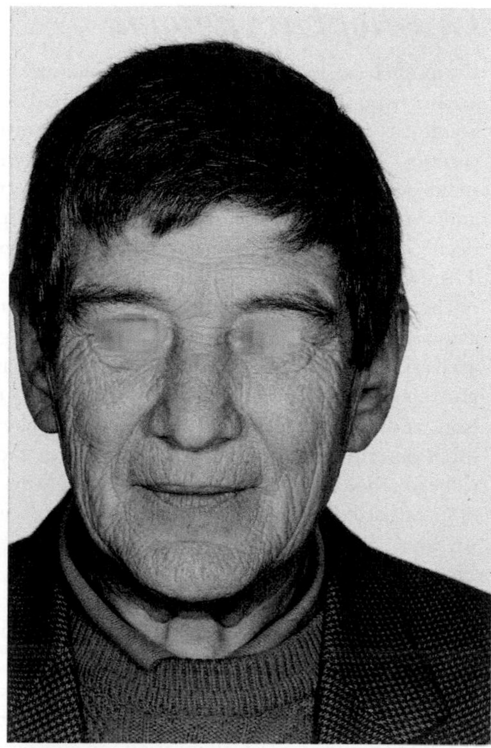

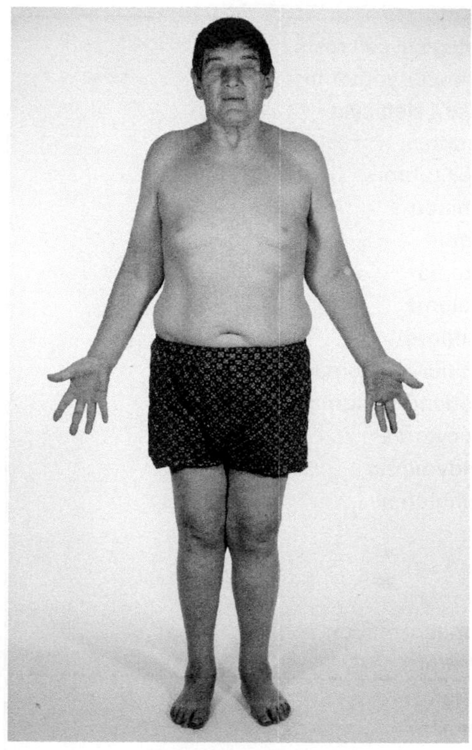

**Figure 1.13**
*Patient with panhypopituitarism secondary to a macroprolactinoma.*

be performed. The presence of diabetes insipidus should raise the likelihood of a different pathology to a pituitary adenoma.

# Lymphocytic hypophysitis

Autoimmune (lymphocytic) hypophysitis[44] (Figure 1.14) is a chronic inflammatory condition that affects the anterior pituitary, posterior pituitary, or both. It has an estimated prevalence of about 9 per million. Isolated involvement of the anterior pituitary has a striking predilection for young females (female:male ratio 6:1), particularly in late pregnancy or in the postpartum period. Involvement of both the anterior and the posterior pituitary occurs about twice as commonly in females, whereas involvement of the pituitary stalk and posterior pituitary (infundibular neurohypophysitis) appears to affect males and females equally. It typically presents with headache, suprasellar pituitary mass, and hypopituitarism. Unlike pituitary adenomas, ACTH secretion is usually affected first, followed by TSH, LH, FSH, and GH and prolactin. Visual field defects are common. Diabetes insipidus occurs with involvement of the posterior pituitary and may be associated with thickening of the pituitary stalk on MRI. Failure of lactation may occur in the postpartum period. Less commonly, hyperprolactinemia may occur, as with other large pituitary tumors, presumably at least in part, due to stalk compression. An important differential diagnosis in the postpartum period is Sheehan's syndrome[42] and granulomatous conditions such as histiocytosis X and sarcoidosis (Figure 1.15). A definitive diagnosis can only be made by biopsy. If the diagnosis is considered to be a possibility and the patient is not at risk from compressive symptoms, then a conservative approach should be adopted, as in some patients the endocrine dysfunction is only transient. High-dose glucocorticoids may be considered in some cases, if interventional therapy is deemed to be necessary.

There is an association between autoimmune hypophysitis and other autoimmune conditions, such as autoimmune thyroid disease (AITD).[45] Circulating antipituitary antibodies occur in autoimmune hypophysitis and in other autoimmune conditions, but their sensitivity and specificity are poor.

| |
|---|
| Embryological cell rests |
| Craniopharyngioma |
| Rathke's cleft cyst |
| Chordoma |
| Germ cell tumors |
| Germinoma |
| Dermoid |
| Teratoma |
| Pinealoma |
| Other tumors |
| Optic nerve glioma |
| Oligodendroglioma |
| Astrocytoma |
| Ependymoma |
| Meningioma |
| Vascular |
| Aneurysm |
| Angioma |
| A-V malformation |
| Inflammatory |
| Sarcoidosis |
| Wegener's granulomatosis |
| Langerhan's cell histiocytosis |
| Autoimmune hypophysitis |
| Lymphocytic adenohypophysitis |
| Lymphocytic infundibuloneurohypophysitis |
| Lymphocytic panhypophysitis |
| Infectious diseases |
| Tuberculosis |
| Abscess |
| Metastatic (e.g., breast, bronchus) |
| Miscellaneous |
| Arachnoid cyst |
| Sphenoid sinus mucocele |

***Table 1.9***
*Differential diagnosis of sellar and suprasellar lesions from pituitary adenomas.*

There are many possible diagnoses to be considered with suprasellar lesions. Craniopharyngiomas, meningiomas (Figures 1.16 and 1.17), and optic gliomas are the most common lesions that are likely to come to the attention of the endocrinologist.

## *Craniopharyngioma*

Craniopharyngiomas[46] are rare embryological remnants, arising from the path of the craniopharyngeal duct. They account for ~10% of childhood intracranial tumors. There is a bimodal distribution, with peak incidences between 5 and 14 years and between 50 and 74 years. Two main histological subtypes have been described: adamantinomatous and papillary. The adamantinomatous subtype occurs at all ages and is the most common subtype in young patients. It is associated with mutations in the α-catenin gene and activation of the Wnt pathway. The tumors have cystic and solid components, with fibrous tissue, calcification, and necrotic debris. The content may be viscous, often described as being like engine oil, or more fluid, rich in cholesterol crystals. The epithelium consists of keratinized squamous cells. The tumors are often invasive. In contrast, the papillary subtype almost exclusively occurs in adults. It consists of mature squamous epithelium, with solid and cystic components. The cyst fluid is usually viscous. Calcification is uncommon. Papillary tumors tend to be less invasive than the adamantinomatous subtype. Calcification in craniopharyngiomas gives rise to typical appearances on CT scan (Figure 1.17). Calcification can also occasionally occur in pituitary tumors. Rathke's cleft cysts are usually small and asymptomatic, but they may present with similar features to craniopharyngiomas, although calcification is not a feature. Craniopharyngiomas are frequently adherent to surrounding structures and can give rise to problems during surgical removal. They are associated with a significant morbidity and mortality. They can have aggressive growth characteristics and tend to recur. A progression rate of ~60% has been reported in patients with residual tumor on imaging, compared with ~20% recurrence in patients who have not. Recurrence was also found to be associated with male sex, intracranial hypertension, onset in childhood before the age of 10 years, and surgery using the pterional approach.[47] Patients usually present with features of hypopituitarism, frequently in association with visual field defects. In children, there is the additional problem of growth failure. Unlike pituitary tumors, diabetes insipidus may also be present. Rarely, patients may also be adipsic, resulting in serious management problems. Large craniopharyngiomas may be associated with headaches and raised intracranial pressure. They are usually clearly suprasellar in their localization, but occasionally they may be intrasellar, mimicking pituitary tumors. Craniopharyngiomas elaborate β-human chorionic gonadotrophin (β-HCG) in the cyst fluid. This gonadotrophin is present in high

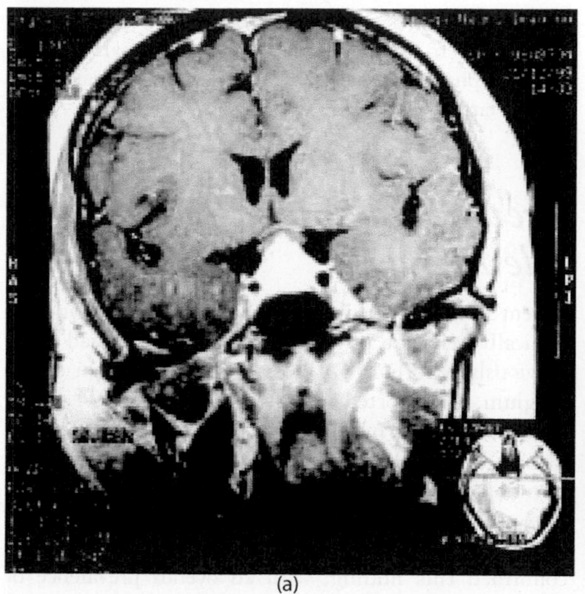

(a)

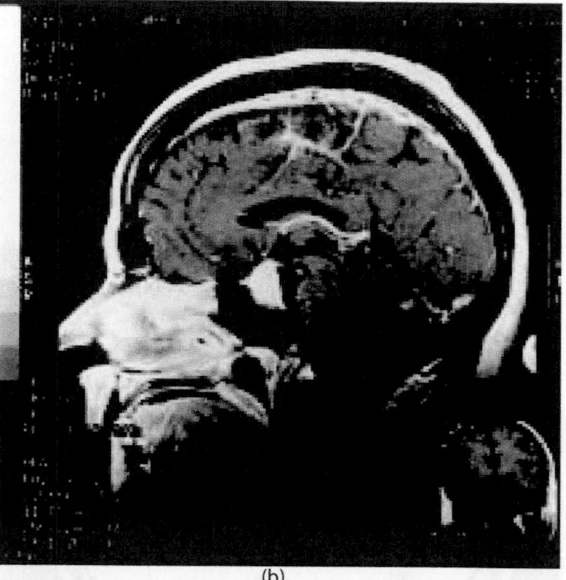

(b)

***Figure 1.14***
*MRI scan (T1-weighted) of lymphocytic hypophysitis. (a) Coronal section demonstrating homogenous enhancement of the pituitary mass with gadolinium, with suprasellar extension. Note the thickening of the pituitary stalk. (b) Sagittal section demonstrating tongue-like extension of the enhancing tissue along the base of the hypothalamus. This extension is typically seen in granulomatous disease and in lymphocytic hypophysitis.*

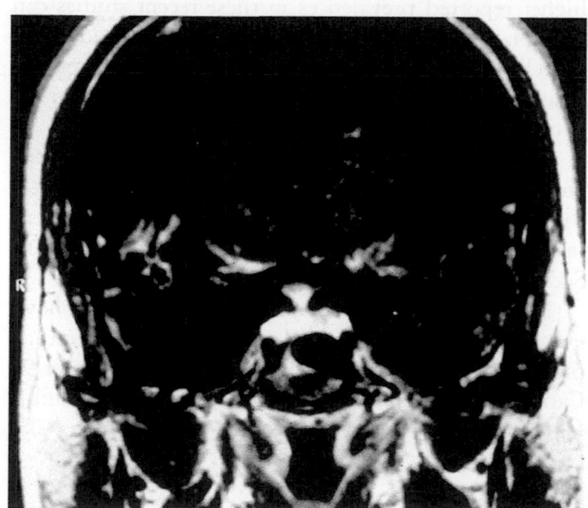

***Figure 1.15***
*Coronal MRI scan (T1-weighted) of pituitary sarcoidosis. Note the thickening of the pituitary stalk, with enhancing tissue extending along the base of the hypothalamus.*

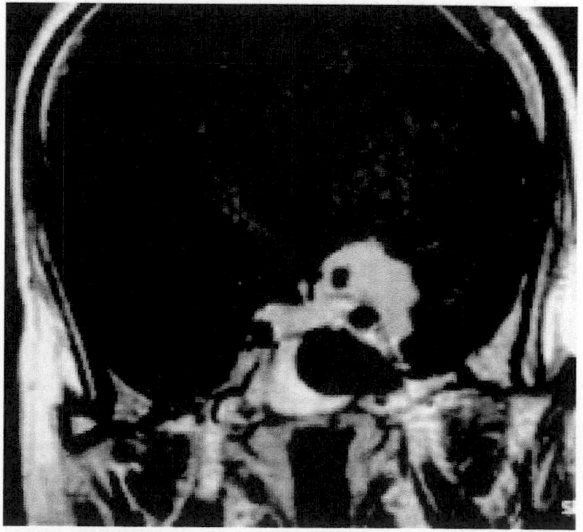

***Figure 1.16***
*Coronal MRI scan (T1-weighted) demonstrating a left-sided suprasellar meningioma.*

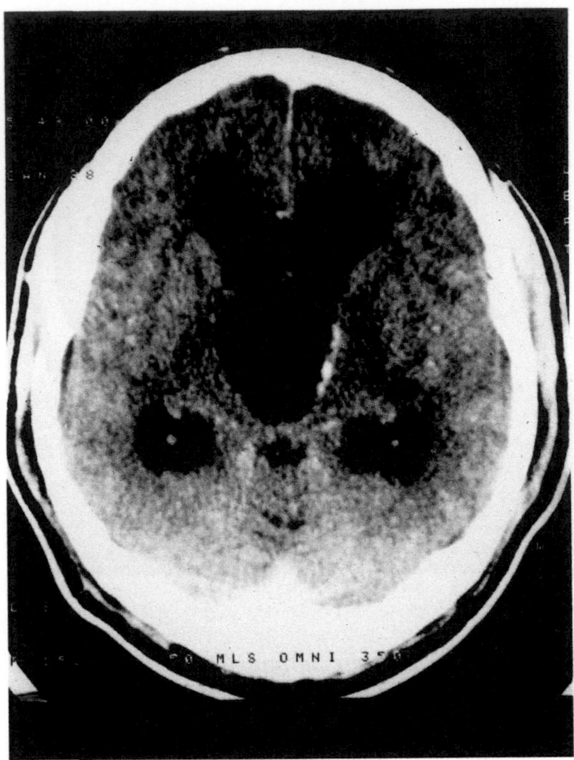


**Figure 1.17**
*Axial CT scan of a craniopharyngioma. There is a central hypodense mass with a surrounding ring of calcification. There is associated hydrocephalus and effacement of the brain, indicative of raised intracranial pressure.*

concentrations and provides a useful diagnostic marker. Occasionally, the β-HCG may also be measurable in the cerebrospinal fluid (CSF).[48]

The treatment of choice is surgical excision. This excision often needs to be carried out using a transcranial approach. Incomplete removal is frequent, particularly if the tumor is closely adherent to surrounding structures. Radiotherapy reduces tumor recurrence and should be considered in such patients. Stereotactic radiosurgery may be considered for small lesions, well-delineated surgical remnants, or recurrences. Some tumors continue to grow in spite of surgery and radiotherapy. In addition, cystic fluid reaccumulation can be a recurrent problem. In this situation, a reservoir can be implanted to facilitate repeated cyst aspiration. Persistently raised intracranial pressure may require ventricular shunting. Other approaches to deal with recurrent disease include intracystic implantation of a β-emitting radioactive source and the use of cytotoxic substances, such as alcohol, during surgery in an attempt to destroy the cyst lining. In spite of these measures, a small number of craniopharyngiomas continue to grow and are ultimately fatal.

## Prevalence of pituitary adenomas

Recent data have demonstrated a higher prevalence of clinically relevant pituitary adenomas than had been previously reported.[49] A cross-sectional study in Liege, Belgium, has reported an overall prevalence of 94 ± 19.3 per 100,000. The mean age at diagnosis was 40.3 years. Macroadenomas comprised 43% of adenomas. The most common tumor was prolactinoma (66%), of which 80% were microadenomas occurring in females.[50] A subsequent cross-sectional study in the United Kingdom has confirmed this finding, with an overall prevalence of 77.6 per 100,000. The mean age of diagnosis was 37 years. The distribution of pituitary adenomas was also confirmed. The proportion and prevalence per 100,000 of each subtype were, respectively, prolactinoma, 44 (57%); nonfunctioning pituitary adenoma (NFPA), 22.2 (28%); somatotroph adenoma, 8.6 (11%); corticotroph adenoma 1.2 (2%); and unknown functional status, 1.2 (2%). The marked female preponderance in prolactinomas was confirmed, with 89% occurring in females and 81% being microadenomas.[51] Part of the reasons for the higher reported prevalences in these recent studies can be explained by the systematic methodologies followed in well-defined populations, together with an increasing awareness of pituitary disease in primary care and in the general population.

Incidental pituitary adenomas are sometimes detected on imaging studies that are carried out for unrelated reasons. Guidelines for the management of pituitary incidentalomas have recently been published by the Endocrine Society.[52]

Most pituitary tumors are sporadic. They may however occur as part of familial syndromes such as multiple endocrine neoplasia type 1 (MEN1) (see Chapter 9), Carney complex, and the more recently identified familial isolated pituitary adenomas (FIPAs) (see Chapter 2).[53]

## Non-functioning pituitary adenomas

Non-functioning pituitary adenomas form part of a spectrum of phenotypes, ranging from the truly null cell adenoma to the gonadotrophinoma that may be associated with elevated serum gonadotrophin levels. As such, NFPAs and gonadotrophinomas are almost certainly derived from the same gonadotroph cell lineage. The majority of NFPAs express mRNA, immunostain, or both for glycoprotein hormone subunits. Similarly, a majority will secrete one or more of these subunits *in vitro*. Gonadotrophinomas secrete intact FSH more frequently than LH, which may be biologically active. More commonly, tumors secrete biologically inactive β-subunits. In addition, paradoxical LHβ and FSHβ responses to thyrotropin-releasing hormone (TRH) are present in a large proportion of these tumors. There is often associated hypersecretion of glycoprotein hormone α-subunit. A proportion of NFPAs secrete α-subunit alone.[54]

Unlike other types of pituitary tumors, most NFPAs and gonadotrophinomas present with pressure symptoms, hypopituitarism, or both, rather than with clinical syndromes related to hormone hypersecretion. Impaired visual acuity and visual field defects are common presenting symptoms.[40] Occasionally, they may be associated with clinical evidence of gonadotrophin hypersecretion.[55] Macroadenomas are frequently associated with hyperprolactinemia due to stalk compression.[56] Consequently, they may be mistaken for prolactinomas and vice versa. Any patient presenting as an emergency with visual disturbance *must* have serum prolactin measured as a matter of urgency.

It is important that the rare, but highly aggressive, "silent corticotroph adenoma" is not misdiagnosed as NFPA at this stage. These tumors may be associated with elevated serum ACTH levels, but no clinical or biochemical evidence of hypercortisolemia. They tend to have aggressive growth characteristics and may present at a later stage with clinical Cushing's syndrome.[57,58]

NFPAs are frequently invasive, with extension into the cavernous sinuses. As such, they present a particular challenge to the surgeon. The standard treatment for NFPAs is transsphenoidal surgery. Visual impairment can be expected to improve in the majority of patients who undergo surgery within a year of the onset of symptoms.[40] A recent study has demonstrated improved surgical outcome at 1 year, after endoscopic surgery, compared with conventional microscopic surgery.[59] The problem is that even with good surgical clearance, there is a high recurrence rate. This high rate may in part be due to dural invasion, microscopic evidence of which has been demonstrated in 88% of intrasellar macroadenomas and in 94% of suprasellar tumors.[60] A recent retrospective review of 155 patients in Oxford, United Kingdom, who underwent

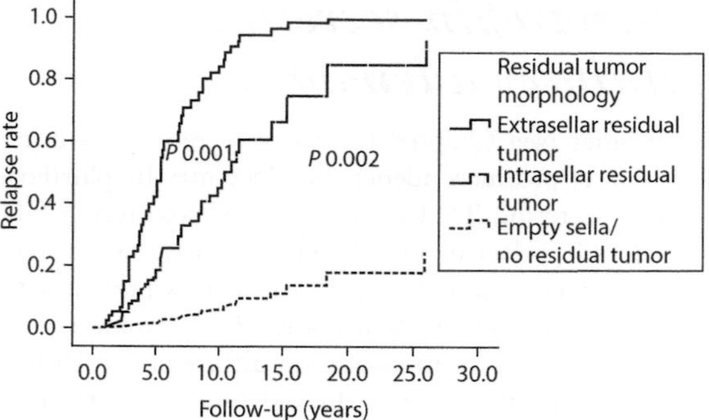


***Figure 1.18***
*Relapse rates with three subgroups of patients according to post-operative scan classification. (From Reddy R et al.,* Eur J Endocrinol *165, 739–44, 2011. With permission.)*

surgical treatment between 1984 and 2007 demonstrated relapse rates of 23%, 47%, and 68% at 5, 10, and 15 years, respectively, indicating the need for prolonged follow-up. Recurrence rates were higher in patients with visible residual tumor after surgery and in younger patients[61] (Figure 1.18). Radiotherapy reduces tumor recurrence after surgery and may be considered for patients at high risk of recurrence.[62]

The abnormal secretion of gonadotrophins or their glycoprotein subunits provides a useful additional means of monitoring individual tumor responses to treatment. Medical therapy of these tumors is largely ineffective. Tumors often express DA receptors, and there are case reports of patients who have responded to DA analogs.[63] Similarly, tumors frequently express SS receptors as demonstrated by radiolabeled scintigraphy. As for DA analogs, there have been case reports of patients demonstrating variable responses to SS analogs.[64] Ophthalmologic responses are sometimes seen in patients without observable effects on tumor size, suggesting that SS analogs may be acting on the optic pathways through different mechanisms.[65] Analogs of gonadotropin-releasing hormone (GnRH) have been found to be unhelpful and may, in fact, stimulate glycoprotein production by tumors.[66]

The development of an effective, safe, and well-tolerated antiproliferative medical therapy for NFPAs is one of the major challenges in pituitary disease. The availability of such a therapeutic option would dramatically change the treatment paradigm for these patients.

## Thyrotropin-secreting pituitary adenomas

TSH-omas (see Chapter 14) are very rare, accounting for ~1% of pituitary adenomas. They may be plurihormonal, secreting TSH alone (72%) or cosecreting GH (16%) and prolactin (11%).[67] These tumors are characteristically large and invasive. Patients may present with local pressure effects, symptoms of thyrotoxicosis, or both. There may be an associated diffuse goiter. Unlike primary hyperthyroidism, thyroid function tests demonstrate elevated levels of thyroid hormones in association with inappropriately normal or elevated serum TSH levels. Thyrotropin-secreting adenomas characteristically secrete glycoprotein α-subunit, with an elevated molar α-subunit to TSH ratio of >1 (α-subunit μg/L ÷ TSH mU/L × 10).[68] An important differential diagnosis is the syndrome of thyroid hormone resistance.

Surgery is the treatment of choice for TSH-omas. Due to the size and invasiveness of many of these tumors, complete resection can be difficult. These tumors typically express SST (Figure 1.11). Patients who cannot undergo surgery or who are not cured by surgery can be offered SS analog therapy. Most patients will demonstrate a reduction in TSH levels, and levels will normalize in the majority of patients. About 50% of patients demonstrate a variable degree of tumor shrinkage. Radiotherapy should be considered for invasive tumors.

# Hyperprolactinemia

Hyperprolactinemia is a common clinical problem. Several different types of clinicians are likely to see patients with hyperprolactinemia, including primary care physicians, urogenital physicians, urologists, obstetricians and gynecologists, and endocrinologists. A guiding principle is that any patient with hyperprolactinemia should be fully investigated by a specialist endocrinologist. Clinical and treatment guidelines have been published recently by the Endocrine Society.[13]

## Clinical features of hyperprolactinemia

The most frequent pathological cause of hyperprolactinemia is the microprolactinoma. Most microprolactinomas remain small. Microprolactinomas typically occur in young women of reproductive age.[69,70] The commonest presentations are oligomenorrhea or amenorrhea. Some patients present with infertility. There may be associated symptoms of estrogen deficiency. Galactorrhea has been reported as having a variable prevalence of 30% upward. It is important to realize, however, that galactorrhea *per se* is not necessarily indicative of hyperprolactinemia.

Although microprolactinomas occur in males, they are less common than in women; most patients present with macroprolactinomas.

Hyperprolactinemia in males tends to present more insidiously than in females, with a reduction in libido and associated erectile dysfunction.[71,72] The patient develops clinical features of hypogonadism. Infertility is a presenting problem in about 10% of patients. Galactorrhea occurs occasionally.

Macroprolactinomas behave quite differently from microprolactinomas. These tumors usually grow, and a small proportion demonstrate aggressive growth characteristics, particularly in males. Apart from the effects of hyperprolactinemia, patients may present with symptoms and signs of other hormone deficiencies. Male patients, in particular, may present with panhypopituitarism. Symptoms and signs resulting from local tumor compression occur frequently. A serum prolactin must always be requested as the priority investigation in any patient presenting with signs of chiasmal compression.

## Investigation of hyperprolactinemia

Normal prolactin levels vary according to the assay used but are about <400 mU/L (20 μg/L) in males and <500 mU/L (25 μg/L) in females. There are several causes in the investigation of hyperprolactinemia (Table 1.10). The history and examination of the patient are particularly important. The possibility of pregnancy should be considered in all amenorrheic women of reproductive age. Clinical features of hypopituitarism, visual disturbance, and acromegaly (50% of patients with acromegaly have associated hyperprolactinemia) should be sought. A detailed drug history is essential. Baseline renal, liver, thyroid, and gonadal function should be assessed.

Stress-induced hyperprolactinemia can be excluded by the measurement of serum prolactin 2 h after cannulation. More than 80% of prolactin circulates as a monomeric form with a molecular mass of 23 kDa. Prolactin also circulates as big prolactin (45–60 kDa). Macroprolactin (big prolactin) refers to high-molecular-weight complexes of prolactin (≥100 kDa). A proportion of macroprolactin is due to immune complex formation. Macroprolactin exhibits lower bioactivity than monomeric prolactin. It occurs in about 15% of patients with serum prolactin <3500 mU/L. Patients with asymptomatic hyperprolactinemia should be checked

| Causes |
|---|
| Physiological |
| Stress |
| Pregnancy |
| Lactation |
| Macroprolactin |
| Pharmacological |
| Major tranquilizers |
| Antiemetics |
| Tricyclic antidepressants |
| Estrogens, e.g., oral contraceptive pill |
| Verapamil |
| Methyl dopa |
| Reserpine |
| Systemic disease/trauma |
| Hypothyroidism |
| Liver disease |
| Renal failure |
| Polycystic ovary syndrome |
| Chest wall trauma |
| Hypothalamic disease/stalk damage |
| Trauma |
| Radiotherapy |
| Infiltrative diseases, e.g., histiocytosis X, sarcoidosis |
| Infection, e.g., tuberculosis |
| Metastatic disease, e.g., breast cancer |
| Craniopharyngioma |
| Glioma |
| Meningioma |
| Astrocytoma |
| Stalk compression from suprasellar extension of pituitary mass |
| Stalk section |
| Pituitary disease |
| Microprolactinoma |
| Macroprolactinoma |
| Mixed lactotroph somatotroph adenoma |
| Mammosomatotroph adenoma |
| Plurihormonal adenoma |
| Lymphocytic hypophysitis |
| Empty sella |

***Table 1.10***
*Causes of and associations with hyperprolactinemia.*

for macroprolactin. Macroprolactin measurement with polyethylene glycol precipitation is now routinely available in most clinics.[73,74]

Some drugs, particularly antipsychotics, may be associated with serum prolactin levels of >4000 mU/L (200 μg/L). There may be associated galactorrhea and hypogonadism. Serum prolactin levels usually return to normal within a few days of stopping the medication. In many patients, however, stopping medication is not possible. Hypogonadism may be treated by estrogen or testosterone supplementation if necessary. If hyperprolactinemia is confirmed and no alternative cause has been identified, hypothalamic–pituitary disease needs to be considered. A serum prolactin of ≥3000 mU/L (150 μg/L) is nearly always indicative of a prolactinoma.[8] Serum prolactin levels generally correlate with prolactinoma size, although there are exceptions.[75] In a retrospective study of histologically verified nonfunctioning pituitary adenomas with suprasellar extensions, 98.7% of patients had serum prolactin levels <2000 mU/L (100 μg/L), indicating that stalk compression is unlikely to be responsible for hyperprolactinemia in patients with higher serum prolactin levels.[76]

An important assay artifact to be aware of is the high-dose "hook" effect that is due to saturation of antibodies in a two-site immunoradiometric assay.[77] This saturation produces erroneously low levels of prolactin and is of critical importance in patients who present with a large macroadenoma with visual impairment. Prolactin should always be checked with serial dilutions. In this situation, if the tumor is nonfunctioning, the patient should undergo surgical decompression. If, however, the patient has a macroprolactinoma, the treatment is medical, with a DA agonist.

All patients should have MRI (T1-weighted) imaging of the hypothalamus and pituitary, with gadolinium enhancement. A high-resolution CT scan with contrast may be performed if the MRI scan is contraindicated. Dynamic assessment of hypothalamic–pituitary–adrenal reserve (see Appendix) is carried out in patients with identifiable abnormalities. GH reserve is assessed in patients with pituitary macroadenomas. Visual fields are performed where appropriate.

The diagnosis of microprolactinomas and most macroprolactinomas is usually straightforward. There remains, however, the gray area where it is unclear whether the patient has a prolactinoma or a nonfunctioning pituitary adenoma. In most cases, these tumors are small macroadenomas. It is often appropriate to consider a trial of a DA agonist. If there is no evidence of tumor shrinkage after 3 months of treatment, the diagnosis of prolactinoma can effectively be discounted and the patient can be referred for consideration of surgery.

Occasionally, larger tumors may cause diagnostic problems, particularly if the MRI scan demonstrates cystic or hemorrhagic areas in the tumor. In the absence of acute compression symptoms and signs and after neurosurgical review, it may be appropriate to consider the trial of a DA agonist, with close monitoring of visual fields.

## *Management of prolactinomas*

The first question to be asked is whether the patient requires any treatment. The majority of microprolactinomas are small benign tumors that will never grow.[78] There will, however, be a small group of tumors that are destined to become macroadenomas. Patients with microprolactinomas that are unassociated with reproductive dysfunction or galactorrhea do not need treatment. A proportion of the population has small pituitary microadenomas unassociated with any clinical abnormality. Postmortem and MRI analyses have demonstrated that these microadenomas occur in up to 30% of the population. The majority are prolactinomas.[52,79,80]

In microprolactinoma patients with amenorrhea, who are not desirous of pregnancy, treatment can be with either cabergoline or an oral contraceptive. Patients who wish to conceive or who have troublesome galactorrhea should be treated with cabergoline. About 18% of macroadenomas and 10% of microadenomas are resistant to DA agonist therapy. Many of the tumors resistant to bromocriptine or to quinagolide are sensitive to cabergoline and demonstrate better tolerability.[11,12] Thus, cabergoline is recommended in preference to other DA agonists.[13] Discordant effects between prolactin response and tumor shrinkage may occur. Some tumors that are resistant to DA agonists have a reduction in D2 receptor expression.[81] In addition, there is a decrease in Gi2$\alpha$ that couples the D2 receptor to adenylyl cyclase.[82]

High-dose cabergoline (mean dose 5 mg/week), with prolonged treatment up to 12 months, has been reported to normalize prolactin in poor-responding patients.[83] Cabergoline doses of 3 mg daily or more, however, have been reported to be associated with cardiac valvular fibrosis in patients with Parkinson's disease.[84,85] There have been several reported studies of cardiac function in patients treated with cabergoline for hyperprolactinemia and acromegaly. Most of these cases are cross-sectional. Although there have been some reports of mild, clinically nonsignificant valvular fibrosis, the evidence indicates that patients treated with the usual doses of cabergoline, ≤2mg/week, are not at risk of cardiac valvular fibrosis.[13,17,86,87] Long-term prospective studies are required to confirm this hypothesis. Periodic echocardiography should be performed in patients who are found to have a cardiac murmur or in those treated with higher doses of cabergoline.

The majority of microprolactinomas (~90%) will respond rapidly to a small dose of DA agonist, with normalization of serum prolactin. The normal starting dose of cabergoline is 0.25 mg twice weekly. Most patients are controlled with doses up to 2 mg/week. A meta-analysis of clinical studies reporting the proportion of patients with persisting normoprolactinemia after withdrawal of DA agonist has demonstrated that normoprolactinemia is achieved in 21% of patients. The probability of treatment success was highest for patients with idiopathic hyperprolactinemia and with treatment of 2 years or more.[88] In practice, most patients recur after treatment withdrawal. Nonrecurrence may be related to tumor apoplexy.

Surgery may be considered in patients who are resistant to, or are unable to tolerate, DA agonists or for whom a DA agonist is considered to be contraindicated, for example, in patients with valvular heart disease or psychiatric disorders. It is also an option for patients with microadenomas who do not wish to take a DA agonist. Microprolactinomas and intrasellar macroadenomas can be successfully managed surgically in specialist centers, with remission rates of 70%–80%.[89–92] Children and adolescents have been shown to respond to medical treatment equally as well as adults.[93,94]

Macroprolactinomas should be managed medically whenever possible. They usually respond to DA agonist therapy, with evidence of tumor shrinkage, and in patients with visual field defects, with an improvement in visual fields within a few days[12,95–98] (Figures 1.19 and 1.20). Even if patients are hypopituitary at presentation, normal endocrine function may return with DA agonist therapy. Continued tumor shrinkage may occur over many months.[98,99] It is therefore important to continue medical therapy alone, without recourse to other treatment modalities, unless there are specific indications. In spite of this therapy, some large invasive macroprolactinomas may only demonstrate a partial response, sometimes discordant, to medical treatment in terms of serum prolactin levels, tumor size, and invasion of surrounding structures.[11,12,95,100] In these situations, it may be necessary to consider surgery, radiotherapy, or both.

Overall, about 10% of patients are resistant to DA agonists, defined as the failure to achieve a normal prolactin with a maximally tolerated dose of DA agonist and/or a failure to achieve at least a 50% reduction in tumor size.[95]

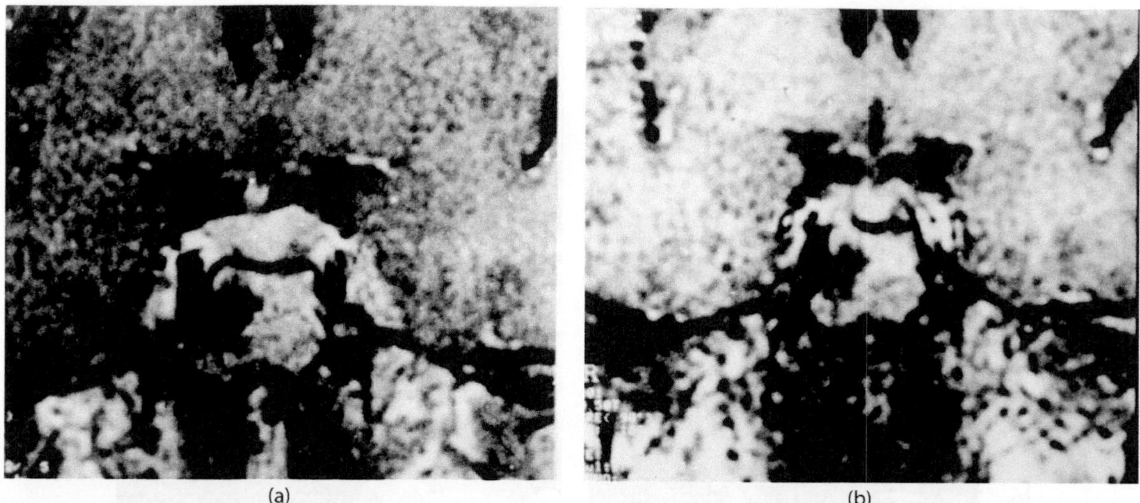


***Figure 1.19***
*Coronal MRI scan (T1-weighted) of an intrasellar macroprolactinoma (a) before and (b) after DA agonist therapy.*

Of course, large macroadenomas do not have such a successful surgical outcome as microadenomas. A recent retrospective study has reported follow-up remission rates of 46% (suprasellar), 12.5% (suprasellar with visual field defects), and 30.8% (parasellar and/or sphenoidal). In addition, there is the risk of new anterior pituitary hormone deficiencies and additional morbidities.[92]

Radiotherapy does not have a place as primary treatment of macroprolactinomas, although it may be used for patients with aggressive macroprolactinomas. The results for both conventional and stereotactic radiotherapies appear to be similar, with normalization of prolactin in up to 30% of patients. There is a long latency over many years before maximal efficacy is achieved with conventional radiotherapy. Stereotactic radiotherapy appears to have the advantage of a more rapid effect.[95]

## *Aggressive prolactinomas*

A subset of macroprolactinomas is particularly aggressive in their behavior, showing only a partial response to DA agonist therapy. These tumors are usually large and invasive. Giant prolactinomas are defined as tumors with a diameter ≥4 cm and/or suprasellar extension ≥2 cm.[95] The suprasellar extension may be associated with hydrocephalus. Lateral extension into the cavernous sinuses may result in cranial nerve palsies, most frequently third nerve palsy. The tumors frequently invade downward into the sphenoid sinus (Figure 1.20). A particular problem with such large tumors is pituitary apoplexy[41] (Figure 1.8) that typically presents with sudden onset of severe headache (see Chapter 24). If there are associated acute compressive effects (e.g., new visual field defects), urgent surgical decompression is required. Serum prolactin levels can be very high, sometimes greater than a million mU/L (>50,000 ng/L). Even if a substantial reduction in serum prolactin levels occurs with DA agonist therapy, the levels often remain markedly elevated. Similarly, tumor shrinkage is very variable. Tumor shrinkage may result in a dural tear, with CSF rhinorrhea. Surgical debulking may be undertaken, but it is rarely curative. Radiotherapy may be required for tumors that continue to grow. Occasionally, growth remains uncontrolled in spite of DA agonist therapy, surgery, and radiotherapy. Very rarely, the tumors become malignant and metastasize[7] (Figure 1.21). Chemotherapy is generally ineffective. If the patient is experiencing severe pain from local tumor invasion, palliation may be obtained from a SS analog.[101] More recently, temozolomide has been demonstrated to be effective in reducing tumor/metastases size and prolactin secretion in some aggressive prolactinomas/carcinomas. Responses are usually seen within the first 3 months of therapy, but relapse may occur a few months later. Current data do not allow a prediction of response, based on MGMT expression or promoter methylation status.[33,102]

Predicting pituitary tumor behavior remains a challenge. A retrospective study of 94 patients who underwent surgical treatment of prolactinomas (54% macroadenoma or giant cell adenoma) classified the tumors as noninvasive, invasive, and aggressive–invasive (corresponding to WHO "atypical adenoma"[5]).

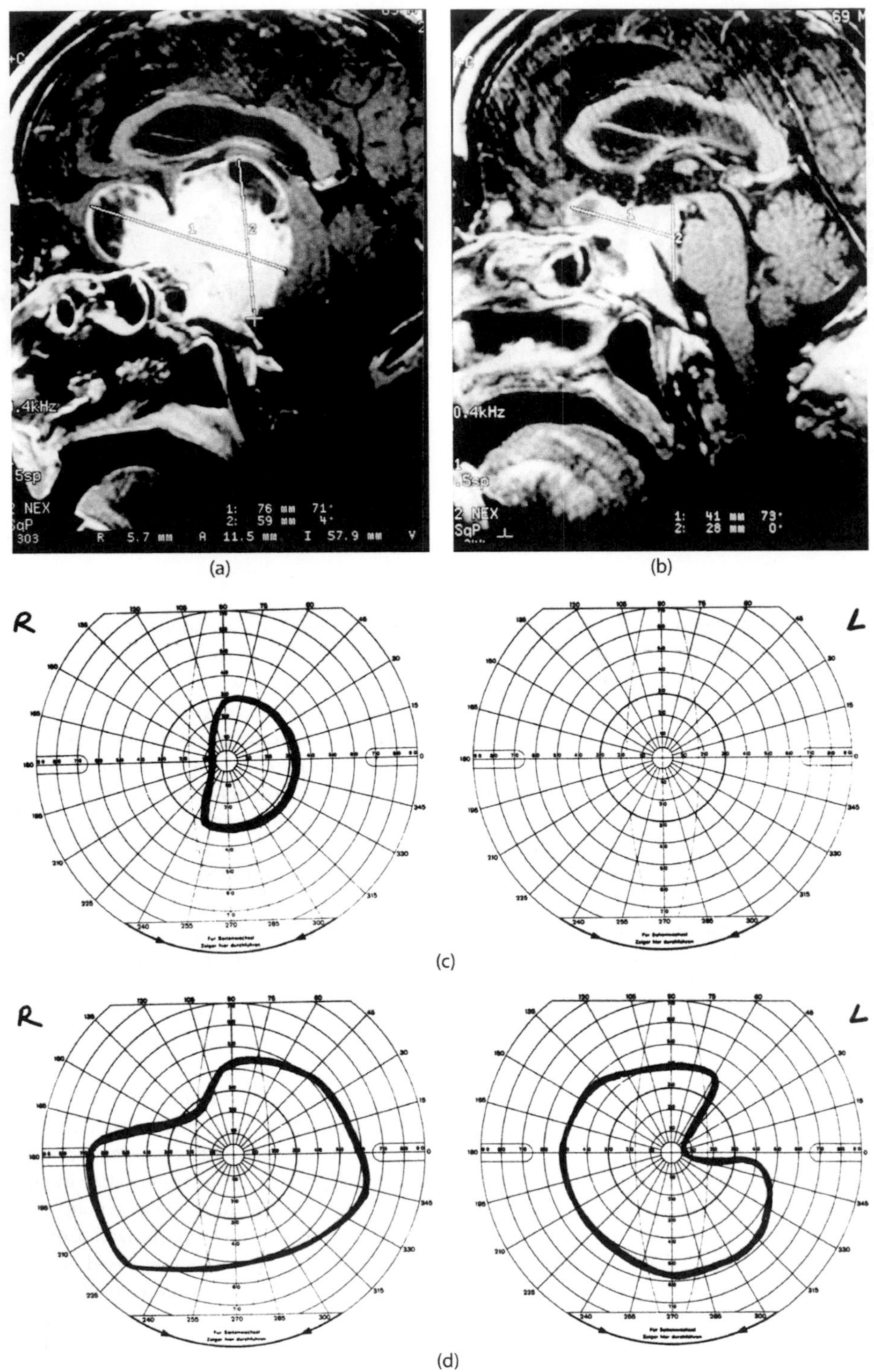


**Figure 1.20**

*Sagittal MRI (T1–weighted) of a giant macroprolactinoma (a) before and (b) after DA agonist therapy. Goldman perimetry (c) before and (d) after DA agonist therapy.*

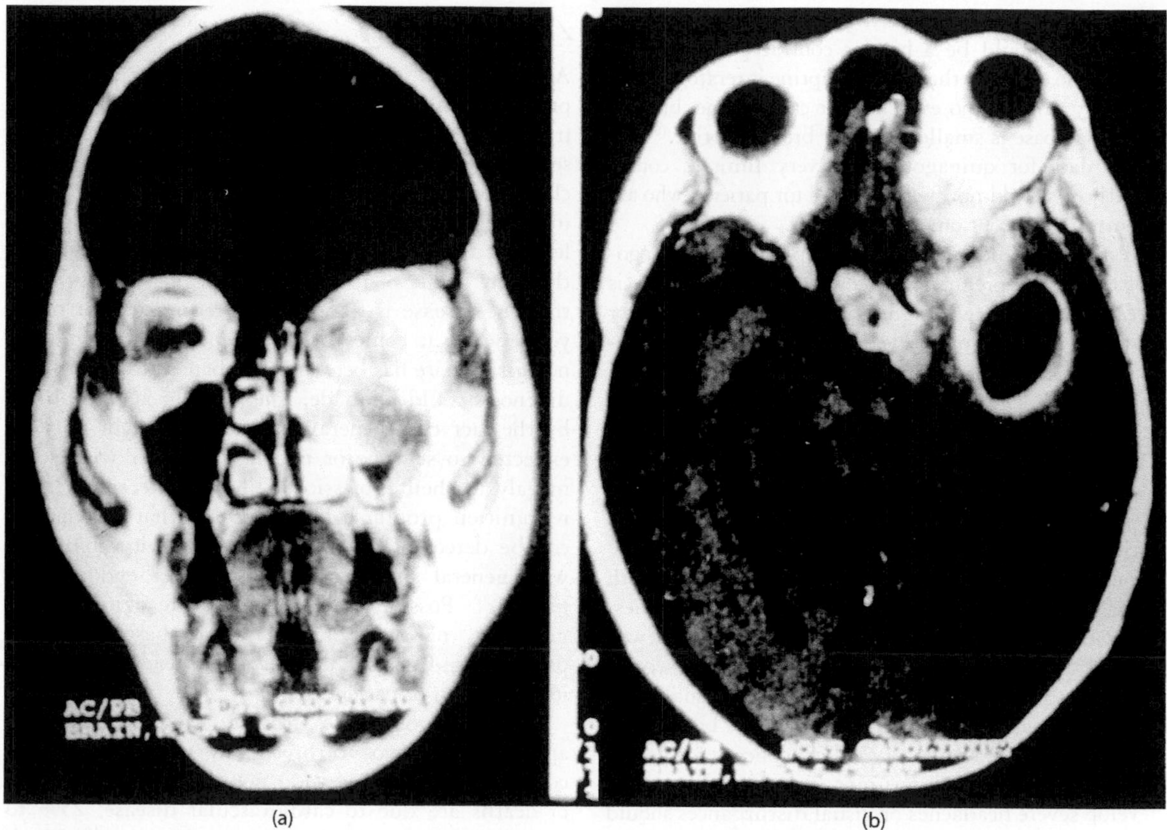


(a) (b)

**Figure 1.21**
*MRI scan (T1-weighted) of a malignant prolactinoma. (a) Coronal section demonstrating extension of the tumor into the right orbit, sphenoid and maxillary sinuses. (b) Axial scan demonstrating extension of the tumor into the right orbit, together with a cystic cerebral metastasis. The tumor had also metastasized to the cervical nodes.*

There was a preponderance of females in the noninvasive group (53/61), 85% of whom remained in long-term remission. In contrast, 18/22 patients in the invasive group were men. All but one patient had persistent disease or progression. All of the invasive aggressive group (five females, six males) demonstrated tumor progression. In addition, based on previous work, seven genes were identified that were associated with tumor recurrence or progression, with five of these genes being highly upregulated in the aggressive-invasive tumors (*ADAMTS6, CRMP1, ASK, CCNB1,* and *CENPE*).[6] Confirmation of these data in a larger cohort of patients would enable a more robust prognostic classification of prolactinomas than is presently available.

## *Prolactinomas in pregnancy*

The management of prolactinomas in pregnancy is covered in the Endocrine Society Clinical Practice Guideline.[13] The normal pituitary gland approximately doubles in size during pregnancy as a result of lactotroph hyperplasia caused by estrogens. This size increase is accompanied by a rise in serum prolactin levels. The increase in prolactin level is very variable but may be as high as 10-fold by term. After delivery, the volume of the gland rapidly decreases, with normalization in size by 6 months, accompanied by a fall in prolactin levels. There is no evidence that estrogens *per se* cause prolactinomas to grow. Microprolactinomas very rarely grow during pregnancy (2.6%). The risk for macroadenomas surgically resected before pregnancy is also low (5%), but medically treated macroadenomas have a higher risk of growth (31%).[75,95] Growth of macroprolactinomas in pregnancy is often associated with pituitary apoplexy that may be estrogen induced. Surgical resection, however, carries the risk of hypopituitarism.

Patients frequently ovulate shortly after starting DA agonist therapy. It is essential that they are warned to take appropriate contraceptive precautions. Ideally, this precaution should be a barrier contraceptive method. There is no evidence that bromocriptine is teratogenic.[103] Similarly, there is no evidence for cabergoline, but the safety database is smaller than for bromocriptine.[16] The safety data for quinagolide are very limited; consequently, it should not be prescribed for patients who are attempting conception.

Patients should immediately stop taking a DA agonist as soon as pregnancy is confirmed, unless there is a real risk of clinically significant tumor expansion, for example, invasive macroadenoma or tumor in proximity to optic chiasm. If the decision is made to treat a patient with a DA agonist throughout pregnancy, the Endocrine Society Guideline recommends the use of bromocriptine.

Because serum prolactin levels normally rise in pregnancy, monitoring of levels in prolactinoma patients is not normally helpful (Table 1.11).[104,105] Patients with microadenomas should be reviewed with clinical examination of visual fields during each trimester. Patients with macroadenomas should be reviewed similarly. If they have not undergone surgical resection before conception, definitive evaluation of visual fields should be made. Visual fields should also be assessed in patients where there is a medical concern for potential clinically significant tumor growth. Patients who develop severe headaches or visual disturbances should have visual field assessment, followed, if indicated, by an MRI scan without contrast. Symptomatic growth of a prolactinoma in pregnancy should be treated with bromocriptine. Cabergoline can be used if bromocriptine is not tolerated. In some circumstances, for instance, if the patient is unable to tolerate DA agonist therapy, if the tumor continues to grow or if there is acute compression from pituitary infarction, surgery may be necessary.

Breastfeeding in prolactinoma patients is generally safe. DA agonists should be avoided because they inhibit lactation. If a patient develops symptomatic growth of a prolactinoma, breastfeeding should be stopped and treatment with a DA agonist reinstated.

## Acromegaly

Acromegaly is insidious in onset and has often been present for many years at the time of diagnosis. It most frequently presents in early middle age, with an equal sex balance. A somatotroph adenoma occurring in childhood/adolescence before epiphysial fusion results in gigantism. Recent data have demonstrated a prevalence for acromegaly that is higher than was previously thought, about 8–13 per 100,000.[50,51] It is apparent that the disease is frequently unrecognized for many years before it comes to the attention of an endocrinologist. There has been much debate as to how earlier diagnosis could be made. The problem is exemplified by the fact that general practitioners might only be expected to see one or two new patients with acromegaly in their professional lifetime. Recently, facial recognition programs have reported that acromegaly can be detected with increased sensitivity compared with general physicians and specialist endocrinologists.[106,107] Possibly, the use of facial recognition programs in national photograph databases, such as passports and driver's licenses, could lead to an earlier identification of patients.

Many retrospective studies have reported an approximately two- to threefold increase in mortality compared with the general population.[1] About 60% of deaths are due to cardiovascular disease, 25% to respiratory disease, and 15% to malignancy.[108] Much of the variability in reported mortality data is likely to be confounded by changes in clinical practice, such as the much lower use of pituitary irradiation, and the more rigorous assessment of adequate control and cure. A recent meta-analysis has reported an overall increase in mortality of 72%. Restriction of the analysis to patients who had undergone transsphenoidal surgery as primary therapy demonstrated an increased mortality of 32%.[109]

Acromegaly is almost invariably caused by a somatotroph adenoma of the pituitary. Most tumors are sporadic. Approximately 40% are associated with activating mutations of Gs (*gsp*),[110,111] and as such they are

| Units | Non-pregnant Female | First Trimester | Second Trimester | Third Trimester |
|---|---|---|---|---|
| ng/mL | 0–20 | 36–213 | 110–330 | 137–372 |
| µg/L | 0–20 | 36–213 | 110–330 | 137–372 |
| pmol/L | 0–859 | 1565–9261 | 4783–14,347 | 5957–16,174 |

***Table 1.11***
*Serum levels of prolactin in non-pregnant female, first, second and third trimesters of pregnancy.*

a feature of the McCune–Albright syndrome (MAS).[112] MAS is an example of a multiple endocrinopathy syndrome. Unlike MEN, however, it is sporadic. Patients have been shown to have widespread tissue expression of the *gsp* oncogene that presumably arises early on in somatic development, providing a mosaic expression in different tissues. The syndrome includes polyostotic fibrous dysplasia of bones, pigmented skin lesions, precocious puberty, autonomous functioning thyroid nodules, pituitary somatotroph adenomas, and adrenal disease, which may be associated with hypercortisolemia. Patients tend to present early on in childhood. The clinical presentation is highly variable.[113] About 20% of patients have GH excess. Excessive growth in childhood may be erroneously ascribed to precocious puberty. Fibrous dysplasia of the skull is a particular problem, because it is often associated with thickening of the skull base and thus may preclude the use of transsphenoidal surgery. In addition, radiotherapy is generally avoided because there is an increased risk of sarcomatous transformation. In consequence, most patients with MAS and acromegaly are treated medically.[114]

Familial syndromes associated with acromegaly include MEN1 (see Chapter 9),[115] FIPA (see Chapter 2),[53] and Carney complex (see "Cushing's syndrome" below).[116] Very rarely, acromegaly is associated with ectopic GHRH or GH production. Thorner et al.[117] and Sassolas et al.[118] originally described two acromegalic patients who had endocrine tumors of the pancreas. Subsequently, GHRH was isolated and characterized from these tumors by Rivier et al.[119] and Guillemin et al.[120] Ectopic production of GHRH has now been described in many cases, most notably in association with carcinoid tumors of the lung and gastrointestinal tract and with islet cell tumors of the pancreas. Occasionally, ectopic production of GHRH has been described in association with intracranial gangliocytomas and other tumors.[121]

| Frequent presenting complaints |
|---|
| Increase in shoe size |
| Increase in ring size |
| Increased linear growth before epiphysial fusion (gigantism) |
| Coarsening of facial features |
| Headaches |
| Carpal tunnel syndrome |
| Arthralgia |
| Snoring |
| Sweating |
| Difficulty with mastication |
| Tongue biting |
| Difficulty with phonation |
| Deepening of voice |

***Table 1.12***
*Frequent presenting complaints in acromegalic patients.*

| Classical signs |
|---|
| Thick, greasy skin |
| Acne |
| Hirsutism |
| Hyperhidrosis |
| Skin tags |
| Soft, "fleshy" hands ("spade-like") |
| Large feet with thickened heel pads |
| Thick "fleshy" lips |
| Prominent supraorbital ridges |
| Rhinomegaly |
| Prognathism |
| Interdental separation |
| Glossomegaly |

***Table 1.13***
*Classical signs of acromegaly.*

## *Clinical features of acromegaly*

Clinical features may relate primarily to the somatic overgrowth engendered by elevated GH and IGF-I levels, to the size of the tumor itself, and/or due to symptoms of associated hypopituitarism. Key features of the condition relate to the somatic overgrowth that results in the characteristic symptoms (Table 1.12) and signs (Table 1.13) of acromegaly. Frequently, the features can best be appreciated by retrospective comparison of the patient's photographs (Figure 1.22). Thickening of the skin is a cardinal physical sign. This thickening can be objectively demonstrated by the measurement of heel pad thickness on x-ray. As a result, venipuncture is often difficult. Skin cuts tend to heal quickly. Patients frequently describe excessive sweating and greasy skin. Skin tags are a common feature, particularly in the axilla and around the nape of the neck. Glossomegaly is also a cardinal sign. The glossomegaly can interfere with mastication that is exacerbated by prognathism and dental malocclusion.

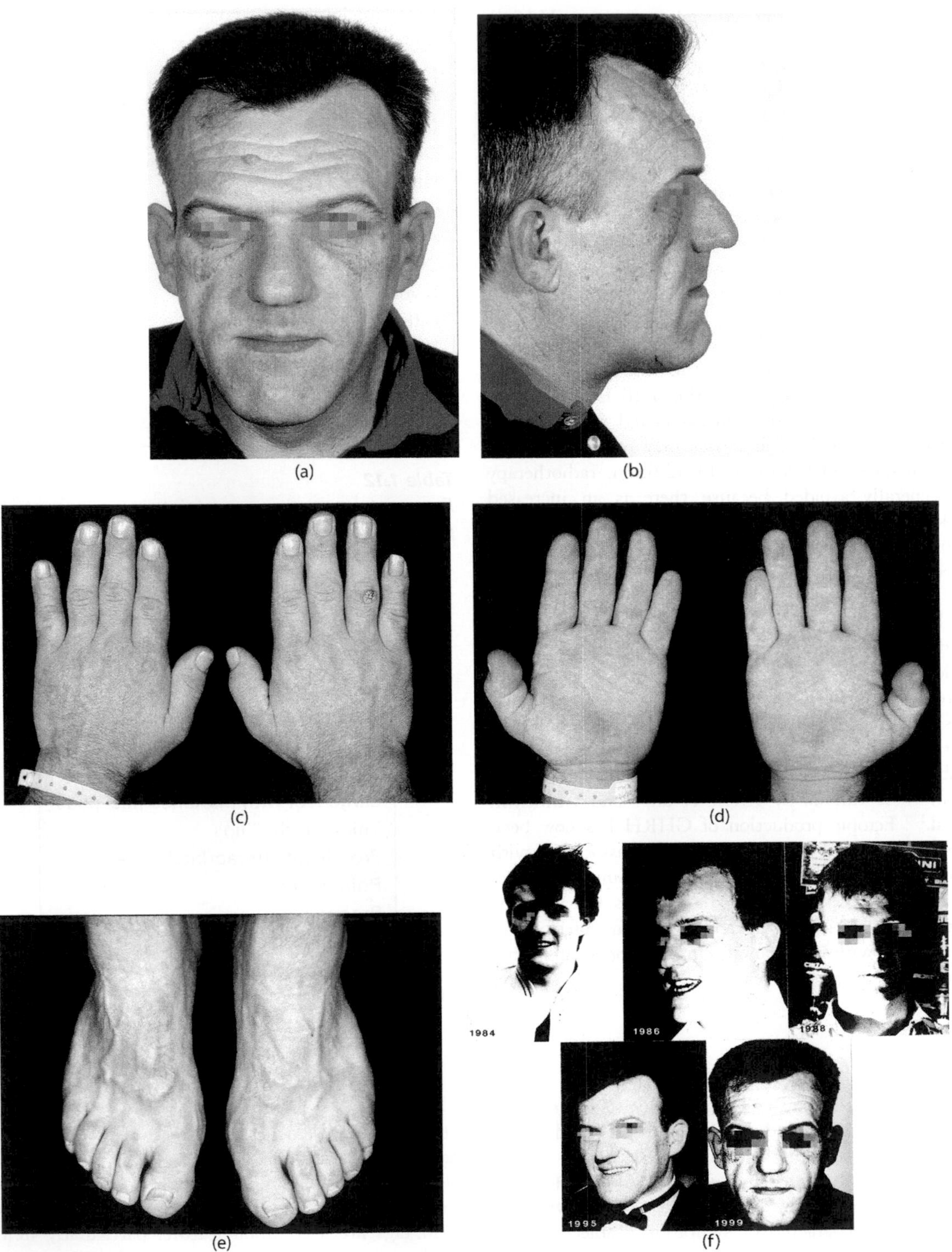


**Figure 1.22**
*(a-e) Patient with acromegaly in 1999. (f) Sequential photographs over time are useful to assess the duration of disease: 1984, 1986, 1988, 1995, 1999.*

There are numerous clinical and metabolic complications arising from acromegaly (Table 1.14).

Glossomegaly, together with pharyngeal and laryngeal swelling, can result in significant upper airway obstruction. Sleep apnea has been reported to be present in up to 80% of patients with acromegaly. It is predominantly obstructive in nature, but there may also be a central component.[108]

Cardiomyopathy is a hallmark of acromegaly and is characterized by biventricular hypertrophy, exacerbated by concomitant hypertension. Over a period of time, diastolic and systolic dysfunction develops. In a retrospective study using Doppler echocardiography in 205 patients with active acromegaly compared with age- and sex-matched nonacromegalic control subjects, the relative risk of developing left ventricular hypertrophy (LVH) was at least 11.9 times higher in the acromegalic patients. Disease duration was found to be the most important criterion for the prevalence and severity of cardiomyopathy. Patients with disease activity of 10 years or more had a threefold higher average relative risk of LVH, associated with diastolic and systolic dysfunction, compared with patients with shorter disease duration. This study also demonstrated an ~1.7-fold increased risk of hypertension and a 4.9-fold increased risk of cardiac arrhythmias.[122] There is an increased prevalence of concomitant valvular heart disease, represented by thickening of the aortic and mitral valves, and resulting in aortic and mitral regurgitation.[123,124]

A causative association between acromegaly and neoplasia remains to be proven. Several studies have reported the occurrence of benign (adenomatous and hyperplastic) colonic polyps in ~45% of patients with acromegaly.[125] The incidence does not differ from that of the general population, using cumulative data from autopsies and screening colonoscopy studies. The polyps are, however, more frequently right-sided, larger, and of advanced histology.[126] The recurrence of adenomatous polyps correlates with serum IGF-I levels.[127] Particular care needs to be taken with patients who have a family history of colon cancer, and a history of previous polyps and multiple skin tags. Current guidelines recommend that all patients with acromegaly should have a colonoscopy at baseline and that patients with colonic polyps should be followed according to the international guidelines for colon cancer.[9] A report has also described an increased incidence of gallbladder polyps in acromegaly.[128]

Degenerative joint disease, affecting both the axial and the appendicular skeletons, is common. In the early stages, where there is thickening of the synovium and articular cartilage, it is potentially reversible.[129] In the

- Pituitary
  - Visual field defects
  - Headaches
  - Hyperprolactinemia
  - Hypopituitarism
- Cardiovascular
  - Cardiomyopathy
  - Arrhythmias
  - Hypertension
- Musculoskeletal
  - Acral enlargement
  - Coarse facial features with prognathism and splayed dentition
  - Enlarged sinuses
  - Excessive long bone growth before epiphysial fusion
  - Degenerative joint disease
  - Mild proximal myopathy
- Neurological
  - Carpal tunnel syndrome
  - Cranial nerve palsies (cavernous sinus invasion by tumor)
  - Headaches
  - Cerebral aneurysms
- Gastrointestinal
  - Colonic polyps with potential risk of malignancy
  - Gall bladder polyps
- Respiratory
  - Upper airways obstruction (macroglossia, pharyngeal)
  - Sleep apnea (obstructive and central)
  - Ventilatory dysfunction
- Metabolic
  - Insulin resistance
  - Impaired glucose tolerance
  - Type 2 diabetes mellitus
  - Dyslipidemia
  - Hypercalciuria—risk of nephrolithiasis
  - Hyperphosphatemia
- Endocrine
  - Multinodular goiter
  - Thyrotoxicosis
  - Oligomenorrhea, amenorrhea
- Impaired quality of life

***Table 1.14***
*Complications of acromegaly.*

majority of patients, however, by the time of diagnosis, irreversible degenerative changes will have occurred. In the spine, intervertebral spaces are typically widened, with vertebral enlargement and osteophyte formation. Axial changes may be present in up to 60% of patients at the time of diagnosis. Severe morphological and structural changes can develop.[130] Clinical symptoms are present in the majority of patients. Long-term uncontrolled disease can lead to severe debilitating arthropathy. Even after disease control, chronic arthropathy remains an important cause of reduced quality of life (QoL).[131]

Headaches are a frequent complaint and are usually unrelated to the size of the pituitary adenoma. The headaches in acromegaly may be rapidly relieved by SS analogs, which are unrelated to the effects on GH secretion. There is an increased prevalence of intracranial saccular aneurysms in acromegaly. A report describes the presence of 40 newly diagnosed aneurysms in 26/152 (17%) of patients who underwent neuroimaging of the Circle of Willis. Ten of the patients had multiple aneurysms. A further two patients had previously undergone aneurysm clipping after subarachnoid hemorrhage. This increased prevalence needs to be borne in mind when patients undergo intracranial imaging.[132]

Carpal tunnel syndrome is associated with edema of the median nerve in the carpal tunnel and is a frequent finding in acromegaly. Approximately 50% of patients have symptoms, but the majority will be found to have evidence of median nerve compression with nerve conduction studies. Although there does not appear to be a relationship with disease duration or GH and IGF-I levels, it may be ameliorated with disease control.[108]

Acromegaly is associated with impaired QoL. A specially designed questionnaire, AcroQol, has been developed to assess the QoL in patients with acromegaly. This questionnaire consists of 22 questions subdivided into two main categories: physical and psychological functions. The psychological category is further subdivided into appearance and personal relationships. Each question is scored out of 5, with a score of 110 representing best possible QoL. A re-evaluation of 56 patients demonstrated that AcroQol is able to demonstrate changes in QoL that would not be detected using generic questionnaires. In addition, a significant negative correlation was demonstrated between change in IGF-I and AcroQol scores.[133,134]

## *Metabolic changes in acromegaly*

Impaired glucose tolerance and diabetes mellitus are well recognized in acromegaly. GH excess leads to hepatic and peripheral insulin resistance. A study of 519 patients in the French Acromegaly Registry estimated the prevalence of diabetes to be 22%.[135] Diabetes was associated with increasing age and weight. There was no significant difference between the levels of GH and IGF-I between diabetic and nondiabetic patients. Diabetes was diagnosed in half the patients at the same time as acromegaly. Diabetes improves with control of acromegaly. This improvement is particularly seen after transsphenoidal surgery or treatment with pegvisomant. SS analogs tend to be relatively neutral in their effects because there is a concomitant inhibition of insulin secretion with improved control of GH.[31,136] An association between hypertension and diabetes was seen, although this association has not been reported in other studies.[137–139] A recent retrospective study of "uncontrolled," "divergent" (high IGF-I, normal GH), and "controlled" patients has reported that in comparison with the controlled group, the divergent group demonstrated higher systolic blood pressure, higher fasting blood glucose, and diabetes mellitus. The total cholesterol was lower in the divergent group than the uncontrolled group, but there was otherwise no difference in lipid profiles between the three groups.[140] There is no consistently abnormal lipid profile that has been identified in acromegaly. Total cholesterol levels have been reported to be low in some studies, returning to normal population levels after treatment with pegvisomant.[141,142] In another study with pegvisomant, cholesterol levels were elevated, and neither cholesterol nor triglyceride levels changed after treatment.[31] Acromegaly has been reported to be associated with hypertriglyceridemia and elevated levels of apolipoprotein E and A-1 and Lp-a.[143]

GH stimulates the activity of 1-α-hydroxylase activity in the kidney, resulting in elevated levels of 1,25-hydroxyvitamin D levels. Hypercalciuria occurs and may result in nephrolithiasis.[144]

## *Diagnosis of acromegaly*

The measurement of GH and age-matched IGF-I concentrations are the key determinants in the diagnosis of acromegaly. The diagnostic criteria for GH levels have changed with the advent of highly sensitive immunoradiometric assays (IRMAs), making comparison with historic data difficult, when the older polyclonal radioimmunoassays (RIAs) were used. A further complicating factor has been the use of different international standards. It is now recommended that the WHO standard 98/574 is used, with the results expressed as micrograms per liter.[145] An additional problem is a lack of uniformity with IGF-I assays, with RIAs as well as IRMAs still in use. In addition, there is a lack of robust age-related normative data available for individual assays.

A single standard is recommended, the IGF-I WHO first international standard (WHO IS 02/254).

GH is secreted in a pulsatile manner. In acromegaly, the GH pulses are increased in frequency about twofold.[146] Random GH levels therefore can be misleading in the diagnosis of acromegaly or in the follow-up of patients posttreatment. Unlike GH that has a half-life of about 22 min, total serum IGF-I has a half-life of about 15 h, and as such provides an integrated reflection of GH secretion over the previous few days. The demonstration of an elevated IGF-I level in the clinic is a useful screen, although it is recommended that this elevation should be confirmed by the oral glucose tolerance test (OGTT). This approach has the added advantage of screening for hyperglycemia. In most cases, the diagnosis is straightforward, with the demonstration of unequivocally elevated GH levels that fail to suppress. In a small proportion of patients, however, the interpretation can be more difficult. The current consensus is that failure to suppress GH below 1 μg/L is diagnostic of acromegaly.[9] This value may however be too high for a small number of individuals. A GH nadir of ≤0.3 μg/L appears to provide adequate discrimination from normal in most cases.[147] This nadir diagnostic detection limit is more of an issue when assessing disease activity after surgery. False positives may occur in diabetes mellitus, liver disease, renal disease, hyperthyroidism, adolescence, anorexia nervosa, and other forms of malnutrition. An elevated serum IGF-I together with failure of suppression of GH on OGTT is required to make the diagnosis of acromegaly. There are, however, also potential confounding factors in which serum IGF-I may be affected.[147] Important variables to be aware of are diabetes mellitus, anorexia nervosa, and malnutrition, all of which can be associated with lower levels of serum IGF-I. Increasing age is also associated with a concomitant reduction is serum IGF-I levels, emphasizing the importance of using well-validated age-dependent normal ranges for a specific assay. Adolescents may have levels that are outside of the quoted normal range for a given assay. Serum IGF-I levels rise throughout pregnancy, under the influence of placental GH.

Serum IGFBP-3 and ALS are additional biomarkers that are usually elevated in acromegaly. IGFBP-3 is a less robust biomarker than ALS. Postsurgically, ALS has been shown to have a sensitivity comparable with IGF-I, with a slightly lower specificity.[148]

The majority of somatotroph adenomas are macroadenomas.[149] In consequence, a proportion of these tumors will have hyperprolactinemia related to stalk compression. Approximately 20% of patients have tumors that also produce prolactin. The majority are mixed somatotroph–lactotroph tumors, with about 5% being mammosomatotrophs. Acidophil cell adenomas are characteristically associated with hyperprolactinemia, often with relatively low GH production[5] (Table 1.4).

All patients must have a full endocrine assessment, including a dynamic assessment of the hypothalamic–pituitary–adrenal (HPA) axis. Ring size provides a simple objective measurement for clinical assessment of treatment efficacy. A generalized enlargement of the pituitary without a discrete tumor being demonstrated on MRI scanning should raise the possibility of ectopic GHRH production.

## Management of acromegaly

Guidelines on the consensus of cure have been published by the Endocrine Society.[145] Optimal disease control is defined as IGF-I level in the age-adjusted normal range, with a random GH measurement ≤1 μg/L. An OGTT has been shown to be inappropriate for patients who are on treatment with SS analogs, where a large proportion of results have been found to be discordant with IGF-I levels.[150] Due to its action of GH receptor antagonism, disease control for patients on pegvisomant therapy can only be assessed using serum IGF-I.[30] Although there is a strong correlation between serum GH and IGF-I levels, a discordance have been reported in >30% of patients with persisting active disease. Most of the discordance is from patients with persistently elevated serum IGF-I with "normal" serum GH. If stricter criteria detailed above are applied using highly sensitive IRMAs for GH, the discrepancies are greatly reduced. Nonetheless, discrepant results remain for some patients. After radiotherapy, some patients demonstrate low serum GH levels, with persistently elevated IGF-I.[151] It is important to exclude potential confounding factors for low IGF-I and elevated GH detailed above. Serum IGF-I levels can take a few months to normalize after surgery. If a persistently elevated IGF-I is seen with apparently normal GH levels, patients should be periodically reassessed for evidence of disease recurrence. The use of IRMAs, together with the stricter definition of disease control, renders the assessment of historical efficacy data for surgery, radiotherapy, and medical therapy in acromegaly difficult.

### Surgery

The first-line treatment of choice is transsphenoidal surgery (see Chapter 3). This approach is particularly the case with readily resectable intrasellar micro- and macroadenomas and where the tumor is causing compressive symptoms. Surgery should also be considered in tumors where total removal is not possible because surgical debulking facilitates subsequent disease control with medical therapy/radiotherapy.[152–154] The key consideration for surgical treatment, as for any pituitary surgery, is performance by an experienced pituitary surgeon. Transsphenoidal surgery is the usual approach. Many surgeons are now using endoscopic surgery, and intraoperative MRIs are being used in a few centers. Overall, biochemical control can now be expected in >70% of patients with surgically resectable tumors. In contrast, biochemical control for macroadenomas is about 50%.[155–158] Surgical pretreatment with SS analogs has been undertaken with the rationale of improved surgical outcome after metabolic control and tumor shrinkage. This approach is unproven at the present time. One prospective randomized study reported biochemical control in 16% of patients with macroadenomas ($n$ = 32), a value that is extremely low, compared with 50% in the pretreated group ($n$ = 30), a value that is in line with the current literature for macroadenomas.[159]

Medical therapy is indicated in the following situations:

1. Failure to achieve control with surgery.
2. Primary medical therapy is an option for patients with tumors that are not considered to be curable by surgery, bearing in mind that surgical debulking facilitates subsequent medical control. It should be considered in patients for whom surgery is contraindicated, for example, serious associated comorbidities and in MAS. Primary medical therapy is not appropriate for patients who have evidence of tumor compression, in particular, visual field defects.
3. Surgical pretreatment, although the effects on surgical outcome remain to be demonstrated.
4. Maintenance of disease control pending the effects of radiotherapy.

## Medical treatment

### DA agonists

Cabergoline has had a limited use in acromegaly.[160] Published data on the efficacy of DA agonists in acromegaly are very variable. A meta-analysis of published data on 149 patients has been performed. None of the studies involved were randomized or placebo-controlled. The meta-analysis demonstrated that the overall efficacy of cabergoline in these studies was dependent upon the basal IGF-I level, although some patients normalized IGF-I from high baseline levels.[161] Hyperprolactinemia was not found to be predictive of response, contrary to previously held views. This finding is not particularly surprising because the majority of somatotroph adenomas express dopamine D2 receptors and demonstrate inhibition of GH secretion to DA agonists *in vitro*. The coexpression of SST2 and D2 receptors by somatotroph adenomas has provided the rationale for the development of SS-DA analog chimeras for the treatment of acromegaly.[28] Overall, 34% of patients achieved normal IGF-I levels, with increasing efficacy over time. There was no clear dose relationship demonstrable. In the responder patients, the mean dose of cabergoline was 2.5 mg/week. There was no evidence of tachyphylaxis. This dose is higher than the dose generally required for patients with prolactinomas (<2 mg/week). It is unknown whether patients with acromegaly are at increased risk of developing cardiac valvular fibrosis with exposure to cabergoline. The dose remains much lower than that used for Parkinson's disease; nevertheless, given the inherent increased risk of cardiac valvular disease in acromegaly, periodic echocardiography should be undertaken.[123,124] Tumor shrinkage may occur and, in contrast to biochemical response, is related to hyperprolactinemia.[161]

In summary, cabergoline therapy may be considered after surgery, for some patients, particularly those with IGF-I levels <150% the upper limit of normal. Cabergoline may also be considered as additional therapy for some patients who remain uncontrolled on SS analogs.[162–164] Its advantages are oral administration and cost. It is not possible to predict whether a patient will respond, so a therapeutic trial is required. The long-term safety in terms of cardiac valvular fibrosis in acromegaly is unknown. It is also important to note that it is not an approved treatment for acromegaly.

### SS analogs

SS analogs are the approved first-line medical therapy for acromegaly. The GH response to an octreotide test dose of 50 μg s.c. can give an indication of the likely responsiveness to long-term treatment, but it is not definitive.[165] In practice, most patients are started on SS analog therapy. A good indication of responsiveness can be obtained within 3 months of treatment, although efficacy continues to improve over time with continued treatment.[166] In addition, unlike functioning carcinoid tumors, tachyphylaxis does not occur.[167]

The true efficacy of SS analogs is difficult to gauge, because most studies have reported data using less stringent criteria of control than are used today. In addition, data have often been on preselected populations. Some studies define a biochemical response as a "safe" GH of ≤2.5 μg/L, together with age-related IGF-I within the normal range. This is, in fact, more generous than the ≤1.0 μg/L defined in the Endocrine Society definition of disease control.[145] Data for studies where patients have not been preselected, using the predefined study

| | Study details | GH ≤2.5 μg/L (%) | Normal age-related IGF-I (%) |
|---|---|---|---|
| Cozzi et al. 2006 | Median follow-up 48 weeks<br>octreotide LAR<br>$n = 67$ | 68.7 | 70.1 |
| Mercado et al. 2007 | 24 weeks<br>48 weeks<br>octreotide LAR<br>$n = 68$ (ITT 98) | 42<br>44 | 38<br>34 |
| Lombardi et al. 2009 | 48–52 weeks<br>lanreotide Autogel<br>$n = 51$ | 63 | 37 |

$n$ = number of patients; ITT, intention to treat; GH, growth hormone; IGF-I, insulin-like growth factor I.

***Table 1.15***
***Efficacies of octreotide LAR and lanreotide Autogel in unselected patients with acromegaly.***

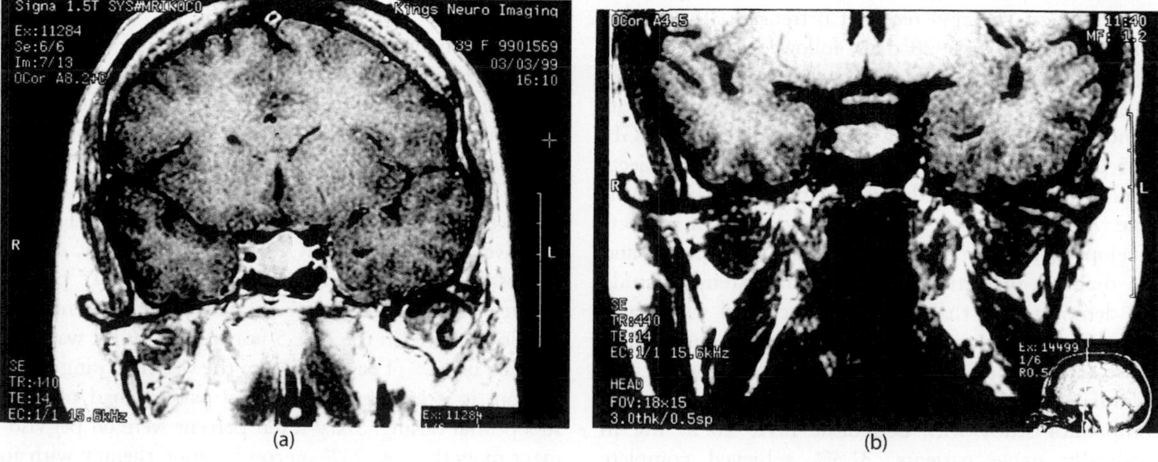


***Figure 1.23***
***Coronal MRI scan (T1-weighted) of a somatotroph adenoma (a) before and (b) after 9 months of treatment with somatostatin analog. Note the high signal hemorrhagic component of the tumor.***

criteria, and with treatment for at least 6 months, are detailed in Table 1.15.[166,168,169] Safe GH levels were obtained in between 42% and 69% of patients, with normal IGF-I levels in between 34% and 70%. The efficacy of SS analogs in *de novo* patients (primary medical therapy) is comparable to that in patients who have first undergone pituitary surgery.[166,168–170] In a recent study (PRIMARYS) of 90 *de novo* patients with acromegaly treated with lanreotide Autogel 120 mg monthly for 48 weeks, 65% achieved GH ≤2.5 μg/L, 39% achieved normal age- and sex-matched IGF-I levels, and 34% achieved normal control with both. Two recent studies have demonstrated similar efficacies for octreotide LAR and lanreotide Autogel (lanreotide depot).[171,172] Control of acromegaly with Autogel may be maintained by increasing dosing intervals between injections.[25,172] SS analogs may also be effective in patients with ectopic production of GH.[173]

Surgery is the definitive means of achieving tumor control and is indicated in patients who have clinical evidence of tumor compression. Somatotroph adenomas demonstrate variable responses in terms of tumor shrinkage to SS analogs (Figure 1.23). The criteria for significant tumor shrinkage varies between studies, ranging from 10% to >45%. A systematic review of studies of pituitary tumor shrinkage during primary medical therapy with SS analogs in patients with acromegaly concluded that overall 37% of patients demonstrated significant shrinkage according to the study criteria. Of these patients, an approximately 50% reduction in tumor mass was seen in patients on primary medical therapy, or before surgery or radiotherapy.[174] There is a wide range of variability between patients, with some demonstrating little or no shrinkage effect and others >60%.[175] The greatest effect is seen in patients who are treated with SS analogs as primary therapy.[176] The recent PRIMARYS study with lanreotide Autogel demonstrated ≥20% tumor volume reduction in 75% of the per protocol population (n = 60). The tumor shrinkage effects and antisecretory effects of SS analogs may not be concordant in individual patients.[20,175,176] Tumor growth may occur in a small proportion (<3%) of patients.[20]

The novel multireceptor ligand SS analog pasireotide has completed clinical development. In a phase II study, 60 patients with active acromegaly (14% *de novo*, 35% prior surgery, 9% prior radiotherapy, 42% prior medical therapy) received octreotide 100 μg s.c. three times daily for 28 days, followed by pasireotide 200, 400, and 600 μg s.c. twice daily in random order for 28 days each. After 3 months of pasireotide treatment, 27% had achieved a biochemical response (GH ≤2.5 μg/L, normal IGF-I). In addition, 39% of subjects demonstrated ≥20% reduction in pituitary tumor volume. After treatment with pasireotide, 7% of subjects developed hyperglycemia, 5% an increase in $HbA_{1c}$, and 5% diabetes mellitus.[26] A subsequent extension study has demonstrated that biochemical control was maintained, with further reductions in tumor volume. The phase III development program has used a long-acting formulation, pasireotide LAR 40/60 mg. In a 12-month comparator study with octreotide LAR 20/30 mg in medically naïve patients, 31.3% achieved complete biochemical control with pasireotide LAR, compared with 19.2% with octreotide LAR. Some patients with low serum IGF-I levels were considered to be noncontrolled. The full response including these patients was 35.8% for pasireotide LAR, compared with 20.9% for octreotide LAR. Mean GH and IGF-I levels plateaued at 3 months, with control being maintained at 12 months. Similar degrees of tumor shrinkage were seen with both treatments. Hyperglycemia-related events were seen in 57.3% of patients treated with pasireotide LAR and in 21.7% of patients treated with octreotide LAR. In a subsequent extension study, patients who were inadequately controlled could switch treatment; 21% of patients inadequately controlled on octreotide LAR achieved full biochemical control after switching to pasireotide LAR, and 2.6% of patients inadequately controlled on pasireotide LAR achieved control after switching to octreotide LAR. Of the patients who continued to receive their randomized therapy, at month 19, full biochemical control was achieved in 45.9% (*n* = 74) with pasireotide LAR and in 45.7% (*n* = 46) with octreotide LAR.

In summary, the phase III data indicate that pasireotide LAR offers a modest improvement in efficacy compared with conventional SS analogs, although at 19 months, there appears to be comparable efficacy with octreotide LAR. This efficacy is at the expense of an increased risk of hyperglycemia and development of diabetes mellitus. Pegvisomant has a clear advantage in this regard. In consequence, the positioning of pasireotide in the medical treatment algorithm of acromegaly remains to be defined.

### *Pegvisomant*

The GH antagonist pegvisomant is indicated for patients who remain uncontrolled on therapy with SS analogs. The U.S. label also allows for the possibility of first-line medical therapy, although most clinicians use it second line.

Pegvisomant is administered as an s.c. injection. The starting dose is 10 mg, and dose can be titrated up to 30–40 mg to achieve normal serum IGF-I. Due to its mechanism of action, GH levels rise two- to threefold during treatment,[30] meaning that measurement of GH levels is not possible to monitor control. In addition, pegvisomant cross-reacts with commercial GH assays. It is highly effective in normalizing IGF-I which, in theory, should be possible in all patients.[31] The ACROSTUDY patient registry, however, has demonstrated that this is not the case in practice. In the first 5-year report, IGF-I was normalized in 62% of patients. From the weekly dosing information, it is apparent that many patients had received suboptimal dosing. Sixty-seven percent were on pegvisomant monotherapy, 23% on combination therapy with an SS analog, 6% on combination therapy with a DA analog, and 4% in combination with an SS analog and a DA analog. Importantly, IGF-I control remained the same, with monotherapy and with the combination therapies.[177]

A safety review of 1288 subjects in the ACROSTUDY registry has reported elevated hepatic transaminases of ≥3 times the upper limit of normal in 2.5% (30) of patients.[32] There were no reports of hepatic failure. Drug-induced hepatitis has been reported in a patient after rechallenge with pegvisomant.[31] Injection site reactions were reported to occur in 2.2% (28) of cases. Lipohypertrophy is a recognized side effect that may occur due to the local effect of GH antagonism at the injection site.[178] Injection site rotation may reduce the risk of lipohypertrophy developing. Increases in pituitary tumor size were confirmed in 3.2% of cases. This increase has been a theoretical concern because unlike SS analogs, pegvisomant does not target the pituitary tumor. Furthermore, GH levels rise on pegvisomant therapy, although this rise should be mitigated by GH receptor antagonism. Tumor growth after conversion of SS analog therapy to pegvisomant may be due to a rebound effect of stopping SS analog therapy. In addition, a small proportion of tumors will grow anyway, as is evidenced in patients on SS analogs.[20] Presently, there are limited long-term follow-up data on patients treated with pegvisomant. Patients who are treated with pegvisomant should continue to have periodic monitoring of tumor size by MRI.

The conversion of treatment from SS analogs to pegvisomant has been shown to be associated with improved insulin sensitivity and glycemic control.[140,179] In a 32-week study of conversion from octreotide LAR to pegvisomant in 53 patients with acromegaly, HbA1c was improved by >1.0% in patients with diabetes. The improved glycemic control in patients treated with pegvisomant is a useful feature to consider in the treatment of patients with impaired glucose tolerance and diabetes mellitus. In this same study, the proportion of patients with normalized IGF-I rose from 29% to 78% at week 32. In the first 3–4 months of conversion, there is an overlapping effect of both drugs. This overlap is demonstrated by the study data in which there was a fall in the proportion of patients with normal IGF-I levels between 3 and 5 months. Thereafter, control improved as the dose of pegvisomant was titrated upward[136]. There was no change in median pituitary volume, although the tumor volume increased ~1 cm in two patients with macroadenomas. One of these patients had previously been treated with pegvisomant without a change in tumor size, and there was no further change in tumor size with continued treatment for a further year. The other patient had a large aggressive tumor that grew despite multiple different treatment modalities, including SS analog therapy.

An alternative approach to conversion is combination therapy with SS analog and pegvisomant. In this case, the patient remains on the same dose of SS analog and additional pegvisomant is added, titrating the dose up until IGF-I is normalized. Dose titration is more straightforward because it is not being done against a waning effect of SS analog. In a head-to-head comparison of pegvisomant monotherapy ($n$ = 27) with octreotide LAR and pegvisomant combination ($n$ = 29) in patients uncontrolled on SS monotherapy, there was no difference in IGF-I normalization rates between the two groups of patients at 40 weeks.[180] The median dose of pegvisomant monotherapy was 20 mg/day and in the combination therapy 15 mg/day. There was improved glycemic control in the pegvisomant monotherapy group. Hepatic transaminases were increased by >10 times upper limit of normal (ULN) in three patients in the combination group. Two of these patients had received high doses of octreotide LAR (60 mg/month). Another patient in the combination group and one in the monotherapy group had increases in hepatic transaminases >3 times ULN. MRI evidence of tumor growth occurred in one patient in the pegvisomant monotherapy group and in one patient in an octreotide LAR safety comparison group. In another study, pegvisomant was administered weekly (40–120 mg) in combination with lanreotide Autogel 120 mg/month for 28 weeks to patients uncontrolled on SS analog monotherapy ($n$ = 92).[181] Normalization of IGF-I occurred in 58% of patients. The median dose of pegvisomant was 60 mg/week. There was no evidence of an overall change in tumor size during treatment. Two patients developed transient elevations in hepatic transaminases (ALT >5 times ULN) that returned to normal after treatment discontinuation. Hepatic transaminases were transiently increased >2 times ULN in a further four patients. Importantly, there was no relationship between diabetic status and elevated hepatic transaminases, a finding that differs from other study data.[182] Another study with patients who were controlled on octreotide LAR or lanreotide Autogel has demonstrated comparable efficacy using low-dose pegvisomant (15–30 mg twice weekly) together with 50% of the previous dose of SS analog.[183] Overall, no efficacy benefit has been demonstrated with combination therapy compared with pegvisomant monotherapy. Liver function needs to be regularly monitored. There are currently no data to suggest an effect on tumor growth compared with patients on pegvisomant monotherapy. There is the potential for dose-sparing and reduced injection frequency. A comparison of the potential advantages and disadvantages of SS analog and pegvisomant therapies is summarized in Table 1.16.

An alternative combination to SS analog and pegvisomant is cabergoline. In the ACROSTUDY registry 5-year report, 6% of patients were treated with DA analog–pegvisomant combination therapy.[32] In a study of 24 patients with acromegaly, cabergoline monotherapy normalized IGF-I in two (8%) of patients, after titrating up to a maximum dose of 3.5 mg/week. The addition of 10 mg of pegvisomant daily for 12 weeks normalized IGF-I in 68% of patients, which compares to 54% with 10-mg monotherapy in the pegvisomant pivotal study. Twelve weeks after cabergoline withdrawal, only 26% of patients maintained a normal IGF-I whilst continuing with pegvisomant.[184] The data are interesting, because the response to cabergoline was much lower than in a previously reported study.[161] In addition, in the pegvisomant pivotal study, 54% of patients normalized IGF-I after 12 weeks treatment with 10 mg.[30]

| | SS analog | Pegvisomant | SS and pegvisomant |
|---|---|---|---|
| Disease control | Normal IGF-I ~50% | Potential for control in most patients | Potential for control in most patients |
| Tumor | Shrinkage ~50% | No evidence of tumor growth | No evidence of tumor growth |
| Glycemic control | Neutral | Improved ++ | Improved + |
| Hepatic | Biliary tract disease ~35%; usually asymptomatic | Elevated transaminases <5% | Biliary tract disease ~35%; usually asymptomatic |
| Gastrointestinal | Intolerance ~10% | Elevated transaminases <10% | Intolerance ~10% |
| Injection site reactions | | Lipohypertrophy | |
| Frequency of administration | Monthly (6–8 weeks, lanreotide Autogel) | Daily (less frequent injections may be possible in well-controlled patients) | Daily to weekly pegvisomant |

***Table 1.16***
*Comparison of the potential advantages and disadvantages of somatostatin (SS) analog therapy, pegvisomant monotherapy, and SS and pegvisomant combination therapy.*

## *Radiotherapy*

Radiotherapy (see Chapter 4) is used much less frequently than in the past. Its most frequent use is the control of tumor growth in aggressive tumors that have not responded to surgery and/or medical therapy. Its utility for biochemical control is much reduced because most patients can now be controlled with SS analogs and pegvisomant. It may be used to avoid potentially expensive long-term medical therapy, but there is a high risk of rendering the patient hypopituitary.

Conventional conformal fractionated radiotherapy can ultimately achieve biochemical control in about 60% of patients at 10 years, rising to >70% at 15 years. Normalization of GH and IGF-I is dependent on the pretreatment levels.[185,186] Stereotactic radiotherapy or single-fraction radiosurgery may be preferred for patients with smaller, more discrete tumors. Presently, there is insufficient evidence to favor one technique over another. Treatment choice is largely dependent upon local facilities and expertise.

## *Pregnancy in acromegaly*

There is little information available on the effects of uncontrolled pregnancy and its treatment in the literature. This discrepancy may be in part because acromegaly is associated with gonadal dysfunction. If a patient is planning pregnancy, the optimal scenario would be to obtain biochemical control by surgery. The management of pregnancy in patients with active disease remains controversial. Many patients will be on medical therapy until conception, but then stop. A recent report has reviewed the outcomes of 47 pregnancies in acromegalic women. Nine patients had no medical treatment, six patients had DA agonist, six patients had combination with DA agonist and SS analog, one patient had pegvisomant SS combination, 24 patients had SS analog alone, and one patient had pegvisomant. After gestation, medical therapy continued in 19 patients, in 10 for <20 weeks: 14 SS analog, three DA agonist, and two pegvisomant. None of the patients developed endocrine or neurological complications. All babies reached full term with normal weights. An extended review of a further 59 pregnancies demonstrated that 81% were without complication; three with gestational diabetes mellitus; seven with preeclampsia; and nine with exacerbations of symptoms of acromegaly, in particular headaches. Eighty-three of the babies were normal weight, seven were microsomic (five SS), and five were macrosomic (two DA).[187] A case report of pegvisomant treatment throughout pregnancy resulted in a normal baby delivered at 40 weeks by caesarian section. Importantly, fetal GH and IGF-I levels remained normal throughout the pregnancy. Fetal pegvisomant levels were minimal. Pegvisomant levels in the breast milk were undetectable.[188] In contrast, a case report of octreotide LAR treatment throughout pregnancy demonstrated evidence of maternal–fetal transfer of drug. The dose of octreotide LAR was reduced from 20 to 10 mg at 21 weeks gestation due to concerns of intrauterine growth retardation. A normal, healthy baby was delivered by caesarian section at 38 weeks, with normal postnatal development, weight, and height reaching the 50th centile at 3 months.[189] In summary, from the limited data that are available, acromegaly is usually associated with normal pregnancy outcomes. Medical therapy should be avoided whenever possible because of the potential effects on fetal size.

### *Aggressive somatotroph adenomas*

These tumors are generally sporadic, but they may occur as a result of an underlying genetic defect, as in MEN1[115] (see Chapter 9), FIPA[53] (see Chapter 2), Carney complex (usually microadenomas),[116] and MAS.[113,114] They are most frequently seen in young adults. It has recently been demonstrated that the aryl hydrocarbon receptor–interacting protein (AIP) mutations seen in some FIPA patients also occur in sporadic tumors.[190] These tumors are often sparsely granulated with a dot-like keratin pattern. There are no predictive molecular markers. They characteristically have a poor response to SS analogs. Pegvisomant can usually provide biochemical control. Radiotherapy may be necessary to control tumor growth.

### *Summary of management*

Surgery remains the first-line therapy in most patients (Figure 1.24). If surgical cure is not obtained, treatment should be started with SS analog. Cabergoline may be considered in patients with mild residual disease. If the patient remains uncontrolled, treatment should be switched to pegvisomant. Pegvisomant combination therapy with SS analog is an alternative option. In patients who have aggressive disease, radiotherapy may be required in addition to medical therapy. The positioning of pasireotide in the medical treatment of patients with acromegaly remains to be defined.

## *Cushing's syndrome*

Harvey Cushing first described the chromophobe pituitary adenoma as being the underlying cause of some cases of the condition,[191] thereafter referred to as Cushing's disease. Although florid cases of Cushing's syndrome are easy to diagnose, subtler cases can be extremely difficult. Alcohol abuse, obesity, and depression can all give rise to "pseudo-Cushing's syndrome," not only mimicking Cushing's syndrome clinically but also, on occasion, biochemically. In addition, some cases of Cushing's disease "cycle" in and out of active disease. A recent review of 201 patients identified 30 (14%) patients with a median intercyclic period of 4 years, although the period can be highly variable.[192] Once the diagnosis of Cushing's syndrome has been confirmed, it is necessary to make a specific etiological diagnosis. Although the differentiation of Cushing's syndrome into ACTH-dependent and ACTH-independent disease is usually straightforward, the identification of the source of ACTH in the former can be very difficult. Neurosurgery should only

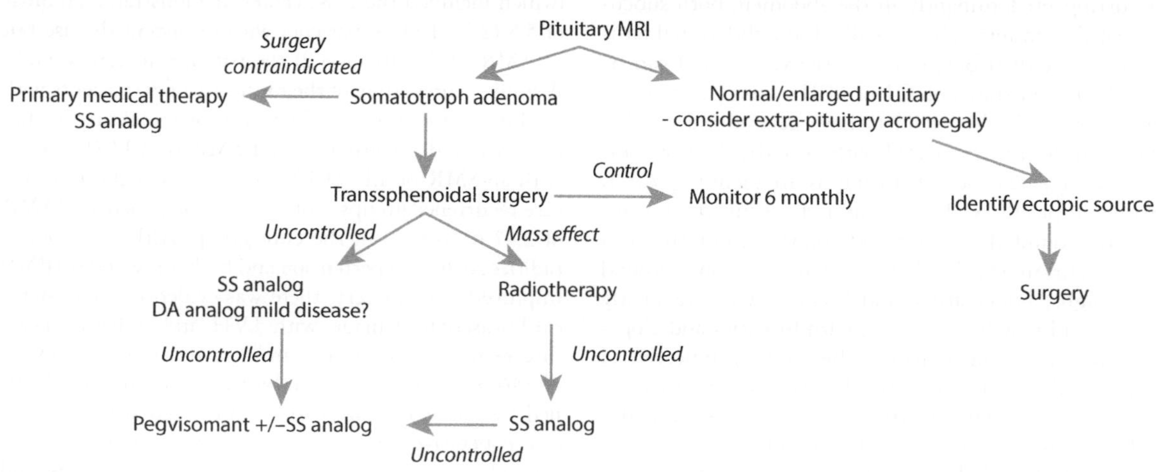


**Figure 1.24**
*Treatment algorithm for patients with acromegaly.*

be carried out by a dedicated neuroendocrine surgeon. An experienced endocrine surgeon should be available for bilateral adrenalectomy, and there should be ready access to thoracic surgery.

## Clinical features of Cushing's syndrome

The clinical signs of Cushing's syndrome are well recognized (Figures 1.25 and 1.26) and are summarized in Table 1.17. Patients most commonly present complaining of rapid weight gain. Growth retardation occurs in >80% of children and adolescents. This growth retardation, together with weight gain, is an important discriminating feature of Cushing's syndrome in this age group. Oligomenorrhea and amenorrhea are commonly associated presentations in women. Some patients complain of weakness, particularly if their work involves a great deal of physical activity. Difficulty with climbing stairs is a frequent complaint. Recurrent infections are occasionally a presenting problem. The majority of patients will have some form of psychological disturbance, ranging from mild symptoms to a severe psychosis.

Cushing's syndrome is associated with severe morbidities (Table 1.18). A 2-year review of 481 patients with Cushing's syndrome from the European Registry on Cushing's syndrome (ERCUSYN) summarizes the morbidities associated with the different etiologies of the disease.[193] Patients characteristically have a rounded, plethoric face. There is typically a central distribution of body fat with contrastingly thin arms and legs. The acquisition of body fat can be rapid, occurring predominantly in the abdomen, both subcutaneously and intra-abdominally. Intra-abdominal fat is particularly distributed around the viscera and can be clearly demonstrated on CT or MRI scans (Figure 1.27). In contrast, children tend to have generalized obesity. The skin is thin compared with an individual of comparable age and sex. Bruising is frequently present. Striae, typically violaceous or red, occur most commonly around the axillae and abdomen, but they can also occur in the lumbar or gluteal regions, around the thighs, upper arms, and breasts. Acne frequently occurs and may be associated with hirsuties and alopecia. Acanthosis nigricans may be present, indicative of hyperinsulinemia. There may be evidence of cutaneous infections with viral warts, oral candidiasis, and fungal infections, reflecting immunosuppression. Proximal myopathy should always be sought and is best assessed by asking the patient to rise from a squat without using a support, with the back kept straight.

Osteoporosis can be extremely rapid in onset, with serious sequelae. The ERCUSYN review found that osteoporosis had a higher prevalence in men, with more vertebral and rib fractures, than women.[193] QoL is severely affected. A disease-specific QoL questionnaire, CushingQoL, has been developed.[194]

Psychiatric complications occur in >60% of patients with Cushing's syndrome, most commonly depression. There are significant associations with increasing age, female sex, and higher urinary free cortisol levels.[195] It is essential that all patients with Cushing's syndrome undergo a formal psychiatric assessment both at presentation and after their treatment. It is important to realize that the psychiatric/psychological component of the disease is often extremely severe and may take many months to remit after curative treatment. It is most important that patients are warned of this before treatment is undertaken.

## Mortality of Cushing's syndrome

The early reports of Cushing's syndrome documented a mortality of about 50% in 5 years.[191,196] These patients almost certainly reflected the extreme end of the spectrum. In a review of 60 Cushing's disease patients at a single U.K. center, the overall SMR was 4.8 (95% CI, 2.8–8.3), with 9/13 deaths due to cardiovascular disease. SMR for persistent disease was 16 (6.7–38.4) and 3.3 (1.7–6.7) for those in remission. Hypertension and diabetes mellitus were associated with significantly poorer survival.[197] Mortality was further analyzed in a meta-analysis in seven studies that demonstrated an overall SMR of 2.2 (1.45–3.41). Data from four of the studies (which included the U.K. center) demonstrated an SMR of 5.5 (2.7–11.3) for patients with persistent disease but an SMR of 1.2 (0.45–3.2) for patients in remission.[197] A single-center study of the mortality of 80 patients with Cushing's disease, treated by transsphenoidal surgery, has demonstrated a similar overall SMR of 3.17 (1.7–5.43), with an SMR of 4.12 (1.12–10.54) in the persistent disease/recurrence groups, but a persistently increased SMR of 2.47 (0.8–5.77) in the cure group. Although comorbidities such as hypertension and body mass index (BMI) improved after surgery, there was evidence of long-term cardiovascular damage with LVH and ischemic heart disease on electrocardiogram.[198] A retrospective review of 346 patients operated on by the same surgeon identified increased mortality to be associated with duration of preoperative symptoms until postoperative remission was achieved by any means, older age at diagnosis, and preoperative ACTH concentration. In the groups who achieved overall (immediate and late) and immediate

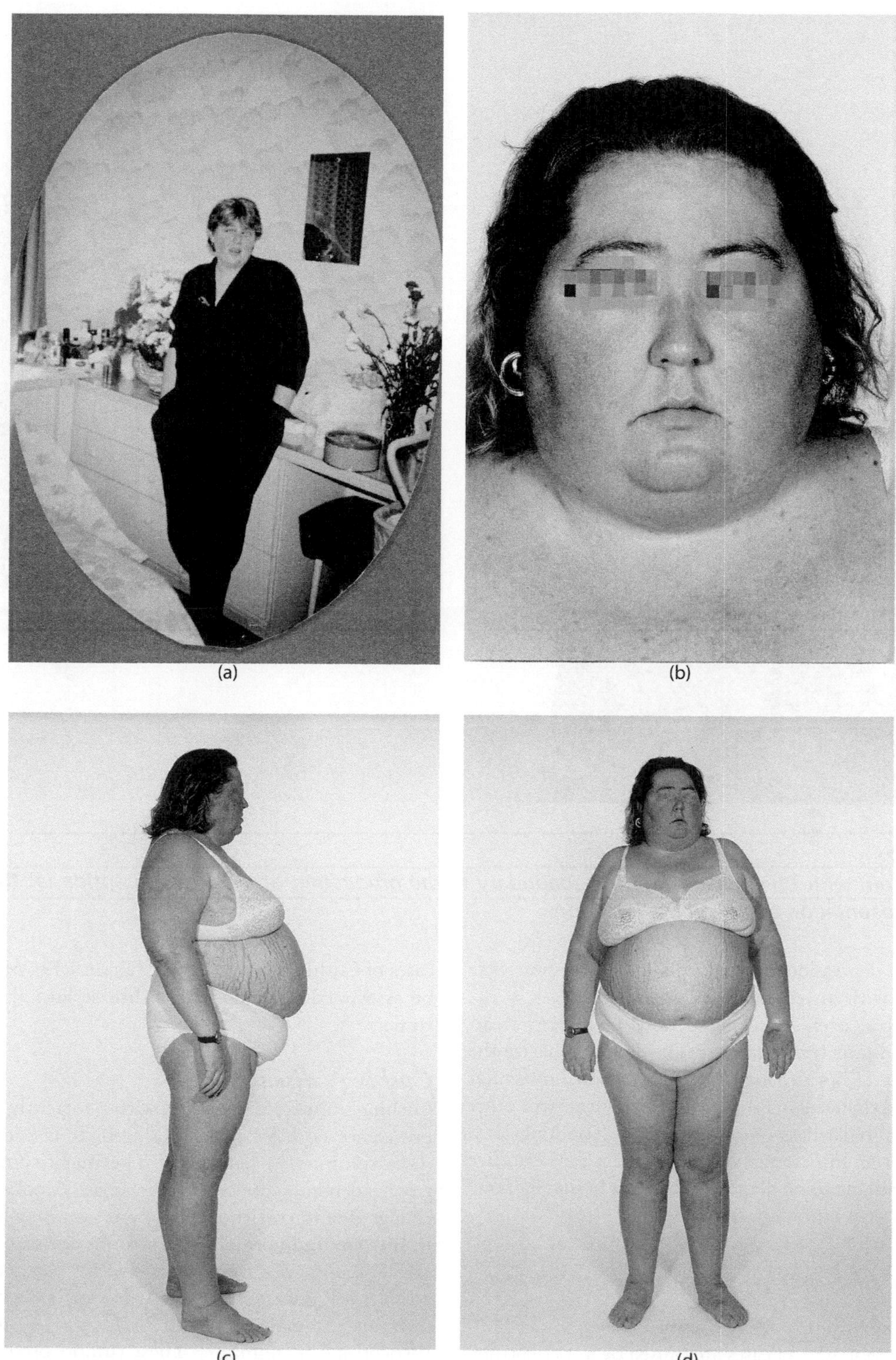

**Figure 1.25**
*Patient with Cushing's disease (a) 2 years before presentation and (b-d) at presentation.*

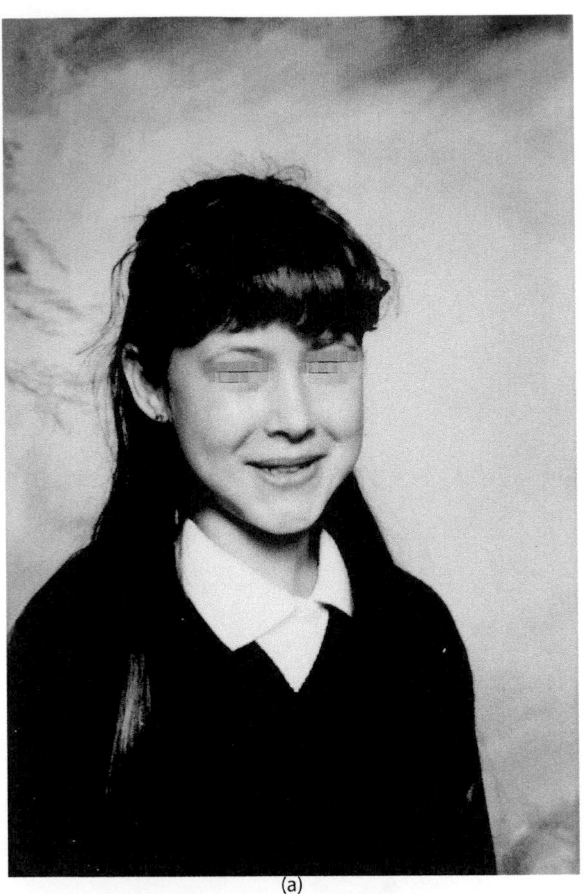

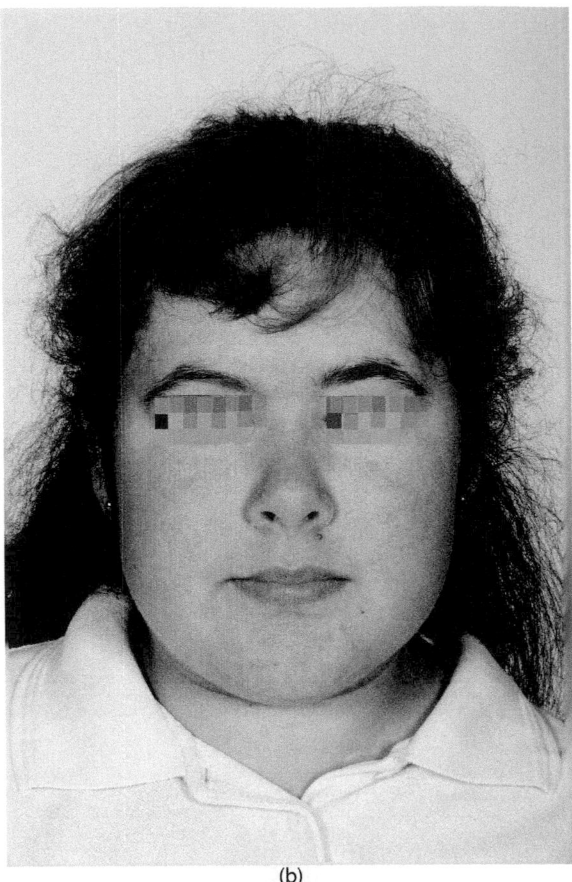

(a) (b)

**Figure 1.26**
*Teenage girl with Cushing's syndrome secondary to the production of a CRH-like peptide (a) 18 months before presentation and (b) at presentation.*

remission, depression at diagnosis and male sex were associated with increased risk of death.[199]

Inevitably, over such long periods of review, treatment paradigms have changed. The data emphasize the importance of optimizing the control of cardiovascular disease and diabetes in all patients after surgery or other treatments, regardless of cortisol status. The long-term mortality risk in patients who have undergone curative surgery remains to be demonstrated in adequately powered long-term follow-up studies.

## Causes of Cushing's syndrome

Cushing's syndrome is ACTH-dependent in about 80% of cases. About 70% of cases are caused by a corticotroph adenoma of the pituitary gland (Cushing's disease), with the remainder being caused by ectopic ACTH production. Primary adrenal disease accounts for about 20% of cases of Cushing's syndrome[200] (Table 1.19). MEN1 may be associated with Cushing's disease and also adrenal tumors.[201]

### Cushing's disease

Cushing's disease is very rare, with a currently estimated prevalence of 1.2–2.4 per 100,000. It is 3 to 4 times more common in females.[202] The majority of corticotroph adenomas are microadenomas. Crooke's hyaline change due to corticotroph suppression may be present in surrounding normal corticotrophs and also occasionally within tumor cells themselves.[203] Macroadenomas are often aggressive in their behavior and occur more frequently in males, particularly for the so-called silent corticotroph adenoma.[57,58] These tumors present as clinically nonfunctioning pituitary adenomas, often with mass effects. Immunostaining of the tumor is positive for ACTH. The tumors tend to be recurrent and

| Best discriminators |
|---|
| Plethoric, rounded face |
| Bruising |
| Livid, purple/red striae |
| Proximal myopathy |
| Other typical features |
| Central distribution of body fat, with correspondingly thin arms and legs |
| "Buffalo" hump (cervical fat pad) |
| Thin skin |
| Poor wound healing, scarring |
| Acne |
| Alopecia |
| Hirsuties |
| Edema |

***Table 1.17***
*Clinical signs of Cushing's syndrome.*

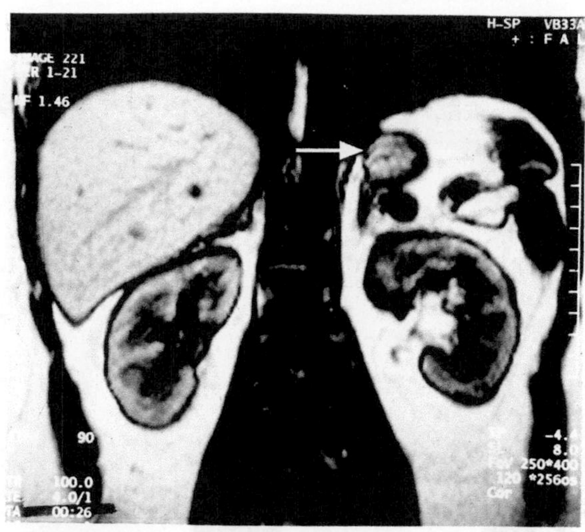

***Figure 1.27***
*Coronal abdominal MRI scan (T1-weighted) of a patient with Cushing's syndrome, demonstrating retroperitoneal fat and an enlarged left nodular adrenal gland (arrow).*

| Clinical associations |
|---|
| Infection |
| Poor wound healing |
| Hypertension |
| Diabetes mellitus |
| Deep venous thrombosis/pulmonary embolism |
| Ischemic heart disease |
| Oligomenorrhea/amenorrhea |
| Myopathy |
| Osteoporosis |
| Glaucoma |
| Reduced QoL |
| Psychiatric |

***Table 1.18***
*Clinical associations with Cushing's syndrome.*

| ACTH dependent | % |
|---|---|
| Corticotroph adenoma (Cushing's disease) | 70 |
| Ectopic ACTH production | 10 |
| ACTH independent | |
| Adrenal adenoma | 10 |
| Adrenal carcinoma | 5 |
| Nodular adrenal hyperplasia | 5 |
| Primary pigmented nodular adrenal disease | |
| Massive macronodular adrenal hyperplasia | |
| Ectopic receptor expression | |

ACTH, adrenocorticotropic hormone.

***Table 1.19***
*Causes of Cushing's syndrome.*

increasingly aggressive in time, associated with increasingly severe Cushing's disease. Rarely the tumors metastasize.[7,58] Nelson's syndrome describes the rapid growth of a corticotroph adenoma after medical or surgical adrenalectomy. The reported incidence varies between 8% and 43% over long-term follow-up. This incidence is associated with a rapid increase in serum ACTH levels, manifested by increasing skin pigmentation[204] (Figure 1.28). Nelson's tumors can be highly aggressive and can become resistant to treatment. They tend to occur in tumors with an underlying propensity for aggressive behavior, such as silent corticotroph adenomas. Prophylactic pituitary irradiation after bilateral adrenalectomy reduces the risk.[205–207]

Corticotroph hyperplasia rather than a corticotroph adenoma is occasionally seen. The presence of

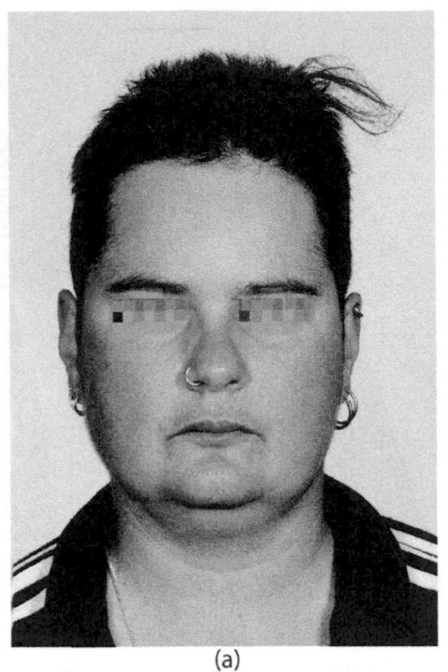
(a)

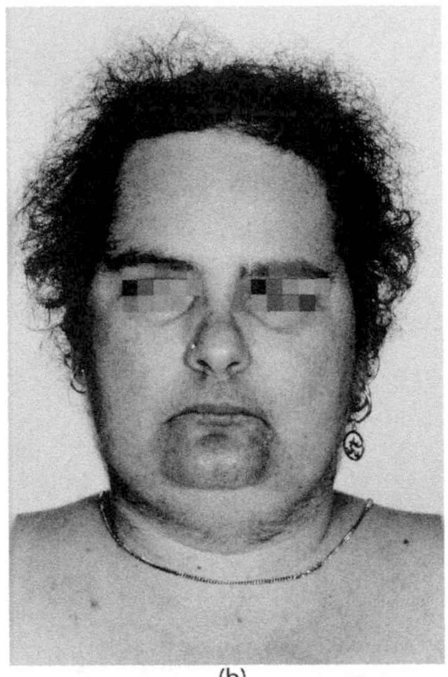
(b)

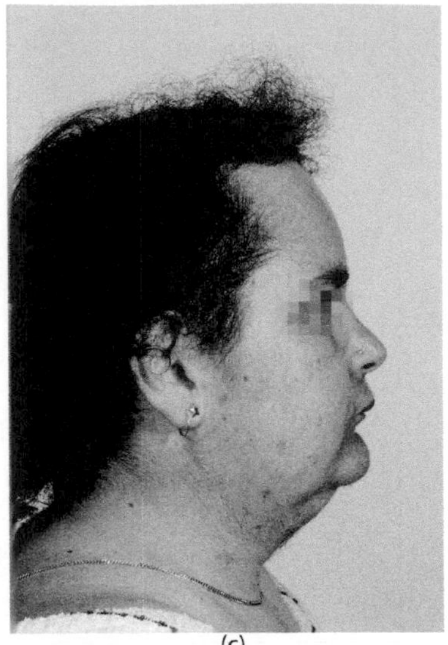
(c)

**Figure 1.28**
*Nelson's syndrome. (a) Patient at presentation with a recurrent corticotroph adenoma. (b and c) Two years later, after bilateral adrenalectomy. The tumor finally developed into a pituitary carcinoma. The patient originally presented with a visual field defect from a silent corticotroph macroadenoma.*

hyperplasia should always raise the possibility of an ectopic source of CRH.

## Ectopic hormone production

Cushing's syndrome secondary to ectopic production of CRH or ACTH is most commonly due to a bronchial carcinoid, but it may be associated with several other tumors, notably gastroenteropancreatic tumors, thymic carcinoid, medullary carcinoma of the thyroid, and pheochromocytoma.[208,209] Ectopic ACTH production by small cell carcinoma of the lung is usually associated with a rapidly progressive wasting disease, with pigmentation and hypokalemic alkalosis.

## Adrenal disease

Adrenal adenomas account for about 60% of cases of ACTH-independent Cushing's syndrome (Figure 1.29). The majority of the remainder is accounted for by adrenal carcinomas.[200] Adenomas range in size from about 1 cm to 7 cm and often present with a relatively prolonged history, sometimes over a few years. Adrenal carcinomas, in contrast, tend to be larger at presentation, often >6 cm. The patients often have typical symptoms of malignant disease, either from the local effects of the tumor or from metastatic disease. The patients may have a short history of rapid onset of Cushing's syndrome, or present with a wasting disease, similar to ACTH-producing small cell carcinoma of the lung.

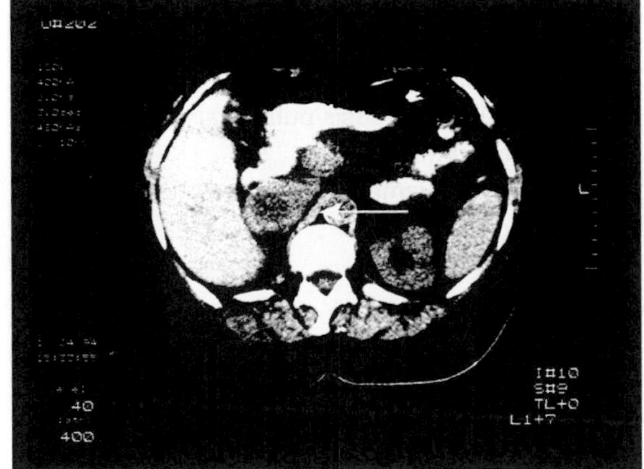


**Figure 1.29**
*CT scan demonstrating an adrenal tumor (arrow) in a patient with Cushing's syndrome.*

The tumors often produce high levels of steroid precursors, resulting in virilization of females, hypertension, and hypokalemic alkalosis.[210]

### Primary pigmented nodular adrenal disease

Patients with primary pigmented nodular adrenal disease (PPNAD) present at a younger age than other causes of Cushing's syndrome. The disease ranges from subclinical or mild to severe. About 50% of patients have autosomal dominant disease, as described by Carney et al.[211] The Carney–myxoma endocrine complex exists in at least two genetically distinct forms, one of which maps to chromosome 17 and the other to chromosome 2. The chromosome 17 form, Carney complex type 1, has been shown to be due to mutations in the protein kinase A regulatory subunit 1$\alpha$.[212] This condition is heterogeneous, typically consisting of pigmented/blue naevi and lentigines, in association with many different tumors, such as somatotroph adenomas, cutaneous myxomas, cardiac myxomas, breast tumors, testicular tumors, and peripheral nerve lesions. Imaging of the adrenal glands can be variable, ranging from apparent normality to bilateral enlargement, or asymmetric nodularity. Pathological examination reveals small, unencapsulated, pigmented adrenal nodules, ranging from 1 cm upward. There is atrophy of the surrounding adrenal tissue, unlike in macronodular adrenal hyperplasia (MAH). Adrenocortical cancer has been reported in a family with Cushing's syndrome due to Carney complex.[213]

### *Macronodular adrenal hyperplasia*

MAH describes a radiological appearance, rather than a distinct disease entity. The adrenal glands exhibit nodules varying in size from 0.5 to 7 cm. Unlike PPNAD, there is hyperplastic adrenal tissue between the nodules. It is not uncommonly seen in patients with Cushing's syndrome and can give rise to diagnostic confusion. Investigations may demonstrate biochemical evidence of ACTH-dependent disease or adrenal autonomy. Between 20% and 40% of patients with Cushing's disease develop adrenal nodular disease (Figure 1.30). It is likely that some patients with Cushing's disease develop a degree of secondary adrenal autonomy.[214] Nodular adrenal autonomy may be seen in the MAS.[112,113,215] Adrenocorticotropic-independent MAH has also been recognized as a result of aberrant expression of G-protein-coupled receptors (GPCRs), first described with aberrant expression of glucose-dependent insulinotropic peptide (gastric inhibitory polypeptide [GIP]) in patients who developed biochemical evidence of hypercortisolemia after food.[216,217] Since then, ectopic expression of other GPCRs such as $\beta$-adrenoreceptor, $V_1$-vasopressin receptor, interleukin-1 receptor, 5-$HT_4$ receptor, and LH receptor has been described, associated with MAH and also with solitary adrenal adenomas.[218] The identification of the ectopic expression of an aberrant GPCR is important because it provides the opportunity to target the receptor with specific medical treatment, for example, propranolol for ectopic $\beta$-adrenoreceptor and GnRH analogs for ectopic LH receptors.

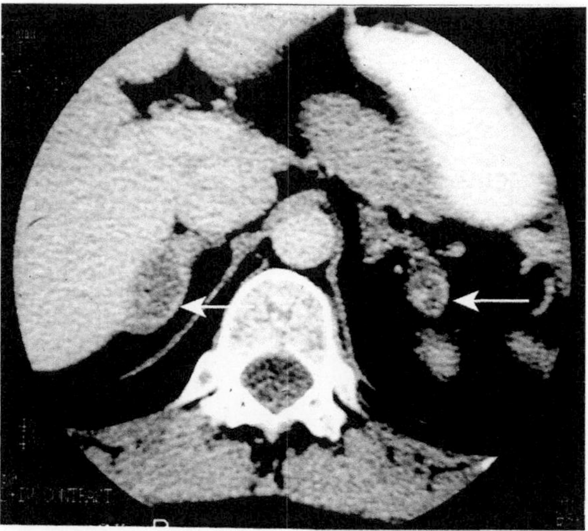

***Figure 1.30***
*Axial CT of abdomen of a patient with ACTH-dependent Cushing's syndrome, demonstrating bilateral macronodular adrenal hyperplasia (arrows) and retroperitoneal fat.*

Occasionally, there may be massive MAH associated with ACTH-independent adrenal function.[219]

## *Investigation of suspected Cushing's syndrome (Figure 1.31)*

A guideline to the diagnosis of Cushing's syndrome has been provided by the Endocrine Society.[220]

A detailed history of medication (oral, inhaled, topical steroids) must be taken. Hypercortisolemia (pseudo-Cushing's) may be associated with chronic excessive alcohol consumption, psychiatric illness, morbid obesity, and poorly controlled diabetes mellitus.

Initial screening is undertaken to demonstrate the presence or absence of hypercortisolemia. One of the following tests is recommended.[221,222]

### *Twenty-four hour urinary free cortisol (UFC)*

UFC provides an integrated measure of cortisol secretion over 24 h. It measures free cortisol, rendering it free from potential confounding factors that may affect cortisol-binding globulin (CBG). UFC excretion in Cushing's syndrome is very variable so that at least two collections should be taken.

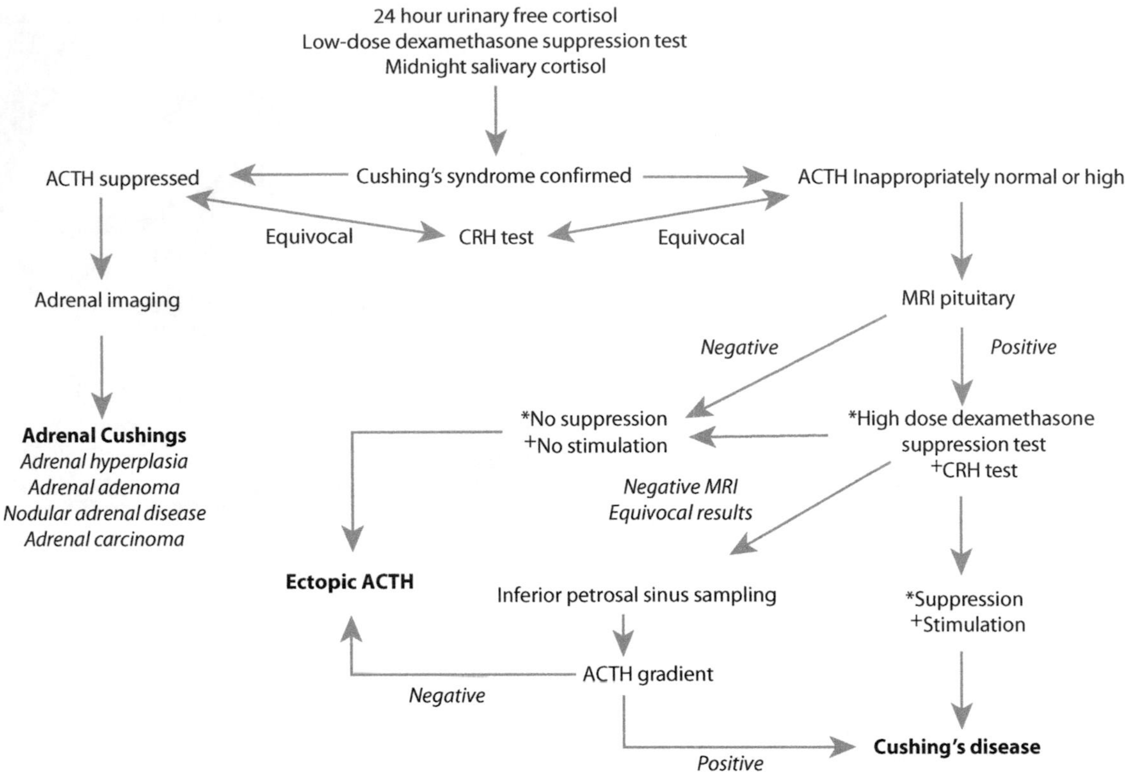


***Figure 1.31***
*Algorithm for the investigation of Cushing's syndrome; * High dose dexamethasone suppression test; + CRH test. See text for biochemical criteria.*

Consistently recorded measurements outside of the normal range have high sensitivity and specificity. This test will effectively exclude normal patients, with the exception of patients who are in the quiescent phase of cycling.[192] If cyclical Cushing's is suspected, patients should carry out repeat urine collections at periodic intervals. It is important to note that UFC measurements may be misleading in patients with renal impairment, as glomerular filtration rate falls below 60 mL/min.

## *Late night salivary cortisol*

Salivary cortisol (SC)[223] is in equilibrium with free blood cortisol (~4% circulating cortisol). It is stable at room temperature for 7 days or refrigerated for several weeks. Loss of cortisol circadian rhythm, with elevated midnight cortisol, is a key feature of Cushing's syndrome, although it can also occur in pseudo-Cushing's states.[214] The measurement of serum cortisol at midnight requires hospitalization and should be done when the patient is stress-free and sleeping, that is, not on the first night in the hospital. A major advantage of SC is the ability to assess midnight cortisol status in a stress-free environment at home. The major disadvantage of SC is that there is presently no standardized assay in use, each assay having its own normal ranges. A potential drawback is the expression of the enzyme 11β-hydroxysteroid dehydrogenase type 2 (11β-HSD2) in the salivary glands, which catalyzes the conversion of cortisol to cortisone. Inhibition of 11β-HSD2 by liquorice or tobacco (contain glycyrrhizic acid) could result in false elevation of SC. Overall, SC appears to have high sensitivity and specificity comparable to UFC.

## *Dexamethasone suppression tests*

The overnight dexamethasone suppression test can be performed in the outpatient clinic: 1 mg of dexamethasone at 2300–2400 hours, with measurement of serum cortisol at 0900 hours the following morning. The optimum sensitivity is achieved using a cut-off of 50 nmol/L (1.8 μg/dL). Women taking the oral contraceptive pill (OCP) should stop for 6 weeks before the test, due to the stimulatory effect of estrogens on CBG. Drugs, in particular anticonvulsants, can induce the hepatic clearance of dexamethasone through CYP3A4, thereby reducing the sensitivity of the test.

The low-dose dexamethasone suppression test is an alternative option: 0.5 mg of dexamethasone 6 hourly for 48 h, with measurement of serum cortisol at 0900 hours after the last dose. The same 50 nmol/L (1.8 μg/dL) criterion can be used. This test is the preferred one to use to exclude pseudo-Cushing's. Patients should abstain from alcohol for at least 2 weeks before the test.

## *Differential diagnosis of Cushing's syndrome (Figure 1.31)*

The first determination to be made is whether the patient has ACTH-dependent disease. Patients with primary adrenal disease will usually have suppressed 0900 hour serum ACTH levels, in contrast to patients with ACTH-dependent disease (Figure 1.32). There may be uncertainty in some patients with nodular adrenal disease. In this situation, a CRH test can be used to differentiate between the two. Patients with suppressed serum ACTH levels should proceed directly to adrenal imaging, and if an adrenal tumor is identifiable, then proceed to surgery. Patients with ACTH-dependent disease require further investigations.

The differential diagnosis of Cushing's disease from ectopic ACTH secretion can be difficult. The most definitive test is inferior petrosal sinus sampling, but this test is not available in all centers. There is no consensus on the optimal approach. Many centers will use the high-dose dexamethasone suppression test, together with the CRH test.

The rationale for the high-dose dexamethasone (2 mg 6 hourly for 48 h) is that the corticotroph adenoma retains a degree of responsiveness to glucocorticoid negative feedback. In Cushing's disease, the serum cortisol should suppress to <50% of baseline values. Dexamethasone suppressibility should be absent in patients with ectopic ACTH production. This test has a sensitivity of >80%, with a specificity of about 60%. Similar results can be obtained using an overnight 8-mg dexamethasone suppression test or a 7-h intravenous dexamethasone suppression test.[224,225]

The CRH test is a useful, well-validated adjunct in the investigation of Cushing's syndrome.[226] Both ovine and human CRHs are available. The response to ovine CRH may be slightly greater due to its longer half-life. Typically, patients with Cushing's disease demonstrate clear rises in cortisol of >20% and in ACTH of >35% over basal values, giving sensitivities and specificities of about 90%.[227] Combined testing with high-dose dexamethasone and CRH improves the diagnostic accuracy of the investigation.[226,227] Patients with Cushing's disease frequently demonstrate ACTH and cortisol responses to desmopressin, but up to 50% of ectopic ACTH-producing tumors can also respond, limiting its use in the differential diagnosis of ACTH-secreting tumors.[227]

A pituitary MRI scan will identify a corticotroph adenoma in about 60% of cases. Cushing's disease is diagnosed in most patients with dexamethasone suppression and CRH testing indicative of pituitary disease, together with a clearly identifiable pituitary adenoma. Because most corticotroph adenomas are small microadenomas, there is a small potential risk of identifying a pituitary "incidentaloma" (usually <5 mm in diameter) as a corticotroph adenoma.[52] More problematic is the patient with the normal MRI scan.

In patients who do not have an identifiable pituitary adenoma, or in whom the diagnosis remains unclear, inferior petrosal sinus sampling (IPSS) with CRH

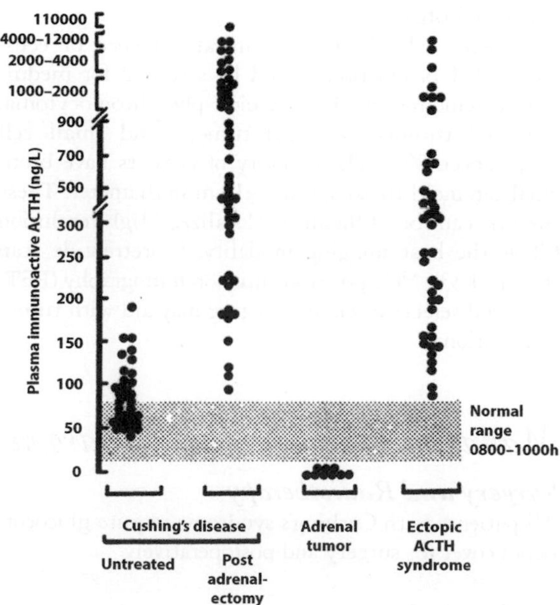


**Figure 1.32**
*Serum ACTH levels in patients with Cushing's syndrome. (From Drury PL, Besser GM. Adrenal cortex. In: Hall R, Besser M (eds),* Fundamentals of Clinical Endocrinology, *Harcourt Publishers, 1989, 153–184. With permission.)*

| | ACTH (ng/L) | | |
|---|---|---|---|
| | Peripheral | LIPS | RIPS |
| Baseline | 64 | 78 | 356 |
| CRF + 5′ | 85 | 110 | 482 |
| CRF + 10′ | 96 | 260 | 595 |

ACTH, adrenocorticotropic hormone; CRH, corticotropin-releasing factor; LIPS, left inferior petrosal sinus; RIPS, right inferior petrosal sinus. The test demonstrates elevated basal serum ACTH levels that clearly rise after CRF. In addition, there is a central-to-peripheral gradient, with lateralization to the RIPS. This patient was found to have a right-sided corticotroph adenoma. False lateralization can, however, occur, due to anomalous venous drainage from the contralateral side.

***Table 1.20***
*Inferior petrosal sinus sampling with CRF (100 μg i.v.).*

offers an additional diagnostic approach.[228] A central-to-peripheral ACTH gradient of >2, or an ACTH rise of >300% over peripheral ACTH values after CRH, is indicative of Cushing's disease (Table 1.20).[229] There are exceptions, with some patients with Cushing's disease, failing to reach the diagnostic threshold and some patients with ectopic ACTH reaching the threshold criteria. It has a sensitivity of about 90%, possibly a lower specificity. A positive test for a pituitary adenoma is highly predictive, whereas a negative test predictive of an ectopic source of ACTH is much lower.[229] Anomalous results can also be obtained in patients with hypoplastic or plexiform inferior petrosal sinuses[230] and also in the rare cases of ectopic CRH production.[231] In a single-center review of 501 consecutive patients with confirmed corticotroph adenomas, IPSS confirmed a pituitary source of ACTH in 491 patients (98%). The 10 patients with false-negative results had peak IPSS ACTH concentrations of <400 ng/L. Interpetrosal ratios were ≥1.4 in 491 (98%) of patients, correctly predicting lateralization in 273/396 (positive predictive value 69%) of patients with a lateral adenoma. When the preoperative MRI was positive, however, the positive predictive value was 85% (171/201). These data indicate that when positive, MRI imaging is superior to IPSS in determining the intrapituitary localization of an adenoma. Lateralization with IPSS can be used to guide an initial pituitary exploration if the MRI is negative, but if an adenoma is not found, the whole pituitary should be explored.[232]

Patients with ectopic production of ACTH often process proopiomelanocortin (POMC) abnormally. In cases where the differential diagnosis remains in doubt, the measurement of serum ACTH precursors may help. Ectopic ACTH-secreting tumors process ACTH precursors less efficiently than corticotroph adenomas, resulting in much higher levels in the circulation that can be measured using two-site immunoradiometric assays.[233]

### *Imaging*

The majority of corticotroph adenomas are microadenomas. Patients suspected of Cushing's disease should undergo a pituitary MRI with and without gadolinium enhancement. The presence of a microadenoma may be due to a pituitary "incidentaloma" rather than to a corticotroph adenoma.

Adrenal imaging should be performed with CT or MRI. Patients with ACTH-dependent disease generally demonstrate adrenal hyperplasia, although the adrenal glands may appear to be normal. Nodular adrenal hyperplasia may be seen in >20% of patients with Cushing's disease (Figure 1.30). Incidental adrenal adenomas have been reported to be present in up to 5% of autopsies (see Chapter 10). A plasma ACTH level is essential to avoid misdiagnosis (Figure 1.32). Some adrenal incidentalomas are associated with subclinical hypercortisolism.[234]

Patients who have biochemical evidence of ectopic ACTH production should be screened for medullary carcinoma of the thyroid, pheochromocytoma, islet cell tumors, carcinoid tumors, and small cell lung cancer.[208,209] The majority of patients have bronchial carcinoid tumors, often <1 cm in diameter. These tumors can be difficult to localize. High-resolution CT is the best imaging modality. Pentetreotide scan (Figure 1.33), $^{68}$Ga positron emission tomography (PET) scan, and selective venous imaging may aid with tumor localization.

## *Management of Cushing's Syndrome*

### *Surgery and Radiotherapy*

All patients with Cushing's syndrome require glucocorticoid cover for surgery and postoperatively.

#### *Cushing's disease*

The treatment of choice is transsphenoidal surgery. Overall, up to approximately 70%–80% of patients can expect to experience remission after surgery.[235–237] Up to 90% of patients with a microadenoma can expect to experience remission after surgery with an experienced surgeon.[235,238] Macroadenomas, in contrast, have

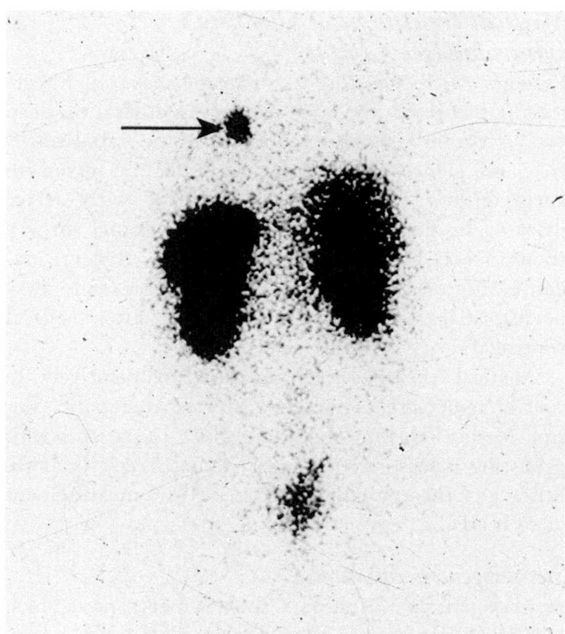

***Figure 1.33***
*[111]In-pentetreotide scan, demonstrating a carcinoid tumor in a patient with ectopic ACTH production.*

lower overall remission, depending on the size of the tumor and extrasellar extension.[235,238] Frequently, at least in part due to the small size of the tumor, a corticotroph adenoma is not identified histologically. In one series, 50% achieved remission, probably due to a reduced rate of surgical removal.[236] The most accurate postoperative assessment of remission remains a subject of debate. In addition, there appears to be a minority of patients, who demonstrate a delayed onset of remission within the first 3 months after surgery, possibly reflecting residual adrenal autonomy.[237] Patients who are biochemically hypoadrenal (0900 hour cortisol <50 nmol/L, <1.8 μg/dL) in the immediate postoperative period have the lowest rate of relapse of approximately 10% at 10 years. Patients with cortisol levels >140 nmol/L (5 μg/dL) within the first 3 months require further evaluation. Patients whose cortisol values are between these two values may be considered to be in remission. A simultaneously measured plasma ACTH of >20 ng/L in the perioperative period has been reported as being highly predictive of future disease recurrence.[239] Overall, recurrence rates over long-term follow-up range from about 9% to 25%.[235–239] Failure of surgery at the first attempt may be followed by a repeat procedure with a success rate of between 50% and 70%.[240] Inevitably, reoperation is associated with an increased risk of postoperative hypopituitarism.

Radiotherapy (see Chapter 4) may be considered in patients who fail control with surgery or who have aggressive, invasive tumors. Pituitary radiotherapy in patients with Cushing's disease reduces the risk of developing Nelson's syndrome after bilateral adrenalectomy. Remission occurs in about 50% of patients, with reports between 42% and 83%.[241] It has a slow onset, but the majority of patients respond within the first 3 years, with a slower ongoing rate of response thereafter. The different radiotherapy modalities, fractionated or single-dose stereotactic, appear to have similar results. Recurrence after radiotherapy is infrequent. Radiosurgery may be used in some centers as first-line treatment, depending on the availability of local expertise. Patients will require medical treatment until remission is achieved, unless the patient is referred for bilateral adrenalectomy.

There is a small group of patients who have relentlessly aggressive pituitary disease that cannot be controlled by repeated surgery and radiotherapy. Occasionally, the tumors undergo malignant transformation.[7,58] Data have demonstrated that a proportion of patients with highly aggressive corticotroph adenomas and carcinomas will respond to temozolomide.[33,102]

Bilateral adrenalectomy provides immediate control of hypercortisolism in patients who have severe disease that has failed to respond to pituitary surgery and medical treatment. It is highly effective when performed by an experienced endocrine surgeon. In the past, bilateral adrenalectomy has tended to be reserved as a last-resort treatment, and patients were often *in extremis*. It should be considered as a third-line treatment option for patients who cannot be controlled by pituitary surgery or medical therapy. Many clinicians now give earlier consideration to bilateral adrenalectomy than in the past. The associated morbidity of surgery can be minimized by endoscopic surgery. An inevitable consequence is life-long hypoadrenalism, with the requirements for both glucocorticoid and mineralocorticoid replacement therapies. Regular pituitary MRI scans and ACTH assays should be undertaken to monitor potential corticotroph progression. Patients who have residual pituitary tumors exhibiting aggressive behavior should be referred for pituitary radiotherapy to minimize the risk of Nelson's syndrome.

## *Adrenal tumors*

It is essential that a clear diagnosis of adrenal autonomy is made before a patient is referred for surgery. Adrenal tumors are treated by unilateral adrenalectomy, generally performed by laparoscopic surgery. Patients will require postoperative glucocorticoid replacement therapy, due to contralateral adrenal suppression, that can take a prolonged period to recover. Massive macronodular hyperplasia requires bilateral adrenalectomy. These conditions are cured by surgery. In contrast, adrenal carcinomas have a poor prognosis, with best results being for patients undergoing adrenalectomy with grade I and grade II disease.[242]

## *Ectopic ACTH/CRF-producing tumors*

The choice of treatment depends on the tumor identification, localization, and staging. Surgical resection is the treatment of choice and can be curative, particularly for small, localized carcinoid tumors. These tumors may remain occult, in spite of strenuous efforts at localization. In this situation, medical therapy can be given to control hypercortisolism, and in those who fail to respond, consideration can be given to bilateral adrenalectomy. Tumor-directed therapy can include SS analogs, interferon-α, molecular-targeted therapies, chemotherapy, embolization, and radiofrequency ablation.

## *Glucocorticoid replacement therapy after surgery*

It is essential that the patient with Cushing's syndrome understands that full recovery often takes many months after successful surgery. Cognitive functioning may take a considerable period to return to premorbid levels. This period of time can be extremely difficult for the patient, and it is most important that the clinician provides particular support and reassurance for the patient and their family.

Regardless of the etiology of the Cushing's syndrome, the patient will require glucocorticoid therapy after successful surgery. The hypothalamic–pituitary axis and the contralateral adrenal gland, in the case of an adrenal tumor, may take many months to return to normal functioning. Ideally, patients should be placed on a low replacement dose of glucocorticoids immediately after surgery, for example, hydrocortisone 20–25 mg daily in a split dose. Many patients, however, have severe symptoms of glucocorticoid deficiency, and it may be necessary for them to have a slightly increased dose for a period of time, for example, 25–30 mg daily, but the dose should be reduced again as soon as possible. The patient should be maintained on as low a replacement dose as possible. Recovery of the HPA axis should be assessed by the short Synacthen (cosyntropin, tetracosactin) test. A cortisol response of ≥500 nmol/L (18 μg/dL) indicates that the replacement therapy can be stopped.

## *Medical treatment of Cushing's syndrome (see Chapter 24)*

Patients with Cushing's syndrome have a hypercoagulable state and are at increased risk of deep venous thrombosis and venous thromboembolism.[243] In consequence, consideration should be given to anticoagulant prophylaxis of patients with active disease. In particular, patients undergoing surgery should receive thromboprophylaxis.[244] Recent evidence suggests that the hypercoagulable state may persist, at least for the first few weeks, after medical control.[245]

Medical therapy may be used preoperatively to control hypercortisolism and improve metabolic control. Medical therapy should be given to patients with persisting disease after surgery, radiotherapy, or both. Efficacy of therapy is usually assessed by measurement of 24 h UFC.

### *Steroidogenesis inhibitors*

Steroidogenesis inhibitors[246] such as metyrapone block cortisol (F) production by inhibiting 11-β-hydroxylase, with a consequent rise in serum 11-deoxycortisol (S) levels. This cross-reacts with some cortisol assays and hence may lead to the erroneous impression that cortisol production is not fully blocked. Although serum ACTH levels rise, the block is not overcome. Aldosterone production is also blocked, but there is an increased production of mineralocorticoid precursors, such as 11-deoxycorticosterone, with the potential development of hypertension, hypokalemia, and edema. Similarly, there is an increased production of androgens that may result in acne and hirsutism. Metyrapone acts rapidly to reduce cortisol levels within 2 h and needs to be given 6–8 hourly with food. Patients should start on 250 mg 8 hourly, increasing as necessary to achieve full blockade. Concomitant replacement therapy may be given with dexamethasone (does not cross-react with cortisol assays) 0.25–0.5 mg.

Ketoconazole is an imidazole that was originally developed as an antifungal agent. It is, however, also a potent inhibitor at several levels of adrenal steroidogenesis. Its most important action is at the 20–22 desmolase step that catalyzes the conversion of cholesterol to pregnenolone. As a result, the accumulation of androgenic steroid metabolites is avoided. The corollary of this is that ketoconazole is potentially teratogenic to male fetuses. Ketoconazole has a slower onset and a more prolonged duration of action than metyrapone. Consequently, it is usually easier to stabilize adrenal blockade, often without the need for concomitant dexamethasone replacement. It may take several weeks for the full effects of ketoconazole to be seen. Unlike metyrapone, ketoconazole is not associated with a compensatory rise in ACTH and may represent an adjustment of the sensitivity of this HPA axis, rather than a direct inhibitory action on ACTH.[240] The most worrying side effect is hepatotoxicity. Biochemical evidence of abnormal liver function occurs in about 10% of patients and is usually reversible. Liver function should be routinely monitored, and the drug should be stopped if abnormalities develop. Some patients develop gastrointestinal disturbances with high doses. Patients should be started on 200 mg daily and the dose adjusted up to 1200 mg daily if necessary, to achieve normal 24 h UFC excretion. Ketoconazole should be avoided in pregnancy.

Mitotane (o,p'DDD) blocks adrenal cortisol production by inhibiting cholesterol side-chain cleavage and 11-β-hydroxylase and, in addition, has a direct cortical adrenolytic action. In consequence, ACTH levels raise about threefold. Its primary use is in adrenal carcinoma, although it may also be used in patients with Cushing's syndrome if control cannot be achieved by other means. It has a slow onset of action over several weeks and similarly has a prolonged action due to its accumulation in adipose tissue. Patients with Cushing's syndrome can be managed with doses of up to about 2.5 g/day, a dose that is much lower than the doses required for adrenal carcinoma patients, in whom the dose is optimized to achieve a therapeutic threshold of >14 mg/L. Intolerance to the dose used in Cushing's disease is about 10%. Side effects include nausea, vomiting and diarrhea, abnormal liver function tests, hypercholesterolemia, and elevated low-density lipoprotein (LDL) cholesterol.[247] Mitotane should be avoided in pregnancy.

Patients who require emergency control of hypercortisolism can be managed with the imidazole derivative etomidate. It has a rapid duration of action and is given intravenously. It is usually given in an intensive care setting, although it has rarely been used for longer term management.[248]

### *Glucocorticoid receptor antagonists*

Mifepristone is the only glucocorticoid receptor antagonist[249] available. It is also a potent antiprogestogen and a weak androgen antagonist. Blockade of the glucocorticoid receptors leads to a marked increase in cortisol and ACTH levels. As a result, stimulation of the mineralocorticoid receptors can lead to profound hypokalemia in about 30% of patients and also to hypertension. Furthermore, because it is not possible to monitor disease control by measurement of serum cortisol and ACTH levels, there is a risk of hypoadrenalism. If hypoadrenalism occurs, the drug should be immediately stopped and dexamethasone given in parallel (0.25 mg for 100 mg of mifepristone over 48 h).

It has a rapid onset of action, with improvement in signs of hypercortisolism, psychiatric symptoms, and hypertension in about 50% of patients. In the pivotal study in the United States of 50 patients who failed or relapsed after surgery, with glucose intolerance or hypertension, 6-month treatment with 300–1200 mg/day resulted in improvement in HbA1c from 7.4% to 6.3%. In the hypertension group, 38% of the 21 patients achieved a ≥5 mm reduction in blood pressure. As a result, it has gained approval for the control of hyperglycemia secondary FDA to hypercortisolism in patients with Cushing's syndrome, who have failed surgery or are not candidates for surgery. Mifepristone is available as 300 mg tablets, once a day. Treatment should be started at the lowest dose, and the dose increased every 2–4 weeks based on clinical efficacy and tolerability. Patients should be closely monitored for hypokalemia and signs of adrenal insufficiency. Endometrial hyperplasia may occur in up to 50% of premenopausal women and may be associated with vaginal bleeding. This condition should be monitored by regular pelvic ultrasound.

### *DA agonists and cabergoline*

Approximately 80% of corticotroph adenomas express D2 receptors. There is evidence that some patients with Cushing's disease respond to cabergoline treatment, although the number of patients is small and one study was retrospective. Long-term control (2–5 years) has been reported in 30%–40% of patients. A proportion of patients (25% in one study) may escape control. Higher doses of cabergoline may be required than those used for hyperprolactinemia and acromegaly.[250–252] The use of high doses of cabergoline has been associated with the development of cardiac valvular fibrosis in patients with Parkinson's disease.[84,85] In consequence, patients should be regularly monitored with echocardiography.

### *SS analogs*

Corticotroph adenomas predominantly express SST5, perhaps explaining why the conventional SS analogs octreotide and lanreotide, which predominantly act via SST2, are ineffective in Cushing's disease. This expression forms the rationale for the treatment of patients with Cushing's disease with the multireceptor-targeted SS analog pasireotide. The pivotal phase III study with pasireotide was in patients with Cushing's disease, with UFC at least 1.5 times the ULN. Patients were randomized to receive pasireotide s.c. at a dose of 600 μg

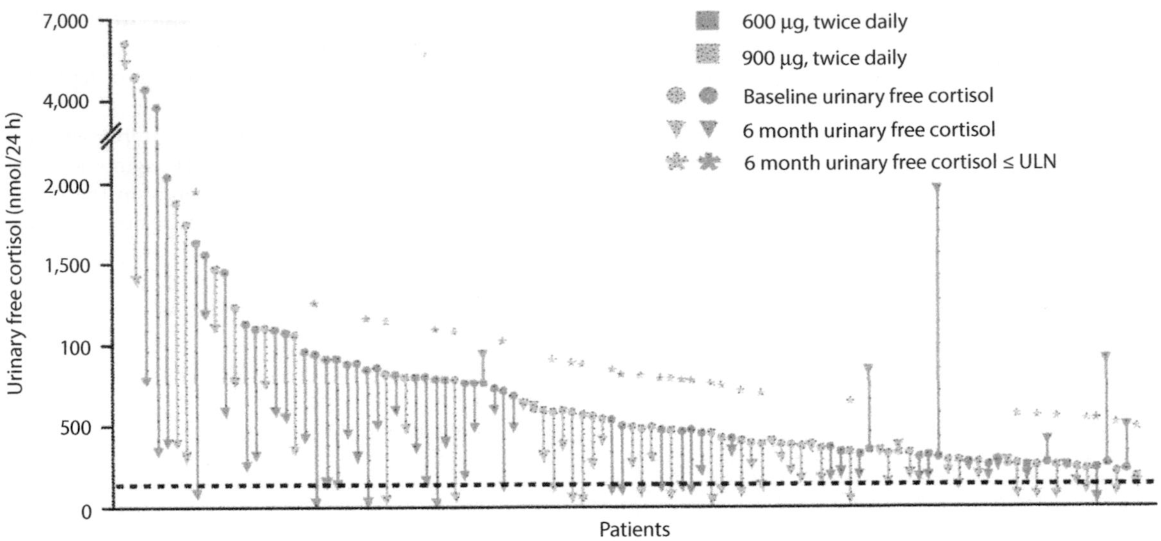


***Figure 1.34***
*Pasireotide treatment in Cushing's disease: absolute changes in urinary free cortisol (UFC) levels from baseline to month 6. UFC at baseline and at 6 months in 103 patients; 61 patients had a reduction of at least 50% in UFC. Black dashed line represents ULN [145 nmol/24 h (52.5 µg/24 h)]. (From Colao AM et al.,* N Engl J Med*, 366, 914–24, 2012.)*

(82 patients) or 900 µg (80 patients) s.c. twice daily. At 6 months, 15% (95% CI, 7–22) patients in the 600 µg group and 26% (95% CI, 17–36) in the 900 µg group achieved normal UFC (Figure 1.34). This response was associated with a concomitant improvement in serum corticotropin levels, symptoms, and signs, including body weight, systolic and diastolic blood pressure, LDL cholesterol, and health-related QoL. Normalization of UFC was more likely to be achieved in patients with relatively low baseline UFC. The effects of pasireotide occurred quickly. Patients who are likely to respond can be identified within the first 2 months of treatment. Pasireotide has the typical class adverse events for SS analogs. In addition, it is associated with hyperglycemia that has been shown to be associated with inhibition of insulin and incretin release. Hyperglycemia occurred soon after the initiation of treatment. Overall, 118/162 (73%) of patients had a hyperglycemic event. Mean HbA1c increased from 5.8% at baseline in both treatment groups to 7.2% in the 600 µg group and 7.4% in the 900 µg group at 6 months. Preexisting diabetes mellitus or impaired glucose tolerance increased the risk of hyperglycemia-related events. New antidiabetic medication was initiated in 74 of the patients.[253] The 24-month efficacy and safety profiles of pasireotide were similar to those seen at 12 months.

Pasireotide offers a new medical therapy for patients with Cushing's disease who have failed to respond to surgery. The most important side effect to be aware of is hyperglycemia, which may respond to hypoglycemic agents.

### *Combination therapies and other approaches*

There have been reports of the use of various drug combinations for the treatment of Cushing's syndrome.

A study of 12 patients with Cushing's disease demonstrated that cabergoline in doses between 2 and 3 mg/week for 6 months normalized UFC in 3 (25%) of the patients. The addition of ketoconazole to the nine uncontrolled patients resulted in normalization of UFC levels in six (66.7%) at doses of between 200 and 400 mg/day.[254]

The stepwise medical therapy using pasireotide (100–250 µg three times daily), cabergoline (0.5–1.5 mg on alternate days), and ketoconazole (300 mg daily) in 17 patients with Cushing's disease resulted in overall biochemical control in 88% of patients, with concomitant improvement in clinical signs.[255]

The combination of high-dose mitotane (3.0–5.0 g/24 h) with metyrapone (3.0–4.5 g/24 h) and ketoconazole (400–1200 mg/24 h), given concomitantly to 11 patients with severe hypercortisolism, resulted in a rapid fall in UFC over 24–48 h. In seven patients, metyrapone and ketoconazole were withdrawn after 3.5 months, with continued control with mitotane. This approach provides a medical approach which may be considered in place of bilateral adrenalectomy.[256]

Although these data are from small, open studies, they demonstrate that combination therapies can be effective in the management of patients with Cushing's syndrome. The medical control of a patient rather than the need for bilateral adrenalectomy could be particularly advantageous.

### *Cushing's syndrome in pregnancy*

Pregnancy in patients with Cushing's syndrome is very uncommon. The signs of Cushing's syndrome can be difficult to detect because of the physiological changes that take place in pregnancy. The majority of cases are due to ACTH-independent adrenal disease. When it occurs, Cushing's syndrome is associated with a high maternal and fetal morbidity, with an increased risk of spontaneous abortion. Surgical treatment should be considered whenever possible. Treatment with adrenal steroidogenesis inhibitors should be avoided if possible because of potential deleterious effects on the fetus. The role of pasireotide in the management of pregnant patients with Cushing's disease remains to be established.[240]

## *Summary*

Cushing's syndrome remains a diagnostic and therapeutic challenge. Surgery is the first-line approach for both adrenal and ACTH-dependent Cushing's syndrome. Even successful surgery in Cushing's disease, however, is associated with a relapse rate of up to 25% over time. Macroadenomas are particularly difficult to manage. Radiotherapy is indicated for tumors with aggressive growth characteristics and maybe used to obtain long-term biochemical control. There are several medical options available, but they all have drawbacks in terms of efficacy and side effects. Bilateral adrenalectomy remains an effective option if surgery and medical therapy fail. In this situation, patients with Cushing's disease need to be carefully monitored for the development of Nelson's syndrome. The risk can be reduced with pituitary radiotherapy.

Surgery is likely to remain the first-line option for most patients with Cushing's syndrome. There is, however, also the need for reliably safe and effective medical therapy(ies), providing biochemical and antiproliferative control. The availability of a robust medical option(s) for patients with Cushing's syndrome would provide a major advance in the optimization of treatment for these patients.

## *References*


1. Sherlock M, Ayuk J, Tomlinson JW, et al. Mortality in patients with pituitary disease. *Endocrine Rev* 2010; 31: 301–42.
2. Asa SL, Scheithauer BW, Bilbao JM, et al. A case for hypothalamic acromegaly: A clinicopathological study of six patients with hypothalamic-gangliocytomas producing growth hormone-releasing factor. *J Clin Endocrinol Metab* 1984; 58: 796–803.
3. Asa SL, Kovacs K, Tindall GT, et al. Cushing's disease associated with an intrasellar gangliocytoma producing corticotrophin-releasing factor. *Ann Intern Med* 1984; 101: 789–93.
4. Plum FC, Uitert RV. Nonendocrine diseases and disorders of the hypothalamus. In: Reichlin S, Baldessarini RJ, Martin JB (eds.), *The Hypothalamus*, Vol. 56. New York: Raven; 1978, 415–74.
5. Al-Shraim M, Asa SL. The 2004 World Health Organization classification of pituitary tumours: What's new? *Acta Neuropathol* 2006; 111: 1–7.
6. Raverot G, Wierinckx A, Dantony E, et al. Prognostic factors in prolactin pituitary tumours: Clinical, histological and molecular data from a series of 94 patients with a long post-operative follow-up. *J Clin Endocrinol Metab* 2010; 95(4): 1708–16.
7. Heaney AP. Pituitary carcinoma: Difficult diagnosis and treatment. *J Clin Endocrinol Metab* 2011; 96(12): 3649–60.
8. Casaneuva FF, Molich ME, Schlechte JA, et al. Guidelines of the Pituitary Society in the diagnosis and management of prolactinomas. *Clin Endocrinol (Oxf)* 2006; 65(2): 265–73.
9. Melmed S, Colao A, Barkan A, et al. Guidelines for acromegaly management: An update. *J Clin Endocrinol Metab* 2009; 94: 1509–17.
10. Webster J. A comparative review of the tolerability profiles of dopamine agonists in the treatment of hyperprolactinaemia and inhibition of lactation. *Drug Saf* 1996; 14(4): 228–38.
11. Colao A, Di Sarno A, Sarnacchiaro F, et al. Prolactinomas resistant to standard dopamine agonists respond to chronic cabergoline treatment. *J Clin Endocrinol Metab* 1997; 82: 876–83.
12. Verhelst J, Abs R, Maiter D, et al. Cabergoline in the treatment of hyperprolactinaemia: A study of 455 patients. *J Clin Endocrinol Metab* 1999; 84: 2518–22.
13. Melmed S, Casaneuva FF, Hoffman AR, et al. Diagnosis and management of hyperprolactinaemia: An Endocrine Society clinical practice guideline. *J Clin Endocrinol Metab* 2011; 96(2): 273–88.
14. Molitch ME. Pituitary disorders during pregnancy. *Endocrinol Metab Clin North Am* 2006; 35: 99–116.
15. Raymond JP, Goldstein E, Konopka P, et al. Follow-up of children born of bromocroptine-treated mothers. *Horm Res* 1985; 22: 239–46.
16. Colao A, Abs R, Bárcena DG, et al. Pregnancy outcomes following cabergoline treatment: Extended results from a 12-year observational study. *Clin Endocrinol (Oxf)* 2008; 68: 66–71.

17. Tan T, Cabrita IZ, Hensman D, et al. Assessment of cardiac valve dysfunction in patients receiving cabergoline treatment for hyperprolactinaemia. *Clin Endocrinol* 2010; 73: 369–74.
18. Lamberts SWJ, Van der Lely A-J, De Herder WW, et al. Octreotide. *N Engl J Med* 1996; 334(4): 246–54.
19. Hoyer D, Bell GI, Berelowitz M, et al. Classification and nomenclature of somatostatin receptors. *Trends Pharmacol Sci* 1995; 16: 86–8.
20. Bevan JS. The anti-tumoral effects of somatostatin analog therapy in acromegaly. *J Clin Endocrinol* 2005; 90(3): 1856–63.
21. Lamberts SWJ, Krenning EP, Reubi JC. The role of somatostatin and its analogues in the diagnosis and treatment of tumors. *Endocr Rev* 1991; 12: 450–82.
22. Plockinger U, Bader M, Hopfenmuller W, et al. Results of somatostatin receptor scintigraphy do not predict pituitary tumour volume- and hormone-response to octreotide therapy and do not correlate with tumour histology. *Eur J Endocrinol* 1997; 136: 369–76.
23. Davies PH, Stewart SE, Lancranjan I, et al. Long-term therapy with long-acting octreotide (Sandostatin LAR) for the management of acromegaly. *Clin Endocrinol* 1998; 48: 311–16.
24. Caron P, Cogne M, Raingeard I, et al. Effectiveness and tolerability of 3-year lanreotide Autogel treatment in patients with acromegaly. *Clin Endocrinol* 2006; 64: 209–14.
25. Lucas T, Astorga R, Spanish-Portuguese Multicentre Autogel Study Group on Acromegaly. Efficacy of lanreotide Autogel administered every 4–8 weeks in patients with acromegaly previously responsive to lanreotide particles 30 mg: A phase III trial. *Clin Endocrinol* 2006; 65: 320–6.
26. Petersenn S, Schopol J, Barkan A, et al. Pasireotide (SOM230) demonstrates efficacy and safety in patients with acromegaly. A randomised multicenter, phase II trial. *J Clin Endocrinol Metab* 2010; 95: 2781–9.
27. Boscaro M, Ludlam WH, Atkinson B, et al. Treatment of pituitary-dependent Cushing's disease with the multireceptor ligand somatostatin analog pasireotide (SOM230): A multicenter phase II trial. *J Clin Endocrinol Metab* 2009; 94(1): 115–22.
28. Saveanu A, Lavaque E, Gunz G, et al. Demonstration of enhanced potency of a chimeric somatostatin-dopamine molecule, BIM23A387 in suppressing growth hormone and prolactin secretion from human pituitary somatotroph adenoma cells. *J Clin Endocrinol Metab* 2002; 87: 5545–52.
29. Kopchick JJ. Discovery and mechanism of action of pegvisomant. *Eur J Endocrinol* 2003; 148: S21–5.
30. Trainer PJ, Drake WM, Katznelson L, et al. Treatment of acromegaly with the growth hormone-receptor antagonist pegvisomant. *N Engl J Med* 2000; 342: 1171–7.
31. van der Lely AJ, Hutson RK, Trainer PJ, et al. Long-term treatment of acromegaly with pegvisomant, a growth hormone receptor antagonist. *Lancet* 2001; 358: 1754–9.
32. van der Lely AJ, Biller BMK, Brue T, et al. Long-term safety of pegvisomant in patients with acromegaly: Comprehensive review of 1288 subjects in ACROSTUDY. *J Clin Endocrinol Metab* 2012; 97: 1589–97.
33. McCormack AI, Wass JAH, Grossman AB. Aggressive pituitary tumours: The role of temozolomide and the assessment of MGMT status. *Eur J Clin Invest* 2011; 41(10): 1133–48.
34. Rosen T, Bengtsson B. Premature mortality due to cardiovascular disease in hypopituitarism. *Lancet* 1990; 336: 285–8.
35. Bates AS, Van't Hoff W, Clayton RN. Life expectancy in hypopituitarism. *J Clin Endocrinol Metab* 1996; 81: 1169–72.
36. Bülow B, Hagmar L, Mikoczy Z, et al. Increased cerebrovascular mortality in patients with hypopituitarism. *Clin Endocrinol* 1997; 46: 75–81.
37. Bates AS, Bullivant B, Sheppard MC, et al. Life expectancy following surgery for pituitary tumours. *Clin Endocrinol* 1999; 50: 315–19.
38. Nilsson B, Gustavsson-Kadaka E, Bengtsson B-Å, et al. Pituitary adenomas in Sweden between 1958 and 1991: Incidence, survival and mortality. *J Clin Endocrinol Metab* 2000; 85(4): 1420–5.
39. Tomlinson JW, Holden N, Hills RK, et al. Association between mortality and hypopituitarism. *Lancet* 2001; 357: 425–31.
40. Harris PE, Afshar F, Coates P, et al. The effects of transsphenoidal surgery on endocrine function and visual fields in patients with functionless pituitary tumours. *Q J Med* 1989; 71(265): 417–27.
41. Kerr JM, Wierman ME. Pituitary apoplexy. New guidelines refine best practice, but some areas remain uncertain. *BMJ* 2011; 342: 668–9.
42. Yen SSC. Chronic anovulation due to CNS-hypothalamic-pituitary dysfunction. In: Yen SSC, Jaffe RB (eds), *Reproductive Endocrinology: Physiology, Pathophysiology and Clinical Management*, 2nd ed. Philadelphia: WB Saunders; 1986, 500–45.
43. Post KD, McCormick PC, Bello JA. Differential diagnosis of pituitary tumors. *Endocrinol Metab Clin North Am* 1997; 16(3): 609–45.
44. Caturegli I, Newschaffer C, Olivi A, et al. Autoimmune hypophysitis. *Endo Rev* 2005; 26: 599–614.
45. Manetti L, Lupi I, Morselli LL, et al. Prevalence and functional significance of antipituitary antibodies in patients with autoimmune and non-autoimmune thyroid diseases. *J Clin Endocrinol Metab* 2007; 92: 2176–81.
46. Karavitaki N, Cudlip S, Adams CBT, et al. Craniopharyngiomas. *Endo Rev* 2006; 27(4): 371–97.

47. Gautier A, Godbout A, Grosheny C, et al. Markers of recurrence and long-term morbidity in craniopharyngioma: A systemic analysis of 171 patients. *J Clin Endocrinol Metab* 2012; 97: 1258–67.
48. Harris PE, Perry L, Chard T, et al. Immunoreactive human chorionic gonadotrophin from the cyst fluid and CSF of patients with craniopharyngioma. *Clin Endocrinol* 1988; 29: 503–8.
49. Beckers A. Higher prevalence of clinically relevant pituitary adenomas confirmed. *Clin Endocrinol* 2010; 72: 290–1.
50. Daly AF, Rixhon M, Adam C, et al. High prevalence of pituitary adenomas: A cross-sectional study in the province of Liege, Belgium. *J Clin Endocrinol Metab* 2006; 91: 4769–75.
51. Fernandez A, Karavitaki N, Wass JAH. Prevalence of pituitary adenomas: A community-based, cross-sectional study in Banbury (Oxfordshire, UK). *Clin Endocrinol* 2010; 72: 37–382.
52. Freda PU, Beckers AM, Katznelson L, et al. Pituitary incidentaloma: An Endocrine Society clinical practice guideline. *J Clin Endocrinol Metab* 2011; 96(4): 894–904.
53. Elston MS, McDonald KL, Clifton-Bligh RJ, et al. Familial pituitary tumor syndromes. *Nat Rev Endocrinol* 2009; 5: 453–61.
54. Harris PE. Biochemical markers for clinically non-functioning pituitary tumours. *Clin Endocrinol* 1998; 49: 163–4.
55. Heseltine D, White MC, Kendall-Taylor P, et al. Testicular enlargement and elevated serum inhibin concentrations in patients with pituitary macroadenomas secreting follicle stimulating hormone. *Clin Endocrinol* 1989; 31: 411–23.
56. Franks S, Nabarro JDN. Prolactin secretion in patients with chromophobe adenomas of the pituitary: Incidence and presentation of hyperprolactinaemia: Results of surgical treatment. *Ann Clin Res* 1978; 10: 157–63.
57. Raverot G, Wierinckx A, Jouanneau E, et al. Clinical, hormonal and molecular characterization of pituitary ACTH adenomas without (silent corticotroph adenomas) and with Cushing's disease. *Eur J Endocrinol* 2010; 163: 35–43.
58. Harris PE. Clinical and genetic changes in a case of a Cushing's carcinoma. *Clin Endocrinol* 1995; 42: 671–2.
59. Messserer M, Battista JCD, Raverot G, et al. Evidence of improved surgical outcome following endoscopy for non-functioning pituitary adenoma removal. *Neurosurg Focus* 2011; 30(4): 1–9.
60. Selman WR, Laws ER, Scheithauer BW, et al. The occurrence of dural invasion in pituitary adenomas. *J Neurosurg* 1986; 64: 402–7.
61. Reddy R, Cudlip S, Byrne JV, et al. Can we ever stop imaging in surgically treated and radiotherapy-naïve patients with non-functioning pituitary adenoma? *Eur J Endocrinol* 2011; 165: 739–44.
62. Dekkers OM, Pereira AM, Romijn JA. Treatment and follow-up of clinically nonfunctioning pituitary macroadenomas. *J Clin Endocrinol Metab* 2008; 93: 3717–26.
63. Pivonello R, Matrone C, Filippella M, et al. Dopamine receptor expression and function in clinically nonfunctioning pituitary tumors: Comparison with the effectiveness of cabergoline treatment. *J Clin Endocrinol Metab* 2004; 89: 1674–83.
64. Borson-Chazot F, Houzard C, Ajzenberg C, et al. Somatostatin receptor imaging in somatotroph and non-functioning pituitary adenomas: Correlation with hormonal and visual responses to octreotide. *Clin Endocrinol* 1997; 47: 589–98.
65. De Bruin TWA, Kwekkeboom DJ, Vant Verlaat JW, et al. Clinically non-functioning pituitary adenoma and octreotide response to long term high dose treatment and studies *in vitro*. *J Clin Endocrinol Metab* 1992; 75: 1310–17.
66. Klibanski A, Jameson JL, Biller BMK, et al. Gonadotropin and α-subunit responses to chronic LHRH analogue administration in patients with pituitary tumors. *J Clin Endocrinol Metab* 1989; 68: 81–6.
67. Beck-Peccoz P, Brucker-Davis F, Persani L, et al. Thyrotropin-secreting pituitary tumors. *Endocrine Rev* 1996; 17(6): 610–38.
68. Brucker-Davis F, Oldfield EH, Skarulis MC, et al. Thyrotropin-secreting pituitary tumors: Diagnostic criteria, thyroid hormone sensitivity and treatment outcome in 25 patients followed at the National Institutes of Health. *J Clin Endocrinol Metab* 1999; 84: 476–86.
69. Franks S, Murray MAF, Jequier AM, et al. Incidence and significance of hyperprolactinaemia in women with amenorrhoea. *Clin Endocrinol* 1975; 4: 597–607.
70. Bachman GA, Kemmann E. Prevalence of oligomenorrhea and amenorrhea in a college population. *Am J Obstet Gynecol* 1982; 144: 98–102.
71. Carter JN, Tyson JE, Tolis G. Prolactin-secreting tumors and hypogonadism in 22 men. *N Engl J Med* 1978; 299: 847–52.
72. Schwartz MF, Baumann JE, Masters WH. Hyperprolactinaemia and sexual disorders in men. *Biol Psychiatr* 1982; 17: 861–76.
73. Olukoga AO, Kane JW. Macroprolactinaemia: Validation and application of the polyethylene glycol precipitation test and clinical characterization of the condition. *Clin Endocrinol* 1999; 51: 119–26.
74. Glezer A, Soares CR, Vieira JG, et al. Human macroprolactin displays low biological activity via its homologous receptor in a new sensitive bioassay. *J Clin Endocrinol Metab* 2006; 91: 1048–55.
75. Mancini T, Casaneuva FF, Giustina A. Hyperprolactinemia and prolactinomas. *Endocrinol Metab Clin North Am* 2008; 37(1): 67–99.

76. Karavitaki N, Thanabalasingham G, Shore HCA, et al. Do the limits of serum prolactin in disconnection hyperprolactinaemia need re-definition? A study of 226 patients with histologically verified non-functioning pituitary macroadenoma. *Clin Endocrinol (Oxf)* 2006; 65(4): 524–9.
77. Barkan AL, Chandler WF. Giant pituitary macroprolactinoma with a falsely low serum prolactin: The pitfall of the 'high dose hook effect': Case report. *Neurosurgery* 1998; 42: 913–15.
78. Molitch ME. Pathologic hyperprolactinaemia. *Endocrinol Metab Clin North Am* 1992; 21(4): 877–901.
79. Molitch ME. Pituitary incidentalomas. *Endocrinol Metab Clin North Am* 1997; 26(4): 725–40.
80. Buurman H, Saeger W. Subclinical adenoma in postmortem pituitaries: Classification and correlations to clinical data. *Eur J Endocrinol* 2006; 154: 753–8.
81. Pellegrini I, Rasolonjanahary R, Gunz G, et al. Resistance to bromocriptine in prolactinomas. *J Clin Endocrinol Metab* 1989; 69: 500–9.
82. Molitch ME. Pharmacological resistance in prolactinoma patients. *Pituitary* 2005; 8: 43–52.
83. Ono M, Miki N, Kawamata T, et al. Prospective study of high-dose cabergoline treatment of prolactinomas in 150 patients. *J Clin Endocrinol Metab* 2008; 93: 4721–7.
84. Schade R, Andersohn F, Suissa S, et al. Dopamine agonists and the risk of cardiac-valve regurgitation. *N Engl J Med* 2007; 356: 29–38.
85. Zanettini R, Antonini A, Gatto G, et al. Valvular heart disease and the use of dopamine agonists for Parkinson's disease. *N Engl J Med* 2007; 356: 39–46.
86. Nachtigall LB, Valassi E, McCarty D, et al. Gender effects on cardiac valvular function in hyperprolactinaemic patients receiving cabergoline; a retrospective study. *Clin Endocrinol (Oxf)* 2010; 72(1): 53–8.
87. Boguszewski CL, Dos Santos CM, Sakamoto KS, et al. A comparison of cabergoline and bromocriptine on the risk of valvular heart disease in patients with prolactinomas. *Pituitary* 2012; 15(1): 44–9.
88. Dekkers OM, Lagro J, Burman P, et al. Recurrence of hyperprolactinaemia after withdrawal of dopamine agonists: Systematic review and meta-analysis. *J Clin Endocrinol Metab* 2010; 95: 43–51.
89. Randall RV, Laws ER Jr, Abboud CF, et al. Transsphenoidal microsurgical treatment of prolactin-producing pituitary adenomas: Results in 100 patients. *Mayo Clin Proc* 1983; 58: 108–21.
90. Hardy J. Transsphenoidal microsurgery of microprolactinomas. In: Black P, Zervas NT, Ridgeway EC, et al. (eds), *Secretory Tumors of the Pituitary Gland*. New York: Raven Press; 1984, 73–81.
91. Thomson JA, Davies DL, McLaren EH, et al. Ten year follow up of microprolactinoma treated by transsphenoidal surgery. *BMJ* 1994; 309: 1409–10.
92. Kreutzer J, Buslei R, Wallaschofski H, et al. Operative treatment of prolactinomas: Indications and results in a current consecutive series of 212 patients. *Eur J Endocrinol* 2008; 158: 11–18.
93. Acharya S, Gopal RA, Bandgar TR, et al. Clinical profile and long term follow up of children and adolescents with prolactinomas. *Pituitary* 2009; 12: 186–9.
94. Colao A, Loche S, Cappa M, et al. Prolactinomas in children and adolescents. Clinical presentation and long-term follow-up. *J Clin Endocrinol Metab* 1998; 83: 2777–80.
95. Gillam MP, Molitch ME, Lombardi G, et al. Advances in the treatment of prolactinomas. *Endocr Rev* 2006; 27: 485–534.
96. Bevan JS, Webster J, Burke CW. Dopamine agonists and pituitary tumour shrinkage. *Endocr Rev* 1992; 13: 220–40.
97. Mbanya JCN, Mendelow AD, Crawford PJ, et al. Rapid resolution of visual abnormalities with medical therapy alone in patients with large prolactinomas. *Brit J Neurosurg* 1993; 7: 519–27.
98. Biller BMK, Molitch ME, Vance ML, et al. Treatment of prolactin-secreting macroadenomas with the once-weekly dopamine agonist cabergoline. *J Clin Endocrinol Metab* 1996; 81: 2338–43.
99. Colao A, Sarno AD, Landi ML, et al. Long-term and low-dose treatment with cabergoline induces macroprolactinoma shrinkage. *J Clin Endocrinol Metab* 1997; 82: 3574–9.
100. Molitch ME. Dopamine resistance of prolactinomas. *Pituitary* 2003; 6: 19–27.
101. Hurel SJ, Harris PE, McNicol AM, et al. Metastatic prolactinoma: Effect of octreotide, cabergoline, carboplatin and etoposide; immunocytochemical analysis of protooncogene expression. *J Clin Endocrinol Metab* 1997; 82: 2962–5.
102. Raverot G, Castinetti F, Jouanneau E, et al. Pituitary carcinomas and aggressive pituitary tumours: Merits and pitfalls of temozolomide treatment. *Clin Endocrinol* 2012; 76: 769–75.
103. Bronstein MD. Prolactinomas and pregnancy. *Pituitary* 2005; 8: 31–8.
104. Kratz A, Ferraro M, Sluss PM, Lewandrowski KB. Laboratory references values. *N Engl J Med.* 2004; 351(15): 1548–632.
105. Abbassi-Ghanavati M, Greer LG, Cunningham FG. Pregnancy and laboratory studies: A references table for clinicians. *Obstet Gynecol* 2009; 114(6): 1326–31.
106. Miller RE, Learned-Miller EG, Trainer P, et al. Early diagnosis of acromegaly: Computers vs clinicians. *Clin Endocrinol* 2011; 75: 226–31.
107. Schneider HJ, Kosilek RP, Günther M, et al. A novel approach to the detection of acromegaly: Accuracy of diagnosis by automatic face classification. *J Clin Endocrinol Metab* 2011; 96: 2074–80.

108. Colao, A, Ferone D, Marzullo P, et al. Systemic complications of acromegaly: Epidemiology, pathogenesis and management. *Endocrine Rev* 2004; 25: 102–52.
109. Dekkers OM, Biermasz NR, Pereira AM, et al. Mortality in acromegaly: A metaanalysis. *J Clin Endocrinol Metab* 2008; 93: 61–7.
110. Vallar L, Spada A, Giannattasio G. Altered Gs and adenylate cyclase activity in human GH-secreting pituitary adenomas. *Nature* 1987; 330: 566–8.
111. Lyons J, Landis CA, Harsh G, et al. Two G protein oncogenes in human endocrine tumors. *Science* 1990; 249: 655–9.
112. Weinstein LS, Shenker A, Gejman PV, et al. Activating mutations of the stimulatory G protein in the McCune-Albright syndrome. *N Engl J Med* 1991; 325: 1688–95.
113. Lumbroso S, Paris F, Sultan C. Activating Gsα mutations: Analysis of 113 patients with signs of McCune-Albright syndrome – a European collaborative study. *J Clin Endocrinol Metab* 2004; 89: 2107–13.
114. Akintoye SO, Kelly MH, Brillante B, et al. Pegvisomant for the treatment of gsp-mediated growth hormone excess in patients with McCune-Albright syndrome. *J Clin Endocrinol Metab* 2006; 91: 2960–6.
115. Teh BT, Kytölä S, Farnebo F, et al. Multiple analysis of the MEN 1 gene in multiple endocrine neoplasia type 1, familial acromegaly and familial isolated hyperparathyroidism. *J Clin Endocrinol Metab* 1998; 83(8): 2621–6.
116. Boikos SA, Stratakis CA. Carney complex: The first 20 years. *Curr Opin Oncol* 2007; 19(1): 24–9.
117. Thorner MO, Perryman RL, Cronin MJ, et al. Somatotroph hyperplasia. Successful treatment of acromegaly by removal of a pancreatic islet tumour secreting a growth hormone-releasing factor. *J Clin Invest* 1982; 70: 965–77.
118. Sassolas G, Chayvialle JA, Partensky C, et al. Acromegalie, expression clinique de la production de facteurs de liberations de l'hormone de croissance (G.R.F.) par une tumeur pacreatique. *Annales d'Endocrinologie* 1983; 44: 347–54.
119. Rivier J, Speiss J, Thorner M, et al. Characterisation of a growth hormone releasing factor from a human pancreatic tumor. *Nature* 1982; 300: 276–8.
120. Guillemin R, Brazeau P, Bohlen P, et al. Growth hormone releasing factor from a human pancreatic tumor that caused acromegaly. *Science* 1982; 218: 585–7.
121. Faglia G, Arosio M, Bazzoni N. Ectopic acromegaly. *Endocrinol Metab Clin North Am* 1992; 575–95.
122. Colao A, Pivonello R, Grasso LFS, et al. Determinants of cardiac disease in newly diagnosed patients with acromegaly: Results of a 10 year survey. *Eur J Endocrinol* 2011; 165: 713–21.
123. Colao A, Spinelli L, Marzullo P, et al. High prevalence of cardiac valve disease in acromegaly; an observational, analytical case-control study. *J Clin Endocrinol Metab* 2003; 88: 3196–201.
124. Pereira AM, van Thiel SW, Lindner JR, et al. Increased prevalence of regurgitant valvular heart disease in acromegaly. *J Clin Endocrinol Metab* 2004; 89: 71–5.
125. Ben-Shlomo A, Melmed S. Acromegaly. *Endocrinol Metab Clin N Am* 2008; 37(1): 101–22.
126. Renehan AG, Bhaskar P, Painter JE, et al. The prevalence and characteristics of colorectal neoplasia in acromegaly. *J Clin Endocrinol Metab* 2000; 85(9): 3417–24.
127. Jenkins PJ, Frajese V, Jones AM, et al. Insulin-like growth factor I and the development of colorectal neoplasia in acromegaly. *J Clin Endocrinol Metab* 2000; 85(9): 3218–21.
128. Annamalai AK, Gayton EL, Webb A, et al. Increased prevalence of gallbladder polyps in acromegaly. *J Clin Endocrinol Metab* 2011; 96: E1120–5.
129. Colao A, Marzullo P, Vallone G, et al. Ultrasonographic evidence of joint thickening reversibility in acromegalic patients treated with lanreotide for 12 months. *Clin Endocrinol* 1999; 51: 611–18.
130. Scarpa R, De Brasi D, Pivonello R, et al. Acromegalic axial arthropathy: A clinical case-control study. *J Clin Endocrinol Metab* 2004; 89: 598–603.
131. Biermasz NR, Pereira AM, Smit JWA, et al. Morbidity after long-term remission for acromegaly: Persisting joint-related complaints cause reduced quality of life. *J Clin Endocrinol Metab* 2005; 90: 2731–9.
132. Manara R, Maffei P, Citton V, et al. Increased rate of intracranial saccular aneurysms in acromegaly: An MR angiography study and review of the literature. *J Clin Endocrinol Metab* 2011; 96: 1292–300.
133. Webb SM, Prieto L, Badia X, et al. Acromegaly Quality of Life Questionnaire (ACROQOL) a new health-related quality of life questionnaire for patients with acromegaly: Development and psychometric properties. *Clin Endocrinol* 2002; 57: 251–8.
134. Paisley AN, Rowles SV, Roberts ME, et al. Treatment of acromegaly improves quality of life, measured by AcroQol. *Clin Endocrinol* 2007; 67: 358–62.
135. Fieffe S, Morange I, Petrossians P, et al. Diabetes in acromegaly, prevalence, risk factors and evolution: Data from the French acromegaly register. *Eur J Endocrinol* 2011; 164: 877–84.
136. Barkan AL, Burman P, Clemmons DR, et al. Glucose homeostasis and safety in patients with acromegaly converted from long-acting octreotide to pegvisomant. *J Clin Endocrinol Metab* 2005; 90: 5684–91.
137. Nabarro JD. Acromegaly. *Clin Endocrinol* 1987; 26: 481–512.
138. Wass JA, Cudworth AG, Bottazzo GF, et al. An assessment of glucose intolerance in acromegaly and its response to medical treatment. *Clin Endocrinol* 1980; 12: 53–9.

139. Biering H, Knappe G, Gerl H, et al. Prevalence of diabetes in acromegaly and Cushing syndrome. *Acta Medica Austriaca* 2000; 27: 27–31.
140. Matta M, Bongard V, Grunenwald S, et al. Clinical and metabolic characteristics of acromegalic patients with high IGFI/normal GH levels during somatostatin analog treatment. *Eur J Endocrinol* 2011; 164: 885–9.
141. Sesmilo G, Fairfield WP, Katznelson L, et al. Cardiovascular risk factors in acromegaly before and after normalisation of serum IGF-I levels with the GH antagonist pegvisomant. *J Clin Endocrinol Metab* 2002; 87: 1692–9.
142. Parkinson C, Drake WM, Wieringa G, et al. Serum lipoprotein changes following IGF-I normalisation using a growth hormone receptor antagonist in acromegaly. *Clin Endocrinol (Oxf)* 2002; 56: 303–11.
143. Wildbrett J, Hanefeld M, Fücker K, et al. Anomalies of lipoprotein pattern and fibrinolysis in acromegalic patients; relation to growth hormone levels and insulin-like growth factor I. *Exp Clin Endocrinol Diabetes* 1997; 105: 331–5.
144. Hennessey JV, Jackson IMD. Clinical features and differential diagnosis of pituitary tumours with emphasis on acromegaly. *Balliere's Clin Endocrinol Metab* 1995; 9(2): 271–14.
145. Giustina A, Chanson P, Bronstein MD, et al. A consensus on criteria for cure for acromegaly. *J Clin Endocrinol Metab* 2010; 95: 3141–8.
146. Hartman ML, Veldhuis JD, Vance ML, et al. Somatotropin pulse frequency and basal concentrations are increased in acromegaly and are reduced by successful therapy. *J Clin Endocrinol Metab* 1990; 70: 1375–84.
147. Freda PU. Pitfalls in the biochemical assessment of acromegaly. *Pituitary* 2003; 6: 135–40.
148. Arosio M, Garrone S, Bruzzi P, et al. Diagnostic value of the acid-labile subunit in acromegaly: Evaluation in comparison with insulin-like growth factor (IGF) 1, and IGF-binding protein-1,-2, and-3. *J Clin Endocrinol Metab* 2001; 86: 1091–8.
149. Mestron A, Webb SM, Astorga R, et al. Epidemiology, clinical characteristics, outcome, morbidity and mortality in acromegaly based on the Spanish Acromegaly Registry (Registro Español de Acromegalia, REA). *Eur J Endocrinol* 2004; 151: 439–46.
150. Carmichael JD, Bonert VS, Mirocha JM, et al. The utility of oral glucose tolerance testing for diagnosis and assessment of treatment outcomes in 166 patients with acromegaly. *J Clin Endocrinol Metab* 2009; 94: 523–7.
151. van der Klaauw AA, Pereira AM, van Thiel SW, et al. Attenuated pulse size, disorderly growth hormone and prolactin secretion with preserved nyctohemeral rhythm distinguish irradiated from surgically treated acromegaly patients. *Clin Endocrinol (Oxf)* 2007; 66: 489–98.
152. Petrossians P, Borges-Martins L, Espinoza C, et al. Gross total resection or debulking of pituitary adenomas improves hormonal control of acromegaly by somatostatin analogues. *Eur Endocrinol* 2005; 152: 61–6.
153. Colao A, Attanasio R, Pivonello R, et al. Partial surgical removal of growth hormone-secreting pituitary tumors enhances the response to somatostatin analogues in acromegaly. *J Clin Endocrinol Metab* 2006; 91: 85–92.
154. Karavitaki N, Turner HE, Adams CB, et al. Surgical debulking of pituitary macroadenomas causing acromegaly improves control by lanreotide. *Clin Endocrinol (Oxf)* 2008; 68: 970–5.
155. Laws ER, Vance ML, Thapar K. Pituitary surgery for the management of acromegaly. *Horm Res* 2000; 53(Suppl 3): 71–5.
156. De P, Rees DA, Davies N, et al. Transsphenoidal surgery for acromegaly in Wales: Results based on stringent criteria of remission. *J Clin Endocrinol Metab* 2003; 88: 3567–72.
157. Mortini P, Losa M, Barzaghi R, et al. Results of transsphenoidal surgery in a large series of patients with pituitary adenomas. *Neurosurgery* 2005; 56: 1222–33.
158. Nomikos P, Buchfelder M, Fahlbusch R. The outcome of surgery in 668 patients with acromegaly using current criteria of biochemical 'cure'. *Eur J Endocrinol* 2005; 152: 379–87.
159. Carlsen SM, Lund-Johansen M, Schreiner T, et al. Preoperative octreotide treatment in newly diagnosed acromegalic patients with macroadenomas increases short-term postoperative rates: A prospective, randomized trial. *J Clin Endocrinol Metab* 2008; 93: 2984–90.
160. Abs R, Verhelst J, Maiter D, et al. Cabergoline in the treatment of acromegaly: A study in 64 patients. *J Clin Endocrinol Metab* 1998; 83: 374–8.
161. Sandret L, Maison P, Chanson P. Place of cabergoline in acromegaly: A meta-analysis. *J Clin Endocrinol Metab* 2011; 96: 1327–35.
162. Marzullo P, Ferone D, Di Somma C, et al. Efficacy of combined treatment with lanreotide and cabergoline in selected therapy-resistant acromegalic patients. *Pituitary* 1999; 1: 115–20.
163. Cozzi R, Attanasio R, Lodrini S, et al. Cabergoline addition to depot somatostatin analogues in resistant acromegalic patients: Efficacy and lack of prediction of prolactin status. *Clin Endocrinol (Oxf)* 2004; 61: 209–15.
164. Selvarajah D, Webster J, Ross R, et al. Effectiveness of adding dopamine agonist therapy to long-acting somatostatin analogues in the management of acromegaly. *Eur J Endocrinol* 2005; 152: 569–74.
165. Gilbert JA, Miell JP, Chambers SM, et al. The nadir growth hormone after an octreotide test dose predicts the long-term efficacy of somatostatin analogue therapy in acromegaly. *Clin Endocrinol (Oxf)* 2006; 64(4): 475–6.

166. Cozzi R, Montini M, Attanasio R, et al. Primary treatment of acromegaly with octreotide LAR: A long-term (up to nine years) prospective study of its efficacy in the control of disease activity and tumour shrinkage. *J Clin Endocrinol Metab* 2006; 91: 1397–403.
167. Maiza JC, Vezzosi D, Matta M, et al. Long-term (up to 18 years) effects on GH/IGF-I hypersecretion and tumour size of primary somatostatin analogue (SSTa) therapy in patients with GH-secreting pituitary adenoma responsive to SSTa. *Clin Endocrinol (Oxf)* 2007; 67(2): 282–9.
168. Mercado M, Borges F, Bouterfa H, et al. A prospective, multicentre study to investigate the efficacy, safety and tolerability of octreotide LAR (long-acting repeatable octreotide) in the primary therapy of patients with acromegaly. *Clin Endocrinol (Oxf)* 2007; 66: 859–68.
169. Lombardi G, Minuto F, Tamburrano G, et al. Efficacy of the new long-acting formulation of lanreotide (lanreotide Autogel) in somatostatin analogue-naive patients with acromegaly. *J Endocrinol Invest* 2009; 32: 202–9.
170. Colao A, Cappabianca P, Caron P, et al. Octroetide LAR vs surgery in newly diagnosed patients with acromegaly: A randomised, open-label, multicentre study. *Clin Endocrinol* 2009; 70: 757–68.
171. Tutuncu Y, Berker D, Isik S, et al. Comparison of octreotide LAR and lanreotide Autogel as post-operative medical treatment in acromegaly. *Pituitary* 2012; 15: 398–404.
172. Schopohl J, Strasburger CJ, Caird D, et al. Efficacy and acceptability of lanreotide Autogel 120 mg at different dose intervals in patients previously treated with octreotide LAR. *Exp Clin Endocrinol Diabetes* 2011; 119(3): 156–62.
173. Drange MR, Melmed S. Long-acting lanreotide induces clinical and biochemical remission of acromegaly caused by disseminated growth hormone-releasing hormone-secreting carcinoid. *J Clin Endocrinol Metab* 1998; 83: 3104–9.
174. Melmed S, Sternberg R, Cook D, et al. A critical analysis of pituitary tumour shrinkage during primary medical therapy in acromegaly. *J Clin Endocrinol Metab* 2005; 90: 4405–10.
175. Bevan JS, Atkin SL, Atkinson AB, et al. Primary medical therapy for acromegaly: An open, prospective, multicenter study of the effects of subcutaneous and intramuscular slow-release octreotide on growth hormone, insulin-like growth factor-I, and tumor size. *J Clin Endocrinol Metab* 2002; 87: 4554–63.
176. Resmini E, Dadati P, Ravetti J-L, et al. Rapid pituitary tumor shrinkage with dissociation between antiproliferative and antisecretory effects of a long-acting octreotide in an acromegalic patient. *J Clin Endocrinol Metab* 2007; 92: 1592–9.
177. Trainer PJ. ACROSTUDY: The first 5 years. *Eur J Endocrinol* 2009; 161: S19–24.
178. Bonert VS, Kennedy L, Petersenn S, et al. Lipodystrophy in patients with acromegaly receiving pegvisomant. *J Clin Endocrinol Metab* 2008; 93: 3515–18.
179. Drake WM, Rowles SV, Roberts ME, et al. Insulin sensitivity and glucose tolerance improve in patients with acromegaly converted from depot octreotide to pegvisomant. *Eur J Endocrinol* 2003; 149: 521–7.
180. Trainer PJ, Ezzat S, D'Souza GA, et al. A randomized, controlled, multicentre trial comparing pegvisomant alone with combination therapy of pegvisomant and long-acting octreotide in patients with acromegaly. *Clin Endocrinol* 2009; 71: 549–57.
181. van der Lely AJ, Bernabeu I, Cap J, et al. Coadministration of lanreotide Autogel and pegvisomant normalizes IGF 1 levels and is well tolerated in patients with acromegaly partially controlled by somatostatin analogs alone. *Eur J Endocrinol* 2011; 164: 325–33.
182. Neggers SJ, de Herder WW, Janssen JA, et al. Combined treatment for acromegaly with long-acting somatostatin analogues and pegvisomant: Long-term safety for up to 4.5 years (median 2.2 years) of follow-up in 86 patients. *Eur J Endocrinol* 2009; 160: 529–33.
183. Madsen M, Poulsen PL, Ørskov H, et al. Cotreatment with pegvisomant and a somatostatin analog (SA) in SA-responsive acromegalic patients. *J Clin Endocrinol Metab* 2011; 96: 2405–13.
184. Higham CE, Atkinson AB, Aylwin S, et al. Effective combination treatment with cabergoline and low-dose pegvisomant in active acromegaly: A prospective clinical trial. *J Clin Endocrinol Metab* 2012; 97: 1187–93.
185. Barrande G, Pittino-Lungo M, Coste J, et al. Hormonal and metabolic effects of radiotherapy in acromegaly: Long-term results in 128 patients followed in a single center. *J Clin Endocrinol Metab* 2000; 85: 3779–85.
186. Minniti G, Jaffrain-Rea M-L, Osti M, et al. The long-term efficacy of conventional radiotherapy in patients with GH-secreting pituitary adenomas. *Clin Endocrinol* 2005; 62: 210–16.
187. Cheng S, Grasso L, Martinez-Orozco JA, et al. Pregnancy in acromegaly: Experience from two referral centres and systematic review of the literature. *Clin Endocrinol* 2012; 76: 264–71.
188. Brian SR, Bidlingmaier M, Wajnrajch MP, et al. Treatment of acromegaly with pegvisomant during pregnancy: Maternal and fetal effects. *J Clin Endocrinol Metab* 2007; 92: 3374–7.
189. Fassnacht M, Capeller B, Arlt W, et al. Octreotide LAR treatment throughout pregnancy in an acromegalic woman. *Clin Endocrinol* 2001; 55: 411–15.
190. Tichomirowa MA, Barlier A, Daly AF, et al. High prevalence of *AIP* gene mutations following focused

screening in young patients with sporadic pituitary macroadenomas. *Eur J Endocrinol* 2011; 165: 509–15.

191. Cushing H. The basophil adenomas of the pituitary body and their clinical manifestations (pituitary basophilism). *Bull Johns Hopkins Hosp* 1932; 50: 137–95.

192. Alexandraki KI, Kaltsas GA, Isidori AM, et al. The prevalence and characteristic features of cyclicity and variability in Cushing's disease. *Eur J Endocrinol* 2009; 160: 1011–18.

193. Valassi E, Santos A, Yaneva M, et al. The European registry on Cushing's syndrome: 2-year experience. Baseline demographic and clinical characteristics. *Eur J Endocrinol* 2011; 165(3): 389–92.

194. Webb SM, Badia X, Barahona MJ, et al. Evaluation of health-related quality of life in patients with Cushing's syndrome with a new questionnaire. *Eur J Endocrinol* 2008; 158: 623–30.

195. Pereira AM, Tiemensma J, Romijn JA. Neuropsychiatric disorders in Cushing's syndrome. *Neuroendocrinol* 2010; 92(Suppl 1): 65–70.

196. Plotz CM, Knowlton AI, Ragan C. The natural history of Cushing's syndrome. *Am J Med* 1952; 13: 597–614.

197. Clayton RN, Raskauskiene D, Reulen RC, et al. Mortality and morbidity in Cushing's disease over 50 years at Stoke-on-Trent, UK: Audit and meta-analysis of the literature. *J Clin Endocrinol Metab* 2010; 96: 632–42.

198. Hassan-Smith ZK, Sherlock M, Reulen RC, et al. Outcome of Cushing's disease following transsphenoidal surgery in a single center over 20 years. *J Clin Endocrinol Metab* 2012; 97: 1194–201.

199. Lambert JK, Goldberg L, Fayngold S, et al. Predictors of mortality and long-term outcomes in treated Cushing's disease: A study of 346 patients. *J Clin Endocrinol Metab* 2013; 98: 1022–30.

200. Newell-Price J, Bertagna X, Grossman AB, et al. Cushing's syndrome. *Lancet* 2006; 367: 1605–17.

201. Simonds WF, Varghese S, Marx SJ, et al. Cushing's syndrome in multiple endocrine neoplasia type 1. *Clin Endocrinol* 2012; 76: 379–86.

202. Lindholm J, Juul S, Jørgensen JOL, et al. Incidence and late prognosis of Cushing's syndrome: A population-based study. *J Clin Endocrinol Metab* 2001; 86: 117–23.

203. Thapar K, Kovacs K, Muller PJ. Clinical-pathological correlations of pituitary tumours. *Bailliere's Clin Endocrinol Metab* 1995; 9(2): 243–70.

204. Nelson DH, Meakin JW, Thorn GW. ACTH-producing pituitary tumors following adrenalectomy for Cushing's syndrome. *Ann Int Med* 1960; 52: 560–9.

205. Kelly PA, Samandouras G, Grossman AB, et al. Neurosurgical treatment of Nelson's syndrome. *J Clin Endocrinol Metab* 2002; 87: 5465–9.

206. Assié G, Bahurel H, Coste J, et al. Corticotroph tumor progression after adrenalectomy in Cushing's disease: A reappraisal of Nelson's syndrome. *J Clin Endocrinol Metab* 2007; 92: 172–9.

207. Barber TM, Adams E, Ansorge O, et al. Nelson's syndrome. *Eur J Endocrinol* 2010; 163: 495–507.

208. Ilias I, Torpy DJ, Pacak K, et al. Cushing's syndrome due to ectopic corticotropin secretion: Twenty years' experience at the National Institutes of Health. *J Clin Endocrinol Metab* 2005; 90: 4955–62.

209. Isodori AM, Kaltsas GA, Pozza C, et al. The ectopic adrenocorticotropin syndrome: Clinical features, diagnosis, management, and long-term follow-up. *J Clin Endocrinol Metab* 2006; 91: 371–7.

210. Samuels MH, Loriaux DL. Cushing's syndrome and the nodular adrenal gland. *Endocrinol Metab Clin North Am* 1994; 23(3): 555–69.

211. Carney JA, Young WF. Primary pigmented nodular adrenocortical disease and its associated conditions. *Endocrinologist* 1992; 2: 6.

212. Kirschner LS, Sandrini F, Monbo J, et al. Genetic heterogeneity and spectrum of mutations of the *PRKAR1A* gene in patients with the Carney complex. *Hum Mol Genet* 2000; 9(20): 3037–46.

213. Anselmo J, Medeiros S, Carneiro V, et al. A large family with Carney complex caused by the S147G *PRKAR1A* mutation shows a unique spectrum of disease including adrenocortical cancer. *J Clin Endocrinol Metab* 2012; 97: 351–9.

214. Trainer PJ, Grossman A. The diagnosis and differential diagnosis of Cushing's syndrome. *Clin Endocrinol* 1991; 34: 317–30.

215. Brown RJ, Kelly MH, Collins MT. Cushing syndrome in the McCune-Albright syndrome. *J Clin Endocrinol Metab* 2010; 95: 1508–15.

216. Lacroix AL, Bolté E, Tremblay J, et al. Gastric inhibitory poypeptide-dependent cortisol hypersecretion – a new cause of Cushing's syndrome. *N Engl J Med* 1992; 327: 974–80.

217. Resnik Y, Allali-Zerah V, Chayvialle JA, et al. Food-dependent Cushing's syndrome mediated by aberrant adrenal sensitivity to gastric inhibitory polypeptide. *N Engl J Med* 1992; 327: 981–6.

218. Lacroix A, Bourdeau I, Lampron A, et al. Aberrant G-protein receptor expression in relation to adrenocortical overfunction. *Clin Endocrinol* 2010; 73: 1–15.

219. Malchoff CD, Rosa J, DeBold CR, et al. Adrenocorticotropin-independent bilateral macronodular adrenal hyperplasia: An unusual cause of Cushing's syndrome. *J Clin Endocrinol Metab* 1989; 68: 855–60.

220. Nieman LK, Biller BMK, Findling JW, et al. The diagnosis of Cushing's syndrome: An Endocrine Society Clinical Practice Guideline. *J Clin Endocrinol Metab* 2008; 93(5): 1526–40.

221. Pecori GF, Ambrogio AG, De Martin M, et al. Specificity of first-line tests for the diagnosis of Cushing's syndrome: Assessment in a large series. *J Clin Endocrinol Metab* 2007; 92: 4123–9.

222. Elamin MB, Murad HM, Mullan R, et al. Accuracy of diagnostic tests for Cushing's syndrome: A systematic review and metaanalyses. *J Clin Endocrinol Metab* 2008; 93(5): 1553–62.
223. Alexandraki KI, Grossman AB. Novel insights in the diagnosis of Cushing's syndrome. *Neuroendocrinol* 2010; 92(Suppl 1): 35–43.
224. Dichek HL, Nieman LK, Oldfield EH, et al. A comparison of the standard high dose dexamethasone suppression test and the overnight 8-mg dexamethasone suppression test for the differential diagnosis of adrenocorticotropin-dependent Cushing's syndrome. *J Clin Endocrinol Metab* 1994; 78: 418–22.
225. van den Bogaert DPM, de Herder WW, de Jong FH, et al. The continuous 7-hour intravenous dexamethasone suppression test in the differential diagnosis of ACTH-dependent Cushing's syndrome. *Clin Endocrinol* 1999; 51: 193–8.
226. Nieman LK, Oldfield EH, Wesley R, et al. A simplified morning ovine corticotrophin-releasing hormone stimulation test for the differential diagnosis of adrenocorticotropin-dependent Cushing's syndrome. *J Clin Endocrinol Metab* 1993; 77(5): 1308–12.
227. Arnaldi G, Angeli A, Atkinson AB, et al. Diagnosis and complications of Cushing's syndrome; a consensus statement. *J Clin Endocrinol Metab* 2003; 88: 5593–602.
228. Oldfield EH, Doppman JL, Nieman LK, et al. Petrosal sinus sampling with and without corticotropin-releasing hormone for the differential diagnosis of Cushing's syndrome. *N Engl J Med* 1991; 325: 897–905.
229. Swearingham B, Katznelson L, Miller K, et al. Diagnostic errors after inferior petrosal sinus sampling. *J Clin Endocrinol Metab* 2004; 89: 3752–63.
230. Doppman JL, Chang R, Oldfield EH, et al. The hypoplastic inferior petrosal sinus: A potential source of false-negative results in petrosal sampling for Cushing's disease. *J Clin Endocrinol Metab* 1999; 84: 533–40.
231. Young J, Deneux C, Grino M, et al. Pitfall of petrosal sinus sampling in a Cushing's syndrome secondary to ectopic adrenocorticotropin-corticotropin releasing hormone (ACTH-CRH) secretion. *J Clin Endocrinol Metab* 1998; 83: 305–08.
232. Wind JJ, Lonser RR, Nieman LK, et al. The lateralization accuracy of inferior petrosal sinus sampling in 501 patients with Cushing's disease. *J Clin Endocrinol Metab* 2013; 98(6): 2285–93.
233. Oliver RL, Davis JRE, White A. Characterisation of ACTH related peptides in ectopic Cushing's syndrome. *Pituitary* 2003; 6: 119–26.
234. Chiodini I, Morelli V, Salcuni AS, et al. Beneficial metabolic effects of prompt surgical treatment in patients with an adrenal incidentaloma causing biochemical hypercortisolism. *J Clin Endocrinol Metab* 2010; 95: 2736–45.
235. Hammer GD, Tyrrell JB, Lamborn KR, et al. Transsphenoidal microsurgery for Cushing's disease: Initial outcome and long-term results. *J Clin Endocrinol Metab* 2004; 89: 6348–57.
236. Pouratian N, Prevedello DM, Jagannathan J, et al. Outcomes and management of patients with Cushing's disease without pathological confirmation of tumor resection after transsphenoidal surgery. *J Clin Endocrinol Metab* 2007; 92: 3383–88.
237. Valassi E, Biller BMK, Swearingen B, et al. Delayed remission after transsphenoidal surgery in patients with Cushing's disease. *J Clin Endocrinol Metab* 2010; 95: 601–10.
238. Buchfelder M, Schlaffer S. Pituitary surgery for Cushing's disease. *Neuroendocrinol* 2010; 92(Suppl 1): 102–6.
239. Abdelmannan D, Chaiban J, Selman WR, et al. Recurrences of ACTH-secreting adenomas after pituitary adenomectomy can be accurately predicted by perioperative measurement of plasma ACTH levels. *J Clin Endocrinol Metab* 2013; 98: 1458–65.
240. Biller BMK, Grossman AB, Stewart PM, et al. Treatment of adrenocorticotropin-dependent Cushing's syndrome: A consensus statement. *J Clin Endocrinol Metab* 2008; 93: 2454–62.
241. Losa M, Picozzi P, Redaelli MG, et al. Pituitary radiotherapy for Cushing's disease. *Neuroendocrinol* 2010; 92(Suppl 1): 107–10.
242. Allolio B, Hahner S, Weismann D, et al. Management of adrenocortical carcinoma. *Clin Endocrinol* 2004; 60: 273–87.
243. Stuijver DJF, van Zaane B, Feelders RA, et al. Incidence of venous thromboembolism in patients with Cushing's syndrome: A multicenter cohort study. *J Clin Endocrinol Metab* 2011; 96: 3525–32.
244. Bosacro M, Sonino N, Scarda A, et al. Anticoagulant prophylaxis markedly reduces thromboembolic complications in Cushing's syndrome. *J Clin Endocrinol Metab* 2002; 87: 3662–6.
245. van der Pas R, de Bruin C, Leebeek FWG, et al. The hypercoagulable state in Cushing's disease is associated with increased levels of procoagulant factors and impaired fibrinolysis, but is not reversible after short-term biochemical remission induced by medical therapy. *J Clin Endocrinol Metab* 2012; 97: 1303–10.
246. Feelders RA, Hofland LJ, de Herder WW. Medical treatment of Cushing's syndrome: Adrenal-blocking drugs and ketaconazole. *Neuroendocrinol* 2010; 92(Suppl 1): 111–15.
247. Mauclère-Denost S, Leboulleux S, Borget I, et al. High-dose mitotane strategy in adrenocortical carcinoma: Prospective analysis of plasma mitotane measurement during the first 3 months of follow-up. *Eur J Endocrinol* 2012; 166(2): 261–8.
248. Krakoff J, Koch CA, Calis KA, et al. Use of a parenteral propylene glycol-containing etomidate preparation for

the long-term management of ectopic Cushing's syndrome. *J Clin Endocrinol* 2001; 86: 4104–08.
249. Castinetti F, Conte-Devlox B, Brue T. Medical treatment of Cushing's syndrome: Glucocorticoid receptor antagonists and mifepristone. *Neuroendocrinol* 2010; 92(Suppl 1): 125–30.
250. Pivonello R, De Martino MC, Cappabianca P, et al. The medical treatment of Cushing's disease: Effectiveness of chronic treatment with the dopamine agonist cabergoline in patients unsuccessfully treated by surgery. *J Clin Endocrinol Metab* 2009; 94: 223–30.
251. Godbout A, Manavela M, Danilowicz K, et al. Cabergoline monotherapy in the long-term treatment of Cushing's disease. *Eur J Endocrinol* 2010; 163: 709–16.
252. Petrossians P, Thonnard A-S, Beckers A. Medical treatment in Cushing's syndrome: Dopamine agonists and cabergoline. *Neuroendocrinol* 2010; 92(Suppl 1): 116–19.
253. Colao A, Petersenn S, Newell-Price J, et al. A 12-month phase 3 study of pasireotide in Cushing's disease. *N Engl J Med* 2012; 366: 914–24.
254. Vilar L, Naves LA, Azevedo MF, et al. Effectiveness of cabergoline in monotherapy and combined with ketoconazole in the management of Cushing's disease. *Pituitary* 2010; 13: 123–9.
255. Feelders RA, de Bruin C, Pereira AM, et al. Pasireotide alone or with cabergoline and ketoconazole in Cushing's disease. *N Engl J Med* 2010; 362(19): 1846–8.
256. Kamenicky P, Droumaguet C, Salenave S, et al. Mitotane, metyrapone, and ketoconazole combination therapy as an alternative to rescue adrenalectomy for severe ACTH-dependent Cushing's syndrome. *J Clin Endocrinol Metab* 2011; 96: 2796–804.

# 2

# Familial isolated pituitary adenomas

*Vladimir Vasilev, Renata S. Auriemma, Adrian F. Daly, Albert Beckers*

## Introduction

Pituitary adenomas are generally benign tumors with diverse functional characteristics, and they can have a significant impact on patients and medical specialists. Their prevalence in the population has long been a matter of debate because of controversial data coming from pathological and imaging studies and earlier clinical series. A meta-analysis of autopsy and magnetic resonance imaging (MRI) studies suggests that pituitary tumors occur quite frequently at 14.4% and 22.5% in unselected populations, respectively.[1] Conversely, the few epidemiological studies performed in the past estimated their prevalence to be as low as 19–28 cases per 100,000 inhabitants.[2] The issue was addressed by a large community-based cross-sectional study in the province of Liège, Belgium, revealing that clinically relevant pituitary adenomas are present in 94 of every 100,000 individuals.[3] These data were later confirmed in Banbury, United Kingdom, where similar prevalence was observed: 78 cases per 100,000 individuals.[4] Such comparatively high prevalence, together with the variable clinical presentation, unpredictable growth, and the complex and expensive management, raises the need for in-depth understanding of the pathological processes that underlie their development.

Pituitary adenomas are generally considered to originate from clonal expansion of a single mutated cell,[5] and molecular studies have identified several genetic and epigenetic abnormalities that may have a possible causative role in pituitary tumorigenesis. These abnormalities include somatic mutations in *gsp* oncogene, disruptions in cell cycle regulation and intracellular signaling pathways, and rarely mutations of classic oncogenes.[6,7] The majority of pituitary adenomas occur sporadically, and inherited germline mutations that are responsible for familial presentation are quite infrequent. Altogether, familial/genetically inherited pituitary tumors account for approximately 5% of all pituitary adenomas.[8] Traditionally, inherited genetic susceptibility can be expected when pituitary pathology is associated with extrapituitary presentations typical for some multiple endocrine neoplasia syndromes. Multiple endocrine neoplasia type 1 (MEN1) is by far the most common condition with familial pituitary adenomas and accounts for approximately 3% of all pituitary tumors.[9] In addition to pituitary pathology, it is also associated with primary hyperparathyroidism and entero-pancreatic neuroendocrine tumors, and >70% of the cases may be attributed to inactivating mutations of the tumor suppressor gene *MEN1* on chromosome 11q13.[10,11] Carney complex (CNC) is another syndromic disease that presents infrequently with pituitary adenomas, mostly acromegaly.[12] The majority of cases can be related to germline mutations of the gene encoding type 1A regulatory subunit of protein kinase A (*PRKAR1A*).[13,14] Familial pituitary adenomas can also develop as a part of multiple endocrine neoplasia type 4 (MEN4) characterized by inactivating mutations of the *CDKN1B* gene. This condition, however, seems to be extremely rare with only few cases documented in literature so far[15,16] (Table 2.1).

Apart from syndromic diseases, there has been evidence for familial pituitary adenomas arising in an isolated setting, from the beginning of the 20th century (Figure 2.1). By the 1990s, only occasional cases of familial pituitary tumors unrelated to MEN1 or CNC were described, with

| Disease | Gene and location | Mode of inheritance | Associated pathology |
|---|---|---|---|
| MEN1 | *MEN1*, 11q13 (>80% of cases) | AD with high penetrance | Hyperparathyroidism<br>Gastroenteropancreatic tumors<br>Pituitary adenomas<br>Adrenal adenomas<br>Carcinoid tumors<br>Facial angiofibromas<br>Lipomas<br>Collagenomas |
| CNC | *PRKAR1A*, 17q22–24 (>70% of cases) | AD with high penetrance | Spotty skin pigmentation<br>Lentiginosis<br>Myxomas<br>Primary pigmented nodular adrenal dysplasia (PPNAD)<br>Large cell calcifying Sertoli cell tumors (LCCSCT)<br>Acromegaly<br>Thyroid nodules<br>Schwannomas |
| MEN4 | CDKN1B, 12p13 | AD, unknown penetrance | Hyperparathyroidism<br>Acromegaly<br>Corticotropinoma<br>Testicular tumor<br>Renal angiolipoma<br>Cervical carcinoma |
| FIPA | *AIP*, 11q13 (25% of cases) | AD with incomplete penetrance | All kinds of pituitary adenomas<br>No known extrapituitary pathology |

MEN1, multiple endocrine neoplasia type 1; CNC, Carney complex; MEN4, multiple endocrine neoplasia type 4; FIPA, familial isolated pituitary adenomas; AD, autosomal dominant.

***Table 2.1***
*Conditions associated with familial pituitary adenomas.*

most of them presenting with acromegaly.[17] Initially, the condition was termed isolated familial somatotropinomas, but with the accumulation of cases it became obvious that although less common, other functional types may also be present.[18–21] The first single-center study to specifically search for cases of familial pituitary adenomas was performed in Liège, Belgium, in the late 1990s and led to the identification of an initial cohort of 27 patients that included both familial somatotropinomas and other pituitary tumor phenotypes.[22] To accurately reflect this more complex presentation of the condition, the term familial isolated pituitary adenomas (FIPA) was coined to describe families with two or more related members with pituitary adenomas in the absence of MEN1 and CNC.[23–25] Because FIPA encompasses a broader clinical spectrum, cases with familial acromegaly could now be referred to a subgroup of the new condition. The definition of FIPA expanded the search internationally, and by 2012, >200 affected families were reported.[26,27] FIPA is currently considered to be as frequent a cause for inherited pituitary pathology as MEN1 and accounts for approximately 2% of pituitary adenomas.[28]

## Clinical characteristics of FIPA (see Chapter 1)

The syndrome of FIPA is defined as the hereditary presentation of any type of pituitary adenoma in the

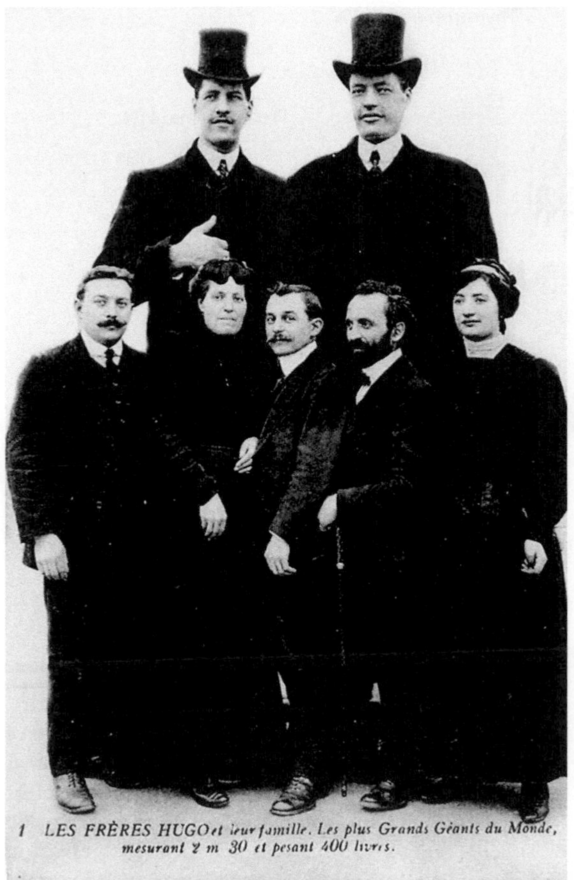
1 LES FRÈRES HUGO et leur famille. Les plus Grands Géants du Monde,
mesurant 2 m 30 et pesant 400 livres.

**Figure 2.1**
*The famous brothers Baptiste and Antoine Hugo and their family in the beginning of the 20th century. Antoine Hugo was found to harbor a giant pituitary adenoma after his death.*

absence of clinical and genetic evidence for MEN1 and CNC.[29] After the initial description of the condition, the clinical characteristics of a large international cohort of 64 families made up of >140 patients from 22 tertiary referral centers were reported in 2006.[28] Genealogical information suggested that FIPA is inherited in an autosomal dominant pattern with low or variable penetrance. According to the tumor phenotype in the individual families, FIPA can be divided in two almost equal subgroups: homogeneous when all affected members harbor the same type of adenomas, and heterogeneous when different pituitary tumors arising within the family. Altogether, prolactinomas and somatotropinomas encompass >70% of all tumors, and although in heterogeneous FIPA all functional types can be observed, there is at least one prolactin- or growth hormone (GH)–secreting adenoma in almost all affected families. Females tend to be more frequently affected (62%) because prolactinomas are the most common phenotype. Prolactin-secreting adenomas make up 40% of all FIPA patients, and their features are usually similar to matched sporadic patients in terms of sex, age at diagnosis, and proportion of microadenomas. In heterogeneous FIPA families, however, they exhibit more aggressive behavior with significantly higher rates of suprasellar expansion and cavernous sinus invasion than sporadic prolactinomas. GH-secreting adenomas account for 30% of FIPA tumors, and mixed secretion of GH and prolactin is observed in another 7% of them. They are equally distributed between homogeneous and heterogeneous families, but unlike FIPA prolactinomas, somatotropinomas are more aggressive when occurring in a homogeneous setting. In homogeneous FIPA, acromegaly is usually diagnosed 10 years earlier, with tumors more frequently displaying extrasellar growth compared with heterogeneous kindreds and sporadic populations.[29] Nonsecreting adenomas are predominantly associated with heterogeneous families and account for 13% of FIPA patients. They are also characterized by more aggressive evolution, being diagnosed earlier and exhibiting more invasive properties than sporadic adenomas. Gonadotropinomas, corticotropinomas, and thyrotropinomas are rare in FIPA (Figure 2.2). They are usually associated with other adenoma types in heterogeneous kindreds, although individual families with homogeneous presentation have been reported previously.[29] The descendants in FIPA families with multiple affected generations are diagnosed considerably earlier than their parents/grandparents.

# *Molecular genetics of FIPA*

The elucidation of the responsible genetic causes of FIPA started with the identification of loss of heterozygosity in locus 11q13 in kindreds with familial acromegaly who lacked mutations in the *MEN1* gene.[30,31] Further research in a Finnish cohort of patients with familial pituitary tumors revealed inactivating mutations in the gene for aryl hydrocarbon receptor (AhR)–interacting protein (AIP).[32] The causative role of *AIP* in FIPA was soon confirmed with the discovery of new germline mutations in a large series of 73 families.[33] Loss of heterozygosity in tumor tissues suggests a tumor suppressor function for *AIP*, but the exact molecular mechanisms leading to pituitary tumorigenesis are not completely known.

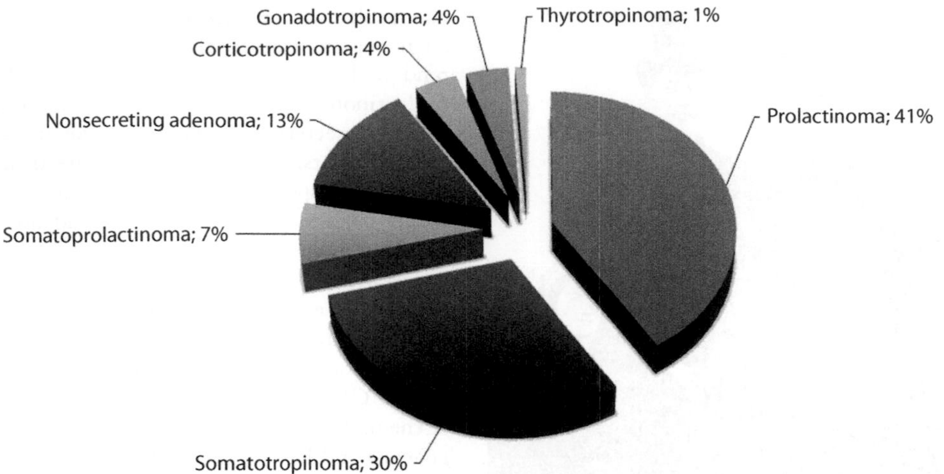


***Figure 2.2***
*Frequency distribution of the different functional tumor types in patients with familial isolated pituitary adenomas.*

The *AIP* gene is universally expressed in various tissues throughout the body, and in normal pituitary, it is associated with secretory granules in somatotrope and lactotrope cells. In sporadic pituitary adenomas, *AIP* is expressed in all tumor types, but in prolactinomas, nonsecreting adenomas, and corticotropinomas it can only be identified in the cytoplasm, whereas in somatotropinomas it is localized within secretory vesicles.[34] Homozygous $AIP^{-/-}$ knockout mice die in the early embryonic period of severe cardiovascular abnormalities, suggesting that AIP may play a role in cardiovascular development.[35] Heterozygous $AIP^{+/-}$ animals, however, develop a phenotype that is very similar to human pituitary disease, with the majority of the mice presenting with aggressive somatotropinomas.[36] The *AIP* gene consists of six exons and codes a 330 amino acid protein whose sequence is highly conserved among different species.[37] AIP takes part in numerous protein–protein interactions, mediated through its C-terminal end that contains three tetratricopeptide repeats (TPRs) and a terminal $\alpha$-helix. Among the first identified partners of AIP was the AhR, a ligand-inducible transcription factor that modulates cellular responses to various xenobiotic toxins, such as dioxins, as well as some endogenous compounds, such as cAMP.[38] In the absence of ligands, the AhR binds to two molecules of the 90 kDa heat-shock protein (hsp90), acting as chaperone, with AIP and p23 proteins, acting as cochaperones, to form a multiprotein complex in the cytoplasm.[39] The activation of the complex by its xenobiotic ligand results in nuclear translocation where AhR binds to the AhR nuclear translocator (ARNT) and promotes the transcription of specific genes coding various drug-metabolizing enzymes as well as other proteins, such as the cyclin-dependent kinase inhibitor $p27^{Kip1}$.[40] The effect of AIP on the functional status of AhR is still not clear because conflicting results have been reported, but it seems that it maintains the stability of the complex by protecting AhR from ubiquitin-dependent degradation.[41] Data on the effect of AhR activation on cell proliferation are controversial, but it has been shown that reduced AIP expression in pituitary adenomas, positive for *AIP* mutations, is associated with decreased AhR activity, suggesting an inhibitory function of AhR in pituitary tumorigenesis.[42] Furthermore, AIP overexpression in cell cultures including pituitary cell lines slows down cell proliferation rates.[34] Another possible pathophysiological link between AIP and pituitary tumorigenesis lies in the interaction with two specific types of phosphodiesterases: PDE4A5 and PDE2A. These enzymes inactivate cyclic nucleotides such as cAMP by disrupting the phosphodiester bond in their molecules. Thus, they may participate in the regulation of the various signaling pathways using cAMP as intracellular second messenger, including the growth hormone–releasing hormone (GHRH) receptor cascade in pituitary cells. Disruptions in signal transduction that lead to abnormally high cAMP concentrations are associated with pituitary hyperplasia and adenoma formation in some conditions such as Carney complex and McCune–Albright syndrome.[43] AIP binding to PDE4A5 reduces its catalytic activity. It is unclear whether this interaction plays a role in pituitary tumorigenesis, because loss of AIP would presumably result in low cAMP levels. The interaction with PDE2A interrupts the nuclear translocation of the AhR complex, possibly by local reduction in cAMP levels.[44] AIP was recently shown to interact with the tyrosine kinase receptor, encoded by the RET protooncogene. Depending on the presence or the absence of its specific ligand glial cell line–derived neurotropic factor (GDNF), RET promotes cell growth and migration or induces apoptosis, respectively. Moreover, the domain responsible for the proapoptotic activity is the same that is responsible for AIP interaction.[40] This RET–AIP binding presumably prevents the formation of a complex between AIP and surviving, a recently identified inhibitor of apoptosis and cell cycle regulator. Without the stabilizing role of AIP, survivin is degraded rapidly, with consequent increase in apoptosis.[45] These effects, however, are contrary to the proposed tumor suppressor role of AIP, and their true relevance is unclear. Apart from stabilizing the AhR complex, AIP may also bind to a set of nuclear receptors including the peroxisome proliferator-activated receptor α (PPARα), glucocorticoid receptor, and α-thyroid hormone receptor 1 (TRα1). Furthermore, AIP has been proposed to have a role in virus-induced tumorigenesis as a potential partner of hepatitis B virus X antigen and Epstein–Barr virus-encoded nuclear antigen 3 (EBNA-3).[40] The significance of these interactions, however, still remains to be fully elucidated.

More than 50 different mutations in the *AIP* sequence have been identified in FIPA families worldwide, and they are spread through the entire length of the gene[37,46] (Figure 2.3). Most of them affect the C-terminal end and the TPR motifs, supporting their essential role in AIP function. Nonsense and frameshift mutations lead to premature stop codons with resultant truncated protein, whereas missense mutations tend to affect the TPR domains and the terminal α-helix. Whole gene deletions have also been identified, suggesting the use of multiple ligation-dependent probe amplification (MLPA) method in FIPA patients in whom sequencing fails to identify abnormalities.[47,48] Mutations in codons R304, R271, and R81 have been

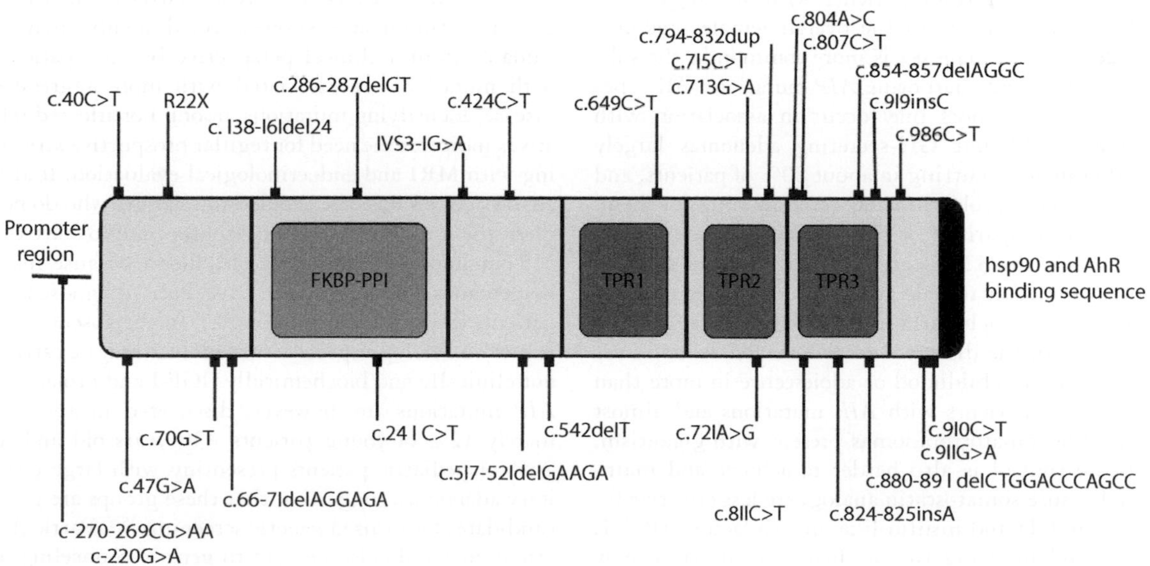


***Figure 2.3***
*AIP gene and some of the known mutations. AhR, aryl hydrocarbon receptor; FKBP-PPI, FK506 binding protein-type peptidyl-propyl cis-trans isomerase; TPR, tetratricopeptide repeat domain; hsp90, heat-shock protein 90.*

reported in independent FIPA kindreds, indicating possible hot spots.[37] No genotype–phenotype correlati ons have been observed to date in *AIP*-mutated FIPA patients, although some observations may imply a less aggressive character for mutations with conserved C-terminal part of AIP.[49]

Mutations in *AIP* gene, however, are found only in approximately 25% of all FIPA patients and in 40%–50% in the subgroup of patients with acromegaly from homogeneous FIPA families.[26] The genetic cause for the rest of the cases is still unknown, but several other loci, such as 2p16, 3q28, 4q32, 8q12, 19q13, and 21q22, may be involved in the development of the syndrome, although no particular genes have been yet identified at this sites.[50] In contrast, the penetrance of *AIP* mutations is estimated at about 30% in the largest reported families,[29,48,51] implying that other genetic or environmental modifying factors may also be present.

## Clinical features of AIP-mutated FIPA patients

*AIP*-related pituitary adenomas are also shown to exhibit some specific clinical characteristics that differentiate them from patients with wild-type *AIP* alleles.[52] In contrast to the overall female predominance in FIPA, male sex is more common in the subgroup of patients harboring *AIP* mutations. All types of pituitary tumors may occur in association with mutated *AIP*, but GH-secreting adenomas largely predominate, occurring in about 80% of patients, and cosecretion of prolactin is observed in >50% of them. A direct comparison of 75 *AIP*-mutated somatotropinomas with 232 mutation-negative control subjects with acromegaly revealed that *AIP* anomalies are associated with much earlier onset and more aggressive evolution of the disease. Invasive macroadenomas are manifested in childhood or adolescence in more than half of the patients with *AIP* mutations and almost a third of somatotropinomas present with gigantism. Disease control is also harder to achieve and maintain because somatostatin analogs are less effective for lowering GH and insulin-like growth factor I (IGF-I) levels and inducing tumor shrinkage in acromegaly due to *AIP* mutations. Moreover, these patients have significantly worse long-term therapeutic control, although they frequently receive multiple surgeries and radiotherapy. *AIP*-mutated prolactinomas also present with large tumors size and invasive features. Resistance to dopamine agonists may be observed in 50% of them, resulting in the need for surgery, radiotherapy, or both.

## Clinical management

Treatment of familial pituitary adenomas practically does not differ from the management of their sporadic counterparts regarding indications and therapeutic approaches. The identification of an underlying genetic susceptibility, however, may provide significant benefits for the patients and their relatives in terms of early diagnosis and treatment, as well as preventive screening for associated pathological conditions in syndromic diseases (Figure 2.4). Moreover, pituitary tumors developing as a part of MEN1 and FIPA, especially in patients with *AIP* mutations, have more aggressive evolution, present earlier, and often respond poorly to therapy, thus constituting additional challenge for endocrinologists and neurosurgeons. Thorough physical examination for extrapituitary involvement and comprehensive family history should be initially performed, and any suspicion for syndromic conditions or FIPA should be appropriately confirmed before referring patients to genetic screening. Currently, there are no consensus protocols for the management of *AIP*-mutated FIPA patients, and although mutations of *AIP* gene are observed in only a quarter of the cases, genetic testing in at least one affected member may be valuable from a clinical perspective because patients with mutations are associated with more aggressive disease. Identifying mutations among nonaffected relatives indicates the need for regular prospective screening with MRI and endocrinological evaluation. It also enables screening to be avoided in relatives who do not carry the mutation. It may be appropriate to start the MRI monitoring from early childhood because macroadenomas and gigantism have been diagnosed in patients as young as 6–8 years.[48,52] In the absence of a tumor on MRI, prospective surveillance may be carried out clinically and biochemically (IGF-I and prolactin). *AIP* mutations are, however, discovered in approximately 12% of young patients <30 years old and in 20% of pediatric patients presenting with large pituitary adenomas, suggesting that these groups are good candidates for focused genetic screening.[46,53] Particular attention should also be paid to genetic counseling of FIPA patients and their relatives because of the relatively low prevalence of *AIP* mutations and the uncertain degree of penetrance. Widespread screening for *AIP* mutations among apparently sporadic pituitary adenomas may not be warranted because the prevalence of *AIP* alterations is low.[54]

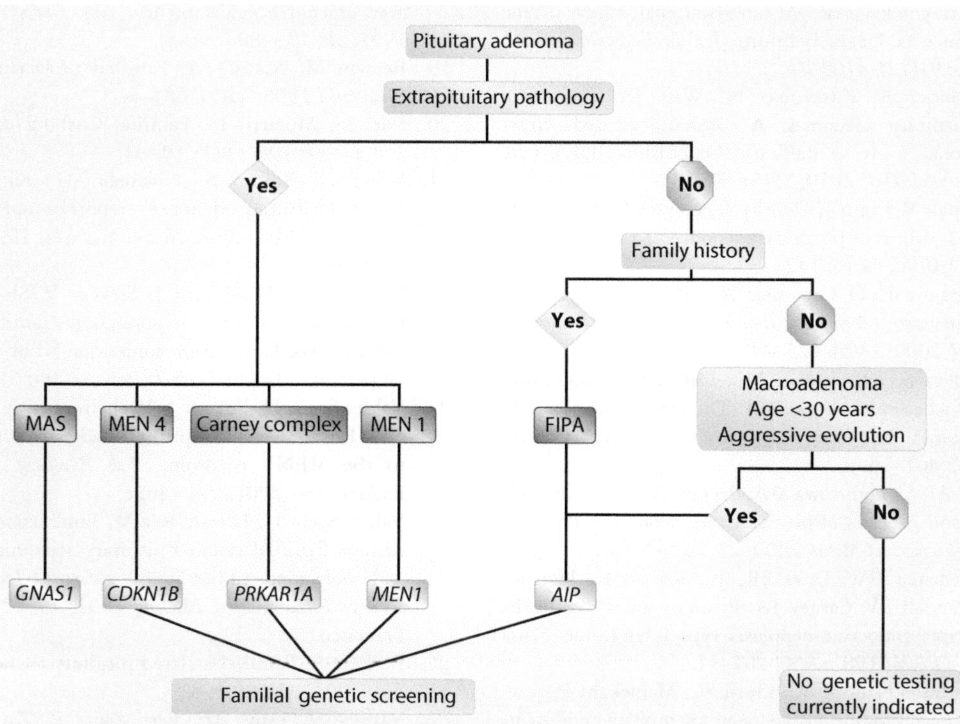


***Figure 2.4***
*Flowchart for selecting patients with genetic susceptibility for pituitary adenomas in whom genetic testing is appropriate. MAS is caused by postzygotic mutations of the* GNAS1 *gene, and no familial cases have been described to date. Diagnostic testing for mutations in* MEN1 *gene is available in several genetic laboratories worldwide.* AIP, CDKN1B, *and* PRKAR1A *testings are undertaken in several reference centers. MAS, McCune–Albright syndrome; MEN1, multiple endocrine neoplasia type 1; MEN4, multiple endocrine neoplasia type 4; FIPA, familial isolated pituitary adenomas.*

# Conclusions

Genetic predisposition to pituitary adenomas is increasingly being recognized, and the array of the known familial pituitary pathology has recently been enriched with the definition of FIPA. Thanks to the collaborative efforts from different centers around the world, the clinical features of the new condition have been characterized. The identification of *AIP* gene mutations as the underlying molecular defects in a proportion of FIPA patients has provided the opportunity for genetic screening in affected families. Consensus guidelines concerning the management and follow-up of FIPA patients are still lacking but will hopefully be developed with the accumulation of data from large international cohorts and long-term monitoring studies. Further research is also needed for the elucidation of the genetic defects in the subset of patients with no *AIP* mutations. The thorough understanding of the molecular pathophysiology of familial pituitary tumors may provide basis for the future development of specifically targeted therapeutic tools and translate in better prevention and appropriate management of individual patients.

# References

1. Ezzat S, Asa SL, Couldwell WT, et al. The prevalence of pituitary adenomas: A systematic review. *Cancer* 2004; 101(3): 613–19.
2. Davis JR, Farrell WE, Clayton RN. Pituitary tumours. *Reproduction* 2001; 121(3): 363–71.
*3. Daly AF, Rixhon M, Adam C, Dempegioti A, Tichomirowa MA, Beckers A. High prevalence of

* Key or Classic references.

pituitary adenomas: A cross-sectional study in the province of Liege, Belgium. *J Clin Endocrinol Metab* 2006; 91(12): 4769–75.

4. Fernandez A, Karavitaki N, Wass JA. Prevalence of pituitary adenomas: A community-based, cross-sectional study in Banbury (Oxfordshire, UK). *Clin Endocrinol (Oxf)* 2010; 72(3): 377–82.
5. Herman V, Fagin J, Gonsky R, Kovacs K, Melmed S. Clonal origin of pituitary adenomas. *J Clin Endocrinol Metab* 1990; 71(6): 1427–33.
6. Dworakowska D, Grossman AB. The pathophysiology of pituitary adenomas. *Best Pract Res Clin Endocrinol Metab* 2009; 23(5): 525–41.
7. Vandeva S, Jaffrain-Rea ML, Daly AF, Tichomirowa M, Zacharieva S, Beckers A. The genetics of pituitary adenomas. *Best Pract Res Clin Endocrinol Metab* 2010; 24(3): 461–76.
8. Daly AF, Tichomirowa MA, Beckers A. The epidemiology and genetics of pituitary adenomas. *Best Pract Res Clin Endocrinol Metab* 2009; 23(5): 543–54.
9. Scheithauer BW, Laws ER, Jr., Kovacs K, Horvath E, Randall RV, Carney JA. Pituitary adenomas of the multiple endocrine neoplasia type I syndrome. *Semin Diagn Pathol* 1987; 4(3): 205–11.
10. Chandrasekharappa SC, Guru SC, Manickam P, et al. Positional cloning of the gene for multiple endocrine neoplasia-type 1. *Science* 1997; 276(5311): 404–7.
11. Lemos MC, Thakker RV. Multiple endocrine neoplasia type 1 (MEN1): Analysis of 1336 mutations reported in the first decade following identification of the gene. *Hum Mutat* 2008; 29(1): 22–32.
12. Carney JA, Hruska LS, Beauchamp GD, Gordon H. Dominant inheritance of the complex of myxomas, spotty pigmentation, and endocrine overactivity. *Mayo Clin Proc* 1986; 61(3): 165–72.
13. Kirschner LS. PRKAR1A and the evolution of pituitary tumors. *Mol Cell Endocrinol* 2010; 326(1–2): 3–7.
14. Rothenbuhler A, Stratakis CA. Clinical and molecular genetics of Carney complex. *Best Pract Res Clin Endocrinol Metab* 2010; 24(3): 389–99.
15. Pellegata NS, Quintanilla-Martinez L, Siggelkow H, et al. Germ-line mutations in p27Kip1 cause a multiple endocrine neoplasia syndrome in rats and humans. *Proc Natl Acad Sci U S A* 2006; 103(42): 15558–63.
16. Agarwal SK, Mateo CM, Marx SJ. Rare germline mutations in cyclin-dependent kinase inhibitor genes in multiple endocrine neoplasia type 1 and related states. *J Clin Endocrinol Metab* 2009; 94(5): 1826–34.
17. Verloes A, Stevenaert A, Teh BT, Petrossians P, Beckers A. Familial acromegaly: Case report and review of the literature. *Pituitary* 1999; 1(3–4): 273–7.
18. Linquette M, Herlant M, Laine E, Fossati P, Dupont-Lecompte J. Adenome a prolactine chez une jeune fine dont la mere etait porteuse d'un adenome hypophysaire avec amenorrheegalactorrhee. *Ann Endocrinol (Paris)* 1997; 28: 773–80.
19. Berezin M, Karasik A. Familial prolactinoma. *Clin Endocrinol* 1995; 42(5): 483–6.
20. Salti IS, Mufarrij IS. Familial Cushing disease. *Am J Med Genet* 1981; 8(1): 91–4.
21. Yuasa H, Tokito S, Nakagaki H, Kitamura K. Familial pituitary adenoma—report of four cases from two unrelated families. *Neurol Med Chir* 1990; 30(13): 1016–19.
22. Valdes Socin H, Poncin J, Stevens V, Stevenaert A, Beckers A. Adenomes hypophysaires familiaux isoles non lies avec la mutation somatique NEM-1. Siuvi de 27 patients. *Ann Endocrinol (Paris)* 2000; 61: 301.
23. Valdes Socin H, Poncin J, Vanbelinghen J, et al., editors. Familial isolated pituitary adenomas not related to the MEN1 syndrome. *5th European Congress of Endocrinology* 2001, 9–13 June.
24. Valdes Socin H, Jaffrain Réa M, Tamburrano G, et al., editors. Familial isolated pituitary adenomas: Clinical and molecular studies in 80 patients. *The Endocrine Society's 84th Annual Meeting* 2002; 19–22 June; San Francisco.
25. Beckers A. Familial isolated pituitary adenomas. *J Int Med* 2004; 255(6): 698.
26. Vasilev V, Daly AF, Petrossians P, Zacharieva S, Beckers A. Familial pituitary tumor syndromes. *Endocr Pract* 2011; 17(Suppl 3): 41–6.
27. Beckers A, Aaltonen LA, Daly AF, Karhu A. Familial isolated pituitary adenomas (FIPA) and the pituitary adenoma predisposition due to mutations in the aryl hydrocarbon receptor interacting protein (AIP) gene. *Endocr Rev.* 2013; 34(2): 239–77.
*28. Daly AF, Jaffrain-Rea ML, Ciccarelli A, et al. Clinical characterization of familial isolated pituitary adenomas. *J Clin Endocrinol Metab* 2006; 91(9): 3316–23.
29. Beckers A, Daly AF. The clinical, pathological, and genetic features of familial isolated pituitary adenomas. *Eur J Endocrinol* 2007; 157(4): 371–82.
30. Yamada S, Yoshimoto K, Sano T, et al. Inactivation of the tumor suppressor gene on 11q13 in brothers with familial acrogigantism without multiple endocrine neoplasia type 1. *J Clin Endocrinol Metab* 1997; 82(1): 239–42.
31. Gadelha MR, Prezant TR, Une KN, et al. Loss of heterozygosity on chromosome 11q13 in two families with acromegaly/gigantism is independent of mutations of the multiple endocrine neoplasia type I gene. *J Clin Endocrinol Metab* 1999; 84(1): 249–56.
*32. Vierimaa O, Georgitsi M, Lehtonen R, et al. Pituitary adenoma predisposition caused by germline mutations in the AIP gene. *Science* 2006; 312(5777): 1228–30.
*33. Daly AF, Vanbellinghen JF, Khoo SK, et al. Aryl hydrocarbon receptor-interacting protein gene mutations in

familial isolated pituitary adenomas: Analysis in 73 families. *J Clin Endocrinol Metab* 2007; 92(5): 1891–6.
34. Leontiou CA, Gueorguiev M, van der Spuy J, et al. The role of the aryl hydrocarbon receptor-interacting protein gene in familial and sporadic pituitary adenomas. *J Clin Endocrinol Metab* 2008; 93(6): 2390–401.
35. Lin BC, Sullivan R, Lee Y, Moran S, Glover E, Bradfield CA. Deletion of the aryl hydrocarbon receptor-associated protein 9 leads to cardiac malformation and embryonic lethality. *J Biol Chem* 2007; 282(49): 35924–32.
*36. Raitila A, Lehtonen HJ, Arola J, et al. Mice with inactivation of aryl hydrocarbon receptor-interacting protein (Aip) display complete penetrance of pituitary adenomas with aberrant ARNT expression. *Am J Pathol* 2010; 177(4): 1969–76.
37. Ozfirat Z, Korbonits M. AIP gene and familial isolated pituitary adenomas. *Mol Cell Endocrinol* 2010; 26(1–2): 71–9.
38. Oesch-Bartlomowicz B, Huelster A, Wiss O, et al. Aryl hydrocarbon receptor activation by cAMP vs. dioxin: Divergent signaling pathways. *Proc Natl Acad Sci U S A* 2005; 102(26): 9218–23.
39. Kazlauskas A, Poellinger L, Pongratz I. Evidence that the co-chaperone p23 regulates ligand responsiveness of the dioxin (Aryl hydrocarbon) receptor. *J Biol Chem* 1999; 274(19): 13519–24.
40. Trivellin G, Korbonits M. AIP and its interacting partners. *J Endocrinol* 2011; 210(2): 137–55.
41. Kazlauskas A, Poellinger L, Pongratz I. The immunophilin-like protein XAP2 regulates ubiquitination and subcellular localization of the dioxin receptor. *J Biol Chem* 2000; 275(52): 41317–24.
*42. Jaffrain-Rea ML, Angelini M, Gargano D, et al. Expression of aryl hydrocarbon receptor (AHR) and AHR-interacting protein in pituitary adenomas: Pathological and clinical implications. *Endocr Relat Cancer* 2009; 16(3): 1029–43.
43. Horvath A, Stratakis CA. Clinical and molecular genetics of acromegaly: MEN1, Carney complex, McCune-Albright syndrome, familial acromegaly and genetic defects in sporadic tumors. *Rev Endocr Metab Disord* 2008; 9(1): 1–11.
44. de Oliveira SK, Hoffmeister M, Gambaryan S, Muller-Esterl W, Guimaraes JA, Smolenski AP. Phosphodiesterase 2A forms a complex with the co-chaperone XAP2 and regulates nuclear translocation of the aryl hydrocarbon receptor. *J Biol Chem* 2007; 282(18): 13656–63.
45. Vargiolu M, Fusco D, Kurelac I, et al. The tyrosine kinase receptor RET interacts in vivo with aryl hydrocarbon receptor-interacting protein to alter survivin availability. *J Clin Endocrinol Metab* 2009; 94(7): 2571–8.
46. Jaffrain-Rea M-L, Daly AF, Angelini M, Petrossians P, Bours V, Beckers A. Genetic susceptibility in pituitary adenomas: From pathogenesis to clinical implications. *Expet Rev Endocrinol Metab* 2011; 6(2): 195–214.
47. Georgitsi M, Heliovaara E, Paschke R, et al. Large genomic deletions in AIP in pituitary adenoma predisposition. *J Clin Endocrinol Metab* 2008; 93(10): 4146–51.
*48. Igreja S, Chahal HS, King P, et al. Characterization of aryl hydrocarbon receptor interacting protein (AIP) mutations in familial isolated pituitary adenoma families. *Hum Mutat* 2010; 31(8): 950–60.
49. Cazabat L, Guillaud-Bataille M, Bertherat J, Raffin-Sanson ML. Mutations of the gene for the aryl hydrocarbon receptor-interacting protein in pituitary adenomas. *Horm Res* 2009; 71(3): 132–41.
50. Toledo RA, Lourenco DM, Jr., Toledo SP. Familial isolated pituitary adenoma: Evidence for genetic heterogeneity. *Front Horm Res* 2010; 38: 77–86.
51. Naves LA, Daly AF, Vanbellinghen JF, et al. Variable pathological and clinical features of a large Brazilian family harboring a mutation in the aryl hydrocarbon receptor-interacting protein gene. *Eur J Endocrinol* 2007; 157(4): 383–91.
*52. Daly AF, Tichomirowa MA, Petrossians P, et al. Clinical characteristics and therapeutic responses in patients with germ-line AIP mutations and pituitary adenomas: An international collaborative study. *J Clin Endocrinol Metab* 2010; 95(11): E373–83.
*53. Tichomirowa MA, Barlier A, Daly AF, et al. High prevalence of AIP gene mutations following focused screening in young patients with sporadic pituitary macroadenomas. *Eur J Endocrinol* 2011; 165(4): 509–15.
54. Barlier A, Vanbellinghen JF, Daly AF, et al. Mutations in the aryl hydrocarbon receptor interacting protein gene are not highly prevalent among subjects with sporadic pituitary adenomas. *J Clin Endocrinol Metab* 2007; 92(5): 1952–5.

# 3

# Surgical management of pituitary adenomas

*Garni Barkhoudarian, Edward R. Laws, Jr.*

## *Introduction*

Pituitary lesions are a relatively common finding among neurosurgical patients. Autopsy studies have demonstrated that up to 20% of individuals harbor pituitary tumors or cysts, with many of them asymptomatic and incidentally discovered upon autopsy. Among symptomatic intracranial lesions, pituitary surgery accounts for approximately 20% of neurosurgical procedures. Given the intersection of the pituitary gland, cerebral vasculature, cranial nerves, and the optic apparatus in the sellar and parasellar region, the management of lesions in this location can be quite complex and involves a multidisciplinary approach.

Sellar and parasellar lesions can be superficially categorized as lesions arising from cells within the pituitary gland as opposed to extrapituitary origins secondarily affecting the pituitary gland and surrounding structures. The types of lesions in this region are numerous and have a wide range of pathophysiology (Table 3.1). The most common lesions include pituitary adenomas, Rathke cleft cysts (RCCs), arachnoid cysts, and craniopharyngiomas. Among pituitary adenomas, there are numerous subtypes and clinical scenarios, including hormonally active lesions, lesions primarily causing mass effect, lesions causing pituitary insufficiency, and a combination of these effects (see Chapter 5).

This chapter focuses on the management of pituitary adenomas, evaluating the various hormone-secreting subtypes, nonfunctioning adenomas, medical and surgical management of these lesions, and pitfalls using each therapeutic modality.

## *Clinical presentation (see Chapter 1)*

Pituitary adenomas can present with various clinical signs and symptoms, many of which are often subtle or overlooked. Given the size and pathological characteristics of these tumors, primary complaints can vary from headaches—both acute and chronic—to visual loss, endocrine dysfunction, or hormone hypersecretion. Various other signs and symptoms have been reported with these lesions (Table 3.2).

Headaches can be a common symptom in patients harboring pituitary lesions. It can sometimes be difficult to associate the lesion with the patient's headaches. Numerous patients suffer from chronic headaches due to other etiologies, such as migraines or tension headaches, and undergo imaging identifying a small pituitary lesion. It is important to counsel these patients preoperatively regarding the chance of headache improvement postoperatively. Headaches associated with pituitary tumors tend to radiate to the vertex or remain retro-orbital in location. Often, the pain lateralizes to one side of the head, reflecting cavernous sinus involvement.

In the setting of headaches with acute or abrupt onset, pituitary tumor apoplexy should be suspected. Depending on the size of the hemorrhage, the presentation can vary. Often, these are isolated symptoms that spare vision. Acute visual loss with or without headache can be a surgical emergency (see Chapter 24).

Visual complaints are another common finding with pituitary adenomas. Bitemporal hemianopsia or other visual field deficits can occur. Other associated findings such as decreased visual acuity, diplopia, and

| | | |
|---|---|---|
| ***Adenomas*** | ***324*** | ***76.6%*** |
| Nonfunctional adenoma | 154 | 47.5% |
| Acromegaly | 51 | 15.7% |
| Prolactinoma | 46 | 14.2% |
| Cushing's disease | 33 | 10.2% |
| Silent ACTH adenoma | 17 | 5.2% |
| GH/prolactinoma | 15 | 4.6% |
| Mammosomatotroph | 6 | 1.9% |
| Pituitary hyperplasia | 1 | 0.3% |
| Pituitary carcinoma | 1 | 0.3% |
| ***Cysts*** | ***50*** | ***11.8%*** |
| Rathke cleft cyst | 39 | 78.0% |
| Arachnoid cyst | 8 | 16.0% |
| Pituitary cyst | 2 | 4.0% |
| Colloid cyst | 1 | 2.0% |
| ***Nonadenomatous tumors*** | ***31*** | ***7.3%*** |
| Craniopharyngioma | 18 | 58.1% |
| Metastases | 4 | 12.9% |
| Chordoma | 3 | 9.7% |
| Oncocytoma | 2 | 6.5% |
| Granular cell tumor | 1 | 3.2% |
| Lymphoma | 1 | 3.2% |
| Meningioma | 1 | 3.2% |
| Pituitary carcinoma | 1 | 3.2% |
| ***Inflammatory disease*** | ***8*** | ***1.9%*** |
| Lymphocytic hypophysitis | 4 | 50.0% |
| Wegener's granulomatosis | 1 | 12.5% |
| Giant reparative granuloma | 1 | 12.5% |
| Granulomatous lesion | 1 | 12.5% |
| Pituitary inflammation | 1 | 12.5% |
| ***Bone lesions*** | ***3*** | ***0.7%*** |
| Fibrous dysplasia | 1 | 33.3% |
| Basilar invagination | 1 | 33.3% |
| Lipomatous bone cyst | 1 | 33.3% |
| ***Miscellaneous*** | ***6*** | ***1.4%*** |
| Nondiagnostic | 3 | 50.0% |
| Spontaneous CSF leak | 2 | 33.3% |
| Aneurysm | 1 | 16.7% |
| ***Total*** | ***423*** | |

***Table 3.1***
*Typical lesions of the sellar and parasellar region—experience at the Brigham and Women's Hospital (April 2008–January 2012).*

| |
|---|
| Hormone oversecretion |
| Prolactin |
| Growth hormone |
| Adrenocorticotropic hormone |
| Thyroid-stimulating hormone |
| Mass effect |
| Headaches |
| Optic nerve compression |
| Cavernous sinus |
| Third ventricle |
| Hypopituitarism |
| Anterior lobe dysfunction |
| Diabetes insipidus |
| Other |
| Cerebrospinal fluid rhinorrhea |
| Incidental finding |

***Table 3.2***
*Signs and symptoms of pituitary adenomas.*

nystagmus should be evaluated. Close communication with a neuro-ophthalmologist can help discern ocular from chiasmal etiology of the visual deficits.

Among the anterior pituitary gland cells that secrete hormones, most can be involved in hypersecretion syndromes. The most common hypersecreted hormone is prolactin. This oversecretion can be due to lactotroph cell adenomas (prolactinomas) or disinhibition from infundibular compression (pseudoprolactinomas). Adrenocorticotropic hormone (ACTH) hypersecretion results in excessive cortisol production and Cushing's disease. Growth hormone (GH) oversecretion results in acromegaly or gigantism, depending on the age of onset. Thyroid-stimulating hormone (TSH) oversecretion is rare, but when present, it can result in central hyperthyroidism. These syndromes, along with secretion of gonadotrophs, are described in detail in subsequent sections.

Either because of mass effect compressing the normal gland or from hormonal inhibition, various levels of pituitary insufficiency can occur, sometimes in conjunction with hypersecretion syndromes. In particular, elevated prolactin can inhibit the gonadotropes producing luteinizing hormone (LH) and follicle-stimulating hormone (FSH) insufficiency, resulting in hypogonadism, decreased libido, amenorrhea, and infertility. It is important to identify hypothyroidism and hypocortisolism in the preoperative setting because significant deficiencies can result in clinical complications if not repleted.

In the age of advanced neuroimaging and frequent use of magnetic resonance imaging (MRI), the incidental pituitary adenoma is becoming increasingly common and can pose as a dilemma for the clinician for its management. It is important to obtain a baseline pituitary endocrine laboratory evaluation and baseline visual field examination. Patients may harbor subclinical pituitary hypofunction or visual loss. If conservative management is chosen, any change in these studies can help guide more definitive therapies.

## *Prolactinoma (see Chapter 1)*

The prolactin-secreting pituitary adenoma, or prolactinoma, is the most common type of pituitary adenoma. These tumors can present with hypogonadism and galactorrhea. In women, this results in amenorrhea and infertility. Men typically present with erectile dysfunction and decreased libido. Galactorrhea is rare in men and pregravid women. Prolactinomas can often be macroadenomas causing mass effect, visual loss, and pituitary insufficiency.

It is critically important to differentiate prolactinoma from pseudoprolactinoma. Given that prolactin secretion is tonically inhibited by dopamine produced in the hypothalamus, compression or disruption of the pituitary infundibulum results in a modest hyperprolactinemia. "Stalk effect," as it is otherwise known, can result in serum prolactin levels ranging from 20 to 200 μg/L (400–4000 mU/L). Generally, a microprolactinoma typically has prolactin levels less than <100 μg/L (2000 mU/L) and a macroprolactinoma has levels greater than >200 μg/L (4000 mU/L), although exceptions occur.

The decision to treat a prolactinoma medically or surgically relies on accurate laboratory information. A known diagnostic phenomenon with the prolactin assay is the "Hook effect."[1] This effect is commonly seen with many radiometric immunoassay, such as for prostate-specific antigen (PSA) and β-human choriogonadotropin hormone (βHCG). The high concentrations of antigen overwhelm the bound and soluble antibodies, resulting in the formation of fewer antibody–antigen complexes. This effect is circumvented by serial dilutions of the serum that should routinely be used in the laboratory diagnosis of prolactinomas.[2,3]

Currently, prolactinoma is the pituitary adenoma that can most successfully be treated with medical therapy. Dopamine agonist therapy has been well established as a primary strategy to treat prolactinomas. This treatment is more efficacious for microadenomas (85%–90%) than macroadenomas (65%–70%).

The two most commonly used dopamine agonists are bromocriptine and cabergoline. Bromocriptine is a fast-acting agent with a short half-life, necessitating daily dosing. Its effect on tumor size can be seen within hours and may restore vision rapidly. Given its pharmacokinetics, too rapid dose escalation of bromocriptine may result in adverse effects such as nausea, orthostatic hypotension, headache, and other systemic effects. Hence, the use of cabergoline, a long-acting but less toxic dopamine agonist, allows for weekly or biweekly dose schedules and improved medication tolerance. Cabergoline has been found to normalize prolactin levels more reliably than bromocriptine.[4] Typically, patients must remain on dopamine agonist therapy for life-long tumor suppression.

Despite the advances in medical therapy, surgical intervention may be necessary in some scenarios. These scenarios include medication side effect intolerance, tumor resistance to treatment, cerebrospinal fluid (CSF) rhinorrhea due to tumor shrinkage, persistent mass effect from cystic lesions, and lesions that are not histologically prolactinomas. By far, the most common of these scenarios is medication intolerance. Headaches, orthostatic hypotension, fatigue, and mood changes are frequent detractors of patient compliance. High doses of dopamine agonists may produce cardiac valvular disease (23%–28.6%).[5,6] Frequent echocardiograms are necessary to detect this serious complication.

Prolactinomas can be resistant to the dopamine agonist effect and continue to grow despite medical therapy. The likely mechanism for resistance is decreased transcription of the dopamine receptor ($D_2$) gene and its associated G protein.[7] Frequently, these tumors will be more susceptible to cabergoline than bromocriptine, but resistance can exist to all agents, and may require surgical resection.[8]

In the setting of large pituitary adenomas that have eroded the floor of the sella turcica and the sellar dura, occasionally treatment with dopamine agonists can result in CSF rhinorrhea. In a series of 114 patients with macroprolactinomas treated without surgery, CSF rhinorrhea was encountered in 8.7% of patients. The incidence of spontaneous CSF rhinorrhea was 2.6%, and dopamine agonist–induced CSF rhinorrhea was 6.1%. There was no CSF rhinorrhea seen in their cohort of nonfunctional adenomas (181 patients).[9]

Prolactinomas that have cystic components are less likely to respond to dopamine agonist therapy.[10,11] If the cysts are causing mass effect, the patient's symptoms may not be alleviated with medical therapy alone. Occasionally, associated cysts can be extratumoral, such as RCCs and arachnoid cysts. When symptomatic, surgery is the definitive therapy for these cysts.

Medical therapy has significantly reduced the frequency of surgical indications for prolactinomas. Regardless, the role of surgery is still an important part of tumor management, as indicated above. The most common indication is medication intolerance. In addition, in the setting of an ambiguous tumor size and prolactin correlation (e.g., a 10 mm adenoma with a prolactin level of 150 μg/L–3000 mU/L), surgical resection may be considered as a first-line therapy. Pituitary apoplexy of known prolactinomas with acute visual loss or other neurological deficit remains a third surgical indication. The mass effect of the hematoma decreases the efficacy of dopamine agonists to reduce tumor size and improve visual symptoms.

The goals of surgery are to achieve a gross total resection (when safely possible) or significant cytoreduction of the prolactinoma, to obtain a diagnosis of the tumor (when in question), and to normalize serum prolactin levels. The latter is most necessary when the patient presents with amenorrhea, infertility, or galactorrhea.

Overall, dopamine agonist therapy of prolactinomas has been shown to achieve normalization of prolactin levels and restoration of gonadal function in 85%–90% of microadenomas and 65%–70% of macroadenomas. In addition, >50% decrease in tumor size can be seen in more than half of presenting prolactinomas.

Surgical resection of prolactinomas can normalize prolactin levels and restore gonadal function in 60%–87% of microadenomas and 40%–60% of macroadenomas.[12] Gross total resection as measured by MRI has been reported in 98% of microadenomas, 64% of macroadenomas, and 24% of giant adenomas.[13] The overall rate of major complications is approximately 5%, with epistaxis and sinus infection the most common.

Stereotactic radiosurgery and stereotactic fractionated radiotherapy are alternatives for the management of prolactinomas. These modalities are typically prescribed in the setting of medically or surgically refractory tumors. Frequently, these tumors can invade the cavernous sinus. Clinical remission from radiosurgery is achieved in approximately 25% of patients, although higher remission rates have been reported in select series.[14,15]

## *Cushing's disease (see Chapter 1)*

Cushing's disease occurs in the setting of a pituitary adenoma secreting ACTH. It is a rare disorder occurring in approximately one to two cases for 1 million people. The clinical syndrome of weight gain, truncal obesity, moon facies, dorsocervical and supraclavicular fat-pad deposition, abdominal striae, hirsutism, hypertension, and diabetes can have serious deleterious effects on overall health and survival. Cognitive deficits and cerebral atrophy have also been reported.[16]

The diagnosis of Cushing's disease is made in the setting of clinical suspicion affirmed with laboratory results of hypercortisolemia. Typically, serum cortisol is elevated with an inappropriately normal or moderately elevated ACTH level. Given the daily fluctuations of cortisol levels, the midnight serum or salivary cortisol levels are more sensitive in confirming hypercortisolemia. Elevated 24 h urine free cortisol (UFC) is the standard to establish Cushing's syndrome. The dexamethasone suppression test can help differentiate Cushing's disease from nonpituitary sources of elevated circulating cortisol.

Neuroimaging of the pituitary gland will often demonstrate a microadenoma (90%) or macroadenoma (10%). Dynamic MRI with contrast can help differentiate microadenomas from the surrounding gland by varying the timing of contrast in the sella. In the setting of ambiguous imaging or laboratory findings, direct sampling of the cavernous sinus via inferior petrosal sinus sampling (IPSS) can confirm the source of ACTH secretion.

Currently, the optimal primary therapy for Cushing's disease is surgical resection of the pituitary tumor. Postoperative remission rates have been reported in 70%–93% of patients. Remission rates are higher in microadenomas (82%–93%) than in macroadenomas (40%–86%). Tumor recurrence has been detected in up to 26% of cases with long-term (20 year) follow-up.[17,18] Favorable factors predicting remission include the identification of a microadenoma on MRI.[19,20] Negative pathological findings for ACTH immunoreactivity were associated with a 66% remission rate.[21] Baseline serum cortisol and ACTH levels do not predict surgical outcomes.[22] Macroadenomas are more likely to invade the cavernous sinus and are more difficult to cure surgically.[23,24]

Operative mortality is relatively low (0.9%), but overall complication rates can be as high as 15%.[25] The increased rate of morbidity compared with other pituitary lesions is due to the increased medical comorbidities that occur in Cushing's disease patients. Obesity, diabetes, hypertension, and coronary artery disease contribute to these factors. Deep vein thrombosis (DVT) is disproportionately present postoperatively in these patients relative to other pituitary disorders.[26]

Diligent postoperative care is critical to prevent these medical complications. DVT prophylaxis with aspirin or other anticoagulants can be useful and is initiated as early as the first postoperative day.

Frequent serum cortisol measurement is necessary to confirm the expected hypocortisolemia, and replacement therapy should begin before symptomatic hypocortisolemia occurs.[27] Tight blood-sugar control can help prevent wound healing complications. It is important to obtain daily weight measurement to assess the patient's fluid status. This measurement can be helpful in the management of postoperative sodium fluctuations and diabetes insipidus.

Cushing's disease can be difficult to cure. Any amount of residual tumor can result in persistence of disease without clinical improvement. Remission of Cushing's disease does not guarantee recurrence free survival. Postoperative data suggest disease recurrence in 5%–27% of patients with long follow-up (33–59 months) who had achieved clinical remission after pituitary adenectomy.[22,28–32] In a long-term study with a mean follow-up of 49 months, Patil et al.[33] report a recurrence rate of 17.4%. The mean time-to-recurrence was 39 months.

Reoperative management of patients with recurrent Cushing's disease from an ACTH-secreting tumor, when possible, is ideal. Locatelli et al.[34] advocate immediate postoperative management when the postoperative cortisol remains above 2 μg/dL (56 nmol/L). They report 12 patients with such management, of which eight achieved clinical remission without additional therapy.[34] Others report 53%–70% remission with this approach.[31,35] In specific settings, hemi-hypophysectomy or total hypophysectomy may be indicated. Tumors demonstrating invasion on imaging or histopathology are not likely to benefit from hypophysectomy.[36,37]

If reoperation is not an option, radiosurgery/radiation therapy or medical therapy are viable options and can be used in tandem. Radiosurgery is a safe and efficacious option.[38] Sheehan et al.[39] report a 63% clinical remission at 12 months after gamma-knife radiosurgery. In their series of 43 patients, they encountered new endocrine deficits in 16% of patients and one patient with new visual loss (see Chapter 5).

Medication treatment options include cortisol synthesis inhibition in the adrenal cortex, neuromodulator agents acting on the hypothalamic–pituitary system, and glucocorticoid antagonists. Metyrapone and ketoconazole are well-established cortisol synthesis inhibitors. They inhibit 11β-hydroxylase necessary for converting 11-deoxycortisol to cortisol. Metyrapone works well to decrease cortisol levels, but it has significant androgenous side effects, including hirsutism and acne. Although efficacious in decreasing cortisol levels, ketoconazole is associated with a 5%–10% risk of reversible hepatotoxicity with occasional serious hepatic injury.[40] Etomidate is a parenterally administered imidazole derivative anesthetic. Although its uses are limited, it remains an option for severe, life-threatening Cushing's disease.[41,42] Newer suppressive agents such as mifepristone and paseriotide have been used in clinical trials and now have Food and Drug Administration (FDA) approval for treatment of Cushing's disease.

Neuromodulator agents, such as octreotide and bromocriptine, exert effect on the hypothalamic pituitary axis to decrease cortisol secretion. Octreotide is a synthetic long-acting somatostatin analog that has applications for numerous neuroendocrine tumors. This class of medications has been shown to effectively decrease ACTH secretion in Nelson's syndrome, although its efficacy in Cushing's disease has been equivocal.[43,44] Pasireotide has recently been approved for Cushing's disease. It provides control in approximately 20% of patients but is associated with aggravation of diabetes mellitus.[45] The dopamine agonist bromocriptine has been used to treat refractory Cushing's disease. Its efficacy varies widely among published reports. Corticotrophic hyperplasia and "normal gland" variants of Cushing's disease appear to be more responsive to this therapy.[46]

Potent glucocorticoid antagonism is seen with the abortifacient agent mifepristone. This agent blocks cortisol systemically at the cellular level. As a result, the clinical effects of Cushing's disease can be reversed with a subsequent rise in circulating ACTH and cortisol.[47,48] Because there are no biochemical markers to monitor this therapy, close clinical follow-up is necessary for safe administration of this agent.[49]

In the setting of persistent disease despite hypophysectomy, radiosurgery, and/or medication therapy, the option of bilateral adrenalectomy remains. When this operation is possible, circulating cortisol levels diminish consistently. Patients do report increased fatigue, and cortisol replacement is necessary. Because this operation can be performed laparoscopically, complication rates have diminished with significant morbidity at 7.5%–12%.[50,51]

Nelson's syndrome can occur once the negative feedback of cortisol is removed with bilateral adrenalectomy.[52] Residual tumor cells are uninhibited and tumor growth can be seen in 15%–50% of patients.[53,54] Smith et al.[55] report 40 patients who had undergone bilateral adrenalectomy. Of these patients, 33% developed ACTH levels >200 ng/mL. Seven of these patients (54%) required further therapy to the pituitary gland. De Tommasi et al.[56] affirm the difficult management of Nelson's syndrome with one patient (of six) achieving disease remission with a variety of interventions.

## Acromegaly (see Chapter 1)

Acromegaly is a well-described condition that occurs in the setting of excess GH exposure. The disease is typically due to a pituitary adenoma secreting GH. GH and its effector hormone insulin-like growth factor I (IGF-I) have an effect on every organ in the body. The most common findings include bony and soft-tissue enlargement in the face and extremities. Hand and foot size can increase. Hyperhidrosis and increased fluid retention can occur. Facial features include frontal bossing, increased jaw size, increased tooth spacing and bite mismatch, and increased tongue size. Obstructive sleep apnea can occur and can result in sleep disorders and pulmonary hypertension in more severe cases. Arthritic changes can occur, as well as nerve entrapment syndromes, most commonly carpal tunnel syndrome.

Systemically, these patients often have diabetes mellitus with insulin resistance and hypertension. Skin tags are common. Colonoscopy can demonstrate polyp formation. In growing children, elevated GH can result in gigantism, because the epiphyseal plates have not yet fused. If left untreated, acromegaly can result in a shortened life expectancy, with a 1.6–3.3-fold increase in age-matched mortality.[57]

The diagnosis of acromegaly is established with a laboratory evaluation. GH levels >5 μg/L that do not suppress below 1 μg/L with the oral glucose tolerance test (OGTT) are indicative of acromegaly. IGF-I levels greater than age- and sex- specific levels are indicative of acromegaly as well. Frequently, the GH level is equivocal and can fluctuate widely throughout the day. Hence, IGF-I levels are more reliable for diagnosis and management of acromegaly.

It is important to obtain echocardiograms to evaluate for hypertrophic cardiomegaly. Frequent colonoscopy is necessary to screen for colonic polyps.

At present, the optimal primary therapy for acromegaly is surgical resection of the offending adenoma. Surgical series demonstrate a 70% normalization of IGF-I at 1 year postresection.[58] This outcome is higher for microadenomas at upwards of 85%–91%.[59,60] Factors that determine tumor recurrence include dural invasion and involvement of surrounding structures such as the cavernous sinus. Significantly elevated preresection GH predicts higher recurrence rates.[61]

Surgical nuances for the transsphenoidal approach for these adenomas vary from other tumors. Because of the effect of acromegaly, the nasal mucosa is engorged and thickened. The paranasal structures are enlarged with more atypical sphenoid sinus architecture. Often, these tumors erode the floor of the sella with growth inferiorly (Figure 3.1). Increased bleeding can occur from the mucosa, necessitating meticulous hemostasis to achieve adequate visualization of the tumor. In the postoperative setting, these patients can diurese much of their excess interstitial fluid, mimicking diabetes insipidus. In patients with obstructive sleep apnea, continuous

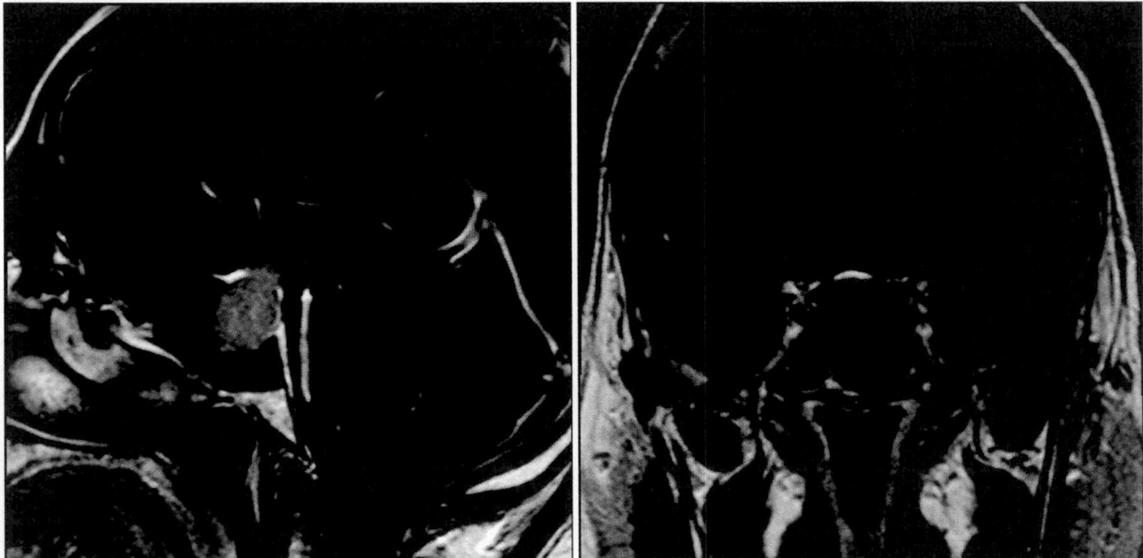

**Figure 3.1**
*Sagittal and coronal postcontrast MRI of a patient with acromegaly demonstrating sellar floor remodeling without significant suprasellar extension.*

positive airway pressure (CPAP) machines should be avoided in the setting of an intraoperative CSF leak. Close monitoring and treatment of the patient's blood pressure and blood sugars is necessary and may require intensive care unit (ICU) management.

The goal of surgery is to achieve a gross total resection of the adenoma when possible and maximal cytoreduction if there is invasive disease. Any reduction of the postoperative IGF-I can help with medical and radiosurgical management. Yearly monitoring of IGF-I levels after resection is necessary as recurrence rates can be as high as 8% at 10 years. Persistent postoperative acromegaly occurs in 10%–40% of patients, more commonly with macroadenomas and invasive tumors. In this situation, there are several options. If an obvious postoperative residual or recurrent tumor that is safe to resect is seen on imaging, then reoperation may be indicated. If surgery is not feasible, nonsurgical management is possible with medications and/or radiation.

Medications for acromegaly include somatostatin analogs, dopamine agonists, and GH receptor antagonists. Somatostatin analogs, such as octreotide or lanreotide, are agonists of the somatostatin receptor (SSTR). Because these analogs are peptides, they must be given parenterally. Freda et al.[62] demonstrated 67% normalization of IGF-I and 80% normalization of GH levels with medical therapy using a somatostatin analog. Pretreatment of a *de novo* acromegaly adenoma can decrease tumor size in approximately 50% of patients; however, overall outcomes are no different if treatment is initiated after surgery[63] (Figure 3.2).

A subset of patients with acromegaly will have elevation in prolactin levels. Often, immunohistochemistry will demonstrate coexisting lactotrope adenoma cells (Figure 3.3). Dopamine agonists may be a helpful adjunct in some patients. Bromocriptine and cabergoline have been reported to normalize IGF-I levels in 10% and 40%, respectively, of patients with acromegaly.[64]

The most effective medical agent is the GH receptor antagonist pegvisomant. This injectable molecule prevents dimerization of the GH receptor, hence decreasing its effect on target tissues. As a result, the IGF-I can be normalized in 89%–97% of patients.[65,66] There is an expected concomitant increase in GH levels. In addition to the cost of this medication, side effects include the risk of liver dysfunction and lipohypertrophy at injection sites.

Stereotactic radiosurgery (SRS) or stereotactic radiation therapy is an occasionally useful adjunct to treat persistent or recurrent acromegaly. A recent prospective study demonstrated normalization of IGF-I and GH levels in 23% and 37% of patients, respectively.[67] Similar results have been reported in retrospective series.[68,69] The average time to normalization of GH occurred at 1.4 years after stereotactic radiosurgery (SRS). Conventional radiation therapy has a higher incidence of complications (optic nerve, pituitary function) and a slower rate to normalization (7 years). Because of the effectiveness

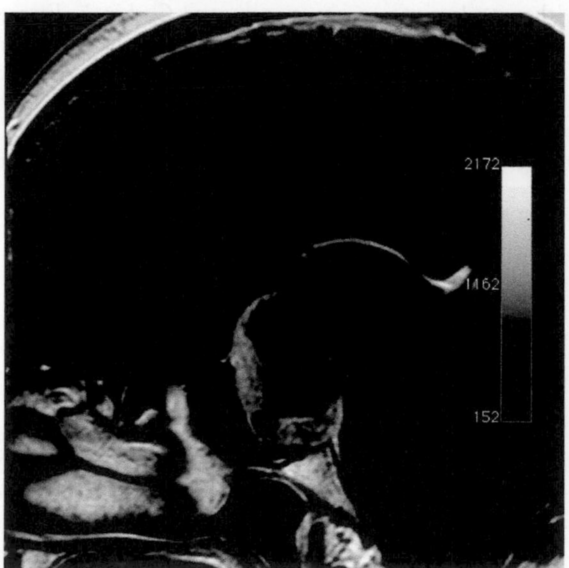


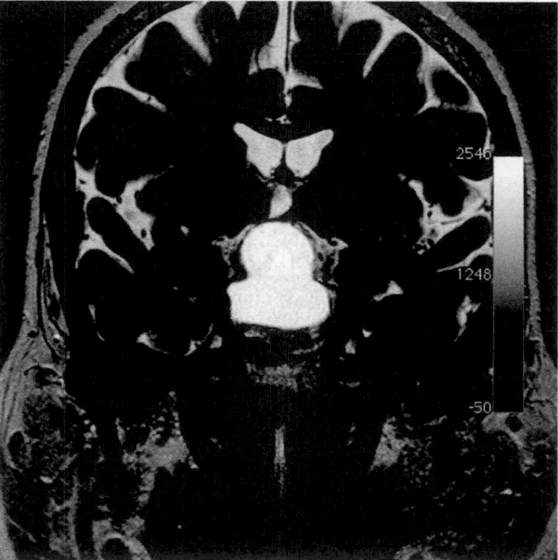


**Figure 3.2**
*Pre- and posttreatment contrast-enhanced MRI of a patient with acromegaly treated preoperatively with octreotide.*

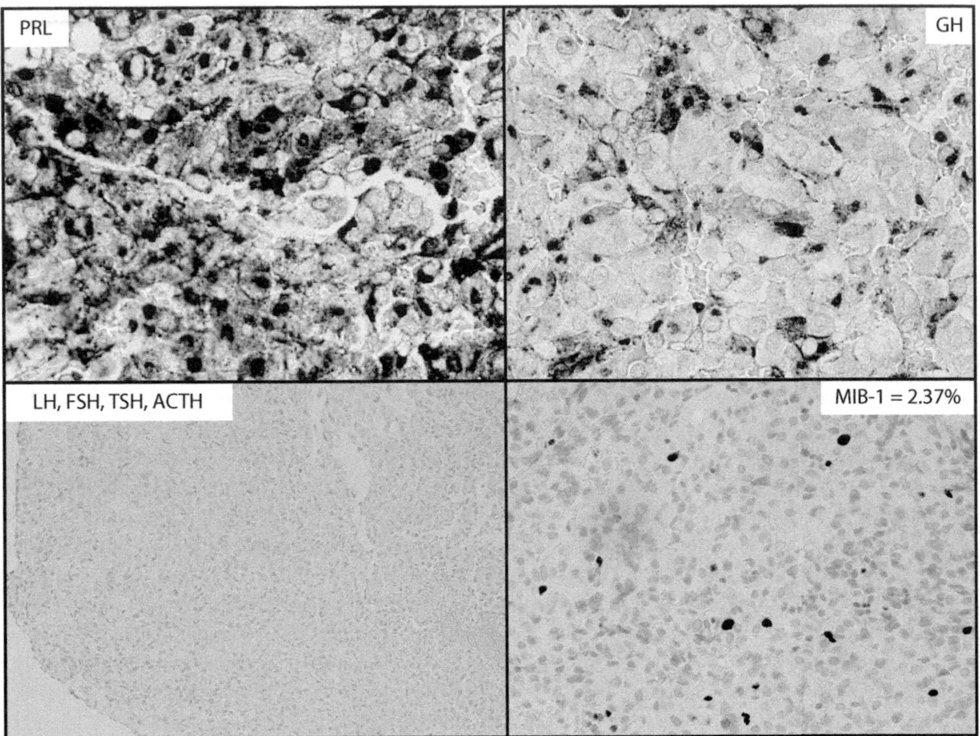


***Figure 3.3***
*Immunohistopathology of a patient with a mammosomatotroph adenoma causing both acromegaly and amenorrhea due to elevated IGF-I and prolactin.*

of medical therapy, fewer patients with acromegaly are being referred for radiotherapy or radiosurgery.

Reoperation for recurrent acromegaly is a well-established option. As with *de novo* tumors, the goals of surgery are to achieve gross total resection when safely possible and maximal cytoreduction with invasive tumors. The overall remission rate ranges from 19% to 56%.[70–73]

The ultimate goal for the management of acromegaly is normalization of IGF-I levels. This normalization is associated with amelioration of the signs and symptoms of acromegaly, improved quality of life, and normalization of mortality data.[74,75] Carefully balancing the risks, benefits, and costs of the various therapeutic modalities is critical and should be done on a case-by-case basis.

# Other hormone-secreting adenomas

As expected, adenomas secreting thyrotropin and gonadotropins have been described, but they are much rarer than prolactinomas, acromegaly, and Cushing's disease. These adenomas often present with mass effect or vision loss, and the patients may be asymptomatic from their hypersecretion syndrome. It is prudent to routinely check all the anterior pituitary gland laboratory markers and target gland hormones. Even if subclinical, these can serve as biomarkers to track tumor recurrence.

## Thyroid-stimulating hormone–secreting adenomas (see Chapters 1, 14)

Patients with hyperthyroidism have been reported to harbor pituitary adenomas secreting thyrotropin (TSH). As this is quite a rare condition, many these patients have had thyroidectomy under the assumption of primary hyperthyroidism. The primary differentiating factor is an elevated TSH as opposed to a suppressed TSH with elevated free T3 and free T4 levels. Occasionally, these can present with cosecretion of other pituitary hormones such as ACTH or prolactin.[76–78]

Surgery remains the mainstay treatment for these adenomas. Goals of surgery include establishing a diagnosis with immunohistochemical analysis and normalizing thyroxine levels. Remission rates range from 23% to 62.5%, with further improvement achieved with adjuvant medical therapy (somatostatin analogs). Similar to other tumors, remission rates in microadenomas are superior to macroadenomas.[76,77,79,80]

Persistent disease can occur after surgery. Octreotide and similar compounds have been used to normalize thyroxine levels. This treatment has been quite successful, with almost all patients responding to treatment and up to 73% with normal thyroid hormone levels.[81] In some cases, somatostatin analog therapy was used primarily with comparable results. Radiation therapy and radiosurgery have been reported to be somewhat efficacious for these tumors (62.5%).[82]

## Gonadotropin-secreting adenomas

Although symptomatic gonadotropin-secreting adenomas are exceedingly rare, frequently adenomas demonstrate immunoreactivity for FSH, LH, or the α-subunit. These adenomas are typically grouped with the nonfunctioning adenomas, and the secreted proteins are thought to be dysfunctional and not bioactive.[83–85] In one series, 35% of patients had elevation in at least one of these proteins (45% men and 25% premenopausal women). There were no obvious related clinical manifestations of hypersecretion.[85]

Ovarian hypersecretion syndrome has been described in the setting of gonadotropic pituitary adenomas. These patients present with pelvic pain, multicystic ovaries, and metromenorrhagia. Pituitary adenoma resection can reverse these symptoms.[86–89]

In men, a similar syndrome of testosterone hypersecretion has been reported.[90,91] The clinical effects of elevated testosterone are unclear in these patients, but elevated sperm count has been noted. In these rare cases, hypogonadism is a potential complication after resection of the gonadotropin-secreting adenoma.

## Multiple hormone-secreting adenomas

Within adenomas themselves, coexpression of multiple cell types has been reported. Often, these adenomas are detected at the histopathological level without hormonal consequences. Sometimes, there may be normal pituitary gland cells trapped within the adenoma. The most common hormonally active combined lesion is the mammosomatotroph. This adenoma secretes both prolactin and GH from the same cell line, resulting in symptoms of both syndromes.[92] A similar clinical scenario is the finding of GH and prolactin expressed by an adenoma with dual cell lines.[93,94] If surgical therapy is not successful, combined medical therapy with somatostatin analogs and dopamine agonists is somewhat successful.

## Nonfunctional adenomas (see Chapter 1)

Nonfunctional adenomas can present with headaches, visual loss, hypopituitarism, or other neurological deficits. A subset of these tumors is found incidentally. It is key to evaluate all the pituitary hormone axes because subclinical hypopituitarism or hypersecretion syndromes can be seen. Preoperative replacement of cortisol and thyroid hormone is critical to prevent cardiac complications when there is profound hypopituitarism. Formal visual field evaluation is helpful in patients where visual deficits are suspected. These evaluations can be used to detect subclinical deficits before surgery and to follow visual recovery after surgery.

Primary indications for tumor resection include visual deficits and pituitary insufficiency. If headaches are the presenting symptom, one must differentiate typical tension and migrainous headache symptoms from tumor-related headaches because these symptoms can often overlap. Typical differentiating factors include headaches upon awakening, retro-orbital or vertex in location, and lateralizing to one side. Although many patients' headaches improve after surgery, preoperative counseling is necessary to caution against the converse. Incidentally found tumors, if truly asymptomatic, may be managed conservatively until evidence of tumor growth, new visual symptoms, or endocrine deficits appear.

Surgical results for nonfunctional adenomas are excellent, with symptomatic improvement common and a relatively low recurrence rate. Visual symptoms are normalized or improved in up to 64%–91% of patients.[95–98] Headache improvement is seen in most patients with preoperative headaches. Some studies report up to 100% of patients with improvement or resolution of headaches.[99] Pituitary insufficiency improvement is less consistent, with studies reporting 15%–57% improvement.[96,100–103] This variability may be due to laboratory assay differences and criteria for establishing hormone deficiency, along with age of the patient and duration of preoperative hypopituitarism.

In the immediate postoperative period, serial visual examinations are the most sensitive tests to diagnose postoperative optic apparatus compression. Cortisol and sodium levels are obtained to diagnose hypocortisolism, diabetes insipidus, and syndrome of inappropriate antidiuretic hormone secretion (SIADH), each of which could have life-threatening consequences if left untreated. These assays should be repeated at the 1-week follow-up as delayed hypopituitarism and SIADH can occur. Routine MRI should be performed yearly at first to monitor for recurrent adenoma. Recurrence in grossly resected tumor occurs between 10% and 21% at 10 years.[96,103] Tumors with atypical features (Ki-67 >3%) tend to be more invasive with a higher recurrence rate. They should be monitored with more frequent neuroimaging.

There are two distinct scenarios of postresection tumor management. The first scenario is tumor recurrence after a gross total resection and no evidence of tumor on initial postoperative imaging (typically performed at 3 months). The second scenario is known tumor residual left behind due to invasion into surrounding structures (cavernous sinus, carotid artery), adherence to critical structures (cranial nerves), or tumor not visualized at initial exposure.

If there is tumor recurrence after gross total resection, then surgical reoperation is the ideal first therapy for noninvasive tumors. If residual tumor is detectable in initial postoperative scans and is surgically accessible, then reoperation may be indicated. A different surgical approach may be necessary (endoscopic, endonasal, or craniotomy). In our experience, reoperation for recurrent tumor is associated with similar complication rates as *de novo* tumors with comparable tumor resection outcomes.

For aggressive tumors such as atypical adenomas and pituitary carcinomas, radiotherapy/radiosurgery or medical therapy such temozolomide may be efficacious.[104,105] In one series, three of eight patients responded to temozolomide therapy with three cycles of therapy necessary to determine response. Radiosurgery or stereotactic radiotherapy is a safe option for residual tumor. The control rate for these tumors ranges from 92% to 100%. The major detriment is anterior pituitary insufficiency that is mainly dose-volume dependent. Tumors >4 cc in volume had a 58% risk of endocrine dysfunction at 5 years.[106]

## Combined lesions

Often, lesions in the pituitary gland can be a combination of two differing pathologies. Because RCCs and arachnoid cysts are common sellar abnormalities, they can be associated with pituitary adenomas as well[107] (Figure 3.4). Arachnoid cysts, in particular, can develop as the tumor erodes through the dura or after tumor

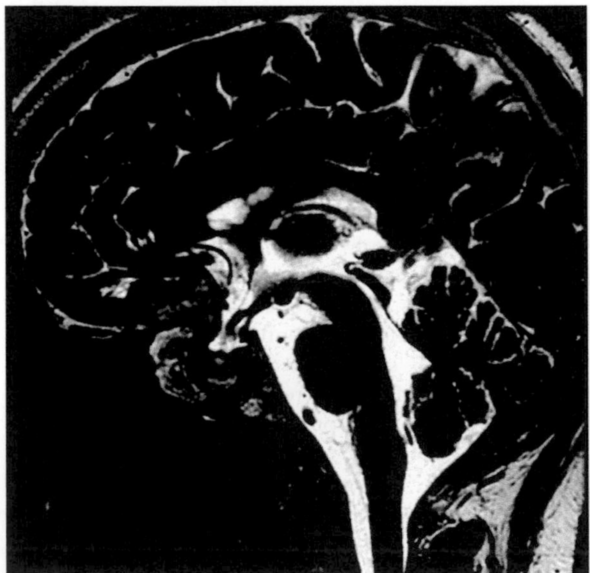

Pretreatment

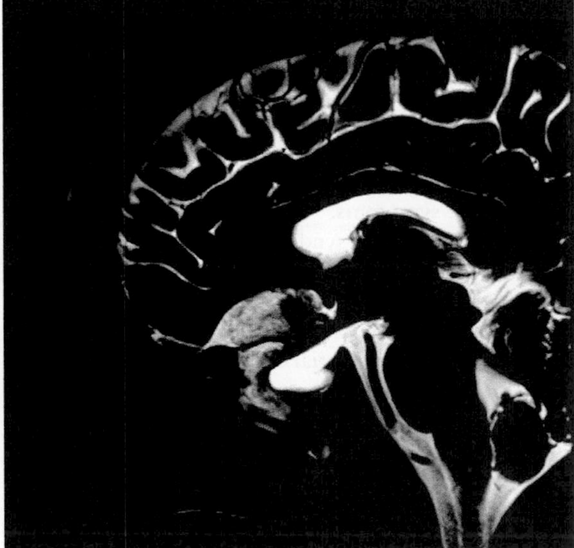

Posttreatment

***Figure 3.4***
*Sagittal postcontrast MRI and coronal T2 MRI of a patient with bitemporal hemianopsia harboring a cystic macroadenoma. Intraoperative findings confirmed a posterior dural defect confirming the source of the arachnoid cyst.*

shrinkage with medical therapy. Hence, it is important to always inspect the walls of a cyst to ensure that occult tumors are fully resected.

A rare intrasellar finding is the gangliocytoma.[108] To date, fewer than 80 reported cases of this tumor have been reported. When intrasellar, these tumors are usually associated with pituitary adenomas. Most are hormonally active (75%), with GH secretion in the majority of cases. Cushing's disease and prolactinomas are less common.[109] Occasionally, the neuronal cells demonstrate immunoreactivity for releasing hormones, such as growth hormone-releasing hormone (GHRH). The paracrine stimulation of adenohypophysial cells is one proposed mechanism for the development of these combined lesions.[110] Treatment is surgical resection of the combined lesion and close monitoring in the postoperative phase. Long-term outcomes have not been reported with this disease.

## *Hypopituitarism (see Chapter 5)*

Hypopituitarism can be encountered in the preoperative evaluation. This condition can improve or worsen postoperatively. Hypopituitarism has been associated with a long-term risk of increased vascular disease and morbidity.[111] In a large retrospective study, Nomikos et al.[112] characterized the incidence of hypopituitarism before and after tumor resection; 85% of patients with macroadenomas had insufficiency in at least one pituitary axis. Gonadotroph deficiency was the most common (76%), followed by ACTH deficiency (31%) and TSH deficiency (19%). After transsphenoidal surgery, pituitary deficiency normalized in 19.6%, improved in 30%, and worsened in 1.4%. Forty-nine percent had persistent deficits. In patients with normal preoperative endocrine function, only 4% developed postoperative insufficiency. Factors predicting pituitary hypofunction include tumor size, prolactin level, and age. Transcranial surgery had a much higher incidence of postoperative hypopituitarism.

## *Visual deficits*

Given the unique anatomy of the suprasellar region, visuals disturbances are a common finding with pituitary tumors. The classic presentation is a bitemporal hemianopsia resulting from optic chiasm compression, which may be asymmetric. Fibers from the medial retina that reflect the temporal visual field decussate in the optic chiasm. Hence, the nasal fields are often spared (see Chapter 1).

In the setting of chronic optic apparatus compression or with a large intracranial mass, these patients can also have an enlarged central scotoma, which often can be overlooked. Homonymous hemianopsia, monocular blindness, and junctional scotomas can also be found, depending on the portion of the optic apparatus affected. Preoperative, formal, quantified visual fields are necessary to evaluate patients with visual loss or a macroadenoma with significant suprasellar extension. Optical coherence tomography (OCT) can be helpful to determine the severity and longevity of optic nerve damage. Because of cortical compensation, some patients will not notice visual field loss, and a thorough preoperative exam can often detect subtle visual deficits. Without coexisting ocular pathology such as glaucoma or cataracts, visual acuity can be preserved even with severe hemianopsia. A pin hole–corrected visual exam can elucidate this finding. The duration of visual loss can help guide the urgency of treatment. Pituitary apoplexy with acute onset visual loss is an emergency that necessitates rapid surgical intervention.[113,114]

Postoperative outcomes of visual recovery vary based on patient age and duration of visual symptoms. Various studies with objective visual evaluations demonstrated 74%–80% improvement of visual fields after tumor resection.[115,116] Comparing transcranial and transsphenoidal surgery for macroadenomas with visual impairment, outcomes are significantly better with the transsphenoidal approach (57% vs. 83%).[117] Typically, visual improvement stabilizes at the 3-month time point.

Diplopia can occur when there is tumor involvement of the cavernous sinus. The most common finding is an abducens nerve paresis, causing lateral gaze diplopia. Oculomotor and trochlear nerve diplopia can also occur. Hemifacial hypesthesia can also occur due to trigeminal nerve-based involvement. Cavernous sinus compression or invasion is the etiology of these findings. In one series, 9 of 64 patients with pituitary macroadenomas were diagnosed with extraocular muscle weakness.[118] Seven of these patients had full recovery of their diplopia at 6 months after surgery.

## *Pitfalls of surgery*

The key for successful surgical results is vetted in appropriate patient selection. It is important to weigh the risks and benefits for each patient, taking in to account the chances of complications and cure. Occasionally, medical intervention or optimization may need to precede surgical resection of a tumor. A second operation can be the better option over radiosurgery. This selection process can also be applied in the operating room, deciding between transsphenoidal and transcranial approaches to reach suprasellar pathology.

In addition to the goal of gross total resection of the tumor, complication avoidance is crucial. Complication avoidance is accomplished with careful analysis of the neuroimaging before surgery, including identifying the optic chiasm, normal gland, and carotid arteries in relationship to the tumor. Intraoperative neuronavigation is helpful and essentially necessary for recurrent tumors, where the anatomy may be distorted and surgical planes altered. Patient positioning should not be overlooked. Ideally, the head should be elevated and the neck neutral to reduce venous bleeding. Preoperative hypocortisolemia should be treated with stress-dose steroids during and after surgery. Adequate repair of CSF fistulae should be addressed and monitored postoperatively. Early surgical repair of a postoperative CSF fistula can shorten hospital stay and reduce temporizing procedures.

The postoperative management of patients is as important as the attention in the operating room. Close monitoring of fluid status, including body weight and sodium levels, should be performed to aid in the diagnosis and management of SIADH or diabetes insipidus. Early ambulation can help prevent DVT, pulmonary embolism, atelectasis, and pneumonia. Because delayed SIADH can occur in up to 10% of patients, typically at around 5–7 days after surgery, routine early postoperative laboratory evaluation is necessary for early identification.[119]

# Conclusions

The diagnosis, treatment, and perioperative management of pituitary adenomas lie at the intersection of multiple disciplines. Cohesive collaboration among fellow clinicians can help deliver the best possible care to these patients. A thorough discussion with the patient regarding all treatment options, risks, and benefits is necessary. Frequent follow-up with neuroimaging or laboratory evaluation is necessary to monitor treatment efficacy, remissions, and recurrence.

# References


1. Petakov, M.S., Damjanovic, S.S., Nikolic-Durovic, M.M., et al. Pituitary adenomas secreting large amounts of prolactin may give false low values in immunoradiometric assays. The hook effect. *J Endocrinol Invest*, 1998; 21(3): p. 184–8.
2. Smith, T.P., Kavanagh, L., Healy, M.L., et al. Technology insight: Measuring prolactin in clinical samples. *Nat Clin Pract Endocrinol Metab*, 2007; 3(3): p. 279–89.
3. Barkan, A.L. and Chandler, W.F. Giant pituitary prolactinoma with falsely low serum prolactin: The pitfall of the "high-dose hook effect": Case report. *Neurosurgery*, 1998; 42(4): p. 913–15; discussion 915–16.
4. Webster, J., Piscitelli, G., Polli, A., et al. A comparison of cabergoline and bromocriptine in the treatment of hyperprolactinemic amenorrhea. Cabergoline Comparative Study Group. *N Engl J Med*, 1994; 331(14): p. 904–9.
5. Zanettini, R., Antonini, A., Gatto, G., et al. Valvular heart disease and the use of dopamine agonists for Parkinson's disease. *N Engl J Med*, 2007; 356(1): p. 39–46.
6. Horvath, J., Fross, R.D., Kleiner-Fisman, G., et al. Severe multivalvular heart disease: A new complication of the ergot derivative dopamine agonists. *Mov Disord*, 2004; 19(6): p. 656–62.
7. Molitch, M.E. Pharmacologic resistance in prolactinoma patients. *Pituitary*, 2005; 8(1): p. 43–52.
8. Molitch, M.E. The cabergoline-resistant prolactinoma patient: New challenges. *J Clin Endocrinol Metab*, 2008; 93(12): p. 4643–5.
9. Suliman, S.G., Gurlek, A., Byrne, J.V., et al. Nonsurgical cerebrospinal fluid rhinorrhea in invasive macroprolactinoma: Incidence, radiological, and clinicopathological features. *J Clin Endocrinol Metab*, 2007; 92(10): p. 3829–35.
10. Inder, W.J. and Macfarlane, M.R. Hyperprolactinaemia associated with a complex cystic pituitary mass: Medical versus surgical therapy. *Intern Med J*, 2004; 34(9–10): p. 573–6.
11. Bahuleyan, B., Menon, G., Nair, S., et al. Non-surgical management of cystic prolactinomas. *J Clin Neurosci*, 2009; 16(11): p. 1421–4.
12. Massoud, F., Serri, O., Hardy, J., et al. Transsphenoidal adenomectomy for microprolactinomas: 10 to 20 years of follow-up. *Surg Neurol*, 1996; 45(4): p. 341–6.
13. Gokalp, H.Z., Deda, H., Attar, A., et al. The neurosurgical management of prolactinomas. *J Neurosurg Sci*, 2000; 44(3): p. 128–32.
14. Landolt, A.M. and Lomax, N. Gamma knife radiosurgery for prolactinomas. *J Neurosurg*, 2000; 93(Suppl 3): p. 14–18.
*15. Sheehan, J.P., Pouratian, N., Steiner, L., et al. Gamma Knife surgery for pituitary adenomas: Factors related to radiological and endocrine outcomes. *J Neurosurg*, 2011; 114(2): p. 303–9.
16. Patil, C.G., Lad, S.P., Katznelson, L., et al. Brain atrophy and cognitive deficits in Cushing's disease. *Neurosurg Focus*, 2007; 23(3): p. E11.


* Key or Classic references.

17. Leinung, M.C., Kane, L.A., Scheithauer, B.W., et al. Long term follow-up of transsphenoidal surgery for the treatment of Cushing's disease in childhood. *J Clin Endocrinol Metab*, 1995; **80**(8): p. 2475–9.
18. Estrada, J., Boronat, M., Mielgo, M., et al. The long-term outcome of pituitary irradiation after unsuccessful transsphenoidal surgery in Cushing's disease. *N Engl J Med*, 1997; **336**(3): p. 172–7.
19. Semple P.L., D.M., Vance, M.L., Findling, J., et al. Transsphenoidal surgery for Cushing's disease: Outcome in patients with a normal magnetic resonance imaging scan. *Neurosurgery*, 2000; **46**(3): p. 553–8; discussion 558–9.
*20. Prevedello, D.M., Pouratian, N., Sherman, J., et al. Management of Cushing's disease: Outcome in patients with microadenoma detected on pituitary magnetic resonance imaging. *J Neurosurg*, 2008; **109**(4): p. 751–9.
21. Sheehan, J.M., Lopes, M.B., Sheehan, J.P., et al. Results of transsphenoidal surgery for Cushing's disease in patients with no histologically confirmed tumor. *Neurosurgery*, 2000; **47**(1): p. 33–6; discussion 37–9.
22. Bochicchio, D., Losa, M., and Buchfelder, M. Factors influencing the immediate and late outcome of Cushing's disease treated by transsphenoidal surgery: A retrospective study by the European Cushing's Disease Survey Group. *J Clin Endocrinol Metab*, 1995; **80**(11): p. 3114–20.
23. Monteith, S.J., Starke, R.M., Jane, J.A., Jr., et al. Use of the histological pseudocapsule in surgery for Cushing disease: Rapid postoperative cortisol decline predicting complete tumor resection. *J Neurosurg*, 2012; **116**(4): p. 721–7.
24. Jagannathan, J., Smith, R., DeVroom, H.L., et al. Outcome of using the histological pseudocapsule as a surgical capsule in Cushing disease. *J Neurosurg*, 2009; **111**(3): p. 531–9.
25. Semple, P.L. and Laws, E.R., Jr. Complications in a contemporary series of patients who underwent transsphenoidal surgery for Cushing's disease. *J Neurosurg*, 1999; **91**(2): p. 175–9.
26. Hofmann, B.M., Hlavac, M., Martinez, R., et al. Long-term results after microsurgery for Cushing disease: Experience with 426 primary operations over 35 years. *J Neurosurg*, 2008; **108**(1): p. 9–18.
27. Simmons, N.E., Alden, T.D., Thorner, M.O., et al. Serum cortisol response to transsphenoidal surgery for Cushing disease. *J Neurosurg*, 2001; **95**(1): p. 1–8.
28. Hammer, G.D., Tyrrell, J.B., Lamborn, K.R., et al. Transsphenoidal microsurgery for Cushing's disease: Initial outcome and long-term results. *J Clin Endocrinol Metab*, 2004; **89**(12): p. 6348–57.
29. Utz, A.L., Swearingen, B., and Biller, B.M. Pituitary surgery and postoperative management in Cushing's disease. *Endocrinol Metab Clin North Am*, 2005; **34**(2): p. 459–78, xi.
30. Chen, J.C., Amar, A.P., Choi, S., et al. Transsphenoidal microsurgical treatment of Cushing disease: Postoperative assessment of surgical efficacy by application of an overnight low-dose dexamethasone suppression test. *J Neurosurg*, 2003; **98**(5): p. 967–73.
31. Ram, Z., Nieman, L.K., Cutler, G.B., Jr., et al. Early repeat surgery for persistent Cushing's disease. *J Neurosurg*, 1994; **80**(1): p. 37–45.
32. Rees, D.A., Hanna, F.W., Davies, J.S., et al. Long-term follow-up results of transsphenoidal surgery for Cushing's disease in a single centre using strict criteria for remission. *Clin Endocrinol (Oxf)*, 2002; **56**(4): p. 541–51.
*33. Patil, C.G., Prevedello, D.M., Lad, S.P., et al. Late recurrences of Cushing's disease after initial successful transsphenoidal surgery. *J Clin Endocrinol Metab*, 2008; **93**(2): p. 358–62.
*34. Locatelli, M., Vance, M.L., and Laws, E.R. Clinical review: The strategy of immediate reoperation for transsphenoidal surgery for Cushing's disease. *J Clin Endocrinol Metab*, 2005; **90**(9): p. 5478–82.
35. Trainer, P.J., Lawrie, H.S., Verhelst, J., et al. Transsphenoidal resection in Cushing's disease: Undetectable serum cortisol as the definition of successful treatment. *Clin Endocrinol (Oxf)*, 1993; **38**(1): p. 73–8.
36. Thomas, J.P. and Richards, S.H. Long term results of radical hypophysectomy for Cushing's disease. *Clin Endocrinol (Oxf)*, 1983; **19**(5): p. 629–36.
37. Robert, F. and Hardy, J. Cushing's disease: A correlation of radiological, surgical and pathological findings with therapeutic results. *Pathol Res Pract*, 1991; **187**(5): p. 617–21.
38. Jagannathan, J., Sheehan, J.P., Pouratian, N., et al. Gamma Knife surgery for Cushing's disease. *J Neurosurg*, 2007; **106**(6): p. 980–7.
39. Sheehan, J.M., Vance, M.L., Sheehan, J.P., et al. Radiosurgery for Cushing's disease after failed transsphenoidal surgery. *J Neurosurg*, 2000; **93**(5): p. 738–42.
40. Lewis, J.H., Zimmerman, H.J., Benson, G.D., et al. Hepatic injury associated with ketoconazole therapy. Analysis of 33 cases. *Gastroenterology*, 1984; **86**(3): p. 503–13.
41. Drake, W.M., Perry, L.A., Hinds, C.J., et al. Emergency and prolonged use of intravenous etomidate to control hypercortisolemia in a patient with Cushing's syndrome and peritonitis. *J Clin Endocrinol Metab*, 1998; **83**(10): p. 3542–4.
42. Krakoff, J., Koch, C.A., Calis, K.A., et al. Use of a parenteral propylene glycol-containing etomidate preparation for the long-term management of ectopic Cushing's syndrome. *J Clin Endocrinol Metab*, 2001; **86**(9): p. 4104–8.

43. de Herder, W.W. and Lamberts, S.W. Is there a role for somatostatin and its analogs in Cushing's syndrome? *Metabolism*, 1996; 45(8 Suppl 1): p. 83–5.
44. De Herder, W.W. and Lamberts, S.W. Octapeptide somatostatin-analogue therapy of Cushing's syndrome. *Postgrad Med J*, 1999; 75(880): p. 65–6.
45. Boscaro, M., Ludlam, W.H., Atkinson, B., et al. Treatment of pituitary-dependent Cushing's disease with the multireceptor ligand somatostatin analog pasireotide (SOM230): A multicenter, phase II trial. *J Clin Endocrinol Metab*, 2009; 94(1): p. 115–22.
46. Croughs, R.J., Koppeschaar, H.P., van't Verlaat, J.W., et al. Bromocriptine-responsive Cushing's disease associated with anterior pituitary corticotroph hyperplasia or normal pituitary gland. *J Clin Endocrinol Metab*, 1989; **68**(2): p. 495–8.
47. Healy, D.L., Chrousos, G.P., Schulte, H.M., et al. Increased adrenocorticotropin, cortisol, and arginine vasopressin secretion in primates after the antiglucocorticoid steroid RU 486: Dose response relationships. *J Clin Endocrinol Metab*, 1985; **60**(1): p. 1–4.
48. Nieman, L.K., Chrousos, G.P., Kellner, C., et al. Successful treatment of Cushing's syndrome with the glucocorticoid antagonist RU 486. *J Clin Endocrinol Metab*, 1985; **61**(3): p. 536–40.
49. Sartor, O. and Cutler, G.B., Jr. Mifepristone: Treatment of Cushing's syndrome. *Clin Obstet Gynecol*, 1996; 39(2): p. 506–10.
50. Henry, J.F., Defechereux, T., Raffaelli, M., et al. Complications of laparoscopic adrenalectomy: Results of 169 consecutive procedures. *World J Surg*, 2000; 24(11): p. 1342–6.
51. Gagner, M., Pomp, A., Heniford, B.T., et al. Laparoscopic adrenalectomy: Lessons learned from 100 consecutive procedures. *Ann Surg*, 1997; **226**(3): p. 238–46; discussion 246–7.
52. Nelson, D.H., Meakin, J.W., and Thorn, G.W. ACTH-producing pituitary tumors following adrenalectomy for Cushing's syndrome. *Ann Intern Med*, 1960; **52**: p. 560–9.
53. Jenkins, P.J., Trainer, P.J., Plowman, P.N., et al. The long-term outcome after adrenalectomy and prophylactic pituitary radiotherapy in adrenocorticotropin-dependent Cushing's syndrome. *J Clin Endocrinol Metab*, 1995; **80**(1): p. 165–71.
54. Assie, G., Bahurel, H., Coste, J., et al. Corticotroph tumor progression after adrenalectomy in Cushing's disease: A reappraisal of Nelson's syndrome. *J Clin Endocrinol Metab*, 2007; 92(1): p. 172–9.
*55. Smith, P.W., Turza, K.C., Carter, C.O., et al. Bilateral adrenalectomy for refractory Cushing disease: A safe and definitive therapy. *J Am Coll Surg*, 2009; **208**(6): p. 1059–64.
*56. De Tommasi, C., Vance, M.L., Okonkwo, D.O., et al. Surgical management of adrenocorticotropic hormone-secreting macroadenomas: Outcome and challenges in patients with Cushing's disease or Nelson's syndrome. *J Neurosurg*, 2005; **103**(5): p. 825–30.
57. Clemmons, D.R., Chihara, K., Freda, P.U., et al. Optimizing control of acromegaly: Integrating a growth hormone receptor antagonist into the treatment algorithm. *J Clin Endocrinol Metab*, 2003; **88**(10): p. 4759–67.
*58. Kreutzer, J., Vance, M.L., Lopes, M.B., et al. Surgical management of GH-secreting pituitary adenomas: An outcome study using modern remission criteria. *J Clin Endocrinol Metab*, 2001; **86**(9): p. 4072–7.
59. Shimon, I., Cohen, Z.R., Ram, Z., et al. Transsphenoidal surgery for acromegaly: Endocrinological follow-up of 98 patients. *Neurosurgery*, 2001; **48**(6): p. 1239–43; discussion 1244–5.
60. Ahmed, S., Elsheikh, M., Stratton, I.M., et al. Outcome of transsphenoidal surgery for acromegaly and its relationship to surgical experience. *Clin Endocrinol (Oxf)*, 1999; **50**(5): p. 561–7.
61. Bourdelot, A., Coste, J., Hazebroucq, V., et al. Clinical, hormonal and magnetic resonance imaging (MRI) predictors of transsphenoidal surgery outcome in acromegaly. *Eur J Endocrinol*, 2004; **150**(6): p. 763–71.
62. Freda, P.U. Somatostatin analogs in acromegaly. *J Clin Endocrinol Metab*, 2002; **87**(7): p. 3013–18.
63. Cozzi, R., Montini, M., Attanasio, R., et al. Primary treatment of acromegaly with octreotide LAR: A long-term (up to nine years) prospective study of its efficacy in the control of disease activity and tumor shrinkage. *J Clin Endocrinol Metab*, 2006; **91**(4): p. 1397–403.
64. Abs, R., Verhelst, J., Maiter, D., et al. Cabergoline in the treatment of acromegaly: A study in 64 patients. *J Clin Endocrinol Metab*, 1998; **83**(2): p. 374–8.
65. Trainer, P.J., Drake, W.M., Katznelson, L., et al. Treatment of acromegaly with the growth hormone-receptor antagonist pegvisomant. *N Engl J Med*, 2000; 342(16): p. 1171–7.
66. van der Lely, A.J., Hutson, R.K., Trainer, P.J., et al. Long-term treatment of acromegaly with pegvisomant, a growth hormone receptor antagonist. *Lancet*, 2001; **358**(9295): p. 1754–9.
67. Attanasio, R., Epaminonda, P., Motti, E., et al. Gamma-knife radiosurgery in acromegaly: A 4-year follow-up study. *J Clin Endocrinol Metab*, 2003; **88**(7): p. 3105–12.
68. Castinetti, F., Taieb, D., Kuhn, J.M., et al. Outcome of gamma knife radiosurgery in 82 patients with acromegaly: Correlation with initial hypersecretion. *J Clin Endocrinol Metab*, 2005; **90**(8): p. 4483–8.
69. Landolt, A.M., Haller, D., Lomax, N., et al. Stereotactic radiosurgery for recurrent surgically

treated acromegaly: Comparison with fractionated radiotherapy. *J Neurosurg*, 1998; **88**(6): p. 1002–8.
70. Kurosaki, M., Luedecke, D.K., and Abe, T. Effectiveness of secondary transnasal surgery in GH-secreting pituitary macroadenomas. *Endocr J*, 2003; **50**(5): p. 635–42.
71. Laws, E.R., Jr., Fode, N.C., and Redmond, M.J. Transsphenoidal surgery following unsuccessful prior therapy. An assessment of benefits and risks in 158 patients. *J Neurosurg*, 1985; **63**(6): p. 823–9.
72. Long, H., Beauregard, H., Somma, M., et al. Surgical outcome after repeated transsphenoidal surgery in acromegaly. *J Neurosurg*, 1996; **85**(2): p. 239–47.
73. Abe, T. and Ludecke, D.K. Recent results of secondary transnasal surgery for residual or recurring acromegaly. *Neurosurgery*, 1998; 42(5): p. 1013–21; discussion 1021–2.
74. Bates, A.S., Van't Hoff, W., Jones, J.M., et al. An audit of outcome of treatment in acromegaly. *Q J Med*, 1993; **86**(5): p. 293–9.
*75. Swearingen, B., Barker, F.G., 2nd, Katznelson, L., et al. Long-term mortality after transsphenoidal surgery and adjunctive therapy for acromegaly. *J Clin Endocrinol Metab*, 1998; **83**(10): p. 3419–26.
76. Brucker-Davis, F., Oldfield, E.H., Skarulis, M.C., et al. Thyrotropin-secreting pituitary tumors: Diagnostic criteria, thyroid hormone sensitivity, and treatment outcome in 25 patients followed at the National Institutes of Health. *J Clin Endocrinol Metab*, 1999; **84**(2): p. 476–86.
77. Losa, M., Giovanelli, M., Persani, L., et al. Criteria of cure and follow-up of central hyperthyroidism due to thyrotropin-secreting pituitary adenomas. *J Clin Endocrinol Metab*, 1996; **81**(8): p. 3084–90.
*78. Laws, E.R., Vance, M.L., and Jane, J.A., Jr. TSH adenomas. *Pituitary*, 2006; 9(4): p. 313–15.
79. Hamilton, C.R., Jr., Adams, L.C., and Maloof, F. Hyperthyroidism due to thyrotropin-producing pituitary chromophobe adenoma. *N Engl J Med*, 1970; **283**(20): p. 1077–80.
80. Socin, H.V., Chanson, P., Delemer, B., et al. The changing spectrum of TSH-secreting pituitary adenomas: Diagnosis and management in 43 patients. *Eur J Endocrinol*, 2003; **148**(4): p. 433–42.
81. Chanson, P., Weintraub, B.D., and Harris, A.G. Octreotide therapy for thyroid-stimulating hormone-secreting pituitary adenomas. A follow-up of 52 patients. *Ann Intern Med*, 1993; 119(3): p. 236–40.
82. Caron, P., Arlot, S., Bauters, C., et al. Efficacy of the long-acting octreotide formulation (octreotide-LAR) in patients with thyrotropin-secreting pituitary adenomas. *J Clin Endocrinol Metab*, 2001; **86**(6): p. 2849–53.
83. Rishi, A., Sharma, M.C., Sarkar, C., et al. A clinicopathological and immunohistochemical study of clinically non-functioning pituitary adenomas: A single institutional experience. *Neurol India*, 2010; **58**(3): p. 418–23.
84. Young, W.F., Jr., Scheithauer, B.W., Kovacs, K.T., et al. Gonadotroph adenoma of the pituitary gland: A clinicopathologic analysis of 100 cases. *Mayo Clin Proc*, 1996; 71(7): p. 649–56.
85. Ho, D.M., Hsu, C.Y., Ting, L.T., et al. The clinicopathological characteristics of gonadotroph cell adenoma: A study of 118 cases. *Hum Pathol*, 1997; **28**(8): p. 905–11.
86. Gryngarten, M.G., Braslavsky, D., Ballerini, M.G., et al. Spontaneous ovarian hyperstimulation syndrome caused by a follicle-stimulating hormone-secreting pituitary macroadenoma in an early pubertal girl. *Horm Res Paediatr*, 2010; 73(4): p. 293–8.
87. Kihara, M., Sugita, T., Nagai, Y., et al. Ovarian hyperstimulation caused by gonadotroph cell adenoma: A case report and review of the literature. *Gynecol Endocrinol*, 2006; 22(2): p. 110–13.
88. Cooper, O., Geller, J.L., and Melmed, S. Ovarian hyperstimulation syndrome caused by an FSH-secreting pituitary adenoma. *Nat Clin Pract Endocrinol Metab*, 2008; 4(4): p. 234–8.
89. Murakami, T., Higashitsuji, H., Yoshinaga, K., et al. Management of ovarian hyperstimulation due to follicle-stimulating hormone-secreting gonadotroph adenoma. *Bjog*, 2004; **111**(11): p. 1297–300.
90. Dizon, M.N. and Vesely, D.L. Gonadotropin-secreting pituitary tumor associated with hypersecretion of testosterone and hypogonadism after hypophysectomy. *Endocr Pract*, 2002; **8**(3): p. 225–31.
91. Zarate, A., Fonseca, M.E., Mason, M., et al. Gonadotropin-secreting pituitary adenoma with concomitant hypersecretion of testosterone and elevated sperm count. Treatment with LRH agonist. *Acta Endocrinol (Copenh)*, 1986; **113**(1): p. 29–34.
92. Felix, I.A., Horvath, E., Kovacs, K., et al. Mammosomatotroph adenoma of the pituitary associated with gigantism and hyperprolactinemia. A morphological study including immunoelectron microscopy. *Acta Neuropathol*, 1986; 71(1–2): p. 76–82.
93. Lloyd, R.V., Cano, M., Chandler, W.F., et al. Human growth hormone and prolactin secreting pituitary adenomas analyzed by *in situ* hybridization. *Am J Pathol*, 1989; **134**(3): p. 605–13.
94. Li, J., Stefaneanu, L., Kovacs, K., et al. Growth hormone (GH) and prolactin (PRL) gene expression and immunoreactivity in GH- and PRL-producing human pituitary adenomas. *Virchows Arch A Pathol Anat Histopathol*, 1993; 422(3): p. 193–201.
95. Bevan, J.S., Adams, C.B., Burke, C.W., et al. Factors in the outcome of transsphenoidal surgery for prolactinoma and non-functioning pituitary tumour, including pre-operative bromocriptine therapy. *Clin Endocrinol (Oxf)*, 1987; **26**(5): p. 541–56.

96. Ebersold, M.J., Quast, L.M., Laws, E.R. Jr., et al. Long-term results in transsphenoidal removal of non-functioning pituitary adenomas. *J Neurosurg*, 1986; 64(5): p. 713–19.
97. Salmi, J., Grahne, B., Valtonen, S., et al. Recurrence of chromophobe pituitary adenomas after operation and postoperative radiotherapy. *Acta Neurol Scand*, 1982; 66(6): p. 681–9.
98. Sassolas, G., Trouillas, J., Treluyer, C., et al. Management of nonfunctioning pituitary adenomas. *Acta Endocrinol (Copenh)*, 1993; 129(Suppl 1): p. 21–6.
*99. Losa, M., Mortini, P., Barzaghi, R., et al. Endocrine inactive and gonadotroph adenomas: Diagnosis and management. *J Neurooncol*, 2001; 54(2): p. 167–77.
100. Petruson, B., Jakobsson, K.E., Elfverson, J., et al. Five-year follow-up of nonsecreting pituitary adenomas. *Arch Otolaryngol Head Neck Surg*, 1995; 121(3): p. 317–22.
101. Shone, G.R., Richards, S.H., Hourihan, M.D., et al. Non-secretory adenomas of the pituitary treated by trans-ethmoidal sellotomy. *J R Soc Med*, 1991; 84(3): p. 140–3.
102. Arafah, B.M. Reversible hypopituitarism in patients with large nonfunctioning pituitary adenomas. *J Clin Endocrinol Metab*, 1986; 62(6): p. 1173–9.
103. Comtois, R., Beauregard, H., Somma, M., et al. The clinical and endocrine outcome to trans-sphenoidal microsurgery of nonsecreting pituitary adenomas. *Cancer*, 1991; 68(4): p. 860–6.
104. Raverot, G., Sturm, N., de Fraipont, F., et al. Temozolomide treatment in aggressive pituitary tumors and pituitary carcinomas: A French multicenter experience. *J Clin Endocrinol Metab*, 2010; 95(10): p. 4592–9.
105. Losa, M., Mazza, E., Terreni, M.R., et al. Salvage therapy with temozolomide in patients with aggressive or metastatic pituitary adenomas: Experience in six cases. *Eur J Endocrinol*, 2010; 163(6): p. 843–51.
106. Medel, R., Williams, B., and Sheehan, J.P. Stereotactic radiosurgery, in *Sellar and Parasellar Tumors: Diagnosis, Treatments and Outcomes*, E.R. Laws Jr. and J.P. Sheehan, editors. New York: Thieme, 2011; p. 216–28.
107. Ring, B.A. and Waddington, M. Primary arachnoid cysts of the sella turcica. *Am J Roentgenol Radium Ther Nucl Med*, 1966; 98(3): p. 611–15.
108. Puchner, M.J., Ludecke, D.K., Saeger, W., et al. Gangliocytomas of the sellar region—a review. *Exp Clin Endocrinol Diabetes*, 1995; 103(3): p. 129–49.
109. Saeger, W., Puchner, M.J., and Ludecke, D.K. Combined sellar gangliocytoma and pituitary adenoma in acromegaly or Cushing's disease. A report of 3 cases. *Virchows Arch*, 1994; 425(1): p. 93–9.
110. Kontogeorgos, G., Mourouti, G., Kyrodimou, E., et al. Ganglion cell containing pituitary adenomas: Signs of neuronal differentiation in adenoma cells. *Acta Neuropathol*, 2006; 112(1): p. 21–8.
111. Bulow, B., Hagmar, L., Mikoczy, Z., et al. Increased cerebrovascular mortality in patients with hypopituitarism. *Clin Endocrinol (Oxf)*, 1997; 46(1): p. 75–81.
*112. Nomikos, P., Ladar, C., Fahlbusch, R., et al. Impact of primary surgery on pituitary function in patients with non-functioning pituitary adenomas—a study on 721 patients. *Acta Neurochir (Wien)*, 2004; 146(1): p. 27–35.
113. Agrawal, D. and Mahapatra, A.K. Visual outcome of blind eyes in pituitary apoplexy after transsphenoidal surgery: A series of 14 eyes. *Surg Neurol*, 2005; 63(1): p. 42–6; discussion 46.
114. Reid, R.L., Quigley, M.E., and Yen, S.S. Pituitary apoplexy. A review. *Arch Neurol*, 1985; 42(7): p. 712–19.
*115. Cohen, A.R., Cooper, P.R., Kupersmith, M.J., et al. Visual recovery after transsphenoidal removal of pituitary adenomas. *Neurosurgery*, 1985; 17(3): p. 446–52.
116. Laws, E.R., Jr., Trautmann, J.C., and Hollenhorst, R.W. Jr., Transsphenoidal decompression of the optic nerve and chiasm. Visual results in 62 patients. *J Neurosurg*, 1977; 46(6): p. 717–22.
117. Wichers-Rother, M., Hoven, S., Kristof, R.A., et al. Non-functioning pituitary adenomas: Endocrinological and clinical outcome after transsphenoidal and transcranial surgery. *Exp Clin Endocrinol Diabetes*, 2004; 112(6): p. 323–7.
118. Robert, C.M., Jr., Feigenbaum, J.A., and Stern, E.W. Ocular palsy occurring with pituitary tumors. *J Neurosurg*, 1973; 38(1): p. 17–9.
*119. Kelly, D.F., Laws, E.R., Jr., and Fossett, D. Delayed hyponatremia after transsphenoidal surgery for pituitary adenoma. Report of nine cases. *J Neurosurg*, 1995; 83(2): p. 363–7.

# 4

# Pituitary radiotherapy

*Thankamma Ajithkumar, Michael Brada*

## *Introduction*

External beam radiotherapy (RT) remains an important component of management of patients with pituitary adenoma, and a significant proportion of patients receive it during the course of their illness.

Traditional policy had been to use RT for all patients with residual nonfunctioning pituitary adenoma (NFPA) after surgery because the majority were considered to progress, achieving tumor control in >90% of patients at 10 years and in 85%–92% of patients in 20 years.[1–9] With improvement in surgical techniques and access to magnetic resonance (MR) imaging, postoperative RT is no longer routinely used, even in the presence of residual tumor. The use of RT is based on relative risk assessment, generally withholding further treatment until progression, unless there is a perceived threat to function, particularly vision, or further surgery is risky if the tumor were to progress. Currently, RT is used in patients with progressive NFPA demonstrated on interval imaging.

RT remains an integral component of treatment of patients with secreting adenoma who fail to achieve biochemical cure after surgery and optimal medical treatment and for patients with progressive/recurrent tumor mass, regardless of the status of hypersecretion. The slow rate of decline in hormone levels means that normalization takes months to years and that the delay is primarily related to pretreatment hormone levels.[10] Nevertheless, RT leads to normalization of excess hormone secretion in the majority of patients.

The past two decades has seen improvements in RT that can largely be considered as refinement of existing technology. The principal aim of modern high-precision RT is to treat the tumor with a uniform therapeutic dose with least possible dose to surrounding normal tissues, thereby minimizing the risk of normal tissue injury. The higher precision relies on increased accuracy of tumor delineation using modern imaging and improved immobilization techniques during treatment. The overall success of modern high-precision treatment is more likely to be related to the treatment center infrastructure and expertise and the accuracy in identifying the tumor than to the exact equipment used.

## *Review of modern RT techniques*

### *Three-dimensional conformal radiotherapy*

The current standard of care is the use of three-dimensional (3D) conformal radiotherapy (CRT) using computed tomography (CT) and MR imaging, computerized 3D planning, and the use of multiple shaped beams. The practical steps before treatment delivery include noninvasive method of patient immobilization, coregistered 3D imaging with CT and magnetic resonance imaging (MRI), and 3D computerized treatment planning followed by quality assurance (QA) procedures in the form of image guidance to ensure the accuracy of the whole process both before and during treatment.

Immobilization is critical to the accuracy of treatment, and the device should be comfortable and reproducible, and should minimize movement during the preparation steps and during treatment. Patients are usually immobilized in a custom-made closely fitting plastic mask made of lightweight thermoplastic material applied directly to the face in a single procedure. The repositioning accuracy is in the region of 3–5 mm[11] and can be reduced to 2–3 mm with a more closely fitting though frequently less comfortable mask.[12]

Imaging for the purpose of treatment planning is performed in the immobilization device and includes an unenhanced thin-slice MRI and a coregistered CT scan. The extent of the pituitary adenoma visible tumor on MRI is outlined in all orthogonal planes. It should take into account all previous imaging, particularly preoperative scans, to ensure that all areas of uncertainty, which may contain residual tumor, are included. It is not standard practice to include the whole extent of tumor before a debulking procedure, especially when normal anatomical structures have returned to their normal position. The outline of the visible and presumed tumor is defined as the gross tumor volume (GTV). A margin of 5–10 mm is added in the treatment planning process to account for the technical uncertainty of immobilization, treatment planning, and delivery, and this is defined as the planning target volume (PTV). The exact margin applied should be based on the measurement of uncertainty specific to each center and the system used. Surrounding normal structures, such as the optic chiasm and optic nerves, the brain stem, and the hypothalamus, may also be outlined.

The computerized treatment planning process defines the number, shaping, and orientation of radiation beams to achieve uniform dose within the PTV and as low a dose as possible to the surrounding normal tissue. With conventionally fractionated RT, the dose to the adenoma is below the radiation tolerance of the surrounding neural structures, with the exception of hypothalamus, and in fractionated CRT no specific measures are generally taken to avoid the optic apparatus, hypothalamus, and brain stem, particularly because in many patients requiring RT some or all of the structures are within or in proximity to the adenoma. Nevertheless, the preferred beam paths tend to avoid the eyes.

The usual CRT arrangement is three fixed radiation beams shaped to conform to the PTV with a multileaf collimator (MLC). The MLC leaves are automatically preset to the shape of the PTV as defined in the planning process. Radiation dose intensity can also be altered across the beam by MLC leaves placed in the beam path, and this is described as intensity-modulated radiotherapy (IMRT). IMRT is a form of CRT that can spare critical structures within a concave PTV. This is rarely required for pituitary adenomas, and IMRT offers neither technical nor clinical advantage compared with CRT for most sellar and suprasellar tumors.[13]

## *Stereotactic CRT and radiosurgery*

Stereotactic techniques are a refinement of CRT with improved immobilization, more accurate image coregistration, and high-precision treatment delivery. The term "stereotactic," derived from neurosurgery, denotes the method of determining the position of a lesion within a space defined by coordinates based on the immobilization system, usually a stereotactic frame.

Stereotactic irradiation can be given in multiple doses as fractionated stereotactic radiotherapy (fSRT) and as fractionated stereotactic conformal radiotherapy (fSCRT), or in a single dose when it is described as stereotactic radiosurgery (SRS), although despite the terminology, this remains a radiation and not a surgical procedure. fSRT/fSCRT is generally delivered using a linear accelerator. SRS can be delivered using either a multiheaded cobalt unit (gamma-knife [GK]) or a linear accelerator. The precision of modern linear accelerators does not require modification for stereotactic irradiation. Smaller linear accelerators have been mounted on a robotic arm (CyberKnife) that allows for nonisocentric movement. However, the access to the lesion is restricted by the robotic arm geometry, and the small size of the accelerator produces smaller beams at a lower dose rate. In comparative studies, the robotic arm–mounted linear accelerator does not offer better target and normal tissue dose distribution[14] and no advantage in the accuracy of treatment delivery compared with other high-precision techniques.

## *Fractionated treatment*

For fSRT patients are immobilized in a noninvasive relocatable frame with a relocation accuracy of 1–2 mm[15,16] or a precisely fitting mask system with an accuracy of 2–3 mm.[12] As in conventional RT, GTV is outlined on MRI coregistered with a CT scan. The PTV margin is smaller than for conventional RT, usually in the region of 3 mm, and this is based on the overall accuracy of the system of which the principal determinant is the repositioning accuracy of the patient in the immobilization device.[17] The most important aspect of treatment preparation is precise definition of the tumor. This precision is essential to avoid treatment failure due to exclusion of a part of the tumor from the high-dose radiation.

SRT uses larger number of beams than conventional RT (usually four to six), each conforming to the shape of the tumor using a narrow leaf MLC (5-mm width described as mini MLC or 3 mm width as micro MLC). fSRT/fSCRT combine the precision of the stereotactic positioning and treatment delivery, treating less normal neural tissue, with fractionation that preferentially spares damage to normal tissue. In addition, complete avoidance of critical structures such as the optic apparatus is not necessary, especially because the dose fractionation schemes as used for conventional RT are below radiation tolerance of normal brain structures. fSRT technique is therefore suitable for pituitary adenomas of all sizes, regardless of the relationship to critical structures.

## Single-fraction treatment

For single-fraction SRS, patients are immobilized in an invasive neurosurgical frame fixed to the skull. It requires all the preparation procedures and treatment to be done in 1 day.

GK delivers a spherical dose distribution of 6–18 mm in diameter. Larger nonspherical tumors, representing the majority of pituitary adenomas, are treated by combining several radiation spheres, and this is defined using a 3D computerized treatment planning system similar to that used for linear accelerator RT. The use of multiple isocenters results in dose inhomogeneity within the target with small areas of high radiation dose (hot spots) in the region of overlap of the radiation dose spheres. The dose delivered to the periphery of a target is approximately half the dose delivered to the geometric center of the target, and the dose prescription in gamma-knife radiosurgery (GKS) is the dose delivered to the margin of the target. This may lead to radiation damage if critical normal structures such as cranial nerves are within the hot spots of the target.

Linear accelerator–based radiosurgery can be carried out either in a relocatable or a fixed stereotactic frame. Computerized treatment planning defines the arrangement of beams as in SRT/SCRT. At the inception, this was as multiple arcs of rotation, simulating GK treatment, producing small spherical dose distributions and such techniques are no longer in use. Treatment is usually given as for fSRT using multiple fixed fields, although single-fraction SRS is rarely used using linear accelerator.

Because of the potential damaging effect of large single radiation doses to normal neural structures, SRS is only suitable for small pituitary adenomas 3–5 mm away from the optic chiasm.

CyberKnife can be used for single-fraction and fractionated treatment. The robotic arms linked with real-time image guidance using linked orthogonal X-rays can apply adjustments based on patient setup variation. The treatment uses multiple small beams with conformality similar to GKS and linear accelerator fSRT. Because the dose rate is relatively low, each treatment session takes longer compared with other linear accelerator–based RT, and the course of treatment tends to be given in fewer fractions (described as hypofractionated RT).

## Proton therapy

The biological effect of protons is equivalent to the ionization damage caused by photons. The principal benefit is more localized deposition of energy of a monoenergetic proton beam described as the Bragg peak, with little ionizing radiation beyond the peak.[18] The preparation steps are as would be used for other conformal RT techniques. The principal dose-sparing effect of modulated proton beams is beyond the target.

## Dose fractionation of RT

The therapeutic benefit of RT in malignant tumors is considered to be due to cell attrition either as apoptosis or reproductive cell death as a consequence of radiation-induced DNA damage. The time taken to manifest radiation effects is related to the rate of cell proliferation in the tissue irradiated. In rapidly proliferating cells, radiation effects are expressed either during or immediately after the course of RT, whereas in slowly proliferating cell population, they take months or years to manifest. It is assumed that the beneficial effects of radiation in pituitary adenomas conform to the same mechanism with depletion of tumor cells where adenomas are considered as slowly proliferating tissue. The surrounding normal brain parenchyma is also considered to consist largely of slow proliferating cell population, although critical cell populations with faster turnover, such as blood vessels, are also present and affected by radiation.

Conventional RT/CRT and fractionated SCRT are given to total dose of 45–50 Gy at 1.8 Gy per fractionation, once a day, 5 days per week. The dose is below the tolerance of the central nervous system, and the risk of structural damage is <1%.

Although single large doses of radiation may result in higher cell kill than the same dose given in a small number of fractions, this is also true for normal tissue cell population leading to toxicity that may not be acceptable if affecting eloquent regions such as optic chiasm. Because the majority of pituitary adenomas requiring radiation lie in proximity to the optic apparatus and the nerves in the cavernous sinus, radiosurgery is suitable only for small lesions located away from the critical structures, and dose to the optic apparatus should not exceed beyond 8–10 Gy.

# *Indications for RT in pituitary adenoma (see Chapter 1)*

## *Nonfunctioning pituitary adenoma*

There is no consensus on the optimal postoperative management of NFPA after subtotal excision. After gross resection of tumor, 17% of NFPAs recur and the rate of recurrence after incomplete resection is 43%.[19] A recent study of NFPA reported relapse rate of 23% at 5 years, 47% at 10 years, and 68% at 15 years after surgery alone.[20] The 5-year recurrence rate was 53% with extrasellar compared with 20% with intrasellar residual tumor, and younger patients had a higher risk of recurrence (HR, 0.975; 95% CI, 0.974–0.998; $p = 0.034$). Brochier reported a postoperative relapse rate of 25% at 5 years, 43% at 10 years, and 61% at 15 years in patients with NFPA in a cohort of 142 patients. At a mean follow-up of 7 years, the risk of recurrence was higher in those with residual tumor (47%) compared with those who had a complete macroscopic resection (24%). Invasion of cavernous sinus and absence of immediate postoperative RT were independent risk factors for recurrence.[21,22]

In summary, young age, cavernous sinus invasion, extent of suprasellar extension, and macroscopic residual disease are associated with increased risk of recurrence/progression, and the risk also increases with longer follow-up.[19,21–23] In the absence of randomized controlled trials evaluating the role of routine postoperative RT in pituitary adenoma, it is not clear whether patients with or without the risk factors for recurrence should receive immediate postoperative treatment or be treated at the time of progression. With the routine use of MRI, the previous policy of routine postoperative RT has largely been replaced by a risk-based approach. Currently, RT is reserved for aggressive tumors, significant residual tumors near eloquent structures, and progressive tumors on imaging.

## *Secretory pituitary adenoma*

### *Acromegaly*

Surgery remains the first-line treatment followed by somatostatin analogs to correct hypersecretion of growth hormone (GH)/insulin-like growth factor I (IGF-I). Optimal management of the 10%–50% of patients with GH-secreting tumors who fail to achieve a biochemical remission after surgery and the 20% who develops biochemical recurrence remains unclear.[24,25] The current options include prolonged use of somatostatin analogs, GH receptor antagonists in patients resistant to somatostatin analogs, and RT. The indications for RT include poor tolerance and resistance to systemic treatment and progressive tumor mass threatening function, particularly vision.[10]

### *Cushing's disease*

Persistent Cushing's disease after surgery is a frequent indication for RT because medical treatment is a less effective option.[26]

### *Prolactinoma*

Prolactinoma are successfully treated with medical management with or without surgical resection. RT is reserved for patients who fail medical management or recur after surgery and medical treatment,[27] although in this setting it is not as effective in normalizing hormone levels as in other secretary tumors.[28]

# *Assessing clinical outcome of pituitary RT*

The clinical efficacy of RT for pituitary adenoma should be assessed in terms of survival, actuarial tumor control [progression-free survival (PFS)], and quality of life. The commonly reported endpoints for nonfunctioning pituitary adenoma are local tumor control measured as PFS and long-term morbidity, and in patients with secreting pituitary adenoma, normalization of elevated hormone levels. The rate of hormonal decline after RT varies with the type of secreting tumor, and the time to reach normal levels is dependent on the initial hormone level. The appropriate comparative measure for each hormone is the time to reach 50% of pretreatment hormone level, and this should be corrected for the confounding effect of medical treatment. Surrogate endpoints such as "control rate" without indication of time and duration of follow-up and the proportion of patients achieving normal hormone levels without a clear relationship to pre-RT values do not provide comparative information on the efficacy of different treatment approaches and are potentially misleading.[29]

The reporting of efficacy of various techniques of RT is also subject to selection bias. Although fractionated RT is suitable for all pituitary tumors, irrespective of size, shape, or proximity to critical structures, radiosurgery is only suitable for small tumors away from the optic chiasm. Studies reporting efficacy of SRS therefore mostly deal with small tumors that are often associated with lower hormone levels. Varying biochemical endpoints, length of follow-up, differing indications, and evolution of RT over time make comparison of different RT techniques difficult.

# *Efficacy and toxicity of conventional RT*

## *Tumor control*

The long-term results after conventional fractionated RT are listed in Table 4.1.[30,31] The actuarial PFS is in the region of 80%–90% at 10 years and 75%–90% at 20 years.[30,31] The largest series of patients with pituitary adenoma treated at The Royal Marsden Hospital in the 1970s and 1980s reported a 10-year PFS of 92% and a 20-year PFS of 88%.[3]

## *Endocrine control*

Fractionated irradiation leads to normalization of excess hormone secretion in the majority of patients, albeit with delay. Using a strict remission criteria of GH below 2 ng/mL and/or normalized IGF-I, normalization is achieved in 30%–50% of acromegalic patients at 5–10 years and in 75% of patients at 15 years after treatment[30,31] (Table 4.1), and the time to normalization of GH is related to pretreatment of GH. Patients with higher initial levels of GH and IGF-I take longer to achieve a remission and have a lower remission rate.[24]

| Authors | Type of adenoma | Number of patients | Follow-up Median (years) | Actuarial PFS % | Late toxicity (%) Visual | Late toxicity (%) Hypopituitarism |
|---|---|---|---|---|---|---|
| Grigsby et al 1989 | NFA, SA | 121 | 11.7 | 89.9 at 10 years | 1.7 | NA |
| McCollough et al. 1991 | NFA, SA | 105 | 7.8 | 95 at 10 years | NA | NA |
| Brada et al. 1993 | NFA, SA | 411 | 10.8 | 94 at 10 years<br>88 at 20 years | 1.5 | 30 at 10 years |
| Tsang et al. 1994 | NFA, SA | 160 | 8.7 | 87 at 10 years | 0 | 23[c] |
| Zierhut et al. 1995 | NFA, SA | 138 | 6.5 | 95 at 5 years | 1.5 | 27[c] |
| Estrada et al. 1997 | SA (ACTH) | 30 | 3.5 | 73 at 2 years[b] | 0 | 48[c] |
| Rush et al. 1997 | NFA, SA | 70 | 8 | NA | NA | 42[c] |
| Breen et al. 1998 | NFA | 120 | 9 | 87.5 at 10 years | 1 | NA |
| Gittoes et al. 1998 | NFA | 126 | 7.5 | 93 at 10 and 15 years | NA | NA |
| Barrande et al. 2000 | SA (GH) | 128 | 11 | 53 at 10 years[b] | 0 | 50 at 10 years |
| Biermasz et al. 2000 | SA (GH) | 36 | 10 | 60 at 10 years[b] | 0 | 54 at 10 years |
| Sasaki et al. 2000 | NFA, SA | 91 | 8.2 | 93 at 10 years | 1 | NA |
| Epaminonda et al. 2001 | SA (GH) | 67 | 10 | 65 at 15 years[b] | 0 | NA |
| Minniti et al. 2005 | SA (GH) | 45 | 12 | 52 at 10 years[b] | 0 | 45 at 10 years |
| Langsenlehner et al. 2007 | NFA, SA | 87 | 15 | 93 at 15 years | 0 | 88 at 10 years |
| Minniti et al. 2007 | SA (ACTH) | 40 | 9 | 78 and 84 at 5 and 10 years[b] | 0 | 62 at 10 years |

NFA, nonfunctioning adenoma; SA, secreting adenoma; NA, not assessed, ACTH—Cushings, GH—acromegaly.
[a] For details of individual papers, please see references [19] and [20].
[b] Hormone concentration normalization.
[c] no time specified.

***Table 4.1***
*Summary of results of published series on conventional RT for pituitary adenomas.*[a]

The rate of decline is log-normal, with an apparent initial faster drop followed by a slower decline. The time to achieve a 50% reduction of GH is in the region of 2 years, with IGF-I reaching half of pretreatment levels over a longer period.[32,33]

After conventional fractionated RT in Cushing's disease, urinary free cortisol (UFC) reduces to 50% of pretreatment value in 6–12 months and plasma cortisol in 12 months.[34] The median time to reaching normal cortisol level is in the region of 24 months.[34] The reported tumor and hormone control at a median follow-up of 8 years are 97% and 74%, respectively (Table 4.1).

The majority of patients with prolactinoma are treated with surgery and optimal medical management. Less than 10% of patients do not achieve hormonal normalization after surgery and medical management.[35] Following with fractionated RT, the 10-year tumor and biochemical control is in the region of 90% and 50%, respectively.[36–38]

## Toxicity of conventional RT

The toxicity of modern fractionated RT with doses of 45–50 Gy at <2 Gy per fraction is low. The reported incidence of presumed radiation optic neuropathy resulting in visual deficit is 1%–3%,[3,4] and risk of necrosis of normal brain structures is almost unknown, although reported in 0.2% of patients.[39] Hypopituitarism represents the most commonly reported late complication, occurring in 30%–60% of patients 10 years after RT.[3,4,31] GH secretion appears to be most frequently affected, followed by gonadotrophin, adrenocorticotrophin (ACTH), and thyroid-stimulating hormone (TSH) deficiency. Long-term routine testing for pituitary deficiency of all pituitary axes is therefore an essential component of management of patients after all types of pituitary RT.

An increased incidence of cerebrovascular accidents and excess cerebrovascular mortality have been reported in patients with pituitary adenoma treated with conventional RT. The cause is multifactorial, including the metabolic and cardiovascular consequences of hypopituitarism, the effects of individual endocrine syndromes, the consequences of surgical intervention, and vascular effects of RT. The relative contribution of radiation to its frequency remains to be determined.[40–43]

Radiation is associated with the development of a second, radiation-induced brain tumor. The reported cumulative incidence of development of gliomas and meningiomas after treatment of pituitary adenoma is in the region of 2% at 20 years, and the median time interval between RT and second intracranial tumor was 17 years.[43–46]

RT to large volumes of normal brain, particularly in children, is associated with neurocognitive impairment. The effect of small-volume irradiation on neurocognitive function in adults is not clear, particularly because the effect of RT cannot be clearly differentiated from the effect of other interventions and the tumor itself.[47,48] Some studies found clear worsening of cognitive function,[49,50] whereas others did not.[47–49,51–53] Most of the studies consisted of small sample sizes and heterogeneous study population.

# Efficacy and toxicity of GKS

## Tumor control

The published results of SRS in patients with nonfunctioning and secreting pituitary adenomas are summarized in systematic reviews[30,31] and are shown in Table 4.2.[30,31,54,55] The majority of published reports provide information on control rate without specifying a time and provide little useful information on the efficacy of SRS. In a study of 380 patients, for both secretory and nonsecretory tumors, the tumor control rate (defined as unchanged or smaller tumor volume) was 90% at a median follow-up of 31 months.[56] In this study, cessation of antisecretory medication was not associated with better tumor control. The summary figure of the actuarial 5-year control rate (PFS) after SRS for nonfunctioning adenomas is in the region of 94% (there are few reliable 10-year results). This rate of tumor control, when only small tumors suitable for SRS are treated, is below that reported after fractionated RT for adenomas of all sizes.

## Endocrine control

The outcome of GK-SRS in acromegaly is shown in Table 4.3.[24,30,31,54,55,57–59] In the summary of published literature, 40% of patients achieved normalization of serum GH, at a median follow-up of 39 months. The time to reach 50% of baseline serum GH, reported in only three studies, is in the region of 1.5–2 years with a slower reduction in IGF-I levels,[60–62] similarly to the rate reported after conventional fractionated RT, suggesting the rate of decline in GH level after SRS is no faster than after conventional RT. Lower pretreatment levels of GH and IGF-I levels, higher total

| Authors | Number of patients | Follow-up Median (months) | Tumor growth control rate (%) | Late toxicity % Visual | Hypopituitarism |
|---|---|---|---|---|---|
| Martinez et al. 1998 | 14 | 26–45 | 100 | 0 | 0 |
| Pan L et al. 1998 | 17 | 29 | 95 | 0 | 0 |
| Ikeda et al. 1998 | 13 | 45 | 100 | 0 | 0 |
| Mokry et al. 1999 | 31 | 20 | 98 | NA | NA |
| Sheehan et al. 2002 | 42 | 31[b] | 97 | 2.3 | 0 |
| Wowra & Stummer 2002 | 45 | 55 | 93 at 3 years | 0 | 14 |
| Petrovich et al. 2003 | 56 | 36 | 94 at 3 years | 4 | NA |
| Pollock & Carpenter 2003 | 33 | 43 | 97 at 5 years | 0 | 28 and 41 at 2 and 5 years |
| Losa et al. 2004 | 56 | 41[b] | 88 at 5 years | 0 | 24 |
| Iwai et al. 2005 | 34 | 60 | 93 at 5 years | 0 | 6 |
| Mingione et al. 2006 | 100 | 45[b] | 92 | 0 | 25 |
| Liscak et al. 2007 | 140 | 60 | 100 | 0 | 2 |
| Pollock et al. 2008 | 62 | 64 | 95 at 3 and 7 years | 0 | 32 at 5 years |
| Kobayashi 2009 | 60 | >3 years | 97 | 4.3 | 8.2 worsening |

NA, not assessed.
[a] For details of individual papers, please see references: [19] and [20].
[b] Mean follow-up.

***Table 4.2***
*Summary of results of published series on SRS for nonfunctioning pituitary adenomas.*[a]

integral dose, higher maximal dose to the adenoma, and small tumor size are predictors of earlier normalization.[59,61,63] IGF-I level of <2.5 times the upper limit was also reported to predict the likelihood of remission (HR, 2.9).[24] A recent systematic review of radiosurgery in patients with new, persistent, and recurrent acromegaly reported a biochemical remission rate of 44.5% in patients who were off medical therapy and 60.3% in those still on medical therapy although this rate was not related to initial hormone levels, and the persistent use of medical treatment may simply represent a group of tumors with higher initial values.[64,65]

Fifty-one percent of patients with Cushing's disease achieved biochemical remission (as defined by plasma cortisol and 24 h UFC level) at a corrected median follow-up of 42 months after SRS[24,30,31,54,55,57,58] (Table 4.4). The reported time to hormonal response ranged from 3 months to 3 years, with no clear difference in the rate of decline of hormone level compared with fractionated RT. SRS for Cushing's disease recorded a remission rate of 54%, with 20% of patients who achieved remission subsequently relapsing, suggesting a higher failure rate than after fractionated treatment.[66]

Hormonal normalization in patients with prolactinoma treated with SRS ranges from 5 months to 40 months[24,30,31,54,55,67,68] (Table 4.5). At a corrected median follow-up of 29 months (median range, 6–55 months), 33% of patients had normalization of serum prolactin concentrations after SRS.[31] One study of 35 patients reported a hormonal normalization of 80% at a median of 96 months and a tumor control of 97%.[68] Large-volume tumors are associated with low probability of remission.[69] There is insufficient information to assess the rate of decline of prolactin in comparison with fractionated RT.

Early studies of linear accelerator SRS report a small number of patients, and the results are broadly equivalent to those reported for GK-SRS.[13] The largest study of 175 patients with pituitary adenoma treated

| Authors | Number of patients | Follow-up Median (months) | Hormone normalization[b] (%) | Late toxicity (%) Visual | Hypopituitarism |
|---|---|---|---|---|---|
| Thoren M et al. 1991 | 21 | 64 | 10 | 0 | 15 |
| Martinez et al. 1998 | 7 | 26–45 | NA | 0 | 0 |
| Pan L et al. 1998 | 15 | 29 | NA | 0 | 0 |
| Morange Ramos et al. 1998 | 15 | 20 | 20 | 6 | 16 |
| Lim et al. 1998 | 20 | 26 | 30 | 5 | 5 |
| Kim et al. 1999 | 11 | 27 | 35 | NA | NA |
| Landolt et al. 1998 | 16 | 17 | 50 | 0 | 16 |
| Mokry et al. 1999 | 16 | 46 | 31 | 0 | NA |
| Hayashi et al. 1999 | 22 | >6 | 41 | 0 | 0 |
| Inoue et al. 1999 | 12 | >24 | 58 | 0 | 0 |
| Zhang et al. 2000 | 68 | >12 | 40 | NA | NA |
| Izawa et al. 2000 | 29 | >6 | 41 | 0 | 0 |
| Pollock et al. 2002 | 26 | 36 | 47 | 4 | 16 |
| Attanasio et al. 2003 | 30 | 46 | 23 | 0 | 6 |
| Choi et al. 2003 | 12 | 43 | 30 | 0 | 0 |
| Jane et al. 2003 | 64 | >18 | 36 | 0 | 28 |
| Petrovich et al. 2003 | 6 | 36 | 100 | 0 | NA |
| Castinetti et al. 2005 | 82 | 49.5[b] | 17 | 0 | 18 |
| Gutt et al. 2005 | 44 | 22 | 48 | NA | NA |
| Kobayashi et al. 2005 | 67 | 63 | 17 | 0 | NA |
| Jezkova et al. 2006 | 96 | 54 | 50 | 0 | 26 |
| Pollock et al. 2007 | 46 | 63 | 11 and 60 at 2 and 5 years | 0 | 33 at 5 years |
| Jagannathan et al. 2009 | 95 | 57 (mean) | 53 | 5[c] | 34 (new) |
| Kobayashi 2009 | 49 | 63 | 17 (normal or nearly normal) | 11 | 15 |
| Wan 2009 | 103 | 60 (minimum) | 37 | 0 | 1.7[d] |
| Castinetti 2009 | 27 | 60 (minimum) | 42 at 50 months | 1.3[d] | 23[d] |
| Iwai 2010 | 26 | 84 | 38 | 0 | 8 |
| Hayashi 2010 | 25 | 36 (mean) | 40 | 0 | 0 |
| Erdur 2011 | 22 | 60 | 55 | 0 | 29 |
| Sheehan 2011 | 130 | 30 | 53 at 30 months | 0 | 34 |

NA, not assessed.
[a] For details of individual papers, please see references [19] and [20].
[b] Mean follow-up.
[c] 3 had previous RT.
[d] Whole series.

**Table 4.3**
*Summary of results of published series on SRS for growth hormone–secreting pituitary adenomas.*[a]

| Authors | Number of patients | Follow-up Median (months) | Tumor growth control rate (%) | Hormone normalization[b] (%) | Late toxicity (%) | |
|---|---|---|---|---|---|---|
| | | | | | Visual | Hypopituitarism |
| Degerblad et al. 1986 | 29 | 3–9 years | 76 | 48 | NA | 55 |
| Ganz et al. 1993 | 4 | 18 | NA | NA | 0 | NA |
| Seo et al. 1995 | 2 | 24 | 100 | NA | 0 | NA |
| Martinez et al. 1998 | 3 | 26–45 | 100 | 100 | 0 | 0 |
| Pan L et al.1998 | 4 | 29 | 95 | NA | 0 | 0 |
| Morange Ramos et al. 1998 | 6 | 20 | 100 | 66 | 0 | 16 |
| Lim et al. 1998 | 4 | 26 | NA | 25 | 2 | 2 |
| Mokry et al.1999 | 5 | 26 | 93 | 20 | 0 | 2 |
| Kim et al. 1999 | 8 | 26 | 100 | 60 | NA | NA |
| Hayashi et al. 1999 | 10 | >6 | 100 | 10 | 0 | 5% |
| Inoue et al.1999 | 3 | >24 | 100 | 100 | 0 | 0 |
| Izawa et al. 2000 | 12 | >6 | 100 | 17 | NA | 0 |
| Sheehan et al. 2000 | 43 | 44 | 100 | 63 | 2 | 16 |
| Hoybye et al. 2001 | 18 | 17 yr | 100 | 83 | 0 | 66 |
| Kobayashi et al. 2002 | 20 | 60 | 100 | 35 | NA | NA |
| Pollock et al. 2002 | 11 | 36 | 85 | 35 | 35 | 8 |
| Choi et al. 2003 | 9 | 43 | 100 | 55 | 0 | 0 |
| Jane et al. 2003 | 45 | >18 | 100 | 63 | 1 | 31 |
| Petrovich et al. 2003 | 4 | 36 | NA | 50 | 0 | NA |
| Devin et al. 2004 | 35 | 35 | 91 | 49 | 0 | 40 |
| Castinetti et al. 2007 | 40 | 54 | 100 | 42 | 0 | NA |
| Jagannathan et al. 2009 | 90 | 45 | 96 | 54 | 5 | 22 |
| Kobayashi 2009 | 25 | 64 (mean) | 100 | 35 | NA | NA |
| Wan 2009 | 68 | 60 (minimum) | 90 | 28 | 0 | 1.7 |
| Castinetti 2009 | 18 | 60 (minimum) | – | 50 at 28 months | 1.3[c] | 23[c] |
| Hayashi 2010 | 13 | 36 (mean) | 97 | 38 | 0 | 0 |
| Sheehan 2011 | 82 | 30 | – | 54 | 0 | 22 |

NA, not assessed.
[a] For details of individual papers, please see references [19] and [20].
[b] Time not specified.
[c] Whole series.

***Table 4.4***
*Summary of results of published series on SRS for ACTH-secreting pituitary adenomas.*[a]

| Authors | Number of patients | Follow-up Median (months) | Hormone normalization (%) | Late toxicity (%) Visual | Hypopituitarism |
|---|---|---|---|---|---|
| Ganz et al. 1993 | 3 | 18 | 0 | 0 | NA |
| Martinez et al. 1998 | 5 | 26–45 | 0 | 0 | 0 |
| Pan L et al. 1998 | 27 | 29 | 30 | 0 | 0 |
| Morange Ramos et al. 1998 | 4 | 20 | 0 | 0 | 16 |
| Lim et al. 1998 | 19 | 26 | 50 | NA | NA |
| Mokry et al. 1999 | 21 | 31 | 57 | 0 | 19 |
| Kim et al. 1999 | 18 | 27 | 16 | NA | NA |
| Hayashi et al. 1999 | 13 | >6 | 15 | NA | 5 |
| Inoue et al. 1999 | 2 | >24 | 50 | 0 | 0 |
| Landolt 2000 | 20 | 29 | 25 | 0 | NA |
| Pan L et al. 2000 | 128 | 33 | 41 | 0 | NA |
| Izawa et al. 2000 | 15 | >6 | 16 | 0 | NA |
| Polllock et al. 2002 | 7 | 26 | 29 | 14 | 16 |
| Choi et al. 2003 | 21 | 43 | 23 | 0 | 0 |
| Jane et al. 2003 | 19 | >18 | 11 | 0 | 21 |
| Petrovich et al. 2003 | 12 | 36 | 83 | 0 | NA |
| Pouratian et al. 2006 | 23 | 55 | 26 | 7 | 28 |
| Jezkova et al. 2009 | 35 | 96 | 80 | NA | NA |
| Kabayashi 2009 | 27 | 37 (mean) | 17 | 0 | 0 |
| Wan 2009 | 176 | 60 (minimum) | 23 | 0 | 1.7 |
| Castinetti 2009 | 15 | 60 (minimum) | 46 at 24 months | 1.3[b] | 23[b] |
| Sheehan 2011 | 32 | 30 | 26 at 25 months | – | 38 |

NA, not assessed.
[a] For details of individual papers, please see references [19] and [20].
[b] Whole series.

***Table 4.5***
*Summary of results of published series on SRS for prolactin-secreting pituitary adenomas.*[a]

with linear accelerator SRS with a single dose of 20 Gy reported local tumor control rate of 97% at a minimum of 12 months follow-up.[70] Actuarial 5-year PFS is not reported. Hormonal normalization rates were 47% for GH-secreting adenomas, 65% with Cushing's disease, and 39% with prolactinomas, with a mean time for hormone normalization of 36 ± 24 months. Within the limited follow-up, 12% developed additional pituitary dysfunction, 3% radiation-induced tissue damage, and 1% radiation-induced neuropathy. These results are difficult to evaluate but are broadly similar to those achieved with GK-SRS.

## Toxicity of GK-SRS

The most commonly observed complication after SRS is hypopituitarism, with a crude incidence ranging from 0% to 66%[30,31]; the actuarial incidence is not fully defined. Some reports suggest a lower incidence of hypopituitarism with GKS, most likely a reflection of selection of patients with small intrasellar tumors. In patients who had previous transphenoidal surgery, lack of enhancing tumor on MRI and pituitary stalk dose of >7.7 Gy are associated with a higher risk of hypopituitarism.[71,72] The doses to the residual pituitary gland and to the distal infundibulum are independent factors for predicting the risk of hypopituitarism.[73,74] In NFPA, the risk of new pituitary deficiency is also correlated with adenoma volume.[75]

The frequency of visual complications should be low if SRS is only offered to patients with adenoma at a safe distance from the optic chiasm and nerves (≥5 mm). Only 10 studies of radiosurgery in acromegaly report visual complications.[65] Optic nerve deficit and cranial nerves palsies were reported in up to 11% of cases.[76,77] Patients with Cushing's disease have a reported 10% incidence of new cranial nerve deficit, with 6% incidence of optic neuropathy, and patients with prolactinoma have 10% incidence of cranial nerve deficit, a high incidence not seen after fractionated treatment.[66,78] Long-term risks of cerebrovascular events and the incidence of second tumors are not yet defined.

A small study of 14 patients of which five received GKS reported no impairment of neurocognitive function.[79]

## *Efficacy and toxicity of CyberKnife radiosurgery/RT*

A study of 100 patients with NFPA treated with CyberKnife to a dose of 21 Gy in three fractions or 25 Gy in five fractions reported a 3-year survival of 98% and local control rate of 98%. Three patients developed transient cystic enlargement, and one patient developed new visual problem.[80] Cho et al.[81] reported a tumor control rate of 92% in 26 patients treated with CyberKnife radiosurgery at a mean of 30 months. Hormonal normalization was achieved in four of the nine (44%) patients, within a mean duration of 16 months; two patients (7.6%) developed worse visual acuity due to cystic enlargement of tumor. A small study of nine patients with acromegaly reported 44% biochemical remission.[82] Other studies also report a tumor control of 95%–100% with radiosurgery or hypofractionated radiotherapy.[83,84] However, long-term follow-up is needed to establish the safety and efficacy of this technique.

## *Efficacy and toxicity of fSCRT*

A review of the efficacy and toxicity of fSCRT in pituitary adenoma is shown in Table 4.6.[13,30,31,85–87] At a corrected median follow-up of 39 months (median range, 10–60 months), tumor control was achieved in 98% of patients. The 5-year actuarial PFS of 92 patients (67 nonfunctioning, 25 secreting) treated at The Royal Marsden Hospital was 97%.[88] The results are similar to patient cohorts treated with conventional RT (Table 4.1).

In the Royal Marsden series, 6 of 18 acromegalic patients (35%) had normalization of GH/IGF-I at a median follow-up of 39 months.[88] Similarly, in a study of 20 patients treated with SCRT, normalization of GH levels was reported in 70% and local control in 100% at a median follow-up of 26 months.[89] Data on the rate of decline are not available, although it is expected to be similar to that seen after conventional RT because the same dose fractionation is used. There is limited data on SCRT in patients with Cushing's disease. In a small series of 12 patients, control of elevated cortisol was reported in nine of 12 patients (75%) at a median time of 29 months.[90]

In a study of 34 patients with acromegaly, SCRT results in 50% hormonal normalization at 30 months.[85] Tumor was stable or reduced in size in 91%; 29% patients developed new pituitary deficiency.

Hypopituitarism was reported in 20%–30% of patients at an overall corrected median follow-up of 60 months. Other late complications were rarely recorded. Although the incidence appears low, longer follow-up is necessary to detect toxicity appearing many years after treatment.

In summary, SCRT achieves tumor control and normalization of hormone hypersecretion at rates similar to the reported rates after conventional fractionated RT. Longer follow-up is required to demonstrate the presumed lower incidence of long-term morbidity compared with conventional CRT.

## *Efficacy and toxicity of proton treatment*

An early study of 30 patients with acromegaly reported 80% decrease in GH at 4.5 years, whereas pituitary deficiency and oculomotor nerve palsies were more common.[91] The use of proton SRS in 22 patients with acromegaly reported 59% normalization of GH at a median of 42 months. New pituitary deficiency was reported in 38% of patients.[92] A study of 47 patients treated with fractionated proton RT reported tumor stabilization in only 41 (87%) patients at a minimum 6 months follow-up; one patient developed temporal lobe necrosis, three developed new significant visual deficits, and 11

| Authors | Number of patients | Follow-up Median (months) | Tumor growth control rate (%) | Late toxicity (%) Visual | Hypopituitarism |
|---|---|---|---|---|---|
| Coke et al. 1997 | 19[b] | 9 | 100 | 0 | 0 |
| Mitsumori et al. 1998 | 30[b] | 33 | 86 at 3 years | 0 | 20 |
| Milker-Zabel et al. 2001 | 68[b] | 38 | 93 at 5 years | 7 | 5 |
| Paek et al. 2005 | 68 | 30 | 98 at 5 years | 3 | 6 |
| Colin et al. 2005 | 110[b] | 48 | 99 at 5 years | 2 | 29 at 4 years |
| Minniti et al. 2006 | 92[b] | 32 | 98 at 5 years | 1 | 22 |
| Selch et al. 2006 | 39[b] | 60 | 100 | 0 | 15 |
| Kong et al. 2007 | 64[b] | 37 | 97 at 4 years | 0 | 11 |
| Snead et al. 2008 | 100[b] | 6.7 years | 98 at 10 year for NFA and 73 SA | 1 | 35 |
| Roug 2010 | 34[b] | 34 | 91(50% hormonal normalization) | – | – |
| Schalin-Jantti 2010 | 30 | 5.3 years | 100 | 0 | 23 |
| Weber 2011 | 27[b] | 72.4 | 96 | 4 | 8 |

[a] For details of individual papers, please see references [19] and [20].
[b] Series include secreting pituitary adenomas.

***Table 4.6***
*Summary of results on published studies on SCRT for pituitary adenomas.*[a]

developed hypopituitarism.[93] The available peer review reports of protons for pituitary adenoma demonstrate disappointing efficacy and toxicity.

# *Factors affecting the efficacy of radiation*

## *Hormone levels and tumor size*

There are no studies demonstrating dose response for conventional RT, with no clear improvement in tumor control after higher radiation doses beyond 45–50 Gy. With radiosurgery, the suggestion is that the tumor margin dose correlates with tumor control, although this correlation may also be related to the size of the residual tumor.[57]

With conventional RT in acromegalic patients, the proportion of patients achieving hormonal remission increases with time, and this is a function of the steady rate of decline in hormone hypersecretion. Consequently, patients with lower initial hormone levels reach normalization earlier,[94] and this is also seen after radiosurgery.[95]

Smaller tumors associated with lower levels of pretreatment hormones are also associated with better response.[56,67,78,82,96,97] The rate of endocrine remission was increased by a factor of 1.30 (95% CI, 1.05–1.61), with each 1 cc reduction in treatment volume.[56]

## *Medical treatment during radiation*

Some studies suggest an increased rate of biochemical response in secretory adenoma irradiated while off medical treatment,[56,78,97,98] although this is not substantiated and may simply reflect the suppressed hormone levels with medical treatment not reflective of the true level. Hence, the time to reach normal level may appear longer than would be the case for similar levels in patients not on medical therapy.

## *Dose of radiosurgery*

A higher margin dose while using GKS results in a better chance of endocrine remission and control of tumor growth.[56] The odds ratio (OR) of adenoma volume control for each 1 Gy increase in margin dose was 1.062 (95% CI, 1.008–1.118) for all tumors and 1.15 (95% CI, 1.022–1.294) for secretory adenoma. Tumor margin dose was also correlated with time to remission. A 5 Gy reduction in dose increased the time to remission by a factor of 1.36 (95% CI, 1.05–1.79).

# Re-irradiation for recurrent pituitary adenoma

Re-irradiation for progression of pituitary adenoma after RT is considered risky because of the presumed cumulative radiation damage to optic apparatus, cranial nerves, and normal brain. Fractionated re-irradiation using conventional or stereotactic techniques is feasible with acceptable toxicity,[29] providing there is 3–4 year gap from primary RT to doses of 45 Gy at <1.8 Gy fraction. SRS has also been used for small recurrent lesions[99] with hormonal normalization in some patients with acromegaly and a proportion of patients with ACTH-secreting adenoma.[28,99] Although the impression is that late toxicity of re-irradiation is uncommon, there are insufficient long-term data to demonstrate it.

# Choice between radiosurgery and RT

Many arguments have been put in favor of radiosurgery, such as convenient single-day treatment, shorter period to achieve biochemical remission, lower incidence of new hormonal deficits, and lower risk of radiation-induced tumors.[100] Although there are no direct comparative studies of RT with radiosurgery, the retrospective RT and radiosurgery cohorts corrected for confounding factors such as the technique, dose, pretreatment hormone levels, and tumor size should provide some information on which to base an informed judgment.

An example of inappropriate comparison is an apparently superior results of an early report of radiosurgery in patients with acromegaly treated between 1994 and 1996 when compared with a cohort of patients treated at another institution between 1973 and 1992 with low-dose conventional RT who had higher GH levels and likely larger tumors than those suitable for radiosurgery. In addition, the measure for comparative efficacy was time to reach normalization, which is not the appropriate comparative endpoint to provide a measure of rate of GH decline in the different cohorts.[101] Although the unfounded belief in faster decline of GH levels persists, the majority of published studies and systematic reviews fail to show superiority of radiosurgery over fractionated irradiation in terms of rate of hormone decline.[30,31]

Loss of pituitary function is cumulative over a period of 10–15 years.[102] Although there are many studies reporting long-term pituitary dysfunction with RT, radiosurgery data have not been reported in cumulative actuarial manner and are frequently not mature enough to assess long-term effect on pituitary function. The only study with minimum 10-year follow-up reported 46% endocrine remission in acromegaly patients with 50% developing new pituitary insufficiency where the majority of hypopituitarism appeared >5 years after radiosurgery.[103] Currently, there is therefore no evidence that radiosurgery results in lower incidence of new hypopituitarism. A similar argument exists for the incidence of second tumors, where radiosurgery series do not have sufficient length of follow-up and are generally not large enough to detect a change from the low 20-year rate reported for fractionated RT.

In conclusion, although patients with small residual pituitary adenomas away from critical structures can be treated with single-fraction radiosurgery as safely as with fractionated treatment, the tumor control results are inferior to fractionated RT, and it remains unclear whether this group, particularly with NFPA, should be treated at all. In patients with larger tumors requiring RT, fractionated high-precision conformal radiation remains the treatment of choice.

# Conclusions

Fractionated RT is an effective treatment achieving excellent disease control and normalization of hormone levels. Although overall safe, it is not devoid of side effects, and it should only be used when the risks from the disease itself are considered to outweigh the risks from the treatment. The balance of risks should consider not only early consequences of the disease and treatment, measured in terms of disease control and immediate morbidity, but also late effects, particularly the effect on survival and quality of life, both of which are not so well defined.

Residual tumors, most of which have indolent natural history, pose little threat to function, unless close to the optic apparatus, or when destructively invading surrounding structures, which is an uncommon event. The risks are therefore minimal and in the absence of progression or hormone hypersecretion, there is currently little justification to offer adjuvant treatment whether in the form of fractionated or single-fraction treatment. However, the policy of surveillance requires close monitoring, usually in the form of annual MRI proceeding with timely irradiation, before the need for further surgery. The aim is to arrest tumor growth without the additional risks of reoperation.

In secreting tumors, irradiation is generally offered to patients with persistent hormone elevation that is not decreasing at the expected rate after previous intervention. That generally means persistent elevation in patients with acromegaly, Cushing's disease, and other secreting adenomas, regardless of the actual level, as the aim in most instances is to reach normalization. In patients with acromegaly treated with somatostatin analogs, the expense and inconvenience of protracted systemic treatment would also argue for early RT to allow for gradual withdrawal of medical treatment. The alternative is to continue medical management indefinitely without RT. It is not clear which policy is associated with better long-term survival and quality of life, and this should ideally be tested in a prospective randomized trial. The proposed phase II RTOG trial 0930 is planned to evaluate radiosurgery for the treatment of persistent acromegaly after transphenoidal surgery.

The current practice is therefore to offer treatment to patients with progressive nonfunctioning (or secretory) adenomas considered to be of threat to function and to patients with secretory adenomas with persistent hypersecretion. On the evidence available, single-fraction radiosurgery, although apparently more convenient, is less effective in achieving long-term disease control of adenoma tumor masses and without faster decline in hormone levels in secreting tumors. In addition, single-fraction treatment of larger adenomas close to critical structures carries a significant risk of radiation-induced damage. Fractionated irradiation either as CRT or SCRT therefore remains the standard of care with SRS considered as an experimental and in some instances less effective treatment.

The availability of radiosurgery has in some centers led to the policy of adjuvant single-fraction radiosurgery in patients with small residual tumors. It is not clear that such practice is appropriate because the risks from small nonfunctioning adenomas are unlikely to be greater than the risks of SRS. Similarly, some patients with slow decline in hormone levels, particularly in acromegaly, have been offered additional SRS. There is no clear evidence that further irradiation significantly speeds up the hormone decline while carrying additional morbidity of re-irradiation.

Modern conformal techniques of fractionated irradiation have become standard practice, with many centers offering the additional accuracy of high-precision treatment with "stereotactic" guidance. Such practice relies on the expertise of accurate target definition using modern imaging, on the precision of the system based on exhaustive QA program, and infrastructure, particularly in the form of expertise of staff in complex techniques of treatment planning and delivery. In the final analysis, it is likely that the expertise at all levels of staff is more important to the success of pituitary RT than the equipment and the precise technique of treatment. Although proton therapy is currently under investigation and may have a potential of treating less normal brain, the complexity of the technology and the limitation in our understanding of the biological and clinical effects mean that carefully designed prospective studies are required before accepting it as an effective and safe alternative to photon irradiation.

## References


1. Grigsby PW, Simpson JR, Emami BN, Fineberg BB, Schwartz HG. Prognostic factors and results of surgery and postoperative irradiation in the management of pituitary adenomas. *Int J Radiat Oncol Biol Phys*. 1989;16(6):1411–17.
2. McCollough WM, Marcus RB, Jr., Rhoton AL, Jr., Ballinger WE, Million RR. Long-term follow-up of radiotherapy for pituitary adenoma: The absence of late recurrence after greater than or equal to 4500 cGy. *Int J Radiat Oncol Biol Phys*. 1991;21(3):607–14.
3. Brada M, Rajan B, Traish D, Ashley S, Holmes-Sellors PJ, Nussey S, et al. The long-term efficacy of conservative surgery and radiotherapy in the control of pituitary adenomas. *Clin Endocrinol (Oxf)*. 1993;38(6):571–8.
4. Tsang RW, Brierley JD, Panzarella T, Gospodarowicz MK, Sutcliffe SB, Simpson WJ. Radiation therapy for pituitary adenoma: Treatment outcome and prognostic factors. *Int J Radiat Oncol Biol Phys*. 1994;30(3):557–65.
5. Zierhut D, Flentje M, Adolph J, Erdmann J, Raue F, Wannenmacher M. External radiotherapy of pituitary adenomas. *Int J Radiat Oncol Biol Phys*. 1995; 33(2):307–14.
6. Rush S, Cooper PR. Symptom resolution, tumor control, and side effects following postoperative radiotherapy for pituitary macroadenomas. *Int J Radiat Oncol Biol Phys*. 1997;37(5):1031–4.
7. Breen P, Flickinger JC, Kondziolka D, Martinez AJ. Radiotherapy for nonfunctional pituitary adenoma: Analysis of long-term tumor control. *J Neurosurg*. 1998;89(6):933–8.

8. Gittoes NJ, Bates AS, Tse W, Bullivant B, Sheppard MC, Clayton RN, et al. Radiotherapy for non-function pituitary tumours. *Clin Endocrinol (Oxf)*. 1998;48(3):331–7.
9. Sasaki R, Murakami M, Okamoto Y, Kono K, Yoden E, Nakajima T, et al. The efficacy of conventional radiation therapy in the management of pituitary adenoma. *Int J Radiat Oncol Biol Phys*. 2000;47(5):1337–45.
10. Chanson P, Salenave S, Kamenicky P, Cazabat L, Young J. Pituitary tumours: Acromegaly. *Best Pract Res Clin Endocrinol Metab*. 2009;23(5):555–74.
11. Khoo VS, Oldham M, Adams EJ, Bedford JL, Webb S, Brada M. Comparison of intensity-modulated tomotherapy with stereotactically guided conformal radiotherapy for brain tumors. *Int J Radiat Oncol Biol Phys*. 1999;45(2):415–25.
12. Karger CP, Jakel O, Debus J, Kuhn S, Hartmann GH. Three-dimensional accuracy and interfractional reproducibility of patient fixation and positioning using a stereotactic head mask system. *Int J Radiat Oncol Biol Phys*. 2001;49(5):1493–504.
13. Ajithkumar T, Brada M. Stereotactic linear accelerator radiotherapy for pituitary tumors. *Treat Endocrinol*. 2004;3(4):211–16.
14. Cozzi L, Clivio A, Bauman G, Cora S, Nicolini G, Pellegrini R, et al. Comparison of advanced irradiation techniques with photons for benign intracranial tumours. *Radiother Oncol*. 2006;80(2):268–73.
15. Gill SS, Thomas DG, Warrington AP, Brada M. Relocatable frame for stereotactic external beam radiotherapy. *Int J Radiat Oncol Biol Phys*. 1991;20(3):599–603.
16. Graham JD, Warrington AP, Gill SS, Brada M. A non-invasive, relocatable stereotactic frame for fractionated radiotherapy and multiple imaging. *Radiother Oncol*. 1991;21(1):60–2.
17. Kumar S, Burke K, Nalder C, Jarrett P, Mubata C, A'Hern R, et al. Treatment accuracy of fractionated stereotactic radiotherapy. *Radiother Oncol*. 2005;74(1):53–9.
18. Greco C, Wolden S. Current status of radiotherapy with proton and light ion beams. *Cancer*. 2007;109(7):1227–38.
19. Greenman Y, Stern N. Non-functioning pituitary adenomas. *Best Pract Res Clin Endocrinol Metab*. 2009;23(5):625–38.
20. Reddy R, Cudlip S, Byrne JV, Karavitaki N, Wass JA. Can we ever stop imaging in surgically treated and radiotherapy-naive patients with non-functioning pituitary adenoma? *Eur J Endocrinol*. 2011;165(5):739–44.
21. Brochier S, Galland F, Kujas M, Parker F, Gaillard S, Raftopoulos C, et al. Factors predicting relapse of nonfunctioning pituitary macroadenomas after neurosurgery: A study of 142 patients. *Eur J Endocrinol*. 2010;163(2):193–200.
22. O'Sullivan EP, Woods C, Glynn N, Behan LA, Crowley R, O'Kelly P, et al. The natural history of surgically treated but radiotherapy-naive nonfunctioning pituitary adenomas. *Clin Endocrinol (Oxf)*. 2009;71(5):709–14.
23. Chang EF, Zada G, Kim S, Lamborn KR, Quinones-Hinojosa A, Tyrrell JB, et al. Long-term recurrence and mortality after surgery and adjuvant radiotherapy for nonfunctional pituitary adenomas. *J Neurosurg*. 2008;108(4):736–45.
24. Castinetti F, Nagai M, Morange I, Dufour H, Caron P, Chanson P, et al. Long-term results of stereotactic radiosurgery in secretory pituitary adenomas. *J Clin Endocrinol Metab*. 2009;94(9):3400–7.
25. Laws ER. Surgery for acromegaly: Evolution of the techniques and outcomes. *Rev Endocr Metab Disord*. 2008;9(1):67–70.
26. Vance ML. Cushing's disease: Radiation therapy. *Pituitary*. 2009;12(1):11–14.
27. Sheplan Olsen LJ, Robles Irizarry L, Chao ST, Weil RJ, Hamrahian AH, Hatipoglu B, et al. Radiotherapy for prolactin-secreting pituitary tumors. *Pituitary*. 2012; 15(2):135–45.
28. Swords FM, Monson JP, Besser GM, Chew SL, Drake WM, Grossman AB, et al. Gamma knife radiosurgery: A safe and effective salvage treatment for pituitary tumours not controlled despite conventional radiotherapy. *Eur J Endocrinol*. 2009;161(6):819–28.
29. Brada M, Jankowska P. Radiotherapy for pituitary adenomas. *Endocrinol Metab Clin North Am*. 2008;37(1):263–75.
30. Brada M, Ajithkumar TV, Minniti G. Radiosurgery for pituitary adenomas. *Clin Endocrinol (Oxf)*. 2004;61(5):531–43.
31. Minniti G, Gilbert DC, Brada M. Modern techniques for pituitary radiotherapy. *Rev Endocr Metab Disord*. 2009;10(2):135–44.
32. Biermasz NR, Dulken HV, Roelfsema F. Postoperative radiotherapy in acromegaly is effective in reducing GH concentration to safe levels. *Clin Endocrinol (Oxf)*. 2000;53(3):321–7.
33. Minniti G, Jaffrain-Rea ML, Osti M, Esposito V, Santoro A, Solda F, et al. The long-term efficacy of conventional radiotherapy in patients with GH-secreting pituitary adenomas. *Clin Endocrinol (Oxf)*. 2005;62(2):210–16.
34. Minniti G, Osti M, Jaffrain-Rea ML, Esposito V, Cantore G, Maurizi Enrici R. Long-term follow-up results of postoperative radiation therapy for Cushing's disease. *J Neurooncol*. 2007;84(1):79–84.
35. Oh MC, Aghi MK. Dopamine agonist-resistant prolactinomas. *J Neurosurg*. 2011;114(5):1369–79.
36. Tsagarakis S, Grossman A, Plowman PN, Jones AE, Touzel R, Rees LH, et al. Megavoltage pituitary irradiation

in the management of prolactinomas: Long-term follow-up. *Clin Endocrinol (Oxf)*. 1991;34(5):399–406.
37. Johnston DG, Hall K, Kendall Taylor P, Ross WM, Crombie AL, Cook DB, et al. The long-term effects of megavoltage radiotherapy as sole or combined therapy for large prolactinomas: Studies with high definition computerized tomography. *Clin Endocrinol (Oxf)*. 1986;24(6):675–85.
38. Mehta AE, Reyes FI, Faiman C. Primary radiotherapy of prolactinomas. Eight- to 15-year follow-up. *Am J Med.* 1987;83(1):49–58.
39. Becker G, Kocher M, Kortmann RD, Paulsen F, Jeremic B, Muller RP, et al. Radiation therapy in the multimodal treatment approach of pituitary adenoma. *Strahlenther Onkol*. 2002;178(4):173–86.
40. Brada M, Ashley S, Ford D, Traish D, Burchell L, Rajan B. Cerebrovascular mortality in patients with pituitary adenoma. *Clin Endocrinol (Oxf)*. 2002;57(6):713–17.
41. Brada M, Burchell L, Ashley S, Traish D. The incidence of cerebrovascular accidents in patients with pituitary adenoma. *Int J Radiat Oncol Biol Phys*. 1999;45(3):693–8.
42. Tomlinson JW, Holden N, Hills RK, Wheatley K, Clayton RN, Bates AS, et al. Association between premature mortality and hypopituitarism. West Midlands Prospective Hypopituitary Study Group. *Lancet*. 2001;357(9254):425–31.
43. Erfurth EM, Bulow B, Svahn-Tapper G, Norrving B, Odh K, Mikoczy Z, et al. Risk factors for cerebrovascular deaths in patients operated and irradiated for pituitary tumors. *J Clin Endocrinol Metab*. 2002;87(11):4892–9.
44. Tsang R, Laperriere N, Simpson W, Brierley J, Panzarella T, Smyth H. Glioma arising after radiation therapy for pituitary adenoma: A report of four patients and estimation of risk. *Cancer*. 1993;72:2227–33.
45. Brada M, Ford D, Ashley S, Bliss JM, Crowley S, Mason M, et al. Risk of second brain tumour after conservative surgery and radiotherapy for pituitary adenoma. *Br Med J*. 1992;304(6838):1343–6.
46. Norberg L, Johansson R, Rasmuson T. Intracranial tumours after external fractionated radiotherapy for pituitary adenomas in northern Sweden. *Acta Oncol*. 2010;49(8):1276–82.
47. Peace KA, Orme SM, Padayatty SJ, Godfrey HP, Belchetz PE. Cognitive dysfunction in patients with pituitary tumour who have been treated with transfrontal or transsphenoidal surgery or medication. *Clin Endocrinol (Oxf)*. 1998;49(3):391–6.
48. Guinan EM, Lowy C, Stanhope N, Lewis PD, Kopelman MD. Cognitive effects of pituitary tumours and their treatments: Two case studies and an investigation of 90 patients. *J Neurol Neurosurg Psychiatry*. 1998;65(6):870–6.
49. McCord MW, Buatti JM, Fennell EM, Mendenhall WM, Marcus RB, Jr, Rhoton AL, et al. Radiotherapy for pituitary adenoma: Long-term outcome and sequelae. *Int J Radiat Oncol Biol Phys*. 1997;39(2):437–44.
50. Noad R, Narayanan KR, Howlett T, Lincoln NB, Page RC. Evaluation of the effect of radiotherapy for pituitary tumours on cognitive function and quality of life. *Clin Oncol (R Coll Radiol)*. 2004;16(4):233–7.
51. Brummelman P, Elderson MF, Dullaart RP, van den Bergh AC, Timmer CA, van den Berg G, et al. Cognitive functioning in patients treated for nonfunctioning pituitary macroadenoma and the effects of pituitary radiotherapy. *Clin Endocrinol (Oxf)*. 2011;74(4):481–7.
52. van den Bergh AC, van den Berg G, Schoorl MA, Sluiter WJ, van der Vliet AM, Hoving EW, et al. Immediate postoperative radiotherapy in residual nonfunctioning pituitary adenoma: Beneficial effect on local control without additional negative impact on pituitary function and life expectancy. *Int J Radiat Oncol Biol Phys*. 2007;67(3):863–9.
53. Peace KA, Orme SM, Sebastian JP, Thompson AR, Barnes S, Ellis A, et al. The effect of treatment variables on mood and social adjustment in adult patients with pituitary disease. *Clin Endocrinol (Oxf)*. 1997;46(4):445–50.
54. Kobayashi T. Long-term results of stereotactic gamma knife radiosurgery for pituitary adenomas. Specific strategies for different types of adenoma. *Prog Neurol Surg*. 2009;22:77–95.
55. Wan H, Chihiro O, Yuan S. MASEP gamma knife radiosurgery for secretory pituitary adenomas: Experience in 347 consecutive cases. *J Exp Clin Cancer Res*. 2009;28:36.
56. Sheehan JP, Pouratian N, Steiner L, Laws ER, Vance ML. Gamma Knife surgery for pituitary adenomas: Factors related to radiological and endocrine outcomes. *J Neurosurg*. 2011;114(2):303–9.
57. Jagannathan J, Yen CP, Pouratian N, Laws ER, Sheehan JP. Stereotactic radiosurgery for pituitary adenomas: A comprehensive review of indications, techniques and long-term results using the Gamma Knife. *J Neurooncol*. 2009;92(3):345–56.
58. Hayashi M, Chernov M, Tamura N, Nagai M, Yomo S, Ochiai T, et al. Gamma Knife robotic microradiosurgery of pituitary adenomas invading the cavernous sinus: Treatment concept and results in 89 cases. *J Neurooncol*. 2010;98(2):185–94.
59. Poon TL, Leung SC, Poon CY, Yu CP. Predictors of outcome following Gamma Knife surgery for acromegaly. *J Neurosurg*. 2010;113(Suppl):149–52.
60. Attanasio R, Epaminonda P, Motti E, Giugni E, Ventrella L, Cozzi R, et al. Gamma-knife radiosurgery in acromegaly: A 4-year follow-up study. *J Clin Endocrinol Metab*. 2003;88(7):3105–12.

61. Castinetti F, Taieb D, Kuhn JM, Chanson P, Tamura M, Jaquet P, et al. Outcome of gamma knife radiosurgery in 82 patients with acromegaly: Correlation with initial hypersecretion. *J Clin Endocrinol Metab*. 2005;90(8):4483–8.
62. Jagannathan J, Sheehan JP, Pouratian N, Laws ER, Jr, Steiner L, Vance ML. Gamma knife radiosurgery for acromegaly: Outcomes after failed transsphenoidal surgery. *Neurosurgery*. 2008;62(6):1262–9;
63. Castinetti F, Regis J, Dufour H, Brue T. Role of stereotactic radiosurgery in the management of pituitary adenomas. *Nat Rev Endocrinol*. 2010;6(4):214–23.
64. Yang I, Kim W, De Salles A, Bergsneider M. A systematic analysis of disease control in acromegaly treated with radiosurgery. *Neurosurg Focus*. 2010;29(4):E13.
65. Stapleton CJ, Liu CY, Weiss MH. The role of stereotactic radiosurgery in the multimodal management of growth hormone-secreting pituitary adenomas. *Neurosurg Focus*. 2010;29(4):E11.
66. Jagannathan J, Sheehan JP, Pouratian N, Laws ER, Steiner L, Vance ML. Gamma Knife surgery for Cushing's disease. *J Neurosurg*. 2007;106(6):980–7.
67. Pollock BE, Brown PD, Nippoldt TB, Young WF Jr. Pituitary tumor type affects the chance of biochemical remission after radiosurgery of hormone-secreting pituitary adenomas. *Neurosurgery*. 2008;62(6):1271–6; discussion 6–8.
68. Jezkova J, Hana V, Krsek M, Weiss V, Vladyka V, Liscak R, et al. Use of the Leksell gamma knife in the treatment of prolactinoma patients. *Clin Endocrinol (Oxf)*. 2009;70(5):732–41.
69. Tanaka S, Link MJ, Brown PD, Stafford SL, Young WF Jr, Pollock BE. Gamma knife radiosurgery for patients with prolactin-secreting pituitary adenomas. *World Neurosurg*. 2010;74(1):147–52.
70. Voges J, Kocher M, Runge M, Poggenborg J, Lehrke R, Lenartz D, et al. Linear accelerator radiosurgery for pituitary macroadenomas: A 7-year follow-up study. *Cancer*. 2006;107(6):1355–64.
71. Rowland NC, Aghi MK. Radiation treatment strategies for acromegaly. *Neurosurg Focus*. 2010;29(4):E12.
72. Feigl GC, Bonelli CM, Berghold A, Mokry M. Effects of gamma knife radiosurgery of pituitary adenomas on pituitary function. *J Neurosurg*. 2002;97(5 Suppl):415–21.
73. Marek J, Jezkova J, Hana V, Krsek M, Bandurova L, Pecen L, et al. Is it possible to avoid hypopituitarism after irradiation of pituitary adenomas by the Leksell gamma knife? *Eur J Endocrinol*. 2011;164(2):169–78.
74. Leenstra JL, Tanaka S, Kline RW, Brown PD, Link MJ, Nippoldt TB, et al. Factors associated with endocrine deficits after stereotactic radiosurgery of pituitary adenomas. *Neurosurgery*. 2010;67(1):27–32.
75. Pollock BE, Cochran J, Natt N, Brown PD, Erickson D, Link MJ, et al. Gamma knife radiosurgery for patients with nonfunctioning pituitary adenomas: Results from a 15-year experience. *Int J Radiat Oncol Biol Phys*. 2008;70(5):1325–9.
76. Kobayashi T, Mori Y, Uchiyama Y, Kida Y, Fujitani S. Long-term results of gamma knife surgery for growth hormone-producing pituitary adenoma: Is the disease difficult to cure? *J Neurosurg*. 2005;102(Suppl):119–23.
77. Tinnel BA, Henderson MA, Witt TC, Fakiris AJ, Worth RM, Des Rosiers PM, et al. Endocrine response after gamma knife-based stereotactic radiosurgery for secretory pituitary adenoma. *Stereotact Funct Neurosurg*. 2008;86(5):292–6.
78. Pouratian N, Sheehan J, Jagannathan J, Laws ER Jr, Steiner L, Vance ML. Gamma knife radiosurgery for medically and surgically refractory prolactinomas. *Neurosurgery*. 2006;59(2):255–66.
79. Tooze A, Hiles CL, Sheehan JP. Neurocognitive changes in pituitary adenoma patients after gamma knife radiosurgery: A preliminary study. *World Neurosurg*. 2012;78(1–2):122–8.
80. Iwata H, Sato K, Tatewaki K, Yokota N, Inoue M, Baba Y, et al. Hypofractionated stereotactic radiotherapy with CyberKnife for nonfunctioning pituitary adenoma: High local control with low toxicity. *Neuro Oncol*. 2011;13(8):916–22.
81. Cho CB, Park HK, Joo WI, Chough CK, Lee KJ, Rha HK. Stereotactic radiosurgery with the CyberKnife for pituitary adenomas. *J Korean Neurosurg Soc*. 2009;45(3):157–63.
82. Roberts BK, Ouyang DL, Lad SP, Chang SD, Harsh GRt, Adler JR Jr, et al. Efficacy and safety of CyberKnife radiosurgery for acromegaly. *Pituitary*. 2007;10(1):19–25.
83. Killory BD, Kresl JJ, Wait SD, Ponce FA, Porter R, White WL. Hypofractionated CyberKnife radiosurgery for perichiasmatic pituitary adenomas: Early results. *Neurosurgery*. 2009;64(2 Suppl):A19–25.
84. Kajiwara K, Saito K, Yoshikawa K, Kato S, Akimura T, Nomura S, et al. Image-guided stereotactic radiosurgery with the CyberKnife for pituitary adenomas. *Minim Invasive Neurosurg*. 2005;48(2):91–6.
85. Roug S, Rasmussen AK, Juhler M, Kosteljanetz M, Poulsgaard L, Heeboll H, et al. Fractionated stereotactic radiotherapy in patients with acromegaly: An interim single-centre audit. *Eur J Endocrinol*. 2010;162(4):685–94.
86. Schalin-Jantti C, Valanne L, Tenhunen M, Setala K, Paetau A, Sane T, et al. Outcome of fractionated stereotactic radiotherapy in patients with pituitary adenomas resistant to conventional treatments: A 5.25-year follow-up study. *Clin Endocrinol (Oxf)*. 2010;73(1):72–7.
87. Weber DC, Momjian S, Pralong FP, Meyer P, Villemure JG, Pica A. Adjuvant or radical fractionated stereotactic radiotherapy for patients with pituitary

functional and nonfunctional macroadenoma. *Radiat Oncol*. 2011;6:169.

88. Minniti G, Traish D, Ashley S, Gonsalves A, Brada M. Fractionated stereotactic conformal radiotherapy for secreting and nonsecreting pituitary adenomas. *Clin Endocrinol (Oxf)*. 2006;64(5):542–8.
89. Milker-Zabel S, Debus J, Thilmann C, Schlegel W, Wannenmacher M. Fractionated stereotactically guided radiotherapy and radiosurgery in the treatment of functional and nonfunctional adenomas of the pituitary gland. *Int J Radiat Oncol Biol Phys*. 2001;50(5):1279–86.
90. Colin P, Jovenin N, Delemer B, Caron J, Grulet H, Hecart AC, et al. Treatment of pituitary adenomas by fractionated stereotactic radiotherapy: A prospective study of 110 patients. *Int J Radiat Oncol Biol Phys*. 2005;62(2):333–41.
91. Ludecke DK, Lutz BS, Niedworok G. The choice of treatment after incomplete adenomectomy in acromegaly: Proton—versus high voltage radiation. *Acta Neurochir (Wien)*. 1989;96(1–2):32–8.
92. Petit JH, Biller BM, Coen JJ, Swearingen B, Ancukiewicz M, Bussiere M, et al. Proton stereotactic radiosurgery in management of persistent acromegaly. *Endocr Pract*. 2007;13(7):726–34.
93. Ronson BB, Schulte RW, Han KP, Loredo LN, Slater JM, Slater JD. Fractionated proton beam irradiation of pituitary adenomas. *Int J Radiat Oncol Biol Phys*. 2006;64(2):425–34.
94. Jenkins PJ, Bates P, Carson MN, Stewart PM, Wass JA. Conventional pituitary irradiation is effective in lowering serum growth hormone and insulin-like growth factor-I in patients with acromegaly. *J Clin Endocrinol Metab*. 2006;91(4):1239–45.
95. Iwai Y, Yamanaka K, Yoshimura M, Kawasaki I, Yamagami K, Yoshioka K. Gamma knife radiosurgery for growth hormone-producing adenomas. *J Clin Neurosci*. 2010;17(3):299–304.
96. Kobayashi T, Kida Y, Mori Y. Gamma knife radiosurgery in the treatment of Cushing disease: Long-term results. *J Neurosurg*. 2002;97(5 Suppl):422–8.
97. Castinetti F, Nagai M, Dufour H, Kuhn JM, Morange I, Jaquet P, et al. Gamma knife radiosurgery is a successful adjunctive treatment in Cushing's disease. *Eur J Endocrinol*. 2007;156(1):91–8.
98. Pollock BE, Jacob JT, Brown PD, Nippoldt TB. Radiosurgery of growth hormone-producing pituitary adenomas: Factors associated with biochemical remission. *J Neurosurg*. 2007;106(5):833–8.
99. Edwards AA, Swords FM, Plowman PN. Focal radiation therapy for patients with persistent/recurrent pituitary adenoma, despite previous radiotherapy. *Pituitary*. 2009;12(1):30–4.
100. Pollock BE. Comparing radiation therapy and radiosurgery for pituitary adenoma patients. *World Neurosurg*. 2012;78(1–2):58–9.
101. Landolt AM, Haller D, Lomax N, Scheib S, Schubiger O, Siegfried J, et al. Stereotactic radiosurgery for recurrent surgically treated acromegaly: Comparison with fractionated radiotherapy. *J Neurosurg*. 1998;88(6):1002–8.
102. Oldfield EH. Editorial: Unresolved issues: Radiosurgery versus radiation therapy: Medical suppression of growth hormone production during radiosurgery: And endoscopic surgery versus microscopic surgery. *Neurosurg Focus*. 2010;29(4):E16.
103. Ronchi CL, Attanasio R, Verrua E, Cozzi R, Ferrante E, Loli P, et al. Efficacy and tolerability of gamma knife radiosurgery in acromegaly: A 10-year follow-up study. *Clin Endocrinol (Oxf)*. 2009;71(6):846–52.

# 5

# Replacement therapy in adult hypopituitarism

*Anna G. Nilsson, Gudmundur Johannsson*

## *Introduction*

The function of the hypothalamic–pituitary axis is essential for the regulation of key endocrine systems[1] (Figure 5.1). Already in the third century B.C., Aristotle concluded that the brain was necessary for the maintenance of the body.[2] The experimental evidence of the role of the hypothalamus and the pituitary in the regulation of several endocrine systems is, however, relatively recent.[3,4] It was not until the beginning of the 20th century that the role of the pituitary as a regulator of growth and maturation was described when injections of pituitary extracts in rodents resulted in stimulation and maturation of peripheral glands.[5] The clinical syndrome of hypopituitarism was first described in 1914.[6] The history of the management of hypopituitarism has been influenced by the availability of the hormone used for replacement therapy. Desiccated thyroid hormone became available in 1891, synthetic estrogen and testosterone became available in the third decade of the 20th century, synthetic hydrocortisone (HC) became available in 1948, and the first placebo-controlled trials of growth hormone (GH) replacement therapy in adults were published in 1989.[7,8]

In the early 1990s, it was described that the mortality rate in adults with hypopituitarism was twofold in men and nearly threefold in women[9] (Figure 5.2). The reason for this observation was that GH was not replaced in adults with hypopituitarism because its importance for adults was not generally recognized. Another putative possibility is that other hormones were not adequately replaced, in particular, an unphysiological or inappropriately high dose with glucocorticoids because a similar increased mortality rate was later described in patients with Addison's disease.[10]

The scope of this chapter is to summarize today's management of pituitary insufficiency, from a clinically practical point of view. The importance of an individualized approach for each of the hormones to be replaced is emphasized, together with the importance of considering different phases of the patient's life in the overall management of patients with hypopituitarism.

## *Hypopituitarism (see Chapter 1)*

Hypopituitarism occurs when the pituitary gland is unable to produce its hormones, either due to a disease in the pituitary or due to inadequate stimulation of the pituitary from the hypothalamus. Patients with hypothalamic pituitary disease may develop anterior pituitary hormone deficiency due to the underlying disease or its treatment. Some of these patients will also develop posterior pituitary hormone deficiency with loss of arginine vasopressin (AVP) secretion, causing diabetes insipidus (DI). The management of these patients requires treatment and monitoring of their pituitary hormone deficiencies and monitoring of the underlying cause of their hypopituitarism, often by a hypothalamic–pituitary tumor. The clinical syndrome of adult hypopituitarism includes fatigue, infertility, loss of muscle mass and strength, abdominal adiposity, and osteoporosis. The symptoms depend on which of the pituitary hormones are affected. When there is deficiency of all the hormones of the adenohypophysis, it is termed panhypopituitarism.

Because most adult patients with hypopituitarism have multiple pituitary hormone deficiencies, the treatment requires knowledge of hormone–hormone

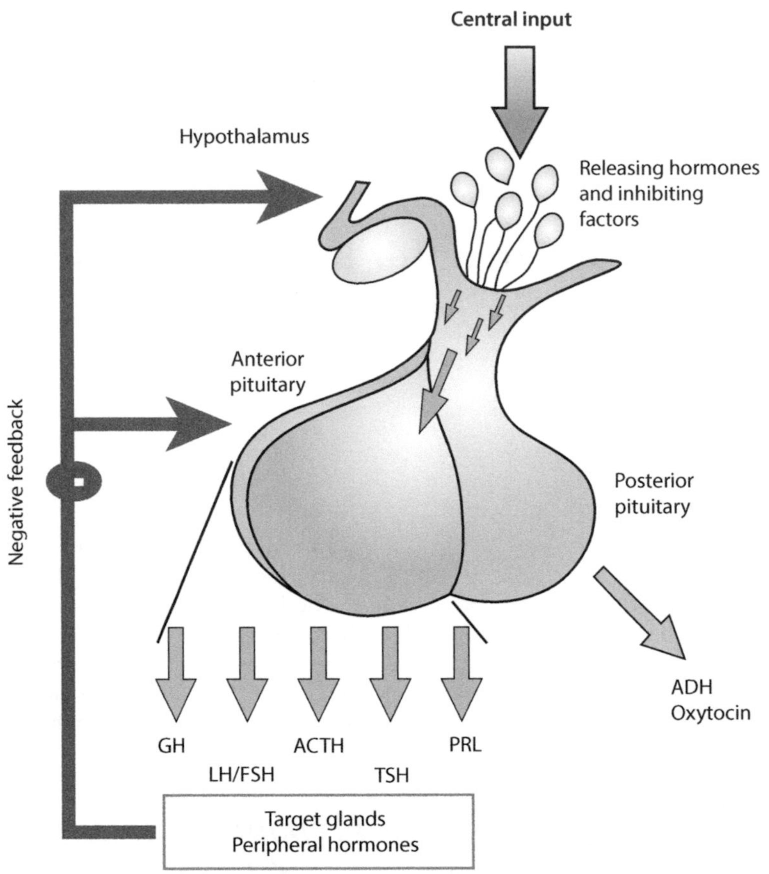


**Figure 5.1**

*Overview of the hypothalamic–pituitary–target gland system. Hypopituitarism may occur due to loss of function in the hypothalamus or the pituitary or due to processes disturbing the pituitary stalk function. The anterior pituitary (adenohypophysis) produces ACTH, TSH, LH, FSH, PRL (prolactin), and GH in response to hypothalamic factors and is under negative feedback from their peripheral hormones. The posterior pituitary (neurohypophysis) stores and releases the hypothalamic hormones ADH and oxytocin. (Reprinted from Schneider HJ et al.,* The Lancet, *369, 1461–70, 2007. Copyright (2007), with permission from Elsevier.)*

interactions, such as between thyroid hormones and glucocorticoids. Another important feature in the management of these patients is the fertility because a large proportion of patients are at an age when family planning occurs. Patients with hypopituitarism need to be informed of the possible and specific managements that may be offered related to fertility.

## Causes of hypopituitarism (Table 5.1)

The major cause of hypopituitarism is a disorder in the hypothalamic–pituitary area. The majority of patients will have a benign tumor in this area, but other reasons for hypopituitarism are traumatic, as a consequence of radiotherapy involving the hypothalamic–pituitary region, infiltrative disorders, and autoimmune mechanisms.

Identification of genetic causes of hypopituitarism is becoming more frequent because the knowledge of mutations causing hypopituitarism is growing rapidly[11] and because genetic tests are becoming easier to perform, are more readily available, and cost less. The diagnosis is usually established during childhood in a child with growth failure. The importance of genetic testing and a correct diagnosis is evident for some of the genetic disorders that lead to progressive and sequential loss of the anterior pituitary function that often follows a specific pattern. When such a mutation is known, the surveillance of that patient can be tailored accordingly.

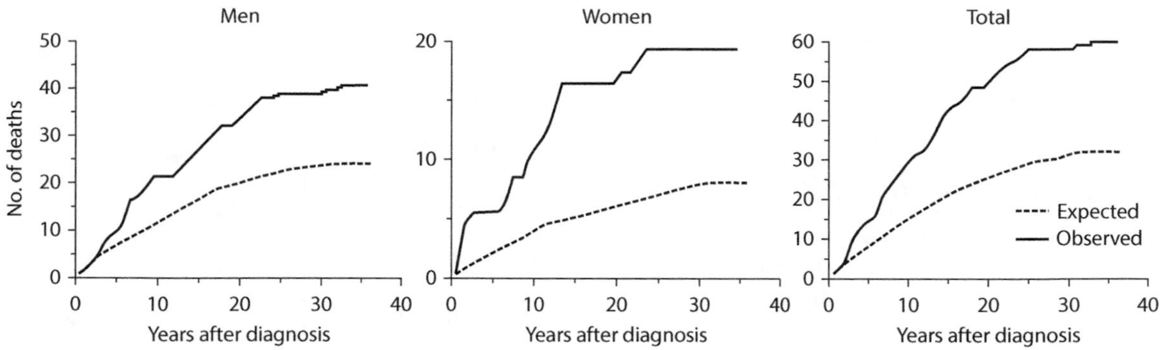


***Figure 5.2***
*Death rates from vascular disorders in patients with hypopituitarism and in age- and sex-matched controls. Solid lines represent observed death rates and dotted lines represent the expected death rates in men (the left panel), women (the middle panel), and the total study population (the right panel) (Reprinted from Rosén T and Bengtsson B-Å,* The Lancet, *336, 285–8, 1990, Copyright 1990, with permission from Elsevier.)*

| *Causes* | *Estimated Percentage* |
|---|---|
| Nonfunctioning pituitary adenoma | 26–57 |
| Craniopharyngioma | 4–12 |
| Prolactinoma | 9–13 |
| Idiopathic | 11–15 |
| Empty sella syndrome | 2–7 |
| Parasellar lesions/tumors | 3–5 |
| Other pituitary tumors; acromegaly, Cushing's disease, gonadotropinomas, TSH-secreting tumors, pituitary apoplexy, pituicytoma/choristoma | <20 |
| Infiltrative; sarcoidosis, eosinophllic granuloma, tuberculosis, syphilis, Wegener's granulomatosis, Langerhans cell histiocytosis, basilar meningitis | ? |
| Traumatic | ? |
| Autoimmune: lymphocytic hypophysitis | <1 |
| Radiation therapy (linked to underlying tumor) | ? |
| Genetic | ? |
| Other: Sheehan's syndrome | |

*Source:* Adapted from Sherlock M et al., *Endocr Rev*, 31, 301–42, 2010.
*Note:* ?, unknown

***Table 5.1***
*Causes of hypopituitarism in adults.*

The most common genetic cause in hypopituitarism is the *PROP1* mutation. At presentation, GH and central hypothyroidism are present, hypogonadotropic hypogonadism is usually detected when the patient enters puberty, and finally adrenal insufficiency may develop later in life.

There is also increased awareness of the risk of hypopituitarism in patients suffering from traumatic brain injury (TBI) and subarachnoid hemorrhage (SAH). In these patients, an unrecognized hypopituitarism may lead to death due to adrenal crisis or influence the rehabilitation potential and long-term morbidity. The true frequency of hypopituitarism in TBI and SAH is not known, but data indicate that any type of anterior pituitary hormone deficiency may be found in 30% or more in these patients.[1]

## Epidemiology of hypopituitarism

The epidemiology of hypopituitarism is not very well studied. Data have been collected before the increased awareness of hypopituitarism in TBI and SAH, suggesting that published data may underestimate the true prevalence of hypopituitarism.

There is only one study that has estimated both incidence and prevalence of hypopituitarism. This study examined an average population sample of 146,000 adult inhabitants in South Galicia, Spain.[12] The study demonstrated an increase in the prevalence from 29 to 45.5/100,000 between 1992 and 1999, with an average annual incidence rate of 4.21 cases/100,000. A Swedish study on the incidence of pituitary adenomas, the most common cause of hypopituitarism in adults, demonstrated an increased incidence from 0.6 to 1.1 cases/100,000 between 1975 and 1991.[13] The combined results from these studies indicate an increase in the prevalence of hypopituitarism. Whether this is a true increase in the prevalence or an increased awareness of hypopituitarism is not known.

## Mortality in adults with hypopituitarism

The first indication of excess mortality in hypopituitary adults came from a retrospective study by Rosén et al.[9] showing doubled overall standardized mortality rate in hypopituitary patients compared with the normal population (Figure 5.2). Several additional retrospective studies, and one prospective study, have confirmed that overall mortality rate is increased by twofold and even higher in the women with hypopituitarism[14,15] (Figure 5.3). Another study more specifically investigating the impact of GH deficiency on mortality rate also demonstrated that young age at diagnosis was associated with a more marked increase in the standardized mortality rate.[16]

Several studies have shown that the observed excess mortality rate in hypopituitarism was mainly due to an increased rate of death of cardiovascular causes. These studies have not been able to show in a consistent pattern that the increased mortality is due to any specific hormone deficiency. Some studies have suggested that untreated GH deficiency may be the most important

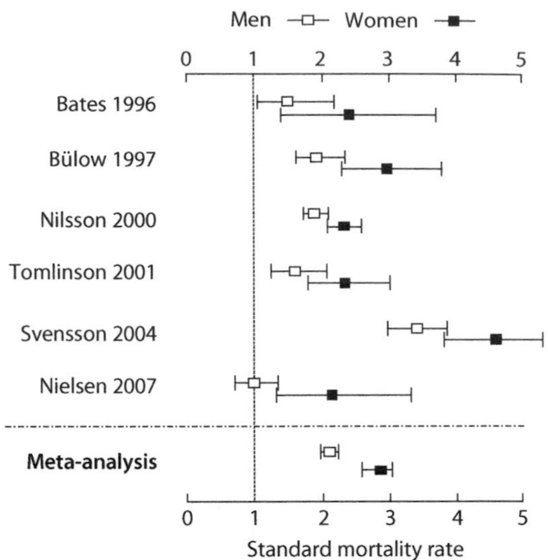


***Figure 5.3***
*Standard mortality rates (SMRs) and 95% confidence intervals (CIs) in individual studies on patients with nonmalignant pituitary diseases not associated with excess ACTH or GH secretion, and in the weighted meta-analysis (bottom line). Results are shown for men (open boxes) and women (black boxes) separately. Weighted SMR values for men (SMR = 2.06; CI 1.94–2.20) and women (SMR = 2.80; CI 2.59–3.02) were calculated using the inverse variance method. (Reprinted from Nielsen EH et al.,* Clin Endocrinol (Oxf)*, 67, 693–7, 2007. With permission. Copyright 2007, Blackwell.)*

contributor to the increased mortality rate. Other likely contributing factors are unphysiological replacement with glucocorticoids, both in terms of the actual dose and the cortisol exposure time profile; poor replacement of sex steroids in women; the presence of DI; underlying disease, such as craniopharyngioma; and previous treatment with radiotherapy.[17] Some studies have in fact demonstrated that the presence of adrenal insufficiency and the actual daily dose of glucocorticoids is associated with the excess mortality rate.[18,19]

## Symptoms and signs

The initial clinical presentation varies considerably due to the numerous underlying causes of hypopituitarism, the speed at which the pituitary insufficiency develops, and what hormones are lost. Because most patients have an insidious and slow onset of the disease, nonspecific complaints are common, such as weakness, lethargy, fatigue, reduced muscle strength, reduced energy and vitality, and reduced exercise tolerance. More specific symptoms or signs indicating hypopituitarism may also be found.

Pituitary tumors are the most common cause of hypopituitarism and may present either with symptoms due to expansion—headache, visual field defects, and even obstructive hydrocephalus, if the tumor obstructs the third ventricle—or with symptoms and signs associated with hypopituitarism. Patients without tumors will, however, only present with symptoms and signs of hypopituitarism. These symptoms and signs are in most cases slowly progressive over years. The initial symptoms and signs are therefore vague, are not easily detected, and are often even ignored by the patients and nonspecialist physicians. In consequence, therefore, there is frequently a delay in the time of diagnosis, which may thus be very prolonged. A few causes of hypopituitarism have, however, a very rapid onset, such as in postpartum pituitary necrosis, where absence of lactation is associated with a rapid decline in general health.

In some cases, hypopituitarism presents itself as loss of only one hormone deficiency. This is most commonly seen in isolated growth hormone deficiency (GHD) with short stature in childhood or isolated hypogonadotropic hypogonadism. Other isolated losses may occur, but clinical hypopituitarism in adults usually presents itself as combined deficiencies, making the initial presentation more complex and at the same time more ambiguous. In general, the order of loss of anterior pituitary function is predictable, particularly if the cause is a tumor or due to the radiotherapy. The order of loss is usually GH, the gonadotropins luteinizing hormone (LH) and follicle-stimulating hormone (FSH), thyroid-stimulating hormone (TSH) or adrenocorticotropic hormone (ACTH), and finally prolactin. A notable exception to this occurs in patients with lymphocytic hypophysitis where ACTH secretion is often lost first followed by TSH, gonadotropins, and prolactin.

## General considerations

In the initial diagnosis of hypopituitarism, an underlying tumor should always be suspected because this is by far the most common cause in adults. This means that early in the diagnostic process visual field and visual acuity should be assessed because if there is indication of optic nerve compression, neurosurgical decompression is required. Symptoms of an expansive process, a history of severe head trauma, and symptoms of pituitary hormone deficiency should be sought (Table 5.2). It is important to early gain insight into whether the patient has symptoms or signs that could be associated with adrenal insufficiency because this may need urgent attention. If adrenal insufficiency is suspected, the patient should be supplied with HC tablets that should be taken in case of an intercurrent illness, together with steroid cards and bracelet, if medical attention is needed before the final diagnosis is made.

| *Hormone deficiency* | *Symptoms* | *Signs* |
|---|---|---|
| ACTH | Weakness, dizziness, lethargy, fatigue, anorexia, weight loss, infections | Pallor, wasting, loss of body hair |
| TSH | Fatigue, weight gain, cold intolerance, constipation | Bradycardia, sallow complexion, slow-relaxing reflexes |
| FSH/LH | Men: reduced libido, erectile dysfunction, infertility, reduced muscle and strength, fatigue | Fine wrinkling of skin, loss of beard, loss of bodily hairs (male pattern), muscle atrophy, abdominal obesity, reduced or soft testes |
| | Women: oligo/amenorrhea, infertility, loss of libido, dyspareunia | Fine wrinkling of skin, breast atrophy |
| GH | Reduced energy and vitality, reduced exercise tolerance | Reduced muscle mass, central adiposity |
| ADH | Polyuria and polydipsia | |

***Table 5.2***
*Common symptoms and signs seen in patients with hypopituitarism.*

## Secondary adrenal insufficiency (see also Appendix)

Secondary adrenal insufficiency or ACTH deficiency is estimated to occur among approximately 60%–80% of adults with hypopituitarism.[14] Because this pituitary hormone deficiency often occurs late in the order of loss of anterior pituitary deficiency, it usually occurs in combination with other pituitary hormone deficiencies.

The symptom and signs occurring in hypopituitarism (Table 5.2) are therefore present in most of the patients with adrenal insufficiency. More specific symptoms and signs may be fatigue, pallor, anorexia, and weight loss. Glucocorticoid deficiency may also mask the presence of DI so that when replaced, diuresis and thirst develop.

A specific and important situation in adrenal insufficiency is the occurrence of an intercurrent infection or major physical stress that may trigger the development of an adrenal crisis. Adrenal crisis occurs in patients with secondary adrenal insufficiency, although the frequency is lower than seen in patients with Addison's disease.[21] Patients with secondary adrenal insufficiency may develop severe hyponatremia during an illness if not adequately replaced with glucocorticoids.

## Definition and diagnosis

Secondary adrenal insufficiency is when there is a hypothalamic–pituitary reason for the adrenal insufficiency, that is, ACTH deficiency. In contrast to primary adrenal insufficiency, these patients have a functioning renin–angiotensin–aldosterone system and therefore no mineralocorticoid deficiency and they have no need for such replacement therapy. The women with hypogonadotropic hypogonadism and ACTH deficiency have very low circulating androgens levels, due to insufficient ovarian and adrenal androgen secretion, that may contribute to their symptoms and signs.

The diagnostic approach to a patient with hypothalamic–pituitary disease and suspected adrenal insufficiency is somewhat different from the approach used in patients with primary adrenal insufficiency. The first line of evidence is to demonstrate low serum morning cortisol concentration in combination with a serum ACTH that is not elevated. The second line of evidence, if needed, is the short Synacthen test (SST). Finally, the reference test used for secondary adrenal insufficiency is the insulin tolerance test (ITT) (Box 5.1). In the event of a clearly low serum cortisol concentration without any other confounders, such as concomitant synthetic steroid use (topical, inhalation, oral), further testing may not be necessary. In other situations, further testing should be performed. The SST dose has been debated, but there is no evidence that the low dose (1 μg) is superior to the high dose (250 μg) despite the theoretical possibility that the low dose may be more appropriate in testing for secondary adrenal insufficiency.[22] Because the SST test only evaluates the responsiveness of the adrenal cortex, there is a risk for a false-negative test, particularly in patients with short duration of secondary adrenal insufficiency (<3 months).

## Management

The aims of glucocorticoid replacement therapy (Box 5.2) are to mimic the circadian serum steroid profile and to respond to the increased need for cortisol during physical and physiological stimulation. Most patients receive HC or cortisone acetate for replacement, although synthetic steroids are still used in a minority of patients.[23] In patients with secondary adrenal insufficiency, the most common dose is 30 mg, but the trend is to use lower doses. This is based on data on cortisol production rate that is lower than previously thought, corresponding to approximately 15.5–19 mg/day in an average adult subject,[24] and the outcome data showing an increase in cardiovascular risk factors among patients with a mean daily HC equivalent dose >20 mg/day[25] (Figure 5.4). Moreover, because most patients with hypopituitarism

**Box 5.1** *Assessment of secondary adrenal insufficiency*

- Morning serum cortisol (0700–0900 hours)
  - <100 nmol/L: hypocortisolism
  - >550 nmol/L: hypocortisolism excluded
- Morning ACTH
  - Normal or low
- Short Synacthen test (250 or 1 μg i.v.)
  - Cortisol <550 nmol/L: hypocortisolism
- Insulin tolerance test
  - Cortisol <550 nmol/L: hypocortisolism

**Box 5.2** *Glucocorticoid replacement therapy*

Preferred glucocorticoid is HC that is chemically identical to endogenous cortisol.

The daily dose should be individualized using the lowest dose to maintain well-being without increasing the risk of adrenal insufficiency and crisis.

An appropriate daily dose is likely to be between 10 and 20 mg in most patients.

The treatment regimen should consider that cortisol exposure is highest in the morning and low during evening and night.

The daily dose should be divided, and three daily doses may have benefit over two daily doses.

During intercurrent illness, there should be a high awareness of the risk of developing acute adrenal insufficiency.

- For milder clinical conditions, the normal daily replacement dose must be increased temporarily—at least doubled.
- Parenteral administration of glucocorticoids is warranted during transient illnesses such as infections, in particular gastroenteritis; high fever of any etiology; or extensive physical stress such as surgery under general anesthesia when oral administration is not possible.
- The patient must be carefully informed and also advised to immediately seek medical attention should an acute deterioration occur, especially in cases of gastroenteritis, vomiting, and/or diarrhea.
- Some patients may be taught to self-administer parenteral HC.
- To minimize risk during an emergency, patients should carry a "steroid treatment" card that gives clear guidance on the precautions to be taken during an intercurrent illness or any emergency situation where extra administration of HC is urgently needed.

and adrenal insufficiency also have GHD, it is likely that they are particularly sensitive to glucocorticoids because there is an increased local 11β-hydroxysteroid dehydrogenase (HSD) type 1 activity in adipose tissues, resulting in increased local cortisol exposure in GHD that is reduced after GH replacement.[26,27] This adds further to the unfavorable metabolic features associated with hypopituitarism in patients being replaced for adrenal insufficiency. The diagnosis of adrenal insufficiency may also be affected in such a manner that the patient may pass tests for adrenal insufficiency before GH replacement and fail after commencement of GH therapy.[28]

Another indication that current replacement therapy may be inadequate is the outcome data of patients with primary and secondary adrenal insufficiency showing increased mortality rate from cardiovascular disorder and infectious diseases.[10,18] A possible explanation for this increased mortality rate is inappropriate glucocorticoid replacement therapy with excessive maintenance doses, unphysiological glucocorticoid exposure, and inadequate glucocorticoid exposure in response to stress and intercurrent illness.

The previously recommended dose of 30 mg/day HC is probably too high for most patients with adrenal insufficiency.[29] The daily dose should therefore be lower and the dose divided in such a manner that the normal cortisol exposure time profile more resembles the endogenous serum cortisol profile, with the largest dose in the morning and less during the day and afternoon. For example, HC 10+5+5 mg is preferable over 10+10 mg. An oral dose too late during the day results in excessive exposure during late evening that may affect sleepiness and the sleep quality during the night. This may occur in particular if the dose is administered together with a meal because this will increase bioavailability and delay the exposure time profile. Exciting new developments for the treatment of adrenal insufficiency has been presented, where a more physiological cortisol exposure is achieved[30,31,32]. The outcome data of these new hydrocortisone preparations suggest that outcome can be improved.

Adrenal insufficiency also leads to androgen deficiency, including dehydroepiandrosterone (DHEA) deficiency.[33] Studies on DHEA replacement have been performed in patients with secondary adrenal insufficiency, and some but not all studies have shown beneficial effects on well-being and sexuality.[34,35] Addition of 20–50 mg DHEA may be considered in female patients with hypopituitarism and low serum levels of DHEA who report reduced well-being and libido. Side effects that may occur are increased sweating, acne, and undesired hair growth.

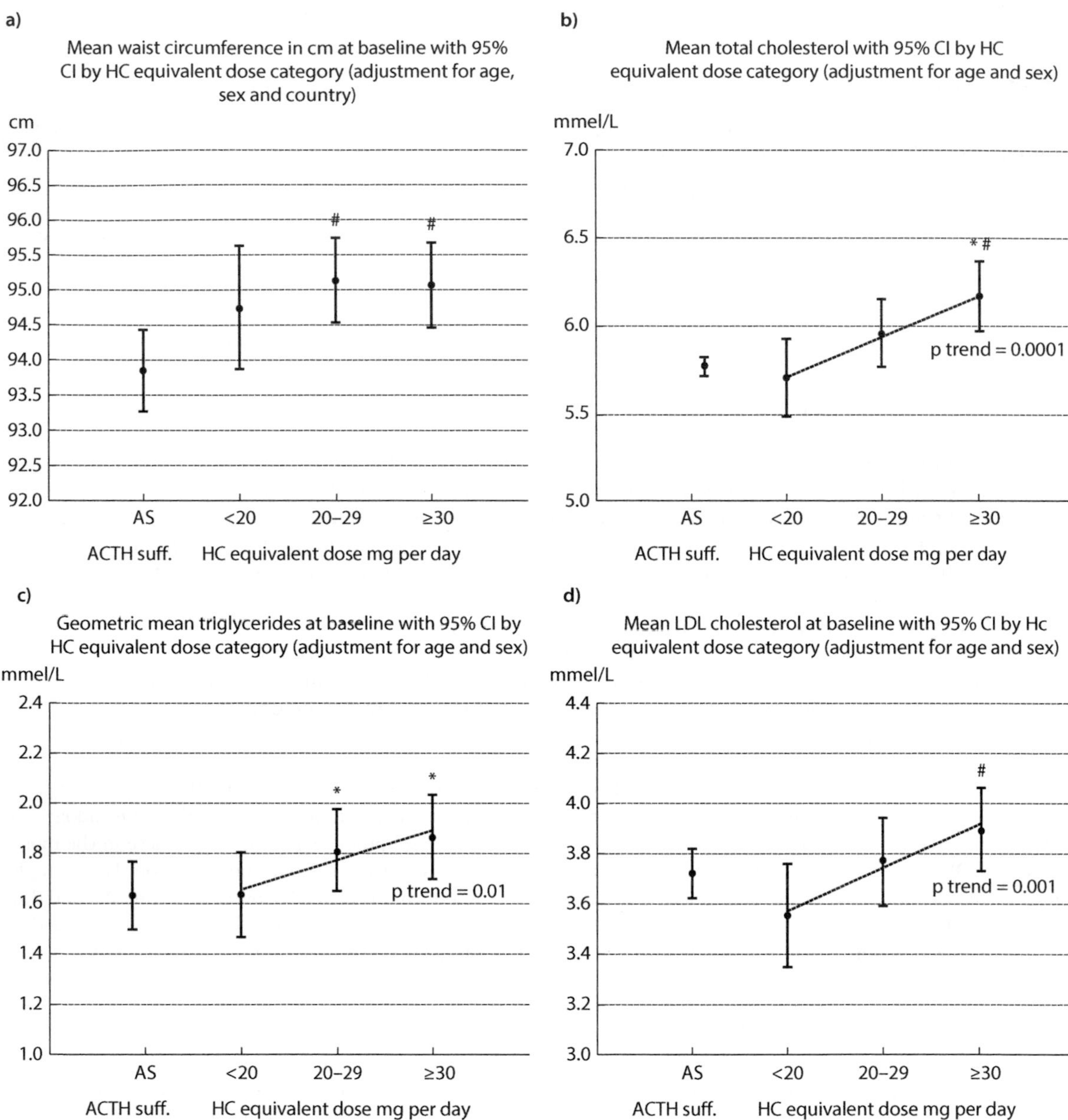


***Figure 5.4***
*Hydrocortisone equivalent dose categories in ACTH-deficient and ACTH-sufficient (AS) hypopituitary patients. The broken line represents a dose–response analysis within the glucocorticoid-treated groups. (a) Waist, #, $p < 0.001$ versus AS. (b) Total cholesterol, *, $p < 0.0001$ versus AS; #, $p < 0.0001$ versus <20 mg/day. (c) Triglycerides, logarithmic-transformed triglycerides are provided to achieve a normal distribution. *, $p < .001$ versus AS. (d) LDL cholesterol, #, $p < 0.05$ versus <20 mg/day. (Reprinted from Filipsson H et al.,* J Clin Endocrinol Metab, *91, 3954–61, 2006. With permission. Copyright 2006, The Endocrine Society.)*

## *Central hypothyroidism (see also Appendix)*

TSH deficiency or central hypothyroidism is considered to occur late in the development of hypopituitarism, in particular when the underlying lesion is a pituitary tumor or due to radiotherapy. Among the general symptoms seen in hypopituitarism, more specific symptoms and signs related to hypothyroidism are cold intolerance, constipation, dry skin, hoarseness, cognitive slowing, weight gain, and bradycardia.

### *Diagnosis*

In central hypothyroidism, the bioactivity of circulating TSH is reduced because the pituitary gland secretes an abnormally glycosylated TSH. TSH in this form has a longer half-life than normal TSH,[33] explaining the normal or sometimes slightly elevated concentrations of TSH that may be seen in central hypothyroidism.[34] This is a common pitfall in the diagnosis of central hypothyroidism because the expected reduction in TSH is frequently not seen. A reduced serum free T4 concentration in combination with a low, normal, or slightly elevated TSH is the single best criterion for diagnosis of central hypothyroidism. Dynamic testing such as the thyrotropin-releasing hormone (TRH) stimulation test and the evaluation of the nocturnal surge of TSH does not, in general, add to the diagnostic reliability.

The correct diagnosis may however sometimes be difficult. For example, in mild central hypothyroidism free T4 may be within the lower normal range due to the large intraindividual variation of the measurement.[35] Patients with untreated GHD have higher free T4 levels than those on GH replacement, which may unmask central hypothyroidism. This is supported by data from hypopituitary patients with thyroid hormone concentrations in the lower range of normal, who often need L-thyroxine replacement when commenced on GH replacement.[36] Hypopituitary patients with free T4 concentration in the lower part of the normal range should be carefully evaluated clinically and have thyroid hormone status repeated regularly. Patients with nonthyroid illness may have a similar thyroid hormone pattern as patients with mild central hypothyroidism, except that they may have higher T3 concentrations. The thyroid hormone data should therefore always be evaluated in their clinical context.

### *Management*

Central hypothyroidism is treated with L-thyroxine (T4) replacement (Box 5.3). The commencement of therapy should be individualized based on the patients' overall medical state and the degree of insufficiency. Therefore, the initial dose should be lower and dose titration done more carefully in the elderly and in those patients who have a very severe insufficiency. In patients with central hypothyroidism, it should be recognized that the degree of insufficiency cannot be defined as well as in patients with primary hypothyroidism where the increase in TSH reflects the severity of the insufficiency. Moreover, it is of particular importance in hypopituitary patients with central hypothyroidism that the status of the hypothalamic–pituitary–adrenal (HPA) axis is assessed and adrenal

**Box 5.3** *Thyroid hormone replacement therapy*

Initial starting dose 12.5–50 µg depending on age, clinical condition, and severity of deficiency.

Patients >60 years of age and those with known or suspected ischemic heart disease should get a low initial dose, and slow dose titration should be done.

Always correct concomitant adrenal insufficiency before commencing thyroid hormone replacement therapy.

Maintenance dose is individual and should be guided by

- Serum free T4 in the upper range of normal
- Serum TSH concentration low or suppressed (<0.1 mIU/L)
- Total daily dose 1.6 µg/kg/day in patients <60 years of age
- Clinical response

Commencement of GH replacement reduces serum free T4.

Simultaneous intake of oral calcium and iron reduces gastrointestinal absorption of L-thyroxine.

Some antidepressive medications increase the peripheral catabolism of thyroxine.

insufficiency is corrected before initiating treatment with L-thyroxine. Failure to do this may trigger an adrenal crisis in patients with untreated adrenal insufficiency, due to the accelerated metabolic clearance of cortisol and the general increase in the overall metabolic rate after T4 replacement.

Monitoring serum TSH concentrations for judging the appropriate L-thyroxine replacement dose in central hypothyroidism is not very useful, making the fine-tuning of the therapy difficult. This is supported by a large trial of hypopituitary adults with GH deficiency, where it could be anticipated that the replacement dose was in many cases arbitrary, based on available tablet strengths.[37] The study also indicated that patients with an average L-thyroxine dose of 1.4 μg/kg/day had the most appropriate replacement dose, whereas patients with lower doses had increased body mass index (BMI) and waist circumference and patients with higher doses had lower BMI and waist circumference, compared with TSH-sufficient hypopituitary patients. These results are in agreement with previous careful dose-titrating studies suggesting that free T4 should be in the upper range of normal, TSH levels should be low or suppressed, and the target dose of L-thyroxine should be dependent on the patient's age. The dose titration studies have found the most appropriate mean L-thyroxine dose to be 1.6 μg/kg/day.[38–40] The optimal dose may also be age-dependent, with an L-thyroxine dose between 1.1 and 1.4 μg/kg/day if >60 years and between 1.41 and 1.7 μg/kg/day in patients <60 years.[40] Other studies have also suggested that TSH should be suppressed (<0.1 mIU/L)[38,41] and serum free T4 concentrations should be in the upper part of the normal range[39,42] to achieve euthyroidism.

The importance of adequate dose titration of L-thyroxine is demonstrated by data showing increased cardiovascular disease, increased fractures, and dysrhythmias in patients with primary hypothyroidism with high or suppressed TSH concentration.[43]

GH replacement increases the conversion of T4 to T3.[8] Therefore, careful monitoring of thyroid function is mandatory during GH treatment because it may induce changes in the dose of L-thyroxine or uncover central hypothyroidism.

# *Hypogonadotropic hypogonadism (see also Appendix)*

## *Women*

Hypogonadotropic hypogonadism is common in pituitary disease. Disturbed secretion of gonadotropin-releasing hormone (GnRH) and/or LH/FSH typically results in dysmenorrhea and amenorrhea, which in fertile women often are among the first signs of hypothalamic or pituitary disease. Infertility is another symptom that may lead to the diagnosis of secondary hypogonadism.

Gonadotropin synthesis is dynamically regulated via pulsatile secretion of GnRH from the hypothalamus. Pulsatility is needed for stimulation of LH/FSH synthesis and secretion, whereas continuous stimulation with GnRH results in reduced gonadotropic activity.

### *Diagnosis*

The diagnosis of hypogonadotropic hypogonadism in women is based on clinical history and the presence of low estrogen levels in the circulation and normal or reduced levels of FSH and LH. In postmenopausal women, the diagnosis is based on the absence of elevated levels of FSH and LH. Hyperprolactinemia needs to be excluded as prolactin per se suppresses the hypothalamic–pituitary–gonadal axis.

### *Management*

Oral replacement of estrogen with cyclic addition of progestin is the most common replacement modality. Typically, the younger adult woman with pituitary insufficiency will be treated with an oral contraceptive pill with a combination of estrogen and progestin. In the middle-aged woman approaching the age of the physiological menopause, oral formulations with lower dose of estrogen may be preferred. If the patient has a uterus, cyclic treatment with progestin is necessary for regular bleeding.[44]

It has been suggested that transdermal estrogen is advantageous because the first passage metabolism of the liver is avoided, thereby reducing the negative effects on lipids, coagulation factors, and systemic inflammation seen in oral estrogen treatment. Insulin-like growth factor I (IGF-I) production in the liver is suppressed by oral estrogens,[45] which may explain the need for higher replacement doses of GH in women.

Estrogen replacement therapy in hypopituitarism is, in general, not subject to individual dose titration. The dose is somewhat reduced in middle-aged women, with a switch to preparations used for perimenopausal estrogen replacement therapy. After the age of 50 years, when menopause may be expected in most women, estrogen treatment is usually withdrawn. The rationale for this is based on the increased morbidity from malignancies in large studies of postmenopausal women using estrogen in higher age groups.[46]

Ovulation and fertility may be achieved in women with hypopituitarism via pulsatile GnRH or gonadotropin therapy. The outcome of such therapy in hypopituitary women is not well documented, but limited data in a selection of patients suggest a good likelihood of inducing ovulation and a successful pregnancy.[47]

## Men

In contrast to women, men suffer from less distinct symptoms from their hypogonadotropic hypogonadism. The symptoms and signs of testosterone deficiency include fatigue, decreased muscle strength, decreased body hair, decreased libido, erectile dysfunction, osteoporosis, anemia, and infertility.

### Diagnosis

In hypogonadotropic hypogonadism, serum testosterone concentrations are low and serum FSH and LH are normal or lower than normal. In panhypopituitarism, serum testosterone concentrations may be unmeasurable, whereas in partial hypopituitarism they may be only slightly below normal levels. If the clinical symptoms are vague, expectance and repeated measure of testosterone may be needed before the correct diagnosis is made. Hyperprolactinemia as a cause of the hypogonadotropic hypogonadism needs to be excluded.

### Management

Before the start of testosterone replacement, prostate cancer needs to be excluded. Digital rectal examination, measurement of serum prostate-specific antigen (PSA), and in selected cases referral to an urologist are recommended, in particular, in middle-aged and elderly men. During testosterone replacement, repeated measurements of PSA (more frequent in middle-aged or elderly men) should be performed. The increased risk of polycythemia and sleep apnea should also be considered.

The aim of testosterone replacement therapy in hypogonadotropic hypogonadism is to provide as near physiological exposure as possible.[48] Intramuscular injections have for long been the preferred modality for testosterone replacement. Depot formulations allow periods for up to 12 weeks between injections. Transdermal preparations are also available with patches and gels. Transdermal testosterone requires daily application and may in some men cause irritation to the skin. The instructions to the patient are important and must include information to secure absorption of the hormone as well as safety for family members because there is a risk that testosterone on the skin can be transferred to a female or a child. Oral preparations are available in some countries, but some have significant hepatic toxicity and others result in fluctuating levels of serum testosterone and need multiple daily dosing.[49]

To induce spermatogenesis in a man with hypogonadotropic hypogonadism (Box 5.4), testosterone treatment needs to be stopped and replaced with pulsatile GnRH or human chorionic gonadotropin (hCG) and/or FSH.[50,51] Though it is possible to achieve sperm production with hCG and FSH injections in most men with hypopituitarism, it may take months and in some cases even 2–3 years. Small testicular volume is a negative predictor for achieving spermatogenesis.[52] Doses of hCG and FSH are guided partly by the serum testosterone levels achieved, and treatment is monitored by regular testicular palpation and sperm counts (in most cases every third month).

## Growth hormone deficiency (see also Appendix)

In the beginning of the 1990s, it was proposed that GHD was one of the reasons for the increased mortality rate seen in hypopituitary patients. This led to insights of the role of GH for several cardiovascular risk factors in adults, such as hypercholesterolemia, abdominal adiposity, and increased body fat mass.[10,53] Furthermore, untreated GHD patients have a higher risk for osteoporosis and reduced quality of life compared to healthy subjects.[54] Studies on GH replacement have demonstrated increased psychological well-being, improvement in several cardiovascular risk factors, and

**Box 5.4** *Stimulation of spermatogenesis in hypogonadotropic hypogonadism*

- Withdraw testosterone replacement
- Sperm count at baseline and every third month until spermatogenesis has been achieved
- Serum testosterone and serum sex hormone-binding globulin (SHBG) every third month
- hCG injections 1500–3000 IU s.c. 2–3 times/week
- Testicular volume below 4 mL or no effect on spermatogenesis after 6 months: add FSH injections 150–225 IU s.c. 2–3 times/week
- In case of pregnancy, switch to maintenance dose of hCG alone (to maintain spermatogenesis until decision regarding further pregnancies)

increased bone mineral density.[55] Insulin resistance is slightly increased but the net effect on cardiovascular risk of GH replacement is considered to be positive.[56,57]

## Symptoms and signs

The symptoms of GHD in adults include fatigue, increased abdominal adiposity, mild depression, and anxiety. These symptoms are not specific, and it is therefore recommended that the clinical diagnosis and investigation of GHD is performed in patients with stable replacement treatment for other hormonal deficiencies.[57]

## Diagnosis

The diagnosis of GH deficiency in adults is based on stimulation tests. Insulin-induced hypoglycemia (ITT) stimulates both ACTH and GH[22] and provides information on both hormonal axes. It is very important to note that ITT is contraindicated in patients with epilepsy, cardiovascular disease, or untreated hypocortisolism. In recent years, the combined stimulation with arginine and GH-releasing hormone (Arg-GHRH) has been validated as a diagnostic test in adult GH deficiency.[58] Arg-GHRH stimulation does not test the function of the hypothalamus and can be misleading in patients with a recent hypothalamic injury because the pituitary may still respond. The best validated tests for adult GH deficiency are the ITT, Arg-GHRH, Arg-GH-releasing peptides, and glucagon.[56] The cut-off values for the diagnosis of GHD vary between the tests, and the response may be influenced by age and adiposity. The Arg-GHRH test has BMI-dependent cut-offs, and higher cut-off values for the diagnosis of GHD may be applicable in young adults who have previously been diagnosed with childhood onset GHD.[59] It is recommended that the retesting in young adults after childhood GH replacement is performed after withdrawal of GH for at least 1 month.

Serum IGF-I can be low but can also be within the age-adjusted reference range in adult hypopituitarism and is therefore not useful for the diagnosis of GHD in adults. However, low IGF-I levels in a patient with three or more deficiencies in other pituitary hormones are considered enough for establishment of the diagnosis.[56]

## Management

In adults, the goal of GH replacement is to improve well-being, to reduce cardiovascular risk, to increase bone density, and to normalize body composition. GH is available as subcutaneous injections. In adults, the treatment with daily subcutaneous injections needs to be initiated at a low dose with dose increments every second to fourth week (Box 5.5). If the dose is increased too fast, there is a substantial risk that the patient will suffer from fluid retention with muscle and joint stiffness and/or pain and in some cases edema. The same symptoms may occur if the replacement dose is too high. To relieve the symptoms of fluid retention, GH injections can be withdrawn for 3–5 days and then restarted at a lower dose.

Serum IGF-I concentrations and the clinical effect on well-being and body composition are the variables that need to be taken into account in the individual dose titration.[60] Other biomarkers, for example, IGF-binding protein 3 and its acid-labile subunit (ALS), have been investigated but have not proven useful.[61] Positive effects on psychological well-being and quality of life are often detectable by the patient after 3–12 months of therapy, and a disease-specific quality of life questionnaire allowing objective assessment of treatment response has been developed.[62]

With advancing age[56] the dose of GH needs to be reduced because the IGF-I levels should not exceed the age- and sex-adjusted reference range. Oral estrogen replacement increases the GH dose needed for the same IGF-I response, and withdrawal of estrogen replacement may elicit side effects due to fluid retention and overly high serum IGF-I concentrations unless the GH dose is reduced. Commencement of GH replacement may unmask central hypothyroidism and secondary adrenal insufficiency as discussed above, and in some patients, dose adjustment of the L-thyroxine may be needed.[28,36]

GH is mitogenic and it has been feared that GH replacement may increase the risk for *de novo* cancer or tumor growth. The presence of malignant disease is a contraindication for GH replacement. If a patient with GH replacement treatment is diagnosed with a malignant disease, GH should be withdrawn. Current data do not suggest increased risk of *de novo* malignancies during long-term GH replacement in adults.[63] Many patients with hypopituitarism have residual pituitary tumor. Long-term follow-up studies have not shown any increased risk for progress or regrowth of pituitary tumors during GH replacement.[20,64] Long-term studies of GH replacement have shown that the beneficial effect on cardiovascular risk factors is sustained with time.[65] Also, the increase in bone mineral density remains after long-term follow-up,[66] but the fracture risk may still be elevated in the male patients.[67] Several factors may influence the risk of fracture in these patients besides GHD and GH replacement, such as long-standing untreated hypogonadism and excessive replacement therapy with glucocorticoid and/or thyroxine.

**Box 5.5** *Suggested approach to GH replacement therapy in adults*

Start with 0.1–0.2 mg s.c. before bedtime.
Increase the dose with 0.1 mg every second to fourth week, after:

- monitoring of side effects indicating overreplacement, mainly symptoms of fluid retention (peripheral edema, muscle and joint stiffness and/or pain)
- measuring serum IGF-I concentration

Individualize the maintenance dose according to:

- serum IGF-I (should be within the normal range, usually in the upper part of the age-adjusted reference range)
- effects on psychological well-being and body composition after 6–12 months of GH replacement
- reducing the dose if symptoms or signs of fluid retention occur (mild symptoms may be transient during the first days after dose increment)

The maintenance dose is usually higher in young adults and in women with (oral) estrogen replacement therapy (0.6–1.0 mg/day).

Dose adjustment is to be expected when route of estrogen replacement is changed, replacement commenced, or discontinued.

During long-term GH replacement, serum IGF-I and glucose metabolism should be monitored at least yearly, and regular assessment of body composition and bone health preferably using DEXA should be done regularly.

Withdraw GH replacement if a malignant disease is suspected or diagnosed.

*Source:* Ho KK, *Eur J Endocrinol*, 157, 695–700, 2007.

# Diabetes insipidus (see Chapter 24)

## Definition and etiology

The primary stimuli of AVP secretion from the posterior pituitary are stimuli from pressure receptors sensing reduced pressure and osmotic receptors sensing increased serum osmolality. DI comes in two forms: central DI due to AVP deficiency; and renal DI due to renal insensitivity to the action of AVP. AVP binds to its receptor (AVP receptor subtype 2 [$V_2$]) in the renal distal tubule and collecting duct.

Central DI has three distinct clinical features: an inappropriately dilute urine (aquaresis) despite strong osmotic or nonosmotic stimuli for AVP secretion, absence of renal disease, and an increase in urine osmolality after the administration of AVP.[68]

The causes of DI are similar to those of hypopituitarism, with the majority of patients having an underlying hypothalamic lesion, or it develops after surgery for a pituitary tumor (Table 5.1). It is uncommon for a patient with a pituitary tumor to present *de novo* with DI. A significant number of patients however have idiopathic causes at the initial presentation. It is recommended in these cases that a careful and continuous re-evaluation of the etiology is performed, because the underlying cause may appear later. A rare form of central DI is a hereditary autosomal dominant form that is caused by a mutation in the AVP-neurophysin gene.

Approximately 90% of the hypothalamic–pituitary AVP containing neurons need to be lost before symptoms of DI appear. This is the most likely reason why most patients with pituitary disease and panhypopituitarism do not have DI.

## Symptoms and signs

The primary symptoms of DI are persistent polyuria (increased aquaresis, electrolyte-free urine), with thirst and polydipsia as a consequence. The volume of urine may vary from 3 to 6 L/day in most cases to a maximum of about 18 L/day, the average volume of glomerular filtrate delivered to collecting ducts in the total absence of AVP. The urinary concentration is typically below that found in serum (<280 mOsm/kg).

Most patients with central DI have an abrupt onset of polyuria and polydipsia with a debut they can trace back to a certain time of a particular day. Patients with severe untreated DI who are unable to drink, do not have access to enough fluid, or have impaired thirst sensation develop volume depletion with hypertonic hypernatremia. Subjects with normal thirst and free access to fluid usually have normal sodium and volume status.

Patients with partial central DI have milder symptoms that are less troublesome. Particularly of importance in the older patients is to differentiate partial DI from nocturia and pollakiuria due to urological conditions. Patients with DI may report thirst during night time, which is less often reported in patients with pollakiuria without polyuria.

## Diagnosis

The diagnosis of DI in a patient with polyuria and polydipsia requires documentation of elevated levels of serum sodium and osmolality and low urine osmolality. In some instances, the criteria are met without formal water deprivation, such as in the clinical setting of a large pituitary tumor with multiple pituitary insufficiency. In these instances, a therapeutic trial of desmopressin (1-desamino-8-D-arginine vasopressin) is all that is required. In other instances, particularly in patients with partial DI, water deprivation test (Box 5.6) is needed. The test should be done in a controlled setting where blood pressure and clinical status can be monitored because patients with complete AVP deficiency may become dehydrated quickly.

Maximal dehydration is typically achieved when the patient has lost 3%–5% of total body weight. In patients with central DI during a water deprivation test, weight is lost due to loss of water, urine osmolality does not exceed serum osmolality, sodium concentration increases, and plasma AVP concentration will be low or undetectable. After administration of desmopressin, urine osmolality levels increase by 50% or above 800 mOsm, urine volume will decrease, and the thirst will improve. Patients with nephrogenic DI do not respond to desmopressin.

## Replacement therapy

Desmopressin is a modified form of the normal human hormone AVP, a peptide containing nine amino acids. Desmopressin can be administered subcutaneously, intramuscularly, or intravenously (Box 5.7).

For maintenance therapy, tablets or nasal preparations are used. Most patients require 0.2–0.8 mg divided into two or three daily doses when using conventional tablets or 60–120 μg per dose when using rapidly soluble tablets. Standard nasal preparations are available in a bottle with a rhinal catheter or as a nasal spray. The rhinal catheter has the benefit of allowing fine-tuning of the dose, whereas the spray gives a fixed dose at each dosing, but it is easier to use. The usual dose of intranasal administration is 10–20 μg one or two times daily. The parenteral form is more potent and usually administered in doses of 1–2 μg divided over the day. Initiation of therapy is done by titrating and finding the most appropriate evening dose. The duration of antidiuresis after nasal administration varies from 6 to 12 h, whereas the oral dose may have shorter duration. A second morning dose is added if the antidiuretic action is insufficient during the day and early evening.

**Box 5.6** *Water deprivation test*

The test is initiated early morning after free availability to fluid overnight. Careful surveillance is needed for monitoring compliance and risk of rapid dehydration.

The test is performed for 8 h or until body weight has reduced by 3%–5%.

- Body weight, blood pressure every hour.
- Serum sodium, urea, and plasma osmolality every 2 h.
- Urine volume and urinary osmolality every 2 h.
- Plasma AVP collected before and at termination of the test.
- Desmopressin 2–4 μg i.m./i.v. is administered after 8 h or when body weight has reduced by 3%–5%.

In overt DI, urinary osmolality will be <300 mOsm/kg or below the serum osmolality; and after desmopressin, the urinary osmolality will increased by >50% or exceed 800 mOsm/kg.

**Box 5.7** *Treatment of DI*

Desmopressin with oral or nasal administration.

The dose and dose frequency are highly individualized.

Orally administered desmopressin is usually delivered three times daily.

- Dose span with conventional tablets 0.2–0.8 mg/day.
- Dose span using rapidly soluble tablets is 60–120 µg/dose occasion.

Nasal administration using spray or rhinal catheter is usually delivered in a dose of 10–20 µg one or two times daily.

Biochemical monitoring can be done using serum sodium and urea measurements as indicators of serum osmolality.

Patient education to recognize:

- Overdosing resulting in hypotonic hyponatremia with headache
- Underdosing with increased urinary output and thirst

Initiation of any drug that may cause syndrome of inappropriate ADH secretion (SIADH) should be done under surveillance.

Most patients require twice-a-day dosing. Patients should learn to sense signs and symptoms indicating lack of efficacy such as increased thirst and increased urinary output and also signs suggesting overdosing such as headache, fatigue (hyponatremia), and low urinary output. Biochemical monitoring is simply done by measuring serum sodium and urea concentrations.

A difficult group of patients are those with DI and a hypothalamic lesion that has resulted in loss of thirst sensation. These patients may develop severe hypertonic hypernatremia within a short period. The solution of this problem is very individual but often best managed by keeping a constant intake of desmopressin each day and at the same time securing a minimum amount of fluid intake per day that can be achieved by filling a container of water each day in the morning (1–1.5L) and ensuring that it has been finished in the evening. Frequent and regular monitoring of serum sodium/urea is needed in these patients, in particular in the beginning.

# Endocrine aspects of pituitary surgery

## Preoperative considerations

In parallel with the evaluation and decision on treatment for a tumor in or close to the hypothalamic/pituitary area, endocrine investigations need to be conducted with two main purposes: (1) to exclude pituitary hormone deficiency, in particular ACTH deficiency; and (2) to diagnose a hormone-producing tumor (Box 5.8). The patients with endocrine active tumors need special considerations, and surgical intervention may be deemed insufficient or unnecessary in these cases. This applies in particular to patients with prolactinomas but also to patients with Cushing's disease and acromegaly, in whom the therapeutic strategy is different compared with patients with nonfunctioning pituitary adenomas. Deficiency in ACTH and TSH secretion is of particular importance to detect and manage preoperatively to avoid increased peri- and postoperative complications.

## Perioperative and postoperative considerations

Some neurosurgical units routinely administer perioperative parenteral glucocorticoids to patients undergoing pituitary surgery or peripituitary surgery followed by oral HC tapered to a replacement dose during postoperative recovery (Box 5.8).[69] Special algorithms for determining which patients need perioperative glucocorticoid treatment have been produced.[70] The routine use of perioperative use of glucocorticoids has however been questioned,[71] but the mainstay of overall management is to prevent an adrenal crisis.

It is essential that pituitary function is tested postoperatively because both recovery and loss of pituitary

**Box 5.8** *Endocrine preoperative testing in patients with pituitary and peripituitary tumors*

Free T4, TSH

Testosterone, estradiol, SHBG, FSH, LH

IGF-I

Cortisol 0800 hours, 24 h urinary free cortisol, ACTH

Prolactin (with serial dilution)

If an endocrine active tumor is suspected, further testing may be required.

**Box 5.9** *Advanced endocrine care after pituitary surgery*

Move the patient from the neurosurgical department to the endocrine ward when stable from surgery/anesthesia.

Postoperative monitoring of fluid status to detect DI and/or SIADH

- Urinary output (fractionated or 24 h)
- U-osmolality (specific gravity) 1–2 times per day
- Serum sodium (urea) 1–2 times per day

Attempt to withdraw peri- and postoperative HC replacement

Monitor 0800 hour serum cortisol concentrations

Repeat the preoperative testing of other pituitary hormones:

Free T4, TSH, FSH, LH, testosterone, estradiol, prolactin, IGF-I

Neuro-ophthalmologic consultation

Otorhinolaryngeal consultation (if transsphenoidal approach)

function may occur (Box 5.9). ACTH, TSH, and AVP production need particular attention in the immediate postoperative phase, whereas deficient FSH/LH and GH production may become overt and symptomatic only with time. The recovery of pituitary function may occur in up to half of patients in one or more of the pituitary hormone axis.[72] Careful monitoring of patients during the first few months after surgery is therefore essential to detect recovery of pituitary function sparing the patient life-long replacement therapy.

## *Postoperative and posttraumatic DI (see Chapter 24)*

Central DI is rapidly detected in the postoperative phase if urine volume, urinary osmolality (specific gravity), and serum sodium (urea) concentrations are monitored. This monitoring needs to be performed several times during the first postoperative day. DI after surgery or trauma to the pituitary or hypothalamus may be transient, permanent, or triphasic. Transient DI usually has an abrupt onset and then resolves within a few days. This is the most common pattern of postoperative and posttraumatic DI. Permanent or prolonged DI is less common and has also an abrupt early onset. In the triphasic form, there is an immediate onset of DI lasting a few days followed by an interphase during which urine osmolality rises and serum osmolality decreases, sometimes producing a period of hypotonic hyponatremia (SIADH), which then turns into a more prolonged or permanent period of DI. These first and last periods need treatment with desmopressin, whereas the interphase period is treated with water deprivation or with vaptans, a vasopressin receptor 2 antagonist. The mechanism for the triphasic postoperative response has been explained by a direct trauma toward the posterior pituitary that inhibits the secretion of the AVP. This is then followed by a period when the stored AVP in the neurons is passively released. Because this release is not regulated serum osmolality may either normalize or become too low due to excess AVP (SIADH). When the neurons have emptied their AVP content, a DI develops again. All patients undergoing surgery close to the hypothalamic–pituitary area should be monitored for DI in the postoperative phase, and if DI occurs, treatment and monitoring during the following days should be done in such manner that a transient period of SIADH can be detected and managed. Because postoperative DI may be a self-limiting condition, patients may be advised to omit one dose of desmopressin on a regular basis particularly in the time period (months) after surgery to determine whether polyuria returns.

## *Hypopituitarism and pregnancy*

Before conception, hormonal replacement therapy in the woman with hypopituitarism should be optimized regarding all axes, and close collaboration with the gynecologists and the fertility clinic should be secured. Patients with large pituitary tumors require special advice. If possible, pituitary surgery should be performed before conception.

Women with FSH/LH deficiency need ovulation stimulation therapy and *in vitro* fertilization to achieve conception after withdrawal of estrogen replacement therapy. As the ovulation stimulation therapy is initiated, the L-thyroxine dose should be increased by approximately 25%–50% and the free T4 levels should be monitored regularly, at least once a month. The need for a higher dose of L-thyroxine comes from increased levels of thyroxine-binding globulin as a result of increased estradiol concentrations.[73]

The placental production of variant GH (GH-V)[74] is clinically evident in women with GH deficiency as their need for GH substitution therapy diminishes after the 20th week of gestation. In women with normal GH secretion, this is the time when pituitary-derived GH secretion is suppressed as GH-V in concert with placental lactogen stimulates maternal IGF-I production. The replacement dose of GH can be maintained until the 20th week of gestation and then reduced gradually until the 30th week of gestation when GH can be withdrawn completely.[47]

In women who plan for conception, a careful evaluation of the HPA axis should be done because this is difficult to perform during pregnancy, due to the marked increase in binding proteins carrying cortisol in the circulation. Women with intact HPA axis may undergo labor without complications. Patients with partial hypopituitarism, where the adrenal function testing has been borderline or ambiguous, may need careful follow-up during pregnancy for symptoms and signs of adrenal insufficiency. It is often necessary to provide extra supervision during labor, and if any clinical event suggests the need of HC, HC should be administered. In women with known ACTH deficiency, the administration of HC during labor follows the routine for surgery (in our unit 50–100 mg i.v. every 4–6 h).

In the postpartum period, the women should return to their pregestational doses of the hormonal replacement. Lactation may occur in patients with partial hypopituitarism,[47] but the patients should be prepared that lactation may not be achievable.

A few studies have reported the experience from women with hypopituitarism who have given birth. The number of births is small, but hitherto there are no indications that the offspring suffers from any malformations. There are however some studies suggesting lower implantation rates after fertility stimulation in patients with hypopituitarism.[75,76]

## *Hypopituitarism and long-term outcome*

An increased morbidity and mortality rate in cardiovascular disease was described in patients with hypopituitarism in studies from the late 1980s and early 1990s. Since then, hormonal replacement therapy has changed; GH has been added and individualized dosing is used for several of the other hormones. It is also plausible that the knowledge of an increased risk of cardiovascular disease has led to more active prevention measures in these patients, such as more aggressive management of blood hypertension and hyperlipidemia. Indeed, the mortality rate in patients with pituitary disease is falling.[15] Some studies even indicated that the mortality rate is near to normal for adult patients with hypopituitarism.[77,78] Subgroups that still demonstrate increased mortality rate are those who have received radiotherapy toward the hypothalamic–pituitary area, patients with craniopharyngioma, and those with an underlying malignancy as cause of their hypopituitarism.[79]

Fracture rate is increased in patients with hypopituitarism. Bone density improves with GH replacement therapy, but to a larger extent in men than in women. However, the fracture rate and the prevalence of osteoporosis is higher in women than in men, and further studies are needed to elucidate how to optimize hormonal replacement further with regard to bone health. Individualized dosing of estradiol replacement and more physiological glucocorticoid replacement may be some of the ways to improve bone quality in women with hypopituitarism.

## Summary

Hypopituitarism is a complex endocrine disease, often with serious underlying conditions, such as a tumor and a complex multiple pituitary hormone insufficiency. Data demonstrate that although endocrine replacement therapy is performed, outcome in terms of morbidity and mortality is compromised. These patients have high frequency of the metabolic syndrome and compromised quality of life. There is an increased knowledge of individualized management of each of the hormone axes and of their hormone–hormone interactions. There is also an increasing trend of managing patients in multidisciplinary teams, including endocrinologists with special interest in pituitary diseases, neuroradiology, and neurosurgery. A core feature in the management of hypopituitarism is also patient education, particularly concerning their glucocorticoid replacement for adrenal insufficiency and desmopressin therapy for DI. All the above-mentioned changes and trends are likely to contribute to the improvements in outcome of patients with hypopituitarism as seen in more recent studies.

## References

*1. Schneider HJ, Aimaretti G, Kreitschmann-Andermahr I, Stalla G-K, Ghigo E. Hypopituitarism. *Lancet*. 2007;369:1461–70.
2. Harris GW. Humours and hormones. *J Endocrinol*. 1972;53:2–23.
3. Toni R. Ancient views on the hypothalamic-pituitary-thyroid axis: An historical and epistemological perspective. *Pituitary*. 2000;3:83–95.
4. Lindholm J, Nielsen EH. Pituitary-gonadal axis: Historical notes. *Pituitary*. 2009;12:226–35.
5. Smith PE, Engle ET. Experimental evidence regarding the role of anterior pituitary in development and regulation of genital system. *Am J Anat*. 1927;40:159–217.

* Key or Classic references.

6. Simmonds M. Uber hypophysisschwund mit todlichem augang. *Dtsch Med Wschr*. 1914;40:322–3.
7. Salomon F, Cuneo RC, Hesp R, Sonksen PH. The effects of treatment with recombinant human growth hormone on body composition and metabolism in adults with growth hormone deficiency. *N Engl J Med*. 1989;321:1797–803.
8. Jorgensen JO, Pedersen SA, Laurberg P, Weeke J, Skakkebaek NE, Christiansen JS. Effects of growth hormone therapy on thyroid function of growth hormone-deficient adults with and without concomitant thyroxine-substituted central hypothyroidism. *J Clin Endocrinol Metab*. 1989;69:1127–32.
9. Rosén T, Bengtsson BA. Premature mortality due to cardiovascular disease in hypopituitarism. *Lancet*. 1990;336:285–8.
10. Bergthorsdottir R, Leonsson-Zachrisson M, Oden A, Johannsson G. Premature mortality in patients with Addison's disease: A population-based study. *J Clin Endocrinol Metab*. 2006;91:4849–53.
11. Brooke AM, Kalingag LA, Miraki-Moud F, Camacho-Hübner C, Maher KT, Walker DM, et al. Dehydroepiandrosterone improves psychological well-being in male and female hypopituitary patients on maintenance growth hormone replacement. *J Clin Endocrinol Metab*. 2006;91:3773–9.
12. Regal M, Paramo C, Sierra SM, Garcia-Mayor RV. Prevalence and incidence of hypopituitarism in an adult Caucasian population in northwestern Spain. *Clin Endocrinol (Oxf)*. 2001;55:735–40.
13. Nilsson B, Gustavsson-Kadaka E, Bengtsson BA, Jonsson B. Pituitary adenomas in Sweden between 1958 and 1991: Incidence, survival, and mortality. *J Clin Endocrinol Metab*. 2000;85:1420–5.
*14. Sherlock M, Ayuk J, Tomlinson JW, Toogood AA, Aragon-Alonso A, Sheppard MC, et al. Mortality in patients with pituitary disease. *Endocr Rev*. 2010;31:301–42.
15. Nielsen EH, Lindholm J, Laurberg P. Excess mortality in women with pituitary disease: A meta-analysis. *Clin Endocrinol (Oxf)*. 2007;67:693–7.
16. Stochholm K, Gravholt CH, Laursen T, Laurberg P, Andersen M, Kristensen LO, et al. Mortality and GH deficiency: A nationwide study. *Eur J Endocrinol*. 2007;157:9–18.
17. Tomlinson JW, Holden N, Hills RK, Wheatley K, Clayton RN, Bates AS, et al. Association between premature mortality and hypopituitarism. West Midlands Prospective Hypopituitary Study Group. *Lancet*. 2001;357:425–31.
18. Mills JL, Schonberger LB, Wysowski DK, Brown P, Durako SJ, Cox C, et al. Long-term mortality in the United States cohort of pituitary-derived growth hormone recipients. *J Pediatr*. 2004;144:430–6.

19. Sherlock M, Reulen RC, Alonso AA, Ayuk J, Clayton RN, Sheppard MC, et al. ACTH deficiency, higher doses of hydrocortisone replacement, and radiotherapy are independent predictors of mortality in patients with acromegaly. *J Clin Endocrinol Metab*. 2009;94:4216–23.
20. Herring R, Russell-Jones D. The effect of growth hormone on pituitary tumour growth. *Curr Opin Endocrinol Diabetes Obes*. 2010;17:365–8.
*21. Hahner S, Loeffler M, Bleicken B, Drechsler C, Milovanovic D, Fassnacht M, et al. Epidemiology of adrenal crisis in chronic adrenal insufficiency: The need for new prevention strategies. *Eur J Endocrinol*. 2010;162:597–602.
22. Dorin RI, Qualls CR, Crapo LM. Diagnosis of adrenalin sufficiency. Ann Intern Med 2003;139:194-204
23. Forss M, Batcheller G, Skrtic S, Johannsson G. Current practice of glucocorticoid replacement therapy and patient-perceived health outcomes in adrenalin sufficiency – a worldwide patient survey. BMC EndocrDisord 2012;12:8
24. Kraan GP, Dullaart RP, Pratt JJ, Wolthers BG, Drayer NM, De Bruin R. The daily cortisol production reinvestigated in healthy men. The serum and urinary cortisol production rates are not significantly different. *J Clin Endocrinol Metab*. 1998;83:1247–52.
*25. Filipsson H, Monson JP, Koltowska-Haggstrom M, Mattsson A, Johannsson G. The impact of glucocorticoid replacement regimens on metabolic outcome and comorbidity in hypopituitary patients. *J Clin Endocrinol Metab*. 2006;91:3954–61.
26. Weaver JU, Thaventhiran L, Noonan K, Burrin JM, Taylor NF, Norman MR, et al. The effect of growth hormone replacement on cortisol metabolism and glucocorticoid sensitivity in hypopituitary adults. *Clin Endocrinol (Oxf)*. 1994;41:639–48.
27. Swords FM, Carroll PV, Kisalu J, Wood PJ, Taylor NF, Monson JP. The effects of growth hormone deficiency and replacement on glucocorticoid exposure in hypopituitary patients on cortisone acetate and hydrocortisone replacement. *Clin Endocrinol (Oxf)*. 2003;59:613–20.
28. Giavoli C, Libe R, Corbetta S, Ferrante E, Lania A, Arosio M, et al. Effect of recombinant human growth hormone (GH) replacement on the hypothalamic-pituitary-adrenal axis in adult GH-deficient patients. *J Clin Endocrinol Metab*. 2004;89:5397–401.
29. Besser GM, Jeffcoate WJ. Endocrine and metabolic diseases. Adrenal diseases. *Br Med J*. 1976;1:448–51.
30. Lovas K, Husebye ES. Continuous subcutaneous hydrocortisone infusion in Addison's disease. *Eur J Endocrinol*. 2007;157:109–12.
31. Debono M, Ghobadi C, Rostami-Hodjegan A, Huatan H, Campbell MJ, Newell-Price J, et al. Modified-release hydrocortisone to provide circadian cortisol profiles. *J Clin Endocrinol Metab*. 2009;94:1548–54.
32. Johannsson G, Nilsson AG, Bergthorsdottir R, Burman P, Dahlqvist P, Ekman B, et al. Improved cortisol exposure-time profile and outcome in patients with adrenal insufficiency: A prospective randomized trial of a novel hydrocortisone dual-release formulation. *J Clin Endocrinol Metab*. 2012;97:473–81.
33. Miller KK, Sesmilo G, Schiller A, Schoenfeld D, Burton S, Klibanski A. Androgen deficiency in women with hypopituitarism. *J Clin Endocrinol Metab*. 2001;86:561–7.
34. Arlt W, Callies F, van Vlijmen JC, Koehler I, Reincke M, Bidlingmaier M, et al. Dehydroepiandrosterone replacement in women with adrenal insufficiency. *N Engl J Med*. 1999;341:1013–20.
35. Johannsson G, Burman P, Wiren L, Engstrom BE, Nilsson AG, Ottosson M, et al. Low dose dehydroepiandrosterone affects behavior in hypopituitary androgen-deficient women: A placebo-controlled trial. *J Clin Endocrinol Metab*. 2002;87:2046–52.
36. Persani L. Hypothalamic thyrotropin-releasing hormone and thyrotropin biological activity. *Thyroid*. 1998;8:941–6.
37. Patel YC, Burger HG. Serum thyrotropin (TSH) in pituitary and-or hypothalamic hypothyroidism: Normal or elevated basal levels and paradoxical responses to thyrotropin-releasing hormone. *J Clin Endocrinol Metab*. 1973;37:190–6.
38. Andersen S, Pedersen KM, Bruun NH, Laurberg P. Narrow individual variations in serum T(4) and T(3) in normal subjects: A clue to the understanding of subclinical thyroid disease. *J Clin Endocrinol Metab*. 2002;87:1068–72.
*39. Agha A, Walker D, Perry L, Drake WM, Chew SL, Jenkins PJ, et al. Unmasking of central hypothyroidism following growth hormone replacement in adult hypopituitary patients. *Clin Endocrinol (Oxf)*. 2007;66:72–7.
40. Filipsson Nystrom H, Feldt-Rasmussen U, Kourides I, Popovic V, Koltowska-Haggstrom M, Jonsson B, et al. The metabolic consequences of thyroxine replacement in adult hypopituitary patients. *Pituitary*. 2011;14:208–16.
41. Alexopoulou O, Beguin C, De Nayer P, Maiter D. Clinical and hormonal characteristics of central hypothyroidism at diagnosis and during follow-up in adult patients. *Eur J Endocrinol*. 2004;150:1–8.
42. Slawik M, Klawitter B, Meiser E, Schories M, Zwermann O, Borm K, et al. Thyroid hormone replacement for central hypothyroidism: A randomized controlled trial comparing two doses of thyroxine (T4) with a combination of T4 and triiodothyronine. *J Clin Endocrinol Metab*. 2007;92:4115–22.

*43. Ferretti E, Persani L, Jaffrain-Rea ML, Giambona S, Tamburrano G, Beck-Peccoz P. Evaluation of the adequacy of levothyroxine replacement therapy in patients with central hypothyroidism. *J Clin Endocrinol Metab.* 1999;84:924–9.
44. Shimon I, Cohen O, Lubetsky A, Olchovsky D. Thyrotropin suppression by thyroid hormone replacement is correlated with thyroxine level normalization in central hypothyroidism. *Thyroid.* 2002;12:823–7.
45. Carrozza V, Csako G, Yanovski JA, Skarulis MC, Nieman L, Wesley R, et al. Levothyroxine replacement therapy in central hypothyroidism: A practice report. *Pharmacotherapy.* 1999;19:349–55.
46. Flynn RW, Bonellie SR, Jung RT, MacDonald TM, Morris AD, Leese GP. Serum thyroid-stimulating hormone concentration and morbidity from cardiovascular disease and fractures in patients on long-term thyroxine therapy. *J Clin Endocrinol Metab.* 2010;95:186–93.
47. Van Aken MO, Lamberts SWJ. Diagnosis and treatment of hypopituitarism: An update. *Pituitary.* 2005;8:183–91.
48. Leung KC, Johannsson G, Leong GM, Ho KK. Estrogen regulation of growth hormone action. *Endocr Rev.* 2004;25:693–721.
49. Schairer C, Lubin J, Troisi R, Sturgeon S, Brinton L, Hoover R. Menopausal estrogen and estrogen-progestin replacement therapy and breast cancer risk. *JAMA.* 2000;26:485–91.
*50. Wiren L, Boguszewski CL, Johannsson G. Growth hormone (GH) replacement therapy in GH-deficient women during pregnancy. *Clin Endocrinol (Oxf).* 2002;57:235–59.
*51. Bhasin S, Cunningham GR, Hayes FJ, Matsumoto AM, Snyder PJ, Swerdloff RS, et al. Testosterone therapy in adult men with androgen deficiency syndromes: An Endocrine Society clinical practice guideline. *J Clin Endocrinol Metab.* 2006;91:1995–2010.
52. Howell S, Shalet S. Testosterone deficiency and replacement. *Horm Res.* 2001;56(Suppl 1):86–92.
53. Vicari E, Mongioi A, Calogero AE, Moncada ML, Sidoti G, Polosa P, et al. Therapy with human chorionic gonadotropin alone induces spermatogenesis in men with isolated hypogonadotropic hypogonadism. Long-term follow-up. *Int J Androl.* 1992;15:320–9.
54. Buchter D, Behre HM, Kliesch S, Nieschlag E. Pulsatile GnRH or human chorionic gonadotropin/human menopausal gonadotropin as effective treatment for men with hypogonadotropic hypogonadism: A review of 42 cases. *Eur J Endocrinol.* 1998;139:298–303.
55. Liu PY, Gebski VJ, Turner L, Conway AJ, Wishart SM, Handelsman DJ. Predicting pregnancy and spermatogenesis by survival analysis during gonadotropin treatment of gonadotropin-deficient infertile men. *Hum Reprod.* 2002;17:625–33.
56. Rosén T, Edén S, Larson G, Wilhelmsen L, Bengtsson B-Å. Cardiovascular risk factors in adult patients with growth hormone deficiency. *Acta Endocrinol.* 1993;129:195–200.
57. Nilsson AG, Svensson J, Johannsson G. Management of growth hormone deficiency in adults. *Growth Horm IGF Res.* 2007;17:441–62.
58. Johannsson G. Management of adult growth hormone deficiency. *Endocrinol Metab Clin North Am.* 2007;36:203–20.
*59. Ho KK. Consensus guidelines for the diagnosis and treatment of adults with GH deficiency II: A statement of the GH Research Society in association with the European Society for Pediatric Endocrinology, Lawson Wilkins Society, European Society of Endocrinology, Japan Endocrine Society, and Endocrine Society of Australia. *Eur J Endocrinol.* 2007;157:695–700.
*60. Molitch ME, Clemmons DR, Malozowski S, Merriam GR, Vance ML; Endocrine Society. Evaluation and treatment of adult growth hormone deficiency: An Endocrine Society clinical practice guideline. *J Clin Endocrinol Metab.* 2011;96:1587–609.
61. Corneli G, Di Somma C, Baldelli R, Rovere S, Gasco V, Croce CG, et al. The cut-off limits of the GH response to GH-releasing hormone-arginine test related to body mass index. *Eur J Endocrinol.* 2005;153:257–64.
62. Clayton PE, Cuneo RC, Juul A, Monson JP, Shalet SM, Tauber M. Consensus statement on the management of the GH-treated adolescent in the transition to adult care. *Eur J Endocrinol.* 2005;152:165–70.
63. Johannsson G, Rosén T, Bengtsson B-Å. Individualized dose titration of growth hormone (GH) during GH replacement in hypopituitary adults. *Clin Endocrinol.* 1997;47:571–81.
64. Drake WM, Coyte D, Camacho-Hübner C, Jivanji NM, Kaltsas G, Wood DF, et al. Optimizing growth hormone replacement therapy by dose titration in hypopituitary adults. *J Clin Endocrinol Metab.* 1998;83:3913–19.
65. Wirén L, Whalley D, McKenna S, Wilhelmsen L. Application of a disease-specific, quality-of-life measure (QoL-AGHDA) in growth hormone-deficient adults and a random population sample in Sweden: Validation of the measure by rasch analysis. *Clin Endocrinol (Oxf).* 2000;52:143–52.
66. Child CJ, Zimmermann AG, Woodmansee WW, Green DM, Li JJ, Jung H, et al. Assessment of primary cancers in GH-treated adult hypopituitary patients: An analysis from the Hypopituitary Control and Complications Study. *Eur J Endocrinol.* 2011;165:217–23.
67. Olsson DS, Buchfelder M, Schlaffer S, Bengtsson B-Å, Jakobsson K-E, Johannsson G, et al. Comparing

progression of non-functioning pituitary adenomas in hypopituitarism patients with and without long-term GH replacement therapy. *Eur J Endocrinol.* 2009;161:1–8.

68. Gotherstrom G, Bengtsson BA, Bosaeus I, Johannsson G, Svensson J. A ten-year, prospective study of the metabolic effects of growth hormone replacement in adults. *J Clin Endocrinol Metab.* 2007;6:6.
69. Elbornsson M, Götherström G, Bosæus I, Bengtsson BA, Johannsson G, Svensson J. Fifteen years of growth hormone (GH) replacement increases bone mineral density in hypopituitary patients with adult onset GH deficiency. *Eur J Endocrinol.* 2012;166: 787–95.
70. Holmer H, Svensson J, Rylander L, Johannsson G, Rosen T, Bengtsson BA, et al. Fracture incidence in GH-deficient patients on complete hormone replacement including GH. *J Bone Miner Res.* 2007;22:1842–50.
71. Robertson GL. Diabetes insipidus. Endocrinol MetabClin North Am. 1995;24(3):549–72
*72. Vance ML. Perioperative management of patients undergoing pituitary surgery. *Endocrinol Metab Clin N Am.* 2003;32:355–65.
73. Bahnsali A, Dutta P, Bhat MH, Mukherjee KK, Rajput R, Bhadada S. Rational use of glucocorticoid during pituitary surgery – a pilot study. *Indian J Med Res.* 2008;128:294–9.
74. Wentworth JM, Gao N, Sumithran KP, Maartens NF, Kaye AH, Colman PG, et al. Prospective evaluationof a protocol for reduced glucocorticoid replacement in trans sphenoidal pituitary adenomectomy: Prophylactic glucocorticoid replacement is seldom necessary. *Clin Endocrinol (Oxf)* 2008;68(1): 29–35.
75. Webb SM, Rigla M, Wagner A, Oliver B, Bartumeus F. Recovery of hypopituitarism after neurosurgical treatment of pituitary adenomas. *J Clin Endocrinol Metab* 1999;84(10):3696–700.
76. Arafah BM. Increased need for thyroxine in women with hypothyroidism during estrogen therapy. *N Engl J Med.* 2001;344:1743–9.
77. Handwerger S, Freemark M. The roles of placental growth hormone and placental lactogen in the regulation of human fetal growth and development. *J Pediatr Endocrinol Metab.* 2000;13:343–56.
78. Hall R, Manski-Nankervis J, Goni N, Davies MC, Conway GS. Fertility outcomes in women with hypopituitarism. *Clin Endocrinol.* 2006;65:71–4.
79. Kübler K, Klingmüller D, Gembruch U, Merz WM. High-risk pregnancy management in women with hypopituitarism. *J Perinatol.* 2009;29:89–95.
80. Svensson J, Bengtsson BA, Rosén T, Odén A, Johannsson G. Malignant disease and cardiovascular morbidity in hypopituitary adults with or without growth hormone replacement therapy. *J Clin Endocrinol Metab.* 2004;89:3306–12.
81. van Bunderen CC, van Nieuwpoort IC, Arwert LI, Heymans MW, Franken AAM, Koppeschaar HPF, et al. Does growth hormone replacement therapy reduce mortality in adults with growth hormone deficiency? Data from the Dutch National Registry of Growth Hormone Treatment in adults. *J Clin Endocinol Metab.* 2011;96:3151–9.
82. Gaillard RC, Mattsson AF, Akerblad AC, Bengtsson BÅ, Cara J, Feldt-Rasmussen U, Koltowska-Häggström M, Monson JP, Saller B, Wilton P, Abs R. Overall and cause-specific mortality in GH-deficient adults on GH replacement. *Eur J Endocrinol* 2012;166:1069–77.

# 6

# IGF-I as a metabolic hormone

*David R. Clemmons*

## Introduction

Insulin-like growth factor I (IGF-I) is a polypeptide hormone whose primary structure is highly homologous (48% amino acid sequence identity) with proinsulin. IGF-I and proinsulin evolved from the same primitive precursor molecule whose function was to link nutrient intake with growth and anabolic responses in primitive organisms. Because these organisms had no means for storing calories, there was a direct link between food intake, synthesis of this precursor hormone, and stimulation of protein synthesis, leading to tissue hypertrophy and cell proliferation. With the evolution of vertebrates, there was a need for a system that enabled conversion of calories into fat for long-term energy storage and also mobilized this energy source during times of nutrient deprivation. This led to the evolutionary divergence of insulin and IGF-I as well as the appearance of growth hormone (GH). These three hormones then functioned together to allow vertebrates to respond to changes in nutrient intake with either storage or use of calories and thereby provide an optimal supply of substrate for anabolism and growth. Distinct receptors for insulin and IGF-I also appeared at this time. Insulin receptors are primarily in organs that are important for intermediary metabolism such as fat, liver, and skeletal muscle. In contrast, fat and liver, the principal sites of IGF-I synthesis, have no IGF-I receptors. Skeletal muscle and bone have abundant IGF-I receptors and are the important target tissues. This difference in receptor distribution accounts for many of the differences in insulin and IGF-I actions. The IGFs have also acquired the specialized function of being able to bind to carrier proteins in serum, whereas insulin does not have this characteristic.[1] This results in a prolonged half-life of IGF-I (e.g., 16 h) compared with insulin, which has a half-life of <10 min. The receptors each have distinct affinities for their respective ligands. The affinity of the IGF-I receptor for IGF-I is 1000-fold greater than for insulin, and the affinity insulin receptor for insulin is hundredfold greater than it is for IGF-I.[2] GH has a completely distinct receptor that belongs to the cytokine family.[3] GH is also regulated in a very distinct manner. Its secretion is inhibited by carbohydrate intake, and it is stimulated in response to stress, whereas stress is an important inhibitor or both insulin and IGF-I actions. Coordinate regulation of the metabolic actions of these three hormones provides an important basis for understanding their individual effects on intermediary metabolism and how they function coordinately to maintain growth in response to variations in nutrient intake.

## Regulation of IGF-I secretion

The two predominant variables that regulate plasma IGF-I concentrations are nutrient intake and GH. Of the two, nutrient intake predominates. IGF-I levels decrease during nutrient restriction, even in the face of rising GH levels, and administration of GH is relatively ineffective in achieving an increase in serum IGF-I. Most IGF-I in serum is derived from hepatic synthesis (i.e., 80%), and after severe caloric or protein restriction, there is a marked decrease in the sensitivity of hepatocytes to GH stimulation.[4] Reinstitution of protein intake results in a graded increase in sensitivity of these cells to GH stimulation with concomitant increases in serum IGF-I concentrations.[5] In contrast, restriction of caloric intake below approximately 800–900 cal/day results in an abrupt refractoriness to GH stimulation due to the loss of insulin secretion, which is required for IGF-I gene transcription in response to GH stimulation. Excessive nutrient intake does not result in equivalent changes, although chronic calorie excess results in changes in peripheral tissue sensitivity to IGF-I. Severe caloric restriction results in down regulation of the GH receptor with a concomitant decrease in IGF-I synthesis in the liver.[5]

## IGF-binding proteins

There are six members of the family of IGF-binding proteins, and all six circulate in plasma. IGFBP-3 is the predominant form, and it accounts for >70% of the IGF-binding capacity in serum.[6] IGFBP-3 plasma concentrations are also altered by nutrient intake, and both caloric and protein restrictions result in decreased IGFBP-3 due to reduced secretion and increased proteolysis.[5] IGFBP-3 and IGF-I form a ternary complex with third protein termed acid-labile subunit or ALS. ALS concentrations are also nutrient dependent; therefore, the coordinate regulation of all three proteins by nutrient intake serves to provide a metabolic link between nutrient intake and peripheral tissue anabolic responses.[7] The formation of this complex results in prolongation of IGF-I half-life from <10 min to 16 h. This complex serves as a reservoir of IGF-I and provides a constant supply to tissues under conditions of variable nutrient intake, thereby allowing balanced growth regulation in response to fluctuating availability of calories and protein.

Two other forms of IGF-binding proteins, IGFBP-1 and -2, that do not bind ALS are also highly nutrient dependent. IGFBP-1 gene transcription is directly suppressed by insulin; therefore, carbohydrate restriction results in substantial increases in IGFBP-1.[8] Even minor changes in carbohydrate intake that occur after ingestion of a normal meal result in significant IGFBP-1 suppression. IGFBP-2 is also regulated by insulin, although it fluctuates much less rapidly than IGFBP-1. Both IGFBP-1 and -2 are altered by chronic increases or decreases in caloric intake and reflect changes in body mass index (BMI), as well as fat mass.[9] Because these proteins fluctuate much more than IGFBP-3, they regulate the amount of free IGF-I that is available to bind to receptors. Under normal circumstances, IGFBP-3 is saturated but IGFBP-1 and -2 are unsaturated; therefore, they are able to partition free IGF-I as needed to respond to fluctuating changes in nutrient intake. Other hormones such as cortisol and thyroxine can also regulate IGF-I biosynthesis and bioavailability, and pathophysiologic alterations in these hormones have been shown to change IGF-I secretion and actions.

## Autocrine/paracrine compared with endocrine actions of IGF-I

Unlike insulin, IGF-I is synthesized and secreted in multiple tissues principally by mesenchymal cell precursors. This locally synthesized IGF-I is a major regulator of growth. Furthermore, it is extremely important for preventing apoptosis and stimulating reparative processes after injury. Local synthesis and secretion of IGF-I are stimulated after a variety of injuries and are a necessary component of the reparative response.[10] This locally synthesized IGF-I is under minimal control of systemic factors that regulate endocrine production of IGF-I. However, the system has significant redundancy because overexpression of systemic (endocrine) IGF-I or administration of supraphysiologic concentrations to experimental animals can mimic the effect of the locally produced IGF-I and stimulate similar increases in anabolic responses, growth responses, or both.[11] However, after injury, locally synthesized IGF-I is the major growth regulatory stimulus. In terms of understanding IGF-I's metabolic actions, however, the endocrine source of IGF-I is the predominant determinate. Approximately 80% of the IGF-I in blood is derived from hepatocytes and adipocytes. After systemic metabolic insults, such as severe nutrient deprivation, new onset of type I diabetes, or pathophysiologic increases in GH secretion, the blood concentrations of IGF-I change dramatically, and these changes often alter lipid and protein metabolism.[12] In contrast, changes in local IGF-I synthesis or actions do not result in systemic metabolic changes. Therefore, delineating the variables that regulate endocrine IGF-I secretion is necessary to establish an integrated understanding of how IGF-I functions as a metabolic hormone.

## Metabolic effects of IGF-I (see Growth hormone deficiency, Chapter 5)

The predominant effects of IGF-I on metabolism are to provide a signal to cells that adequate nutrition is available to avoid apoptosis, enhance cellular protein synthesis, enable cells to undergo hypertrophy in response to the appropriate stimulus, and allow cellular replication.

Therefore, even cell types that do not undergo a proliferative response in normal adult, such as neurons and skeletal myoblasts, respond to IGF-I with an increase in protein synthesis and a change in cellular metabolism. IGF-I receptors are ubiquitous; therefore, changes in serum IGF-I concentrations have the potential to alter these responses in all cell types. The signal induced by IGF-I stimulation of its receptor provides a mechanism for coordinating changes in protein, carbohydrate, and fat metabolisms among various cell types, and each of these responses is regulated coordinately with insulin and GH in the appropriate target tissue. Either insulin or IGF-I may be the primary determinant of such responses, and in some situations, GH functions to coordinate the ability of each of these hormones to modulate all three processes. Unlike the insulin receptor, the IGF-I receptor is expressed ubiquitously, and it has been shown to be present in cell types derived from all three embryonic lineages. Receptor number is maintained in a narrow range. GH has been shown to increase IGF-I receptor expression, an important adaptive mechanism for enabling organisms respond to increased metabolic demands that occur at puberty.[13] The IGF-I receptor is heterotetramer (Figure 6.1). It has two ligand-binding subunits and two subunits that contain the transmembrane signaling apparatus.[14] After ligand occupancy, the receptor undergoes tyrosine autophosphorylation. The key sites that are phosphorylated recruit signaling proteins such as IRS-1 and Shc, which leads to stimulation of the phosphoinositide-3 (PI-3) kinase pathway and/or the mitogen-activated protein (MAP) kinase pathway.[15] These processes are tightly regulated, and the degree of phosphorylation and its duration are regulated not only by stimulation of the intrinsic receptor kinase activity but also by protein tyrosine phosphatases that are recruited to the receptor and regulate the degree of activation. IGF-I receptor activation can be influenced by other systemic hormones that regulate metabolism, such as cortisol and thyroxine.

## Protein metabolism

IGF-I is a potent stimulus of protein synthesis in skeletal tissue such as muscle, bone, and cartilage. Although it stimulates protein synthesis in all cell types, these three tissues account for the bulk of the anabolic response after IGF-I administration. The effects on protein synthesis are mediated through the PI-3 kinase pathway.

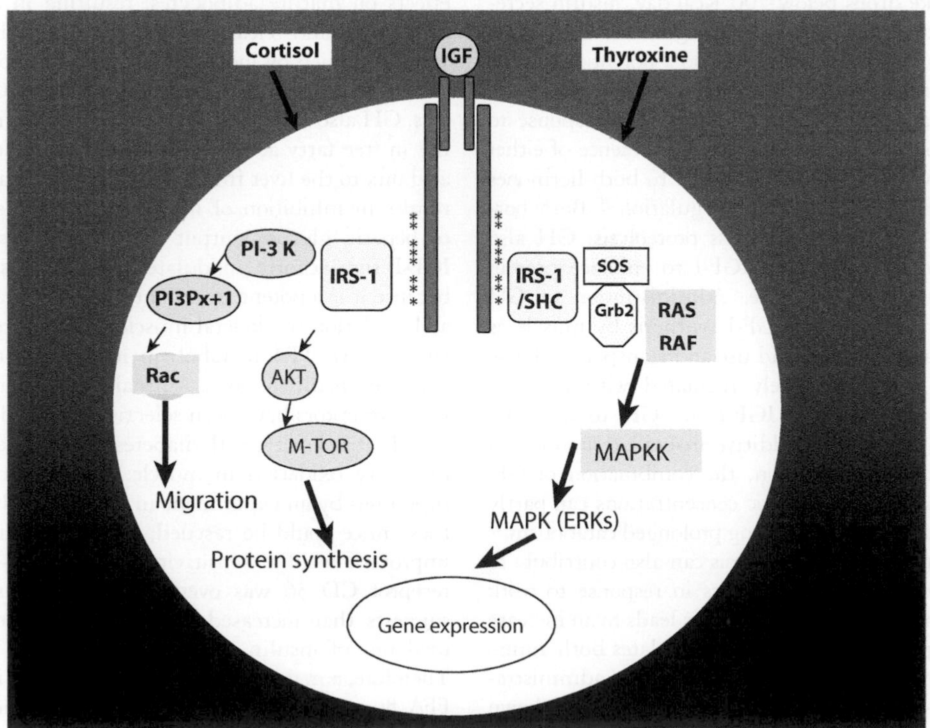


**Figure 6.1**
*IGF-I signaling through the IGF-I receptor.*

Stimulation of this kinase results in AKT activation that then leads to activation of the mTorc-1 complex and phosphorylation of p70S6 kinase as well as E4B1, a translational repressor. These two events then trigger the protein synthesis response.[16] This process is negatively regulated by the nutrient-sensitive AMP kinase that is activated in response to nutrient restriction, thereby limiting the response of tissues such a skeletal muscle to IGF-I if inadequate energy intake is present.[17] Therefore, insufficient energy results not only in decreased serum IGF-I concentrations but also in relative tissue refractoriness to IGF-I stimulation. IGF-I also stimulates amino acid transport as well as inhibition of protein breakdown in muscle. Formation of the atrogen complex that occurs in response to a variety of catabolic stimuli, such as glucocorticoid excess, is antagonized by IGF-I stimulation.[16,18] Conversely, transgenic animals in which formation of this complex is constituently activated are relatively refractory to stimulation of protein synthesis by IGF-I.[19] Glucocorticoid administration during the treatment of inflammatory disorders or due to the presence of endogenous Cushing's syndrome leads to relative IGF-I resistance through this mechanism.[20]

Insulin is also an important coordinate regulator of the ability of IGF-I to stimulate protein synthesis. If energy intake drops below 700 Kcal/day, insulin secretion is markedly attenuated, resulting in decreased IGF-I synthesis in the liver. Insulin is also a potent stimulant of protein translation in skeletal muscle, and its effects are coordinated with those of IGF-I. The response to both hormones is additive and in the presence of either insulin or IGF-I excess, the response to both hormones remains present without down regulation.[21] Both hormones also function to suppress proteolysis. GH also functions coordinately with IGF-I to enhance protein synthesis in skeletal muscle. Administration of GH results in increased local IGF-I synthesis by muscle as well as enhanced amino acid use and transport.[22] These interactions are coordinately regulated with those of IGF-I. Administration of IGF-I and GH to normally fed subjects results in an additive anabolic response, and even after caloric restriction, the combination of GH and IGF-I in supraphysiologic concentrations can partly restore protein synthesis, during prolonged catabolism.[23] Local increases in IGF-I synthesis can also contribute to the anabolic response that occurs in response to work induced hypertrophy. In muscle, this leads to an increase in IGF-I expression that in turn stimulates both amino acid transport and protein synthesis.[24] The administration of IGF-I to experimental animals has been shown to increase skeletal muscle cross-sectional fiber area and muscle force generation.[25] Infusion of IGF-I to normal volunteers increases phenylalanine flux, and this response can be enhanced by simultaneous administration of GH, although GH alone often does not result in an increase.[26] Cardiac hypertrophy results in increased IGF-I expression, and this can occur as a result of either increased pressure or volume overload.[27] Pressure overload in smooth muscle also leads to increased IGF-I and arterial cell hypertrophy. Therefore, the effects of mechanical stimuli on the anabolic response in muscle are coordinated with those of hormones such as GH and insulin, and both use the modification of IGF-I synthesis or its target actions as a final common pathway.

## *Fat metabolism*

Mature adipocytes do not express IGF-I receptors, although preadipocytes express abundant receptors and respond very well to IGF-I stimulation. IGF-I stimulates preadipocyte growth as well as differentiation into mature adipocytes.[28] In contrast, insulin receptors are abundant in mature adipocytes; therefore, IGF-I is only an effective stimulant of lipid synthesis in adipocyte beds in normal subjects, if supraphysiologic concentrations are administered, resulting in stimulation of the insulin receptor by IGF-I. In contrast, GH has direct effects on mature adipocytes, resulting in triglyceride breakdown and release of free fatty acids (FFAs). This is accompanied by increased free fatty acid oxidation in the liver.[29] Hepatocytes also do not have IGF-I receptors. GH also increases lipoprotein lipase activity resulting in free fatty acid release. The increase in free fatty acid flux to the liver from adipose tissue induced by GH results in inhibition of insulin-stimulated suppression of hepatic glucose output and insulin resistance.[29,30] IGF-I significantly modulates this process indirectly because it is a potent stimulant of free fatty acid uptake and oxidation by skeletal muscle.[29] Therefore, it modulates hepatic FFA metabolism in response to GH and enhances insulin actions. Animals in which the insulin/IGF-I receptors have been selectively deleted in skeletal muscle develop type II diabetes due to the decreased free fatty oxidation in muscle.[31] This conclusion was supported by an experiment in which the phenotype of these mice could be rescued; that is, the animals had improved insulin sensitivity if the FFA-mobilizing receptor CD 36 was overexpressed in muscle.[32] This suggests that increased FFA flux is the predominant mediator of insulin resistance under these conditions. Therefore, a major metabolic effect of IGF-I is to reduce FFA flux through the liver, resulting in the ability of insulin to better suppress hepatic glucose output. High concentrations of IGF-I can also suppress insulin secretion, resulting in decreased hepatic gluconeogenesis, but suppression of GH also contributes to decreased hepatic FFA flux. Chronic administration of IGF-I to patients who have genetic mutations in the GH receptor results in increased lipolysis and increased lipid oxidation rates as well as loss of fat mass.[33] Importantly, GH and IGF-I function coordinately by these mechanisms, to maintain both adequate substrate for normal energy use and adequate insulin sensitivity to respond to fluctuations in carbohydrate intake.[34] Interestingly, although differentiated adipocytes have no IGF-I receptors, they express high levels of IGF-I.[35] The exact role of this fat cell-synthesized IGF-I in controlling lipid metabolism is not well defined, but it may contribute to negative feedback regulation of preadipocyte differentiation, as well as regulation of FFA flux through the liver, thus limiting the negative metabolic effects of expansion of the adipocyte beds. IGFBPs also have a modulatory role on the ability of IGF-I to stimulate preadipocyte differentiation. High concentrations of IGFBP-2 that occur in transgenic mice protect mice from age-related changes in glucose intolerance and obesity. In addition, these mice are protected from high-fat diet-induced obesity and insulin resistance.[36] *In vitro*, IGFBP-2 blocked preadipocyte differentiation in response to IGF-I but not insulin. Importantly, in human subjects with obesity, IGFBP-2 levels are suppressed, and they increase in response to caloric restriction.[37] Similarly, IGFBP-1 concentrations are inversely regulated by the presence of obesity and glucose intolerance.[38]

IGF-I may also have important effects on lipid metabolism through regulation of adipokines. Leptin and IGF-I concentrations appear to be directly related.[39] Both leptin and IGF-I levels are significantly reduced in GH deficiency.[40] A recent study demonstrated that leptin injection into the intraventricular fluid resulted in increased serum IGF-I.[41] Leptin and IGF-I levels change in parallel in subjects with caloric restriction and during feeding.[42,43] In contrast, IGF-I is negatively associated with serum adiponectin in multiple pathophysiologic states including type II diabetes.[44] Adiponectin levels are very high in patients with severe IGF-I deficiency.[45] During caloric restriction, infusion of IGF-I to rats was associated with suppression of adiponectin concentrations.[43] Resistin levels have also been shown to be negatively correlated with the IGF-I in healthy women.[46]

## Bone metabolism

IGF-I concentrations are important factor in maintaining normal skeletal mass.[47] Failure to achieve and maintain normal IGF-I concentrations during puberty, as occurs with GH deficiency, results in diminished acquisition of peak bone mass, which cannot be attained in GH- and/or IGF-I-deficient subjects, without supplemental therapy.[48] IGF-I contributes not only to an increase in bone size but also to increased bone mineral density.[47] Both cortical and trabecular bone are stimulated by IGF-I, although endocrine-derived IGF-I appears to be more important for acquisition of normal cortical thickness, whereas autocrine/paracrine IGF-I is important for trabecular bone acquisition.[49] IGF-I functions with GH in a complementary manner to stimulate bone mass acquisition; however, in mice, in which GH was completely deleted, administration of supraphysiologic concentrations of IGF-I rescued normal bone growth and mineral acquisition.[11] Deletion of the IGF-I receptor in mice results in decreased bone mineral density and decreased endosteal bone formation in response to parathyroid hormone.[50,51] IGF-binding proteins also modulate the response to IGF-I in bone. Specifically, IGFBP-2 is required for normal osteoblast replication in response to IGF-I, and the two factors function coordinately to maintain skeletal mass in mice.[52] In osteoporotic humans, IGFBP-2 levels are elevated, leading to the hypothesis that it is inhibiting IGF-I action.[53] However, it is also possible that these elderly individuals are relatively resistant to the growth stimulatory effects of IGFBP-2. The effects of GH on osteoblast proliferation and differentiation are believed to be mediated primarily by IGF-I. IGF-I is able to rescue bone mass expansion and bone strength in young animals that are GH deficient; however, in elderly animals, it is only partially effective.[54,55] IGF-I has been shown to increase bone mineral density in elderly osteoporotic subjects; however, its effects are limited by significant toxicity that occurs, even with slightly supraphysiologic concentrations in this population.[56]

## Carbohydrate metabolism

The ability of IGF-I to modulate carbohydrate metabolism is consistently modified by the influence of both GH and insulin. Supraphysiologic concentrations of IGF-I feedback on the pituitary to reduce GH concentrations, thereby inhibiting the ability of GH to increase insulin resistance. GH-induced insulin resistance in both liver and skeletal muscle are improved. However, these concentrations of IGF-I also suppress insulin secretion, thus negating a part of the beneficial effect. After ingestion of a meal, there is a significant increase in free IGF-I. Portal vein insulin concentrations act directly on the liver to suppress IGFBP-1 synthesis, resulting in an increase in free IGF-I.[57] This change enhances the stimulation of FFA oxidation in muscle and induces suppression of GH secretion. Although infusion of supraphysiologic IGF-I to normal subjects results in stimulation of glucose transport, this degree of increase in free IGF-I does not occur after ingestion of a normal meal in normal subjects. High concentrations of free IGF-I can also directly suppress gluconeogenesis; however, these concentrations are not achieved in normal human subjects; therefore, it is unknown whether the concentrations that are achieved regulate insulin action in the liver.[58] Mice in which serum IGF-I has been lowered by deleting IGF-I expression in liver have impaired glucose tolerance.[59] A major determinant of this effect is stimulation of GH secretion, due to loss of negative feedback regulation, leading to antagonism of insulin action in the liver. Administration of GH receptor antagonist to human subjects with acromegaly resulted in some improvement in insulin sensitivity. However, this response could be further accentuated by administration of supraphysiologic concentrations of IGF-I.[60] Therefore, part of the ability of IGF-I to improve glucose metabolism may be due to its direct effects on skeletal muscle, rather than simply the indirect effect mediated through suppression of GH secretion. Administration of octreotide inhibits GH secretion, and, in type I diabetic patients, results in lowering of glucose; however, concomitant administration of IGF-I further lowers glucose, suggesting that it has additional effects that are GH independent.[61] Interestingly, hepatic glucose output was slightly increased in these subjects, probably due to suppression of insulin secretion, but an overall improvement in glucose homeostasis was maintained, suggesting that the effect of IGF-I on fatty acid metabolism was predominate. Therefore, there appears to be a GH-independent effect of IGF-I to enhance insulin sensitivity, and the suppression of GH secretion functions to exert an additive effect.[62] These responses are attenuated in normal subjects with aging. Aging induces a marked reduction in GH secretion, thus diminishing the actions of IGF-I that are mediated via its suppression. Furthermore, IGF-binding protein concentrations are altered with age, with a decrease in IGFBP-3 in an increase in IGFBP-2. This results in changes in cellular responsiveness to IGF-I administration.[63] IGF-I levels are also significantly influenced by fat mass. When BMI is between 18 and 24, peripheral sensitivity to GH and to IGF-I administration is maintained. However, when BMI ranges between 24 and 36, there is enhanced sensitivity to GH, with substantial increases in IGF-I concentrations.[64] Above a BMI of 37, GH secretion diminishes markedly, and there is enhanced sensitivity suppression of GH by IGF-I. It is possible that this enhanced sensitivity of IGF-I in obesity correlates with increased insulin resistance because some investigators have demonstrated a reciprocal relationship between IGF-I and insulin receptor number in some tissues.[65] In summary, increasing age, BMI, and unknown genetic factors all function to modulate the regulation of both GH and IGF-I and their effects on carbohydrate metabolism. Therefore, the composite interaction of these factors will determine the extent to which changes in IGF-I modulate insulin sensitivity.

## *IGF-I and metabolic syndrome*

IGF-I influences multiple components of the metabolic syndrome, including body composition, both fat and muscle metabolism, vascular tone and vasodilatation, renal function and sodium balance, and carbohydrate metabolism. In addition, several characteristics of the metabolic syndrome also correlate with plasma IGF-I concentrations. In general, patients with a low-normal serum IGF-I concentration who are obese and meet other criteria for metabolic syndrome tend to have a worse cardiovascular disease outcome than those who have serum IGF-I levels that are in the mid-normal range.[66] Many of the subjects also have insulin resistance. Whether the abnormal cytokine profile that accompanies the metabolic syndrome is an etiologic factor accounting for low serum IGF-I has not been definitively determined.[67] Some studies have shown a correlation between low serum IGF-I concentration, waist-to-hip ratios, and impaired glucose tolerance.[68] Although these correlations are robust, the exact determinants of a worse cardiovascular outcome have not been established. Some cytokines such as C-reactive protein (CRP) have been shown to decrease serum IGF-I in experimental animals, and this could contribute to the relationship between low serum IGF-I and a poor cardiovascular prognosis.[67]

Genetic polymorphisms that are associated with lower serum IGF-I have also been shown to correlate with metabolic syndrome parameters. One polymorphism due to a CA dinucleotide repeat in a microsatellite that is one kilobase upstream from the IGF-I transcription start site results in lower serum IGF-I.[69] This polymorphism has been shown to be associated with low birth weight. It occurs in approximately 11% of the Dutch Caucasian population, and when these subjects were analyzed later in life, the relative risk ratio of ischemic heart disease compared with normal individuals was 1.71/1.[70] The subjects were also significantly shorter and had an 18% reduction in serum IGF-I compared with the control group. This polymorphism has also been associated with a threefold increase in the risk of type

II diabetes. However, evaluation of this polymorphism in other populations has not shown the same positive predictive value.[71] IGF-I gene polymorphisms have also been associated with the development of diabetic complications in affected individuals.[72,73]

IGF-binding protein levels are also altered in patients with metabolic syndrome. Recent studies in patients with prediabetes suggest that IGFBP-1 is lower in subjects who will subsequently develop type II diabetes compared with controls that do not develop this problem.[38] This is believed to be due to increased insulin secretion that occurs during the prediabetic phase and results in suppression of IGFBP-1. Petersson et al.[38] hypothesized that as insulin resistance progresses the liver becomes more insulin resistant, leading to reduced suppression of IGFBP-1. IGFBP-2 is also suppressed in obesity and this contributes to the increased free IGF-I found in these subjects.[74] Several studies have shown suppression of IGFBP-2 in obese subjects, and this may be physiologically relevant because transgenic mice that overexpress IGFBP-2 are relatively resistant to the development of obesity during high-fat feeding.[36] Lower IGFBP-1 values are also present in patients with metabolic syndrome who have higher CRP values, and the combination of a high CRP and a low IGFBP-1 is a strong predictor of the presence of this syndrome in middle-age men.[75] The presence of a low IGF-I and high CRP along with low testosterone had a very high predictive value for development of metabolic syndrome.[76] Low IGFBP-2 also predicts the presence of metabolic syndrome and is associated with an elevated fasting glucose.[74] The degree to which IGFBP-2 is directly influencing the insulin-resistant state, or whether its effects are mediated through its ability to suppress preadipocyte differentiation, is unknown. Studies in transgenic mice overexpressing IGFBP-1 have shown that this induces hyperinsulinemia and glucose intolerance and that these changes are accentuated by increased IGFBP-1 phosphorylation, which is also increased.[77] In diabetics after weight loss, there are significant increases in both IGFBP-1 and IGFBP-2 and improvement in insulin sensitivity.[78] Patients with the lowest fasting IGFBP-1 measurements had the highest waist circumference, and those in the lowest quintile had the highest risk of developing diabetes within a year. These patients had not only low-fasting IGFBP-1 but also impaired IGFBP-1 suppression after oral glucose loading.[79] Plasma IGF-I is also associated with insulin sensitivity in prediabetic subjects with different degrees of glucose intolerance. A 5-year follow-up of 615 patients who had IGF-I values in the lower half of the normal range showed that there was an increased predisposition to develop glucose intolerance or type II diabetes and that this change was independently associated with IGFBP-1.[80] Maternal IGF-I/IGFBP-1 ratios predict subsequent risk for gestational diabetes, and IGFBP-1 values >68 ng/mL lower the risk by 57%.[81] A free IGF-I >1 ng/mL also lowers the risk by 69%. In subjects >65 years of age, IGFBP-1 in the lowest quintile predicted increased risk for glucose intolerance.[38] In contrast, IGFBP-1 above the 90th percentile predicted a reduced risk of the development of type II diabetes. Subjects in the lowest quintile of IGFBP-1 had a 12.6% prevalence of diabetes after a 17-year follow-up, whereas those in the highest quintile had only a 1.5% prevalence. IGFBP-1 predicted the development of type II diabetes even when confounding variables such as age, sex, CRP, and waist circumference were taken into consideration.

## Responses to IGF-I in metabolic disorders

### Type I diabetes

In patients with type I diabetes, serum IGF-I concentrations are low due to lack of adequate insulinization of the liver, leading to major suppression of IGF-I biosynthesis. Therefore, acute administration of insulin to type I diabetics results in a 3- to 3.5-fold increase in serum IGF-I due restoration of hepatic synthesis.[82] Administration of insulin through the portal circulation results in an even greater increase in serum IGF-I in type I diabetes compared with peripheral insulin administration. This change in IGF-I concentrations is believed to have significant metabolic consequences in patients with severe IGF-I deficiency due to poorly controlled diabetes. In Mauriac's syndrome, due to very poorly controlled diabetes, the pathophysiology is similar to starvation, and there is major cachexia with loss of protein synthesis in skeletal muscle. This is also accompanied by sodium retention and edema, and these changes resolve when adequate insulin therapy is instituted. Although part of these changes are due solely to insulin deficiency, the combined effects of low insulin and IGF-I result in loss of protein synthesis in peripheral tissues and manifest in extreme cachexia. Even moderate degrees of poor control can affect linear growth in adolescent patients with relatively low serum IGF-I, and children with poor diabetic control do not achieve optimal height.[83] That this change is rate-limiting for growth has been shown in experimental animals with diabetes and low IGF-I concentrations, and administration of IGF-I can restore the normal growth response. These patients also have significant elevation in serum GH concentration that further contributes to induction of insulin resistance in the liver. Even though low levels of insulin are present, they are not adequate to suppress hepatic gluconeogenesis and maintain metabolic control. IGFBP-1 concentrations are also extremely high due to failure of insulin to suppress hepatic IGFBP-1 synthesis and fall abruptly in response to adequate insulin therapy.[82] This contributes to low free IGF-I concentrations. In diabetes, IGFBP-2 concentrations also rise and correlate negatively with a hemoglobin A-1C. The extent to which this rise in IGFBP-2 contributes to loss of the anabolic effect of IGF-I and induction catabolism is unknown. Poorly controlled diabetes is also accompanied by proteolysis of IGFBP-3, resulting in a significant loss of IGF-I carrying capacity in serum and wider fluctuations in free IGF-I concentrations.[84] Treatment of type I diabetics with IGF-I induces significant metabolic improvement. A trial in 223 subjects using IGF-I doses ranging from 20 to 40 μg/kg showed that hemoglobin A-1C improved significantly and insulin requirements decreased.[85] Unfortunately, this was accompanied by significant prevalence of side effects, and four subjects had worsening retinopathy during follow-up after IGF-I administration had been discontinued. Hyperinsulinemic clamp studies have shown that administration of IGF-I enhanced insulin sensitivity and peripheral insulin-stimulated glucose disposal was increased by 34% after IGF-I administration.[86] This was accompanied by a significant lowering of GH concentrations, possibly indicating that GH was the mediator of insulin resistance. However, in another study, octreotide was administered and IGF-I still reduced hepatic glucose production and stimulated glucose uptake without a change in glycerol turnover, suggesting that the effect was due to enhanced insulin sensitivity and not a reduction in GH.[63] IGF-I also improves parameters of lipid metabolism in type I diabetics, lowering LDL cholesterol, triglycerides, and apoprotein B-100.

## *Type II diabetes*

Administration of IGF-I to patients with type II diabetes results in suppression of GH secretion as well as endogenous insulin secretion. Because GH concentrations are quite low basally in these patients, further suppression of GH results in minimal improvement in insulin sensitivity. In spite of this fact, administration of IGF-I (40 μg/kg b.i.d.) results in maintenance of serum IGF-I concentrations that are at the upper range of normal, or slightly above the normal range, and patients with these concentrations invariability show a significant improvement in insulin sensitivity, as evidenced by use of a frequently sampled intravenous glucose tolerance test (Bergman minimal model method).[87] Using this method, investigators were able to show that 6 weeks of IGF-I administration to type II diabetics results in a 3.4-fold improvement in insulin sensitivity. Although the molecular mechanism is unknown, the most likely etiology is improvement in fatty acid use by skeletal muscle, resulting in decreased fatty acid flux to the liver. Indeed, one short-term study using a hyperinsulinemic, hyperglycemic clamp suggested that hepatic glucose output was significantly reduced under these conditions.[58] Because IGF-I does not stimulate hepatocytes directly, this suggests that the responses are the result of IGF-I actions in muscle to reduce FFA flux to liver, thereby enhancing insulin action. Based on these observations, a larger clinical trial in which doses of 10–80 μg/kg/day were administered to 212 adults for 12 weeks showed a dose-dependent reduction in hemoglobin A1C as well as mean daily glucose.[88] Administration of doses in this range to patients who were concomitantly receiving insulin also showed an improvement in their hemoglobin A1C, with a significant reduction in the need for exogenous insulin therapy.[89] The reduction was substantial, 0.8%. However, the side effect profiles were observed with each of these regimens, particularly with the most effective doses, for example, ≥40 μg/kg b.i.d. Because of this, an attempt was made to reduce the excursion of free IGF-I after IGF injections by administering IGF-I with its principle binding IGFBP-3. Forty-eight subjects with type II diabetes were treated with this regimen. Both fasting and postprandial blood glucose fell significantly by 35%–40%, and insulin requirements decreased.[90] This suggests it may be possible to utilize this regimen; however, long-term studies comparing the two types of regimens in inducing side effect profiles have not been undertaken.

## *IGF-I in osteoporosis*

IGF-I has been administered to two types of patients with severe osteopenia. Younger patients with anorexia nervosa respond to short-term IGF-I administration by increasing bone turnover, and there is a significant anabolic effect. Bone mineral density increased by 1.7% after 9 months, whereas it decreased 0.6% in control subjects.[91] IGF-I was also shown to be an effective stimulant of bone formation in men with osteoporosis. Patients with GH deficiency also respond IGF-I with increased bone turnover. Administration of IGF-I to elderly subjects with osteoporosis results in increases in markers of bone resorption and bone formation, indicating that it primarily stimulates turnover.[92] However, none of the studies that have been completed for an extended treatment interval have shown an effect on bone mineral content. A 4-month trial of administration of IGF-I with IGFBP-3 was highly effective in stimulated cortical bone formation in rats.[93] This combination also demonstrated an improvement bone density in osteoporotic patients who were immobilized after a hip fracture.[94] Although there is an association between serum IGF-I concentrations and bone mineral density in elderly adults, even short-term administration of IGF-I has been associated with a significant incidence of side effects.[92] Therefore, the degree of increase in serum IGF-I that can be maintained without side effects for an extended period that would be necessary to achieve significant improvement in bone mineral content has not been established. Clearly, the ability of IGF-I to stimulate bone resorption in parallel with stimulation of bone formation is a limiting factor for the use of this therapy for long-term improvement in bone mineral density in this patient population.

## Catabolic states

Severe catabolic states result in relative resistance to GH and are mediated by increases in cytokines such as tumor necrosis factor (TNF) α and interleukin (IL)-1.[95,96] GH resistance has been demonstrated in patients with human immunodeficiency virus (HIV) wasting disorders, and disorders of inadequate nutrient intake or absorption such as cystic fibrosis and celiac disease. IGF-I has been administered for relatively short intervals to such patients as well as patients with burns, or closed head trauma, who are severely catabolic. These two groups of patients have responded IGF-I with increases in protein synthesis and a positive anabolic response. Administration of the IGF-I/IGFBP-3 complex was also shown to increase protein synthesis in burn patients.[97] One small placebo-controlled subject was completed in patients with myotonic dystrophy and showed that IGF-I stimulated protein synthesis and inhibited protein breakdown.[98] Muscle mass and strength also improved. IGF-I/IGFBP-3 also has an anabolic effect in these patients.[99] Clearly, in these types of patients, variables such as high rates of excretion glucocorticoids result in relative resistance to IGF-I; therefore, its ability to reverse the catabolic process is in part dependent upon how sensitive the anabolic restoring effects are to stimulation compared with stimulation of side effects such as edema, arthralgias, and headaches.

## Summary

IGF-I functions as a key metabolic hormone providing a signal to the cells that adequate nutrient is available for growth. This effect is counterbalanced by hormones that are increased during stress, such as glucocorticoids and thyroxine, which can counteract the effects of IGF-I in stimulating protein synthesis or inhibiting protein breakdown. Although all cells possess IGF-I receptors, cells are differentially programed depending on the cell type and state of differentiation to respond IGF-I. Fully differentiated cell types may respond with increase in protein synthesis, for example, myocytes, or with inhibition of apoptosis, for example, neurons, without undergoing proliferation. In all these cases, however, the response is integrated with the ability of IGF-I to be regulated by adequate nutrients, thus providing a common link between nutrient availability and stimulation of each of these events. The ability to store dietary carbohydrate and to mobilize fat as an energy source is also regulated by IGF-I. This functions as an important modulator of nutrient availability during this time of inadequate calorie intake. However, with excessive energy intake, the balance between GH and IGF-I action is altered, and obesity-induced suppression of GH secretion limits the ability of IGF-I to enhance insulin sensitivity through changes in FFA metabolism. This limitation may be an important contribution to the development of obesity-induced insulin resistance.

## Acknowledgments

I thank Laura Lindsey for help in preparing the manuscript.

## References

1. Duan C. Specifying the cellular responses to IGF signals: Roles of IGF-binding proteins. *J Endocrinol* 2002;175:41–54.
2. Johansson GS, Arngvist HJ. Insulin and IGF-I action on insulin receptors, IGF-I receptors, and hybrid insulin/IGF-I receptors in vascular smooth muscle cells. *Am J Physiol Endocrinol Metab* 2006;291:E1124–30.
3. Brooks AJ, Waters MJ. The growth hormone receptor: Mechanism of activation and clinical implications. *Nat Rev Endocrinol* 2010;6:515–25.
*4. Yakar S, Liu JL, Stannard B, et al. Normal growth and development in the absence of hepatic insulin-like growth factor I. *Proc Natl Acad Sci U S A* 1999;96:7324–9.

* Key or Classic references.

5. Underwood LE, Thissen JP, Lemozy S, et al. Hormonal and nutritional regulation of IGF-I and its binding proteins. *Horm Res* 1994;42:145–51.
6. Baxter RC. Insulin-like growth factor (IGF) binding proteins: Interactions with IGFs and intrinsic bioactivities. *Am J Physiol Endocrinol Metab* 2000;278:E967–76.
7. Boisclair YR, Rhoads RP, Ueki I, et al. The acid-labile subunit (ALS) of the 150 kDa IGF-binding protein complex: An important but forgotten component of the circulating IGF system. *J Endocrinol* 2001;170:63–70.
8. Underwood LE. Nutritional regulation of IGF-I and IGFBPs. *J Pediatr Endocrinol Metab* 1996;3:303–12.
9. Martin RM, Holly JM, Davey Smith G, et al. Associations of adiposity from childhood into adulthood with insulin resistance and the insulin-like growth factor system: 65 year follow up of the Boyd Orr Cohort. *J Clin Endocrinol Metab* 2006;91:3287–95.
10. Philippou A, Maridaki M, Halapas A, et al. The role of the insulin-like growth factor 1 (IGF-1) in skeletal muscle physiology. *In Vivo* 2007;21:45–54.
11. Wu Y, Sun H, Yakar S, et al. Elevated levels of insulin-like growth factor (IGF)-I in serum rescue the severe growth retardation of IGF-I null mice. *Endocrinol* 2009;150:4395–403.
*12. Jones JL, Clemmons DR. Insulin-like growth factors and their binding proteins: Biological actions. *Endocr Rev* 1995;16:3–34.
13. Christoforidis A, Maniadaki I, Stanhope R. Growth hormone/insulin-like growth factor-1 axis during puberty. *Pediatr Endocrinol Rev* 2005;3:5–10.
14. De Meyts P, Gauguin L, Svendsen AM, et al. Structural basis of allosteric ligand-receptor interactions in the insulin/relaxin peptide family. *Ann N Y Acad Sci* 2009;1160:45–53.
15. Myers MJ, White MF. Insulin signal transduction and the IRS proteins. *Ann Rev Pharmacol* 1996;36:615.
*16. Glass DJ. Skeletal muscle hypertrophy and atrophy signaling pathways. *Int J Biochem Cell Biol* 2005;37:1974–84.
17. Ning J, Clemmons DR. AMP-activated protein kinase inhibits IGF-I signaling and protein synthesis in vascular smooth muscle cells via stimulation of insulin receptor substrate 1 S794 and tuberous sclerosis 2 S1345 phosphorylation. *Mol Endocrinol* 2010;24:1218–29.
18. Schakman O, Gilson H, de Conick V, et al. Insulin-like growth factor-I gene transfer by electroporation prevents skeletal muscle atrophy in glucocorticoid-treated rats. *Endocrinol* 2005;146:1789–97.
19. Dehoux M, Van Beneden R, Pasko N, et al. Role of the insulin-like growth factor-I decline in the induction of atrogin-1/MAFbx during fasting and diabetes. *Endocrinol* 2004;245:4806–12.
20. Schakman O, Gilson H, Kalista S, et al. Mechanisms of muscle atrophy induced by glucocorticoids. *Horm Res* 2009;1:36–41.
21. Miers WR, Barrett EJ. The role of insulin and other hormones in the regulation of amino acid and protein metabolism in humans. *J Basic Clin Physiol Pharmacol* 1998;9:235–53.
22. Umpleby AM, Russell-Jones DL. The hormonal control of protein metabolism. *Baillieres Clin Endocrinol Metab* 1996;10:551–70.
23. Kupfer SR, Underwood LE, Baxter RC, et al. Enhancement of the anabolic effects of growth hormone and insulin-like growth factor I by use of both agents simultaneously. *J Clin Invest* 1993;91:391–6.
24. Adamo ML, Farrar RP. Resistance training, and IGF involvement in the maintenance of muscle mass during the aging process. *Aging Res Rev* 2006;5:310–31.
25. Anderson BC, Christiansen SP, Grandt S, et al. Increased extraocular muscle strength with direct injection of insulin-like growth factor-I. *Invest Opthalmol Vis Sci* 2006;47:2461–7.
*26. Liu Z, Long W, Fryburg D, et al. The regulation of body and skeletal muscle protein metabolism by hormones and amino acids. *J Nutr* 2006;136:212S–17S.
27. Catalucci D, Latronico MV, Ellingsen O, et al. Physiological myocardial hypertrophy: How and why? *Front Biosci* 2008;13:312–24.
28. Scavo LM, Karas M, Murray M, et al. Insulin-like growth factor-I stimulates both cell growth and lipogenesis during differentiation of human mesenchymal stem cells into adipocytes. *J Clin Endocrinol Metab* 2004;89:3542–53.
*29. Moller N, Jorgensen JO. Effect of growth hormone on glucose, lipid, and protein metabolism in human subjects. *Endocr Rev* 2009;30:152–77.
30. Krag MB, Gormsen LC, Guo Z, et al. Growth hormone-induced insulin resistance is associated with increased intramyocellular triglyceride content but unaltered VLDL-triglyceride kinetics. *Am J Physiol Endocrinol Metab* 2007;292:E920–7.
31. Fernandez AM, Kim JK, Shoshana Y, et al. Functional inactivation of the IGF-I and insulin receptors in skeletal muscle causes type 2 diabetes. *Genes Dev* 2001;15:1926–34.
32. Heron-Milhavet L, Haluzik M, Yakar S, et al. Muscle-specific overexpression of CD36 reverses the insulin resistance and diabetes of MKR mice. *Endocrinol* 2004;145:4667–76.
*33. Mauras N, Martinez V, Rini J, et al. Recombinant human IGF-I has significant anabolic effects in adults with GH receptor deficiency: Studies on protein, glucose and lipid metabolism. *J Clin Endocrinol Metab* 2000;85:3036–42.
34. Mauras N, O'Brien KO, Welch S, et al. IGF-I and GH treatment in GH deficient humans: Differential effects

on protein, glucose lipid and calcium metabolism. *J Clin Endocrinol Metab* 2000;85:1686–94.
35. Wabitsch M, Heinze E, Debatin KM, et al. IGF-I and IGFBP-3-expression in cultured human preadipocytes and adipocytes. *Horm Metab Res* 2000;32:555–9.
*36. Wheatcroft SB, Kearney MT, Shah MT, et al. IGF-binding protein-2 protects against the development of obesity and insulin resistance. *Diabetes* 2007;56:285–94.
37. Sabin MA, Russo VC, Azar WJ, et al. IGFBP-2 at the interface of growth and metabolism — implications for childhood obesity. *Pediatr Endocrinol Rev* 2011;8:382–93.
*38. Petersson U, Ostegrn CJ, Brudin L, et al. Low levels of insulin-like growth factor binding protein-1 (IGFBP-1) are prospectively associated with the incidence of type 2 diabetes and impaired glucose tolerance (IGT): The Soderakra Cardiovascular Risk Factor Study. *Diabetes Metab* 2009;35:198–205.
39. Iniguez G, Roman R, Avila A, et al. Changes in nocturnal leptin and insulin concentrations in prepubertal low birth weight children after administration of the IGF-I/IGFBP-3 complex. *Horm Res* 2009;72:46–51.
40. Su PH, Chen JY, Yu JS, et al. Leptin expression and leptin receptor gene polymorphisms in growth hormone deficiency patients. *Hum Genet* 2011;129:455–62.
41. Bartell SM, Ravalam S, Ambati S, et al. Central (ICV) leptin injection increases bone formation, bone mineral density, muscle mass, serum IGF-1, and the expression of osteogenic genes in leptin-deficient ob/ob mice. *J Bone Miner Res* 2011;26:1710–20.
42. Grottoli S, Gasco V, Mainolfi A, et al. Growth hormone/insulin-like growth factor I axis, glucose metabolism, and lypolisis but not leptin show some degree of refractoriness to short-term fasting in acromegaly. *J Endocrinol Invest* 2008;31:1103–9.
43. Yamaza H, Komatsu T, To K, et al. Involvement of insulin-like growth factor-1 in the effect of caloric restriction: Regulation of plasma adiponectin and leptin. *J Gerontol A Biol Sci Med Sci* 2007;62:27–33.
44. Kanazawa I, Yamaguchi T, Sugimoto T. Serum insulin-like growth factor-1 is negatively associated with serum adiponectin in type 2 diabetes mellitus. *Growth Horm IGF Res* 2011;21:268–71.
45. Kanety H, Hemi R, Ginsberg S, et al. Total and high molecular weight adiponectin are elevated in patients with Laron syndrome despite marked obesity. *Eur J Endocrinol* 2009;161:837–44.
46. Chen YH, Hung PF, Yao YH. IGF-I downregulates resistin gene expression and protein secretion. *Am J Physiol Endocrinol Metab* 2005;288:E1019–27.
47. Kawai M, Rosen CJ. Insulin-like growth factor-1 and bone: Lessons from mice and man. *Pediatr Nephrol* 2009;24:1277–85.
48. Drake WM, Carroll PV, Maher KT, et al. The effect of cessation of growth hormone (GH) therapy on bone mineral accretion in GH-deficient adolescents at the completion of linear growth. *J Clin Endocrinol Metab* 2003;88:1658–63.
49. Yakar S, Rosen CJ, Bouxsein ML, et al. Serum complexes of insulin-like growth factor-1 modulate skeletal integrity and carbohydrate metabolism. *FASEB J* 2009;23:709–19.
50. Zhang M, Xuan S, Bouxsein ML, et al. Osteoblast-specific knockout of the insulin-like growth factor (IGF) receptor gene reveals an essential role of IGF signaling in bone matrix mineralization. *J Biol Chem* 2002;277:44005–12.
51. Wang Y, Nishida S, Boudignon BM, et al. IGF-I receptor is required for the anabolic actions of parathyroid hormone on bone. *J Bone Miner Res* 2007;22:1329–37.
52. Kawai M, Breggia AC, DeMambro VE, et al. The heparin-binding domain of IGFBP-2 has insulin-like growth factor binding-independent biologic activity in the growing skeleton. *J Biol Chem* 2011;286:14670–80.
53. Amin S, Riggs BL, Atkinson EJ, et al. A potentially deleterious role of IGFBP-2 on bone density in aging men and women. *J Bone Miner Res* 2004;19:1075–83.
54. Fowlkes JL, Thrailkill KM, Liu L, et al. Effects of systemic and local administration of recombinant human IGF-I (rhIGF-I) on *de novo* bone formation in an aged mouse model. *J Bone Miner Res* 2006;21:1359–66.
55. Tanaka H, Wakisaka A, Ogasa H, et al. Effect of IGF-I and PDGF administered in vivo on the expression of osteoblast-related genes in old rats. *J Endocrinol* 2002; 174:63–70.
56. Ghiron LJ, Thompson JL, Holloway L, et al. Effects of recombinant insulin-like growth factor-I and growth hormone on bone turnover in elderly women. *J Bone Miner Res* 1995;10:1844–52.
57. Frystyk J. Free insulin-like growth factors—measurements and relationships to growth hormone secretion and glucose homeostasis. *Growth Horm IGF Res* 2004;14:337–75.
58. Cusi K, DeFronzo R. Recombinant human insulin-like growth factor I treatment for 1 week improves metabolic control in type 2 diabetes by ameliorating hepatic and muscle insulin resistance. *J Clin Endocrinol Metab* 2000;85:3077–84.
59. Yakar S, Liu JL, Fernandez AM, et al. Liver-specific IGF-I gene deletion leads to muscle insulin insensitivity. *Diabetes* 2001;50:1110–18.
60. O'Connell T, Clemmons DR. IGF-I/IGF-binding proteins-3 combination improves insulin resistance by GH-dependent and independent mechanisms. *J Clin Endocrinol Metab* 2002;87:4356–60.
61. Crowne EC, Samra JS, Cheetham T, et al. Recombinant human insulin-like growth factor-I abolishes changes in insulin requirements consequent upon growth hormone pulsatility in young adults with type I diabetes mellitus. *Metabolism* 1998;47:31–8.

62. Simpson HL, Jackson NC, Shojaee-Moradie F, et al. Insulin-like growth factor I has a direct effect on glucose and protein metabolism, but no effect on lipid metabolism in type 1 diabetes. *J Clin Endocrinol Metab* 2004;89:425–32.
63. Rosen CJ, Glowacki J, Craig W. Sex steroids, the insulin-like growth factor regulatory systems, and aging: Implications for the management of older postmenopausal women. *J Nutr Health Aging* 1998;2:39–44.
64. Frystyk J, Freda P, Clemmons DR. The current status of IGF-I assays – a 2009 update. *Growth Horm IGF Res* 2010;20:8–18.
65. Endberding N, San Martin A, Martin-Garrido A, et al. Insulin-like growth factor-1 receptor expression masks the anti-inflammatory and glucose uptake capacity of insulin in vascular smooth muscle cells. *Arterioscler Thromb Vasc Biol* 2009;29:408–15.
66. Saydah S, Ballard-Barbash R, Potischman N. Association of metabolic syndrome with insulin-like growth factors among adults in the US. *Cancer Causes Control* 2009;20:1309–16.
67. Efstratiadis G, Tiaousis G, Athyros VG, et al. Total serum insulin-like growth factor-1 and C-reactive protein in metabolic syndrome with or without diabetes. *Angiology* 2006;57:303–11.
68. Martha S, Pantam N, Thungathurthis S, et al. Study of insulin resistance in relation to serum IGF-I levels in subjects with different degrees of glucose tolerance. *Int J Diabetes Dev Countries* 2008;28:54–9.
69. Arends N, Johnston L, Hokken-Koelega A, et al. Polymorphism in the IGF-I gene: Clinical relevance for short children born small for gestational age (SGA). *J Clin Endocrinol* 2002;87:2720.
*70. Vaessen N, Hautink P, Janssen JA, et al. A polymorphism in the gene for IGF-I:functional properties and risk for type 2 diabetes and myocardial infarction. *Diabetes* 2001;50:637–42.
71. te Velde SJ, van Rossum EF, Voorhoeve PG, et al. An IGF-I promoter polymorphism modifies the relationships between birth weight and risk factors for cardiovascular disease and diabetes at age 36. *BMC Endocr Disord* 2005;5:5.
72. Rietveld I, Hofman A, Pols HA, et al. An insulin-like growth factor-I gene polymorphism modifies the risk of microalbuminuria in subjects with an abnormal glucose tolerance. *Eur J Endocrinol* 2006;154:715–21.
73. Rietveld I, Ikram MK, Vingerling JR, et al. An IGF-I gene polymorphism modifies the risk of diabetic retinopathy. *Diabetes* 2006;55:2387.
74. Heald AH, Haushal K, Siddals KW, et al. Insulin-like growth factor binding protein-2 (IGFBP-2) is a marker for the metabolic syndrome. *Exp Clin Endocrinol Diabetes* 2006;114:371–6.
75. Heald AH, Anderson SG, Ivison F, et al. C-reactive protein and the insulin-like growth factor (IGF) system in relation to risk of cardiovascular disease in different ethnic groups. *Atheroscler* 2003;170: 79–86.
76. Tong PC, Ho CS, Yeung TV, et al. Association of testosterone, insulin-like growth factor-I, and C-reactive protein with metabolic syndrome in Chinese middle-aged men with a family history of type 2 diabetes. *J Clin Endocrinl Metab* 2005;90:6418–23.
77. Sakai K, D'Ercole AJ, Murphy LJ, et al. Physiological differences in insulin-like growth factor binding protein-1 (IGFBP-1) phosphorylation in IGFBP-1 transgenic mice. *Diabetes* 2001;50:32–8.
78. Wabisch M, Blum WF, Muche R, et al. Insulin-like growth factors and their binding proteins before and after weight loss and their associations with hormonal and metabolic parameters in obese adolescent girls. *Int J Obes Relat Metab Disord* 1996;20:103–80.
*79. Lewitt MS, Hilding A, Brismar K, et al. IGF-binding protein 1 and abdominal obesity in the development of type 2 diabetes in women. *Eur J Endocrinol* 2010;163:233–42.
80. Sandhu MS, Heald AH, Gibson JM, et al. Circulating concentrations of insulin-like growth factor-I and development of glucose intolerance: A prospective observational study. *Lancet* 2002;359:1740–5.
81. Qiu C, Vadachkoria S, Meryman L, et al. Maternal plasma concentrations of IGF-I, IGFBP-1, and C-peptide in early pregnancy and subsequent risk of gestational diabetes mellitus. *Am J Obstet Gynecol* 2005; 193:1691–7.
82. Bereket A, Lang CH, Blethen AL, et al. Effect of insulin on the insulin-like growth factor system in children with new onset dependent diabetes. *J Clin Endocrinol Metab* 1995;80:1312–17.
83. Dunger DB, Regan FM, Acerini CL. Childhood and adolescent diabetes. *Endocr Dev* 2005;9:107–20.
84. Bang P, Brismar K, Rosenfeld RG. Increased proteolysis of insulin-like growth factor binding protein-3 (IGFBP-3) in noninsulin-dependent diabetes mellitus serum with elevation of a 29-kilodalton (kDa) glycosylated IGFBP-3 fragment contained in the approximately 130 to 150 kDa ternary complex. *J Clin Endocrinol Metab* 1994;78:1119–27.
85. Quattrin T, Thrailkill K, Baker L, et al. Improvement in HbA1c without increased hypoglycemia in adolescents and young adults with type 1 diabetes mellitus treated with recombinant human insulin-like growth factor-I and insulin. rhIGF-I in IDDM Study Group. *J Pediatr Endocrinol Metab* 2001;14:267–77.
86. Carroll PV, Christ ER, Umpleby AM, et al. IGF-I treatment in adults with type diabetes: Effects on glucose

and protein metabolism in the fasting state and during a hyperinsulinemic-euglycemic amino acid clamp. *Diabetes* 2000;49:789–96.

*87. Moses AC, Young SC, Morrow LA, et al. Recombinant human insulin-like growth factor I increases insulin sensitivity and improves glycemic control in type II diabetes. *Diabetes* 1996;45:91–100.

88. Rh in NIDDM Study Group. Evidence from a dose ranging study that recombinant insulin-like growth factor (RhIGF-I) effectively and safely improves glycemic control in the noninsulin dependent diabetes mellitus. *Diabetes* 1996;45(Suppl 2):27A.

89. RhIGF-I co therapy with insulin subgroup: RhIGF-I improves glucose control in insulin requiring type 2 diabetes mellitus reduces insulin requirements while also lowering fasting glucose. *Proceedings of the 5th Annual Meeting of The American Diabetes Association, San Antonio*, Texas, 1997; abstract: 582.

90. Clemmons DR, Moses AC, Sommer A, et al. Rh/IGF/rhIGFBP-3 administration to patients with type 2 diabetes mellitus reduces insulin requirements while also lowering fasting glucose. *Growth Horm IGF Res* 2005;15:265–74.

91. Grinspoon S, Thomas L, Miller K, et al. Effects of recombinant human IGF-I and oral contraceptive administration on bone density in anorexia nervosa. *J Clin Endocrinol Metab* 2002;87:2883–91.

92. Thompson JL, Butterfield GE, Gylfadottir UK, et al. Effects of human growth hormone, insulin-like growth factor I, and diet and exercise on body composition of obese postmenopausal women. *J Clin Endocrinol Metab* 1998;83:1477–84.

93. Bagi CM, DeLeon E, Brommage R, et al. Treatment of ovariectomized rats with the complex of rhIGF-I/IGFBP-3 increases cortical and cancellous bone mass and improves structure in the femoral neck. *Calcif Tissue* 1995;57:40–6.

94. Boonen S, Rosen C, Bouillon R, et al. Musculoskeletal effects of the recombinant human IGF-I/IGF binding protein-3 complex in osteoporotic patients with proximal femoral fracture: A double blind, placebo-controlled pilot study. *J Clin Endocrinol Metab* 2002;87:1593–9.

95. Gardelis JG, Hatzis TD, Stramogiannou LN, et al. Activity of the growth hormone/insulin-like growth factor-I axis in critically ill children. *J Pediatr Endocrinol Metab* 2005;18:363–72.

96. Cooney RN, Shumate M. The inhibitory effects of interleukin-1 on growth hormone action during catabolic illness. *Vitamin Horm* 2006;74:317–40.

97. Debroy MA, Wolf SE, Zhang XJ, et al. Anabolic effects of insulin-like growth factor in combination with insulin-like growth factor binding protein-3 in severely burned adults. *J Trauma* 1999;47:904–10.

98. Vlackopapdopoulou E, Zachwieja JJ, Gertner JM, et al. Metabolic and clinical response to recombinant human insulin-like growth factor I in myotonic dystrophy—a clinical research center study. *J Clin Endocrinol Metab* 1995;80:3715–23.

99. Heatwole CR, Eichinger KJ, Friedman DL, et al. Open-label trial of recombinant human insulin-like growth factor 1/recombinant human insulin-like growth factor binding protein 3 in myotonic dystrophy type 1. *Arch Neurol* 2011;68:37–44.

# 7

# Radionuclide scanning in the diagnosis and treatment of endocrine disorders

*Rakesh Sajjan, Jamshed Bomanji*

## Introduction

Nuclear medicine has made tremendous progress over the past few decades, and it now plays an important role in the management of many endocrine disorders. With the continuing development and improvement of imaging techniques, including combined modalities such as positron emission tomography–computed tomography (PET–CT) and single-photon emission computed tomography–computed tomography (SPECT–CT), increase in diagnostic accuracy are being achieved. The imaging world has recently gone a step further with the introduction of combined positron emission tomography and magnetic resonance imaging (PET–MRI), which will open a new chapter in the history of imaging.

Radioactivity was first discovered in 1896 by the French scientist Henri Becquerel. Radioactive iodine-131 ($^{131}I$) was discovered by Glenn T. Seaborg and John Livingood at the University of California–Berkeley in the late 1930s. A major breakthrough was achieved in the 1940s when $^{131}I$ was first used to treat patients with thyroid disease.

## Basic principles of nuclear imaging

Nuclear medicine involves the administration of radiotracers or radiopharmaceuticals for the purpose of diagnosis or treatment. Radiopharmaceuticals are pharmaceuticals that have been labeled with a radionuclide, as a result of which they are targeted toward a specific organ.

Nuclear medicine diagnosis determines the cause of a medical problem based on organ or tissue function (physiology) instead of structural appearance. It thus complements the morphological information obtained by radiology.

## Thyroid imaging (see Chapters 13, 14)

The tracers most commonly used for thyroid imaging are iodine-123 ($^{123}I$), technetium-99m ($^{99m}Tc$) pertechnetate, thallium-201 ($^{201}Tl$), $^{99m}Tc$-MIBI, and $^{131}I$. Among these tracers, $^{99m}Tc$-pertechnetate is the most widely used.

### Mechanism of uptake

$^{99m}Tc$ is trapped by the thyroid gland. Pertechnetate ions ($TcO_4^-$) are trapped by the thyroid in the same manner as iodine, but they are not organified; hence, they are not retained in the thyroid for long, and for the same reason, imaging is performed within 15–30 min postadministration.

### Indications

- Graves' disease
- Toxic nodule/autonomous nodule
- Multinodular goiter
- Location of ectopic thyroid tissue
- Differentiation of thyroiditis (subacute or silent) and factitious hyperthyroidism from Graves' disease and other forms of hyperthyroidism

## *Patient preparation and procedure*

1. Ensure that the patient is not pregnant or breast-feeding. Various medications need to be discontinued before scanning, as indicated in Table 7.1.
2. In addition, interfering agents such as iodine-containing food (e.g., kelp) should be avoided, and it may be necessary to avoid other medications (e.g., amiodarone on the advice of a cardiologist and iodinated contrast).

## *Timing of imaging*

When $^{99m}$Tc-pertechnetate is used, imaging should begin 15–30 min after injection.

When $^{123}$I is used, images are obtained at 3–4 h and at 16–24 h after administration.

When $^{131}$I is used, images are obtained at 16–24 h and at 48 h after oral ingestion.

*Advantages of $^{99m}$Tc-pertechnetate over $^{123}$I and $^{131}$I:*

- More readily available
- Short half-life (6 h)
- Lower radiation dose (1 millisieverts[mSv] vs. 4 and 6 mSv, respectively)

*Advantages of $^{123}$I:*

- Trapped and organified by the thyroid gland, allowing overall assessment of thyroid function
- Higher energy and lower background activity

The disadvantages of $^{123}$I are cost, restricted availability, and increased patient radiation dose.

$^{123}$I is both trapped and organified by the thyroid, and because it is stable within the thyroid for a long period, it provides good-quality images.[1]

Examples of the images obtained in various indications are shown in Figures 7.1 through 7.4.

| Medication | Duration (days) medications must be discontinued before scan |
|---|---|
| Levothyroxine (T4) | 28 |
| Tri iodothyronine (T3) | 14 |
| Carbimazole | 5 |
| Propylthiouracil | 5 |

***Table 7.1***
*Medications that must be discontinued before scanning.*

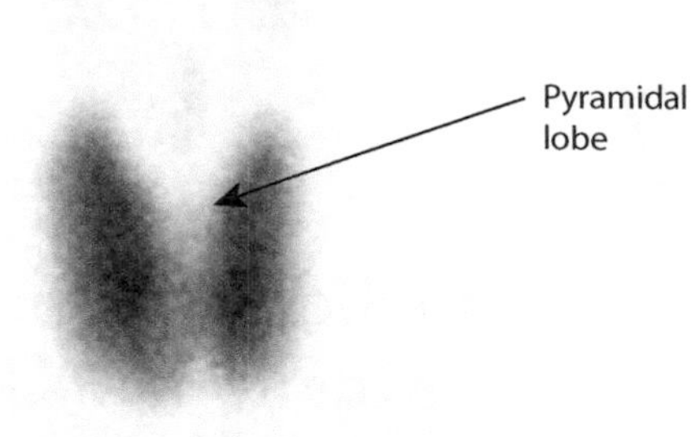


***Figure 7.1***
*This is young lady who presented with hyperthyroidism. Image shows diffuse increased tracer uptake in both thyroid lobes. The arrow shows presence of pyramidal lobe.*

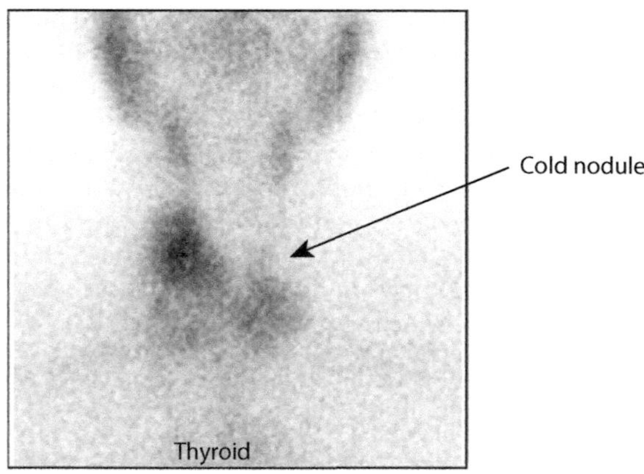


***Figure 7.2***
*Shows heterogeneous tracer uptake bilaterally with photon deficient area on the left side (cold nodule).*

## *Treatment of hyperthyroidism with $^{131}$I*

Radioactive iodine provides the highest rate of cure for thyrotoxicosis. It has the advantages of being simple to administer and cheap. Patients experience no side effects, and no special precautions are needed. The choice of dose depends on several factors, including age of the patient, any associated cardiac problems, and the cause of hyperthyroidism (e.g., Graves' disease, toxic multinodular goiter). The only disadvantage of

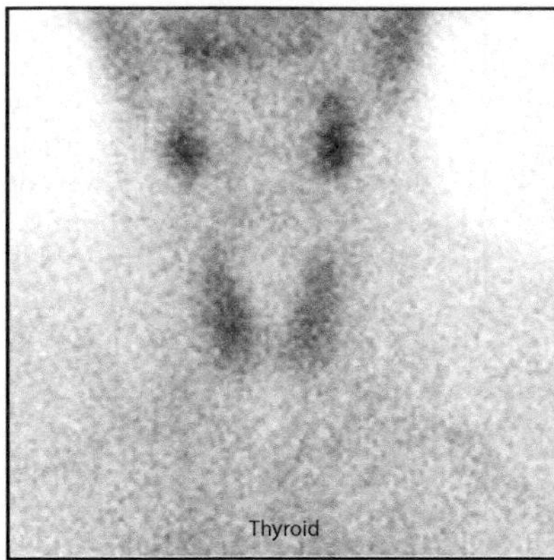


***Figure 7.3***
***This patient was referred with recent onset thyrotoxicosis. Image shows low tracer uptake by thyroid gland which is typical of thyroiditis.***

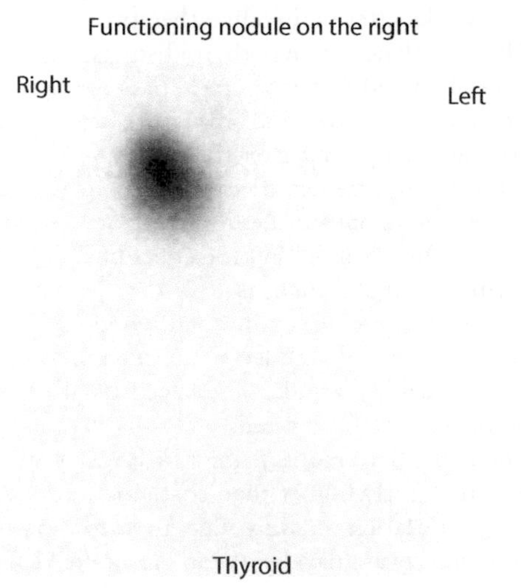


***Figure 7.4***
***This is 30-year-old lady who presented with thyrotoxicosis. Image shows hot functioning nodule on the right with suppressed uptake on the left.***

radioactive iodine treatment is the high incidence of hypothyroidism.

## *Mechanism of uptake and therapeutic effects*

The thyroid takes up the radioiodine in the same way as iodide, by active transport—the iodide transport mechanism. The beta particles cause radiation injury to the thyroid cells, thereby destroying them.

Indications for $^{131}$I therapy and guideline levels of radioactivity are shown in Table 7.2.[2]

## *Contraindications to radioiodine therapy*

*Absolute contraindications:*

- Pregnancy, because radioiodine therapy will damage the fetal thyroid
- Breastfeeding

*Relative contraindications:*

- Situations where it is clear that the safety of other persons cannot be guaranteed
- Allergy to iodine

## *Use in young patients*

Although antithyroid drugs and surgery are generally regarded as the treatments of choice in childhood Graves' disease, radioiodine is effective in this age group. A retrospective study of 116 subjects treated with radioiodine at <20 years old revealed cure of hyperthyroidism without any increased incidence of thyroid cancer, leukemia, or congenital abnormalities in offspring.[3]

## *Role of block and replacement therapy during radioiodine treatment*

A block and replacement therapy strategy may be chosen to avoid thyroid storm after radioiodine therapy. A continuous block-replacement regimen results in a stable thyroid function during $^{131}$I therapy but is hampered by the higher amounts of radioactivity required.[4]

| Thyroid condition | Guide activity (MBq) |
|---|---|
| Uncomplicated Graves' disease | 400–600 |
| Uncomplicated toxic multinodular goiter | 500–800 |
| Toxic adenoma, usually with mild hyperthyroidism | 500 |
| Ablation therapy may be required in patients with severe comorbidity such as heart failure (New York Heart Association [NYHA] grade 3), malignancy, or psychosis and also may be appropriate for those who are intolerant to antithyroid drugs | 500–800 |
| Subclinical hyperthyroidism associated with significant multinodular goiter | 600 |

*Source:* Lazarus JH, *J R Coll Physicians Lond*, 29, 464–9, 1995.

**Table 7.2**
*Indications for $^{131}I$ therapy and guide activities.*

## Ophthalmopathy in hyperthyroid disease

Radioiodine should be avoided, if possible, in patients newly diagnosed with Graves' disease who have active eye disease. Worsening of ophthalmopathy after radioiodine treatment may be caused by the release of thyroid antigen as a result of thyroid injury due to radiation, with subsequent enhancement of the immune response directed toward antigen shared by the thyroid and orbit. Antithyroid drugs are the best first-line treatment in this setting. It is postulated that radioiodine therapy for Graves' disease is followed by the appearance or worsening of ophthalmopathy, but the problem is often transient and can be prevented by administration of prednisolone.[5] One regimen that avoids worsening of eye disease[6] is to give 0.4–0.5 mg of prednisolone per kilogram of body weight starting 2–3 days before radioiodine therapy and continuing for 1 month; the dose is then tapered over a period of 2 months and the drug discontinued. Another regimen involves a lower dose and shorter duration of oral prednisolone, about 0.2 mg/kg/day for 6 weeks.[7]

## Teaching points

- If antithyroid drugs are given before and after radioiodine treatment, they should be discontinued at least 4 days before the treatment and restarted no sooner than 7 days afterward.
- If antithyroid drugs are restarted after radioiodine treatment, they should be withdrawn when the patient is euthyroid, and the thyroid function test should be repeated after 6–8 weeks.
- A thyroid function test should be performed 4–8 weeks after radioiodine therapy.
- The prevalence of hypothyroidism is estimated to be about 90% over a typical patient's lifetime.
- The risk of hypothyroidism with goiter is about 20% and is reduced after treatment.
- Radionuclide treatment is effective in reducing goiter size (small-to-medium size or <100 mL) by 50% at 1 year, half of the effect being evident within the first 3 months.
- In the presence of significant thyroid-associated ophthalmopathy (moderate to severe), radioiodine treatment should be delayed until the eye problem has been treated.
- The mortality among patients with thyroid disease is slightly higher than that among the general population, mainly due to cardiovascular and cerebrovascular disease and low bone density with above-average fracture risk. Mortality is not, however, related to the mode of treatment.[8]

# Thyroid cancer (see Chapter 15)

Thyroid cancer is the most common endocrine cancer and represents 1% of all malignancies. It is among the top 20 cancers in females. The incidence of thyroid cancer has been gradually increasing since 1975 according to Cancer Research UK statistics, and 2154 cases were diagnosed in the United Kingdom in 2008. Nuclear medicine plays an important role in the management of these cancers (Figure 7.5).

The commonest type of thyroid cancer is differentiated thyroid cancer (DTC), accounting for 90%

Thyroid carcinoma

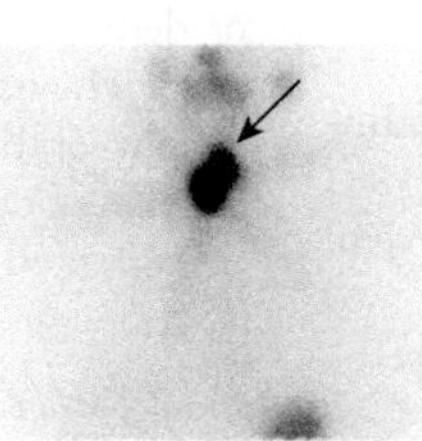

Post I-131 therapy scan
Spot view

Post I-131 therapy scan

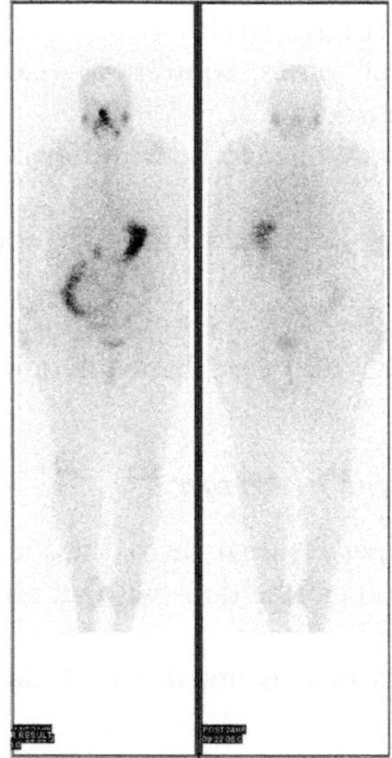

I-123 prognostic scan 6 months postablation

***Figure 7.5***
***This patient was diagnosed with papillary carcinoma, had hemithyroidectomy followed by I-131 ablation. The post therapy scan shows uptake in the residual thyroid (arrows). 6 months after, I-123 scan was performed which showed no residual uptake in thyroid bed (only salivary glands are seen).***

of cases. This cancer is subdivided into two forms: papillary (accounting for 80% of cancer cases) and follicular (accounting for 10% of cancer cases).[9] DTC is highly curable, with a 10-year survival rate of 80%–90%.[10]

# *Differentiated thyroid cancer*[10]

Patients with a papillary thyroid cancer (PTC) >1 cm in diameter or with high-risk follicular thyroid cancer (FTC) should undergo near-total or total thyroidectomy. Patients with low-risk FTC or PTC ≤1 cm in diameter may be treated with thyroid lobectomy alone. After the operation, triiodothyronine 20 μg t.d.s. (normal adult dosage) should be administered. It should be discontinued 2 weeks before $^{131}$I ablation. Thyroglobulin is checked 6 weeks after surgery.

The ablation of thyroid tissue with the help of radioactive iodine is widely used for the following reasons:

1. It may destroy occult microscopic carcinoma within the thyroid.
2. It helps in later detection of recurrence by means of $^{131}$I scanning.
3. It increases the value of serum thyroglobulin measurement. During follow-up, measurement of thyroglobulin is less reliable in patients with a large residual thyroid gland.

## *Indications for $^{131}$I ablation*

*Definite indications:*

1. Distant metastases
2. Incomplete tumor resection
3. Complete tumor resection but high risk of recurrence or mortality (tumor extension beyond the thyroid capsule, or more than ten involved lymph nodes and more than three lymph nodes with extra capsular spread)

*Probable indications:*

1. Less than total thyroidectomy (inferred from operation notes or pathology report, or when an ultrasound scan or isotope scan shows a significant postoperative thyroid remnant)
2. Status of lymph nodes not assessed at surgery
3. Tumor >1 cm and <4 cm in diameter
4. Tumor <1 cm in diameter with unfavorable histology (tall cell, columnar cell, or diffuse sclerosing papillary cancers; widely invasive or poorly differentiated follicular cancers)
5. Multifocal tumors <1 cm

### Patient preparation

1. Low-iodine diet for 2 weeks.
2. Elimination of other sources of excess iodine (e.g., CT contrast).
3. Amiodarone may have to be withdrawn for several months.
4. In females, the possibility of pregnancy must be excluded.
5. In males, pretreatment sperm banking is advised if the patient is having more than two higher dose $^{131}$I treatments.

### Activity of $^{131}$I for ablation

1. If the scan shows residual thyroid tissue only, then thyroid ablation can be done with an ablative dose of 3.7 GBq.[11,12]
2. If distant metastasis is noted, a high dose is given (5–7.4 GBq).[13]

### Role of fluorine-18 fluorodeoxyglucose PET in DTC

Lack of $^{131}$I trapping by metastatic tissue precludes visualization of metastatic spread by means of $^{131}$I scintigraphy. The main indication for fluorine-18 fluorodeoxyglucose ($^{18}$F-FDG) PET scan is in patients who have had total thyroidectomy and $^{131}$I ablation and have detectable thyroglobulin/thyroglobulin antibody with negative $^{131}$I scintigraphy.[14]

Patient follow-up is done by measurement of serum thyroglobulin every 3 months (or annually if the patient is in remission) and by $^{131}$I whole-body scanning 6 months postsurgery. Levothyroxine is the drug of choice to suppress thyroid-stimulating hormone (TSH) on a long-term basis. Dose is adjusted to aim at TSH levels of <0.01 mIU (in low-risk patients, it is adequate to keep serum TSH between 0.01 and 0.05 mIU).

### Oncocytic follicular cancers

Hürthle cell tumors account for 5% of all differentiated follicular carcinomas.[15] These tumors are more common in women. They usually do not take up $^{131}$I, and metastases are frequently undetected. In these cases, $^{201}$Tl, $^{99m}$Tc-MIBI, and $^{99m}$Tc-tetrofosmin are useful.[16] Hürthle cell carcinoma demonstrates intense uptake on $^{18}$F-FDG PET images, and PET improves both disease detection and disease management.[17]

The first-line of treatment is surgery (usually total thyroidectomy) followed by $^{131}$I ablative therapy. Follow-up is done with thyroglobulin assay and $^{131}$I whole-body scan annually. From 15% to 20% of patients with a high serum thyroglobulin level will have a negative $^{131}$I diagnostic whole-body scan.[18,19] In these cases, whole-body scanning is done with $^{201}$Tl or $^{99m}$Tc-MIBI or dedifferentiation therapy with retinoic acid may be used. The usual dose of retinoic acid is 1.18 mg/kg body weight orally for 2 months; this can result in better uptake of radioiodine in tumors and can subsequently be exploited for the purpose of radioiodine treatment.[20]

## Medullary thyroid carcinomas (see Multiple endocrine neoplasia type 2, Chapter 9)

Medullary thyroid carcinomas (MTCs) account for 5%–10% of all thyroid cancers. Twenty-five percent of MTCs are familial (multiple endocrine neoplasia 2A [MEN2A], MEN2B and familial medullary thyroid cancer [FMTC]). These tumors secrete excessive calcitonin, and diagnosis is made with the help of serum calcitonin measurement. Treatment consists of total thyroidectomy as the tumors are multicentric. Postoperatively, serum calcitonin is measured repeatedly for residual or metastatic tumor. If the value is high, then pentavalent DMSA, $^{123}$I-metaiodobenzylguanidine (MIBG), or indium-111 ($^{111}$In) octreotide give good localization of recurrent tumor or metastases. In cases of $^{123}$I-MIBG/$^{111}$In-octreotide/gallium-68 ($^{68}$Ga) DOTATATE-positive disease, therapy with $^{131}$I-MIBG or lutetium-177 ($^{177}$Lu) DOTATATE can be instituted.

Table 7.3 shows the sensitivity of $^{131}$I scintigraphy in detecting metastatic disease due to differentiated thyroid cancers in comparison with other markers. A summary of the management of thyroid cancer (differentiated and medullary) is provided in Figure 7.6.[10]

## Complications of radioiodine treatment for thyroid cancer

1. Radiation thyroiditis occurs in 20% of patients, usually appearing 1 week after $^{131}$I administration. Conservative management with an anti-inflammatory suffices.

| | Sensitivity (%) | Specificity (%) |
|---|---|---|
| $^{131}$I scan | 42–62 | 99–100 |
| Serum thyroglobulin | 55–78 | 55–78 |

**Table 7.3**
*Sensitivity and specificity of $^{131}$I scan and serum thyroglobulin determination.*

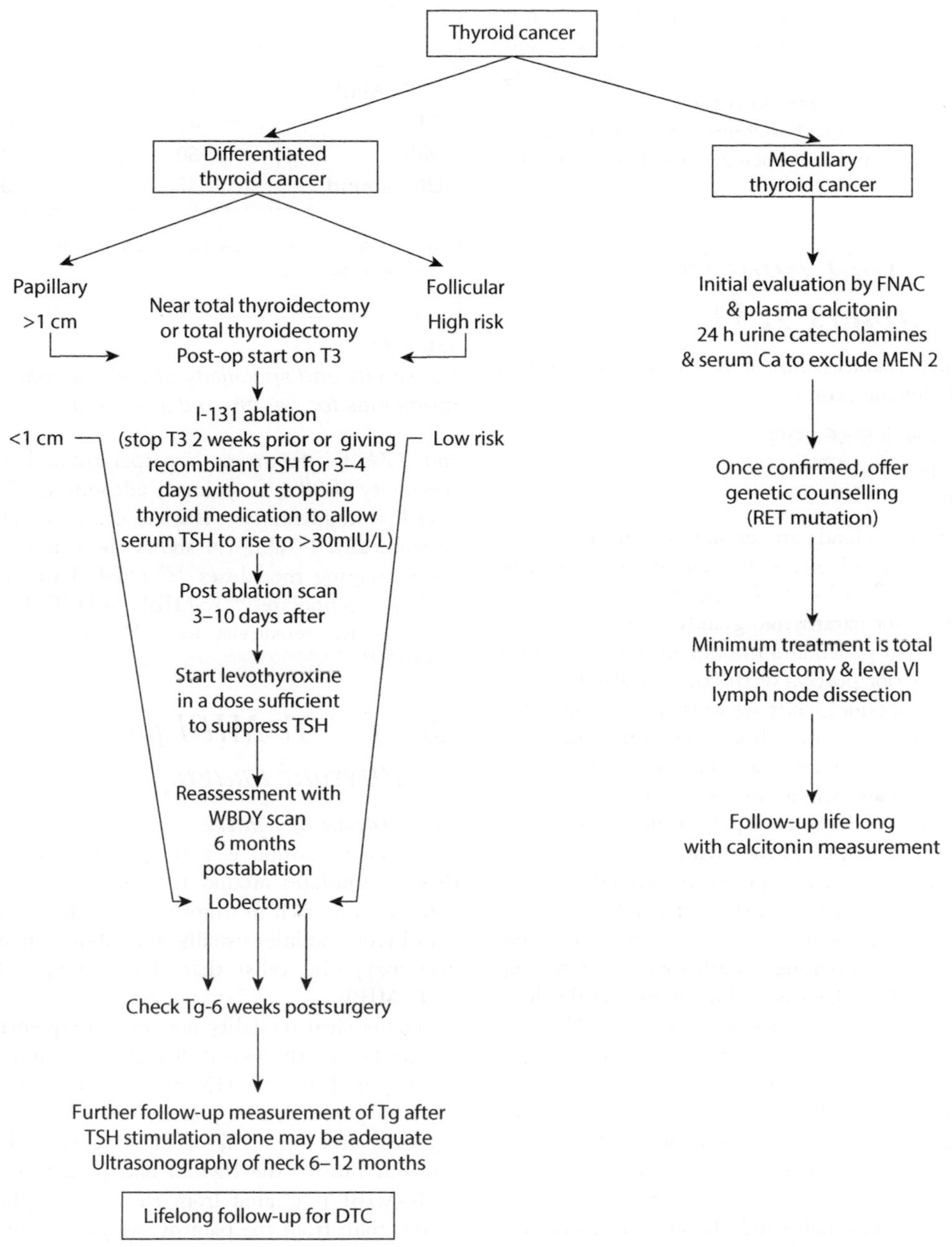


***Figure 7.6***
*Summary of the management of thyroid cancer. (From British Thyroid Association, Royal College of Physicians,* Guidelines for the Management of Thyroid Cancer, *2nd edition, Perros P, (ed). Report of the Thyroid Cancer Guidelines Update Group, Royal College of Physicians, London, 2007.)*

2. Radiation sialadenitis occurs after therapy in 12% of patients and usually involves the parotid or submandibular gland. It can be prevented by giving sour sweets to increase salivation.
3. Acute hematological changes, for example, thrombocytopenia and leukopenia; such changes are rare.

# Parathyroid imaging (see Chapters 9, 11)

Primary hyperparathyroidism is a common condition with the following causes:

1. Adenoma in 80%–85%
2. Hyperplasia in 12%–15%
3. Carcinoma in 1%–3%

The parathyroid glands are situated behind the lateral lobes of the thyroid gland. In general, there are four glands; however, in 10%–13% of people there is a variant number. Superior parathyroid glands originate from the fourth bronchial pouch and migrate in close association with the posterior portion of the thyroid gland, so only <10% of the superior glands are situated ectopically. The inferior parathyroids arise from the third pharyngeal pouch and descend along with the thymus toward the mediastinum (long migration). Approximately 60% of them are found at the inferior pole of the thyroid gland, 39% at the superior pole of the thymus, 2% in the mediastinum, and another 2% anywhere between the angle of the mandible and the level of the aortic arch.

The goal of radionuclide imaging is to localize and lateralize hyperfunctioning parathyroid tissue to help the surgeon to find the lesion, thus shortening the duration of surgery. Focused excision can be achieved by open surgery through a mini-incision, possibly under local anesthesia, or by video-assisted endoscopic surgery under general anesthesia.[21] Most surgeons appreciate having information concerning the whereabouts of the parathyroid glands in the neck before starting dissection and the possibility of locating ectopic parathyroid glands.[22] In the case of a mediastinal gland, the surgeon can proceed directly with first-intention thoracoscopy, avoiding unnecessary initial extensive neck surgery in the search for the elusive gland.[23] Techniques used to ensure completeness of resection include intraoperative parathyroid hormone measurements (68%) and gamma probe (14%).

The first agent used for the parathyroid was thallous chloride in 1980.[24] The most commonly used tracer is $^{99m}$Tc-MIBI. $^{99m}$Tc-MIBI scintigraphy has a sensitivity of 90% for single adenomas, 55% for abnormal glands in patients with multiglandular disease,

| | *Sensitivity (%)* | *Specificity (%)* |
|---|---|---|
| $^{99m}$Tc-MIBI | 70 | 88 |
| CT | 40 | 80 |
| MRI | 60 | 88 |
| Ultrasound | 42 | 92 |

*Source:* Russell Van Husen, Lawrence T. Kim, *World J Surg*, 28, 1122–26, 2004.

***Table 7.4***
*Sensitivity and specificity of various imaging modalities for parathyroid adenomas.*

and 75% for recurrent hyperparathyroidism, and a specificity of 98% for primary adenomas.[25] In general, parathyroid adenomas >500 mg can be detected scintigraphically.[26] Table 7.4 shows the comparison with other imaging modalities.[27,28] Dual-phase, dual-tracer $^{99m}$Tc-pertechnetate/$^{99m}$Tc-MIBI SPECT has further increased the sensitivity to 72.5% and the specificity to 99%.[29]

# Use of $^{99m}$Tc-MIBI for parathyroid imaging

## Mechanism of uptake

MIBI, or sestamibi, is a lipophilic cationic complex that accumulates around the mitochondria and persists in tissue rich in mitochondria. Hyperfunctioning parathyroid nodules usually have abundant mitochondria (oxyphilic cells) that show strong affinity for $^{99m}$Tc-MIBI.

The nuclear modality now most frequently used to image the parathyroids is dual-phase imaging. Images are acquired at early (15 min postinjection) and late (90 min postinjection) phases. The basis for performing early and late $^{99m}$Tc-MIBI imaging is the relative washout rate of the thyroid and parathyroid glands: $^{99m}$Tc-MIBI is cleared from the thyroid gland much earlier than from the parathyroid glands, resulting in visualization of the latter on the delayed image.

In contrast, radionuclide scanning with the $^{201}$Tl/$^{99m}$Tc subtraction technique is now rarely used. The reported sensitivity is highly variable and usually lies between 70% and 90% for parathyroid adenoma.

There is a consensus that the availability of an integrated SPECT/CT/gamma camera system with high spatial resolution, which uses spiral CT for anatomical localization, has improved accuracy and reporter confidence in clinical practice.[30]

## *Patient preparation*

1. No patient preparation is involved for the dual-phase technique. In the case of women of child-bearing age, it must be ensured that the patient is not breastfeeding or pregnant.

## *Imaging technique (dual phase)*

$^{99m}$Tc-MIBI is administered by intravenous injection, followed by imaging. The administered activity is 900 MBq.

The patient must be in the supine position with the arms down. Anterior views of the neck and the upper thorax are obtained using a gamma camera. Early (ideally 10–15 min postinjection, certainly within 30 min) and delayed (1.5–2.5 h postinjection) images are obtained. Further delayed images (4 h postinjection) can be obtained if thyroid washout is poor. Current practice is to obtain SPECT/CT images whenever available to obtain exact anatomical localization.

Examples of the images obtained using $^{99m}$Tc-MIBI are shown in Figures 7.7 through 7.9.

## *Teaching points*

- The main role of parathyroid imaging is the localization of hyperfunctioning parathyroid tissue.
- $^{99m}$Tc-MIBI is now the tracer most commonly used for parathyroid scintigraphy and is used with SPECT-CT when the latter is available.
- Minimally invasive parathyroidectomy is a surgical technique involving a shorter incision (<2–3 cm long). It became popular after suc-

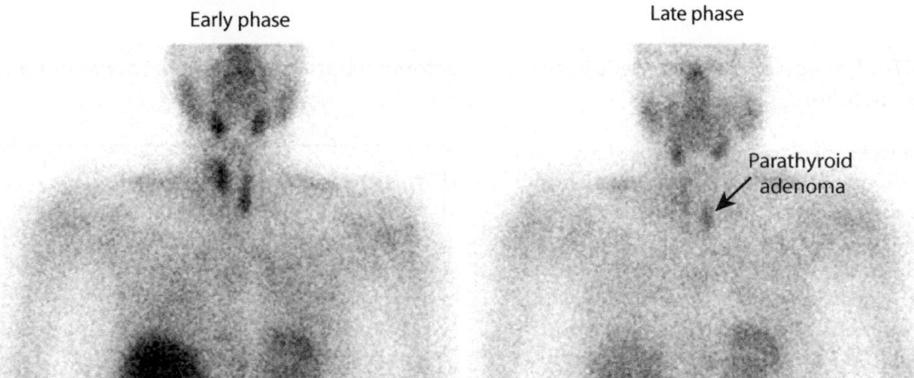


***Figure 7.7***
*This is dual phase Tc-99m sestamibi scan. Early phase shows uptake in thyroid gland and parathyroid adenoma which is difficult to appreciate as there is overlap between the two. But the late phase image shows washout of the tracer from the thyroid revealing parathyroid adenoma on the left side (black arrow).*

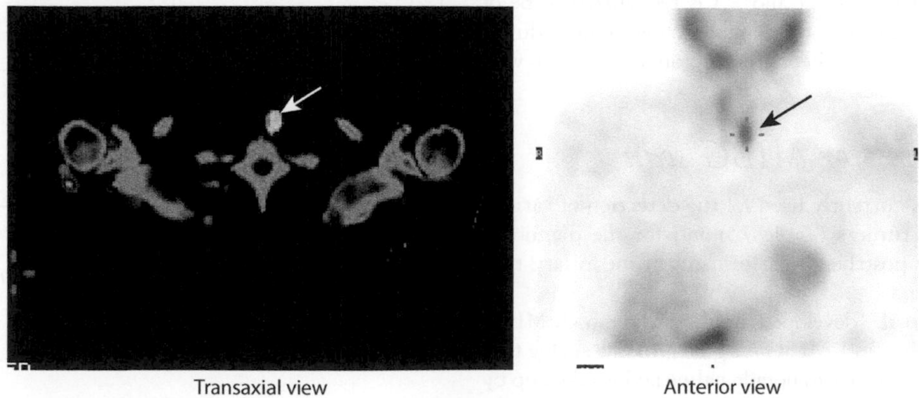


***Figure 7.8***
*This image (same patient as shown in fig. 7.7) shows SPECT image with tracer retention in the left parathyroid gland.*

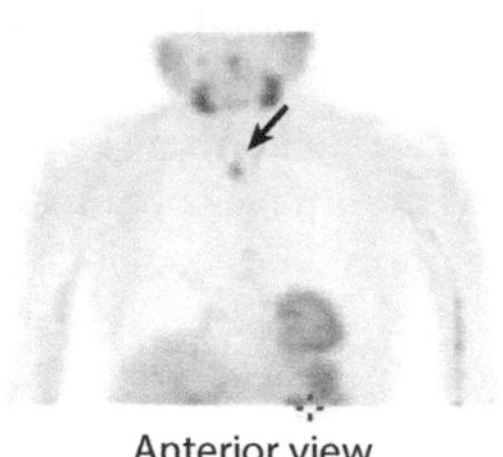


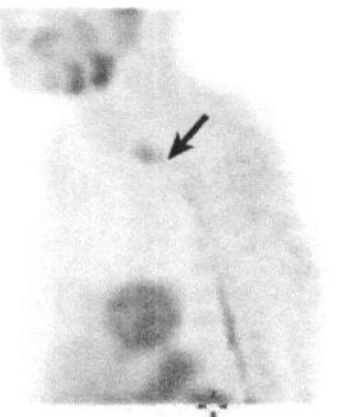


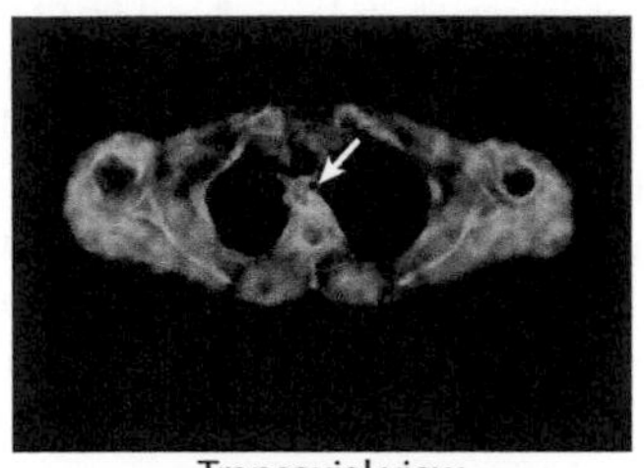


***Figure 7.9***
*This is SPECT-CT image showing tracer uptake in the ectopic parathyroid gland (shown with arrows) in the superior mediastinum.*

cessful preoperative imaging, particularly with $^{99m}$Tc-MIBI scintigraphy and ultrasound.[31] A survey of the members of the International Association of Endocrine Surgeons indicated that minimally invasive parathyroidectomy based on $^{99m}$Tc-MIBI scintigraphy has been adopted by 59% of surgeons.[32] The most popular surgical technique (92%) is the focused approach with a small incision.

| Tumor | MIBG sensitivity (%) |
|---|---|
| Paraganglioma | 89 |
| Pheochromocytoma | 91 |
| Neuroblastoma | 92 |
| Carcinoid | 79 |

***Table 7.5***
*Sensitivity of MIBG scan for various neural crest tumors.*

## Neural crest tumors (see Chapters 8, 9, 21)

MIBG labeled with $^{123}$I and $^{131}$I is recognized to be of value for various diagnostic and therapeutic procedures; indeed, its role in pheochromocytoma has been well known for decades.

## Indications for MIBG scan

$^{123}$I-MIBG is currently used for the detection of various neural crest tumors (Table 7.5) and for the diagnosis, staging, and posttherapy assessment of medullary thyroid carcinoma.

Wieland et al.[33] developed the use of whole-body MIBG scintigraphy in 1980. MIBG is a guanethidine analog that is structurally similar to noradrenaline and is taken up by adrenergic storage vesicles in the adrenal gland and the paraganglia, thus visualizing neuroendocrine tissue.

The sensitivity of MIBG scintigraphy in detecting functioning pheochromocytoma is 91%. Table 7.6 shows the sensitivity and specificity in relation to CT and MRI.[34] Positive MIBG scintigraphy always requires correlation with CT or MRI. In metastatic disease, $^{131}$I-MIBG therapy provides an important palliative therapeutic option.

| | Sensitivity (%) | Specificity (%) |
|---|---|---|
| CT | 90 | 93 |
| MRI | 93 | 93 |
| MIBG scintigraphy | 91 | >95 |

***Table 7.6***
*Sensitivity and specificity of MIBG scintigraphy, CT, and MRI in detecting functioning pheochromocytoma.*

Neuroblastomas also take up MIBG, and in a small group of patients, MIBG scan is more accurate than CT or MRI, usually as a result of showing bony metastases. The main roles of scintigraphy are in staging these tumors at presentation; searching for post-surgical residues; monitoring the effects of treatment; and, frequently, assessing suitability for $^{131}$I-MIBG and $^{177}$Lu-DOTATATE therapy.

## Mechanism of uptake of MIBG

MIBG is an aralkyl guanidine that structurally resembles the neurotransmitter noradrenaline. Owing to this structural similarity, it is taken up by the adrenal medulla via the neuronal uptake 1 mechanism and other tissues that are rich in sympathetic innervations.[35] MIBG is transported into neurosecretory vesicles by an ATPase-dependent proton pump and stored in neurosecretory vesicles.

## Patient preparation

1. If the patient is female and of child-bearing age, it must be ensured that she is not pregnant (if she is pregnant but requires the test, the test *must be justified* taking into account risks and benefits).
2. If the patient is breastfeeding, breastfeeding must be interrupted for at least 48 h.
3. There are medications, such as antihypertensives, tricyclic antidepressants, nasal decongestants, sympathomimetics, and cocaine, that prevent uptake of the tracer, increasing the likelihood of false negatives. The common medications listed in Table 7.7 need to be discontinued prior to MIBG scan.[35]
4. Thyroid blockade should be performed before the $^{123}$I-MIBG scan to prevent iodine uptake by the thyroid gland. The agent usually used for thyroid blockade is potassium iodide 120 mg the night before the scan and 120 mg on the night of $^{123}$I-MIBG administration (other agents used are potassium perchlorate and Lugol's solution).[36]
5. The maximum radioactivity usually administered is 400 MBq. The effective dose is 6 mSv.
6. Once the tracer has been given (over 1–2 min to prevent untoward side effects), imaging is performed at 4 h and again at 24 h.

Figure 7.10 shows an example of imaging findings in a patient with pheochromocytoma.

| *Medication* | *Duration of discontinuation before MIBG administration (h)* |
|---|---|
| Amitriptyline | 48 |
| Amoxapine | 48 |
| Butriptyline | 48 |
| Clomipramine | 24 |
| Desipramine | 24 |
| Diltiazem | 24 |
| Doxepin | 24 |
| Dothiepin/dosulepin | 24 |
| Ephedrine | 24 |
| Imipramine | 24 |
| Iprindole | 24 |
| Isradipine | 48 |
| Labetalol | 72 |
| Lidoflazine | 48 |
| Lofepramine | 48 |
| Loxapine | 48 |
| Methylephedrine | 24 |
| Nicardipine | 48 |
| Nifedipine | 24 |
| Nimodipine | 24 |
| Noradrenaline | 24 |
| Nortriptyline | 24 |
| Phenylephedrine | 48 |
| Phenylpropylamine | 48 |
| Protriptyline | 24 |
| Pseudoephedrine | 24 |
| Reserpine | 72 |
| Trimipramine | 48 |
| Verapamil | 48 |

**Table 7.7**
*Commonly used medications that must be discontinued before MIBG scan.*

## Teaching points

- $^{123}$I-MIBG scan is a well-established technique for imaging of pheochromocytoma and paraganglioma.
- It must be ensured that interfering medications are discontinued to avoid false negatives.
- $^{123}$I-MIBG scintigraphy is an essential step in the selection of patients for $^{131}$I-MIBG therapy.

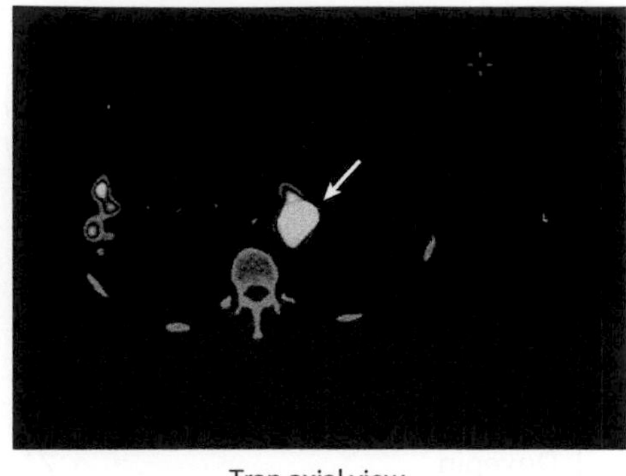

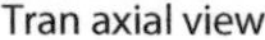

Tran axial view

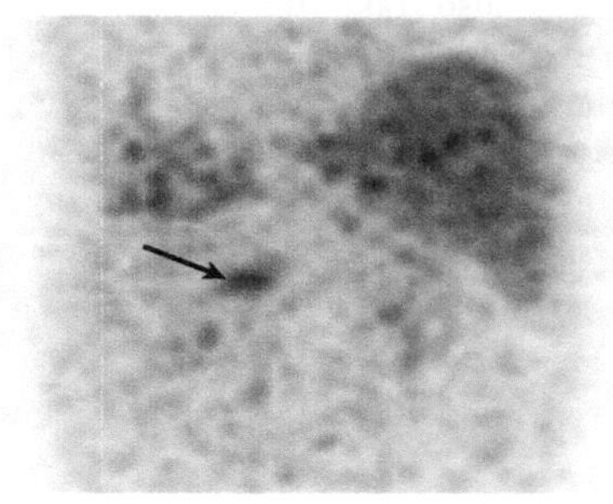

Posterior view

***Figure 7.10***
*The SPECT/CT images show MIBG avid left adrenal mass in keeping with phoeochromocytoma (marked with arrows).*

# Carcinoid tumors/ neuroendocrine tumors (see Chapter 8)

Neuroendocrine tumors (NETs) are rare neoplasms that are characterized by the presence of neuroamine uptake mechanisms and/or peptide receptors at the cell membrane, and these features constitute the basis for the clinical use of specific radiolabeled ligands, both for imaging and for therapy.[37]

Eighty percent of carcinoid tumors are situated in the gastrointestinal tract, out of which 45% are situated in the appendix. Ten percent are found in the lungs and the rest in various organs. The ability of these tumors to concentrate $^{123}$I- or $^{131}$I-MIBG allows scintigraphy to be performed with a cumulative sensitivity of 71%.[38] The main indication for $^{123}$I-MIBG scintigraphy is decision making with regard to the therapeutic dose of $^{131}$I-MIBG.

## $^{111}$In-octreotide scintigraphy

$^{111}$In-labeled octreotide (commercially available as OctreoScan) binds selectively to the somatostatin receptor 2 (SST2), and 80% of carcinoids express somatostatin receptors. $^{111}$In-octreotide scintigraphy is particularly useful for localizing metastases outside the abdomen and can detect metastases sized 0.5–1 cm.

### Common indications[39]

- Sympathoadrenal system tumors (pheochromocytoma, neuroblastoma, ganglioneuroma, and paraganglioma)
- Functioning and nonfunctioning gastroenteropancreatic (GEP) tumors (e.g., carcinoid, gastrinoma, insulinoma, glucagonoma, VIPoma)
- Medullary thyroid carcinoma
- Pituitary adenoma
- Merkel cell carcinoma

$^{111}$In-octreotide is used to localize the primary tumor (Figure 7.11), to detect relapse, to monitor effects of treatment, and to select patients for peptide radionuclide therapy.

### Patient preparation

1. Pregnancy is a relative contraindication—benefits must be weighed against harm.
2. Breastfeeding must be interrupted.
3. $^{111}$In-octreotide should be avoided in patients with renal failure because the kidneys are the route of excretion (if $^{111}$In-octreotide were to be used, images would be nondiagnostic because of activity in the circulation).
4. Somatostatin analog therapy should be temporarily withdrawn when possible.
5. Adequate hydration should be given a day before injection.

### Recommended activity

The recommended activity is 110 MBq and 220 MBq for SPECT.

### Acquisition

Images are acquired at 4 and 24 h postinjection. Delayed views may be required at 24 and 48 h postinjection to clarify suspicious areas. At least one set of SPECT/CT images is acquired when this option is available.

Indium—111 octreotide

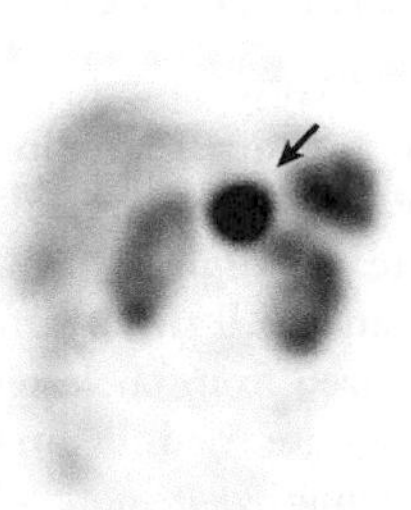

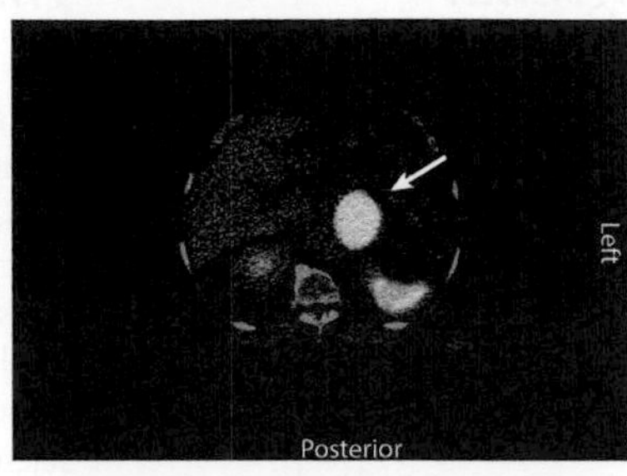


***Figure 7.11***
*59-year-old lady with NET tumour in the tail of pancreas. Uptake in the tail of pancreas on the SPECT (black and white image with black arrow showing the tumour). The corresponding picture on the fused SPECT – CT image is shown on the left hand side (white arrow showing the tumour).*

Gallium octreotate—Pancreatic neuroendocrine tumor with liver & bone metastases

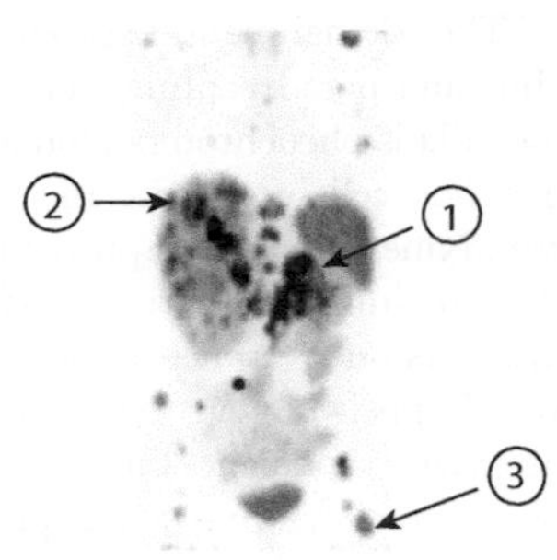


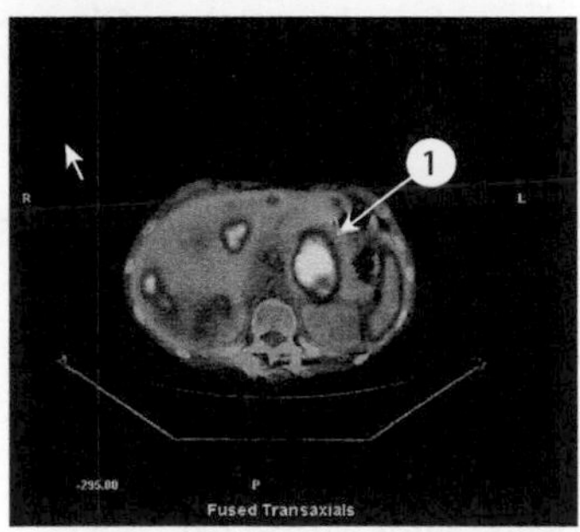


***Figure 7.12***
*This is PET/CT image showing Gallium-68 DOTATAE uptake in the pancreas (1), liver (2) and bone (3).*

# PET tracers

## Gallium-68 DOTA-Tyr$^3$-octreotate ($^{68}$Ga-DOTATATE)

The newer radiopharmaceutical $^{68}$Ga-DOTATATE is known for its excellence in the functional imaging of NETs (Figure 7.12). $^{68}$Ga-DOTATATE PET/CT is a useful novel imaging modality for NETs and is superior to $^{111}$In-octreotide. Functional imaging with both $^{68}$Ga-DOTATATE and $^{18}$F-FDG has the potential to offer more comprehensive assessment of intermediate- and high-grade tumors.[40]

### Indications

- Staging and posttreatment assessment of NETs, and detection of recurrence

### Activity

250 MBq

### Effective dose

1. 8.5 mSv

### Patient preparation

1. It must be checked that the patient is not pregnant or breastfeeding.

## Fluorine-18 3,4-dihydroxy-6-fluoro-dl-phenylananine ($^{18}$F-DOPA)

$^{18}$F-DOPA is another PET tracer used for imaging of NETs. It has been shown that $^{18}$F-DOPA PET detects more lesions, more positive regions, and more lesions per region than combined $^{111}$In-octreotide scintigraphy and CT.[41] However, more studies are needed to confirm this. The practical advantage of $^{18}$F-DOPA PET over MIBG scintigraphy is the lack of uptake in normal adrenal glands, implying that any $^{18}$F-DOPA uptake in the adrenals is abnormal. The specificity of $^{18}$F-DOPA PET seems to be similar to that of MIBG scintigraphy in those tumors.[42]

## $^{18}$F-DOPA in congenital hyperinsulinism

Congenital hyperinsulinism (CHI) causes recurrent hypoglycemia in the newborn/infancy period, posing a high risk of neurological complications.[43] In the past decade, imaging with $^{18}$F-DOPA has revolutionized the way in which infants with CHI are managed (Figure 7.13). $^{18}$F-DOPA PET-CT is a valuable tool to distinguish between focal and diffuse forms of CHI, and in the former case to localize the focus for limited pancreatic surgery.[44]

### Patient preparation

1. The patient should be fasted for 6 h before the injection (because they will be sedated).
2. The patient should be well hydrated.
3. Medications such as diazoxide, octreotide, and glucagon should be stopped for at least 2 days. Glucose infusion should be used to establish euglycemia.

### Activity administered

The administered activity is 4 MBq/kg, with a maximum of 200 MBq.

## Teaching points

- $^{111}$In-octreotide is used in the majority of centers.
- For imaging patients with suspected NET, $^{111}$In-octreotide is the tracer of choice.
- Where PET facilities are available, $^{68}$Ga-DOTATATE is the tracer of choice.
- Somatostatin receptor scintigraphy can be used to stage lesions and select patients for therapy.

## Imaging adrenal glands

The adrenal cortex produces glucocorticoids, mineralocorticoids, and small amounts of sex hormones. Benign tumors of the cortex are called adrenal cortical adenomas, whereas malignant tumors are called adrenal cortical carcinomas. All the aforementioned steroid hormones are synthesized from cholesterol. At present, two cholesterol analogs are used for imaging of the adrenal cortex: $^{131}$I-6β-iodomethyl-19-norcholestrol (NP59) and $^{75}$Se-6β-selenomethyl-19-norcholesterol.[45] Overall, scintigraphy achieves a high sensitivity (71%–100%) with varying specificity (50%–100%) for the differentiation of malignant from benign adrenal masses.[45] The disadvantage of these tracers is the high radiation dose to the adrenals. Currently, the clinical indications for adrenal cortex scintigraphy are very limited because of the development of CT, MRI, and highly sensitive biochemical assays.

The adrenal medulla produces catecholamines (adrenaline and noradrenaline). The commonest tumor in the medulla is pheochromocytoma that arises from the paraganglion cells anywhere in the autonomic nervous system. Ninety percent of pheochromocytomas are sporadic; the remaining 10% are associated with neuroectodermal disorders such as neurofibromatosis, tuberous sclerosis, von Hippel–Lindau syndrome, or multiple endocrine neoplastic syndrome. On $^{123}$I- or $^{131}$I-MIBG scintigraphy, pheochromocytomas are depicted as an abnormal focal area of increased activity. This technique is especially useful for the detection of ectopic pheochromocytomas and also for detection of metastatic or locally recurrent disease because unlike ultrasound, CT, or MRI, it is inherently a whole-body imaging technique. Refer to the section "Neural crest tumors" for further details.

F-DOPA focal hyperinsulinoma

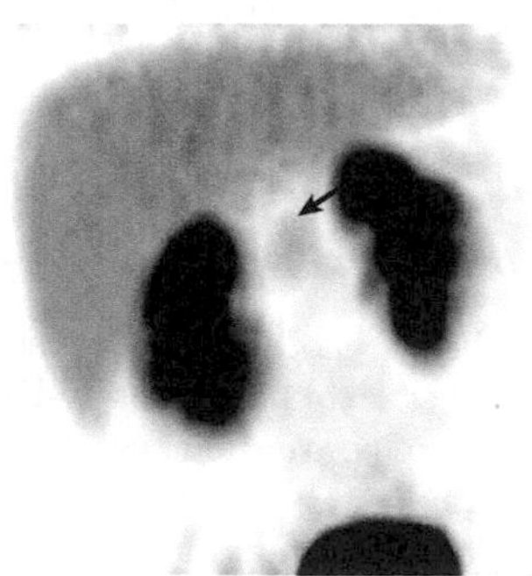


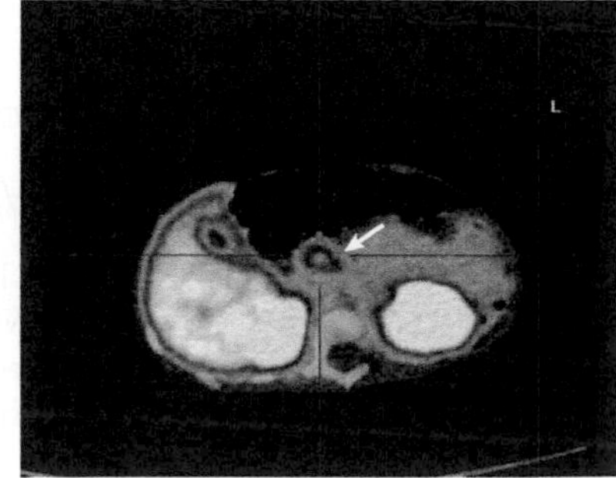


**Figure 7.13**
*These PET/CT images show focal uptake at the head of pancreas (arrows) indicating focal congenital hyperinsulinism.*

## $^{131}$I-MIBG and radionuclide peptide therapy (see Chapters 8, 9, 21)

Since the late 1990s, therapy has played an important role in the management of NETs. Radionuclide therapy works by the principle of internal targeting. The following factors influence radionuclide therapy[46]:

- The more selective and specific the uptake of the radionuclide, the better targeted the therapy.
- The therapeutic effects depend on the release of ionizing radiation, the beta particles (others are alpha particles and electron capture/internal conversion decaying but these are currently not in use).
- The longer the radionuclide stays in the target, the better the therapeutic ratio (to get good therapeutic ratio, it is necessary for the unlabeled radionuclide to be excreted rapidly to get a good target-to-background ratio).

### Indications[47]

- Inoperable malignant pheochromocytoma
- Inoperable malignant paraganglioma
- Neuroblastomas stage III and IV
- Medullary thyroid carcinoma
- Metastatic carcinoid tumors

### Mechanism of localization[46]

1. Internal localization by crossing the cell membrane and bound within cytoplasm or to the nuclear DNA, for example, $^{131}$I in DTC.
2. Uptake in the neurosecretory granules found in neuroendocrine cancer cells, for example, $^{131}$I-MIBG.
3. Binding to the receptors present on some of the tumor cells, for example, somatostatin receptors.

There are no randomized clinical trials available comparing optimal treatment cycle doses, optimal cycle interval, or optimal cumulative dose. Hence, treatment scheme depends on local expertise and clinical judgment.[48]

In the United Kingdom, centers offering peptide therapy are mainly concentrated in London.

Therapies are administered by an Administration of Radioactive Substances Advisory Committee (ARSAC) certificate holder who is either a nuclear medicine physician or oncologist.

## $^{131}$I-MIBG

$^{131}$I-MIBG is a beta-emitting radionuclide with peak energy of 0.61 MeV. It has physical half-life of 8.04 days. MIBG is an analog of noradrenaline. It is indicated in patients who have life expectancy of ≥3 months.

### Contraindications

*Absolute:*

- Pregnancy and breastfeeding
- Life expectancy of <3 months
- Renal insufficiency requiring dialysis

*Relative:*

- Rapidly deteriorating renal function with glomerular filtration rate (GFR) <30 mL
- Unmanageable urinary incontinence
- Myelosuppression

### Patient preparation

1. Patient should have MIBG-positive tumor on $^{123}$I-MIBG diagnostic scan.
2. Prevention of thyroid uptake of free iodide by thyroid blockade using potassium iodide or Lugol's iodine. Treatment begins at 24 h before $^{131}$I-MIBG administration and is continued until 10–15 days.
3. Drugs that interact with MIBG should be stopped (refer to Table 7.7). However, patients with metabolically active catecholamine-secreting tumors (i.e., pheochromocytoma, paraganglioma) are often alpha- and beta-blocked by medical treatment, before MIBG.[47]
4. Good hydration with intravenous fluids.
5. Prophylactic antiemetics.
6. Written informed consent should be obtained.

### Activity administered

Activity administered depends on clinical judgment, and it can range from 3.7 to 14.8 GBq in adults. Three cycles given at three monthly intervals.

*Side effects:*

- Nausea and vomiting
- Myelosuppression
- Flushing in patients with carcinoid

## Peptide receptor radionuclide therapy

There are different isotopes used for peptide receptor radionuclide therapy, mainly, indium-111, lutetium-177, and ytrrium-90, and the peptides used are octreotide (affinity toward somatostatin receptor [SSR] 2, 5, and 3), octreotate (affinity toward SSR 2), lanreotide (affinity toward SSR2, 5, 3, 4, and 1). Normally, the linker is the DOTA.

### Eligibility criteria

Life expectancy >3 months, tumor uptake on the OctreoScan should be at least as high as normal liver uptake and inoperable disease.[48]

Contraindications (both relative and absolute):

- Pregnancy and breastfeeding
- Renal impairment
- Impaired hematological function
- Severe hepatic impairment
- Severe cardiac impairment

### Patient preparation

1. Blood tests including full blood count, urea, and creatinine, and liver function tests should be done routinely before each administration
2. Obtain written informed consent
3. Infusion of amino acids containing lysine and arginine to reduce kidney-absorbed dose

## Lutetium-177 DOTATATE

Lutetium-177 DOTATATE is a beta- and gamma-emitting radioisotope; hence, it has the advantage of scanning on gamma camera posttherapy (for dosimetry and to assess the tumor uptake). It is given in four fractions with 7.4 GBq (total 29.6 GBq) at an interval of 6–9 weeks between each therapy.[49]

## Yttrium-90 DOTATATE

Yttrium-90 is a beta emitter and does not have gamma emission; hence, the patient cannot be imaged. It is given in four fractions of 3–4 GBq.[50]

## Acknowledgments

Special thanks are due to the following colleagues for providing images: Dr. Gill Vivian, Consultant Nuclear Physician, King's College Hospital, London; Dr. Sarah Al-Shahwan, SpR, King's College Hospital, London; Dr. Khalsa Al-Nabhani, Nuclear Medicine Fellow, UCH, London; and Dr. Simon Wan, Year 6 SpR, Nuclear Medicine, UCH, London.

## Useful websites

The following are useful websites with guidelines for reference:

National Institute of Clinical Excellence, www.nice.org.uk

British Nuclear Medicine Society, www.bnms.org.uk

European Association of Nuclear Medicine, www.eanm.org

British Thyroid Association, www.british-thyroid-association.org

Royal College of Physicians, www.rcplondon.ac.uk

European Neuroendocrine Tumour Society, www.enets.org

## References


1. O'Doherty MJ, Kettle AG, Wells PC, et al. Parathyroid imaging with technetium-99m-sestamibi: Preoperative localization and tissue uptake studies. *J Nucl Med* 1992; 33: 313.

*2. Lazarus JH. Guidelines for the use of radioiodine in the management of hyperthyroidism: A summary. The Radioiodine Audit Subcommittee of the Royal College of Physicians Committee on Diabetes and Endocrinology, and the Research Unit of the Royal College of Physicians. *J R Coll Physicians Lond* 1995; 29: 464–9.

3. Read CH, J., Tansey MJ, Menda Y. A 36-year retrospective analysis of the efficacy and safety of radioactive iodine in treating young Graves' patients. *J Clin Endocrinol Metab* 2004; 89: 4229–33.

4. Bonnema SJ, Grupe P, Boel-Jørgensen H, Brix TH, Hegedüs L. A randomized trial evaluating a block-replacement regimen during radioiodine therapy. *Eur J Clin Invest*. 2011; 41(7): 693–702.

5. Bartalena et al. Relation between therapy for hyperthyroidism and the course of Graves' ophthalmopathy. *N Engl J Med.* 1998; 338(2): 73–8.

6. Lai et al. Lower dose prednisone prevents radioiodine-associated exacerbation of initially mild or absent graves' orbitopathy: A retrospective cohort study. *J Clin Endocrinol Metab* 2010; 95(3): 1333–7.

7. Bartalena L, Marcocci C, Bogazzi F, et al. Relation between therapy for hyperthyroidism and the course of Graves' ophthalmopathy. *N Engl J Med* 1998; 338: 73–8.

*8. Franklyn JA, Maisonneuve P, Sheppard MC. Mortality after the treatment of hyperthyroidism with radioactive iodine; *N Engl J Med* 1998; 338: 712–18.

*9. National Institute for Clinical Excellence. *Guidance on Cancer Services: Improving Outcomes in Head and Neck Cancers*. NICE. London, 2004.

*10. British Thyroid Association, Royal College of Physicians. *Guidelines for the Management of Thyroid Cancer*. 2nd ed. Perros P, (ed). Report of the Thyroid Cancer Guidelines Update Group. London: Royal College of Physicians, 2007.


* Key or Classic references.

11. Bal C, Padhy AK, Jana S, et al. Prospective randomized clinical trial to evaluate the optimal dose of 131 I for remnant ablation in patients with differentiated thyroid carcinoma. *Cancer* 1996; 77: 2574–80.
12. Sirisalipoch S, Buachum V, Pasawang P, et al. Prospective randomized trial for the evaluation of the efficacy of low vs high dose 131I for post-operative remnant ablation in differentiated thyroid cancer. *World J Nucl Med* 2004; 3(Suppl 1): S36.
13. Haq MS, McCready RV, Harmer CL. Treatment of advanced differentiated thyroid carcinoma with high activity radioiodine therapy. *Nucl Med Commun* 2004; **25**: 799–805.
14. Nanni C, Rubello D, Fanti S et al. Role of 18-FDG PET and PET CT imaging in thyroid cancer. *Biomed Pharmacother*. 2006; 60(8): 409–13.
15. Al-Abed Y, Gray E, Wolfe K et al. Metastatic Hurthle Cell Carcinoma of the thyroid presenting as a Breast Lump: A Case Report. *Int Sem Surg Oncol* 2008; 5:14.
16. Kasner et al, Thyroid carcinoma: Iodine-131-negative whole-body scan reverses to positive after a combination of thyrogen stimulation and withdrawal. *Clin Nucl Med*. 2002; 27(11):772–80.
17. Lowe et al. 18F-FDG PET of patients with Hürthle cell carcinoma. *J Nucl Med* 2003; 44(9): 1402–6.
18. Baudin E, Do Cao D, Cailleux AF, et al. Positive predictive value of serum thyroglobulin levels, measured during the first year of follow-up after thyroid hormone withdrawal, in thyroid cancer patients. *J Clin Endocrinol Metab* 2003; 88: 1107–11.
19. Wang W, Macapinlac H, Larson SM, et al. [18F]-2-fluro-2-deoxy-D-glucose positron emission tomography localizes residual thyroid cancer in patients with negative diagnostic (131)I whole body scans and elevated serum thyroglobulin levels. *J Clin Endocrinol Metab* 1999; 84: 2291–302.
20. Grünwald F, Pakos E, Bender H, et al. Redifferentiation therapy with retinoic acid in follicular thyroid cancer 1998; 39(9):1555–8.
21. Lee JA, Inabnet WB. The surgeon's armamentarium to the surgical treatment of hyperparathyroidism. *J Surg Oncol* 2005; 89(3): 130–5.
22. Sosa JA, Bowman HM, Tielsch JM, et al. The importance of surgeon experience for clinical and economic outcomes from thyroidectomy. *Ann Surg* 1998; 228: 320–30.
23. Liu RC, Hill ME, Ryan JA Jr. One-gland exploration for mediastinal parathyroid adenomas: Cervical and thoracoscopic approaches. *Am J Surg* 2005; 189(5): 601–5.
24. Ferlin G, Borsato N, Camerani M, et al. New perspectives in localizing enlarged parathyroids by technetium thallium subtraction scan. *J Nucl Med* 1983; 24: 438–4.
25. Pattou F, Huglo D, Proye C. Radionuclide scanning in parathyroid diseases. *Br J Surg*. 1998; 85(12): 1605–16.
*26. Society of Nuclear Medicine. SNM Practice Guideline for Parathyroid Scintigraphy; SNM, published online http://www.snm.org/guidelines. June 2004.
27. Russell Van Husen, Lawrence T. Kim. Accuracy of Surgeon-performed Ultrasound in Parathyroid Localization. *World J. Surg* 2004; **28**: 1122–26.
28. Masatoshi Ishibashi et al. Localization of ectopic parathyroid glands using technetium-99m sestamibi imaging: Comparison with magnetic resonance and computed tomographic imaging. *Eur J Nucl Med* 1997; **24**: 197–201.
29. Lavely et al. Comparison of SPECT/CT, SPECT, and planar imaging with single- and dual-phase (99m) Tc-sestamibi parathyroid scintigraphy. *J Nucl Med*. 2007; **48**(7): 1084–9.
30. Roach PJ, Schembri GP, Ho Shon IA, et al. SPECT/CT imaging using a spiral CT scanner for anatomical localization: Impact on diagnostic accuracy and reporter confidence in clinical practice. *Nucl Med Commun* 2006; 27: 977–87.
*31. EANM AACE/AAES Task Force on Primary Hyperparathyroidism. The American Association of Clinical Endocrinologists and the American Association of Endocrine Surgeons position statement on the diagnosis and management of primary hyperparathyroidism. *Endocr Pract* 2005; 11: 49–54.
32. Sackett WR, Barraclough B, Reeve TS, et al. Worldwide trends in the surgical treatment of primary hyperparathyroidism in the era of minimally invasive parathyroidectomy. *Arch Surg* 2002; 137: 1055–9.
33. Wieland DM, Swanson DP, Brown LE, et al. Imaging the adrenal medulla with an I-131-labeled antiadrenergic agent. *J Nucl Med* 1979; 20: 155–8.
34. Lumachi F, Tregnaghi A, Zucchetta P et al. Sensitivity and positive predictive value of CT, MRI and 123I-MIBG scintigraphy in localizing pheochromocytomas: A prospective study. *Nucl Med Commun* 2006; 27 (7): 583–7.
35. Solanki KK, Bomanji J, Moyes J, et al. A pharmacological guide to medicines which interfere with the biodistribution of radiolabelled MIBG. *Nucl Med Commun* 1992; 13: 513–21.
*36. Solanki KK, Bomanji JB, Waddington WA, et al. Thyroid blocking policy revisited. *Nucl Med Commun* 25(11): 1071–6.
37. Rufini V, Calcagni ML, Baum RP. Imaging of neuroendocrine tumors. *Semin Nucl Med* 2006; 36(3): 228–47.
38. Hoefnagel CA. Metaiodobenzylguanidine and stomatostatin in oncology: Role in the management of neural crest tumours. *Eur J Nucl Med* 1994; 21: 561–81.

39. Bombardieri E, Aktolun C, Richard PB, et al. $^{111}$In-pentetreotide scintigraphy procedure guidelines for tumour imaging. *Eur J Nucl Med Mol Imaging* 2010; 37:1441–48.

*40. Kayani I, Bomanji JB, Groves A, et al. Functional imaging of neuroendocrine tumors with combined PET/CT using 68Ga-DOTATATE (DOTA-DPhe1,Tyr3-octreotate) and 18F-FDG. *Cancer*. 2008; 112(11): 2447–55.

41. Koopmans KP, de Vries EG, Kema IP, et al. Staging of carcinoid tumours with 18F-DOPA PET: A prospective, diagnostic accuracy study. *Lancet Oncol* 2006; 7(9): 728–34.

42. Hoegerle S, Nitzsche E, Altehoefer C, et al. Pheochromocytomas: Detection with 18F DOPA whole body PET – initial results. *Radiology* 2002; 222(2): 507–12.

43. Menni F, de Lonlay P, Sevin C, et al. Neurologic outcomes of 90 neonates and infants with persistent hyperinsulinemic. *Pediatrics* 2001; 107(3): 476–9.

44. Barthlen W, Blankenstein O, Mau H, et al. Evaluation of [18F]fluoro-L-DOPA positron emission tomography-computed tomography for surgery in focal congenital hyperinsulinism. *J Clin Endocrinol Metab*. 2008; 93(3): 869–75.

45. Mansmann G, Lau J, Balk E, et al. The clinically inapparent adrenal mass: Update in diagnosis and management. *Endocr Rev* 2004; 25(2): 309–40.

*46. Bomanji J, Britton K, Clarke S. *Clinicians Guide to Nuclear Medicine Oncology*. 1995. Impact Healthcare, Hatfield.

47. Giammarile F, Chiti A, Lassmann M, et al. EANM procedure guidelines for 131I-mIBG therapy. *Eur J Nucl Med Mol Imaging* 2008; 35: 1039–47.

*48. Kwekkeboom DJ, Krenning EP, Lebtahi R, et al. ENETS Consensus Guidelines for the Standards of Care in Neuroendocrine Tumors: Peptide receptor radionuclide therapy with radiolabeled somatostatin analogs. *Neuroendocrinology*. 2009;90(2): 220–6.

49. Kwekkeboom, de Herder WW, Kam BL, et al. Treatment With the Radiolabeled Somatostatin Analog [177Lu-DOTA0,Tyr3] Octreotate: Toxicity, Efficacy, and Survival. *J Clin Oncol* 2008; 26(13): 2124–30.

50. Cwikla JB, Sankowski A, Seklecka N, Buscombe JR, et al. Efficacy of radionuclide treatment DOTATATE Y-90 in patients with progressive metastatic gastroenteropancreatic neuroendocrine carcinomas (GEP-NETs): A phase II study. *Annals of Oncology* 2010; 21(4): 787–94.

# 8

# Gastroenteropancreatic neuroendocrine tumors (neoplasms)

*Maxime Palazzo, Philippe Ruszniewski, Dermot O'Toole*

## *Introduction*

The field of gastroenteropancreatic (GEP) neuroendocrine neoplasms (NENs) has evolved rapidly over the past decade and this has helped to enhance and understand the epidemiology, genetics, presenting features, and diagnostic capabilities and therapeutics. Several national registries have published interesting data in this field, and although comparisons between countries are sometimes hampered by types of registries and the data recorded (e.g., capture fields used, definition of malignancy, and nomenclature issues), the sheer body of recent work attests to the growing interest in GEP-NENs. Recent data from North America confirm a strong increase in annual incidence in NENs with an annual age adjusted incidence of 1.09/100,000 in 1973 to 5.25/100,000 in 2004[1]. Indeed, these trends in increasing incidence are also found in Europe[2]. Even more significant are the figures pertaining to the high prevalence of GEP-NENs, estimated with a 29-year limited-duration prevalence of NENs of 103,312 in 2004 (35/100,000), making this disease more prevalent than many other gastrointestinal (GI) cancers, including esophageal, gastric, hepatobiliary, and pancreatic.[1] So, although incidence figures assemble GEP-NENs into a so-called "rare tumor" group, enhanced longevity due to the long natural history coupled with enormous improvements in managing symptomatic and oncological disease components means that we are actively seeing more and more patients, underlying the need for proper management resourcing.

Although GEP-NENs are often quite variable, ranging from nonfunctional tumors to those secreting hormones or peptides that are readily identifiable as specific syndromes, such as insulinoma, gastrinoma, and carcinoid syndrome, and emanate from many different organs, they often share common biological and morphological aspects. Most are histologically well differentiated, with a slow progressive pattern, and they express common markers such as synaptophysin and chromogranin. The majority also express membranous somatostatin receptors that allow for specific targets for both diagnostic and therapeutic strategies. A further commonality is the rich vascular network in many of these tumors that has been used to help elucidate biological properties and diagnose and treat these patients. Although surgery for small tumors can be curative, many patients manifest with advanced disease because symptoms are often absent until metastases have occurred, and even when symptomatic, failure of disease recognition is frequent. Therefore, therapies, including surgery, are often aimed at controlling tumor burden and symptoms. Advances in surgery, biotherapy, radionuclide therapy, and more recently specifically targeting membranous or internal cellular molecules (e.g., vascular endothelial growth factor receptor [VEGF-R], tyrosine kinase inhibitors) provide more effective options in treating patients with advanced disease.

## *Histology, tissue markers, and classifications*

"Neuroendocrine" defines the cellular origins of the tumors, which share neuroendocrine markers. Tissue from a GEP-NEN, obtained either by biopsy from a primary tumor or a metastasis (i.e., liver, lymph node) or by surgical resection, is examined histologically for the typical morphology of NEN. It is, however, also crucial to demonstrate neuroendocrine markers such as synaptophysin and chromogranin A (CgA) in the tumor cells.[3,4] Synaptophysin, an integral membrane protein of small clear vesicles (diameter 40–80 nm), occurring in all normal and neoplastic neuroendocrine cells, is diffusely expressed in the cytoplasm of all cells of an NEN. CgA, a protein located in the matrix of large secretory granules (80 nm), in contrast to synaptophysin, is inhomogeneously expressed in the cytoplasm of the tumor cell or can even be lacking because its expression depends on the number of neurosecretory granules present in the cells and on the cell type. CgA may be absent or weak in poorly differentiated tumors or in somatostatin-positive duodenal NEN and rectal NEN. Immunostaining for specific hormones/peptides may also be of help (e.g., serotonin, suggesting a primary in the ileum; gastrin; insulin; pancreatic polypeptide). However, the presence of an individual peptide or hormone upon tissue staining does not necessarily imply that the tumor is "functioning" per se. The issue of functionality of NEN also impacts on nomenclature. Functioning NEN are based on the presence of clinical symptoms due to excess hormone secretion by the tumor and include functioning carcinoid tumors and a variety of other functioning NEN arising in the pancreas or elsewhere. Terms reflecting the clinical syndromes may be applied to these NEN, such as insulinoma, glucagonoma, and gastrinoma, although the term *carcinoid* tumor was formerly used for tumors with or without the carcinoid syndrome and is best avoided.

Once the neuroendocrine nature of the tumor has been established, its proliferative activity has to be determined because it has been shown to provide significant prognostic and therapeutic information. The proliferative activity can be determined by counting the mitoses per high-power field (HPF) and/or more easily by immunostaining for the cell cycle-dependent marker Ki-67 (MIB-1) antigen, expressed in the nucleus. To determine the Ki-67 labeling index, 100 tumor cells have to be assessed in a hot-spot area. In the novel World Health Organization (WHO) 2010 classification for gastrointestinal NEN,[5] all tumors are considered malignant with the potential to metastasize. The Ki-67 proliferative index and the mitotic count then serve as the basis for grading the tumors as G1 (Ki-67: ≤2% or <2 mitoses per HPF), G2 (Ki-67: 3%–20% or 2–20 mitoses per HPF) or G3 (Ki-67: >20% or >20 mitoses per HPF) (Figure 8.1 and Table 8.1). Well-differentiated tumors are called G1 or G2 NEN, and the most malignant tumors, previously classified as poorly differentiated neuroendocrine carcinomas (NEC), are now called large-cell or small-cell type G3 NEC (Table 8.2). The categorization of GEP-NENs according to European Neuroendocrine Tumors Society (ENETS)–based grading has been clearly demonstrated to accurately predict behavior and prognosis in pancreatic tumors in several groups, and limited data for mid- and hindgut tumors as well as gastric tumors suggest the same.[6–8] Two tumor-node-metastasis (TNM)–based staging systems exist for NEN: ENETS 2007[9,10] and Union for International Cancer Control (UICC) 2009.[11] They are site-specific TNM staging of the GEP system (stomach, duodenum, ileum, appendix, colorectum, and pancreas).

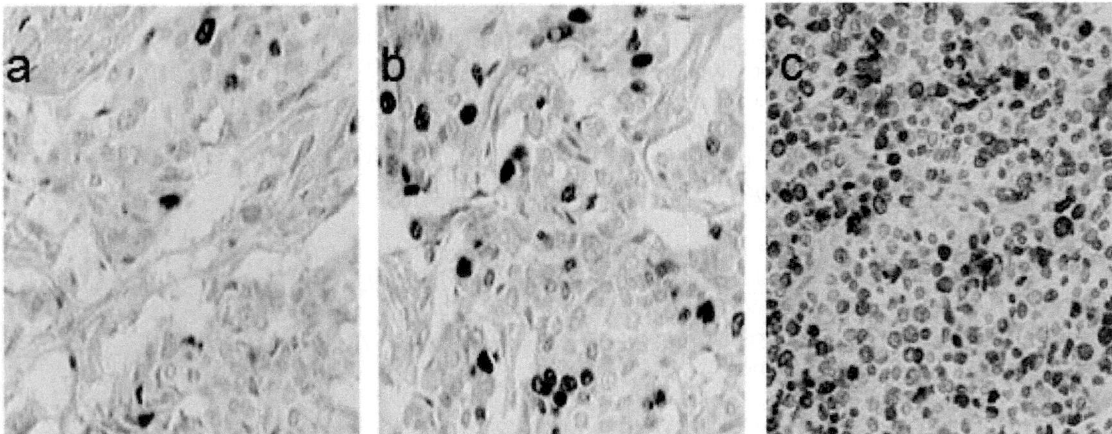


***Figure 8.1***
*Histology form three different well-differentiated pancreatic NETs showing different grades according to Ki-67 proliferative index (using MIB-1 antigen staining): (a) Ki-67 <2% (G1), (b) Ki-67 = 5% (G2), and (c) Ki-67 >80% (G3).*

| *Grading* | *G1* | *G2* | *G3* |
|---|---|---|---|
| Ki-67 index (%)[a] | ≤2 | 3–20 | >20 |
| Mitotic count (10HPF)[b] | <2 | 2–20 | >20 |

[a] Mib1 antibody, percentage of 2000 tumor cells in areas of highest nuclear labeling.
[b] 10HPF, high-power field = 2 mm$^2$, at least 40 fields (at 40× magnification) evaluated in areas of highest mitotic density.

***Table 8.1***
*WHO 2010 grading system.*

| |
|---|
| Neuroendocrine tumor (carcinoid) G1 |
| Neuroendocrine tumor G2 |
| Neuroendocrine carcinoma G3, large-cell or small-cell type |
| Mixed adenoneuroendocrine carcinoma (MANEC) |

***Table 8.2***
*WHO 2010 classification.*

# Clinical presentation

Most GEP-NENs are sporadic, but they can be multiple and part of a familial syndrome such as multiple endocrine neoplasia type 1 (MEN1), von Hippel–Lindau (VHL) syndrome, and neurofibromatosis type 1 (NF1). Clinical presentation depends on the site of the primary tumor and whether they are so-called functioning tumors, that is, whether the peptides secreted produce symptoms. Most GEP-NENs are nonfunctioning and present fairly late, with symptoms of mass effects or distant (usually hepatic) metastases. Gastric NENs are usually discovered incidentally or at the follow-up in patients with chronic atrophic gastritis or more rarely in Zollinger–Ellison syndrome (ZES) during upper digestive endoscopy. Most duodenal NENs are gastrin-secreting, causing ZES. Pancreatic NENs are usually nonfunctioning, and although in the past about 50% were thought to have hepatic metastases at diagnosis,[12] currently incidental discovery of small benign nonfunctional pancreatic NENs is frequent.[13] The general characteristics of pancreatic NENs are shown in Table 8.3.

Functioning pancreatic NENs may secrete several peptide hormones and lead to diverse symptomatology. Insulinomas are typically small benign functioning tumors, and patients present with organic hypoglycemia[14] corresponding to the classical Whipple triad (neuroglucopenic symptoms + fasting glycemia <2.2 mmol/L + reversal of these symptoms when the blood sugar level is restored to normal). Pancreatic gastrinomas are less common than duodenal gastrinomas, but they are usually malignant; about 25% are associated with MEN1.[14] Clinical presentation of gastrinoma is called ZES and combines acid-related mucosal damage in the upper GI tract (classically duodenal ulcers or severe esophagitis) due to chronic hypergastrinemia and diarrhea from high acid output (curiously, the only type of diarrhea likely to respond to proton pump inhibitors, and this simple observation may give an important clue to diagnosis). Diarrhea is not constant in patients with gastrinoma and recurrent upper GI ulceration in *Helicobacter pylori*–negative individuals should prompt the possibility of ZES. Rarer functional pancreatic NENs include *glucagonomas* that result in loss of weight, diabetes, characteristic rash (necrolytic migratory erythema), and thromboembolic manifestations; *VIPomas* are associated with severe watery diarrhea, causing weight loss, dehydration, and severe hypokalemia.[12]

Midgut tumors such as jejuno-ileal, appendiceal, and right colon tumors derive from enterochromaffin cells and are mostly nonfunctioning.[15] Appendiceal NENs are usually small (i.e., confined to the appendix) and identified incidentally during unrelated surgery or during acute appendicitis.

In the presence of liver metastases, serotonin, tachykinins, and other bioactive substances can reach the systemic circulation and cause carcinoid syndrome, characterized by cutaneous flushing, chronic diarrhea, bronchoconstriction, and abdominal pain.[15] A severe form of carcinoid syndrome is called carcinoid crisis and represents a life-threatening situation, associated with prolonged severe flushing, diarrhea, hypotension, tachycardia, dyspnoea, and peripheral cyanosis (see Chapter 24). A further distinct feature of enterochromaffin tumors is their propensity to cause extensive mesenteric fibrosis encasing mesenteric vessels and, occasionally, mesenteric ischemia. Fibrosis may involve the endocardium of the right side of the heart and the tricuspid and pulmonary valves (pulmonary stenosis and tricuspid regurgitation), with impairment of cardiac function. Ten to twenty percent of patients with carcinoid syndrome have heart disease at presentation.

# Genetics associations of GEP-NENs (see Chapter 9)

GEP-NENs can be integrated in several genetic syndromes, such as MEN1, VHL syndrome, and NF1.

| | Size (cm) | Location | Benign (%) | Malignant (%) | Cure (%) | Intra-op. localization | MEN1 (%) |
|---|---|---|---|---|---|---|---|
| Insulinoma | 1 | Pancreas 100% | >90 | <10 | >90 | Possible ++ | <5 |
| Gastrinoma | <0.5 | Duodenum (>60%) | <30 | >70 | Rare | Possible | 25 |
| Nonfunctioning pNET | <2 | | Frequent | – | Frequent | – | |
| | >2 | | – | Frequent | Rare | – | <10 |
| Rare functioning pNET | Large | – | – | Frequent | Rare | – | <10 |

***Table 8.3***
*Characteristics of pancreatic NENs.*

MEN1 is characterized by the association in a same patient of at least two of the following five endocrinopathies:[16] primary hyperparathyroidism (95%–100%), duodeno-pancreatic neuroendocrine neoplasms (30%–75%), pituitary adenoma (15%–65%), adrenocortical hyperplasia or tumor (40%), and thymic or bronchial neuroendocrine tumor (5%–10%). Prevalence is between 1/20,000 and 1/40,000. Transmission is autosomal dominant with a very high penetrance estimated at 45% at 35 years of age, 82% at 50 years of age, and 96% at 70 years of age. The major gene for predisposition is located on 11q13[17] and is a tumor suppressor gene encoding for the 610 amino acid protein menin. Menin is involved in negative regulation of cell proliferation by interacting with transcription-regulating factors, cytoskeleton and extracellular matrix, and replication and repair of genomic DNA. MEN1/GEP-NEN can be functioning or nonfunctioning. Gastrinomas represent the majority of functional MEN1/GEP-NEN (55%–70%), with ~30% being MEN1-related. Insulinomas represent 10% of functional MEN1/GEP-NENs, and only 5% of all insulinoma are MEN1-related. Nonfunctional GEP-NEN represents 15% of all MEN1/GEP-NENs. Genotypic diagnosis of MEN1 mutation is systematically proposed in case of typical MEN1 presentation and in case of one manifestation in a patient aged <50 years.[18]

VHL syndrome variously combines six major involvements:[19] hemangioblastoma of the central nervous system (60%–80%); retinal hemangioblastoma (50%–60%); clear cell renal carcinoma and multiple renal cysts (30%–60%); pancreatic simple cysts, pancreatic serous cystadenoma, and pancreatic NENs (30%–65%); pheochromocytoma (15%); and endolymphatic sac tumors (5%). There are two types of VHL: type 1 without and type 2 with pheochromocytoma. Prevalence is between 1/45,000 and 1/35,000. Transmission is autosomal dominant with an almost complete penetrance at 60 years old. The *VHL* gene is a tumor suppressor gene located on 3p25-26[20] encoding for a 213 amino acid protein interacting with hypoxia-inducible factor (HIF) 1α, leading to its degradation by the proteasome. In the absence of active pVHL, HIF1α is up regulated, leading to the activation of hypoxia-sensitive genes involved in proliferation, angiogenesis, and resistance to apoptosis. Pancreatic NENs in VHL disease are usually nonfunctioning.[21]

Duodenal and pancreatic NENs, especially ampullary and periampullary duodenal somatostatinoma, have been reported to be associated with NF1,[22] but they are not part of the diagnostic criteria.

# Diagnostic measures

## General biological markers

### Chromogranin A

CgA is an acid glycoprotein with 439 amino acids that is present in the secretory dense core granules of most neuroendocrine cells[23] and has been recognized as a general serum marker that can be elevated in both functionally active and nonfunctional NENs.[24] CgA is the most practical and useful general serum tumor marker in patients with NENs. Although performances are limited because specificity for NENs is low in patients with low levels of CgA, very high levels of serum CgA are rarely found outside the setting of NENs, with the exception of patients on gastric acid secretory blockers, especially proton pump inhibitors (PPIs)[25] or those with hypergastrinemia. Specificity of CgA in the diagnosis of NEN depends on the tumor type and burden. Nobels et al.[26] demonstrated a significant positive relation between the serum levels of CgA and the tumor mass in NENs. False-positive elevation of CgA may occur in the following circumstances[27]: impaired renal function; Parkinson's disease; untreated hypertension; pregnancy; steroid treatment or glucocorticoid excess, which can lead to upregulation of CgA mRNA[28]; chronic atrophic gastritis[29]; and treatment with antisecretory medications, especially PPIs.[25] Chronic elevation of gastrin levels provokes hyperplasia of the NE cells of the stomach, and these cells are able to secrete CgA.[30]

Another serum marker that is frequently elevated in NENs includes neuron-specific enolase. Nevertheless, CgA was found to be more sensitive than neuron-specific enolase in all subgroups of a large NEN patient cohort.[31]

### *Urinary 5-hydroxyindole acetic acid and midgut NENs*

NENs originating from the midgut may secrete various peptides and hormones, most notably serotonin (5-hydroxytryptamine, 5-HT). The urinary metabolite of serotonin is urinary 5-hydroxyindole acetic acid (5-HIAA), a metabolite that is particularly useful in the diagnosis and follow-up of NENs with carcinoid syndrome.[24] The overall sensitivity and specificity of urinary 5-HIAA in the presence of the carcinoid syndrome is of the order of 70% and 90%, respectively.[32,33] Foregut and hindgut NENs produce less serotonin than midgut tumors.[32] Urinary 5-HIAA levels may also depend on tumor volume and may be normal in patients with nonmetastatic NENs. Urine should be collected and measured in plastic containers. Acid should be added to ensure sterility and stability. The sample should be stored in a refrigerator until analysis. Intraindividual variation of 5-HIAA is also possible, and this variation may be high; therefore, two consecutive 24 h collections should be performed and the mean value of these two collections taken. Falsely low 5-HIAA levels may be encountered in patients with renal impairment and those on hemodialysis. In addition, 5-HIAA may be increased in untreated patients with malabsorption, who have increased urinary tryptophan metabolites. The following food substances are rich in dietary tryptophan; therefore, patients should abstain from these for 3 days before urinary collection: plums, pineapples, bananas, eggplants, tomatoes, avocados, and walnuts.[34] Patients with NENs are frequently treated with somatostatin analogs (SSAs), and these analogs are known to decrease levels of 5-HIAA; where possible, assays for diagnostic purposes should be made in patients not on SSAs, whereas in the follow-up setting, comparisons should be performed in patients on stable or comparable doses.[24]

## *Insulinoma*

The diagnosis is suggested in the presence of neuroglucopenic symptoms of hypoglycemia, glucose <2.2 mmol/L, and relief of symptoms with administration of glucose.[35] This combination is known as Whipple's triad. The 72 h fast is the standard for diagnosing insulinoma.[24] A 72 h period is recognized as the most appropriate duration.[36] Symptoms appear within 12 h for one-third of patients, 80% within 24 h, 90% within 48 h, approaching 100% within 72 h[37]. Patients should be hospitalized in a specialist unit experienced in performing the test. Patients should stay off all foods except for plain water, black tea, or coffee. Blood analysis should be performed in case of malaise and at the end of test. The endpoint of the test is documented hypoglycemia (blood glucose levels <2.2 mmol/L with concomitant insulin levels >6 μU/L). Differential diagnosis of insulinoma can be self-administration of insulin (low C peptide) or hypoglycemic sulfamids (presence of sulfonylureas in the urine).

## *Gastrinoma: ZES*

The diagnosis of ZES can be established by the demonstration of elevated fasting serum gastrin (FSG) in the presence of low gastric pH. FSG alone is not adequate to make the diagnosis of ZES because hypergastrinemia can be seen in many situations; therefore, gastrin provocative tests are needed to establish the diagnosis. The standard is the secretin test.[38] This hormone, when given intravenously provokes in gastrinoma patients an increase in serum gastrin and secondarily in gastric acid secretion. The test may be repeated during the follow-up after curative surgery. FSG should be performed before the secretin test; if FSG is >1000 pg/mL in the absence of fundic atrophic gastritis, or *H. pylori* infection, and with a basal acid output >15 mmol/h, a secretin test is not necessary. If not, a secretin test should be performed. PPIs should be interrupted 10 days before the test (PPIs must be replaced by H2 blockers); then, H2 blockers should be interrupted for approximately 48 h before the test. However, interruption of all antisecretory medications can be dangerous (certain patients may have to be hospitalized during antisecretory therapy withdrawal). Patients should be warned of reappearance of symptoms and should have sufficient antisecretory medications to start if they become symptomatic. Secretin (2 U/kg body weight) is given as intravenous bolus. Serum gastrin baseline is measured at –15 and –1 min before test and 2, 5, 10, 15, 20, and 30 min after secretin. A delta gastrin of 120 pg/mL seen at any point has a high sensitivity and specificity (94 and 100%, respectively).[38]

## Morphological investigations

Morphological examinations are essential not only for establishing and confirming a diagnosis but also in terms of characterization of the origin of the primary, locoregional, and/or metastatic spread and follow-up. As mentioned, GEP-NENs share certain common characteristics (e.g., rich vascularity; expression of SST receptors, in particular, sst2; dihydroxyphenylalanine [DOPA] decarboxylase activity) that enable specifically directed diagnostic modalities. No technique is 100% sensitive or 100% specific, and multiple imaging modalities are usually required.[39]

## Endoscopy and endoscopic ultrasound

Upper gastrointestinal endoscopy is essential for the detection and characterization of NENs up to the angle of Treitz (esophageal, gastric, and duodenal). Ileo-colonoscopy allows the diagnosis of rectal, colonic, and very occasionally distal ileal lesions. Endoscopic ultrasonography (EUS) is the modality of choice for diagnosing pancreatic NENs and for locoregional staging of esophageal, gastric, duodenal, pancreatic, and rectal NENs. Using EUS neuroendocrine tumors typically appear as well-limited, round-shaped, homogeneous (frequently), hypoechoic lesions with posterior enhancement of the acoustic beam. EUS enables assessment of the degree of parietal extension (invasion of the *muscularis mucosae*) and locoregional lymph node invasion (essential in patients with rectal NENs and gastric tumors approaching 1 cm in size). EUS is the most accurate diagnostic method in the detection and localization of insulinoma,[40] and its combined use with somatostatin receptor scintigraphy permits the detection of gastrinoma in ~90% of patients[41] (Figure 8.2). Contrast-enhanced EUS (with harmonic imaging) takes advantage of the rich vascularity of NENs and appears to enhance diagnostic performance.[42] In addition, transmural sampling of pancreatic NENs or nodes is facilitated by EUS-guided fine-needle aspiration (FNA) (Figure 8.3), allowing cytological and fine cores for histological assessments (including histological grade).[43]

## Gastric, Duodenal and Rectal NENs (Table 8.4)

Gastric NENs (Figure 8.4) are divided into two groups: sporadic tumors and gastric NENs developing in response to enterochromaffin-like cell hyperplasia (ECLoma) from chronic hypergastrinemia. These NENs are classified into three types. Two types are related to chronic hypergastrinemia: type 1 is associated with chronic atrophic gastritis (they are usually

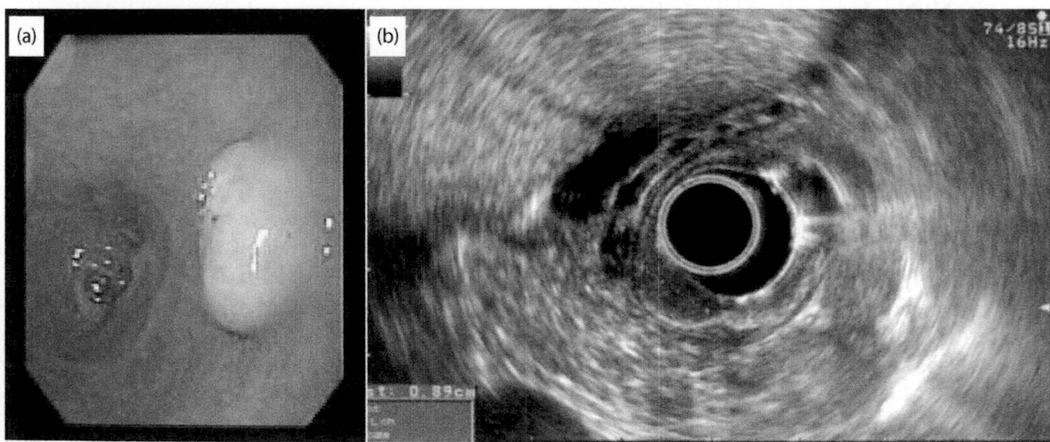


**Figure 8.2**
*Endoscopic (a) and EUS (b) examinations revealing a small (<10 mm) gastrinoma in the lateral wall of the duodenal bulb. The lesion is homogeneous and well demarcated (dotted line) confined to the mucosa and submucosa.*

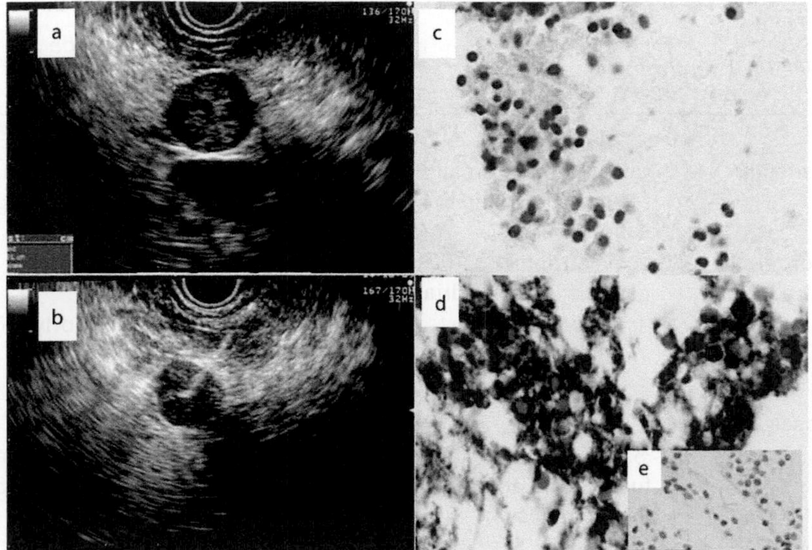

**Figure 8.3**
*EUS (a) and EUS-guided fine needle aspiration and biopsy (b) of small 11-mm incidentally discovered pancreatic NEN in the tail of pancreas. The possibility of an accessory spleen was raised, but the diagnosis was clearly established at biopsy showing typical neuroendocrine cells at haematoxylin and eosin (c) that strongly stain with CgA (d). The Ki-67 proliferative index was <1% (e).*

very low grade lesions with slow growth) and type 2 is in association with a MEN1-related gastrinoma. The sporadic type 3 occurs in the absence of hypergastrinemia. The endoscopic appearance of ECLoma in patients with chronic atrophic gastritis is characterized by the presence of small, often numerous, polypoid tumors (most frequently <1 cm). The type II ECLomas are usually small, even microscopic, and discovered after multiple biopsies of macroscopically normal fundic mucosa. When they are visible, lesions are generally small (<1–2 cm) and multiple.[44,45] Type 3 occurs in a nonatrophic fundic mucosa; they are frequently localized in the antrum and are often unique, large, and clearly aggressive.

Aside from the duodenal gastrinomas, other duodenal NENs are very rare. We distinguish somatostatinomas, nonfunctional NENs (often discovered incidentally during an upper endoscopy), poorly differentiated NECs (including those of the ampulla of Vater), and duodenal paragangliomas.[46] Rectal NENs are not uncommon (1%–2% of rectal tumors) and represent ~12%–20% of all GEP-NEN.[47] Nearly 50% of rectal NENs are discovered incidentally during lower endoscopy.[48] Small tumors often occur in the form of small submucosal polypoid lesion or as a sessile nodule. They are usually yellowish, and 75% of lesions are <8 cm from the anal margin.

## Radiology

With the exception of small gastric and rectal NENs, the use of cross-sectional imaging is almost systematic in the management of GEP-NENs.

### Computed tomography scan

Helical computed tomography (CT), generally multidetector CT scanners, offers very rapid scan times, reducing movement artifacts as well as accurate contrast medium bolus-tracking to ensure optimal timing of the scan, thereby ensuring excellent arterial phase images. Reformatting the images in thinner slices can also be performed, thereby improving resolution and allowing the images to be viewed optimally in multiple anatomical planes. For GEP-NENs, a meticulous technique is very important to optimize performance with high sensitivity. The examination involves unenhanced (for calcifications), and during intravenous contrast, enhancement in an early arterial phase (15–25 s), portal-venous inflow phase (25–30 s), and portal phase (70–90 s). Gastric, duodenal, rectal, and colonic NENs are diagnosed by endoscopy. The role of CT in these cases is to detect regional and distant metastases for staging of the disease. NENs are

| Proportion of gastric NEN (%) | Type 1<br>70–80 | Type 2<br>5–6 | Type 3<br>14–25 |
|---|---|---|---|
| Localization | Body, fundus | Body, fundus, antrum | Antrum |
| Tumor characteristics | Single/multiples, small (<1 cm); polyploid or submucosal | Often multiple, small size (<1–2 cm); polyploid (sessile) | Single, large (>2 cm); occasionally ulcerated |
| Associated disorders | Chronic atrophic gastritis; achlorhydria | Gastrinoma/MEN-1 | Sporadic |
| Histology | Well differentiated | Well differentiated | Poorly differentiated |
| Serum gastrin | ↑ | ↑ | Normal |
| Gastric pH | ↑ | ↓ | Normal |
| Risk of metastases (%) | 2–5 | 10–30 | 50–100 |
| Management | – <5 mm: biopsy of tumors and adjacent gastric mucosa;<br>– 6 to 10 mm: endoscopic resection;<br>– >1 cm or ≥usT2: discussion for surgery | Therapy dictated by the associated gastrinoma and/or its metastases; strict treatment of the gastric NEN is rarely indicated | Surgical resection (oncological resection with lymphadenectomy) |
| Surveillance | Annual upper endoscopy for tumor biopsies and detection of atrophic gastritis-associated dysplasia | Specific for gastrinoma and MEN1 ; annual upper endoscopy | According to histological diagnosis |

***Table 8.4***
*Characteristics of gastric NENs.*

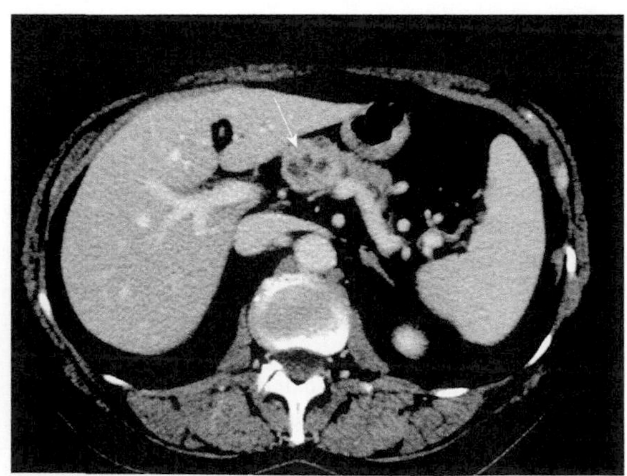

***Figure 8.4***
*CT scan revealing a partially cystic pancreatic NEN (arrow) in the isthmus.*

well vascularized and best depicted during intravenous contrast enhancement in the portal-venous inflow phase where they show up as high enhancing lesions. Functional pancreatic NENs are typically small, sharply delineated and can be multiple in patients with the MEN1 syndrome. Cystic lesions can occur but are rare (≤5%) (Figure 8.4). Nonfunctioning NENs are usually larger; however, the incidental discovery of small benign NENs is increasing in frequency. Larger pancreatic NENs are usually not well vascularized and may comprise areas of necrosis; contrast enhancement is not as pronounced and usually shows an irregular pattern. CT also delineates the position of the tumor in relation to the pancreatic and common bile ducts, evaluates possible vascular encasement and stages the disease with respect to regional lymph node involvement and presence of distant metastases, mainly to the liver.

Small bowel tumors are mostly found in the ileum rather than in the jejunum and are usually small and occasionally multiple. They are best seen with CT enteroclysis. For CT enteroclysis, a naso-jejunal tube is placed downstream to the ligament of Treitz, and 2 L of warmed tap water is administered, preferably by using a pump at 150–200 mL/min. Frequently, midgut tumors present as mesenteric metastasis. At CT, it is typically an irregular soft tissue mass, with one or several areas of calcifications, surrounded by radiating streaks in the mesenteric fat resembling spokes in a wheel (retraction with a fibrous mass) (Figure 8.5). The mesenteric complex may encase the superior mesenteric artery and/or vein or branches/tributaries of these vessels (Figure 8.6). For rectal NENs, the role of CT is for distant staging and not to detect the primary tumor or to appreciate its invasion of the rectal wall, the surrounding mesorectum and adjacent organs that instead is most likely better performed by magnetic resonance imaging (MRI) or EUS.

Generally, NEN liver metastases are well vascularized and best depicted during intravenous contrast enhancement in the portal-venous inflow phase where they show up as high enhancing lesions in the nonenhanced normal liver (Figure 8.7). The CT appearance of NEN lymph node metastases is similar to that from other malignant tumors, although a marked contrast enhancement is frequent. Peritoneal carcinomatosis is occasionally seen, most often in the ventral aspect of the abdomen. Lung metastases from NENs, similarly to those from other malignant tumors, appear as rounded, multiple, and well-delineated dense nodules. NEN bone metastases are often sclerotic (blastic), but they can be osteolytic and sometimes show a mixed appearance.

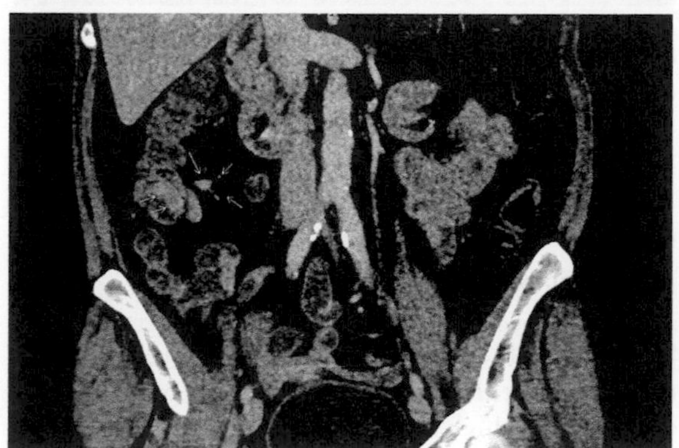

**Figure 8.5**
*CT scan in coronal view showing a primary ileocaecal tumor (double arrows) with a regional node (triple arrows) and some mesenteric retraction (spoke-wheel appearance in mesenteric fat).*

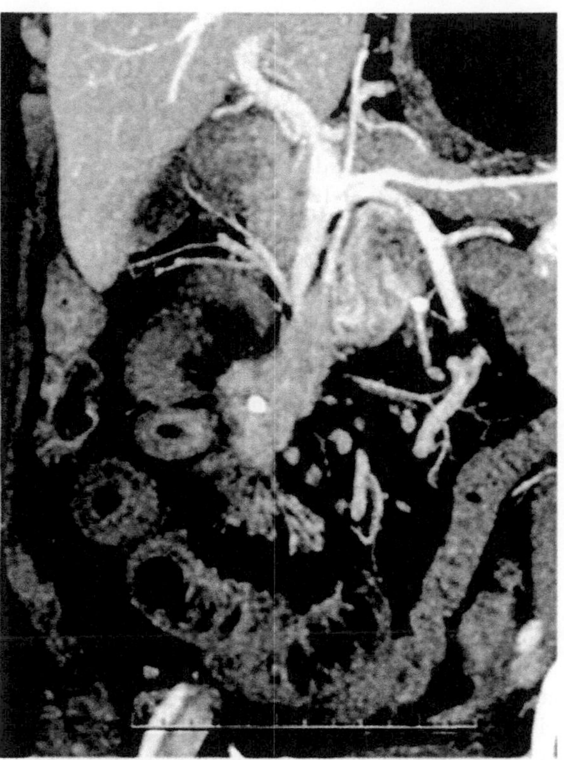

**Figure 8.6**
*CT scan in coronal view showing a mesenteric complex (with a central calcification) resulting in small bowel ischemia (target sign).*

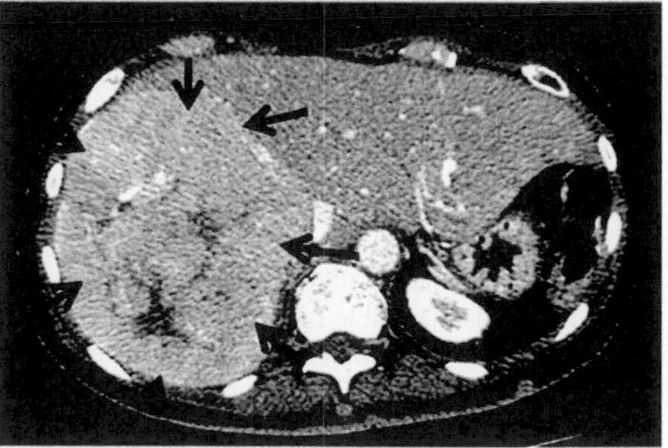

**Figure 8.7**
*CT scan revealing a large metachronous hepatic metastasis of a pancreatic neuroendocrine tumor (hyperdense lesion, arrows on arterial phase).*

The overall diagnostic accuracy in five studies on 162 patients for CT showed a mean sensitivity of 73% (range, 63%–82%) and 96% specificity (range, 83%–100%).[49–53]

In four studies reporting on the detection of NEN liver metastases in 135 patients, the mean sensitivity was 82% (range, 78%–100%), whereas the mean specificity was 92% (range, 83%–100%).[54–57] Performance in the detection of small bowel carcinoids (in 44 patients) with CT enteroclysis showed an impressive sensitivity and specificity of 100% and 96.2%, respectively.[58]

## Magnetic resonance imaging

The advantages of MRI over CT are the lack of ionizing radiation and the use of gadolinium (Gd) chelate contrast agent that has better safety profile in terms of allergic reactions and nephrotoxicity. As with CT, an adequate technique is essential to ensure the best sensitivity. The MRI sequences that are generally recommended for the detection of NENs are fat-saturated transaxial T1-weighted and fat-saturated T2-weighted sequences and optionally fat-saturated transaxial in and out of phase T1-weighted sequences. For MRI of the pancreas, MR cholangiopancreatography (MRCP) should also be performed by coronal radiated T2-weighted thick slice (25-mm) radiated sequences with two ranges including the pancreatobiliary junction and the pancreatic body, respectively, to better evaluate the regional anatomy and the relation of the tumor to the pancreatic duct and the main bile duct. A T2 thin slice MRCP with three-dimensional (3D) acquisition is also accurate. The conventional extracellular Gd-based MRI contrast medium, with a pharmacokinetic pattern similar to that of iodine used for CT, remains the standard for intravenous contrast-enhanced MRI. At MRI, an NEN appears typically as a low signal lesion in T1-weighted images and a high signal lesion in T2-weighted images (Figure 8.8). The MRI appearances of NEN are similar to those of CT concerning tumor delineation and contrast-enhancement characteristics. Although spatial resolution is poorer with MRI than CT, the better soft tissue contrast of MRI facilitates the detection of small NENs. Depiction of small liver metastases is also favorable by MRI using these signal sequences or using diffusion-weighted sequences and/or agents sucg as Primivist-TM. Lesions that are equivocal or contradictory at CT may better be characterized by using the various MRI sequences that should also include dynamic examination with intravenous contrast agent (Figure 8.9).

The diagnostic accuracy in five studies (192 patients) revealed a mean detection rate for pancreatic NENs of 73% (range, 50%–94%).[59–63] In a direct comparison of MRI with somatostatin receptor scintigraphy and CT in 64 patients, MRI detected 95% of liver metastases.[64]

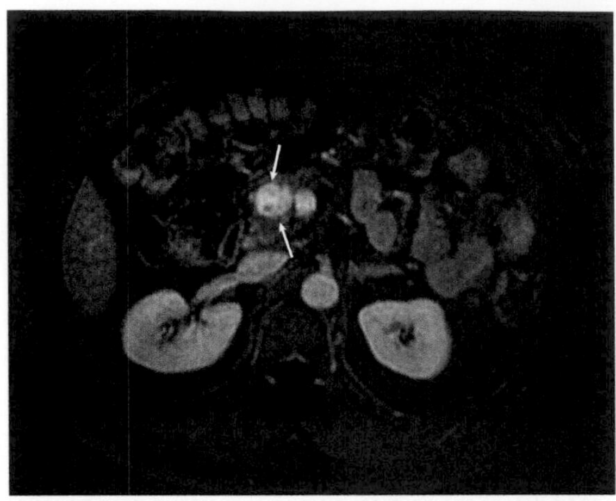

***Figure 8.8***
*Gd-enhanced MRI of pancreas demonstrating a 2 cm pancreatic NEN in the head of pancreas (hyperintense lesion [arrows] with small contrast poor areas representing likely necrotic zones).*

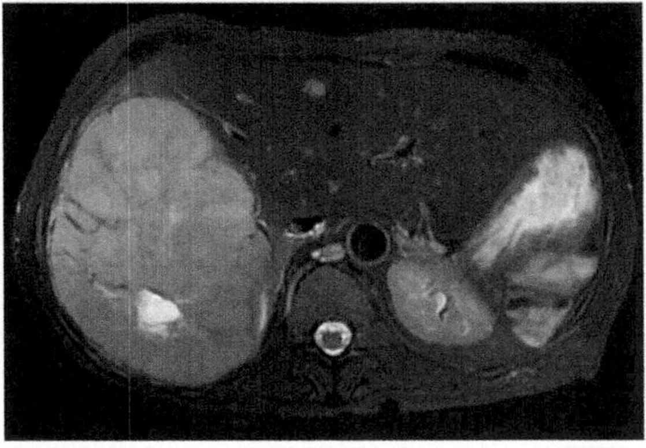

***Figure 8.9***
*MRI revealing a large metachronous hepatic metastasis of a pancreatic neuroendocrine tumor (hyperintensity, T2-weighted phase).*

## Radionuclide imaging

Most GEP-NENs express somatostatin receptors[65,66] and more specifically subtype sst2. Scintigraphy with [$^{111}$In-DTPA-D-Phe1]-octreotide (OctreoScan®) is used to visualize tumors rich in such receptors because octreotide has high affinity for sst2. Normal physiological uptake is seen in the thyroid, spleen, liver, and pituitary due to receptor binding of the peptides, whereas tracer uptake in the kidneys is predominant, secondary to reabsorption of filtered peptides, and bowel uptake is presumably secondary to hepatobiliary clearance. Tumor uptake depends on the overexpression of somatostatin receptors (mainly sst2), and the intensity is related to the density of receptors.[67] Scintigraphy can confirm the known lesions and reveal disease sites not visualized by other imaging techniques. Another major interest of scintigraphy is the prediction of a therapeutic benefit for a possible metabolic radiotherapy (peptide receptor radionuclide therapy, PRRT) using radiolabeled analogs.[68,69] False-positives can occur with a variety of lesions, such as the thyroid gland, accessory spleen, granulomatous or inflammatory tissue, and benign or malignant breast lesions. Other types of neoplasms that demonstrate somatostatin receptor expression include meningiomas and lymphomas. Nonetheless, up until recently, somatostatin receptor scintigraphy was considered the standard in the diagnosis and staging, and occasionally in follow-up of patients with NENs (Figure 8.10); this may have been surpassed by use of more specific tracers using gallium (as discussed below). The recent introduction of single-photon emission computed tomography (SPECT)–CT and positron emission tomography (PET)–CT hybrid systems gives fusion images to correlate anatomical location with function.[70,71] The diagnostic accuracy increased from 65% to 75% for SPECT–scintigraphy, and this increase was further enhanced to 98% for fusion SPECT–CT in a study involving 58 patients with digestive NENs.[72]

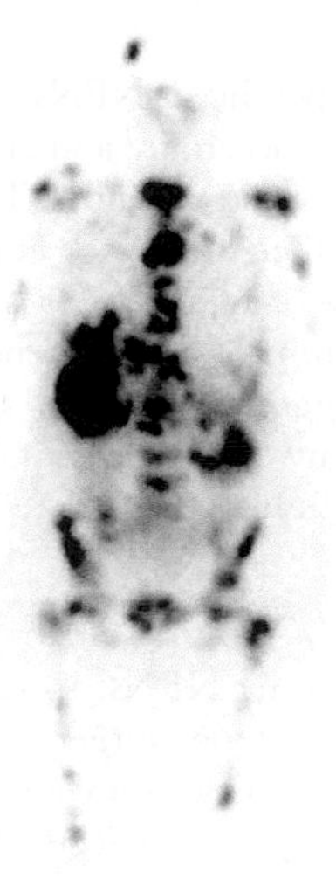

***Figure 8.10***
*Somatostatin receptor scintigraphy of a malignant NEN showing hepatic and multiple bone metastasis.*

It is also possible to perform PET using positron-emitting SSAs (gallium-68-DOTATOC or Ga-68-DOTANOC) with very high affinity for sstl and sst5.[73,74] A large prospective study by Gabriel et al.[75] evaluated the diagnostic value of 68-Ga-DOTATOC PET in 84 patients with known or suspected NENs and demonstrated a sensitivity of 97%, specificity of 92%, and an overall accuracy of 96%, showing significantly higher diagnostic efficacy compared with standard somatostatin/SPECT–CT scintigraphy. In addition, PET-based somatostatin receptor scintigraphy (SRS) detected more tumor sites in the liver, nodes, and bone compared with the other modalities. In several studies, 68-Ga-DOTATOC PET/CT modified treatment strategy 30% compared with management options based on CT and/or MRI alone.[76,77]

The APUD concept describes the ability of neuroendocrine cell types to take up and decarboxylate amino acid precursors. NENs take up monoamine precursors, and thus carbon-11 [$^{11}$C]-labeled and $^{18}$F-labeled monoamine precursors such as serotonin and levodopa can be used.[78,79] In small intestinal NENs, PET labeled with [$^{18}$F]-levodopa performs better than standard scintigraphy[79]; although this type of PET may be limited for nonintestinal NENs. Finally, the use of 18-FDG-PET in NENs is currently controversial; it is certainly positive in very aggressive G3 tumors but tends to be negative or weakly positive in slow-growing, mainly Gl, tumors. There are limited sensitivities overall, but there is emerging evidence that the presence of increased glucose metabolism in tumors, especially G2 NENs, highlights an increased propensity for invasion and metastasis, and overall poorer prognosis.[80] Use of FDG-PET CT may prove useful in selecting patients for therapy.

# Treatment

## General principles (see Figure 1.24)

The oncological principles of management in patients with GEP-NENs depend on many factors and require a multidisciplinary approach. Surgery is the only definitive cure but is rarely possible in patients with metastatic disease, and other approaches are therefore necessary. Antiproliferative treatment decisions depend on several key factors: (1) origin of the primary tumor, (2) histological differentiation, and (3) the tumor's aggressiveness and proliferative capacity or grade. Unlike the case for other solid tumors of the digestive tract, wait-and-see strategies can often be adopted in GEP-NEN patients. Recent data have changed the therapeutic options and the results of biotherapy, traditional chemotherapy, and new targeted agents have opened an exciting volley of therapies in this ever-changing field. Well-coordinated international multicenter trials have afforded the opportunity of pooling resources in a field of rare tumor disease, helping to answer to interesting clinical questions. GEP-NEN is a very heterogeneous group of diseases in terms of origin of the primary tumor, differentiation, disease extent, and functionality. Treatment should therefore be highly individualized.

# Surgery

Surgery is essential in many phases of GEP-NEN management. Surgical resection is the only curative treatment for NENs; nevertheless, most of the cases are detected at an advanced stage. Surgery may be considered in a palliative setting by debulking, to reduce the tumor burden and their related hormonal or obstructive symptoms. It is also recommended that patients undergoing surgery, who will be potentially treated with locoregional therapies and/or SSAs, should undergo cholecystectomy.[81]

## Surgery for specific primary NENs

### Gastric: Type I and type II gastric NENs

Resection is considered in tumors >10 mm, usually with endoscopic resection. In patients with lesions involving the muscularis propria, a wedge resection may be performed. This procedure was formerly associated with antrectomy, to prevent chronic gastrin stimulation.[82]

### Type III gastric NENs

Type III gastric NENs are more aggressive, and the management should be similar to that for gastric adenocarcinomas (partial or total gastrectomy with lymph node dissection).

### Midgut NENs

In localized disease, surgery with curative intent (clearance of all potentially involved lymph nodes) is aimed, to preserve the vascular supply and to limit intestinal resection.[83] Surgery should be considered even if tumors are small, because there is no correlation between size and metastatic potential (vs. pancreatic tumors). In the presence of advanced disease, resection of the jejunal–ileal primary tumor should be considered (even in the absence of symptoms) to prevent intestinal obstruction or ischemic complications, due to the desmoplastic reaction or the primary tumor.[84]

### Duodenopancreatic NENs

In nonfunctioning localized tumors >2 cm, aggressive surgery is recommended due to the risk of metastases when tumors exceed this size.[85] With tumors <2 cm, surgical cure needs to be weighed against the postoperative complications and morbidity. In functioning tumors, resection should always be considered. For gastrinoma, tumors in the pancreatic head area should be enucleated, distal pancreatic resection performed for caudally located tumors, and duodenotomy after transillumination performed routinely to detect small duodenal gastrinomas. In insulinoma, tumor enucleation or limited pancreatic preserving resections are preferred. When the tumor is located in the neck, body, or tail of the pancreas and is anatomically unsuitable for enucleation, central or distal pancreatectomy is safe and effective as an alternative.

### Appendix NENs

The majority of appendiceal NENs are discovered incidentally after appendicectomy and are small (<10 mm), localized to the tip of the appendix. These NENs do not usually require further therapy or follow-up. When the tumor is at the base of appendix, or is >20 mm in diameter, or shows >3 mm of mesoappendiceal invasion, or when histology suggests goblet cell (adenocarcinoid), a right hemicolectomy with locoregional lymphadenectomy is usually indicated.[86]

### Colonic and rectal NENs

Management of colonic NENs, usually highly aggressive tumors, is based on surgery similar to colonic adenocarcinomas with colectomy and oncological resection of lymph drainage.[87] For rectal NENs, smaller T1 lesions are resected using endoscopic methods (either endoscopic mucosal resection or submucosal dissection), but T2 lesions and high Ki-67 are indicators of aggressive behavior that require total mesorectal excision.[88]

### Liver metastasis

Criteria for surgery of hepatic metastasis are (1) resectable well-differentiated liver disease with acceptable morbidity and mortality, (2) absence of right heart insufficiency, (3) absence of extraabdominal metastases, and (4) absence of diffuse peritoneal carcinomatosis.[89] The primary tumor must be resectable (or resected previously).

With unilobar metastases, standard hepatectomy or metastasectomy can be performed. With bilobar metastases, the difficulty is achieving complete resection while maintaining liver function. For that a two-step procedure is needed: the first step corresponds to the resection of the primary tumor and the left liver metastases and ligature of the right branch of the portal vein. The second step is a right hepatectomy 6 weeks later after left liver hypertrophy is obtained.[90] In some cases, total clearance of the liver disease cannot be obtained, and then total hepatectomy followed by liver transplantation may be offered to young patients with very well-differentiated tumors with slow progression and nonresidual extrahepatic disease.

## Medical treatment

### SSAs: Antisecretory effects

Functionally active tumors lead to secretory syndromes that must be rapidly controlled. Any kind of antitumoral treatment (surgery, radiofrequency ablation, transarterial chemoembolization, systemic chemotherapy, targeted therapies, PRRT) may have a potential antisecretory effect by reducing the tumor burden.

SSAs have been shown to be effective in the control of symptoms in functioning pancreatic neuroendocrine neoplasms[91] and this also includes rare functioning tumors[92–94]; in fact, about 80%–90% of patients with VIPoma and glucagonoma improve very promptly, overcoming diarrhea and skin rash, and 60%–80% have a reduction in vasoactive intestinal polypeptide (VIP) and glucagon levels. Symptomatic relief is not always related to reduction in circulating hormone levels, indicating that SSAs have direct effects on the peripheral target organ. Escape from symptomatic control can be seen but an increase in the dose of SSAs can help temporarily. SSAs also effectively reduce hypersecretion-related symptoms in patients with the carcinoid syndrome, namely flushing and diarrhea. The antisecretory effect results in a reduction of biochemical markers in up to 40%–60% and a symptomatic improvement in 40%–80% of patients.[93,95–109] The duration of the effect varies and can be limited due to tachyphylaxis or desensitization, which can be temporarily circumvented by an increase in dose. Tolerance to SSAs and efficacy should be tested individually by initiating therapy with short-acting analogs. Thereafter, depot formulations, usually octreotide long-acting release (LAR) (20, 30 mg) or lanreotide Autogel (60, 90, 120 mg) every 4 weeks can be started and should be individually titrated. In patients with moderate symptoms directly commencing depot preparations by-passing a titration phase is usually possible. The efficacy of lanreotide and octreotide is comparable.[95,100,101] Minor initial side effects include abdominal discomfort, flatulence, and sometimes steatorrhea that usually subside.[97,102,103,110] More than 50% of patients have been reported to develop gallstones; however, virtually all remain asymptomatic.[110] To prevent carcinoid crisis, SSAs should be given intravenously during anesthesia or other interventional procedures. Loperamide and morphine analogs may improve secretory diarrhea. Because diarrhea may have other causes than hormonal (bile acid loss, bacterial overgrowth), other options may be considered, such as cholestyramine and antibiotics.

In addition to SSAs, specific therapy for insulinoma includes diazoxide. It is the first-line drug effective in controlling hypoglycemic symptoms by inhibiting the release of insulin from cells, but with common side effects such as hirsutism and fluid retention, with a need to use thiazidic diuretics. Resistance is common. Everolimus has also been found to normalize plasma glucose levels in metastatic insulinoma.[111]

For patients with gastrinoma and ZES, PPIs are rapidly used because of their ability to block $H^+/K^+$ ATPase proton pump of the parietal cells. Use of omeprazole in ZES was first described in the early 1980s.[112] Patients have been treated for up to 15 years with PPIs with no evidence of tachyphylaxis and no dose-related side effects. The recommended starting dose is equivalent to omeprazole 60 mg per day. Clinical improvement (diarrhea and hyperacidity symptoms) should be obtained quickly. Upper endoscopy should be performed to check the healing of the mucosa. PPI must not be stopped for any reason because of potentially serious complications of rapid hyperacidity with ulcerations and even perforations in some cases.[113]

### Antiproliferative therapy

#### Somatostatin Analogs[114]

Both octreotide and lanreotide are effectively used to control peptide and hormone secretion in patients with functional tumors.[102] Octreotide LAR has also been shown to have antiproliferative effects in patients with slowly progressive small intestinal NENs with limited tumor burden. In patients with a low Ki-67, the PROMID trial demonstrated that monthly injection of octreotide LAR significantly lengthens time to tumor progression compared with placebo in patients with functionally active and inactive metastatic midgut NENs (14.3 vs. 6 months).[115] A second study of another somatostatin analog a broader range of GEP-NEN including pancreatic tumors has also been performed using lanreotide-Autogel (CLARINET trial) and the initial promising results were presented at ESMO 2013.

Recently, analogs that recognize more than one receptor subtype have led to the development of interesting novel agents. Pasireotide is a multireceptor-targeted SSA that has high affinity for four of the five SST receptor subtypes (sst1, -2, -3, and -5) and has therapeutic potential in conditions with tumors of neuroendocrine origin, such as Cushing's disease, acromegaly, and neuroendocrine tumors.[116] Preliminary results showed symptom improvement in 27% of 45 patients with carcinoid syndrome refractory/resistant to octreotide LAR with good tolerance except for episodes of hyperglycemia.[117] The hope is that antiproliferative effects may be mediated via receptor subtypes other than sst2. A recent phase I study of pasireotide in combination with everolimus (a mammalian target of rapamycin [mTOR] inhibitor) demonstrated it to be feasible and associated with preliminary evidence of antitumor activity in patients with advanced neuroendocrine tumors.[118]

Another recent development was use of a possible functional interface of dopamine and somatostatin receptors, when coexpressed in the same cells. Expression of both dopamine receptor, D2R, and somatostatin receptors was recently found in pancreatic and midgut NENs.[119] New experimental drugs developed as hybrid somatostatin–dopamine compounds that have been shown to have interesting activity in experimental and *ex vivo* models in pituitary adenomas[120] have also been tested in both GEP-NENs and patients with pituitary adenomas but formal results are outstanding.

## *Interferon-α*

Interferon-α (IFN-α) exerts an antiproliferation and antisecretory effect on midgut NENs. The standard dose is 3–5 million units subcutaneously, three to five times a week. Symptomatic and biochemical responses have been noted in 50% of patients, with disease stabilization in 60%–80%[121] in phase II studies, with their inherent difficulties to adequately interpret the data. Side effects (flu-like symptoms, bone marrow suppression, thyroid disorders, psychiatric phenomenon, and chronic fatigue syndrome) are common. Side effects of interferon therapy are more pronounced than with SSAs. Therefore, it may be considered as second-line therapy.

## *Systemic cytotoxic chemotherapy*

1. Poorly differentiated NEC (regardless of the primary). Standard regimen is based on etoposide/cisplatin (etoposide 100 mg/m$^2$/day on days 1–3 plus cisplatin 100 mg/m$^2$ on day 1).[122] This results in an overall tumor response rate of 42% with a median overall survival of 15 months, a median progression-free survival (PFS) of 9 months, and a 2-year survival of <20%. Second-line regimen is not consensual, and phase II trials are required.
2. Well-differentiated duodenopancreatic tumor. Standard chemotherapy regimens in well and moderately differentiated pancreatic NENs are streptozotocin/doxorubicin and streptozotocin/5-fluorouracil. With streptozotocin-based regimens, partial response rates of 45%–65% have been reported.[123] An alternative established chemotherapy regimen is dacarbazine with partial response rate of 35% in first-line chemotherapy of pancreatic NEN.[124] Promising data on capecitabine (750 mg/m$^2$ twice a day, days 1–14) and temozolomide (200 mg/m$^2$ once a day at bedtime, days 10–14) every 28 days have been reported[124] with 70% partial response and 27% stable disease, a median PFS of 18 months, and an estimated overall survival of 92% at 2 years. The DNA repair enzyme 0-6-methylguanine DNA methyltransferase (MGMT) is thought to contribute to the resistance of tumor cells against temozolomide.[125] In an immunohistochemical analysis of 97 NENs, 51% of pancreatic NENs, but 0% of small intestine carcinoid tumors, showed MGMT deficiency.[126] This might explain the sensitivity of pancreatic NENs but not of small intestine NENs to temozolomide.
3. Well-differentiated midgut and hindgut tumor. Well-differentiated midgut and hindgut tumors are considered rather insensitive to conventional cytotoxic chemotherapeutics, and as such they have not been recommended by expert groups.[87]

## *Targeted therapies*

1. *Sunitinib*

Sunitinib malate is a small-molecule kinase inhibitor with activity against several tyrosine kinase receptors. In a phase III trial, sunitinib at 37.5 mg/day compared with placebo has shown a significantly prolonged PFS in patients with progressive pancreatic NENs (11.4 vs. 5.5 months).[127] Specific toxicities include fatigue, hair color changes, hypertension, and palmar-plantar erythrodysesthesia.

2. *Everolimus*

Everolimus, an mTor inhibitor, at 10 mg/day compared with placebo significantly prolonged PFS in a phase III among patients with progressive pancreatic NENs (11 vs. 4.6 months).[128] In another recent phase III trial, patients with nonpancreatic NENs associated with carcinoid syndrome (mainly small intestinal tumors), everolimus plus octreotide-LAR compared with placebo plus octreotide-LAR, had improved PFS (16.4 vs. 11.3 months).[129] Specific toxicities include stomatitis, rash, diarrhea, hyperglycemia, and pneumonitis (with possible severe outcome).

# Locoregional treatments

## Radiofrequency ablation

When surgery for liver metastasis is not possible, radiofrequency ablation (RFA) may be considered in the event of a small number of lesions (<5) with a size <5 cm.[130] This therapy may be combined with surgery for lesions that are not easily accessible for surgical resection.

## Transarterial chemoembolization or bland embolization

Transarterial chemoembolization (TACE) is based on the administration of cytotoxic agent (streptozotocin or doxorubicin) directly in the hepatic artery followed by a transient embolization, inducing ischemia in the metastases. TACE may be discussed for patients with inoperable liver metastasis. Tumor response is seen in >50%, a biochemical response of 50%–90%, and symptomatic response with a control of functional syndromes in 60%–95% of cases.[131] Contraindications to TACE are portal venous thrombosis, hepatic insufficiency, or a biliary-digestive anastomosis. A common side effect of TACE is a postembolization syndrome with abdominal pain, nausea, vomiting, fever, and an increase in hepatic transaminases. Severe but rare complications are liver failure, cholecystitis, gastric ulcers, liver abscess, and carcinoid crisis. TACE or bland embolization has recently been demonstrated to yield similar results in a randomized phase II trial[132] and either can be performed in a single session in case of low hepatic burden. In case of a large tumor burden, to limit adverse events, two sessions (4–8 weeks between) should be performed.

## Radioembolization

Radioembolization is based on the administration of yttrium-90 microspheres as a selective internal radiotherapy (SIRT) through hepatic transarterial approach. Tumor response is seen in >50%.[133] Specific complications can occur such as radiation-induced liver disease, hepatic abscess, arterial shunting to the lung, radiation microsphere–induced gastric ulceration and bleeding, acute cholecystitis, or acute pancreatitis.

# Peptide receptor radionuclide therapy (see Chapter 7)

PRRT is currently based on radiolabeled SSAs with high affinity to the sst2, being expressed by 80%–95% of all well-differentiated NENs. The most frequently used radiopharmaceuticals for PRRT are 90-Yttrium-DOTA-Tyr3-octreotide (90-Y-DOTA-TOC), 90-Yttrium-DOTA-Tyr3-octreotate (90Y-DOTA-TATE), and 177-Lutetium-DOTA-Tyr3-octreotate (177-Lu-DOTA-TATE). Adequate tumor uptake in [$^{111}$In-DTPA-D-Phe1]-octreotide scintigraphy is essential when considering PRRT as a therapeutic option. PRRT with 177-Lu-DOTA-TATE has shown excellent results in patients with multisite metastases in a phase II trial, yielding a complete response in 2%, a partial response in 28%, a minor response in 16%, stable disease in 35%, and progressive disease in 20%.[134] The median PFS was 33 months, and the median overall survival from the start of PRRT was 46 months. Nonetheless, this therapy requires prospective comparison with other therapies.

# Conclusions

GEP-NEN represents a mixed group of interesting tumors that involves a vast array of medical and surgical specialists. Their numbers are growing—perhaps in part due to better recognition—but their quite high prevalence ensures the need for dedicated multidisciplinary groups to streamline management of these patients. The field of NEN is rapidly changing from epidemiological and histopathological classifications perspectives; many national and international societies and groups have linked well together to pool patient resources and provide expert opinion and guidelines. Nonetheless, even better and clearer nomenclature will need to be developed to ensure clearer and rapid data capture.

The field of diagnostics has been improved with advances in axial imaging techniques such as CT and MRI but also contrast-enhanced techniques such as endosonography. Radionuclides that are more sensitive and specific for GEP-NENs are also providing better detection rates and allowing for important modifications in therapeutic algorithms. Surgical strategies have become clearer, and pancreatic-sparing procedures have been better defined in high-volume centers to allow for limited resections in certain individuals. Long-acting SSAs, crucial to control symptoms in patients with hormonally active syndromes, have also been shown to have an antiproliferative capacity in some (namely, midgut NENs). Finally, the active pharmacopoeia for systemic agents (better cytotoxics, small targeted molecules and combination therapy) for use in advanced nonoperable cases of GEP-NENs is expanding at a steady pace; this pace has been fuelled by large multicenter trials. Further improvements are required with dedicated strategy-driven protocols; many interesting combinations need to be examined. As with other areas in modern oncology, identification of novel and specific molecular targets capable of predicting therapeutic responses will help streamline and tailor therapies in this field.

## References


*1. Yao JC, Hassan M, Phan A, Dagohoy C, Leary C, Mares JE, et al. One hundred years after "carcinoid": Epidemiology of and prognostic factors for neuroendocrine tumors in 35,825 cases in the United States. *J Clin Oncol*. 2008;26(18):3063–72.
2. Hauso O, Gustafsson BI, Kidd M, Waldum HL, Drozdov I, Chan AK, et al. Neuroendocrine tumor epidemiology: Contrasting Norway and North America. *Cancer*. 2008 15;113(10):2655–64.
3. Lloyd RV. Practical markers used in the diagnosis of neuroendocrine tumors. *Endocr Pathol*. 2003;14(4):293–301.
4. Bussolati G, Volante M, Papotti M. Classic and recent special stains used in differential diagnosis of endocrine tumors. *Endocr Pathol*. 2001;12(4):379–87.
5. Bosman FT, World Health Organization, International Agency for Research on Cancer. *WHO classification of tumours of the digestive system*. 4th ed. Lyon: International Agency for Research on Cancer; 2010.
6. Scarpa A, Mantovani W, Capelli P, Beghelli S, Boninsegna L, Bettini R, et al. Pancreatic endocrine tumors: Improved TNM staging and histopathological grading permit a clinically efficient prognostic stratification of patients. *Mod Pathol*. 2010;23(6):824–33.
7. Jann H, Roll S, Couvelard A, Hentic O, Pavel M, Muller-Nordhorn J, et al. Neuroendocrine tumors of midgut and hindgut origin: Tumor-node-metastasis classification determines clinical outcome. *Cancer*. 2011;117(15):3332–41.
8. La Rosa S, Inzani F, Vanoli A, Klersy C, Dainese L, Rindi G, et al. Histologic characterization and improved prognostic evaluation of 209 gastric neuroendocrine neoplasms. *Hum Pathol*. 2011;42(10):1373–84.
*9. Rindi G, Kloppel G, Alhman H, Caplin M, Couvelard A, de Herder WW, et al. TNM staging of foregut (neuro) endocrine tumors: A consensus proposal including a grading system. *Virchows Arch*. 2006;449(4):395–401.
*10. Rindi G, Kloppel G, Couvelard A, Komminoth P, Korner M, Lopes JM, et al. TNM staging of midgut and hindgut (neuro) endocrine tumors: A consensus proposal including a grading system. *Virchows Arch*. 2007;451(4):757–62.
*11. Edge SB, Compton CC. The American Joint Committee on Cancer: The 7th edition of the AJCC cancer staging manual and the future of TNM. *Ann Surg Oncol*. 2010;17(6):1471–4.
12. Kaltsas GA, Besser GM, Grossman AB. The diagnosis and medical management of advanced neuroendocrine tumors. *Endocr Rev*. 2004;25(3):458–511.
13. Cheema A, Weber J, Strosberg JR. Incidental detection of pancreatic neuroendocrine tumors: An analysis of incidence and outcomes. *Ann Surg Oncol*. 2012; 19(9):2932–6.
14. Oberg K, Eriksson B. Endocrine tumours of the pancreas. *Best Pract Res Clin Gastroenterol*. 2005; 19(5):753–81.
15. Modlin IM, Kidd M, Latich I, Zikusoka MN, Shapiro MD. Current status of gastrointestinal carcinoids. *Gastroenterology*. 2005;128(6):1717–51.
16. Marx S, Spiegel AM, Skarulis MC, Doppman JL, Collins FS, Liotta LA. Multiple endocrine neoplasia type 1: Clinical and genetic topics. *Ann Intern Med*. 1998;129(6):484–94.
17. Lemmens I, Van de Ven WJ, Kas K, Zhang CX, Giraud S, Wautot V, et al. Identification of the multiple endocrine neoplasia type 1 (MEN1) gene. The European Consortium on MEN1. *Hum Mol Genet*. 1997;6(7):1177–83.
18. Jensen RT, Niederle B, Mitry E, Ramage JK, Steinmuller T, Lewington V, et al. Gastrinoma (duodenal and pancreatic). *Neuroendocrinology*. 2006;84(3): 173–82.
19. Couch V, Lindor NM, Karnes PS, Michels VV. von Hippel-Lindau disease. *Mayo Clin Proc*. 2000;75(3): 265–72.
20. Latif F, Tory K, Gnarra J, Yao M, Duh FM, Orcutt ML, et al. Identification of the von Hippel-Lindau disease tumor suppressor gene. *Science*. 1993;260(5112): 1317–20.
21. Hammel PR, Vilgrain V, Terris B, Penfornis A, Sauvanet A, Correas JM, et al. Pancreatic involvement in von Hippel-Lindau disease. The Groupe Francophone d'Etude de la Maladie de von Hippel-Lindau. *Gastroenterology*. 2000;119(4):1087–95.
22. Mayoral W, Salcedo J, Al-Kawas F. Ampullary carcinoid tumor presenting as acute pancreatitis in a patient with von Recklinghausen's disease: Case report and review of the literature. *Endoscopy*. 2003;35(10):854–7.
23. Deftos LJ. Chromogranin A: Its role in endocrine function and as an endocrine and neuroendocrine tumor marker. *Endocr Rev*. 1991;12(2):181–7.
*24. O'Toole D, Grossman A, Gross D, Delle Fave G, Barkmanova J, O'Connor J, et al. ENETS Consensus Guidelines for the Standards of Care in Neuroendocrine Tumors: Biochemical markers. *Neuroendocrinology*. 2009;90(2):194–202.


* Key or Classic references.

25. Sanduleanu S, De Bruine A, Stridsberg M, Jonkers D, Biemond I, Hameeteman W, et al. Serum chromogranin A as a screening test for gastric enterochromaffin-like cell hyperplasia during acid-suppressive therapy. *Eur J Clin Invest*. 2001;31(9):802–11.
26. Nobels FR, Kwekkeboom DJ, Coopmans W, Schoenmakers CH, Lindemans J, De Herder WW, et al. Chromogranin A as serum marker for neuroendocrine neoplasia: Comparison with neuron-specific enolase and the alpha-subunit of glycoprotein hormones. *J Clin Endocrinol Metab*. 1997;82(8):2622–8.
27. Hsiao RJ, Mezger MS, O'Connor DT. Chromogranin A in uremia: Progressive retention of immunoreactive fragments. *Kidney Int*. 1990;37(3):955–64.
28. Rozansky DJ, Wu H, Tang K, Parmer RJ, O'Connor DT. Glucocorticoid activation of chromogranin A gene expression. Identification and characterization of a novel glucocorticoid response element. *J Clin Invest*. 1994;94(6):2357–68.
29. O'Toole D. Current trend: Endocrine tumors of the stomach, small bowel, colon and rectum. *Gastroenterol Clin Biol*. 2006;30(2):276–91.
30. D'Adda T, Corleto V, Pilato FP, Baggi MT, Robutti F, Delle Fave G, et al. Quantitative ultrastructure of endocrine cells of oxyntic mucosa in Zollinger-Ellison syndrome. Correspondence with light microscopic findings. *Gastroenterology*. 1990;99(1):17–26.
31. Baudin E, Gigliotti A, Ducreux M, Ropers J, Comoy E, Sabourin JC, et al. Neuron-specific enolase and chromogranin A as markers of neuroendocrine tumours. *Br J Cancer*. 1998;78(8):1102–7.
32. Meijer WG, Kema IP, Volmer M, Willemse PH, de Vries EG. Discriminating capacity of indole markers in the diagnosis of carcinoid tumors. *Clin Chem*. 2000;46(10):1588–96.
33. Feldman JM. Urinary serotonin in the diagnosis of carcinoid tumors. *Clin Chem*. 1986;32(5):840–4.
34. Mashige F, Matsushima Y, Kanazawa H, Sakuma I, Takai N, Bessho F, et al. Acidic catecholamine metabolites and 5-hydroxyindoleacetic acid in urine: The influence of diet. *Ann Clin Biochem*. 1996;33(Pt 1):43–9.
35. Service FJ. Hypoglycemic disorders. *N Engl J Med*. 1995;332(17):1144–52.
36. de Herder WW, Niederle B, Scoazec JY, Pauwels S, Kloppel G, Falconi M, et al. Well-differentiated pancreatic tumor/carcinoma: Insulinoma. *Neuroendocrinology*. 2006;84(3):183–8.
37. Grant CS. Insulinoma. *Best Pract Res Clin Gastroenterol*. 2005;19(5):783–98.
38. Berna MJ, Hoffmann KM, Long SH, Serrano J, Gibril F, Jensen RT. Serum gastrin in Zollinger-Ellison syndrome: II. Prospective study of gastrin provocative testing in 293 patients from the National Institutes of Health and comparison with 537 cases from the literature. evaluation of diagnostic criteria, proposal of new criteria, and correlations with clinical and tumoral features. *Medicine (Baltimore)*. 2006;85(6):331–64.
39. Sundin A, Vullierme MP, Kaltsas G, Plockinger U. ENETS Consensus Guidelines for the Standards of Care in Neuroendocrine Tumors: Radiological examinations. *Neuroendocrinology*. 2009;90(2):167–83.
40. Khashab MA, Yong E, Lennon AM, Shin EJ, Amateau S, Hruban RH, et al. EUS is still superior to multidetector computerized tomography for detection of pancreatic neuroendocrine tumors. *Gastrointest Endosc*. 2011;73(4):691–6.
41. Cadiot G, Lebtahi R, Sarda L, Bonnaud G, Marmuse JP, Vissuzaine C, et al. Preoperative detection of duodenal gastrinomas and peripancreatic lymph nodes by somatostatin receptor scintigraphy. Groupe D'etude Du Syndrome De Zollinger-Ellison. *Gastroenterology*. 1996;111(4):845–54.
42. Ishikawa T, Itoh A, Kawashima H, Ohno E, Matsubara H, Itoh Y, et al. Usefulness of EUS combined with contrast-enhancement in the differential diagnosis of malignant versus benign and preoperative localization of pancreatic endocrine tumors. *Gastrointest Endosc*. 2010;71(6):951–9.
43. Figueiredo FA, Giovannini M, Monges G, Bories E, Pesenti C, Caillol F, et al. EUS-FNA predicts 5-year survival in pancreatic endocrine tumors. *Gastrointest Endosc*. 2009;70(5):907–14.
44. Rindi G, Bordi C, Rappel S, La Rosa S, Stolte M, Solcia E. Gastric carcinoids and neuroendocrine carcinomas: Pathogenesis, pathology, and behavior. *World J Surg*. 1996;20(2):168–72.
45. Lehy T, Cadiot G, Mignon M, Ruszniewski P, Bonfils S. Influence of multiple endocrine neoplasia type 1 on gastric endocrine cells in patients with the Zollinger-Ellison syndrome. *Gut*. 1992;33(9):1275–9.
46. Burke AP, Federspiel BH, Sobin LH, Shekitka KM, Helwig EB. Carcinoids of the duodenum. A histologic and immunohistochemical study of 65 tumors. *Am J Surg Pathol*. 1989;13(10):828–37.
47. Maggard MA, O'Connell JB, Ko CY. Updated population-based review of carcinoid tumors. *Ann Surg*. 2004;240(1):117–22.
48. Jetmore AB, Ray JE, Gathright JB, Jr., McMullen KM, Hicks TC, Timmcke AE. Rectal carcinoids: The most frequent carcinoid tumor. *Dis Colon Rectum*. 1992;35(8):717–25.
49. Stark DD, Moss AA, Goldberg HI, Deveney CW. CT of pancreatic islet cell tumors. *Radiology*. 1984;150(2):491–4.
50. Rossi P, Baert A, Passariello R, Simonetti G, Pavone P, Tempesta P. CT of functioning tumors of the pancreas. *AJR Am J Roentgenol*. 1985;144(1):57–60.
51. Van Hoe L, Gryspeerdt S, Marchal G, Baert AL, Mertens L. Helical CT for the preoperative localization

of islet cell tumors of the pancreas: Value of arterial and parenchymal phase images. *AJR Am J Roentgenol.* 1995;165(6):1437–9.

52. Procacci C, Carbognin G, Accordini S, Biasiutti C, Bicego E, Romano L, et al. Nonfunctioning endocrine tumors of the pancreas: Possibilities of spiral CT characterization. *Eur Radiol.* 2001;11(7):1175–83.
53. Fidler JL, Fletcher JG, Reading CC, Andrews JC, Thompson GB, Grant CS, et al. Preoperative detection of pancreatic insulinomas on multiphasic helical CT. *AJR Am J Roentgenol.* 2003;181(3):775–80.
54. Chiti A, Fanti S, Savelli G, Romeo A, Bellanova B, Rodari M, et al. Comparison of somatostatin receptor imaging, computed tomography and ultrasound in the clinical management of neuroendocrine gastro-entero-pancreatic tumours. *Eur J Nucl Med.* 1998;25(10):1396–403.
55. Kumbasar B, Kamel IR, Tekes A, Eng J, Fishman EK, Wahl RL. Imaging of neuroendocrine tumors: Accuracy of helical CT versus SRS. *Abdom Imaging.* 2004;29(6):696–702.
56. Hubalewska-Dydejczyk A, Fross-Baron K, Mikolajczak R, Maecke HR, Huszno B, Pach D, et al. 99mTc-EDDA/HYNIC-octreotate scintigraphy, an efficient method for the detection and staging of carcinoid tumours: Results of 3 years' experience. *Eur J Nucl Med Mol Imaging.* 2006;33(10):1123–33.
57. Cwikla JB, Buscombe JR, Caplin ME, Watkinson AF, Walecki J, Gorczyca-Wisniewska E, et al. Diagnostic imaging of carcinoid metastases to the abdomen and pelvis. *Med Sci Monit.* 2004;10(Suppl 3):9–16.
58. Kamaoui I, De-Luca V, Ficarelli S, Mennesson N, Lombard-Bohas C, Pilleul F. Value of CT enteroclysis in suspected small-bowel carcinoid tumors. *AJR Am J Roentgenol.* 2010;194(3):629–33.
59. Ichikawa T, Peterson MS, Federle MP, Baron RL, Haradome H, Kawamori Y, et al. Islet cell tumor of the pancreas: Biphasic CT versus MR imaging in tumor detection. *Radiology.* 2000;216(1):163–71.
60. Shi W, Johnston CF, Buchanan KD, Ferguson WR, Laird JD, Crothers JG, et al. Localization of neuroendocrine tumours with [111In] DTPA-octreotide scintigraphy (Octreoscan): A comparative study with CT and MR imaging. *QJM.* 1998;91(4):295–301.
61. Termanini B, Gibril F, Reynolds JC, Doppman JL, Chen CC, Stewart CA, et al. Value of somatostatin receptor scintigraphy: A prospective study in gastrinoma of its effect on clinical management. *Gastroenterology.* 1997;112(2):335–47.
62. Carlson B, Johnson CD, Stephens DH, Ward EM, Kvols LK. MRI of pancreatic islet cell carcinoma. *J Comput Assist Tomogr.* 1993;17(5):735–40.
63. Owen NJ, Sohaib SA, Peppercorn PD, Monson JP, Grossman AB, Besser GM, et al. MRI of pancreatic neuroendocrine tumours. *Br J Radiol.* 2001;74(886):968–73.
64. Dromain C, de Baere T, Lumbroso J, Caillet H, Laplanche A, Boige V, et al. Detection of liver metastases from endocrine tumors: A prospective comparison of somatostatin receptor scintigraphy, computed tomography, and magnetic resonance imaging. *J Clin Oncol.* 2005;23(1):70–8.
65. Reubi JC, Kvols L, Krenning E, Lamberts SW. Distribution of somatostatin receptors in normal and tumor tissue. *Metabolism.* 1990;39(9 Suppl 2):78–81.
66. Yamada Y, Kagimoto S, Kubota A, Yasuda K, Masuda K, Someya Y, et al. Cloning, functional expression and pharmacological characterization of a fourth (hSSTR4) and a fifth (hSSTR5) human somatostatin receptor subtype. *Biochem Biophys Res Commun.* 1993;195(2):844–52.
67. Hofland LJ, Lamberts SW, van Hagen PM, Reubi JC, Schaeffer J, Waaijers M, et al. Crucial role for somatostatin receptor subtype 2 in determining the uptake of [111In-DTPA-D-Phe1]octreotide in somatostatin receptor-positive organs. *J Nucl Med.* 2003;44(8):1315–21.
68. Krenning EP, Valkema R, Kwekkeboom DJ, de Herder WW, van Eijck CH, de Jong M, et al. Molecular imaging as in vivo molecular pathology for gastroenteropancreatic neuroendocrine tumors: Implications for follow-up after therapy. *J Nucl Med.* 2005;46(Suppl 1):76S–82S.
*69. Kwekkeboom DJ, Teunissen JJ, Bakker WH, Kooij PP, de Herder WW, Feelders RA, et al. Radiolabeled somatostatin analog [177Lu-DOTA0,Tyr3]octreotate in patients with endocrine gastroenteropancreatic tumors. *J Clin Oncol.* 2005;23(12):2754–62.
70. Amthauer H, Ruf J, Bohmig M, Lopez-Hanninen E, Rohlfing T, Wernecke KD, et al. Diagnosis of neuroendocrine tumours by retrospective image fusion: Is there a benefit? *Eur J Nucl Med Mol Imaging.* 2004;31(3):342–8.
71. Moreira AP, Duarte LH, Vieira F, Joao F, Lima JP. Value of SPET/CT image fusion in the assessment of neuroendocrine tumours with 111In-pentetreotide scintigraphy. *Rev Esp Med Nucl.* 2005;24(1):14–18.
72. Gabriel M, Hausler F, Bale R, Moncayo R, Decristoforo C, Kovacs P, et al. Image fusion analysis of (99m) Tc-HYNIC-Tyr(3)-octreotide SPECT and diagnostic CT using an immobilisation device with external markers in patients with endocrine tumours. *Eur J Nucl Med Mol Imaging.* 2005;32(12):1440–51.
73. Hofmann M, Maecke H, Borner R, Weckesser E, Schoffski P, Oei L, et al. Biokinetics and imaging with the somatostatin receptor PET radioligand (68) Ga-DOTATOC: Preliminary data. *Eur J Nucl Med.* 2001;28(12):1751–7.
74. Wild D, Macke HR, Waser B, Reubi JC, Ginj M, Rasch H, et al. 68Ga-DOTANOC: A first compound

for PET imaging with high affinity for somatostatin receptor subtypes 2 and 5. *Eur J Nucl Med Mol Imaging*. 2005;32(6):724.

*75. Gabriel M, Decristoforo C, Kendler D, Dobrozemsky G, Heute D, Uprimny C, et al. 68Ga-DOTA-Tyr3-octreotide PET in neuroendocrine tumors: Comparison with somatostatin receptor scintigraphy and CT. *J Nucl Med*. 2007;48(4):508–18.

76. Frilling A, Sotiropoulos GC, Radtke A, Malago M, Bockisch A, Kuehl H, et al. The impact of 68Ga-DOTATOC positron emission tomography/computed tomography on the multimodal management of patients with neuroendocrine tumors. *Ann Surg*. 2010;252(5):850–6.

77. Ruf J, Heuck F, Schiefer J, Denecke T, Elgeti F, Pascher A, et al. Impact of multiphase 68Ga-DOTATOC-PET/CT on therapy management in patients with neuroendocrine tumors. *Neuroendocrinology*. 2010; 91(1):101–9.

78. Koopmans KP, de Vries EG, Kema IP, Elsinga PH, Neels OC, Sluiter WJ, et al. Staging of carcinoid tumours with 18F-DOPA PET: A prospective, diagnostic accuracy study. *Lancet Oncol*. 2006;7(9):728–34.

79. Montravers F, Grahek D, Kerrou K, Ruszniewski P, de Beco V, Aide N, et al. Can fluorodihydroxyphenylalanine PET replace somatostatin receptor scintigraphy in patients with digestive endocrine tumors? *J Nucl Med*. 2006;47(9):1455–62.

80. Garin E, Le Jeune F, Devillers A, Cuggia M, de Lajarte-Thirouard AS, Bouriel C, et al. Predictive value of 18F-FDG PET and somatostatin receptor scintigraphy in patients with metastatic endocrine tumors. *J Nucl Med*. 2009;50(6):858–64.

81. Norlen O, Hessman O, Stalberg P, Akerstrom G, Hellman P. Prophylactic cholecystectomy in midgut carcinoid patients. *World J Surg*. 2010;34(6):1361–7.

82. Ahlman H. Surgical treatment of carcinoid tumours of the stomach and small intestine. *Ital J Gastroenterol Hepatol*. 1999;31(Suppl 2):S198–201.

83. Ahlman H, Wangberg B, Jansson S, Friman S, Olausson M, Tylen U, et al. Interventional treatment of gastrointestinal neuroendocrine tumours. *Digestion*. 2000;62(Suppl 1):59–68.

84. Eriksson B, Kloppel G, Krenning E, Ahlman H, Plockinger U, Wiedenmann B, et al. Consensus guidelines for the management of patients with digestive neuroendocrine tumors — well-differentiated jejunal-ileal tumor/carcinoma. *Neuroendocrinology*. 2008;87(1):8–19.

85. Norton JA, Kivlen M, Li M, Schneider D, Chuter T, Jensen RT. Morbidity and mortality of aggressive resection in patients with advanced neuroendocrine tumors. *Arch Surg*. 2003;138(8):859–66.

86. Makridis C, Oberg K, Juhlin C, Rastad J, Johansson H, Lorelius LE, et al. Surgical treatment of mid-gut carcinoid tumors. *World J Surg*. 1990;14(3):377–83; discussion 84–5.

87. Ramage JK, Goretzki PE, Manfredi R, Komminoth P, Ferone D, Hyrdel R, et al. Consensus guidelines for the management of patients with digestive neuroendocrine tumours: Well-differentiated colon and rectum tumour/carcinoma. *Neuroendocrinology*. 2008;87(1):31–9.

88. Ramage JK, Davies AH, Ardill J, Bax N, Caplin M, Grossman A, et al. Guidelines for the management of gastroenteropancreatic neuroendocrine (including carcinoid) tumours. *Gut*. 2005;54(Suppl 4):iv1–16.

*89. Steinmuller T, Kianmanesh R, Falconi M, Scarpa A, Taal B, Kwekkeboom DJ, et al. Consensus guidelines for the management of patients with liver metastases from digestive (neuro)endocrine tumors: Foregut, midgut, hindgut, and unknown primary. *Neuroendocrinology*. 2008;87(1):47–62.

90. Kianmanesh R, Sauvanet A, Hentic O, Couvelard A, Levy P, Vilgrain V, et al. Two-step surgery for synchronous bilobar liver metastases from digestive endocrine tumors: A safe approach for radical resection. *Ann Surg*. 2008;247(4):659–65.

91. Plockinger U, Rindi G, Arnold R, Eriksson B, Krenning EP, de Herder WW, et al. Guidelines for the diagnosis and treatment of neuroendocrine gastrointestinal tumours. A consensus statement on behalf of the European Neuroendocrine Tumour Society (ENETS). *Neuroendocrinology*. 2004;80(6):394–424.

92. Gorden P, Comi RJ, Maton PN, Go VL. NIH conference. Somatostatin and somatostatin analogue (SMS 201-995) in treatment of hormone-secreting tumors of the pituitary and gastrointestinal tract and non-neoplastic diseases of the gut. *Ann Intern Med*. 1989;110(1):35–50.

93. Tomassetti P, Migliori M, Corinaldesi R, Gullo L. Treatment of gastroenteropancreatic neuroendocrine tumours with octreotide LAR. *Aliment Pharmacol Ther*. 2000;14(5):557–60.

94. Nikou GC, Toubanakis C, Nikolaou P, Giannatou E, Safioleas M, Mallas E, et al. VIPomas: An update in diagnosis and management in a series of 11 patients. *Hepatogastroenterology*. 2005;52(64):1259–65.

95. Faiss S, Pape UF, Bohmig M, Dorffel Y, Mansmann U, Golder W, et al. Prospective, randomized, multicenter trial on the antiproliferative effect of lanreotide, interferon alfa, and their combination for therapy of metastatic neuroendocrine gastroenteropancreatic tumors—the International Lanreotide and Interferon Alfa Study Group. *J Clin Oncol*. 2003;21(14):2689–96.

96. Eriksson B, Oberg K. Summing up 15 years of somatostatin analog therapy in neuroendocrine tumors: Future outlook. *Ann Oncol*. 1999;10(Suppl 2):S31–8.

97. Wymenga AN, Eriksson B, Salmela PI, Jacobsen MB, Van Cutsem EJ, Fiasse RH, et al. Efficacy and safety of prolonged-release lanreotide in patients with

gastrointestinal neuroendocrine tumors and hormone-related symptoms. *J Clin Oncol*. 1999;17(4):1111.
98. Ducreux M, Ruszniewski P, Chayvialle JA, Blumberg J, Cloarec D, Michel H, et al. The antitumoral effect of the long-acting somatostatin analog lanreotide in neuroendocrine tumors. *Am J Gastroenterol*. 2000;95(11):3276–81.
99. di Bartolomeo M, Bajetta E, Buzzoni R, Mariani L, Carnaghi C, Somma L, et al. Clinical efficacy of octreotide in the treatment of metastatic neuroendocrine tumors. A study by the Italian Trials in Medical Oncology Group. *Cancer*. 1996;77(2):402–8.
100. Arnold R, Trautmann ME, Creutzfeldt W, Benning R, Benning M, Neuhaus C, et al. Somatostatin analogue octreotide and inhibition of tumour growth in metastatic endocrine gastroenteropancreatic tumours. *Gut*. 1996;38(3):430–8.
101. Aparicio T, Ducreux M, Baudin E, Sabourin JC, De Baere T, Mitry E, et al. Antitumour activity of somatostatin analogues in progressive metastatic neuroendocrine tumours. *Eur J Cancer*. 2001;37(8):1014–19.
102. O'Toole D, Ducreux M, Bommelaer G, Wemeau JL, Bouche O, Catus F, et al. Treatment of carcinoid syndrome: A prospective crossover evaluation of lanreotide versus octreotide in terms of efficacy, patient acceptability, and tolerance. *Cancer*. 2000;88(4):770–6.
103. Ruszniewski P, Ducreux M, Chayvialle JA, Blumberg J, Cloarec D, Michel H, et al. Treatment of the carcinoid syndrome with the long acting somatostatin analogue lanreotide: A prospective study in 39 patients. *Gut*. 1996;39(2):279–83.
104. Tomassetti P, Migliori M, Gullo L. Slow-release lanreotide treatment in endocrine gastrointestinal tumors. *Am J Gastroenterol*. 1998;93(9):1468–71.
*105. Rubin J, Ajani J, Schirmer W, Venook AP, Bukowski R, Pommier R, et al. Octreotide acetate long-acting formulation versus open-label subcutaneous octreotide acetate in malignant carcinoid syndrome. *J Clin Oncol*. 1999;17(2):600–6.
106. Ricci S, Antonuzzo A, Galli L, Ferdeghini M, Bodei L, Orlandini C, et al. Octreotide acetate long-acting release in patients with metastatic neuroendocrine tumors pretreated with lanreotide. *Ann Oncol*. 2000;11(9):1127–30.
107. Ruszniewski P, Ish-Shalom S, Wymenga M, O'Toole D, Arnold R, Tomassetti P, et al. Rapid and sustained relief from the symptoms of carcinoid syndrome: Results from an open 6-month study of the 28-day prolonged-release formulation of lanreotide. *Neuroendocrinology*. 2004;80(4):244–51.
108. Khan MS, El-Khouly F, Davies P, Toumpanakis C, Caplin ME. Long-term results of treatment of malignant carcinoid syndrome with prolonged release Lanreotide (Somatuline Autogel). *Aliment Pharmacol Ther*. 2011;34(2):235–42.
109. Bajetta E, Procopio G, Catena L, Martinetti A, De Dosso S, Ricci S, et al. Lanreotide autogel every 6 weeks compared with Lanreotide microparticles every 3 weeks in patients with well differentiated neuroendocrine tumors: A Phase III Study. *Cancer*. 2006;107(10):2474–81.
110. Plockinger U, Dienemann D, Quabbe HJ. Gastrointestinal side-effects of octreotide during long-term treatment of acromegaly. *J Clin Endocrinol Metab*. 1990;71(6):1658–62.
111. Kulke MH, Bergsland EK, Yao JC. Glycemic control in patients with insulinoma treated with everolimus. *N Engl J Med*. 2009;360(2):195–7.
112. Blanchi A, Delchier JC, Soule JC, Payen D, Bader JP. Control of acute Zollinger-Ellison syndrome with intravenous omeprazole. *Lancet*. 1982;2(8309):1223–4.
113. Poitras P, Gingras MH, Rehfeld JF. The Zollinger-Ellison syndrome: Dangers and consequences of interrupting antisecretory treatment. *Clin Gastroenterol Hepatol*. 2012;10(2):199–202.
*114. IPSEN. Study of Lanreotide Autogel in Non-functioning Entero-pancreatic Endocrine Tumours (CLARINET), NCT00353496. Available from: http://clinicaltrials.gov/ct2/show/NCT00353496
*115. Rinke A, Muller HH, Schade-Brittinger C, Klose KJ, Barth P, Wied M, et al. Placebo-controlled, double-blind, prospective, randomized study on the effect of octreotide LAR in the control of tumor growth in patients with metastatic neuroendocrine midgut tumors: A report from the PROMID Study Group. *J Clin Oncol*. 2009;27(28):4656–63.
116. Fleseriu M, Petersenn S. Medical management of Cushing's disease: What is the future? *Pituitary*. 2012;15(3):330–41.
117. Kvols LK, Oberg KE, O'Dorisio TM, Mohideen P, de Herder WW, Arnold R, et al. Pasireotide (SOM230) shows efficacy and tolerability in the treatment of patients with advanced neuroendocrine tumors refractory or resistant to octreotide LAR: Results from a phase II study. *Endocr Relat Cancer*. 2012;19(5):657–66.
118. Chan JA, Ryan DP, Zhu AX, Abrams TA, Wolpin BM, Malinowski P, et al. Phase I study of pasireotide (SOM 230) and everolimus (RAD001) in advanced neuroendocrine tumors. *Endocr Relat Cancer*. 2012;19(5):615–23.
119. O'Toole D, Saveanu A, Couvelard A, Gunz G, Enjalbert A, Jaquet P, et al. The analysis of quantitative expression of somatostatin and dopamine receptors in gastro-entero-pancreatic tumours opens new therapeutic strategies. *Eur J Endocrinol*. 2006;155(6):849–57.

120. Gatto F, Hofland LJ. The role of somatostatin and dopamine D2 receptors in endocrine tumors. *Endocr Relat Cancer*. 2011;18(6):R233–51.
121. Oberg K, Ferone D, Kaltsas G, Knigge UP, Taal B, Plockinger U. ENETS Consensus Guidelines for the Standards of Care in Neuroendocrine Tumors: Biotherapy. *Neuroendocrinology*. 2009;90(2):209–13.
122. Mitry E, Baudin E, Ducreux M, Sabourin JC, Rufie P, Aparicio T, et al. Treatment of poorly differentiated neuroendocrine tumours with etoposide and cisplatin. *Br J Cancer*. 1999;81(8):1351–5.
123. Vilar E, Salazar R, Perez-Garcia J, Cortes J, Oberg K, Tabernero J. Chemotherapy and role of the proliferation marker Ki-67 in digestive neuroendocrine tumors. *Endocr Relat Cancer*. 2007;14(2):221–32.
124. Ramanathan RK, Cnaan A, Hahn RG, Carbone PP, Haller DG. Phase II trial of dacarbazine (DTIC) in advanced pancreatic islet cell carcinoma. Study of the Eastern Cooperative Oncology Group-E6282. *Ann Oncol*. 2001;12(8):1139–43.
125. Dunn J, Baborie A, Alam F, Joyce K, Moxham M, Sibson R, et al. Extent of MGMT promoter methylation correlates with outcome in glioblastomas given temozolomide and radiotherapy. *Br J Cancer*. 2009;101(1):124–31.
126. Kulke MH, Hornick JL, Frauenhoffer C, Hooshmand S, Ryan DP, Enzinger PC, et al. O6-methylguanine DNA methyltransferase deficiency and response to temozolomide-based therapy in patients with neuroendocrine tumors. *Clin Cancer Res*. 2009;15(1):338–45.
*127. Raymond E, Dahan L, Raoul JL, Bang YJ, Borbath I, Lombard-Bohas C, et al. Sunitinib malate for the treatment of pancreatic neuroendocrine tumors. *N Engl J Med*. 2011;364(6):501–13.
*128. Yao JC, Shah MH, Ito T, Bohas CL, Wolin EM, Van Cutsem E, et al. Everolimus for advanced pancreatic neuroendocrine tumors. *N Engl J Med*. 2011;364(6):514–23.
*129. Pavel ME, Hainsworth JD, Baudin E, Peeters M, Horsch D, Winkler RE, et al. Everolimus plus octreotide long-acting repeatable for the treatment of advanced neuroendocrine tumours associated with carcinoid syndrome (RADIANT-2): A randomised, placebo-controlled, phase 3 study. *Lancet*. 2011;378(9808):2005–12.
130. Vogl TJ, Naguib NN, Zangos S, Eichler K, Hedayati A, Nour-Eldin NE. Liver metastases of neuroendocrine carcinomas: Interventional treatment via transarterial embolization, chemoembolization and thermal ablation. *Eur J Radiol*. 2009;72(3):517–28.
131. Nazario J, Gupta S. Transarterial liver-directed therapies of neuroendocrine hepatic metastases. *Semin Oncol*. 2010;37(2):118–26.
132. Maire F, Lombard-Bohas C, O'Toole D, Vullierme MP, Rebours V, Couvelard A, et al. Hepatic arterial embolization versus chemoembolization in the treatment of liver metastases from well-differentiated midgut endocrine tumors: A prospective randomized study. *Neuroendocrinology*. 2012;96(4):294–300.
133. Kennedy AS, Dezarn WA, McNeillie P, Coldwell D, Nutting C, Carter D, et al. Radioembolization for unresectable neuroendocrine hepatic metastases using resin 90Y-microspheres: Early results in 148 patients. *Am J Clin Oncol*. 2008;31(3):271–9.
*134. Kwekkeboom DJ, de Herder WW, Kam BL, van Eijck CH, van Essen M, Kooij PP, et al. Treatment with the radiolabeled somatostatin analog [177 Lu-DOTA 0,Tyr3]octreotate: Toxicity, efficacy, and survival. *J Clin Oncol*. 2008;26(13):2124–30.

# 9

# Hereditary primary hyperparathyroidism and multiple endocrine neoplasia

*Emma Tham, Catharina Larsson*

## *General principles of hereditary cancer syndromes*

Approximately 5% of all cases of primary hyperparathyroidism (pHPTH) are hereditary. Most patients with a hereclitary form of the clisease have a family history suggestive of the disease, however, isolated cases may also have a genetic predisposition due to a *de novo* mutation or a somatic/germline mosaic state. They are generally characterized by pHPTH that affect men as often as women at an earlier age of onset. There may be an association with other (multicentric) tumors (Figure 9.1). Hereditary pHPTH syndromes are outlined below, after a brief introduction to cancer genetics.

## *Tumor genes*

Tumors are the result of a multistep process involving mutations in several different cancer genes that lead to increased cell proliferation, prolonged cell survival, accumulation of mutations, and resistance to programmed cell death or apoptosis. Later, the cells acquire the ability to metastasize. There are two major classes of genes that are involved in almost all types of tumors: tumor suppressor genes (TSGs) and oncogenes.

TSGs inhibit cell proliferation and induce senescence, apoptosis, or both. DNA repair genes are a specific subset of TSGs. Hereditary cancer is almost always caused by inherited mutations in one of two copies of a TSG in all cells of the body (a so-called germline mutation), but the second copy of the TSG needs to be knocked out before a tumor can develop. This forms the basis of the two-hit hypothesis that was first described by Dr. A. G. Knudson.[1] If an individual is born with one mutation in a TSG in all their body cells, then the probability of a second mutation occurring in the same gene in a specific cell type (e.g., parathyroid cell) is the penetrance of the disease and often results in early onset and multicentric tumor development. In sporadic cases, a mutation in a TSG in a single parathyroid cell is acquired. Then, a second mutation in the same gene must occur *in the same cell* for the TSG function to be abolished. This process frequently requires more time (later age of onset), and the overall chance of developing this tumor is less (Figure 9.2). For example, in multiple endocrine neoplasia type 1 (MEN1), there is a 90%–99% risk of pHPTH, whereas in the general population, this risk is 1%–3%.

The other class of cancer genes is oncogenes. They are drivers of cell division; thus, an activating mutation in one copy of the gene is sufficient to stimulate cell growth or survival. Others may induce angiogenesis or metastasis. A handful of oncogenes can cause hereditary cancer syndromes, including MEN2 (see below).

## *Inheritance of tumor predisposition*

Many cancer types are inherited in an autosomal dominant manner. Thus, one mutation in a TSG or oncogene on an autosome (chromosome 1–22) is sufficient to cause a cancer *predisposition*. In these families, tumors are typically present in several generations and affect men and women equally often. Children to an affected parent (mother or father) have a 50% risk of inheriting the mutation and thus the cancer predisposition (Figure 9.3). In some situations the mutation is

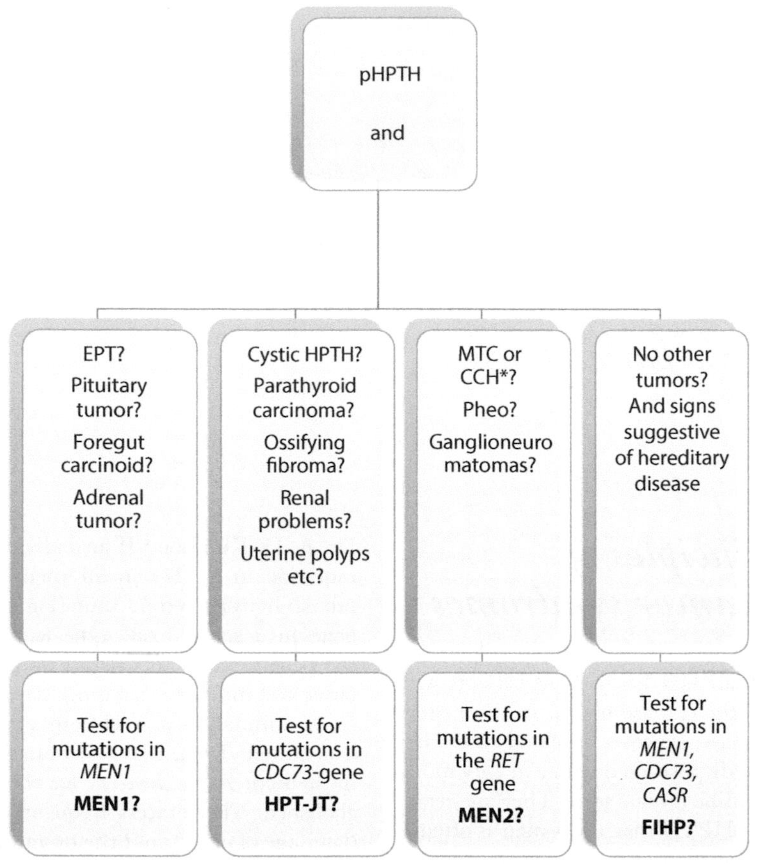


***Figure 9.1***
*Guide to diagnosis of hereditary primary hyperparathyroidism (pHPTH) syndromes. Ascertain whether the same individual or first-degree relatives have any other endocrine tumors or other associated manifestations and perform the appropriate genetic testing. This is done on DNA isolated from peripheral blood in an EDTA-tube. * If C-cell hyperplasia, exclude secondary hyperplasia due to HPTH, chronic lymphocytic thyroiditis, hypergastrinemia, near-follicular–derived tumors, and aging. EPT, enteropancreatic endocrine tumor; HPTH, hyperparathyroidism; MTC, medullary thyroid carcinoma; CCH, C-cell hyperplasia; MEN1, multiple endocrine neoplasia type 1; HPT-JT, hyperparathyroidism and jaw tumor syndrome; MEN2, multiple endocrine neoplasia type 2; FIHP, familial isolated hyperparathyroidism.*

inherited in an autosomal dominant fashion, but the clinical expression depends on the gender of the transmitting parent (so called genomic imprinting).

In some instances, hereditary cancer is autosomal recessive. In these families, the parents are healthy carriers of a mutation in a TSG, and their children have a 25% risk of inheriting two mutations (one from each parent). There is often no known family history suggestive of the disease in older generations; however, several siblings may be affected. The parents may be related. To date, no hereditary endocrine tumor syndromes with an autosomal recessive pattern of inheritance have been identified.

Lastly, tumors may be inherited in an X-linked manner, where a carrier mother has a risk of having an affected son. Several TSGs have been identified on the X-chromosome and confer a tumor risk to boys with multiorgan syndromes, but to date there is no pure cancer syndrome with X-linked inheritance.

## Oncogenetic clinic

If the diagnosis of hereditary pHPTH is suspected, then an oncogenetic clinic can facilitate diagnosis, investigation, and follow-up of the family. The first step is the construction of a detailed pedigree (Figure 9.3).

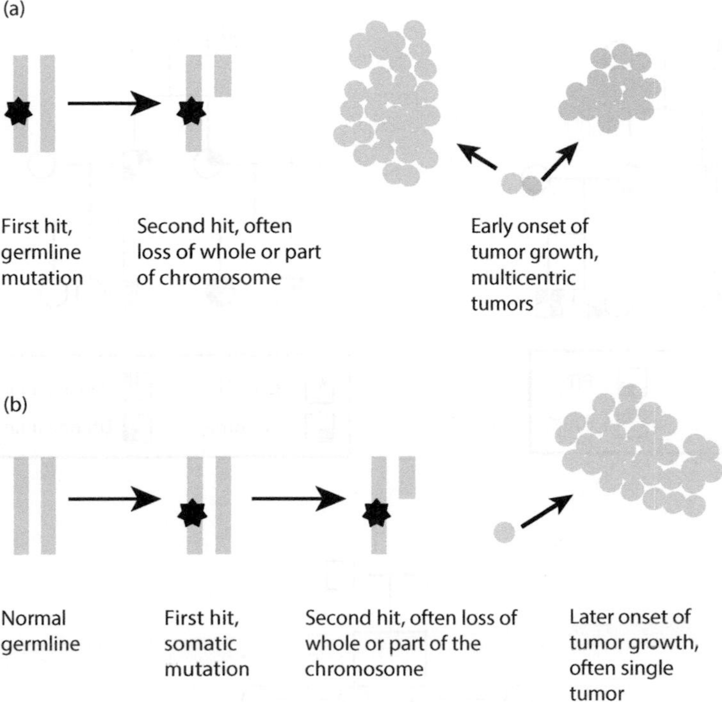


***Figure 9.2***
*Two-hit hypothesis of tumor development. (a) A patient who has inherited a germline mutation in one copy of a TSG in all of their cells, with the second hit occurring as a somatic mutation that results in the cell acquiring a growth advantage. Because there is a high likelihood of the second mutation occurring in several different cells independently of each other, there may be multicentric tumor growth. (b) A patient with two normal germline copies of a TSG, but who acquires two somatic mutations in the same gene in the same cell over time.*

If possible, the diagnoses of the close relatives are confirmed by obtaining their permission to access information from the cancer registry, copies of their medical records, or both. Based on the pedigree information, a genetic diagnosis may be suspected and the appropriate genetic testing offered to an affected individual. Mutation testing for constitutional mutations is performed on peripheral blood sampled in an EDTA-tube. There are several large databases with information on normal variants in genes (e.g., www.ncbi.nlm.gov/SNP or www.ensembl.org). There are also databases over reported patnogenic mutations (www.hgmd.cf.ac.uk). Today mutations are denoted in relation to the first base in the coding sequence (i.e. A in the first ATG is position 1), but in older articles, other nomenclature may be used. Once a mutation is detected, the index patient is urged to spread the information to close relatives at risk of developing the condition. Mutation carriers are offered a surveillance program with the aim of detecting tumors at an early stage where curative therapy is possible. In some instances, prophylactic surgery is possible. Generally, minors are only tested if there is a risk of childhood cancer that will benefit from surveillance as is the case in hereditary endocrine neoplasia (see below).

At-risk family members should be offered genetic counseling with the aim of attaining an informed consent that is voluntary (and not determined by the physician or other family members) and with respect for the patient's autonomy and right not to know. The advantages of presymptomatic genetic testing include optimal treatment of tumors, inclusion in surveillance program/prophylactic measures, and the possibility of prenatal diagnosis (see below). Non-carriers can also be excluded from surveillance programs and unnecessary anxiety. The disadvantages should also be discussed and include anxiety (over the risk of developing a tumor and especially each time a surveillance program is used) and risk of more comprehensive therapy (more side effects, surgical risks) performed at an age with a low risk of tumor development; in some

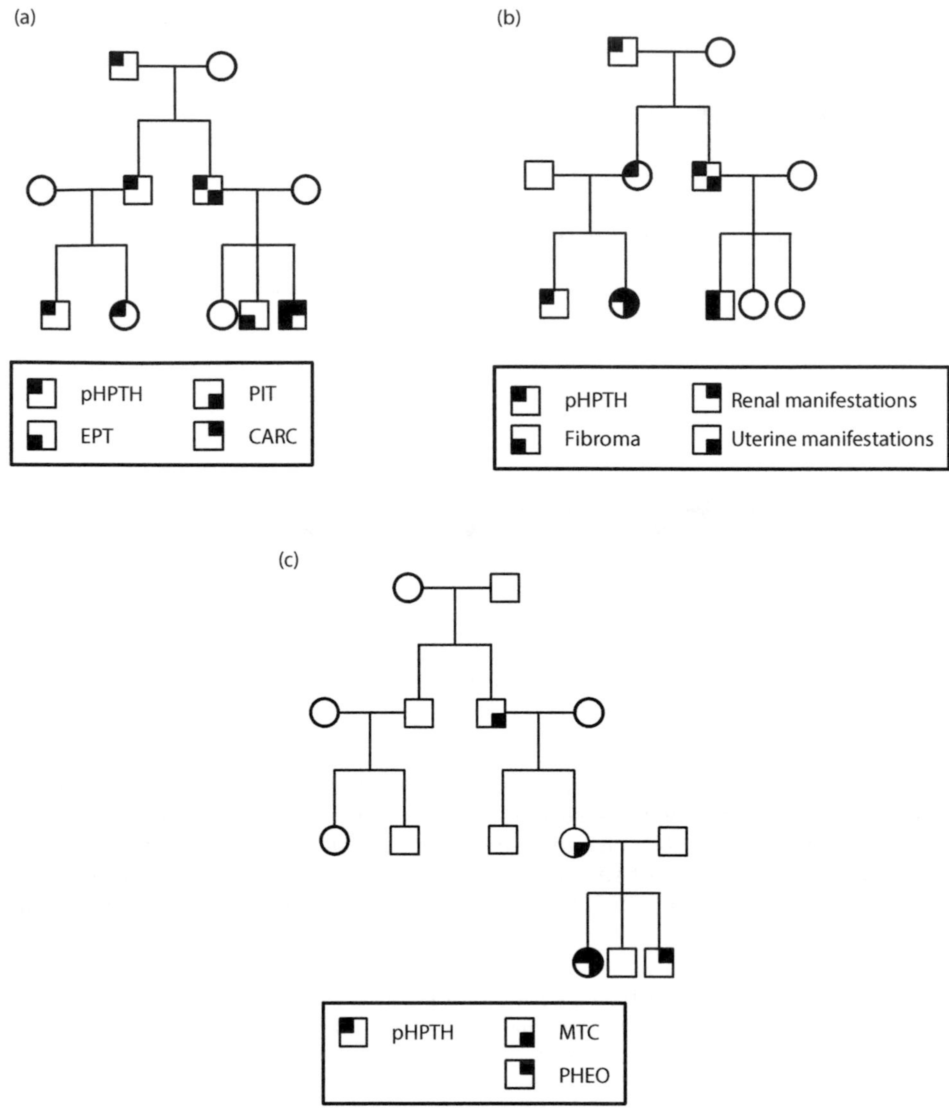


***Figure 9.3***
*Pedigrees demonstrating hereditary endocrine syndromes with reduced penetrance and varying expressivity. (a) Pedigree of a MEN1 family showing reduced penetrance in several individuals who only developed pHPTH, whereas others had the full-blown MEN1 syndrome. (b) Pedigree of a hyperparathyroidism and jaw tumor (HPT-JT) syndrome family. Some members developed only pHPTH, whereas others had ossifying jaw fibromas, renal manifestations, or uterine polyps. (c) Pedigree of a family with MEN2A with a new mutation that arose in the second generation. EPT, enteropancreatic endocrine tumor; PIT, tumors in anterior pituitary; CARC, foregut carcinoids; fibroma, ossifying fibroma of the maxilla or mandible; MTC, medullary thyroid carcinoma; PHEO, pheochromocytoma.*

cases, there may be a lack of evidence to support the benefit of surveillance programs. For instance, in the case of MEN1, a small study has shown that 61% of all patients have been operated on more than three times; 70% are pessimists and they also report lower levels of general health and social functioning,[2] which does raise several ethical issues that need to be discussed with the patients. In addition, stigmatisation in social or work life and/or possible problems with insurance companies (health/life insurance) should be addressed.

If the causative mutation is known, then prenatal diagnosis is possible in cases where the fetus has a risk (usually 25% or 50%) of inheriting the mutation. Prenatal diagnosis entails a chorion villi biopsy in gestation weeks 10–13. DNA is isolated from fetal villi and used for targeted mutation analysis. Simultaneously, a test to exclude maternal cell contamination of the sample is performed using a blood sample from the mother (or results saved from a previous blood sample from the mother). In some countries, preimplantation genetic diagnosis (PGD) is available. PGD requires a conventional *in vitro* fertilization procedure. The embryos are cultured for a few days in the laboratory, and when they reach the eight-cell stage, a single cell can be removed and used for genetic diagnosis. Only healthy embryos are implanted. The method was first introduced in 1990, and so far no major complications have been monitored.[3]

# MEN1 (OMIM 131100)

## Clinical features of MEN1

The combination of pHPTH and/or tumors in the endocrine pancreas or duodenum (enteropancreatic tumors, EPTs) and pituitary tumors was first described in 1903.[4] In 1954, this combination was recognized as being hereditary and was termed Wermer syndrome,[5] but it is now known as MEN1. MEN1 has a prevalence of 1–3/30,000 individuals and has no ethnical predilection.[6]

### pHPTH (see Chapter 11)

pHPTH develops in 90%–100% of all individuals and is usually diagnosed clinically between 20 and 40 years of age, although biochemical evidence of hypercalcemia and raised parathyroid hormone (PTH) levels presents from childhood.[7] Males and females are affected equally often. pHPTH is generally the first lesion in MEN1.[8,9] As a rule, there is polyglandular or multicentric involvement of all four parathyroid glands, although sometimes a single adenoma is found.[6,10] It very rarely progresses into parathyroid carcinoma, although single cases have been reported.[11,12]

### Enteropancreatic endocrine tumors (see Chapter 8)

Enteropancreatic endocrine tumors (EPTs) develop in approximately 60% of all gene carriers and are the cause of death in 15%–33%.[13] In 5% of all cases, they may be the initial MEN1 lesion.[8] Gastrinomas are most frequent, affecting approximately 40%, commonly before 40 years of age. They are usually multiple microadenomas located in the duodenum. It is important to check plasma levels of gastrin and to perform the secretin provocation test before pancreatic surgery because the presence of gastrinomas requires specific surgical procedures. Before the introduction of surveillance programs, metastasis was present upon diagnosis in half of the cases. The overproduction of gastrin causes severe gastric ulcers (Zollinger–Ellison syndrome, ZES), which was previously a major cause of morbidity and mortality.[13] Insulinomas occur in 10%, often before 30 or 40 years of age.[9] They are almost always benign but may cause hypoglycemia and therefore need to be treated surgically. Rare tumors include glucagonomas and VIPomas that also have malignant potential. Up to 55% have nonfunctioning EPTs of which one-third occur before the age of 50 years.[14] The best method of detecting EPTs is by endoscopic ultrasound (EUS), a technique that can detect lesions as small as 5 mm. Complementary assessment of pancreatic hormones may be used (Table 9.1).[6]

### Tumors in the anterior pituitary (see Chapter 1)

Pituitary tumors develop in 40% of all individuals.[10] They are most often solitary macroadenomas with prolactinoma as the most common type, although growth hormone (GH)-, adrenocorticotrophic hormone (ACTH)-, and rarely thyroid-stimulating hormone-secreting tumors may occur. They are generally benign but may recur or grow invasively. The average age of onset is 38 years, but they have been found in children as young as 5 years.[15] Pituitary tumor may be the initial lesion in 17%.[9] Prolactinomas can cause amenorrhea and galactorrhea in females and reduction of libido or impotence in males. ACTH-producing tumors cause Cushing's disease, and GH-producing tumors lead to acromegaly or gigantism in children. Pituitary tumors occur in approximately 1/1000 individuals in the general population[16]; 2.7% of these tumors are caused by MEN1. Differential diagnoses include the chance of occurrence of pHPTH and pituitary tumor in the same individual; familial isolated pituitary adenomas (FIPAs) (3%) or Carney complex (rare). Fifteen percent to 25% of FIPAs are caused by mutations in *AIP* that is especially associated with acromegaly. Ten percent of patients with Carney complex have pituitary tumors in association with spotty skin pigmentation, myxomas, endocrine hyperactivity, and schwannomas, caused by heterozygous mutations in the *PRKAR1A* gene.[16]

| | | Surveillance of presymptomatic individuals[a] | | |
|---|---|---|---|---|
| *Manifestation* | *Penetrance (%)* | *Method* | *Interval* | *From age (year)* |
| pHPTH | 90–99 | *S-Ca²⁺, iPTH* | Annually | 8 |
| EPT | 60 | *fP-gastrin* | Annually | 20 |
| | | *fP-PP* | Annually | 20 |
| | | fP-chromogranin A | Annually | 20 |
| | | fP-glucagon | Annually | 20 |
| | | S-proinsulin | Annually | 5 |
| | | *EUS* | 3 years | 20 |
| Anterior pituitary | 40 | *S-PRL* | Annually | 5 |
| | | S-IGF-1 | Annually | 5 |
| | | *MRI* | 3 years | 5 |
| Foregut carcinoid (thymus, lung, ventricle) | 17 | CT scan of thorax or | 3 years | 20 |
| | | MRI[a] | 3 years | 20 |
| Adrenal gland | 20–40 | *EUS* | 3 years | 20 |

*Source:* Brandi ML et al., *J Clin Endocrinol Metab*, 86, 5658–71, 2001; Waldmann J et al., *World J Surg*, 33, 1208–18, 2009.

[a] Patients with a newly diagnosed lesion should be followed at least annually with the appropriate screening modality. Patients operated for carcinoids or EPTs should be followed annually with CT abdomen, EUS, SRS, and biochemical screening.

*Note:* The features in italics have been suggested to be sufficient for MEN1 surveillance. The initial investigation upon MEN1 diagnosis should include all features as outlined in the 2001 guidelines and follow-up may be individualized according to the findings.

S, serum; fP, fasting plasma; EPT, enteropancreatic endocrine tumor; pHPTH, primary hyperparathyroidism; iPTH, intact parathyroid hormone; PP, pancreatic polypeptide; EUS, endoscopic ultrasound; PRL, prolactin; MRI, magnetic resonance imaging; CT, computerized tomography; SRS, somatostatin receptor scintigraphy.

***Table 9.1***
*MEN1 clinical features and surveillance.*

## *Foregut carcinoids*

Foregut carcinoids arise in the embryonic tissues that develop from the foregut, that is, the thymus, respiratory tract, and ventricle. Foregut carcinoids seldom oversecrete hormones, and the clinical carcinoid syndrome is rarely seen. They occur in 17% of all MEN1 patients, commonly at a later age (44–50 years) and have not been reported as the initial lesion.[9,17] They can be detected using computed tomography (CT), magnetic resonance imaging (MRI), somatostatin receptor scintigraphy (SRS), or a combination. Thymic carcinoids are more common in men, especially if they are smokers and occur in 2.8%–8% of all MEN1 patients.[18] They are often malignant and are a major cause of mortality due to metastatic spread.[10,13] Bronchial carcinoids arise in 1.4%–9.5% of all MEN1 patients.[18] They may be multicentric, but they are more indolent. Ventricle carcinoids develop from the neuroendocrine enterochromaffin-like cells and are sometimes referred to as ECLomas. Their growth is stimulated by hypergastrinemia that, in turn, may be the result of a gastrinoma or gastric achlorhydria induced by proton pump inhibitor treatment. They occur in 21%–37% of all MEN1 patients with ZES.[18] They are generally small, multiple tumors, although 10%–35% may show metastasis upon diagnosis.[18] In contrast, up to 15% are detected incidentally upon endoscopy,[9] and the tumor-related death is <10%.[18]

## *Adrenal tumors (see Chapter 10)*

Adrenocortical tumors are present in 20%–40% of all MEN1 patients and may be bilateral. They are generally diagnosed later (mean age, 46 years) and are the presenting lesion in only 6%. They are generally nonfunctional, although 15% may have oversecretion of cortisol or aldosterone. They are usually benign with slow initial growth.[19] Once they reach 3 cm, there is a risk of malignancy, and adrenocortical carcinomas have been reported in 1%–2% of MEN1 patients. They are diagnosed by CT, MRI, or EUS, and one-third are already present at diagnosis.[20] If an adrenal lesion is found, its functionality should be ascertained by the dexamethasone suppression test, measurements of free cortisol, and metanephrines in 24 hurine and plasma, and aldosterone and renin activity in plasma.

### Other manifestations

Lipomas occur in up to one-third, and multiple facial angiofibromas occur in 40%–80% of all MEN1 patients and may be a cosmetic problem.[6] Collagenomas are also common.[6] Meningioma was found in 8%,[21] whereas ependymoma was reported in 1%.[9] Pheochromocytoma has been rarely reported.[10]

## Diagnostic criteria

MEN1 may be suspected if an individual has at least two of the first three manifestations mentioned above, especially if family history is present. However, MEN1 testing is recommended if there is a young age of onset or multiple tumors in a single organ (Table 9.2).[8]

## Management

### pHPTH

If the diagnosis of MEN1 is suspected (clinical criteria, family history, young age, or multiple gland involvement), genetic diagnosis for MEN1 should be performed before surgery of the parathyroid gland to reduce the risk of postoperative recurrence.[6,22] Generally, pHPTH in MEN1 patients should be treated by subtotal parathyroidectomy with removal of three and a half glands. The viability of the remaining parathyroid remnant (taken from the smallest gland) should be confirmed before removing the other glands. In addition, it should be marked with a suture or clip and sewn away from the laryngeal nerve to reduce risk of hoarseness upon reoperation. Intraoperative measurement of PTH is recommended but needs to be interpreted with caution.[22] Because up to 20% have supernumerary parathyroid glands, surgical exploration along the carotid bifurcation and larynx should be performed. Furthermore, resection of the thymus will reduce the risk of recurrence of pHPTH and pre-empt the development of thymic carcinoids. Because parathyroid remnants may succumb to necrosis, parathyroid tissue should be cryopreserved if possible. Total parathyroidectomy with autotransplantation of parathyroid tissue may be required in cases with advanced involvement of all four glands, but because 35% develop hypoparathyroidism and recurrence occurs in up to 17%, most surgeons do not choose total parathyroidectomy as a first-hand option.[22,23] If only one gland is affected, removal of the two parathyroid glands on the affected side of the throat may be an alternative. Annual postoperative follow-up should be performed to exclude recurrence (Table 9.1).

The timing of parathyroid surgery is controversial. Early intervention will prevent morbidity due to

| *MEN1 manifestations* | *% of cases with mutations if family history* | *% of cases with mutations if no family history* |
|---|---|---|
| pHPTH + EPT + PIT | 73–91 | 31–69 |
| pHPTH + EPT | 60–92 | 5–67 |
| pHPTH + PIT | 46–50 | 0–8 |
| pHPTH | 17–57 | 0–6 |
| EPT | 20–33 | 0 |
| PIT | 0–30 | 0 |
| Familial isolated pHPTH | 17 | Not applicable |

| *Presymptomatic test* | *Age* |
|---|---|
| Individual at risk of MEN1 | From age (3–5 years) |

*Source:* Data from Tham E et al., *J Clin Endocrinol Metab*, 92, 3389–95, 2007.
pHPTH, primary hyperparathyroidism; EPT, enteropancreatic endocrine tumor; PIT, tumor in anterior pituitary.

**Table 9.2**
*Indications for genetic testing of MEN1.*

hypercalcemia, such as severe osteopenia. In addition, removal of the parathyroid glands will ameliorate symptoms of ZES because hypercalcemia stimulates gastrin secretion. In contrast, reoperation (with ensuing increased morbidity) is more likely to be required after early surgery.[22] If there is severe hypercalcemia, cinacalcet hydrochloride, a calcimimetic that binds to the calcium-sensing receptor, may reduce symptoms in inoperable patients.[24] pHPTH during pregnancy should be monitored due to risks to the fetus (intrauterine growth retardation, preterm delivery, intrauterine fetal demise, and/or postpartum neonatal hypocalcemia). If the mother or the fetus develops symptoms, surgical removal of the parathyroid gland is recommended in the second trimester.

### *Enteropancreatic endocrine tumors (see Chapter 8)*

If an EPT is diagnosed synchronously with pHPTH, parathyroidectomy is carried out first because hypercalcemia increases the circulating levels of the EPT hormones. Insulinoma that causes hypoglycemia is an exception and must be removed first.

Medical treatment with proton pump inhibitors, somatostatin analogs, or both is successful against hormone overproduction and may also reduce tumor growth. Chemotherapy may be given in metastatic disease.[25]

The surgical treatment of EPTs is under debate as regards the timing, the choice of procedure, and the effect on mortality and morbidity. For nonfunctioning EPTs (NF-EPTs), most advocate surgical resection when they reach the size of 1–2 cm due to their increased risk of malignancy,[25,26] although some recommend removal of smaller tumors, of which 4% have metastasis.[27] In functioning EPTs, surgery is advocated regardless of size for insulinomas, VIPomas, and glucagonomas. For gastrinomas, there is evidence that some have an indolent course (even after lymph node metastasis), whereas others have rapid tumor progression and poorer prognosis. Therefore, some surgeons advocate operation of lesions 2–3 cm, whereas others recommend intervention at diagnosis of ZES. The surgical procedure that most surgeons recommend is resection of the most affected part of the pancreas with enucleation of tumors >5 mm in the remaining pancreatic tissue and regional lymphadenectomy. Total pancreatectomy has been used for cases with extremely diffuse tumors. Preoperative gastrin levels should be ascertained, because if gastrinoma is present, it is likely to be located in the duodenum (see section "Clinical features"); therefore, surgery should include the duodenum. In this case, there are two main recommended surgical procedures: (1) enucleation of smaller duodenal gastrinomas, or excision of the duodenal wall together with partial pancreatic resection as stated above; or (2) total pylorus-preserving pancreaticoduodenectomy with regional lymphadenectomy. Partial pancreatic resection, with or without duodenectomy, has a higher risk of recurrence (up to 78% in the case of gastrinoma),[25] whereas removal of the entire pancreas causes severe diabetes. Due to the simultaneous loss of insulin, glucagon, and pancreatic polypeptide, the diabetes is difficult to treat and has an increased risk of hypoglycemia and cerebral insult.[14]

All pancreatic surgery, but especially a radical operation, is hampered by postoperative mortality (3.8%–17%) and morbidity (with pancreatic fistulae occurring in 36%, infections, bleeding in a few cases).[25,28] However, studies show that EPTs are the cause of death in 40% of all MEN1 cases[28] and that radical surgery, especially in patients detected presymptomatically, may reduce mortality.[29]

### *Pituitary tumors (see Chapters 1, 3, 4)*

The surgical and medical management follows the conventional approaches for functioning and nonfunctioning pituitary tumors. Prolactinomas are generally treated with dopamine agonists that reduce the levels of prolactin. Transsphenoidal surgery is reserved for dopamine-resistant cases, and radiotherapy may be used after noncurative surgery. For GH-, ACTH-, and nonsecreting tumors, transsphenoidal surgery is the first-line treatment. Somatostatin analogs may normalize serum levels of GH, and radiotherapy may be a postoperative adjuvant.[9,18]

### *Foregut carcinoids and adrenal tumors*

Thymic carcinoids require resection due to the risk of malignancy. The thymus should also be removed prophylactically upon parathyroid surgery. Surgery is also the primary treatment for bronchial carcinoids. Gastric carcinoids >10 mm should be removed surgically. Endoscopic resection may be possible if they do not involve the muscular layer of the stomach wall. Otherwise, local resection is required. Upon recurrence or if malignant, partial or total gastrectomy with lymph node dissection may be performed. Somatostatin analogs may play a role, especially if metastasis is present.[18] Adrenal tumors with malignant potential (usually those >3 cm) are surgically removed.[9,18]

## *MEN1 genetics*

MEN1 is inherited in an autosomal dominant manner; therefore, most cases have a family history. However, 10% are caused by new mutations. Other cases with no apparent family history may be due to reduced penetrance in the parent, later onset in the parent, nonpaternity, or somatic/germline mosaicism.[30] Offspring to an MEN1-affected individual have 50% risk of inheriting the mutation. The penetrance is almost complete for pHPTH but lower for the other manifestations, and there is variable expressivity even within the same family (Figure 9.3). Some families have been initially diagnosed with familial isolated hyperparathyroidism but have later developed other MEN1 manifestations.[8]

MEN1 is caused by a mutation in the *MEN1* gene that was localized to chromosome 11q13 in 1988[31] and identified as the *MEN1* gene in 1997.[32,33] The *MEN1* gene contains ten exons that span 9.8 kb of genomic DNA and produce a major transcript of 2.9 kb. Exons 2–10 encode a 610 amino acid protein called menin. To date, there are >1340 loss-of-function mutations spread across the *MEN1* gene.[34] Most are unique to each family. In some geographical areas, founder *MEN1* mutations have been identified such as in Tasmania, Finland and the Burin peninsula of Newfoundland. The majority are truncating (nonsense and frameshift mutations), but missense, splice, and in-frame mutations are also found. One to four percent have larger deletions of several exons or the whole gene.[9] Clinically, mutation testing is performed on DNA isolated from peripheral blood (EDTA tube). DNA sequencing combined with a test for larger deletions will detect mutations in 31%–65% of all sporadic cases and 90% of all familial MEN1 cases.[8,9] The remaining familial 10% may be phenocopies; have mutations in the *MEN1* gene that cannot be found by conventional methods; or have a mutation in a gene that is involved in the same signaling pathway. To date, mutations have been found in *CDKN1B* (11 published cases, representing up to 2% of all MEN1 cases without a *MEN1* mutation and denoted MEN4, OMIM 610755). Single mutations have also been reported in other cyclin-dependent kinase inhibitors: *CDKN2B*, *CDKN2C*, and *CDKN1A*.[35]

## MEN1 protein functions

The *MEN1* protein menin is predominantly found in the nucleus and is involved in multiple cellular processes that regulate cell division, apoptosis, gene transcription, response to DNA damage and DNA replication, and repair in a cell type–dependent manner.[36] Menin binds to several transcription factors and can repress or enhance their effects. The same pocket in menin binds to JunD (a transcription factor) and to MLL (part of a histone methyltransferase complex). Menin represses the transcriptional activity of JunD, while stimulating the activity of MLL, which in both cases leads to decreased cell proliferation.[37] It can also regulate hormone secretion/production, including that of gastrin (via JunD), PTH (via Smad3), and prolactin (via transforming growth factor-β). It binds nuclear factor-κB (NF-κB) as well as nuclear receptors and controls the subcellular localization of β-catenin. Menin increases the expression of cyclin-dependent kinase inhibitors, including *CDKN1A*, *CDKN1B*, *CDKN2B*, and *CDKN2C* in many different ways, including histone methylation and especially in response to DNA damage.[38] These cyclin-dependent kinase (CDK) inhibitors prevent progression through the cell cycle, and mutations in these genes are a rare cause of MEN1-like syndromes (see above).[35] In mice, knockout of one copy of the *MEN1* gene gives rise to a similar spectrum of endocrine tumors.[39]

There is no genotype–phenotype correlation; thus, patients with a deletion of the whole *MEN1* gene on one allele have the same phenotype as a patient with a missense mutation in the distal part of the gene.[8] This may in part be due to a rapid degradation of menin carrying missense mutations via the ubiquitin-proteasome pathway.[40]

# Hyperparathyroidism-jaw tumor syndrome (HPTH-JT, OMIM 145001)

## Clinical features

HPT-JT syndrome is a rare syndrome characterized by pHPTH, ossifying tumors of the maxilla and mandible, renal lesions, and/or uterine manifestations and was first described in 1958.[41] Approximately 100 affected families have been published. See Table 9.3[42] for clinical details.

### Primary hyperparathyroidism and parathyroid carcinoma in HPT-JT

pHPTH is usually the first manifestation with onset from adolescence to early adulthood (range, 7–71 years).[42] Seventy percent to 80% of affected individuals will develop pHPTH.[43,44] The pHPTH is usually caused by a single adenoma, sometimes with cystic or atypical histology, although an additional adenoma may occur synchronously or months to decades later.[45]

Fifteen percent develop parathyroid carcinoma that is often characterized by intact PTH (iPTH) levels >3 times the upper limit of normal and raised S-$Ca^{2+}$. Ultrasound of the neck is required to detect

| Manifestation | Penetrance (%) | Surveillance of presymptomatic individuals: Method | Interval | From age |
|---|---|---|---|---|
| pHPTH | 70–80 | iPTH, S-$Ca^{2+}$ | 6–12 months | 5–10 years |
| Parathyroid carcinoma | 15 | iPTH, S-$Ca^{2+}$ Parathyroid ultrasound | Periodic May be considered[a] | 5–10 years |
| Ossifying fibroma of maxilla or mandible | 30 | Panoramic jaw x-ray and regular dental care | >every 5 year more often after surgical removal of an ossifying fibroma | 10 years |
| Renal cysts or tumors | 20 | Renal ultrasound (S-creatinine if cysts are present) | At least every 5 years | of diagnosis |
| Uterine polyps tumors or endometrial hyperplasia, etc | 60 | Pelvic ultrasound and gynecological examination | Annual | Reproductive age |

*Source:* Based on Rich TA et al., CDC73-related disorders. In: Pagon RA, Bird TD, Dolan CR, Stephens K, Adam MP, eds. *GeneReviews.* Seattle, WA, 1993.
[a] To exclude nonfunctioning parathyroid carcinoma.
pHPT, primary hyperparathyroidism; iPTH, intact parathyroid hormone; S: serum.

***Table 9.3***
*HPT-JT, clinical features and surveillance.*

the infrequent nonfunctioning carcinoma. Parathyroid carcinoma may present as a palpable neck mass, renal calculi, difficulty speaking or swallowing, or with severe symptoms of hypercalcemia, including muscle weakness, nausea/vomiting, confusion or altered mental status, bone pain, or pathological fractures. Up to 20% have lymph node metastasis upon diagnosis and about one-third develop distant metastases.[46]

## *Ossifying fibromas of the mandible or maxilla*

Ossifying (or cementifying) fibromas of the mandible or maxilla occur in 30% of affected individuals, usually before the third decade of life. They are often diagnosed after pHPTH but may also be the first manifestation of the disorder with onset in early adolescence.[47,48] They may present as a visible or palpable mass or be detected by dental X-ray, often in molar or premolar areas. They are benign tumors but are aggressive and grow if untreated, leading to disruption of dentition, impairment of breathing, and/or considerable cosmetic concern. They may be bilateral or multifocal and may recur after surgery.[49] They should not be confused with the "brown" tumors of severe hyperparathyroidism (osteitis fibrosa cystica) that may appear in the jaw and resolve spontaneously after curative parathyroid surgery.

## *Renal manifestations*

Twenty percent of HPT-JT patients have renal manifestations detected by renal ultrasound. Most have renal cysts that vary in severity from a few minor cysts (as in the normal population) to bilateral polycystic disease with end-stage renal failure.[47,50] Single families with rare benign solid kidney tumors (diagnosed as mixed epithelial-stromal tumors and mesoblastic nephroma) have been described and may be part of the syndrome.[45,50] Wilms tumor has been reported in three unrelated families,[51,52] and single individuals with malignant renal cell carcinomas have also been reported.[44,53]

## *Uterine manifestations*

Sixty percent of all females with HPT-JT have uterine manifestations identified by pelvic ultrasound,[44] commonly uterine polyps or adenomyosis that may cause menorrhagia. Also, adenofibromas, leiomyomas, endometrial hyperplasia, and adenosarcomas have been reported.

Affected women had fewer offspring than expected and had multiple miscarriages, suggesting that the uterine tumors may reduce reproductive fitness.[43]

### Other tumors

Other tumor types have been reported in single patients. In a minority, molecular studies have confirmed a biallelic mutation in *CDC73* in the tumors, as expected for a TSG. Reported tumors include Hürthle cell adenoma of the thyroid, papillary thyroid cancer, colon cancer, clear cell cancer of the pancreas, testicular mixed germ cell tumor, prostate cancer, and cancer of the salivary gland.[43,44,53]

## Diagnostic criteria

The clinical diagnosis of HPT-JT is established if an individual has (a) pHPTH and ossifying fibroma(s) of the mandible/maxilla, (b) pHPTH and a close relative with HPT-JT syndrome, or (c) ossifying fibroma(s) of the mandible/maxilla and a close relative with HPT-JT syndrome. See Table 9.4 for indications for mutation testing of *CDC73*.

## Management

### HPTH

The abnormal gland should be localized preoperatively (e.g., by ultrasound, MRI, or 99mTc-sestamibi scanning). Usually, only one gland is affected; thus, minimally invasive surgery with removal of the abnormal gland is recommended by most surgeons as causing least morbidity.[22,42,44] However, the recurrence rate is about 20% after a mean of 13.7 years, and 15% have parathyroid carcinoma that has led some to advocate subtotal parathyroidectomy.[45,54] Most surgeons do not consider total parathyroidectomy an option due to the risk of postoperative hypoparathyroidism.[42] Intraoperative measurement of iPTH to ensure complete resection may be useful,[42] but measurements need to be interpreted with care in familial pHPTH.[22] Postoperative annual surveillance is required (Table 9.3). Cinacalcet hydrochloride may be an alternative in inoperable patients,[24] and pHPTH during pregnancy should be monitored (see MEN1—management of pHPTH, pg. 185–86).

Parathyroid carcinoma should be resected *en bloc* without damaging the tumor capsule, and this may include the ipsilateral thyroid lobe.[46] Local seeding of the tumor cells may occur if the tumor is broken perioperatively or by biopsy, which should be avoided.[42] Cinacalcet hydrochloride may be an alternative for parathyrotoxicosis or inoperable cases. Radiation of the neck should be avoided.

Jaw tumors should be completely resected if possible, which depends on the size and location of the tumor. Due to the risk of recurrence, patients should be followed annually (Table 9.3).

There are no HPT-JT–specific guidelines for management of kidney or uterine manifestations. These lesions should be followed by a specialist and treatment determined for each individual case.

| *Testing for CDC73 mutations is recommended if the patient has:* | *% of cases with mutations* |
|---|---|
| a) a clinical diagnosis of HPT-JT | 58 |
| b) parathyroid carcinoma regardless of family history | 20–29 |
| c) ossifying fibroma(s) of the jaw | Unknown, 1 of 3 in one study |
| d) familial isolated hyperparathyroidism, especially if at least one individual had cystic or atypical histology and if MEN1 test was normal | 7 (0–33) |
| e) sporadic pHPT <45 years | 1 |
| f) renal cysts/tumor | Unknown |

| *Presymptomatic test* | *Age* |
|---|---|
| Individual at risk of HPT-JT | 5–10 years |

*Source:* Multiple References used to create the table: Including 42, 53, 55-57, 62, 103-112.

***Table 9.4***
*Indications for genetic testing of CDC73.*

## HPT-JT genetics

HPT-JT syndrome is inherited in an autosomal dominant fashion. Most affected individuals have an affected parent, but *de novo* cases have been reported. In some cases, there is no known family history due to missed diagnosis of one parent, later onset in parent, reduced penetrance, or somatic/germline mosaicism.[55]

HPT-JT is caused by a loss-of-function mutation in the *CDC73* gene (previously called *HPRT2*)[52] that is localized on chromosome 1q31.2. *CDC73* spans 1.3 Mb of genomic DNA and encodes a 2.7-kb transcript with 17 coding exons.[56] Most mutations in *CDC73* may be detected by DNA sequencing and are spread across the gene, but with a predilection for exons 1, 2, and 7. The majority of the mutations are unique and 79% are truncating mutations (nonsense or frameshift), whereas 15% are missense or in-frame deletions/insertions and 6% are splice mutations.[57] Single cases with a complete deletion of one copy of the gene have also been reported.[58]

Mutations in *CDC73* can be detected in 58% of patients with a clinical diagnosis of HPT-JT. However, the same mutations can also cause seemingly sporadic parathyroid carcinoma or familial isolated hyperparathyroidism (FIHP); thus, there is no genotype–phenotype correlation, and all mutation carriers should receive the same surveillance[57] (Tables 9.3 and 9.4).

## HPT-JT gene function

The *CDC73* protein parafibromin contains 531 amino acids and is ubiquitously expressed. The parafibromin tumor supressor gene is part of the PAFI protein complex involved in transcription and histone modifications. It regulates gene transcription of genes that regulate cell division. It is proapoptotic and can also regulate the cytoskeleton.[59] Parafibromin is essential for embryonic development and postnatal survival, and loss of its function leads to widespread apoptosis.[60]

# Familial isolated HPT

FIHP is inherited as an autosomal dominant condition that may be true FIHP or one of the above-mentioned syndromes with reduced penetrance. It occurs in approximately 1% of all pHPTH cases.[61] Most cases of FIHP have no known cause (Table 9.5), but genetic testing of *MEN1*, *CASR* (see section "FHH"), and *CDC73* is recommended, even if no other manifestations of these syndromes are apparent. Evidence suggests several alternative gene loci,[62] however, some small kindreds could also represent clustering of cases by chance or have a multifactorial background.

FIHP Differential

| *Diagnosis* | *Gene* | *% of all FIHP* |
|---|---|---|
| MEN1 | *MEN1* | 17 |
| FHH | *CASR* | 7 |
| HPT-JT | *CDC73* | 5 |
| Unknown | ?? | 71 |

*Source:* Multiple References used to create the table: Including 55, 61, 62, 103-105, 107, 110, 113-121.

***Table 9.5***
*Genetic causes of FIHP.*

# Familial benign hypocalciuric hypercalcemia (FBHH, OMIM 145980) (see Chapter 11)

## Clinical features

FBHH (OMIM 145980) was first described in 1966[63] and has a prevalence of at least 1/10,000.[64] In most cases, there is mild hypercalcemia present from birth that does not require treatment. Nonsuppressed PTH, relative hypocalciuria [detected as a ratio of urinary calcium clearance/creatinine clearance (CCCR) <0.01], and normal parathyroid glands establish the diagnosis. However, atypical cases with severe hypercalcemia, raised PTH, CCCR >0.01, and/or nephrolithiasis, chondrocalcinosis, gallstones, or pancreatitis and in some cases hypercalciuria have been reported, sometimes due to concomitant pHPTH that may appear by chance in the family.[64] Thus, genetic testing is essential for diagnosis.[65] This is important because parathyroidectomy is not indicated because it will not normalize calcium levels in classical FBHH.

## Diagnostic criteria

The following diagnostic criteria will correctly diagnose 98% of all FHH cases:

(1) hypercalcemia (average of several measurements with normal vitamin D levels) and (2a) a significant mutation in the *CASR* gene or, if no mutation is found, (2b) a verified autosomal dominant occurrence of hypocalciuria (CCCR < 0.01) with no mutation in *MEN1* or *CDC73*.

## FHH genetics

FHH is an autosomal dominant condition caused by a heterozygous loss-of-function mutation in the calcium-sensing receptor (*CASR*) gene on chromosome 3q.[66,67] Two mutations in the two copies of the CASR gene cause neonatal severe hyperparathyroidism (NSHPT), an autosomal recessive condition with marked symptomatic hypercalcemia. If untreated, the infant will develop severe skeletal, muscular, and neurodevelopmental complications. Usually, the child is born to parents who both have FHH and who therefore have a 25% recurrence risk in the next pregnancy. However, in some cases, the fetal phenotype develops relative to the maternal calcium levels (regulated by the maternal genotype). These cases often have transient and less severe symptoms that respond well to medical treatment.[68] In addition, heterozygous activating mutations in *CASR* cause autosomal dominant hypocalcemia.

The *CASR* gene spans 103 kb and has eight exons, six of which (3234 bp) encode the CASR protein of 1078 amino acids.[68] Mutations are found by DNA sequencing in 18% of cases, and family history more than doubles the likelihood of detecting a mutation.[69] There are 139 different mutations spread across the gene that are known (see http://www.CASRdb.mcgill.ca). To date, no large deletions that cause FHH have been reported.

## CASR function

The CASR protein is a G protein-coupled glycoprotein receptor with seven transmembrane domains. Its functional form is a dimer that binds extracellular ions such as $Ca^{2+}$ and then signals via downstream G proteins. In healthy patients, small increases in extracellular $Ca^{2+}$ are sensed by the CASR, leading to a decrease in PTH from the parathyroid cells; increased renal excretion of $Ca^{2+}$, increased thirst, inhibition of osteoclastic resorption, and increased osteoblastic activity in the bone—all of which lead to a compensatory decrease in serum calcium levels. In FBHH, this response is blunted, thus there is hypercalcemia with normal PTH levels and low renal calcium excretion.[64]

# Multiple endocrine neoplasia type 2 (MEN2)

## Clinical features

MEN2 is characterized by medullary thyroid carcinoma (MTC) in association with pheochromocytoma and/or pHPTH and occurs in 1/30,000 births. An association between thyroid cancer and pheochromocytoma was first described in 1961 by Sipple,[70] but the term MEN2 was coined a few years later.

## Subtypes of MEN2

There are two subtypes of MEN2: (1) >90% are MEN2A (OMIM 171400) and familial MTC (FMTC) (OMIM 155240) and (2) 5% have MEN2B (OMIM 162300). Previously, FMTC was a separate subgroup that comprised 10%–20% of all MEN2 cases, but it is now considered to be MEN2A with reduced penetrance and should therefore have the same follow-up as MEN2A.[71–73]

### MEN2A (and FMTC)

The following manifestations constitute MEN2A.

#### MTC

MTC develops in most individuals, usually by age 20–30 years (range, 9–70 years).[74] MTC is a rare thyroid tumor of the C-cells (<5% of all thyroid tumors). Twenty to 30% are hereditary as part of MEN2 and develop from C-cell hyperplasia, resulting in bilateral/multicentric MTC.[75] Note that C-cell hyperplasia may also be secondary to HPTH, chronic lymphocytic thyroiditis, hypergastrinemia, near follicular derived tumors, and aging and will then not transform to MTC. MTC leads to overproduction of calcitonin, measurement of which may be used as a diagnostic test. Increased calcitonin levels >10 ng/mL may also lead to intractable diarrhea due to increased gastrointestinal secretion and hypermobility. MTC is a therapy-resistant tumor with a 10-year disease-specific survival of about 75%. Seventy percent have spread local disease or lymph node metastasis at clinical diagnosis.[75]

#### *Pheochromocytoma (see Chapter 24)*

Pheochromocytoma is found in 50% of all cases, often before 20–40 years of age. In 13%–27%, pheochromocytoma is the first manifestation of MEN2A.[76] Pheochromocytomas produce adrenalin and noradrenalin that can be measured as metanephrine and normetanephrine in plasma (or urine samples) occasionally dopamine is produced. Symptoms are attacks of hypertension, tachycardia, perspiration, and headache, with a risk of sudden death due to cardiovascular complications. Four percent are diagnosed with malignant pheochromocytoma.[77] Eighty-four percent of all multiple/bilateral pheochromocytomas are hereditary, and 12% of these are due to MEN2. Differential diagnoses of hereditany forms include von Hippel Lindau syndrome (hemangioma and renal cell carcinoma), neurofibromatosis typel (café au lait spots, axillary and inguinal freckling) and the familial pheochromocytoma-paraganglioma syndromes. Altogether, constitutional mutations in 13 susceptibility genes have been described in pheochromocytomas and paragangliomas including: E6LN1/PHD2, EPAS1/HIF2A, KIFIB/3, MAX, MEN1, NF1, RET, SDHA, SDHB, SDHC, SDHD, SDHAF2/SDH5, TMEM127 and VHL.

### *pHPTH*

pHPTH is found in 15%–30%. pHPTH almost always presents after MTC (or pheochromocytoma) and has an average age of onset of 38 years. The hyperparathyroidism is often mild, and typically there is hyperplasia of multiple glands.[74,75]

### *Hirschsprung's disease*

Hirschsprung's disease (HSCR) is characterized by megacolon due to aganglionosis of the gut (not to be confused with the ganglioneuromatosis of MEN2B; see below). It occurs in 1%–16% of all MEN2 cases.[76,78] Conversely, MTC occurs in 4.5% of all HSCR cases.

### *Pruritic cutaneous lichen amyloidosis*

Cutaneous lichen amyloidosis (CLA) occurs in rare families. It is usually located on the upper back and may be the first sign of MEN2A.[79] Most, but not all, cases have been associated with mutations in codon 634[80,81] of the *RET* gene (see below).

### *Unilateral renal agenesis*

A single family with unilateral renal agenesis has been reported.[82]

### *MEN2B*

MEN2B is characterized as follows:

a. An aggressive form of MTC with onset from 2 months of age in all individuals.[74] If untreated, the average age of death is 21 years.[75,83]
b. Pheochromocytoma with average onset 23–28 years, (range, 12–33 years) in 50%; see MEN2A for more information on these tumor types.
c. Ganglioneuromas from infancy/early childhood on tongue, lips, pharynx, eyelids, and intestinal ganglioneuromatosis with abdominal distension, chronic constipation, or diarrhea and megacolon. Up to 86% of all infants with MEN2B are unable to cry tears.
d. Seventy-five percent have musculoskeletal abnormalities, including tall and thin stature (marfanoid habitus), kyphoscoliosis or lordosis, pes cavus, pectus excavatum, hypotonia, proximal muscle weakness, and/or decreased subcutaneous fat.

### *Papillary thyroid cancer*

A few families with MEN2A and MEN2B have an increased risk of papillary thyroid cancer.[84] See table 9.6 for indications for genetic testing of *RET*.

## *MEN2 genetics*

MEN2 is inherited in an autosomal dominant manner. In MEN2A, 95% have an affected parent, whereas 50% of all MEN2B-mutations are *de novo*.[85,86] Healthy parents of a MEN2 patient should be offered genetic testing to exclude missed diagnosis/later onset. In rare instances, there may be nonpaternity or somatic/gonadal mosaicism.[87] The risk of a child acquiring a *de novo* mutation increases with paternal age due to germline selection of *RET*-mutated spermatogonia over time.[86,88]

MEN2 is caused by a gain-of-function mutation in the proto-oncogene REarranged during Transfection (*RET*). *RET* was first discovered 1985.[89] It is located on chromosome 10q21.1[90] and was found to cause MEN2A and MEN2B in 1993–1994.[86,91–93] *RET* contains 21 exons and spans >55 kb genomic DNA. More than 50 different MEN2-causing missense or in-frame mutations have been found[74] (see the *RET* mutation database at http://www.arup.utah.edu/database/MEN2/MEN2_welcome.php[94]). Ninety percent of them are located in exons 10, 11, and 13–16, but if a causative mutation is not found upon analysis of these exons, the other exons should be sequenced to detect rare mutations. MEN 2B patients typically camy a missense mutation of codon 918, which is also somatically mutated in approximately 40% of sporadic MTC tumors. In all, mutations are found in 95% of all cases of familial MEN2A and MEN2B, with a lower detection rate in FMTC (Table 9.6). Inactivating (loss-of-function) mutations in one copy of the *RET* gene cause familial Hirschsprung's disease[95] or renal agenesis/malformation.[96,97] These mutations are spread across the gene.

There is a genotype–phenotype correlation that forms the basis of the current management

| *Testing for mutations in RET is recommended if the patient has:* | *% of cases with mutations* |
|---|---|
| a) a clinical diagnosis of MEN2A or FMTC | 98 |
| b) MEN2B | 95 |
| c) sporadic MTC | 6–9 |
| d) Hirschsprung's disease[a] | 2.5–5 |
| e) renal a/dysgenesis[a] | 4–37 |

| *Presymptomatic test* | *Age* |
|---|---|
| MEN2A/FMTC | Before 5 years |
| MEN2B | As soon as possible after birth |

*Source:* Multiple References used to create the table: Including 6, 75, 78, 96, 97, 122-130.
[a] Exclude gain-of-function mutations in exon 10 as they will confer a risk of MTC and require follow-up.

***Table 9.6***
*Indications for genetic testing of RET: presymptomatic testing.*

recommendations[6,74,76] (Figure 9.4 and Table 9.7)[6–12,34–40,72–74]. These recommendations are updated as new information becomes available.

## *RET protein functions*

RET is a tyrosine kinase receptor that is required for growth and differentiation of neural crest-derived cells. It binds ligands from the glial-derived nerve growth factor family (GDNF). Upon ligand binding, the receptor homodimerizes and phosphorylates intracellular tyrosines that activate various downstream signal pathways, leading to cell growth, motility, survival, and progenitor cell differentiation[98] (Figure 9.4). RET function is required for development of the intestinal nervous system, thyroid C-cells, the kidney, and for spermatogenesis[99] and activated *RET* leads to MTC in mice.[100]

MEN2 mutations are found predominantly in two areas: either in the cysteine-rich extracytoplasmic domain or in the intracellular tyrosine kinase domain, although mutations have infrequently been found in other exons (Figure 9.4 and Table 9.7). Mutations in the extracytoplasmic domain (exons 10 and 11; codons 609–634) lead to loss of intramolecular disulfide bonds that normally stabilize the monomeric protein. Instead, intermolecular bonds are formed between two mutated RET molecules; thus, a constitutively activated receptor is formed that can signal independently of ligand. The most common mutation is in codon 634, which is also associated with CLA, and confers a medium-high risk of young onset MTC and other manifestations.

Mutations in the tyrosine kinase domain (exons 13–16; codons 768–918) cause either a homodimerization of two mutated RET monomers independent of ligand or autophosphorylation of monomers. In both instances, constitutive intracellular signaling is the result.[98] Of note, a mutated codon 804 may display various degrees of severity, partly dependent on the presence of other *RET* variants. In some families, it has been associated with an increased risk of papillary thyroid cancer; in others with CLA. Codon 918 is mutated in 95% of MEN2B. The residual cases often involve codon 883.

At first glance, it seems illogical that a family may have MEN2 and Hirschsprung's disease or renal agenesis because these conditions are caused by mutations with contrasted effects. However, molecular studies have shown that some gain-of-function mutations (e.g., C618 or C620) may create a constitutively active RET receptor but simultaneously cause reduced expression of the RET receptor on the cell surface (e.g., by the mutated RET protein being retained in the Golgi apparatus). Alternatively, the mutation may lead to reduced cell survival in intestinal nerve or renal cells.[78] This is probably dependent on other genetic variations because not all individuals with an HSCR-associated mutation will have HSCR.[76,78]

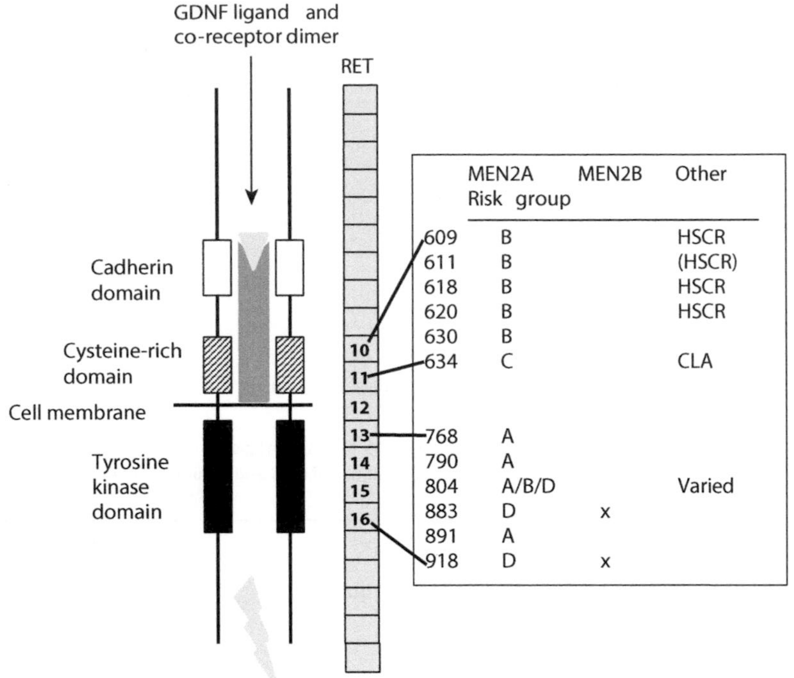


***Figure 9.4***
*Functional domains of the* RET *protein and genotype–phenotype correlations. (Left) Main functional domains of* RET *are depicted, with the extracellular cadherin domain and cysteine-rich domain that bind to the GDNF family of ligands, together with their coreceptor. Binding leads to dimerization of two* RET *monomers and autophosphorylation of tyrosine residues in the tyrosine kinase domain that signal downstream (represented by the lightning symbol). (Middle) The 21 exons of the* RET *gene are represented, with the two major mutation sites (exons 10 and 11 and 13–16). The most commonly mutated MEN2 codons are shown on the far right together with their risk levels and associated phenotypes. Note that mutations in codon 804 causes highly varied phenotypes, from low risk (group A) to MEN2B (group D) depending on whether other genetic variants are present or not (see Table 9.5). CLA = Cutaneous Lichen Amyloidosis; HSCR = Hirschsprung's disease. (Updated and adapted from Plaza-Menacho I,* Trends in Genetics *2006; 22(11): 627–36.)*

# *Management*

## *MTC*

MTC is a chemo- and radiotherapy-resistant tumor. Before genetic testing was available, most MTCs in MEN2 had metastasis at diagnosis, and the prognosis was poor. This is still true for the sporadic MEN2B cases that are often detected at a later age (13–14 years, on average); 50% then have cervical lymph node metastases.[83]

Today, prophylactic total thyroidectomy is advocated for all children with an inherited *RET* mutation. The aim is to operate before lymph node metastasis has arisen but preferably after the age of 3–5 years when postoperative complications, including hypoparathyroidism, are fewer and easier to treat. However, MEN2B mutation carriers require prophylactic operation before 1 year of age. If the child is operated on after the guideline age (Table 9.7), removal of central lymph nodes is recommended, even though this will likely require autotransplantation of at least the inferior parathyroid glands.[75] If there are signs of metastasis, then a comprehensive preoperative evaluation should be carried out and the therapy adapted to minimize morbidity. Before operation of the MTC, pheochromocytoma should be excluded due to the risk of perioperative death due to hypertensive crisis. See Table 9.7 for recommendations of surveillance before and after MTC surgery.

| | RET codons | Youngest age of onset<br>MTC | Surveillance of presymptomatic individuals |
|---|---|---|---|
| A Low risk | 321,515,533,600,603,606,636, 666,768,777,790,804,819,83 3,844,866,891,912 and p531/9bp dup, p.532dup, p635/insert ELRC | 9 years | MTC: Screen from 3 to 5 years, thyroidectomy may be delayed after 5 years if criteria are met[a]<br>PHEO: Screen from 20 years<br>pHPTH: Screen from 20 years |
| B Medium risk | 609, 611,618,620,630,631, and 804+778<br>p633/9bp dup, p.634/12bp dup | 5 years | MTC: Screen from 3 to 5 years, thyroidectomy from 5 years<br>PHEO: Screen from 8 years (codon 630) or 20 years (all other codons)<br>pHPTH: Screen from 8 years (codon 630) or 20 years (all other codons) |
| C Medium-high risk | 634[b] | 13 months | MTC: Screen from 1 to 3 years, thyroidectomy before 5 years<br>PHEO: Screen from 8 years<br>pHPTH: Screen from 8 years |
| D Highest risk, MEN2B | 918, 883<br>804+805/806/904 | 2 months | MTC: Screen as soon as possible, thyroidectomy before 1 years<br>PHEO: Screen from 8 years |

*Source:* Multiple references used to create the table: Including 6, 74-76.

[a] A normal annual basal and/or stimulated serum calcitonin, normal annual neck ultrasound examination, and family history of less aggressive MTC.

[b] Most common MEN2A-mutation.

MTC, medullary thyroid carcinoma, is screened for with serum calcitonin and neck ultrasound; PHEO, pheochromocytoma, is screened for by fasting plasma metanephrine and normetanephrine or adrenalin/noradrenaline in 24 h urine as well as ultrasound or CT examination of the adrenal glands; pHPT, primary hyperparathyroidism, is screened for with serum $Ca^{2+}$, intact PTH and neck ultrasound.

**Table 9.7**
*MEN2 clinical features and surveillance.*

## *Unilateral pheochromocytomas*

Unilateral pheochromocytomas are treated with unilateral adrenalectomy with preoperative antihypertensive treatment. If bilateral disease, cortical-sparing surgery is advocated to minimize the risk of adrenal insufficiency and Addison crisis. Patients with pheochromocytoma should avoid dopamine and adrenergic receptor antagonists as well as monoamine oxidase inhibitors, sympathomimetics (e.g., ephedrine), and certain peptide and corticosteroid hormones. Women should be screened for pheochromocytoma before a planned pregnancy or as early as possible during pregnancy.[75] See Table 9.7 for surveillance.

## *pHPTH*

pHPTH usually presents years after thyroidectomy but should be excluded before thyroid surgery. Preoperative localization is required before excision of the hypertrophied gland or subtotal parathyroidectomy. In both cases, an autotransplant should be performed due to the high risk of recurrent MTC where reoperation often results in hypoparathyroidism. Total parathyroidectomy is reserved for cases with hypertrophy of all four glands.[75] Cinacalcet hydrochloride may be an alternative in inoperable patients.[24]

### *Future developments*

Because RET activation is unique to the cancer cells, several therapeutic agents that block various steps in RET activation or production are being tested in clinical trials. One such group includes tyrosine kinase inhibitors that target RET and other tyrosine kinase receptors [such as vascular endothelial growth factor receptor (VEGFR) 2, epithelial growth factor receptor (EGFR), and hepatocyte growth factor receptor (HGFR)]. One tyrosine kinase inhibitor, vandetanib, has recently been approved in Europe and the United States for treatment of adults with symptomatic or progressive MTC. All have side effects that may limit their use in some patients.[101,102]

## *References*


1. Knudson AG, Jr. Mutation and cancer: Statistical study of retinoblastoma. *Proc Natl Acad Sci U S A.* 1971;68(4):820–3.
2. Berglund G, Liden A, Hansson MG, Oberg K, Sjoden PO, Nordin K. Quality of life in patients with multiple endocrine neoplasia type 1 (MEN 1). *Fam Cancer.* 2003;2(1):27–33.
3. Liebaers I, Desmyttere S, Verpoest W, De Rycke M, Staessen C, Sermon K, et al. Report on a consecutive series of 581 children born after blastomere biopsy for preimplantation genetic diagnosis. *Hum Reprod.* 2010;25(1):275–82.
4. Erdheim J. Zur normalen und pathologischen Histologie der glandula Thyroidea, Parathyroidea und Hypophysis. *Beitr Pathol Anat.* 1903;33:1–234.
5. Wermer P. Genetic aspects of adenomatosis of endocrine glands. *Am J Med.* 1954;16(3):363–71.

*6. Brandi ML, Gagel RF, Angeli A, Bilezikian JP, Beck-Peccoz P, Bordi C, et al. Guidelines for diagnosis and therapy of MEN type 1 and type 2. *J Clin Endocrinol Metab.* 2001;86(12):5658–71.

7. Skogseid B, Eriksson B, Lundqvist G, Lorelius LE, Rastad J, Wide L, et al. Multiple endocrine neoplasia type 1: A 10-year prospective screening study in four kindreds. *J Clin Endocrinol Metab.* 1991;73(2):281–7.
8. Tham E, Grandell U, Lindgren E, Toss G, Skogseid B, Nordenskjold M. Clinical testing for mutations in the MEN1 gene in Sweden: A report on 200 unrelated cases. *J Clin Endocrinol Metab.* 2007;92(9):3389–95.

*9. Falchetti A, Marini F, Brandi ML. *Multiple Endocrine Neoplasia Type 1* Pagon RA, Bird TD et al., editors. GeneReviews, seattle (WA) 1993. [cited August 2012]

10. Machens A, Schaaf L, Karges W, Frank-Raue K, Bartsch DK, Rothmund M, et al. Age-related penetrance of endocrine tumours in multiple endocrine neoplasia type 1 (MEN1): A multicentre study of 258 gene carriers. *Clin Endocrinol (Oxf).* 2007;67(4):613–22.
11. Dionisi S, Minisola S, Pepe J, De Geronimo S, Paglia F, Memeo L, et al. Concurrent parathyroid adenomas and carcinoma in the setting of multiple endocrine neoplasia type 1: Presentation as hypercalcemic crisis. *Mayo Clin Proc.* 2002;77(8):866–9.
12. Shih RY, Fackler S, Maturo S, True MW, Brennan J, Wells D. Parathyroid carcinoma in multiple endocrine neoplasia type 1 with a classic germline mutation. *Endocr Pract.* 2009;15(6):567–72.
13. Doherty GM, Olson JA, Frisella MM, Lairmore TC, Wells SA, Jr., Norton JA. Lethality of multiple endocrine neoplasia type I. *World J Surg.* 1998;22(6):581–6.
14. Triponez F, Dosseh D, Goudet P, Cougard P, Bauters C, Murat A, et al. Epidemiology data on 108 MEN 1 patients from the GTE with isolated nonfunctioning tumors of the pancreas. *Ann Surg.* 2006;243(2):265–72.
15. Agarwal SK, Ozawa A, Mateo CM, Marx SJ. The MEN1 gene and pituitary tumours. *Horm Res.* 2009;71(Suppl 2):131–8.
16. Vasilev V, Daly AF, Petrossians P, Zacharieva S, Beckers A. Familial pituitary tumor syndromes. *Endocr Pract.* 2011;17(Suppl 3):41–6.
17. Gibril F, Chen YJ, Schrump DS, Vortmeyer A, Zhuang Z, Lubensky IA, et al. Prospective study of thymic carcinoids in patients with multiple endocrine neoplasia type 1. *J Clin Endocrinol Metab.* 2003;88(3):1066–81.
18. Pieterman CR, Vriens MR, Dreijerink KM, van der Luijt RB, Valk GD. Care for patients with multiple endocrine neoplasia type 1: The current evidence base. *Fam Cancer.* 2011;10(1):157–71.
19. Waldmann J, Fendrich V, Habbe N, Bartsch DK, Slater EP, Kann PH, et al. Screening of patients with multiple endocrine neoplasia type 1 (MEN-1): A critical analysis of its value. *World J Surg.* 2009;33(6):1208–18.
20. Gatta-Cherifi B, Chabre O, Murat A, Niccoli P, Cardot-Bauters C, Rohmer V, et al. Adrenal involvement in MEN1. Analysis of 715 cases from the Groupe d'etude des Tumeurs Endocrines database. *Eur J Endocrinol.* 2012;166(2):269–79.
21. Asgharian B, Chen YJ, Patronas NJ, Peghini PL, Reynolds JC, Vortmeyer A, et al. Meningiomas may be a component tumor of multiple endocrine neoplasia type 1. *Clin Cancer Res.* 2004;10(3):869–80.
22. Stalberg P, Carling T. Familial parathyroid tumors: Diagnosis and management. *World J Surg.* 2009;33(11):2234–43.


* Key or Classic references.

23. Pieterman CR, van Hulsteijn LT, den Heijer M, van der Luijt RB, Bonenkamp JJ, Hermus AR, et al. Primary hyperparathyroidism in MEN1 patients: A cohort study with longterm follow-up on preferred surgical procedure and the relation with genotype. *Ann Surg*. 2012;255(6):1171–8.
24. Messa P, Alfieri C, Brezzi B. Clinical utilization of cinacalcet in hypercalcemic conditions. *Expert Opin Drug Metab Toxicol*. 2011;7(4):517–28.
*25. Akerstrom G, Stalberg P. Surgical management of MEN-1 and -2: State of the art. *Surg Clin*. 2009;89(5): 1047–68.
26. Tonelli F, Giudici F, Fratini G, Brandi ML. Pancreatic endocrine tumors in multiple endocrine neoplasia type 1 syndrome: Review of literature. *Endocr Pract*. 2011;17(Suppl 3):33–40.
27. Triponez F, Goudet P, Dosseh D, Cougard P, Bauters C, Murat A, et al. Is surgery beneficial for MEN1 patients with small (< or = 2 cm), nonfunctioning pancreaticoduodenal endocrine tumor? An analysis of 65 patients from the GTE. *World J Surg*. 2006;30(5):654–62; discussion 63–4.
28. Goudet P, Murat A, Binquet C, Cardot-Bauters C, Costa A, Ruszniewski P, et al. Risk factors and causes of death in MEN1 disease. A GTE (Groupe d'Etude des Tumeurs Endocrines) cohort study among 758 patients. *World J Surg*. 2010;34(2):249–55.
29. Ramundo V, Milone F, Severino R, Savastano S, Di Somma C, Vuolo L, et al. Clinical and prognostic implications of the genetic diagnosis of hereditary NET syndromes in asymptomatic patients. *Horm Metab Res*. 2011;43(11):794–800.
30. Klein RD, Salih S, Bessoni J, Bale AE. Clinical testing for multiple endocrine neoplasia type 1 in a DNA diagnostic laboratory. *Genet Med*. 2005;7(2):131–8.
31. Larsson C, Skogseid B, Oberg K, Nakamura Y, Nordenskjold M. Multiple endocrine neoplasia type 1 gene maps to chromosome 11 and is lost in insulinoma. *Nature*. 1988;332(6159):85–7.
32. Chandrasekharappa SC, Guru SC, Manickam P, Olufemi SE, Collins FS, Emmert-Buck MR, et al. Positional cloning of the gene for multiple endocrine neoplasia-type 1. *Science*. 1997;276(5311):404–7.
33. Lemmens I, Van de Ven WJ, Kas K, Zhang CX, Giraud S, Wautot V, et al. Identification of the multiple endocrine neoplasia type 1 (MEN1) gene. The European Consortium on MEN1. *Hum Mol Genet*. 1997;6(7):1177–83.
34. Lemos MC, Thakker RV. Multiple endocrine neoplasia type 1 (MEN1): Analysis of 1336 mutations reported in the first decade following identification of the gene. *Hum Mutat*. 2008;29(1):22–32.
35. Agarwal SK, Mateo CM, Marx SJ. Rare germline mutations in cyclin-dependent kinase inhibitor genes in multiple endocrine neoplasia type 1 and related states. *J Clin Endocrinol Metab*. 2009;94(5):1826–34.
36. Wu X, Hua X. Menin, histone h3 methyltransferases, and regulation of cell proliferation: Current knowledge and perspective. *Curr Mol Med*. 2008;8(8):805–15.
37. Huang J, Gurung B, Wan B, Matkar S, Veniaminova NA, Wan K, et al. The same pocket in menin binds both MLL and JUND but has opposite effects on transcription. *Nature*. 2012;482(7386):542–6.
38. Balogh K, Patocs A, Hunyady L, Racz K. Menin dynamics and functional insight: Take your partners. *Mol Cell Endocrinol*. 2010;326(1–2):80–4.
39. Bertolino P, Tong WM, Galendo D, Wang ZQ, Zhang CX. Heterozygous Men1 mutant mice develop a range of endocrine tumors mimicking multiple endocrine neoplasia type 1. *Mol Endocrinol*. 2003;17(9):1880–92.
40. Yaguchi H, Ohkura N, Takahashi M, Nagamura Y, Kitabayashi I, Tsukada T. Menin missense mutants associated with multiple endocrine neoplasia type 1 are rapidly degraded via the ubiquitin-proteasome pathway. *Mol Cell Biol*. 2004;24(15):6569–80.
41. Jackson CE. Hereditary hyperparathyroidism associated with recurrent pancreatitis. *Ann Intern Med*. 1958;49(4):829–36.
*42. Rich TA, Hu MI, Martin JW, Perrier ND, Waguespack SG. CDC73-related disorders. In: Pagon RA, Bird TD, Dolan CR, Stephens K, Adam MP, eds. *GeneReviews*. University of Washington, Seattle 1993–2012. Accessed 2012-08-01.
43. Bradley KJ, Hobbs MR, Buley ID, Carpten JD, Cavaco BM, Fares JE, et al. Uterine tumours are a phenotypic manifestation of the hyperparathyroidism-jaw tumour syndrome. *J Intern Med*. 2005;257(1):18–26.
44. Iacobone M, Masi G, Barzon L, Porzionato A, Macchi V, Ciarleglio FA, et al. Hyperparathyroidism-jaw tumor syndrome: A report of three large kindred. *Langenbecks Arch Surg*. 2009;394(5):817–25.
45. Sarquis MS, Silveira LG, Pimenta FJ, Dias EP, Teh BT, Friedman E, et al. Familial hyperparathyroidism: Surgical outcome after 30 years of follow-up in three families with germline HRPT2 mutations. *Surgery*. 2008;143(5):630–40.
46. Wei CH, Harari A. Parathyroid carcinoma: Update and guidelines for management. *Curr Treat Options Oncol*. 2012;13(1):11–23.
47. Cavaco BM, Barros L, Pannett AA, Ruas L, Carvalheiro M, Ruas MM, et al. The hyperparathyroidism-jaw tumour syndrome in a Portuguese kindred. *Q J Med*. 2001;94(4):213–22.
48. Frank-Raue K, Haag C, Schulze E, Keuser R, Raue F, Dralle H, et al. CDC73-related

hereditary hyperparathyroidism: Five new mutations and the clinical spectrum. *Eur J Endocrinol.* 2011;165(3):477–83.

49. Chen JD, Morrison C, Zhang C, Kahnoski K, Carpten JD, Teh BT. Hyperparathyroidism-jaw tumour syndrome. *J Intern Med.* 2003;253(6):634–42.
50. Teh BT, Farnebo F, Kristoffersson U, Sundelin B, Cardinal J, Axelson R, et al. Autosomal dominant primary hyperparathyroidism and jaw tumor syndrome associated with renal hamartomas and cystic kidney disease: Linkage to 1q21-q32 and loss of the wild type allele in renal hamartomas. *J Clin Endocrinol Metab.* 1996;81(12):4204–11.
51. Kakinuma A, Morimoto I, Nakano Y, Fujimoto R, Ishida O, Okada Y, et al. Familial primary hyperparathyroidism complicated with Wilms' tumor. *Intern Med.* 1994;33(2):123–6.
52. Szabo J, Heath B, Hill VM, Jackson CE, Zarbo RJ, Mallette LE, et al. Hereditary hyperparathyroidism-jaw tumor syndrome: The endocrine tumor gene HRPT2 maps to chromosome 1q21-q31. *Am J Hum Genet.* 1995;56(4):944–50.
53. Haven CJ, Wong FK, van Dam EW, van der Juijt R, van Asperen C, Jansen J, et al. A genotypic and histopathological study of a large Dutch kindred with hyperparathyroidism-jaw tumor syndrome. *J Clin Endocrinol Metab.* 2000;85(4):1449–54.
54. Kutcher MR, Rigby MH, Bullock M, Trites J, Taylor SM, Hart RD. Hyperparathyroidism-jaw tumor syndrome. *Head Neck.* 2012;35(6):E175–7.
55. Villablanca A, Calender A, Forsberg L, Hoog A, Cheng JD, Petillo D, et al. Germline and de novo mutations in the HRPT2 tumour suppressor gene in familial isolated hyperparathyroidism (FIHP). *J Med Genet.* 2004;41(3):e32.
56. Carpten JD, Robbins CM, Villablanca A, Forsberg L, Presciuttini S, Bailey-Wilson J, et al. HRPT2, encoding parafibromin, is mutated in hyperparathyroidism-jaw tumor syndrome. *Nat Genet.* 2002;32(4):676–80.
57. Newey PJ, Bowl MR, Cranston T, Thakker RV. Cell division cycle protein 73 homolog (CDC73) mutations in the hyperparathyroidism-jaw tumor syndrome (HPT-JT) and parathyroid tumors. *Hum Mutat.* 2010;31(3):295–307.
58. Caron P, Simonds WF, Maiza JC, Rubin M, Cantor T, Rousseau L, et al. Nontruncated amino-terminal parathyroid hormone overproduction in two patients with parathyroid carcinoma: A possible link to HRPT2 gene inactivation. *Clin Endocrinol (Oxf).* 2011;74(6):694–8.
59. Newey PJ, Bowl MR, Thakker RV. Parafibromin—functional insights. *J Intern Med.* 2009;266(1):84–98.
60. Wang P, Bowl MR, Bender S, Peng J, Farber L, Chen J, et al. Parafibromin, a component of the human PAF complex, regulates growth factors and is required for embryonic development and survival in adult mice. *Mol Cell Biol.* 2008;28(9):2930–40.
61. Simonds WF, James-Newton LA, Agarwal SK, Yang B, Skarulis MC, Hendy GN, et al. Familial isolated hyperparathyroidism: Clinical and genetic characteristics of 36 kindreds. *Medicine (Baltimore).* 2002; 81(1):1–26.
*62. Warner J, Epstein M, Sweet A, Singh D, Burgess J, Stranks S, et al. Genetic testing in familial isolated hyperparathyroidism: Unexpected results and their implications. *J Med Genet.* 2004;41(3):155–60.
63. Jackson CE, Boonstra CE. Hereditary hypercalcaemia and parathyroid hyperplasia without definite hyperparathyroidism. *J Lab Clin Med.* 1966;68:883.
64. Christensen SE, Nissen PH, Vestergaard P, Mosekilde L. Familial hypocalciuric hypercalcaemia: A review. *Curr Opin Endocrinol Diabetes Obes.* 2011;18(6):359–70.
65. Frank-Raue K, Leidig-Bruckner G, Haag C, Schulze E, Lorenz A, Schmitz-Winnenthal H, et al. Inactivating calcium-sensing receptor mutations in patients with primary hyperparathyroidism. *Clin Endocrinol (Oxf).* 2011.
66. Brown EM, Gamba G, Riccardi D, Lombardi M, Butters R, Kifor O, et al. Cloning and characterization of an extracellular Ca(2+)-sensing receptor from bovine parathyroid. *Nature.* 1993;366(6455):575–80.
67. Pollak MR, Brown EM, Chou YH, Hebert SC, Marx SJ, Steinmann B, et al. Mutations in the human Ca(2+)-sensing receptor gene cause familial hypocalciuric hypercalcemia and neonatal severe hyperparathyroidism. *Cell.* 1993;75(7):1297–303.
68. Hendy GN, Guarnieri V, Canaff L. Calcium-sensing receptor and associated diseases. *Prog Mol Biol Transl Sci.* 2009;89:31–95.
69. Nissen PH, Christensen SE, Heickendorff L, Brixen K, Mosekilde L. Molecular genetic analysis of the calcium sensing receptor gene in patients clinically suspected to have familial hypocalciuric hypercalcemia: Phenotypic variation and mutation spectrum in a Danish population. *J Clin Endocrinol Metab.* 2007;92(11):4373–9.
70. Sipple J. The association of pheochromocytoma with carcinomas of the thyroid gland. *Am J Med.* 1961;31:163–6.
71. Aiello A, Cioni K, Gobbo M, Collini P, Gullo M, Della Torre G, et al. The familial medullary thyroid carcinoma-associated RET E768D mutation in a multiple endocrine neoplasia type 2A case. *Surgery.* 2005;137(5):574–6.
72. Jimenez C, Habra MA, Huang SC, El-Naggar A, Shapiro SE, Evans DB, et al. Pheochromocytoma and medullary thyroid carcinoma: A new genotype-phenotype correlation of the RET protooncogene 891 germline mutation. *J Clin Endocrinol Metab.* 2004;89(8):4142–5.

73. Nilsson O, Tisell LE, Jansson S, Ahlman H, Gimm O, Eng C. Adrenal and extra-adrenal pheochromocytomas in a family with germline RET V804L mutation. *JAMA*. 1999;281(17):1587–8.
*74. Raue F, Frank-Raue K. Update multiple endocrine neoplasia type 2. *Fam Cancer*. 2010;9(3):449–57.
*75. Kloos RT, Eng C, Evans DB, Francis GL, Gagel RF, Gharib H, et al. Medullary thyroid cancer: Management guidelines of the American Thyroid Association. *Thyroid*. 2009;19(6):565–612.
*76. Moline J, Eng C. Multiple endocrine neoplasia type 2: An overview. *Genet Med*. 2011;13(9):755–64.
77. Modigliani E, Vasen HM, Raue K, Dralle H, Frilling A, Gheri RG, et al. Pheochromocytoma in multiple endocrine neoplasia type 2: European study. The Euromen Study Group. *J Intern Med*. 1995;238(4):363–7.
78. Moore SW, Zaahl MG. Multiple endocrine neoplasia syndromes, children, Hirschsprung's disease and RET. *Pediatr Surg Intl*. 2008;24(5):521–30.
79. Verga U, Fugazzola L, Cambiaghi S, Pritelli C, Alessi E, Cortelazzi D, et al. Frequent association between MEN 2A and cutaneous lichen amyloidosis. *Clin Endocrinol (Oxf)*. 2003;59(2):156–61.
80. Gagel RF, Levy ML, Donovan DT, Alford BR, Wheeler T, Tschen JA. Multiple endocrine neoplasia type 2a associated with cutaneous lichen amyloidosis. *Ann Intern Med*. 1989;111(10):802–6.
81. Rothberg AE, Raymond VM, Gruber SB, Sisson J. Familial medullary thyroid carcinoma associated with cutaneous lichen amyloidosis. *Thyroid*. 2009;19(6):651–5.
82. Lore F, Talidis F, Di Cairano G, Renieri A. Multiple endocrine neoplasia type 2 syndromes may be associated with renal malformations. *J Intern Med*. 2001;250(1):37–42.
83. Skinner MA, DeBenedetti MK, Moley JF, Norton JA, Wells SA, Jr. Medullary thyroid carcinoma in children with multiple endocrine neoplasia types 2A and 2B. *J Pediatr Surg*. 1996;31(1):177–81; discussion 81–2.
84. Shifrin AL, Xenachis C, Fay A, Matulewicz TJ, Kuo YH, Vernick JJ. One hundred and seven family members with the rearranged during transfection V804M proto-oncogene mutation presenting with simultaneous medullary and papillary thyroid carcinomas, rare primary hyperparathyroidism, and no pheochromocytomas: Is this a new syndrome—MEN 2C? *Surgery*. 2009;146(6):998–1005.
85. Schuffenecker I, Ginet N, Goldgar D, Eng C, Chambe B, Boneu A, et al. Prevalence and parental origin of de novo RET mutations in multiple endocrine neoplasia type 2A and familial medullary thyroid carcinoma. Le Groupe d'Etude des Tumeurs a Calcitonine. *Am J Hum Genet*. 1997;60(1):233–7.
86. Carlson KM, Dou S, Chi D, Scavarda N, Toshima K, Jackson CE, et al. Single missense mutation in the tyrosine kinase catalytic domain of the RET protooncogene is associated with multiple endocrine neoplasia type 2B. *Proc Natl Acad Sci U S A*. 1994;91(4):1579–83.
87. Komminoth P, Kunz EK, Matias-Guiu X, Hiort O, Christiansen G, Colomer A, et al. Analysis of RET protooncogene point mutations distinguishes heritable from nonheritable medullary thyroid carcinomas. *Cancer*. 1995;76(3):479–89.
88. Choi SK, Yoon SR, Calabrese P, Arnheim N. Positive selection for new disease mutations in the human germline: Evidence from the heritable cancer syndrome multiple endocrine neoplasia type 2B. *PLoS Genet*. 2012;8(2):e1002420.
89. Takahashi M, Ritz J, Cooper GM. Activation of a novel human transforming gene, ret, by DNA rearrangement. *Cell*. 1985;42(2):581–8.
90. Mathew CG, Chin KS, Easton DF, Thorpe K, Carter C, Liou GI, et al. A linked genetic marker for multiple endocrine neoplasia type 2A on chromosome 10. *Nature*. 1987;328(6130):527–8.
91. Mulligan LM, Kwok JB, Healey CS, Elsdon MJ, Eng C, Gardner E, et al. Germ-line mutations of the RET proto-oncogene in multiple endocrine neoplasia type 2A. *Nature*. 1993;363(6428):458–60.
92. Donis-Keller H, Dou S, Chi D, Carlson KM, Toshima K, Lairmore TC, et al. Mutations in the RET proto-oncogene are associated with MEN 2A and FMTC. *Hum Mol Genet*. 1993;2(7):851–6.
93. Hofstra RM, Landsvater RM, Ceccherini I, Stulp RP, Stelwagen T, Luo Y, et al. A mutation in the RET proto-oncogene associated with multiple endocrine neoplasia type 2B and sporadic medullary thyroid carcinoma. *Nature*. 1994;367(6461):375–6.
94. Margraf RL, Crockett DK, Krautscheid PM, Seamons R, Calderon FR, Wittwer CT, et al. Multiple endocrine neoplasia type 2 RET protooncogene database: Repository of MEN2-associated RET sequence variation and reference for genotype/phenotype correlations. *Hum Mutat*. 2009;30(4):548–56.
95. Carlomagno F, De Vita G, Berlingieri MT, de Franciscis V, Melillo RM, Colantuoni V, et al. Molecular heterogeneity of RET loss of function in Hirschsprung's disease. *EMBO J*. 1996;15(11):2717–25.
96. Jeanpierre C, Mace G, Parisot M, Moriniere V, Pawtowsky A, Benabou M, et al. RET and GDNF mutations are rare in fetuses with renal agenesis or other severe kidney development defects. *J Med Genet*. 2011;48(7):497–504.
97. Skinner MA, Safford SD, Reeves JG, Jackson ME, Freemerman AJ. Renal aplasia in humans is associated with RET mutations. *Am J Hum Genet*. 2008;82(2):344–51.
98. de Groot JW, Links TP, Plukker JT, Lips CJ, Hofstra RM. RET as a diagnostic and therapeutic target in sporadic and hereditary endocrine tumors. *Endocr Rev*. 2006;27(5):535–60.

99. Schuchardt A, D'Agati V, Larsson-Blomberg L, Costantini F, Pachnis V. Defects in the kidney and enteric nervous system of mice lacking the tyrosine kinase receptor Ret. *Nature*. 1994;367(6461):380–3.
100. Michiels FM, Chappuis S, Caillou B, Pasini A, Talbot M, Monier R, et al. Development of medullary thyroid carcinoma in transgenic mice expressing the RET protooncogene altered by a multiple endocrine neoplasia type 2A mutation. *Proc Natl Acad Sci U S A*. 1997;94(7):3330–5.
101. Lodish MB, Stratakis CA. RET oncogene in MEN2, MEN2B, MTC and other forms of thyroid cancer. *Expert Rev Anticanc*. 2008;8(4):625–32.
102. Almeida MQ, Hoff AO. Recent advances in the molecular pathogenesis and targeted therapies of medullary thyroid carcinoma. *Curr Opin Oncol*. 2012; 24(3):229–34.
103. Bradley KJ, Cavaco BM, Bowl MR, Harding B, Cranston T, Fratter C, et al. Parafibromin mutations in hereditary hyperparathyroidism syndromes and parathyroid tumours. *Clin Endocrinol (Oxf)*. 2006;64(3):299–306.
104. Cetani F, Pardi E, Borsari S, Viacava P, Dipollina G, Cianferotti L, et al. Genetic analyses of the HRPT2 gene in primary hyperparathyroidism: Germline and somatic mutations in familial and sporadic parathyroid tumors. *J Clin Endocrinol Metab*. 2004;89(11):5583–91.
105. Cetani F, Pardi E, Ambrogini E, Lemmi M, Borsari S, Cianferotti L, et al. Genetic analyses in familial isolated hyperparathyroidism: Implication for clinical assessment and surgical management. *Clin Endocrinol (Oxf)*. 2006;64(2):146–52.
106. Cetani F, Ambrogini E, Viacava P, Pardi E, Fanelli G, Naccarato AG, et al. Should parafibromin staining replace HRTP2 gene analysis as an additional tool for histologic diagnosis of parathyroid carcinoma? *Eur J Endocrinol*. 2007;156(5):547–54.
107. Mizusawa N, Uchino S, Iwata T, Tsuyuguchi M, Suzuki Y, Mizukoshi T, et al. Genetic analyses in patients with familial isolated hyperparathyroidism and hyperparathyroidism-jaw tumour syndrome. *Clin Endocrinol (Oxf)*. 2006;65(1):9–16.
108. Pimenta FJ, Gontijo Silveira LF, Tavares GC, Silva AC, Perdigão PF, Castro WH, et al. HRPT2 gene alterations in ossifying fibroma of the jaws. *Oral Oncol*. 2006;42(7):735–9.
109. Shattuck TM, Välimäki S, Obara T, Gaz RD, Clark OH, Shoback D, et al. Somatic and germ-line mutations of the HRPT2 gene in sporadic parathyroid carcinoma. *N Engl J Med*. 2003;349(18):1722–9.
110. Simonds WF, Robbins CM, Agarwal SK, Hendy GN, Carpten JD, Marx SJ, et al. Familial isolated hyperparathyroidism is rarely caused by germline mutation in HRPT2, the gene for the hyperparathyroidism-jaw tumor syndrome. *J Clin Endocrinol Metab*. 2004;89(1):96–102.
111. Starker LF, Akerström T, Long WD, Delgado-Verdugo A, Donovan P, Udelsman R, et al. Frequent germline mutations of the MEN1, CASR, and HRPT2/CDC73 genes in young patients with clinically nonfamilial primary hyperparathyroidism. *Horm Cancer*. 2012;3(1–2):44–51.
112. Vierimaa O, Villablanca A, Alimov A, Georgitsi M, Raitila A, Vahteristo P, et al. Mutation analysis of MEN1, HRPT2, CASR, CDKN1B, and AIP genes in primary hyperparathyroidism patients with features of genetic predisposition. *J Endocrinol Invest*. 2009; 32(6):512–18.
113. Bergman L, Teh B, Cardinal J, Palmer J, Walters M, Shepherd J, et al. Identification of MEN1 gene mutations in families with MEN 1 and related disorders. *Br J Cancer*. 2000;83(8):1009–14.
114. Cardinal JW, Bergman L, Hayward N, Sweet A, Warner J, Marks L, et al. A report of a national mutation testing service for the MEN1 gene: Clinical presentations and implications for mutation testing. *J Med Genet*. 2005;42(1):69–74.
115. Pannett AA, Kennedy AM, Turner JJ, Forbes SA, Cavaco BM, Bassett JH, et al. Multiple endocrine neoplasia type 1 (MEN1) germline mutations in familial isolated primary hyperparathyroidism. *Clin Endocrinol (Oxf)*. 2003;58(5):639–46.
116. Perrier ND, Villablanca A, Larsson C, Wong M, Ituarte P, Teh BT, et al. Genetic screening for MEN1 mutations in families presenting with familial primary hyperparathyroidism. *World J Surg*. 2002;26(8):907–13.
117. Teh BT, Kytölä S, Farnebo F, Bergman L, Wong FK, Weber G, et al. Mutation analysis of the MEN1 gene in multiple endocrine neoplasia type 1, familial acromegaly and familial isolated hyperparathyroidism. *J Clin Endocrinol Metab*. 1998;83(8):2621–6.
118. Villablanca A, Wassif WS, Smith T, Höög A, Vierimaa O, Kassem M, et al. Involvement of the MEN1 gene locus in familial isolated hyperparathyroidism. *Eur J Endocrinol*. 2002;147(3):313–22.
119. Teh BT, Esapa CT, Houlston R, Grandell U, Farnebo F, Nordenskjöld M, et al. A family with isolated hyperparathyroidism segregating a missense MEN1 mutation and showing loss of the wild-type alleles in the parathyroid tumors. *Am J Hum Genet*. 1998;63(5):1544–9.
120. Kassem M, Kruse TA, Wong FK, Larsson C, Teh BT. Familial isolated hyperparathyroidism as a variant of multiple endocrine neoplasia type 1 in a large Danish pedigree. *J Clin Endocrinol Metab*. 2000;85(1):165–7.
121. Szabo E, Carling T, Hessman O, Rastad J. Loss of heterozygosity in parathyroid glands of familial hypercalcemia with hypercalciuria and point mutation in calcium receptor. *J Clin Endocrinol Metab*. 2002;87(8): 3961–5.
122. Caron P, Attié T, David D, Amiel J, Brousset F, Roger P, et al. C618R mutation in exon 10 of the RET

proto-oncogene in a kindred with multiple endocrine neoplasia type 2A and Hirschsprung's disease. *J Clin Endocrinol Metab*. 1996;81(7):2731–3.

123. Chatterjee R, Ramos E, Hoffman M, VanWinkle J, Martin DR, Davis TK, et al. Traditional and targeted exome sequencing reveals common, rare and novel functional deleterious variants in RET-signaling complex in a cohort of living US patients with urinary tract malformations. *Hum Genet*. 2012;131:1725–38.
124. Eng C, Clayton D, Schuffenecker I, Lenoir G, Cote G, Gagel RF, et al. The relationship between specific RET proto-oncogene mutations and disease phenotype in multiple endocrine neoplasia type 2. International RET mutation consortium analysis. *JAMA*. 1996;276(19):1575–9.
125. Hansford JR, Mulligan LM. Multiple endocrine neoplasia type 2 and RET: From neoplasia to neurogenesis. *J Med Genet*. 2000;37(11):817–27.
126. Romei C, Cosci B, Renzini G, Bottici V, Molinaro E, Agate L, et al. RET genetic screening of sporadic medullary thyroid cancer (MTC) allows the preclinical diagnosis of unsuspected gene carriers and the identification of a relevant percentage of hidden familial MTC (FMTC). *Clin Endocrinol (Oxf)*. 2011;74(2):241–7.
127. Sijmons RH, Hofstra RM, Wijburg FA, Links TP, Zwierstra RP, Vermey A, et al. Oncological implications of RET gene mutations in Hirschsprung's disease. *Gut*. 1998;43(4):542–7.
128. Wiench M, Wygoda Z, Gubala E, Wloch J, Lisowska K, Krassowski J, et al. Estimation of risk of inherited medullary thyroid carcinoma in apparent sporadic patients. *J Clin Oncol*. 2001;19(5):1374–80.
129. Wohllk N, Cote GJ, et al. Relevance of RET proto-oncogene mutations in sporadic medullary thyroid carcinoma. *J Clin Endocrinol Metab*. 1996;81(10):3740–5.
130. Zedenius J, Wallin G, Hamberger B, Nordenskjöld M, Weber G, Larsson C, et al. Somatic and MEN 2A de novo mutations identified in the RET proto-oncogene by screening of sporadic MTC:s. *Hum Mol Genet*. 1994;3(8):1259–62.
131. Plaza-Menacho I, Burzynski GM, de Groot JW, Eggen BJ, Hofstra RM. Current concepts in RET-related genetics, signaling and therapeutics. *Trends Genet*. 2006;22(11):627–36.

# 10

# Coincidental adrenal masses and adrenal cancer

*Marinella Tzanela, Dimitra Argyro Vassiliadi, Stylianos Tsagarakis*

## Introduction

With the widespread use of sophisticated imaging modalities, adrenal masses are routinely discovered coincidentally during the course of imaging investigations performed for reasons unrelated to suspicion of adrenal disease. They are commonly defined as adrenal incidentalomas and are among the most frequently encountered endocrine tumors, with a prevalence that depends on patient's age and ranges from 0.2% in younger persons to 4%–5% in middle age to 6.9% in those >70 years old.[1,2] Most are unilateral, but bilateral lesions either in the form of solitary well-defined adenomas or less frequently in the form of bilateral macronodular hyperplasia are encountered in 9%–17%.[3] The clinical consequences of incidentally discovered adrenal lesions remain relatively unclear, and their discovery poses diagnostic and therapeutic challenges to physicians and anxiety to patients who face both an unexpected diagnosis and the ensuing additional workup.[4] The diagnostic approach involves two major questions: Is the mass malignant and is it functional? Overall, the patient's history and physical examination, the imaging characteristics of the lesion, and a proper hormonal evaluation provide significant clues to the differential diagnosis among adrenocortical adenomas, adrenocortical cancer, and other nonadenomatous lesions and guide further management.

## Etiology of coincidental adrenal masses

The majority of coincidental adrenal masses are benign adrenocortical adenomas with a considerable low probability of malignancy. Occasionally, other lesions might present as adrenal incidentalomas[5,6] (Table 10.1). The incidence of cancer among consecutive, unselected asymptomatic patients without a known history of malignancy, corresponding to the typical patient who is referred for endocrinological consultation, approximates 1.9%.[7] The likelihood that an adrenal mass is a metastasis is extremely low in these patients (0.7%)[7] but rises significantly, up to 20%, in patients with known extra-adrenal malignancies.[5,8] Even in these patients, however, an adrenal mass does not necessarily represent metastasis.[9,10] Thus, patients with extra-adrenal malignancies should be evaluated with caution not only because a diagnosis of metastasis may alter their staging but also because large bilateral metastases may compromise the adrenal gland function, leading to adrenal insufficiency.

## Diagnostic evaluation

The first step in the investigation of an incidentally discovered adrenal mass is the characterization of its imaging phenotype. Current radiological and scintigraphic techniques are able to discriminate between benign and malignant lesions and/or provide insight on the nature of the underlying lesion. Furthermore, although in the early days adrenal incidentalomas were considered to be nonfunctioning, it is now well established that a substantial proportion exhibit autonomous hormonal secretion.[2,5] The most frequently encountered endocrine disorder is autonomous cortisol production, with a frequency that varies substantially between 1% and 47%, depending on the criteria used to define it. Primary hyperaldosteronism is also diagnosed in 1.1%–10% of

- Adrenocortical adenoma (80%–90%) or, rarely adrenocortical carcinoma
  - Nonfunctional
  - Cortisol-producing
  - Aldosterone-producing
  - Androgen- or estrogen-producing (rare)
- Pheochromocytoma
- Other nonfunctional lesions
  - Myelolipoma
  - Cyst
  - Ganglioneuroma
  - Oncocytoma
  - Hemangioma
- Extra-adrenal infiltrative lesions
  - Metastasis
  - Granuloma
  - Amyloidosis

***Table 10.1***
*Etiology of coincidental adrenal masses.*

patients, whereas a proportion of about 4%–7% may harbor pheochromocytomas.[2]

# *Radiological imaging*

The size of the lesion used to be considered as a major predictor of malignancy, and surgery is usually recommended for lesions >4–6 cm. The prevalence of adrenocortical carcinoma (ACC) is thought to be 2% among tumors that are ≤4 cm, 6% among tumors that are 4.1–6.0 cm, and 25% among larger tumors.[11] Size has both a low specificity and low sensitivity for the detection of cancer because 75% of tumors >6 cm are not malignant, and also small ACCs have been reported. In lesions of <4 cm, a repeat imaging evaluation at 3–6 months, depending on the size and imaging characteristics of the mass, is usually advocated. A rapid and significant (usually >5 mm) change in size may occasionally indicate malignancy, but again it is not an accurate predictor of adrenal cancer.[7,12] The role of further repeat imaging has been challenged recently by Cawood et al.[7] who raised concerns that the risk of inducing cancer from the ionizing radiation delivered from multiple computed tomography (CT) scans outweighs the possible benefits, given the substantially small probability of malignant transformation of these tumors.

The imaging phenotype of the mass, using current imaging techniques, determines with much more accuracy the nature of the adrenal lesion.[6,13] CT before and after intravenous contrast administration is the modality of choice.[6] Narrow collimation is preferred, with thin slices of 3–5 mm, because tumors as small as 5 mm can be detected. Benign adenomas are usually rounded, homogeneous, with smooth contour, and well-delineated margins clearly separated from adjacent structures (Figure 10.1a). The unenhanced images provide information about the density of the mass expressed in Hounsfield unit (HU). By definition, 0 HU represents the radiodensity of distilled water at standard pressure and temperature (STP), whereas the radiodensity of air at STP is defined as –1000 HU. Most adrenal adenomas, due to their high fat

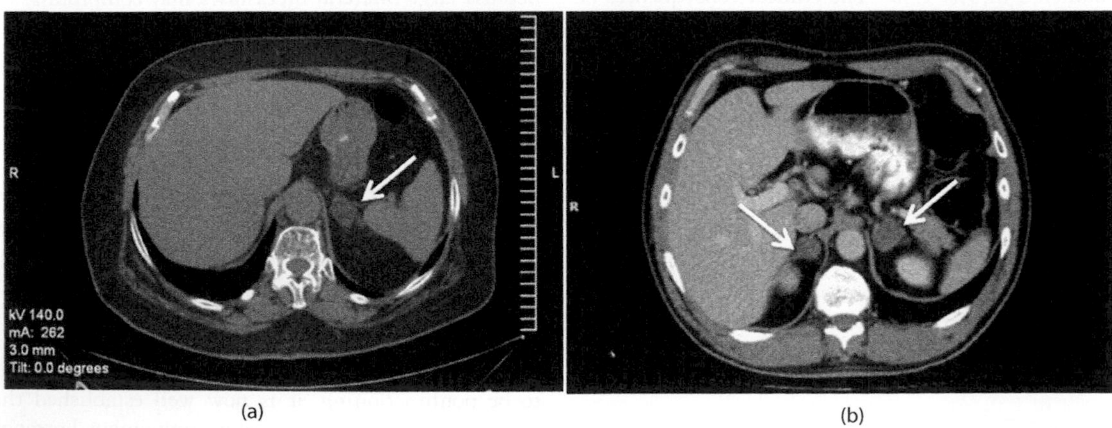


***Figure 10.1***
*(a) Unenhanced CT scan showing a well-defined, unilateral ovoid lesion in the left adrenal (arrow). The lesion is quite hypodense relative to the liver and spleen (attributed to the presence of microscopic fat), being suggestive of a benign adenoma. (b) Contrast-enhanced CT scan (portal-venous phase) depicting bilateral discrete well-defined benign adrenal adenomas (arrows).*

content, have low attenuation values of <10 HU. However, attenuation values >10 HU can be encountered in lipid-poor adenomas that represent 25%–30% of all adenomas. Adenomas show early enhancement after contrast administration, greater than normal adrenal tissue, with an early washout of the contrast media (Figure 10.1b). Thus, an absolute (compared with unenhanced images) washout of >60% and a relative washout (compared with early, at 60 s enhanced images) of >40% indicate a benign adenoma, with a sensitivity of 98% and a specificity of 92%.

In case of indeterminate lesions, magnetic resonance imaging (MRI) may provide additional information using T1-weighted, T2- weighted, and chemical shift imaging (CSI) (Figure 10.2). Benign adenomas are homogenous, have low or equal signal intensity compared with the liver on T2-weighted images, and enhance only mildly after contrast administration. The washout characteristics after administration of gadolinium are similar as those of CT. Moreover, on out-of-phase CSI, benign adenomas lose at least 30% of their signal intensity compared with the in-phase images due to their high intracellular lipid content. Pheochromocytomas may be homogeneous or inhomogeneous, with a high density of 40–50 HU in unenhanced CT scans (Figure 10.3) and characteristically high signals on T2-weighted MRI images without signal loss on CSI.[6] Other benign lesions with distinct imaging characteristics include myelolipomas that are usually distinguishable by their very low attenuation values (–30 to –100 HU) due to very high fat content and cysts that present as clearly defined lesions, hypodense on T1-weighted MRI images and markedly hyperdense on T2-weighted MRI images (Figure 10.4).

## Scintigraphic imaging

Besides localization, radionuclear imaging and, more recently, imaging with positron emission tomography (PET) provide metabolic information of the adrenal lesions. The traditional nuclear medicine imaging of the adrenal cortex uses either $^{131}$I-6b-iodomethyl-norcholesterol (NP-59) or $^{75}$Se-selenomethyl-19-norcholesterol as radiotracers. There are three distinct scintigraphic patterns that can be observed in patients with adrenal incidentalomas: (1) a discordant pattern, that is, absent or decreased or distorted uptake on the side of the adrenal lesion; (2) "normal" symmetrical adrenal uptake; and (3) concordant uptake, that is, predominant or exclusive uptake from the adrenal mass. A discordant pattern suggests a space-occupying, nonfunctioning mass, such as ACC or metastatic lesion, or other destructive lesion.[14] Most studies on adrenal incidentalomas consider a concordant unilateral exclusive uptake to be indicative of a functional adenoma[14,15] (Figure 10.5). However, functioning ACCs are likely to show uptake.[15] Although there is some correlation of tracer uptake with the results of endocrine testing, several patients with unilateral uptake do not have biochemical evidence of subclinical hypercortisolism and vice versa.[16] In practice,

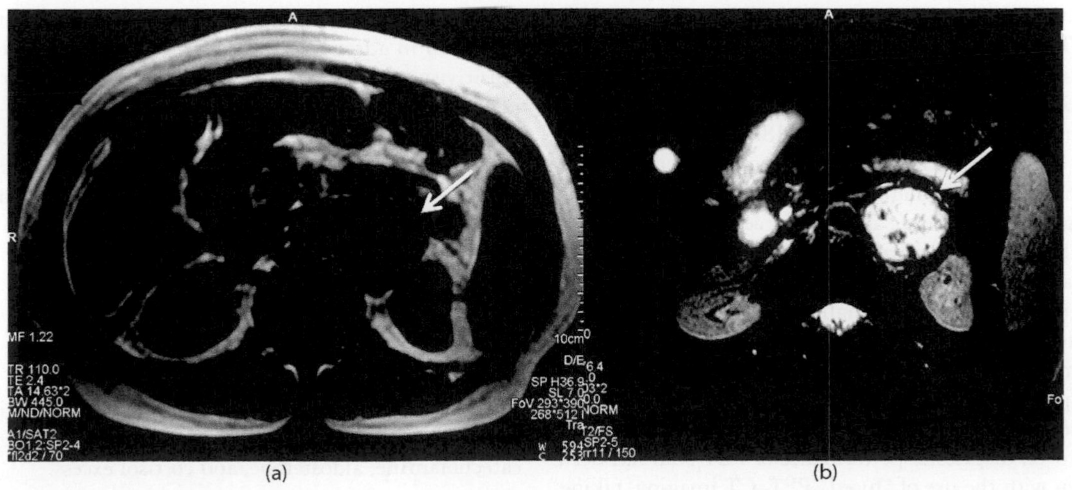


***Figure 10.2***
*(a) Axial MRI T1-weighted image, using chemical shift imaging-opposed phase (out-of-phase) image. The lesion in the left adrenal does not show significant signal drop-off (arrow). (b) Axial MRI T2-weighted, fat-suppressed image. The lesion in the left adrenal (arrow) is inhomogeneously hyperintense, with some linear and nodular hypointense regions. These imaging findings are consistent with either an adrenocortical carcinoma or a pheochromocytoma.*

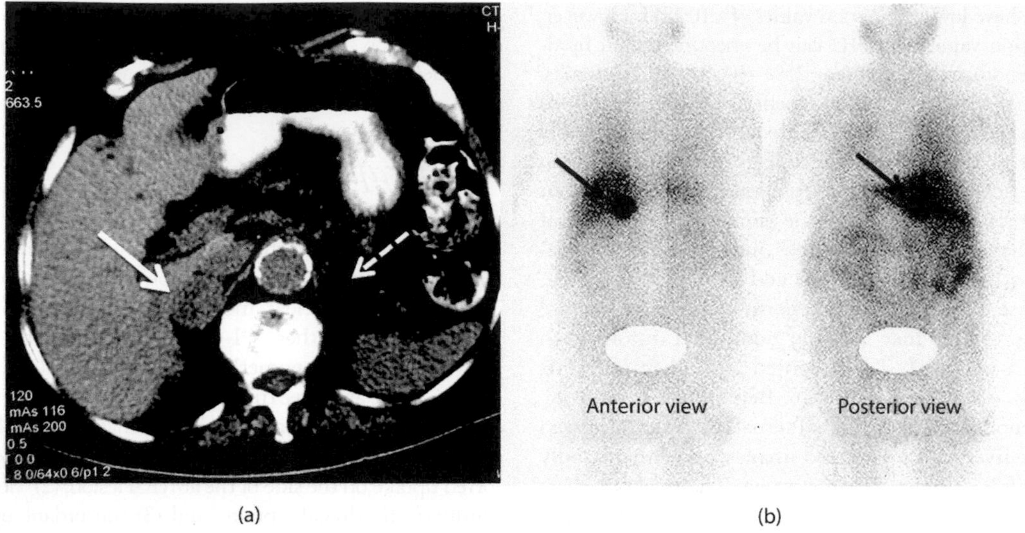


***Figure 10.3***
*Coexistence of an incidentally detected pheochromocytoma (right) and adenoma (left). (a) Unenhanced CT scan showing a round, inhomogeneously high-density lesion in the right adrenal (white arrow) and a hypodense, well-defined ovoid lesion in the left adrenal (dashed arrow). The latter is suggestive of a benign adenoma. (b) $^{131}$I-meta-Iodobenzylguanidine (MIBG, a selective radiotracer for catecholamine secreting tumors) scan, showed unilateral uptake by the right adrenal mass (arrows).*

scintigraphy rarely provides additional information relative to radiological imaging and hormonal evaluation. Its use is also limited because it is a cumbersome and expensive procedure that involves a relatively high level of radiation and is no longer widely available.

The usefulness of PET scanning is increasingly evaluated in various adrenal pathologies.[17,18] In one study of 13 patients[17] and another study of 54 patients[18] with nonfunctioning adrenal tumors, increased 18F-fluorodeoxyglucose PET ($^{18}$F-FDG PET) uptake was seen in all primary or secondary adrenal malignant lesions and in none of the benign lesions, yielding a diagnostic accuracy of 100%.[17,18] In other studies, however, a small number of benign adenomas also showed $^{18}$F-FDG PET uptake.[19] Overall, in patients without known malignancy, $^{18}$F-FDG PET has an excellent sensitivity (99%–100%) to identify ACC but a somewhat lower specificity, depending on the applied interpretative criterion.[19] In patients with known cancer, the reported specificity for metastatic disease is higher.[20] Improved diagnostic performance of PET scan has been shown with the use of "fused" PET–CT imaging, taking advantage of the combined information provided by the CT attenuation measurements plus the intensity of FDG uptake. In a large cohort of 150 patients.[21] PET alone had 99% sensitivity and 92% specificity for the diagnosis of malignancy, whereas the corresponding values for PET-CT were 100% and 98%.

Besides the use of $^{18}$F-FDG as a tracer, the use of etomidate derivatives, such as iodometomidate (IMTO), is currently being explored. These are highly specific tracers for adrenocortical tissue because they have high specificity and avidity to CYP11B enzymes exclusively expressed in adrenocortical cells.[22] A study[22] reported a sensitivity of 83.3% and a specificity of 86.4% for the identification of benign or malignant, functional or not, adrenocortical lesions based on a cutoff value for the tumor-to-liver ratio of 1.3. Setting specificity to 100%, a sensitivity of 61.1% was reached at a cutoff value of tumor-to-liver ratio of 3.8.

# *Hormonal evaluation (see Chapters 1, 21)*

The recommended hormonal evaluation in patients with a coincidental adrenal mass includes testing for catecholamine, aldosterone, and cortisol excess.

### *Catecholamines*

Because it represents a potentially life-threatening condition, pheochromocytoma should be sought in all patients with an adrenal incidentaloma. A study of 174 patients with adrenal incidentalomas reported that routine screening may not be necessary[23] in those with

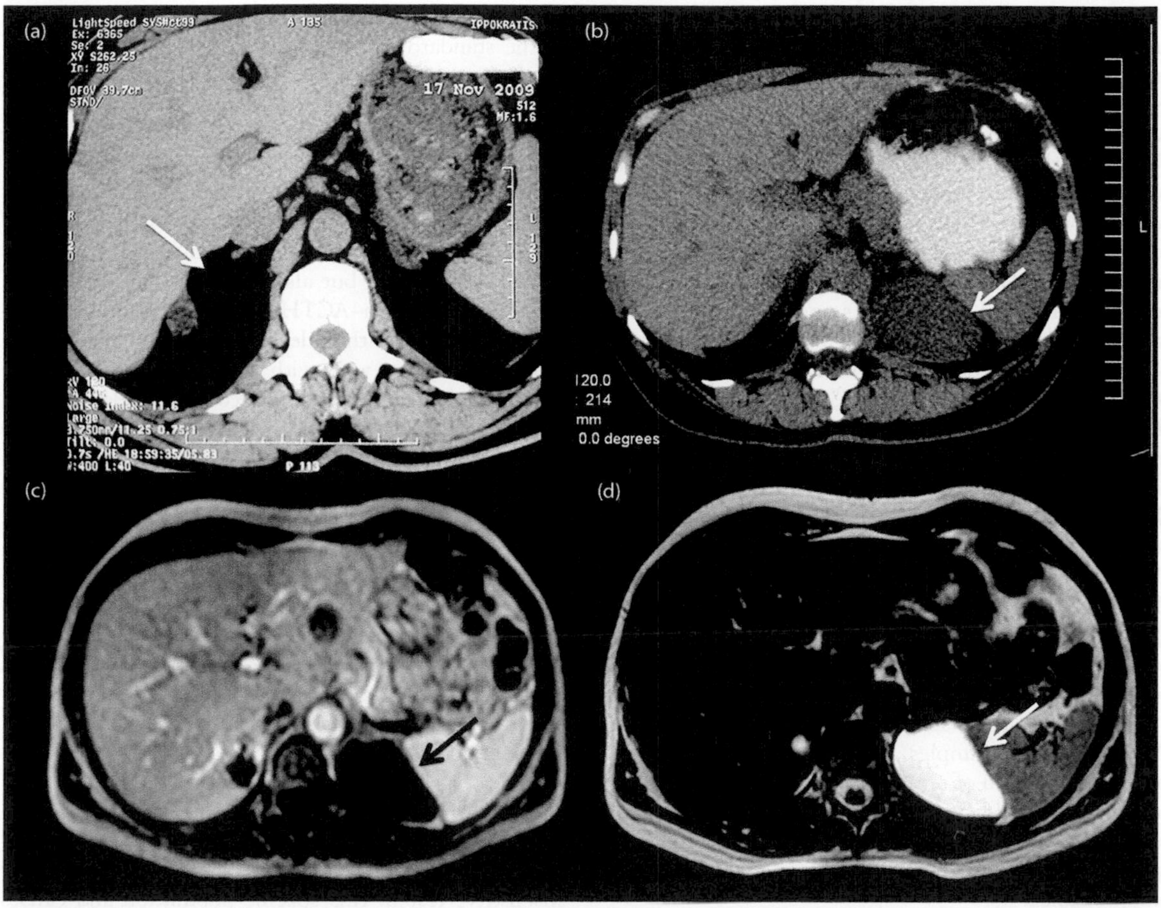

**Figure 10.4**
*(a) CT scan of a markedly hypodense mass in the right adrenal (white arrow). There is evidence of macroscopic fat density, characteristic of a myelolipoma. (b) CT scan of a well-defined homogenous mass with fluid density (white arrow). The same lesion appears hypointense on (c) the T1-weighted (black arrow) and markedly hyperintense on (d) the T2-weighted MR image, compatible with the presence of fluid (cyst) (white arrow).*

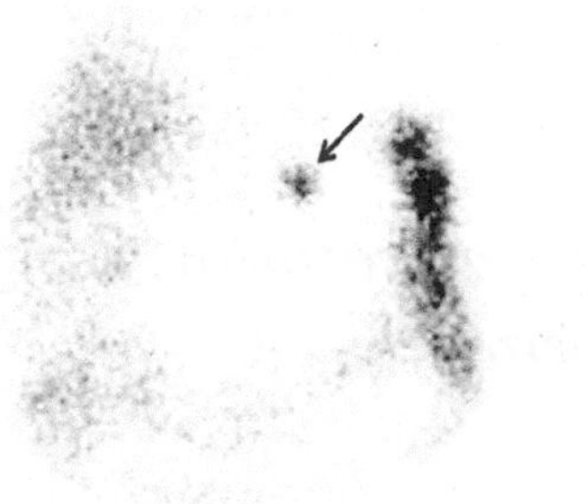

**Figure 10.5**
*Imaging with NP-59 showing exclusive unilateral uptake of the radiotracer by a left adrenal adenoma (arrow).*

small homogenous adrenal lesions characterized by an unenhanced HU value <10.

The preferred screening test with optimal sensitivity is the measurement of fractionated metanephrines in urine or plasma.[24]

### Aldosterone

Screening for primary hyperaldosteronism is recommended in hypertensive patients with adrenal incidentalomas, due to the high prevalence of this disorder in this particular group.[25] In a study of 269 patients with adrenal incidentaloma, 14 of the 169 patients with hypertension had increased aldosterone-to-plasma renin activity ratio and elevated aldosterone levels, and further testing confirmed primary hyperaldosteronism in 4%.[26] In the same study, hyperaldosteronism was not found in any of the patients without hypertension, so screening for hyperaldosteronism in patients without hypertension is not routinely advocated. It should be noted that hypokalemia is not an outcome for the diagnosis because most patients with confirmed hyperaldosteronism are normokalemic.[25] The currently recommended screening test is the aldosterone-to-renin ratio (ARR). Antihypertensive medications that markedly affect the ARR, such as spironolactone, eplerenone, amiloride, triamterene, and potassium-wasting diuretics, should be discontinued for at least 4 weeks. Other interfering medications, such as β-adrenergic blockers, angiotensin-converting enzyme inhibitors, angiotensin receptor blockers, central α-2-agonists, renin inhibitors, dihydropyridine calcium channel blockers, and nonsteroidal anti-inflammatory drugs, may also need to be discontinued for at least 2 weeks. Blood pressure should be managed with medications known to have minimal effects on ARR (verapamil, hydralazine, doxazosin, prazosin, terazosin).[25] Blood collection should be performed with the patient in the upright position for at least 1 h and then seated for 5–15 min. Caution should be taken to ensure proper handling of the samples, depending on the assay used for determination of renin.[25,27] The finding of an abnormal ARR should be followed by further confirmatory testing. Confirmatory tests are saline infusion, captopril challenge, oral sodium loading, and fludrocortisone suppression tests.[28]

### *Cortisol*

Autonomous cortisol secretion is the most prevalent biochemical, albeit clinically silent, disorder among patients with adrenal incidentalomas, and in the recent guidelines of the Endocrine Society, routine biochemical testing for its detection has been recommended.[29] The optimal test however remains debatable. The diagnostic tests that are currently recommended are the same that are used for the diagnosis of overt Cushing's syndrome: increased midnight serum or salivary cortisol levels, increased urinary free cortisol levels and nonsuppression of cortisol levels after dexamethasone administration. The most widely used and easy-to-perform test, even in an outpatient basis, is the 1 mg overnight dexamethasone suppression test (DST). In patients with adrenal incidentalomas, cortisol levels above the traditionally recommended cutoff of 138 nmol/L (5 μg/dL) have a low sensitivity for the detection of hypercortisolism, whereas the use of a lower cutoff of 50 nmol/L (1.8 μg/dL) increases the sensitivity, making it more appropriate as a screening test,[29] but decreases the specificity.[30] A test that is likely to be more appropriate is the standard 48 h, 2 mg/day DST (low-dose dexamethasone suppression test, LDDST). It involves administration of higher doses of dexamethasone, aiming to fully suppress pituitary adrenocorticotropic hormone (ACTH) levels, resulting in a much better specificity.[31] After dexamethasone administration, a wide range of cortisol levels, from undetectable to >138 nmol/L (5 μg/dL), is obtained,[31] and this value demonstrates not only a qualitative defect but also a quantitative measure of the degree of non–ACTH-dependent residual cortisol production by the adenoma.[2] Cortisol levels post-LDDST correlate well with other indices of cortisol excess, namely higher midnight cortisol levels and lower ACTH and dehydroepiandrosterone sulfate (DHEA-S) levels, and also with the size of the adenoma.[32] The most commonly used cutoff is 50 nmol/L (1.8 μg/dL), but the optimal cutoff of this test for the diagnosis of subclinical hypercortisolism remains debatable.[30,33]

Most clinicians currently recommend an additional positive test to support the diagnosis of subclinical hypercortisolism, including an elevated midnight cortisol level or 24 h urinary free cortisol level and/or a low ACTH level.[30] Inappropriately high midnight cortisol levels are commonly observed in patients with adrenal incidentalomas. Although the measurement of late-night salivary cortisol is a recommended approach to screen for Cushing syndrome,[29] its utility in the diagnosis of subclinical hypercortisolism has been questioned.[34] Urinary free cortisol is considered a rather insensitive test in this specific population and carries many technical and diagnostic pitfalls.[29] Measurements of ACTH and DHEA-S levels are of some value in these patients because low values indicate adrenal cortisol autonomy.[29]

To summarize, most experts recommend the DST as a prerequisite for the demonstration of cortisol autonomy, followed by additional tests to consolidate the diagnosis.[29] However, so far no consensus on the best cutoff value for the DST exists.

## *Benign adrenocortical adenomas*

The majority of coincidental adrenal masses demonstrate an imaging phenotype consistent with a benign adrenocortical adenoma. Current trends in the management of these apparently benign tumors depend on our understanding about the natural history and the possible implications relevant to their hormonal secretory activity.

## Natural history

Two main issues have been addressed in the few available long-term observational studies regarding the natural history of lesions consistent with benign adrenocortical adenomas: whether a lesion initially classified as benign can harbor malignancy and whether overt Cushing's syndrome can develop during follow-up. So far, the evidence suggests an extremely low rate of malignant transformation of less than 1 out of 1000.[7,8,35,36] A significant proportion, however, ranging from 5% to 20%, may show a >1 cm increase in size and/or appearance of another lesion in the contralateral gland.[8,35–37] In addition, decrease in size or even disappearance of the mass may be occasionally seen.

The appearance of hormonal hypersecretion in the form of catecholamine or aldosterone excess with time is extremely unusual.[5] Progression to overt Cushing's syndrome is also encountered in <1% of cases.[5] New development or worsening of preexisting subclinical autonomous cortisol secretion may occur in up to 11% and is usually associated with an increase in the size of the lesion. Larger lesions and those with a prevalent scintigraphic pattern are more prone to display cortisol secretion alterations with time.[8] Although this usually happens within the first 4 years of follow-up, it may occur even later.[8] In many patients, however, repeat endocrine tests may be inconsistent, and intermittent cortisol secretion with spontaneous normalization has been documented in many patients.[38]

## Clinical implications

Several studies have reported a clustering of disorders such as hypertension, central obesity, impaired glucose tolerance, or diabetes and dyslipidemia, conditions associated with increased insulin resistance and cardiovascular risk, in patients with adrenal incidentalomas harboring a benign imaging phenotype.[5,30,39] As a matter of fact, in the first description of adrenal nodules that was made in 1889 in an autopsy study by Letulle,[40] it was noted that adrenal nodules were more prevalent in those who had died from cardiovascular disease. Given that these features are common in patients with overt Cushing's syndrome, it has been hypothesized that even subtle cortisol autonomy exhibited by many adrenal incidentalomas may underlie the increased prevalence of metabolic disorders. Several studies have shown this association, but what is more intriguing is the fact that even patients without biochemical evidence of subclinical hypercortisolism also have an unfavorable metabolic phenotype. In a study by Garrapa et al.,[41] the body composition and metabolic profile in patients with adrenal nodules and no evidence of cortisol autonomy were intermediate between normal controls and patients with overt Cushing's syndrome. Besides metabolic disorders, osteoporosis and more importantly the incidence of new vertebral fractures is considerably increased in patients with incidentally discovered benign adrenal adenomas, especially those with biochemical evidence of subclinical hypercortisolism.[42] Even though most studies agree that there exists an increased prevalence of metabolic disorders in patients with adrenal incidentalomas, it remains unknown whether this chronic exposure to even subtle glucocorticoid excess affects mortality. Data from small studies with relatively short follow-up focusing mainly on the potential for malignant transformation or progression to overt Cushing's syndrome suggest that the main cause of death in such patients is cardiovascular disease. However, mortality has not been addressed as the main outcome in any of the studies so far and has not been compared with that of the general population.

## Management

Currently, there are no straightforward and widely accepted guidelines regarding the management of patients with incidentally discovered apparently benign adrenocortical adenomas.[2] Surgery is the treatment of choice in case of large (>4–6 cm) lesions, those significantly increasing in size, or those with suspicious imaging characteristics. However, it remains debatable whether surgery is more beneficial compared with the most commonly adopted conservative approach in patients with radiologically benign lesions and subclinical hypercortisolism. The desired benefit of reversing subclinical hypercortisolism would be to improve the associated metabolic disorders and, optimistically, decrease the cardiovascular risk.[7] Although in all studies surgery fully restores the preoperative endocrine abnormalities in all patients,[2] improvement of metabolic parameters is not universal. Blood pressure has been consistently shown to improve, as well as glucose metabolism or insulin sensitivity, but changes in body weight and lipids are heterogeneous. Notably, improvement is also seen in patients operated on the basis of tumor size without biochemical evidence of subclinical hypercortisolism.[2] Most of the available data, however, come from small retrospective uncontrolled studies. In the few studies that included a conservatively managed control group, including one prospective randomized study, worsening of the metabolic profile was noted in the nonoperated patients.[2,39,43,44] However, medical management in the observational groups was not standardized in any of these studies. Moreover, all studies focused on metabolic parameters, whereas outcome of other symptoms including proximal myopathy, fatigue, or cognitive impairment has not been systematically addressed. Overall, the existing studies have several limitations, providing inconclusive evidence that should be interpreted with caution having in view that even laparoscopic adrenalectomy carries significant risks with a complication rate of 9% and a low albeit existing mortality rate of 0.2%.[13] Until there is more evidence, most published recommendations adopt a practical approach, offering surgery to younger patients with clear biochemical evidence of autonomous cortisol secretion, especially those with recently developed or worsening metabolic or bone disease[39] (Figure 10.6).

# Adrenocortical carcinoma

ACC is a rare malignancy with an estimated incidence of 1–2 per million population per year[45] and follows a bimodal age distribution, with peaks in early childhood and in the fourth to fifth decades of life.[45] Women are more often affected than men (1.5:1), and tumor aggressiveness is higher in adults than in children.[46] Interestingly, an increased occurrence of ACCs has been reported on the left side rather than the right side of the body.[47] Most cases are of sporadic origin; however, some occur as part of hereditary cancer predisposition syndromes.[48] ACC also has been identified in patients with Carney complex.[49,50]

## Pathogenesis

The rare genetic syndromes associated with ACC (Table 10.2) have offered a great opportunity to understand the molecular genetics of this disease. Gene defects observed in germline DNA of hereditary syndromes have also been identified in somatic DNA in sporadic cases.[51] Several chromosomal alterations are identified by comparative genomic hybridization in ACC; interestingly, a positive correlation between the size of the tumor and the number of chromosomal alterations has been demonstrated.[52]

### TP53

*TP53* is a tumor suppressor gene involved in cell proliferation, located at 17p13, and plays a role in ACC pathogenesis. Germline mutations characterized most families with Li–Fraumeni syndrome that present susceptibility to breast cancer, soft tissue sarcoma, osteosarcoma, brain tumors, leukemia, and ACC.[53] A germline mutation in exon 10 of the TP53 gene has been found in almost all pediatric ACCs in southern Brazil, where the incidence of the disease is 10-fold higher than in the rest of the

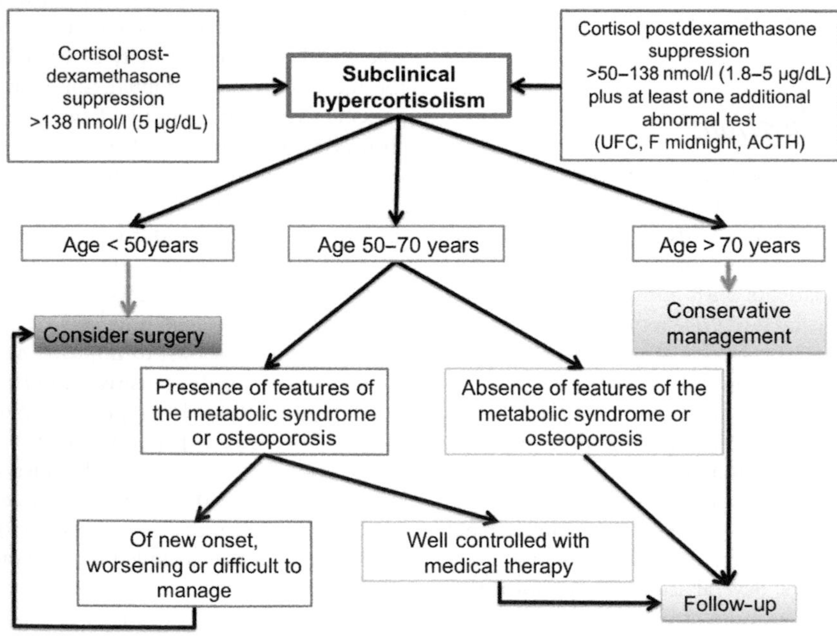


**Figure 10.6**
*Approach to a patient with subclinical hypercortisolism.*

| Genetic syndrome | Gene | Location | Manifestations |
|---|---|---|---|
| Li–Fraumeni | *TP53* | 17p13 | Soft tissue sarcoma, breast cancer, brain tumors, leukemia, ACC |
| Beckwith–Wiedemann | *CDKN1C; IGF-2; H19* | 11p15 | Omphalocele, macroglossia, macrosomia, Wilms tumor |
| MEN1 | *menin* | 11q13 | Parathyroid, pituitary, pancreas tumors, adrenal adenomas, rarely ACC |
| Carney complex | *PRKAR1A* | 17q22-24 | Myxomas, testicular neoplasms, primary pigmented nodular adrenocortical disease (PPNAD), pituitary tumors, thyroid cancer |

**Table 10.2**
*Genetic syndromes with ACC.*

world;[54] other germline mutations of this gene were demonstrated in 50%–80% of children with apparently sporadic ACC.[55] Somatic *TP53* mutations are found in up to 70% of ACCs,[56] and loss of heterozygosity (LOH) at 17p13 is a common finding. Thus, LOH at 17p13 has been proposed as a molecular marker of malignancy in adrenal tumors. Interestingly, 17p13 LOH correlates with Weiss score, and tumors with 17p13 LOH are more susceptible to recurrence after surgery.[57]

### *Insulin-like growth factor-II*

Insulin-like growth factor II (IGF-II) is overexpressed in approximately 90% of ACCs.[57,58] The underlying mechanism is paternal isodisomy (loss of the maternal allele and duplication of the paternal allele) of the 11p15 region where the IGF-II gene is located. The 11p15 paternal isodisomy correlates with the Weiss score and a higher risk of tumor recurrence.[57]

Various other growth factors that regulate growth and function of normal adrenal are also overexpressed in ACC. Thus, vascular endothelial growth factor (VEGF)[58] and epidermal growth factor receptor (EGFR)[59] are overexpressed in ACC compared with adrenal adenomas, but the clinical significance of these findings is not validated so far.

### *Steroidogenic factor 1*

Steroidogenic factor 1 (SF-1) is a transcription factor expressed primarily in the steroidogenic organs and plays a key role in their development.[60] SF1 overexpression has been found[61] in most cases of childhood onset but also in many cases of adult onset ACCs.[62] Interestingly, strong SF-1 protein expression in the tumor significantly correlates with a poor clinical outcome.[63]

### *Wnt-β-catenin*

The protein β-catenin stimulates and/or maintains proliferation of adrenal cortical cells during embryonic development and is required for cell renewal in the adult adrenal cortex.[64] The Wnt-β-catenin signaling pathway is involved in the pathogenesis of a variety of cancers. Mutations of β-catenin (*CTNNB1*) that lead to constitutive activations of the protein are found in 15%–27% of adrenocortical adenomas and in up to 31% of ACC.[65]

### *Transcriptome analysis*

Quantification of gene expression (transcriptome) of adrenocortical tumors is made possible by modern molecular biology techniques.[66] Such a tissue-specific transcriptome signature might help discriminate between benign adenomas and ACC because a large number of genes are differentially expressed in benign versus malignant tumors, and between primary and secondary adrenal cancer. Adrenal-specific malignancy signature includes growth factor pathways, such as the insulin-like growth factor (IGF)-II and fibroblast growth factor receptor (FGFR) 1 and 4. Using transcriptome analysis, two different groups of ACCs in terms of overall survival were identified.[67] The group with worse prognosis overexpresses many transcription factors, whereas the group with better prognosis expresses genes involved in cell metabolism, apoptosis, and cell differentiation. These data may lead to a development of a molecular predictor of prognosis for ACC.[66]

### *Gene methylation*

Several epigenetic alterations of DNA, which modify gene expression without altering gene sequence, are present in ACC tissues. Data suggest that gene methylation status may be an important regulator of gene expression in ACC.[68] Interestingly, studies of the whole genome demonstrated that hypermethylation of genomic regions rich to CpG dinucleotides, usually found in the promoter of genes, is associated with worse prognosis in ACC patients.[69] Further confirmation of these results will expand our understanding of the molecular mechanisms involved in the pathogenesis of ACC, and they will also offer an additional marker of disease aggressiveness.[70]

## Clinical presentation

More than 60% of patients with ACC seek medical advice because of symptoms and signs of Cushing's syndrome.[71] Cushing's syndrome develops over a few months, and usually, due to the rapid onset of hypercortisolism, profound muscle atrophy, severe hypertension, hypokalemia, and diabetes mellitus are prominent features. In women, signs and symptoms of androgen excess (acne, hirsutism, menstrual abnormalities) and virilization coexist, depending on the secretory potential of the tumor. Excess androgens can counteract the catabolic effects of hypercortisolemia.[72] Rarely, ACC with mineralocorticoid excess leads to severe hypertension and hypokalemia.[73] In the exceptional case of estrogen secretion, gynecomastia in men and excessive uterine bleeding in women can be provoked.[71,73] As mentioned, IGF-II is frequently overexpressed in ACCs, and its release from the tumor may occasionally result in hypoglycemia.[73] In about 40%, the ACCs are nonsecretory or they secrete biologically inactive precursors (such as 17OH-progesterone). These tumors are discovered by symptoms of mass effect (local discomfort, retroperitoneal hemorrhage). A substantial and increasing proportion of nonsecretory ACCs are discovered incidentally during abdominal imaging studies.[74] Interestingly, the revealed pattern of predominantly immature, early-stage steroidogenesis in ACC implies that the study of urine steroid metabolites (metabolomics) may provide a novel, highly sensitive, and specific biomarker tool for discriminating benign from malignant adrenal tumors.[75]

## Diagnostic evaluation and staging of ACCs

The European Network for the Study of Adrenal Tumors (ENSAT) recommends a comprehensive diagnostic hormonal and imaging evaluation in all patients with suspected or confirmed ACC (Table 10.3).[76]

### Imaging studies

The CT and MRI imaging phenotype of a malignant adrenal mass have been extensively described in a previous session. ACCs commonly metastasize in the liver, lung, and bones. Complementary radiological evaluation is required to exclude dissemination of the disease at these sites. $^{18}$F-FDG PET, besides its differentiating role between malignant and benign lesions, also provides accurate staging in a single-imaging modality because it also reveals distant tumor spread in case of metastases[17,18] (Figure 10.7). However, small metastatic lesions may occasionally be missed.[77] An important clinical scenario of false-positive $^{18}$F-FDG PET scan has been recently pointed out;[78] 14%–29% of patients followed up for ACC may show transient FDG uptake in the remaining adrenal gland for up to 24 months after adrenalectomy and onset of o',p'-DDD treatment. This uptake is hypothesized to be related to a trophic adrenal effect of ACTH levels that show a compensatory increase upon initiation of the adrenolytic o',p'-DDD.[78]

### Histopathology

Pathological diagnosis of ACC is essential both to differentiate between adenoma and carcinoma and to predict disease outcome. It is based on several morphological criteria and requires evaluation by an experienced pathologist. The most widely used Weiss score[79] (Table 10.4) is graded from 0 to 9 according to the presence or absence of the following histological features: (i) high mitotic rate, (ii) atypical mitoses, (iii) high nuclear grade, (iv) low percentage of clear cells, (v) necrosis, (vi) diffuse architecture of tumor, (vii) capsular invasion, (viii) sinusoidal invasion, and (ix) venous invasion. A score >3 indicates a malignant tumor.[79] The expression of several potential discriminatory markers between adenoma and carcinoma, such as Ki-67 of p53, IGF-II, and cyclin E has also been applied with limited efficacy.[46,71,72]

Several criteria have been used to predict outcome of ACC. Worse outcome is characterized by high mitotic rate (>20 mitoses per 40 high-power field [HPF])[79] and a high Ki-67 index.[71,80] The predictive value of SF-1 has been confirmed; strong SF-1 protein expression significantly correlated with poor clinical outcome in a large cohort study on tissue samples from 167 ACCs.[63] The extent of surgical resection and the status of tumor capsule must be reported because they

| *Diagnostic workup Hormonal evaluation* | *Treatment* |
|---|---|
| Glucocorticoid excess (minimum 3 of 4 tests) | • Dexamethasone suppression test (1 mg, 2300 hours)<br>• Excretion of free urinary cortisol (24-h urine)<br>• Basal cortisol (serum)<br>• Basal ACTH (plasma) |
| Sex steroids and steroid precursors | • DHEA-S (serum)<br>• 17-OH-Progesterone (serum)<br>• Androstenedione (serum)<br>• Testosterone (serum)<br>• 17-β-Estradiol (serum, only in men and postmenopausal women) |
| Mineralocorticoid excess | • Potassium (serum)<br>• Aldosterone/renin ratio (only in patients with arterial hypertension and/or hypokalemia) |
| Exclusion of a pheochromocytoma | • Catecholamine or metanephrine excretion (24 h urine)<br>• Metanephrines and normetanephrines (plasma) |
| Imaging studies | • CT or MRI of abdomen and CT thorax<br>• Bone scintigraphy (when suspecting skeletal metastases)<br>• FDG-PET (optional) |
| Follow-up | • CT or MRI of abdomen and CT thorax every 2–3 months (depending on treatment) |

*Source:* European Network for the Study of Adrenal Tumors 2010. Available from: http://www.ensat.org/ with permission.

***Table 10.3***
*Recommendations of the diagnostic workup in patients with suspected or proven ACC.*

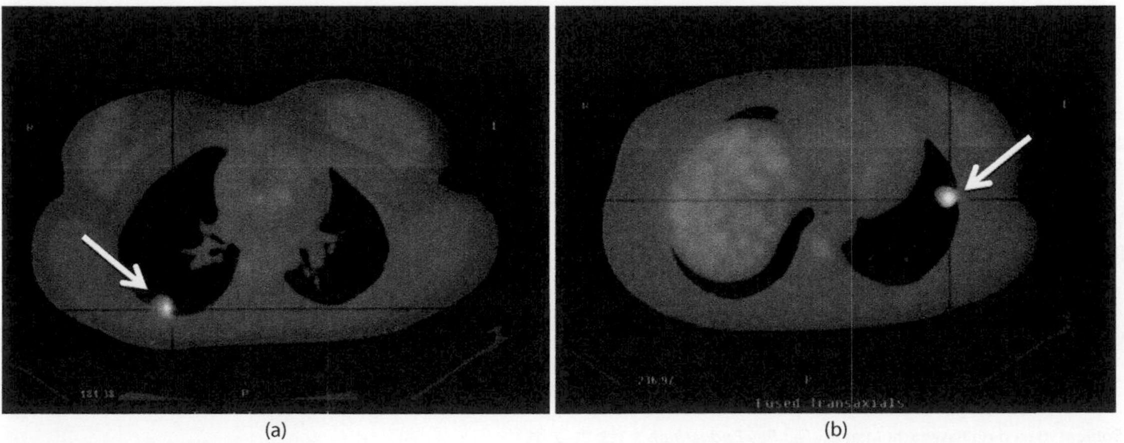

(a) (b)

***Figure 10.7***
*$^{18}$F-FDG PET in a patient with adrenocortical carcinoma: There are two lung nodules exhibiting high radiotracer uptake, consistent with metastases in the (a) right (arrow) and (b) left lung (arrow).*

both are major predictors of the disease outcome.[71] Finally, studies of cell regulatory genes expression (such as *DGL7* that is increased in aggressive ACC, and *PINK1* that is decreased in most aggressive ACCs) are promising and may lead to the development of useful molecular prognostic markers when validated with clinical data.[67]

### Staging

Staging is essential for the treatment of ACC as it allows stratification of the patients and predicts prognosis. At present, the ENSAT staging system (Table 10.5)[71,81] offers the best prognostic potential. Analysis of survival data of the German ACC cohort[81] revealed that patients without distant metastases had an improved survival compared with patients who had metastatic disease. Therefore, stage IV is restricted to patients with distant metastases, and stage III included patients with tumor invasion in adjacent organs or infiltration in surrounding tissue because they both express similar mortality ratio.[81] According to the study of North America ACC cohort, the ENSAT staging system showed higher accuracy (83.0%) in predicting 3-year mortality rates, relative to the 2004 Union International Contre le Cancer staging system (79.5%).[82]

## Treatment of ACC

The choice of treatment for ACC depends largely on the presumed staging of the patient at the time of diagnosis (Figure 10.8). Patients with stage I or II

| *Histological criteria* | *Score grade 0* | *Score grade 1* |
|---|---|---|
| Mitotic rate | ≤5 per 50 HPF | ≥6 per 50 HPR:1 |
| Atypical mitoses | Absent | Present |
| High nuclear grade | 1 and 2 | 3 and 4 |
| Percentage of clear cells | >25 | ≤25 |
| Necrosis | Absent | Present |
| Diffuse architecture of tumor | ≤33% of surface | >33% of surface |
| Capsular invasion | Absent | Present |
| Sinusoidal invasion | Absent | Present |
| Venous invasion | Absent | Present |

**Table 10.4**
*Weiss histopathological criteria for the diagnosis of ACC.*

| *Stage* | *Size* | *Lymph nodes* | *Local invasion* | *Metastases* | *TNM* | *5-year disease-free survival (%)* |
|---|---|---|---|---|---|---|
| I | <5 cm | No | No | No | T1, N0, M0 | 82 |
| II | >5 cm | No | No | No | T2, N0, M0 | 51 |
| III | Any | No/yes | Yes | No | T1–2, N1, M0; T3–4, N0–1, M0 | 60 |
| IV | Any | No/yes | No/yes | Yes | T1–4, N0–1, M1 | 13 |

*Source:* Based on Fassnacht M et al., *Nat Rev Endocrinol*, 7, 323–35, 2011.

**Table 10.5**
*ENSAT staging system for ACC.*

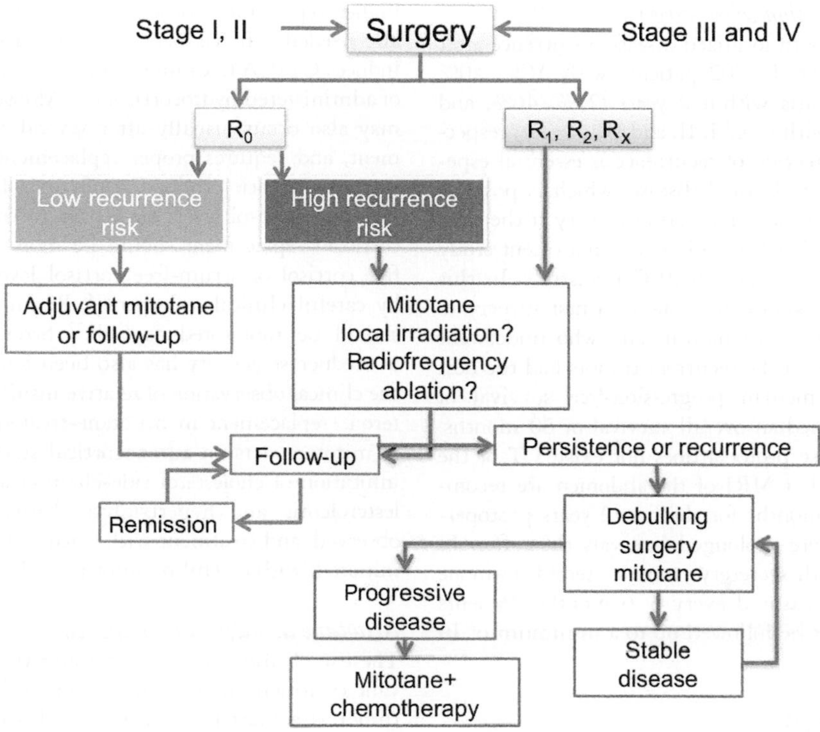


***Figure 10.8***
*Treatment algorithm for adrenocortical carcinoma. $R_0$, complete surgical resection; $R_1$, microscopic residual tumor; $R_2$, macroscopic residual tumor; $R_x$, unknown resection status.*

will be offered surgery as first-line treatment. If complete resection is achieved, recurrence risk must be assessed according to staging, histology features, and tumor markers, and adjuvant mitotane therapy needs to be considered. Low risk of recurrence is characterized by Ki-67 <10%, fewer than five mitoses per 50 HPF, tumor size <8 cm, and no microscopic evidence of invasion of blood vessels or tumor capsule.[71] If residual tumor is detected postsurgery, local treatment modalities such as reoperation, radiofrequency ablation, or irradiation should be considered.[71,72,83] In patients with advanced disease (stage III and IV) at the time of initial diagnosis, complete surgical resection is not usually achievable. In secreting tumors, partial resection (debulking) may help to control the clinical symptoms, offering thus a better performance status for systematic therapy (mitotane and/or chemotherapy); however, the final effect on survival is questionable.[46,83] Similarly, in patients with recurrent disease, reoperation is an option, depending upon the clinical status of the patient and the site of recurrence, the aim being to remove as much as possible of the malignant tissue. The approach for patients with recurrent ACC is similar to the patients with advanced disease.[71,72,83]

## *Surgery*

Surgery offers both the possibilities of complete cure and definite diagnosis with staging of the disease, which is an essential predictor of patient's outcome. Complete surgical resection with clear margins leads to a 5-year survival of 40%–50%, whereas patients with incomplete resection have a median survival <1 year.[84] It is important that all patients with clinical, biochemical, and imaging characteristics of malignancy must be referred to experienced surgeons with a volume of at least >20 adrenalectomies per year.[71] The role of laparoscopic surgery for malignant adrenal tumors is controversial. Although a worse outcome has been reported when laparoscopic approach was used,[46,83] recent data demonstrated similar results of laparoscopic vs open adrenalectomy performed by experienced surgeons for localized tumors <10 cm.[85] As most of the patients with ACC have cortisol hypersecretion from the tumor[71] they require peri- and postoperative glucocorticoid cover to avoid adrenal insufficiency that may occur after complete tumor removal.

### Follow-up evaluation after surgery

Even in patients with localized disease, recurrence after surgery is frequent. In 202 patients with ACC, 40% developed metastasis within 2 years (27%, 46%, and 63% of patients with stage I, II, and III disease, respectively).[74] Early detection of recurrence is essential especially in the case of limited disease, which is possibly amenable to reoperation. The role of surgery at the time of first recurrence has been addressed in a recent study in patients from the German ACC Registry.[86] In this study, patients in whom the time from first surgery to first recurrence was >12 months and who underwent complete resection of the recurrent tumors had the best prognosis, with median progression-free survival of 24 months and median overall survival of 60 months. Although a precise protocol does not exist, CT of the chest and CT and/or MRI of the abdomen are recommended every 3 months for the first 2 years postoperatively and in more prolonged intervals thereafter. In those patients with secretory tumors, steroid hormone levels must be measured every 3–6 months. Patients in remission must be followed up to a minimum of 10 years.[71,72,83]

## Mitotane therapy

Mitotane (o,p-DDD) is an adrenolytic drug with a well-known efficacy in ACC, controlling both hormonal hypersecretion and tumor growth.[73] This drug acts by inhibition of cholesterol side-chain cleavage (human cytochrome P450, cholesterol desmolase, or 20,22 desmolase) and 11β-hydroxylase (P450 11β or CYP11β1).[87] At initiation of therapy, adipose tissue accumulation delays achievement of therapeutic serum levels for 12–14 weeks. Conversely, after discontinuation of mitotane, its slow release from adipose tissue results in measurable serum levels for months.[88] After initiation of treatment, mitotane levels should be monitored at 4–8-week intervals until therapeutic levels are reached and subsequently every 3 months.[89] As body stores saturate, lower doses are needed. In patients who receive long-term therapy, mitotane doses should be adjusted every 4–8 weeks on the basis of serum levels until a stable level on a stable dose is achieved with tolerable adverse effects.[90]

Unfortunately, mitotane effectiveness is limited by its side effects (Table 10.6) that include gastrointestinal toxicity (anorexia, nausea, vomiting, and diarrhea), and neuromuscular manifestations and skin rash may appear. Occasionally, side effects are attributed to the inhibition of glucocorticoid secretion, and hydrocortisone replacement should always be administered in patients receiving mitotane treatment. As the drug increases the clearance of exogenously administered hydrocortisone, higher replacement doses (two- to threefold) are usually needed.[91] It has been demonstrated that mitotane induces CYP3A4, leading to rapid inactivation of >50% of administered hydrocortisone.[92] Aldosterone deficiency may also occur, usually after several months of treatment, and requires proper replacement.[72] As mitotane increases hepatic production of cortisol binding globulin, total cortisol levels are falsely increased and glucocorticoid replacement should be monitored by urinary free cortisol or serum-free cortisol levels[93] and mainly by careful clinical judgment.[90] Renin and electrolytes should be monitored as well.[72] Strong inhibition of 5α-reductase activity has also been found, in line with the clinical observation of relative insufficiency of testosterone replacement in mitotane-treated men.[92] Finally, as mitotane acts on adrenocortical steroid synthesis by inhibition of cholesterol side-chain cleavage, hypercholesterolemia and hypertriglyceridemia are commonly observed, and treatment with statins or fibrates must be initiated, with careful monitoring of hepatic function.

### Mitotane as adjuvant treatment

The use of mitotane in stage I and II patients as adjuvant treatment after complete removal of a malignant tumor is a matter of controversy because randomized controlled studies do not exist. A retrospective study of 177 ACC patients in 8 Italian and 47 German centers demonstrated that the group on adjuvant mitotane had a better outcome in terms of disease-free survival and deaths.[94] Therefore, most specialists recommend adjuvant mitotane either to every patient with ACC[72] or to those at higher risk of recurrence, based on size of initial tumor, presence of vascular invasion, and Ki-67 >10%.[46] The recommended mitotane dose for adjuvant therapy is 0.5 g twice daily with meals with gradual increase to reach a final dose of 2 g/day within 2 weeks with a target of 14–20 μg/mL.[72] The duration of adjuvant mitotane treatment in most centers is between 2 and 5 years.[72,83]

### Mitotane treatment in advanced ACC

In patients with advanced ACC, the recommended first-line treatment regimen is mitotane alone or in combination with chemotherapeutic agents, depending on the growth velocity of the tumor and the experience and preference of the treating center. Mitotane control of hormonal hypersecretion is reported in 75% and tumor regression in 30%.[46,72,74,95] Effectiveness is correlated with serum mitotane levels, and toxicity is more common with levels >20 μg/mL.[95] Therapeutic levels are 14–20 μg/mL.[96] A protocol by Fassnacht et al.[71] proposes to start with 1.5 g daily and increase the dose within 4–6 days to 6.0 g/day, depending on

| Toxicity/manifestation | Side effects |
|---|---|
| Gastrointestinal | Anorexia, nausea, vomiting, diarrhea |
| Neuromuscular | Ataxia, speech disturbance, confusion, somnolence, muscle tremors, vertigo, depression |
| Hepatotoxicity | Abnormalities in liver function tests, hyperbilirubinemia |
| Biochemical | Hypercholesterolemia, hypertriglyceridemia |
| Endocrinological | Increased hepatic production of sex hormone-, thyroxine-, cortisol-, and vitamin D-binding globulins |
| | Increased total hormone levels and impaired free hormone bioavailability |
| | Gynecomastia |
| | Sexual Dysfunction |
| | Reduction in free thyroxine |
| Hematological | Cytopenias, prolongation of bleeding time |
| Renal abnormalities | Hematuria cystitis |
| Other | Skin rash |

***Table 10.6***
*Side effects of mitotane.*

the general health status and tolerability of the patient. After 3 weeks, the dose is adapted according to tolerability and mitotane blood levels. With this regimen, about 50% of patients achieve target levels within 3 months.[71] The maximum mitotane dose in this group of patients is 12 g daily, but most patients do not tolerate doses >8 g. If with the maximum tolerable dose therapeutic levels could not be reached, cytotoxic therapy must be added.[71]

## Treatment of hormonal hypersecretion

Most patients with ACC have symptoms of cortisol or androgen hypersecretion.[71] Mitotane is a potent inhibitor of hormonal production from the adrenal malignant tumor; thus, the use of other drugs is needed only when the tolerable dose of mitotane is not sufficient to control hormonal production.[90] Ketoconazole acts by inhibiting C17-20 desmolase, cholesterol side-chain cleavage, 11β-hydroxylation, and 18-hydroxylation. The initial dose is 200 mg three or four times per day with titration by 400 mg/d every 1–2 days to a final dose of 3600–6400 mg/day.[72] The most common adverse effects are hepatotoxicity, nausea, vomiting, abdominal pain, fever, weakness, hypertension, hypothyroidism, gynecomastia, and hypertriglyceridemia.[90] Frequent monitoring of liver function tests is mandatory; in case of abnormal liver function tests withdrawal or reduction of ketoconazole can normalize them within days to weeks. Ketoconazole can also affect the metabolism and toxicity of chemotherapeutic agents, and it should be discontinued 24–48 h before chemotherapy and resume administration after the end of the treatment.[90] Metyrapone inhibits 11β-hydroxylation in the adrenals and therefore decreases cortisol but increases androgens and steroid precursors such as 11-deoxycortisol. The initial dose is 250 mg two or four times per day, with titration by 0.5–1 g/day every few days to a final dose 4–6 g/day. The most common adverse effects are hypertension (due to increase of 11-deoxycortisol), alopecia, hirsutism, acne (due to increase of androgens), nausea, abdominal discomfort, headache, weakness, and leucopenia. Etomidate is the only parenteral steroidogenesis inhibitor of cholesterol side-chain cleavage (at high doses) and 11-hydroxylase (at lower doses)[97]; its administration is only advocated in an intensive care unit (ICU) setting. The glucocorticoid antagonist mifepristone also was approved for the treatment of intractable glucocorticoid excess.

## Chemotherapy

Systemic chemotherapy in combination with mitotane is used in patients with advanced ACC. So far, the most effective protocol has been proposed by Berruti et al.[98] They demonstrated in a phase II trial of 72 patients that treatment with etopocide, doxorubicin, and cisplatin (EDP) in combination with mitotane led to a complete response of the disease in five patients and partial response in 30 (overall response rate, 49%). The average time to progression in responding patients was 24 months, and surgical resection of residual disease subsequent to chemotherapy led to a more favorable outcome.[98] The combination of mitotane and streptozotocin[99] is less effective; a partial or complete response was found in 36% of patients, and the 2- and 5-year survival rates were 70% and 33%, respectively. The First International Randomized Trial in locally advanced and Metastatic Adrenocortical Cancer Treatment (FIRM-ACT) study has been designed to compare the efficacy of EDP plus mitotane versus streptozotocin plus mitotane as first-line treatment in patients with locally advanced or metastatic disease. The results of this study were published in 2012.[100] Rates of response and progression-free survival were significantly better with EDP plus mitotane than with streptozotocin plus mitotane as first-line therapy. More specifically, the response rate with EDP plus mitotane was 23%, compared with 9.2% in the streptozotocin–mitotane group, and the median progression-free survival was 5.0 months versus 2.1 months, respectively. However, no significant difference in overall survival was noted (14.8 and 12.0 months, respectively). The two regiments showed similar rates of toxic events.[100]

### Radiotherapy

After reviewing the available literature, German ACC experts recommended adjuvant radiotherapy to the tumor bed in patients with ENSAT stage I–III tumors at high risk for local recurrence (incomplete or uncertain/resection status or patients with complete resection but >8 cm in size, invasion of blood vessels, or a Ki-67 index >10%) in addition to mitotane therapy. A total dose of >40 Gy with single fractions of 1.8–2 Gy should be administered.[71,101] However, a retrospective study in 48 patients from the MD Anderson ACC cohort[102] demonstrated that adjuvant radiotherapy did not improve clinical outcomes.[102] In advanced disease, radiotherapy can be used in a palliative setting for symptomatic metastases to bone, brain, or vena cava obstruction.[71,101] However, prospective trials on adjuvant or palliative treatment must be conducted to investigate its effectiveness on final outcome. Equally unknown is the long-term effectiveness of percutaneous radiofrequency ablation. Short-term local control of an unresectable tumor or small metastases (<5 cm in diameter) has been reported with this technique.[103]

### Future therapies

The aggressiveness of advanced ACC and the limited effectiveness of therapies have led to an effort toward the development of novel therapeutic molecules. Because IGF-II is the single highest up regulated transcript in ACC, it offers an obvious target for new drugs development. So far, the most promising results have been shown with IGF-1R antagonists. These molecules cause significant dose-dependent growth inhibition in ACC cell lines. Furthermore, mitotane results in enhanced growth inhibition when used in combination with the IGF-1R antagonists.[104] In a phase I trial with an orally available IGF-1 receptor inhibitor, stabilization of progressive ACC was demonstrated; hyperglycemia was the most common adverse event.[105] Tyrosine kinase inhibitors (TKIs) have been applied in the treatment of endocrine tumors and are currently under phase II trials for advanced ACC.[106] Finally, in a study of 11 patients with advanced ACC, targeted radiation therapy with [$^{131}$I]iodometomidate was used with promising results that have to be further evaluated.[107]

## Summary

Adrenal incidentalomas are lesions discovered coincidentally during abdominal imaging for reasons unrelated to adrenal disease. They are among the most frequently encountered endocrine tumors, with a prevalence of 0.4%–7%. Incidentally discovered lesions cover a wide range of pathologies. Modern imaging techniques can usually distinguish between benign and malignant lesions. The majority (90%–95%) are benign adrenocortical adenomas, with a substantial proportion exhibiting autonomous hormonal hypersecretion. Subclinical hypercortisolism is the most common hormonal abnormality and is associated with features of the metabolic syndrome (hypertension, obesity, glucose intolerance) and an increased risk for osteoporotic fractures. Optimal management of subclinical hypercortisolism remains elusive. Surgery is currently reserved for younger patients with unequivocal evidence of subclinical hypercortisolism and metabolic or bone disease. Adrenocortical carcinomas (ACCs) are rare but extremely aggressive tumors. Most cases are of sporadic origin; however, some occur as part of hereditary cancer predisposition syndromes. They are usually functional (60%), most often secreting cortisol alone (45%) or in combination with androgens (25%). Nonfunctioning ACCs are diagnosed either because of tumor effects (e.g., flank abdominal pain) or as adrenal incidentalomas. Histological confirmation of ACCs may be challenging; the most widely used criterion is the Weiss score. Molecular markers are helpful for risk stratification. Surgery is the treatment of choice. Complete resection offers the best survival rates; however, even in patients with localized disease, recurrence after surgery is frequent. Mitotane (o,p-DDD) is a specific antitumor drug for ACCs, controlling both hormonal hypersecretion and tumor growth. Monitoring mitotane levels is essential to achieve therapeutic levels and avoid side effects. In patients with advanced ACC, systemic chemotherapy in combination with mitotane is used. Adjuvant mitotane therapy, radiotherapy, or both may be used in tumors at high risk for local recurrence. In view of the limited effectiveness of available therapies, there is a great need for ongoing efforts through multicenter studies toward the development of novel therapeutic modalities.

## References


1. Kloos RT, Gross MD, Francis IR, et al. Incidentally discovered adrenal masses. *Endocr Rev* 1995; 16: 460–84.
*2. Vassiliadi DA, Tsagarakis S. Endocrine incidentalomas-challenges imposed by incidentally discovered lesions. *Nat Rev Endocrinol* 2011; 7: 668–80.
3. Vassiliadi DA, Ntali G, Vicha E, et al. High prevalence of subclinical hypercortisolism in patients with bilateral adrenal incidentalomas: A challenge to management. *Clin Endocrinol (Oxf)* 2011; 74: 438–44.
4. Stone JH. Incidentalomas—clinical correlation and translational science required. *N Engl J Med* 2006; 354: 2748–9.
5. Terzolo M, Stigliano A, Chiodini I, et al. AME position statement on adrenal incidentaloma. *Eur J Endocrinol* 2011; 164: 851–70.
6. Ilias I, Sahdev A, Reznek RH, et al. The optimal imaging of adrenal tumours: A comparison of different methods. *Endocr Relat Cancer* 2007; 14: 587–99.
7. Cawood TJ, Hunt PJ, O'Shea D, et al. Recommended evaluation of adrenal incidentalomas is costly, has high false-positive rates and confers a risk of fatal cancer that is similar to the risk of the adrenal lesion becoming malignant; time for a rethink? *Eur J Endocrinol* 2009; 161: 513–27.
8. Barzon L, Sonino N, Fallo F, et al. Prevalence and natural history of adrenal incidentalomas. *Eur J Endocrinol* 2003; 149: 273–85.
9. Frilling A, Tecklenborg K, Weber F, et al. Importance of adrenal incidentaloma in patients with a history of malignancy. *Surgery* 2004; 136: 1289–96.
10. Buurman H, Saeger W. Abnormalities in incidentally removed adrenal glands. *Endocr Pathol* 2006; 17: 277–82.
11. Mantero F, Terzolo M, Arnaldi G, et al. A survey on adrenal incidentaloma in Italy. Study Group on Adrenal Tumors of the Italian Society of Endocrinology. *J Clin Endocrinol Metab* 2000; 85: 637–44.
12. Pantalone KM, Gopan T, Remer EM, et al. Change in adrenal mass size as a predictor of a malignant tumor. *Endocr Pract* 2010; 16: 577–87.
*13. Nieman LK. Approach to the patient with an adrenal incidentaloma. *J Clin Endocrinol Metab* 2010; 95: 4106–13.
14. Gross MD, Shapiro B, Francis IR, et al. Scintigraphic evaluation of clinically silent adrenal masses. *J Nucl Med* 1994; 35: 1145–52.
15. Barzon L, Scaroni C, Sonino N, et al. Incidentally discovered adrenal tumors: Endocrine and scintigraphic correlates. *J Clin Endocrinol Metab* 1998; 83: 55–62.
16. Fagour C, Bardet S, Rohmer V, et al. Usefulness of adrenal scintigraphy in the follow-up of adrenocortical incidentalomas: A prospective multicenter study. *Eur J Endocrinol* 2009; 160: 257–64.
17. Tenenbaum, F, Groussin L, Foehrenbach H, et al. 18F-fluorodeoxyglucose positron emission tomography as a diagnostic tool for malignancy of adrenocortical tumours? Preliminary results in 13 consecutive patients. *Eur J Endocrinol* 2004; 150: 789–92.
18. Maurea, S, Klain M, Mainolfi C, et al. The diagnostic role of radionuclide imaging in evaluation of patients with nonhypersecreting adrenal masses. *J Nucl Med* 2001; 42: 884–92.
19. Groussin L, Bonardel G, Silvera S, et al. 18F-Fluorodeoxyglucose positron emission tomography for the diagnosis of adrenocortical tumors: A prospective study in 77 operated patients. *J Clin Endocrinol Metab* 2009; 94: 1713–22.
20. Yun M, Kim W, Alnafisi N, et al. 18F-FDG PET in characterizing adrenal lesions detected on CT or MRI. *J Nucl Med* 2001; 42: 1795–9.
21. Metser U, Miller E, Lerman H, et al. 18F-FDG PET/CT in the evaluation of adrenal masses. *J Nucl Med* 2006; 47: 32–7.
22. Hahner S, Kreissl MC, Fassnacht M, et al. Functional characterization of adrenal lesions ising [123I]IMTO-SPECT/CT. *J Clin Endocrinol Metab* 2013; 98(4): 1508–18.
23. Sane T, Schalin-Jantti C, Raade M. Is biochemical screening for pheochromocytoma in adrenal incidentalomas expressing low unenhanced attenuation on computed tomography necessary? *J Clin Endocrinol Metab* 2012; 97: 2077–83.
*24. Pacak K, Eisenhofer G, Ahlman H, et al. Pheochromocytoma: Recommendations for clinical practice from the First International Symposium. October 2005. *Nat Clin Pract Endocrinol Metab* 2007; 3: 92–102.
*25. Funder JW, Carey RM, Fardella C, et al. Case detection, diagnosis, and treatment of patients with primary aldosteronism: An endocrine society clinical


* Key or Classic references.

practice guideline. *J Clin Endocrinol Metab* 2008; 93: 3266–81.

26. Vierhapper H. Determination of the aldosterone/renin ratio in 269 patients with adrenal incidentaloma. *Exp Clin Endocrinol Diabetes* 2007; 115: 518–21.
27. Rossi GP. A comprehensive review of the clinical aspects of primary aldosteronism. *Nat Rev Endocrinol* 2011; 7: 485–95.
28. Rossi GP, Seccia TM, Pessina AC. Adrenal gland: A diagnostic algorithm-the holy grail of primary aldosteronism. *Nat Rev Endocrinol* 2011; 7: 697–9.

*29. Nieman LK, Biller BM, Findling JW, et al. The diagnosis of Cushing's syndrome: An Endocrine Society Clinical Practice Guideline. *J Clin Endocrinol Metab* 2008; 93: 1526–40.

30. Tsagarakis S, Vassiliadi D, Thalassinos N. Endogenous subclinical hypercortisolism: Diagnostic uncertainties and clinical implications. *J Endocrinol Invest* 2006; 29: 471–82.
31. Tsagarakis S, Kokkoris P, Roboti C, et al. The low-dose dexamethasone suppression test in patients with adrenal incidentalomas: Comparisons with clinically euadrenal subjects and patients with Cushing's syndrome. *Clin Endocrinol (Oxf)* 1998; 48: 627–33.
32. Tsagarakis S, Roboti C, Kokkoris P, et al. Elevated post-dexamethasone suppression cortisol concentrations correlate with hormonal alterations of the hypothalamo-pituitary adrenal axis in patients with adrenal incidentalomas. *Clin Endocrinol (Oxf)* 1998; 49: 165–71.

*33. Young WF, Jr., Clinical practice. The incidentally discovered adrenal mass. *N Engl J Med* 2007; 356: 601–10.

34. Nunes ML, Vattaut S, Corcuff JB, et al. Late-night salivary cortisol for diagnosis of overt and subclinical Cushing's syndrome in hospitalized and ambulatory patients. *J Clin Endocrinol Metab* 2009; 94: 456–62.
35. Grossrubatscher E, Vignati F, Possa M, et al. The natural history of incidentally discovered adrenocortical adenomas: A retrospective evaluation. *J Endocrinol Invest* 2001; 24: 846–55.
36. Libe R, Dall'Asta C, Barbetta L, et al. Long-term follow-up study of patients with adrenal incidentalomas. *Eur J Endocrinol* 2002; 147: 489–94.
37. Lam KY, Lo CY. Metastatic tumours of the adrenal glands: A 30-year experience in a teaching hospital. *Clin Endocrinol (Oxf)* 2002; 56: 95–101.
38. Vassilatou E, Vryonidou A, Michalopoulou S, et al. Hormonal activity of adrenal incidentalomas: Results from a long-term follow-up study. *Clin Endocrinol (Oxf)* 2009; 70: 674–9.

*39. Terzolo M, Pia A, Reimondo G. Subclinical Cushing's syndrome: Definition and management. *Clin Endocrinol (Oxf)* 2012; 76: 12–18.

40. Letulle M. Note sur la degenerescence graisseuse de la capsule surrenale. *Bull Mem Soc Anat Paris* 1889; 3: 264–7.
41. Garrapa GG, Pantanetti P, Arnaldi G, et al. Body composition and metabolic features in women with adrenal incidentaloma or Cushing's syndrome. *J Clin Endocrinol Metab* 2001; 86: 5301–6.
42. Morelli V, Eller-Vainicher C, Salcuni AS, et al. Risk of new vertebral fractures in patients with adrenal incidentaloma with and without subclinical hypercortisolism: A multicenter longitudinal study. *J Bone Miner Res* 2011; 26: 1816–21.
43. Chiodini I, Morelli V, Salcuni AS, et al. Beneficial metabolic effects of prompt surgical treatment in patients with an adrenal incidentaloma causing biochemical hypercortisolism. *J Clin Endocrinol Metab* 2010; 95: 2736–45.
44. Iacobone M, Citton M, Viel G, et al. Adrenalectomy may improve cardiovascular and metabolic impairment and ameliorate quality of life in patients with adrenal incidentalomas and subclinical Cushing's syndrome. *Surgery* 2012; 152: 991–7.
45. Wajchenberg BL, Albergaria Pereira MA, Medonca BB, et al. Adrenocortical carcinoma: Clinical and laboratory observations. *Cancer* 2000; 88: 711–36.

*46. Fassnacht M, Allolio B. Clinical management of adrenocortical carcinoma. *Best Pract Res Clin Endocrinol Metab* 2009; 23: 273–89.

47. Bilimoria KY, Shen WT, Elaraj D, et al. Adrenocortical carcinoma in the United States: Treatment utilization and prognostic factors. *Cancer* 2008; 113: 3130–6.
48. Soon PS, McDonald KL, Robinson BG, et al. Molecular markers and the pathogenesis of adrenocortical cancer. *Oncologist* 2008; 13: 548–61.
49. Morin E, Mete O, Wasserman JD, et al. Carney complex with adrenal cortical carcinoma. *J Clin Endocrinol Metab* 2012; 97: E202–6.
50. Anselmo J, Medeiros S, Carneiro V, et al. A large family with Carney complex caused by the S147G PRKAR1A mutation shows a unique spectrum of disease including adrenocortical cancer. *J Clin Endocrinol Metab* 2012; 97: 351–9.
51. Libe R, Bertherat J. Molecular genetics of adrenocortical tumours, from familial to sporadic diseases. *Eur J Endocrinol* 2005; 153: 477–87.
52. Sidhu S, Marsh DJ, Theodosopoulos G, et al. Comparative genomic hybridization analysis of adrenocortical tumors. *J Clin Endocrinol Metab* 2002; 87: 3467–74.
53. Hisada M, Garber JE, Fung CY, et al. Multiple primary cancers in families with Li-Fraumeni syndrome. *J Natl Cancer Inst* 1998; 90: 606–11.
54. Ribeiro RC, Sandrini F, Figueiredo B, et al. An inherited p53 mutation that contributes in a tissue-specific

manner to pediatric adrenal cortical carcinoma. *Proc Natl Acad Sci U S A* 2001; 98: 9330–5.
55. Varley JM, McGown G, Thorncroft M, et al. Are there low-penetrance TP53 alleles? evidence from childhood adrenocortical tumors. *Am J Hum Genet* 1999; 65: 995–1006.
56. Barzon L, Chilosi M, Fallo F, et al. Molecular analysis of CDKN1C and TP53 in sporadic adrenal tumors. *Eur J Endocrinol* 2001; 145: 207–12.
57. Gicquel C, Bertagna X, Gaston V, et al. Molecular markers and long-term recurrences in a large cohort of patients with sporadic adrenocortical tumors. *Cancer Res* 2001; 61: 6762–7.
58. de Fraipont F, El Atifi M, Cherradi N, et al. Gene expression profiling of human adrenocortical tumors using complementary deoxyribonucleic acid microarrays identifies several candidate genes as markers of malignancy. *J Clin Endocrinol Metab* 2005; 90: 1819–29.
59. Adam P, Hahner S, Hartmann M, et al. Epidermal growth factor receptor in adrenocortical tumors: Analysis of gene sequence, protein expression and correlation with clinical outcome. *Mod Pathol* 2010; 23: 1596–604.
60. Crawford PA, Sadovsky Y, Milbrandt J. Nuclear receptor steroidogenic factor 1 directs embryonic stem cells toward the steroidogenic lineage. *Mol Cell Biol* 1997; 17: 3997–4006.
61. Figueiredo BC, Cavalli LR, Pianovski MA, et al. Amplification of the steroidogenic factor 1 gene in childhood adrenocortical tumors. *J Clin Endocrinol Metab* 2005; 90: 615–19.
62. Almeida MQ, Soares IC, Ribeiro TC, et al. Steroidogenic factor 1 overexpression and gene amplification are more frequent in adrenocortical tumors from children than from adults. *J Clin Endocrinol Metab* 2010; 95: 1458–62.
63. Sbiera S, Schmull S, Assie G, et al. High diagnostic and prognostic value of steroidogenic factor-1 expression in adrenal tumors. *J Clin Endocrinol Metab* 2010; 95: E161–71.
64. Kim AC, Reuter AL, Zubair M, et al. Targeted disruption of beta-catenin in Sf1-expressing cells impairs development and maintenance of the adrenal cortex. *Development* 2008; 135: 2593–602.
65. Tissier F, Cavard C, Groussin L, et al. Mutations of beta-catenin in adrenocortical tumors: Activation of the Wnt signaling pathway is a frequent event in both benign and malignant adrenocortical tumors. *Cancer Res* 2005; 65: 7622–7.
66. Assie G, Guillaud-Bataille M, Ragazzon B, et al. The pathophysiology, diagnosis and prognosis of adrenocortical tumors revisited by transcriptome analyses. *Trends Endocrinol Metab* 2010; 21: 325–34.
67. de Reynies A, Assie G, Rickman DS, et al. Gene expression profiling reveals a new classification of adrenocortical tumors and identifies molecular predictors of malignancy and survival. *J Clin Oncol* 2009; 27: 1108–15.
68. Rechache NS, Wang Y, Stevenson HS, et al. DNA methylation profiling identifies global methylation differences and markers of adrenocortical tumors. *J Clin Endocrinol Metab* 2012; 97: E1004–13.
69. Barreau O, Assie G, Wilmot-Roussel H, et al. Identification of a CpG island methylator phenotype in adrenocortical carcinomas. *J Clin Endocrinol Metab* 2013; 98: E174–84.
70. Liu-Chittenden Y, Kebebew E. CpG island methylator phenotype in adrenocortical carcinoma: Fact or fiction? *J Clin Endocrinol Metab* 2013; 98: 48–50.
*71. Fassnacht M, Libe R, Kroiss M, et al. Adrenocortical carcinoma: A clinician's update. *Nat Rev Endocrinol* 2011; 7: 323–35.
*72. Lacroix A. Approach to the patient with adrenocortical carcinoma. *J Clin Endocrinol Metab* 2010; 95: 4812–22.
73. Luton JP, Cerdas S, Billaud L, et al. Clinical features of adrenocortical carcinoma, prognostic factors, and the effect of mitotane therapy. *N Engl J Med* 1990; 322: 1195–201.
74. Abiven G, Coste J, Groussin L, et al. Clinical and biological features in the prognosis of adrenocortical cancer: Poor outcome of cortisol-secreting tumors in a series of 202 consecutive patients. *J Clin Endocrinol Metab* 2006; 91: 2650–5.
75. Arlt W, Biehl M, Taylor AE, et al. Urine steroid metabolomics as a biomarker tool for detecting malignancy in adrenal tumors. *J Clin Endocrinol Metab* 2011; 96: 3775–84.
76. European Network for the Study of Adrenal Tumors 2010. (online) http://www.ensat.org
77. Mackie GC, Shulkin BL, Ribeiro RC, et al. Use of [18F]fluorodeoxyglucose positron emission tomography in evaluating locally recurrent and metastatic adrenocortical carcinoma. *J Clin Endocrinol Metab* 2006; 91: 2665–71.
78. Leboulleux S, Deandreis D, Escourrou C, et al. Fluorodesoxyglucose uptake in the remaining adrenal glands during the follow-up of patients with adrenocortical carcinoma: Do not consider it as malignancy. *Eur J Endocrinol* 2010; 164: 89–94.
79. Weiss LM, Medeiros LJ, Vickery AL, Jr., Pathologic features of prognostic significance in adrenocortical carcinoma. *Am J Surg Pathol* 1989; 13: 202–6.
80. Morimoto R, Satoh F, Murakami O, et al. Immunohistochemistry of a proliferation marker Ki67/MIB1 in adrenocortical carcinomas: Ki67/MIB1 labeling index is a predictor for recurrence of adrenocortical carcinomas. *Endocr J* 2008; 55: 49–55.

81. Fassnacht M, Johanssen S, Quinkler M, et al. Limited prognostic value of the 2004 International Union Against Cancer staging classification for adrenocortical carcinoma: Proposal for a revised TNM classification. *Cancer* 2009; 115: 243–50.
82. Lughezzani G, Sun M, Perrotte P, et al. The European Network for the Study of Adrenal Tumors staging system is prognostically superior to the international union against cancer-staging system: A North American validation. *Eur J Cancer* 2010; 46: 713–19.
83. Schteingart DE, Doherty GM, Gauger PG, et al. Management of patients with adrenal cancer: Recommendations of an international consensus conference. *Endocr Relat Cancer* 2005; 12: 667–80.
84. Icard P, Goudet P, Charpenay C, et al. Adrenocortical carcinomas: Surgical trends and results of a 253-patient series from the French Association of Endocrine Surgeons study group. *World J Surg* 2001; 25: 891–7.
85. Porpiglia F, Fiori C, Daffara F, et al. Retrospective evaluation of the outcome of open versus laparoscopic adrenalectomy for stage I and II adrenocortical cancer. *Eur Urol* 2010; 57: 873–8.
86. Erdogan I, Deutschbein T, Jurowich C, et al. The role of surgery in the management of recurrent adrenocortical carcinoma. *J Clin Endocrinol Metab* 2013; 98: 181–91.
87. Young RB, Bryson MJ, Sweat ML, et al. Complexing of DDT and o,p'-DDD with adrenal cytochrome P-450 hydroxylating systems. *J Steroid Biochem* 1973; 4: 585–91.
88. Moolenaar AJ, van Slooten H, van Seters AP, et al. Blood levels of o,p'-DDD following administration in various vehicles after a single dose and during long-term treatment. *Cancer Chemother Pharmacol* 1981; 7: 51–4.
89. Terzolo M, Pia A, Berruti A, et al. Low-dose monitored mitotane treatment achieves the therapeutic range with manageable side effects in patients with adrenocortical cancer. *J Clin Endocrinol Metab* 2000; 85: 2234–8.
90. Veytsman I, Nieman L, Fojo T. Management of endocrine manifestations and the use of mitotane as a chemotherapeutic agent for adrenocortical carcinoma. *J Clin Oncol* 2009; 27: 4619–29.
91. Hague RV, May W, Cullen DR. Hepatic microsomal enzyme induction and adrenal crisis due to o,p'-DDD therapy for metastatic adrenocortical carcinoma. *Clin Endocrinol (Oxf)* 1989; 31: 51–7.
92. Chortis V, Taylor AE, Schneider P, et al. Mitotane therapy in adrenocortical cancer induces CYP3A4 and inhibits 5alpha-reductase, explaining the need for personalized glucocorticoid and androgen replacement. *J Clin Endocrinol Metab* 2013; 98: 161–71.
93. Alexandraki KI, Kaltsas GA, le Roux CW, et al. Assessment of serum-free cortisol levels in patients with adrenocortical carcinoma treated with mitotane: A pilot study. *Clin Endocrinol (Oxf)* 2010; 72: 305–11.
94. Terzolo M, Angeli A, Fassnacht M, et al. Adjuvant mitotane treatment for adrenocortical carcinoma. *N Engl J Med* 2007; 356: 2372–80.
95. Baudin E, Pellegriti G, Bonnay M, et al. Impact of monitoring plasma 1,1-dichlorodiphenildichloroethane (o,p'-DDD) levels on the treatment of patients with adrenocortical carcinoma. *Cancer* 2001; 92: 1385–92.
96. Hermsen IG, Fassnacht M, Terzolo M, et al. Plasma concentrations of o,p'-DDD, o,p'-DDA, and o,p'-DDE as predictors of tumor response to mitotane in adrenocortical carcinoma: Results of a retrospective ENS@T multicenter study. *J Clin Endocrinol Metab* 2011; 96: 1844–51.
97. Lamberts SW, Bons EG, Bruining HA, et al. Differential effects of the imidazole derivatives etomidate, ketoconazole and miconazole and of metyrapone on the secretion of cortisol and its precursors by human adrenocortical cells. *J Pharmacol Exp Ther* 1987; 240: 259–64.
98. Berruti A, Terzolo M, Sperone P, et al. Etoposide, doxorubicin and cisplatin plus mitotane in the treatment of advanced adrenocortical carcinoma: A large prospective phase II trial. *Endocr Relat Cancer* 2005; 12: 657–66.
99. Khan TS, Imam H, Juhlin C, et al. Streptozocin and o,p'-DDD in the treatment of adrenocortical cancer patients: Long-term survival in its adjuvant use. *Ann Oncol* 2000; 11: 1281–7.
100. Fassnacht M, Terzolo M, Allolio B, et al. Combination chemotherapy in advanced adrenocortical carcinoma. *N Engl J Med* 2012; 366: 2189–97.
101. Polat B, Fassnacht M, Pfreundner L, et al. Radiotherapy in adrenocortical carcinoma. *Cancer* 2009; 115: 2816–23.
102. Habra MA, Ejaz S, Feng L, et al. A retrospective cohort analysis of the efficacy of adjuvant radiotherapy after primary surgical resection in patients with adrenocortical carcinoma. *J Clin Endocrinol Metab* 2013; 98: 192–7.
103. Wood BJ, Abraham J, Hvizda JL, et al. Radiofrequency ablation of adrenal tumors and adrenocortical carcinoma metastases. *Cancer* 2003; 97: 554–60.
104. Barlaskar FM, Spalding AC, Heaton JH, et al. Preclinical targeting of the type I insulin-like growth factor receptor in adrenocortical carcinoma. *J Clin Endocrinol Metab* 2009; 94: 204–12.
105. Haluska P, Worden F, Olmos D, et al. Safety, tolerability, and pharmacokinetics of the anti-IGF-1R monoclonal antibody figitumumab in patients with refractory adrenocortical carcinoma. *Cancer Chemother Pharmacol* 2010; 65: 765–73.
106. Ye L, Santarpia L, Gagel RF. The evolving field of tyrosine kinase inhibitors in the treatment of endocrine tumors. *Endocr Rev* 2010; 31: 578–99.
107. Hahner S, Kreissl MC, Fassnacht M, et al. [131I] Iodometomidate for targeted radionuclide therapy of advanced adrenocortical carcinoma. *J Clin Endocrinol Metab* 2012; 97(3): 914–22.

# 11

# Disorders of calcium regulation

*Dolores Shoback*

## *Introduction*

This chapter summarizes the development of the calcium-sensing receptor (CaSR) as a molecular mechanism responsible for parathyroid cell $Ca^{2+}$ sensing and for extracellular $Ca^{2+}$-regulated renal $Ca^{2+}$ excretion. The CaSR is acknowledged as the prime regulator of parathyroid hormone (PTH) secretion and parathyroid cell proliferation, although it is appreciated that 1,25-dihydroxyvitamin D and fibroblast growth factor 23(FGF23) also regulate PTH secretion and biosynthesis. Genetic disorders of CaSR function include familial benign hypercalcemia, neonatal severe primary hyperparathyroidism (HPTH), and autosomal dominant hypocalcemia. Primary HPTH is associated with reduced CaSR mRNA and protein expression, thereby underscoring blunted $Ca^{2+}$ sensing as an underlying pathogenic feature of this condition also. The differential diagnosis of hypercalcemia is broad, and the evaluation requires careful laboratory testing. Hypocalcemia, although far less common, requires a thorough clinical evaluation and may require genetic testing eventually to arrive at a definitive diagnosis.

## *Biology of calcium sensing*

### *Background on identification of extracellular CaSR*

The paradigm had developed throughout the 1970s and 1980s that tissues with the specialized function of responding to minute but physiologically highly relevant changes in the extracellular concentration of calcium ($[Ca^{2+}]_e$) by a change in signal transduction were likely to be expressing membrane $Ca^{2+}$-sensing molecules. At that point, the repertoire of cell systems thought to use such extracellular Ca-sensing mechanisms included chief cells in the parathyroid gland, parafollicular cells in the thyroid, and renal tubular cells—controlling PTH secretion, calcitonin secretion, and urinary Ca excretion, respectively. The identification and molecular characterization of the extracellular CaSR changed that paradigm in many ways.

Cloning of the CaSR was reported in 1993[1] by Brown and Hebert and colleagues through the use of an expression cloning strategy in the *Xenopus laevis* oocyte model system. The insights that flowed from that initial cloning and pharmacologic verification that the extracellular Ca-sensing properties of tissues such as the parathyroid glands and kidneys were accomplished through this receptor have been remarkable over the subsequent 20 years of investigation. Although the signaling studies of a putative CaSR, before its cloning, had strongly supported the notion that the molecule was a G-protein–coupled receptor (GPCR), proof for that hypothesis came in the form of the structural details, membrane topography, and signal transduction capabilities of the receptor. The effect of a deeper understanding of the CaSR, its pattern of expression, and its functions within tissues that regulate Ca and mineral homeostasis, and the impact of this knowledge on our understanding of human diseases that involve altered $Ca^{2+}$ sensing are summarized in this chapter.

## *Molecular properties of CaSR: Ion sensing, signal transduction, and dimerization*

The CaSR is a member of family C of the GPCR superfamily. The human receptor cDNA encodes a protein of 1078 amino acids. Its gene is located on chromosome 3q21.1. Structural features of the CaSR include the signature seven transmembrane spanning domains; an extracellular domain; and three extracellular loops, three intracellular loops, and a cytoplasmic carboxyterminal tail (Figure 11.1).[1] The CaSR is notable for the very large size of its extracellular domain (~612 amino acids). This domain has the critical function of sensing minute changes in the extracellular or serum-ionized [$Ca^{2+}$] and coupling to intracellular signaling pathways that are remarkable for their diversity and number, depending on the target cell. It is intriguing that such a large and complicated structure for the extracellular domain, modeled as a "Venus flytrap," is one that has been used by evolution to fine-tune the sensing of a small physiologic ligand, namely $Ca^{2+}$.

Although the initial work of the CaSR cloning and other studies that followed[1–6] made it clear that $Ca^{2+}$ was the critical physiologic ligand for the CaSR, the receptor is also capable of being a divalent, trivalent, and even polyvalent cation sensor. Studies further showed that the CaSR could sense changes in the concentrations of amino acids, polyamines, and even aminoglycoside antibiotics, perhaps offering clues as to some of the functions that this receptor might be mediating in specialized microenvironments in the gut, brain, kidney, and other tissues where the CaSR is expressed.[1–6] The critical importance of the three-dimensional structure of the large extracellular domain of the CaSR and its intramolecular interactions, in determining the ability of the molecule to sense minute differences in $[Ca^{2+}]_e$ with great precision, helps the clinician to understand how a point mutation that alters a single residue in this domain can have such a profound impact on physiologic function of the CaSR to cause human disease.[7] The extracellular loops of the CaSR (Figure 11.1) are also functionally important in its ion-sensing function.[1–6] The transmembrane domains anchor the receptor and allow for signal recognition by the extracellular domain to be transduced to activation of G proteins and ultimately effector systems within the cytoplasm and nucleus of the cell. The variety of G proteins that couple to the CaSR is extensive and depends on the target cell.[5] Intracellular signaling pathways that are coupled to receptor activation are similarly diverse. They include the activation of phospholipase C and mitogen-activated protein kinase cascades, inhibition of adenylate cyclase activity, intracellular $Ca^{2+}$ mobilization, opening of membrane ion channels, and phospholipase A and D activation, depending on the cell system being studied.[1–3,5,6]

The intracellular network of interacting proteins that bind to and mediate downstream CaSR functions is still being unraveled. The intracellular tail of the CaSR appears to play an essential role in tethering to proteins such as filamin A and others,[3,5] such that specific receptor activities are mediated within the appropriate cell types. The second and third intracellular loops of the CaSR are key for coupling to phospholipase C activation and intracellular $Ca^{2+}$ mobilization[8,9] in transfected cell systems that have been used to study the signaling of the CaSR. How exactly these different pathways mediate the diverse functions that are likely to be CaSR-mediated in different cell types (Table 11.1)[4] remains to be fully elucidated. There are relatively fewer naturally occurring mutations within the intracellular loops and the C-terminal tail of the CaSR that have been shown to be involved in human diseases of $Ca^{2+}$ sensing, perhaps underscoring the essential functional importance of these receptor domains.

An analysis of the CaSR sequence placed this receptor in family C of the GPCR superfamily. This family includes a sizeable number of metabotropic glutamate receptor subtypes, the mGluRs 1–8, that are strongly expressed in the central nervous system, the type B (or metabotropic) $\gamma$-aminobutyric acid (GABA) receptors (GABA-B-Rs), a large family of olfactory receptors across many species, and orphan receptors whose functions are still being elucidated (Table 11.2).[6] It is clear from work with other GPCRs, including the mGluRs and the GABA-B-Rs, that receptors in family C dimerize as part of their signal transduction pathway.[10,11] CaSRs also have the capacity to form homodimers or multimers.[5,12] This capacity is thought to be one explanation by which a heterozygous point mutation in the CaSR can mitigate the normal signaling functions of the remaining wild-type CaSR and cause disordered $Ca^{2+}$ sensing *in vivo*. Careful biochemical experiments in this area indicates that there are dominant-negative effects that certain mutant CaSR proteins can exert on the sensing and or signaling capacity of the wild-type receptor counterparts in a dimeric molecular complex on the membranes of target cells (e.g., parathyroid chief cells, renal tubular cells).[12] In addition, in transfected cell model systems and neurons, CaSRs have the capacity to associate (i.e., heterodimerize) with mGluR[10] and

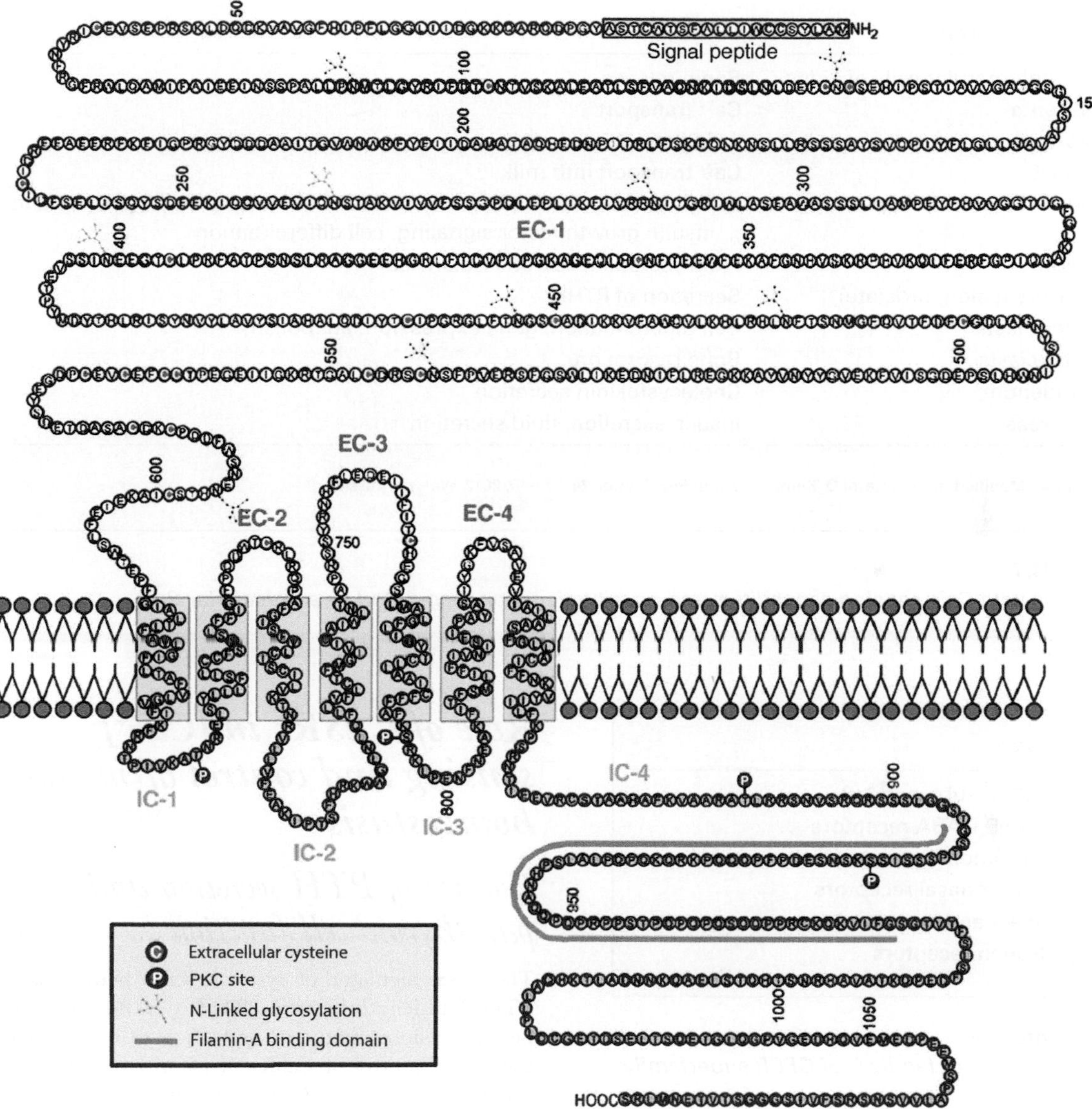


***Figure 11.1***
*Schematic diagram of the CaSR, a GPCR in family C, demonstrating the large extracellular domain (EC-1), the three extracellular loops (EC-2, EC-3, EC-4), the seven transmembrane-spanning domains anchoring the CaSR in the membrane, and the three interconnecting intracellular loops (IC-1 to IC-3) and the C-terminal tail or IC-4. The receptor is glycosylated at the sites shown. This modification is important for receptor function, and the CaSR interacts with multiple intracellular proteins, among them filamin A. (Modified from Brown EM et al.,* Nature, *366, 575–80, 1993; Chang W, Shoback D,* Cell Calcium, *35, 183–96, 2004. With permission.)*

| Tissue or cell type | Function |
|---|---|
| Juxtaglomerular cells of kidney | Renin release |
| Placenta | $Ca^{2+}$ transport |
| Stomach | Acid secretion |
| Breast | $Ca^{2+}$ transport into milk |
| Growth plate cartilage | Longitudinal growth, interaction with PTH-related protein (PTHrP) and insulin growth factor signaling, cell differentiation |
| Colon | Fluid secretion, secretory diarrhea |
| Cancers (colon, prostate) | Secretion of PTHrP |
| Osteoblasts | Cell differentiation, gene expression, anabolism |
| Osteoclasts | Bone resorption |
| Duodenum | Cholecystokinin secretion |
| Pancreas | Insulin secretion, fluid secretion |

*Source*: Modified from Riccardi D, Kemp PJ, *Annu Rev Physiol*, 74, 271–97, 2012. With permission.

***Table 11.1***
*Tissues with $Ca^{2+}$-sensing capabilities and possible functions regulated by extracellular $Ca^{2+}$.*

| CaSR |
|---|
| mGluR subtypes 1–8 |
| Type B GABA receptors |
| Pheromone receptors |
| Vomeronasal receptors |
| Sweet and amino acid taste receptors |
| Orphan receptors |

***Table 11.2***
*Members of family C of GPCR superfamily.*

the type 1 or 2 GABA-B-Rs.[13,14] This latter association affects both trafficking of the CaSR to the cell membrane and the signaling properties of the CaSR in cells expressing high levels of these different receptors.[13,14] Receptor trafficking to the cell surface and receptor number on the cell surface are thought to be important components of determining the sensitivity of a given cell type to changes in the $[Ca^{2+}]_e$. Whether the molecular identity of the partner in the receptor dimer (or multimer) will ultimately determine specialized $Ca^{2+}$-sensing properties in tissues of interest (e.g., in different regions of the brain) remains to be further investigated.

# *Role of CaSRs in $[Ca^{2+}]_e$ sensing and control of mineral homeostasis*

## *Control of PTH secretion and parathyroid cell function*

The chief regulator of systemic $Ca^{2+}$ homeostasis is PTH. Full-length bioactive PTH is an 84 amino acid peptide whose synthesis and exocytosis are under the direct control of CaSRs in parathyroid chief cells (Figure 11.2).[1–3,6,15,16] CaSRs also control the overall proliferation of parathyroid cells. High $[Ca^{2+}]_e$ rapidly inhibit synthesis and release of PTH into the bloodstream. That inhibition of production and secretion has been linked to pathways activated by CaSR-induced signal transduction. Thus, in contrast to countless other GPCRs that are stimulated to release hormone when the secretagogue is applied, the CaSR is activated by high $[Ca^{2+}]_e$, but CaSR activation is coupled to inhibition (not stimulation) of hormone release. Long-term responses to chronic hypercalcemia involve decreased rates of cell proliferation and reduced PTH mRNA stability within the glands. Conversely, low $[Ca^{2+}]_e$ enhances PTH secretion by promoting a relatively inactive receptor conformational state (less $Ca^{2+}$ bound) such that hormone may

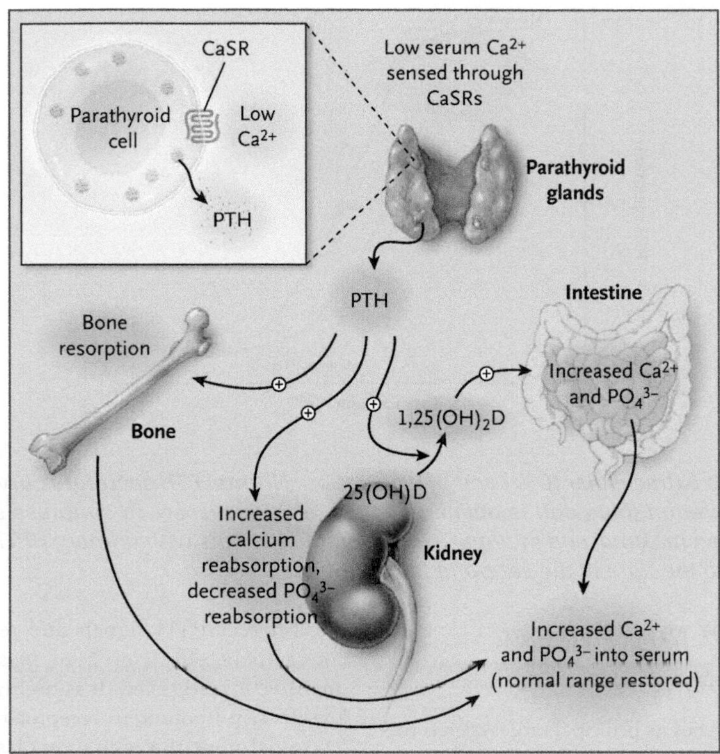


***Figure 11.2***
*Control of PTH secretion by CaSRs expressed on the parathyroid cell. Low serum [$Ca^{2+}$] is sensed by CaSR, leading to increased release of PTH. PTH acts on renal PTH-Rs to promote conversion of 25(OH) D (25-hydroxyvitamin D) to 1,25-D (1,25-dihydroxyvitamin D). 1,25-D mediates $Ca^{2+}$ and phosphate absorption via the intestine. PTH also enhances $Ca^{2+}$ reabsorption in the distal tubule. PTH increases bone resorption and releases $Ca^{2+}$ and phosphate into the bloodstream. High [$Ca^{2+}$]$_e$ feeds-back and inhibits PTH secretion through activating signal transduction by the CaSR. (Reproduced from Shoback D,* N Engl J Med, *359, 391–403, 2008. With permission.)*

be constitutively released. Rapid responses to hypocalcemia up regulate secretion, whereas chronic responses to hypocalcemia require increased cell proliferation and ultimately hyperplasia of the parathyroid glands.

The dynamics of PTH secretion has been described in terms of several secretory parameters. One such parameter is maximal PTH release, that is, the level of secretion under hypocalcemic conditions (Figure 11.3). Although mild elevations in the [$Ca^{2+}$]$_e$ produce prompt inhibitory responses in parathyroid cells, moderate and severe hypercalcemia are associated with negligible or the most minimal rates of PTH secretion that have sometimes been characterized as "$Ca^{2+}$-nonsuppressible" secretion (Figure 11.3). Minimal PTH release is thus the second key secretory parameter. Depending on the sensitivity of the intact PTH assay used in a clinical situation, patients with nonparathyroid-dependent hypercalcemia (discussed below) may have essentially no detectable PTH level in the circulation. Therefore, this component of secretion is often negligible both *in vivo* and *in vitro*. The third secretory parameter is the $Ca^{2+}$ set-point. Fortuitously, the sensitivity of PTH secretion is most acute over a narrow range of physiologically relevant [$Ca^{2+}$]$_e$. This narrow range of [$Ca^{2+}$]$_e$ constitutes the steepest portion of the secretion curve both *in vivo* and *in vitro*.[2,3,6,15,16] Operationally, the half-maximal rate of PTH release has been called the set-point for secretion and is defined as the [$Ca^{2+}$]$_e$ that is halfway (50%) between maximal and minimal rates of PTH release either *in vitro* or *in vivo* (Figure 11.3). A variety of signal transduction pathways and G proteins couple to CaSR activation in parathyroid cells; however, it is unclear which pathway(s) couples to inhibition of secretion and which to dampening proliferation,[1–3,5,8,15,16] and these responses may require the integrated actions of multiple intracellular effectors.

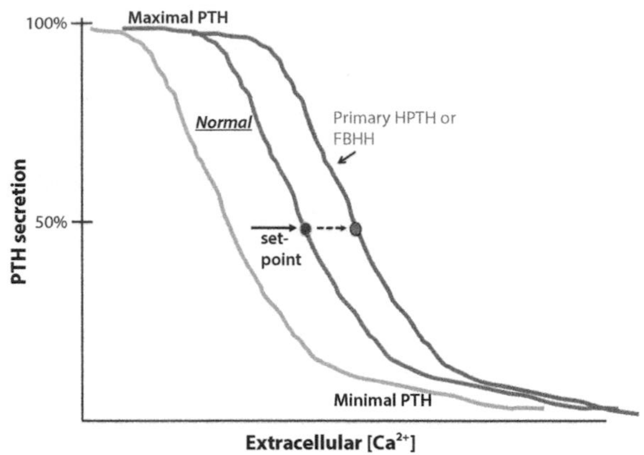


***Figure 11.3***
*Relationship between extracellular [$Ca^{2+}$] and PTH secretion. Normal PTH secretory curve shown in red. The set-point for PTH secretion (blue dot) is defined as the [$Ca^{2+}$]$_e$ necessary to suppress secretion by 50% of the difference between maximal and minimal PTH secretion. Patients with primary HPTH or FBHH generally demonstrate a shift to the right in the set-point for secretion.*

## *PTH actions in target tissues: Bone (see Chapter 12)*

Once released, PTH reaches its principal target organs the bone and kidney via the circulation (Figure 11.2).[17,18] At those sites, the hormone interacts with high-affinity type 1 PTH receptors (PTH-R1s). In bone, PTH-R1s activate multiple signaling pathways in cells of the osteoblast and stromal cell lineages. PTH-R1s increase adenylate cyclase activity, which generates cyclic AMP, and results in increased protein kinase A activity and phosphorylation of intracellular substrates. PTH-R1 activation in bone leads to the expression of receptor activator of nuclear factor-κB ligand (RANK-L). RANK-L interacts with RANK on the surfaces of osteoclast precursors and mature osteoclasts to enhance their differentiation to bone-resorbing cells and to increase their resorptive capacity, respectively. RANK signaling via several signaling mechanisms within the osteoclast determines the cell's phenotypic properties and actions on bone. RANK-L/RANK signaling is the means by which chronically elevated PTH levels stimulate bone resorption. Osteoclast-mediated bone resorption delivers $Ca^{2+}$ (and phosphate as well) into the circulation to restore the [$Ca^{2+}$]$_e$ into the normal range.

Chronically high unremitting PTH levels have a catabolic effect on bone mass. Intermittent low-dose PTH administration in the form of recombinant human PTH (1–34)[19,20] and PTH (1–84)[21] can be anabolic, building up trabecular connectivity and cortical thickness and improving bone strength sufficient to lower fracture risk in individuals with osteoporosis. Exactly how target cells in bone distinguish the different PTH signals and result in anabolic and not catabolic effects on bone mass remains an area of intensive investigation. It is highly likely that the Wnt low-density lipoprotein receptor-related protein (LRP) 5/6 signaling pathway in osteoblast and osteoblast precursors (e.g., mesenchymal progenitors and stem cells) is critically involved in the recruitment of cells into the osteoblastic lineage, stimulating their differentiation to mature matrix-synthesizing and -mineralizing osteoblasts. Anabolic doses of PTH also reduce apoptosis of osteoblastic cells. By these different means, it is thought that intermittent low-dose PTH therapy can increase bone mass and strength and reduce fractures in women and men.[17–21]

## *PTH and CaSR actions in other tissues involved in mineral homeostasis: Kidney and intestine*

Actions of CaSRs and PTH-R1s outside the bone are also critical in the control of systemic $Ca^{2+}$ and bone homeostasis, particularly in their actions in the kidney and intestine.[1–6,15,22] CaSRs play an essential role in the excretion of $Ca^{2+}$ by the kidney and, potentially, in other functions including the production of 1,25-dihydroxyvitamin D [1,25-$(OH)_2$D] and the excretion of phosphate. CaSRs are widely expressed throughout the nephron, including the proximal tubule, thick ascending limb, distal tubule, and collecting ducts.[5,15,22] The main action of the renal CaSRs is to promote $Ca^{2+}$ excretion in response to high [$Ca^{2+}$]$_e$ in the thick ascending limb and the medullary collecting ducts. The CaSR also regulates the activity of the aquaporin-2 water channels by inhibiting their trafficking to the membrane. Aquaporin-2 channels allow the kidney to reabsorb water. CaSR activation also inhibits vasopressin-induced aquaporin-2 expression, thereby interfering with a key means of maintaining water balance *in vivo* through the vasopressin receptor system.[5] CaSR activation induced by high $[Ca^{2+}]_e$ thus promotes $Ca^{2+}$ excretion as well as a water diuresis, thereby contributing to the dehydration attendant to hypercalcemia and creating a vicious cycle for worsening the hypercalcemic state in humans.

PTH-R1s are expressed at several sites in the kidney where PTH plays key roles in the maintenance of serum $Ca^{2+}$, phosphate, and bone homeostasis. The rapid effects of PTH to defend the $[Ca^{2+}]_e$ result from its ability to activate high-affinity adenylate cyclase-coupled receptors in the distal tubule. $Ca^{2+}$ is transported across the renal membrane, thereby conserving $Ca^{2+}$ to restore systemic homeostasis (Figure 11.2). PTH also stimulates the conversion of 25-hydroxyvitamin D (25-OH D) to 1,25-D through its proximal tubule PTH-R1.[23,24] This pathway is part of the long-term response to hypocalcemia and secondary HPTH in that the distal effects of 1,25-D generation require genomic effects on the intestine to up regulate the overall absorption of $Ca^{2+}$ and phosphate chronically by the intestine. PTH also affects the proximal tubular handling of phosphate, promoting its excretion by inhibiting the insertion of the sodium-dependent phosphate cotransporters (NaPi-2a and -2c) into the renal brush border (Figure 11.4).[25] These transporters return phosphate back into the bloodstream. PTH-induced inhibition of phosphate transport allows for the excretion of this mineral via the kidney.

In addition to PTH, FGF23 is another circulating factor that promotes renal phosphate excretion via effects on these same transporters (Figure 11.4).[26,27] Unlike PTH, FGF23 reduces 1,25-D production by inhibiting 1-α-hydroxylase activity and stimulates 1,25-D catabolism by increased renal 24 hydroxylase activity. To complete the feedback mechanisms to maintain homeostasis, 1,25-D inhibits PTH synthesis as does FGF23. Through the actions of these two hormones, serum concentrations of $Ca^{2+}$ and phosphate are maintained.

PTH does not have direct effects on intestinal $Ca^{2+}$ transport; rather, its effects on $Ca^{2+}$ transport by the gut are mediated indirectly through 1,25-D as described below. The CaSR is strongly expressed in the stomach and small and large intestine.[5] Most of the studies on its actions in the intestine are of the colon cells and epithelia and not the small intestine—the organ where most of the active $Ca^{2+}$ transport in response to 1,25-D and other mediators takes place.[28] In studies of colon physiology, it appears the CaSR plays an important role in fluid transport. In mouse models of CaSR deletion, the

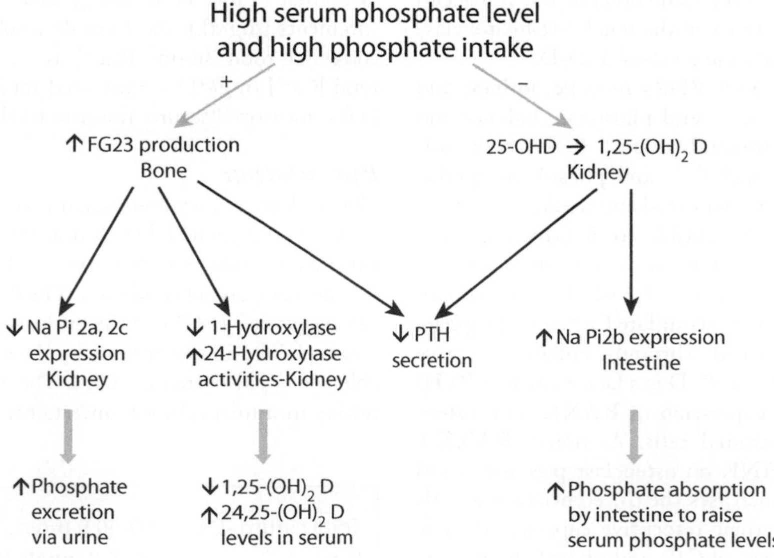


***Figure 11.4***
*Phosphate homeostasis is regulated by FGF23, produced by bone. FGF23 acts on kidney and parathyroid glands as shown. 1,25-D production in the kidney is also regulated by FGF23 and phosphate. 1,25-D mediates phosphate and $Ca^{2+}$ absorption by the intestine. 1,25-D also stimulates FGF23 production by bone (not shown).*

serum [$Ca^{2+}$] is completely dependent on the amount of $Ca^{2+}$ in the diet supporting a role for intestinal CaSRs in $Ca^{2+}$ transport.[29,30]

## Vitamin D production and actions in target tissues (see Chapter 12)

Vitamin D is ingested through the diet from a limited number of foods (e.g., fortified dairy products, fish, mushrooms, and egg yolks).[31] Vitamin D is also generated through the actions of ultraviolet light and heat on the skin.[31–33] Advanced age, skin pigmentation, and the use of sunscreens and clothing all interfere with this important reaction in the skin. Alternatively, multivitamin supplements can supply the daily requirement for vitamin D. Once vitamin D is made or ingested, it travels through the circulation to the liver where the first step in bioactivation occurs. The 25-hydroxylase, a high-capacity enzyme, converts vitamin D (cholecalciferol) to 25-OH D. Thereafter, under tight physiologic control, circulating 25-OH D is taken up by proximal tubular cells in the kidney and converted by the 1-α-hydroxylase to 1,25-D. This naturally occurring vitamin D metabolite has the very high affinity and potency at the vitamin D receptor (VDR). The circulating levels of PTH, ionized $Ca^{2+}$, phosphate, FGF23, and other factors impact on the expression and activity of the renal 1-α-hydroxylase and thereby the circulating levels of 1,25-D.

1,25-D interacts with VDRs in bone, kidney, and intestine to regulate $Ca^{2+}$ and phosphate balance and ultimately matrix mineralization.[31–33] Without sufficient 1,25-D–mediated $Ca^{2+}$ and phosphate uptake, bone matrix is undermineralized and weak. In growing individuals, bone is susceptible to deformity causing rickets. In the adult skeleton, weak bone predisposes to fractures due to osteomalacia. 1,25-D has its primary effects on the intestine to stimulate $Ca^{2+}$ and phosphate absorption accomplished through enhanced active transport. In the bone, 1,25-D is a factor (such as PTH) that stimulates the expression of RANK-L on osteoblast and marrow stromal cells. As noted, RANK-L interacting with RANK on osteoclast precursors and mature osteoclasts increases the differentiation of cells in this lineage and their resorptive capacity, thereby prompting the delivery of $Ca^{2+}$ and phosphate into the circulation. 1,25-D also promotes renal reabsorption of $Ca^{2+}$. Together, these actions of 1,25-D amplify, in terms of serum $Ca^{2+}$ homeostasis, the actions of PTH to defend the serum [$Ca^{2+}$] in a tight normal range.

In addition to the kidney, many other tissues express the 1-α-hydroxylase and generate 1,25-D within them. These tissues include breast, colon, prostate gland, lymph nodes, lung, skin, bone, cartilage, and others. Whether and to what degree these nonrenal tissues contribute to the circulating 1,25-D levels under normal physiologic circumstances is a debatable point. It is thought, however, that the 1,25-D made locally interacts with VDRs and their nuclear receptor partners (e.g., retinoid X receptor, RXR) in these tissues to achieve the actions of 1,25-D on cell growth and differentiation as opposed to the classic actions that 1,25-D mediates via the VDR on $Ca^{2+}$ and mineral metabolism. Specialized cells within these tissues (such as T lymphocytes present in lymph nodes) can generate excessive quantities of 1,25-D, in cases of granulomatous disease (e.g., sarcoid, tuberculosis) or in certain lymphomas, and cause hypercalcemia due to the elevated levels and unregulated production of 1,25-D.

## Disorders of Ca regulation and Ca sensing

### Hypercalcemia (see Severe hypercalcaemia, Chapter 24)

Hypercalcemia is defined as an albumin-corrected total serum [$Ca^{2+}$] or an ionized [$Ca^{2+}$] above the upper limits of normal (Table 11.3). Using total serum [$Ca^{2+}$] measurements (mg/dL), the formula to obtain an albumin-corrected total serum [$Ca^{2+}$] is as follows: corrected total [$Ca^{2+}$] (mg/dL) = measured total [$Ca^{2+}$] (mg/dL) + [4.0 – measured serum albumin (G/dL) × 0.8].

#### Presentation

Hypercalcemia can present as a mild laboratory abnormality with no demonstrable clinical symptoms or as a life-threatening endocrine emergency with acute renal failure, hypotension, and obtundation. The differential diagnosis can be extensive,[34,35] but the evaluation has been refined and expedited in recent years by the development of reliable and rapid hormone assays. The availability of rapid testing minimizes clinical uncertainty so that appropriate

| | |
|---|---|
| Total serum [$Ca^{2+}$] | 9.0–10.5 mg/dL (2.2–2.6 mmol/L) |
| Ionized [$Ca^{2+}$] | 4.5–5.6 mg/dL (1.1–1.35 mmol/L) |

***Table 11.3***
*Normal ranges for the serum total and ionized [$Ca^{2+}$].*

management can be instituted efficiently. Advances in imaging techniques allow for the reliable localization of parathyroid tumors, thereby further improving management of hypercalcemic patients with primary HPTH.

## *Symptoms and signs*

Hypercalcemia is a systemic disorder whose clinical manifestations are strongly influenced by the etiology, age of the patient, severity of the disturbance, and rapidity of its onset. Hypercalcemia occurs when the counter-regulatory mechanisms such as the suppression of PTH secretion by high $[Ca^{2+}]_e$ and the capacity of the kidney to excrete $Ca^{2+}$ are overwhelmed. This occurs when potent hormones such as the PTH-related protein (PTHrP) or 1,25-D are produced ectopically in an uncontrolled manner by malignant tumors.[34–37]

Systemically, hypercalcemia can cause a wide variety of symptoms and signs related to central nervous system, renal, neuromuscular, gastrointestinal, skeletal, and psychiatric functions (Table 11.4).[34] These signs vary from case to case depending on patient factors (e.g., age, comorbidities, chronicity of process) as well as the underlying diagnosis. For example, it is common for patients with hypercalcemia of malignancy, due to a solid tumor, for example, of the head and neck, to present with fairly acute onset of altered mental status, dehydration, hypotension, poor appetite, and weight loss.[36,37] Patients with hypercalcemia due to multiple myeloma may have bone pain, pathologic fractures, anemia, and chronic kidney disease of recent onset that dominate the clinical picture. Primary HPTH, in contrast, may present with a several year history of recurrent kidney stones or simply with biochemical abnormalities (high serum $[Ca^{2+}]$ and intact PTH) and a low bone mineral density by dual-energy x-ray absorptiometry (DXA) scanning or less commonly with fragility fractures.[38–41] Therefore,

- Central nervous system
  - Altered mental status, confusion
  - Reduced memory and concentration
  - Depression
  - Fatigue
  - Progressive obtundation, coma
- Gastrointestinal
  - Constipation
  - Peptic ulcer disease, gastroesophageal reflux
  - Nausea and/or vomiting
  - Pancreatitis
- Skeletal
  - Bone pain, fractures, bone cysts (if HPTH is etiology)
  - Osteopenia or osteoporosis (if chronic)
- Renal
  - Thirst
  - Polyuria
  - Dehydration
  - Reduced renal function
  - Stones
  - Nephrocalcinosis
- Other
  - Proximal muscle weakness (especially if primary HPTH)
  - Hypertension
  - Itching (especially if severe HPTH)
  - Band keratopathy (if chronic)

***Table 11.4***
*Signs and symptoms of hypercalcemia.*

the variety of presentations underscores the heterogeneity of the causes for hypercalcemia.[34,35]

## Evaluation

The typical laboratory profiles for several of the main presentations for hypercalcemia are shown in Table 11.5. The treating clinician obtains the history and performs the physical examination on the patient. Armed with this information and basic laboratory screening tests (e.g., serum total [$Ca^{2+}$], albumin, phosphate, electrolytes, and creatinine), the decision is then made to obtain intact PTH, thyroid-stimulating hormone (TSH), 25-OH D, 1,25-D, or PTHrP levels in a stepwise and logical manner (Figure 11.5). These tests are in general highly reliable and provide a strong level of diagnostic certainty, once they are combined with more disease-specific laboratory tests and imaging (e.g., serum and urine protein electrophoreses, quantitative immunoglobulins and bone marrow examination in multiple myeloma; bone marrow biopsy in lymphoma; CT scans of chest in possible sarcoidosis, fungal infection, and lung cancer). Tissue biopsies are vital in these nonendocrine conditions to confirm the etiology and direct definitive management.

## Differential diagnosis

When evaluating the patient with an elevated total serum or ionized [$Ca^{2+}$], the two most common disorders to be considered are primary HPTH and malignancy-associated hypercalcemia (Figure 11.5). Measurement of the intact PTH is the first diagnostic step. If the PTH is elevated or inappropriately normal (i.e., not suppressed in the presence of hypercalcemia), the differential diagnosis includes all causes of PTH-dependent hypercalcemia. These conditions include primary HPTH, due to a parathyroid adenoma or hyperplasia in 85%–90% or 10%–15% of cases, respectively. Parathyroid carcinoma is quite rare, being responsible for <1% of cases of primary HPTH.[39,42] A palpable neck mass in ~50% of patients and a serum total [$Ca^{2+}$] >14.0 mg/dL are often the first clues that the patient may have this form of cancer.[34,42,43]

When the serum total [$Ca^{2+}$] is elevated and the intact PTH level is normal or mildly elevated, that is, no more than 25% above the upper limit of normal usually, the

| Disorder | S-$Ca^{2\pm}$ | S-Phos | Intact PTH | 25-OH D | 1,25-D | PTHrP | Other lab tests |
|---|---|---|---|---|---|---|---|
| Primary HPTH | ↑ | ↓ or nl | ↑ or nl | ↓ or nl | ↑ or nl | ↓ | U-$Ca^{2+}$ >100 mg/24 h<br>$Ca^{2+}$/creatinine clearance ratio[a] >0.02 |
| Familial benign hypercalcemia | ↑ | ↓ or nl | ↑ or nl | ↓ or nl | ↑ or nl | ↓ | U-$Ca^{2+}$ <100 mg/24 h<br>$Ca^{2+}$/creatinine clearance ratio <0.01<br>CaSR mutation |
| Thyrotoxicosis | ↑ | nl | ↓ | nl | nl | — | suppressed TSH, elevated free T4<br>U-$Ca^{2+}$ ↑ |
| Hypercalcemia of malignancy | ↑ | ↓ | ↓ | ↓ or nl | ↓ or nl | ↑ | U-$Ca^{2+}$ ↑↑↑ |
| Granulomatous disease or sarcoid | ↑ | ↑ or nl | ↓ | ↓ or nl | ↑ or nl | ↓ | U-$Ca^{2+}$ ↑↑↑ |
| Osteolytic metastases | ↑ | ↑ or nl | ↓ | nl | nl | ↓ | U-$Ca^{2+}$ ↑↑↑ |

nl, normal; U, urine.

[a] This clearance ratio is calculated from simultaneous fasting serum and urine $Ca^{2+}$ and creatinine measurements. The urine sample can be from a spot or a 24 h collection. The clearance ratio is calculated as follows:
Urinary Ca (mg/24 h) × plasma creatinine (mg/dL)/plasma Ca (mg/dL) × urinary creatinine (mg/24 h).

**Table 11.5**
*Biochemical profiles in common causes of hypercalcemia.*

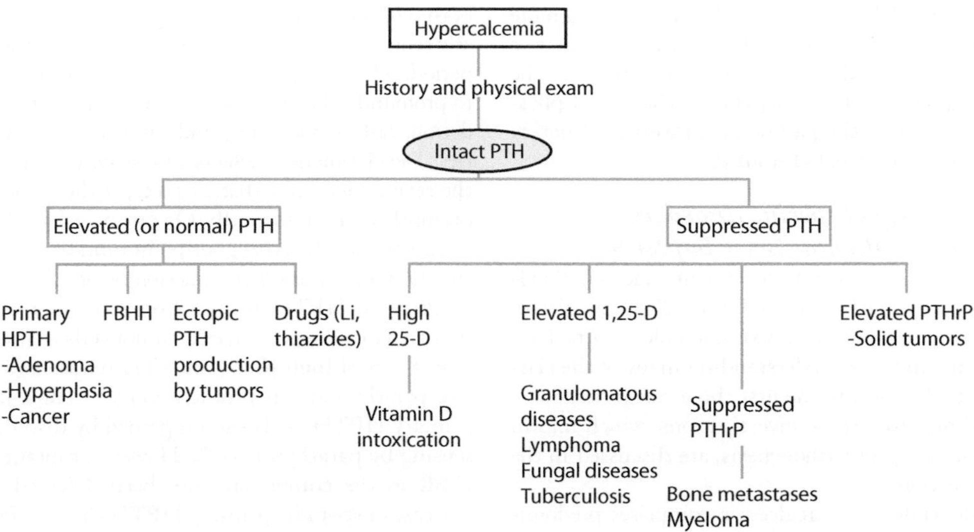


***Figure 11.5***
***Algorithm for the evaluation of patients with hypercalcemia. PTH, Parathyroid hormone; PTHrP, Parathyroid hormone-related protein.***

diagnosis of familial benign hypocalciuric hypercalcemia (FBHH) must be considered (Table 11.5).[44–47] An assessment of urinary $Ca^{2+}$ excretion is mandatory as well as family history review and possibly screening for the presence of usually mild hypercalcemia in the family. The inheritance of the disorder is autosomal dominant. The serum [$Mg^{2+}$] may also be elevated in patients with FBHH. In general, the $Ca^{2+}$/creatinine clearance ratio helps to distinguish cases of FBHH from mild primary HPTH slightly better than does the 24 h urinary $Ca^{2+}$ excretion (Table 11.5).[45,48] There is often overlap between these diagnoses biochemically, hormonally, and clinically. Primary HPTH is often diagnosed in a mild asymptomatic form.[39–42] The clinician may even decide to perform CaSR genetic analysis in a kindred with autosomal dominant hypercalcemia to determine whether there is a mutation present that is known to cause loss of function in the CaSR based on prior reports. Given that the hypercalcemia is often mild, and there are frequently no symptoms present, such an individual can often be followed clinically without genetic testing and the need for surgical intervention.

Other etiologies for PTH-dependent hypercalcemia are the rare instances of ectopic production of PTH by a nonparathyroid malignancy[34,36] and the use of lithium or thiazide diuretics. Hereditary causes of primary HPTH are discussed in Chapter 9 and include multiple endocrine neoplasia (MEN) types 1 and 2a and the HPTH jaw tumor syndrome. A family history including any of the associated tumors and findings would point the clinician to the consideration of one of those syndromes.

PTH-independent hypercalcemia may be due to several etiologies, including 1,25-D overproduction; PTHrP hypersecretion; and miscellaneous disorders, such as vitamin A intoxication, immobilization, acute renal failure, and milk-alkali syndrome (Figure 11.5).[34,35] In 1,25-D–mediated hypercalcemia, the differential diagnosis includes granulomatous diseases (e.g., sarcoidosis, tuberculosis, blastomycosis, cryptococcosis) and lymphomas.[34] 25-OH D levels are elevated in the rare cases of vitamin D intoxication, and this metabolite is thought to mediate the hypercalcemia rather than 1,25-D.

In malignancy-associated hypercalcemia, PTHrP is ectopically produced by solid tumors of the head, neck, lung, pancreas, and many other sites.[34,36,37] Tumors that originate in the bone marrow such as multiple myeloma and leukemia, in certain lymphomas, or with tumors metastatic to the skeleton, the mechanism for hypercalcemia is local osteolysis due to direct tumor cell–mediated bone resorption usually involving cytokines like interleukin 6. In such instances, the calciotropic hormones (i.e., 1,25-D, PTH, PTHrP) are suppressed, whereas the serum $Ca^{2+}$ and sometimes serum phosphate levels are elevated. Any clinical situation in which the responsible factor is not PTH or PTHrP, both of which activate PTH-R1s in the kidney and promote phosphate loss, such as 1,25-D or cytokines, there is increased phosphate delivery into the circulation. The serum phosphate level will depend on the rate of phosphate release due to the pathologic process and dietary intake, balanced by renal clearance.

## *Pathophysiology of specific disorders causing hypercalcemia (see Chapter 9)*

The pathogenesis of hypercalcemia includes (1) PTH-dependent, (2) PTHrP-mediated, (3) 1,25-D–mediated, and (4) other mechanisms. Considerable efforts have been invested in better understanding many of the classic disorders that fit into the first three categories. Some of the findings from those investigations, which inform the understanding of pathogenesis, are discussed in the following section.

PTH-dependent hypercalcemia comprises predominantly primary HPTH and FBHH. FBHH is an inherited disorder of $Ca^{2+}$ sensing.[44–47] It is typically due to heterozygous loss of function mutations in one allele of the CaSR gene. Approximately 70% of the mutations are in the coding sequence of the receptor. These mutations can be point mutations or deletions of small or considerable amounts of genetic material leading to the substitution of a critical amino acid with a nonsense/missense residue or to the truncation of the CaSR, respectively. Well over 100 mutations in the CaSR have been reported, and many of them have been characterized from the standpoint of their functional effects on CaSR signaling in transfected cell lines.[46,47] CaSR mutations in FBHH are carried in the germ cells. Hence, all cells in the body that express CaSRs will bear the mutant allele. Yet, the phenotype in FBHH is only clearly evident in terms of parathyroid and renal function. The sensitivity of PTH secretion to suppression by high $[Ca^{2+}]_e$ is blunted in FBHH (Figure 11.3). The set-point is shifted to the right, which is why hypercalcemia occurs. The degree of that shift to the right in the PTH suppression curve may influence the severity of the hypercalcemia in affected patients. In general, however, hypercalcemia is mild in most cases of FBHH. This misperception of the serum $[Ca^{2+}]$ is accompanied by higher PTH levels that act on target tissues bone and kidney to maintain the elevated serum $[Ca^{2+}]$. In the kidney, reduced $Ca^{2+}$ sensing leads to inadequate excretion of the higher filtered load of $Ca^{2+}$. Thus, the kidney defect maintains and exacerbates, rather than corrects, the parathyroid $Ca^{2+}$-sensing defect.

In some affected kindreds, where there is parental consanguinity, offspring are born with two mutant CaSR alleles, typically resulting in neonatal severe primary HPTH (NSHPTH).[34,44,46,47] These children are born with often life-threatening hypercalcemia and usually require total parathyroidectomy early in the neonatal period. Their bones are severely undermineralized, due to profound PTH hypersecretion. There is growth retardation, failure to thrive, and often respiratory difficulties. Developmental defects can arise, presumably from the severe metabolic disturbances, if the disorder is not promptly treated surgically. On rare occasions, NSHPTH can be due to a heterozygous point mutation in the CaSR that profoundly alters its function *in vivo*.[34,44,46]

Primary HPTH results from both a reduction in sensitivity of the parathyroid tumor cells to the suppressive effects of high $[Ca^{2+}]_e$ on PTH release and to excessive parathyroid cell proliferation.[34,49] Thus, in a sense primary HPTH is also accompanied by disordered $Ca^{2+}$ sensing by parathyroid cells. However, mutations in the CaSR in the tumor have not been detected in nearly any case of sporadic primary HPTH that has been studied. Tissues removed at surgery from patients with primary HPTH tend to display a shift to the right in their $Ca^{2+}$ set-points when PTH secretion is studied in vitro (Figure 11.3). This shift is accompanied by a reduction in CaSR protein and mRNA of ~50% on average. CaSR expression does vary significantly among the tumors, depending on how receptor expression is graded perhaps (immunoblotting, immunocytochemistry, polymerase chain reaction [PCR]); however, variations in CaSR expression may also be due to the heterogeneous pathogenesis of sporadic adenomas.

Approximately 20%–40% of parathyroid adenomas overexpress the cyclin D1 gene, a known growth promoter for parathyroid cells and a critical regulator of the cell cycle.[49] In ~25%–40% of parathyroid tumors, there is somatic loss of one MEN type 1 (MEN1) allele.[49] The MEN1 gene encodes for menin, a protein that is also involved in growth regulation in many endocrine cells, including the parathyroid. The MEN1 tumor syndrome includes early onset parathyroid tumors as one of its most penetrant features (see Chapter 9). In mouse models of both parathyroid cell targeted MEN1 gene deletion[50] and cyclin D1 gene overexpression,[51] there is loss of CaSR expression in the parathyroid glands as the mice age and develop primary HPTH. These models suggest a strong connection between hyperproliferation in the parathyroid and loss of CaSR expression, but the molecular mechanism(s) that links proliferation and control of CaSR expression has not been identified nor has the environmental or genetic triggers for the remainder of the cases of primary HPTH.

PTHrP-dependent hypercalcemia results from the overproduction of PTHrP in a dysregulated manner by an expanding tumor mass.[34,36,37] Tumor burden is generally extensive and evident clinically when PTHrP production reaches levels sufficient to cause hypercalcemia. Clinical prognosis is often poor at that point, and therapeutic options are limited. The responsible tumors vary greatly in their locations and cells of origin, although they are heavily represented by tumors of epithelial cell origin, including squamous cell tumors of the head, neck, and lung; renal cell cancer; breast cancer; and certain gastrointestinal cancers. The actions of PTHrP *in vivo* result from its ability to interact potently with PTH-R1s in bone and kidney. These receptors mediate the hypercalcemic and hypophosphatemic effects of PTHrP, just as they do PTH. PTHrP may interact with other specific receptors specific for it, but PTHrP's biologic actions in causing the hypercalcemia of malignancy syndrome can be explained by interactions with the classic PTH-R1.

1,25-D–mediated hypercalcemia explains <1% of the hypercalcemia in patients with cancer. Approximately 60%–70% of malignancy-associated hypercalcemia is due to humoral mechanisms (predominantly PTHrP). The other 30%–40% is due to local osteolytic disease.[34,36] Lymphomas (typically non-Hodgkin) can overproduce 1,25-D by virtue of the expression of the 1-α-hydroxylase in lymphoid cells. Similarly, in granulomatous diseases in which 1,25-D is overproduced, the lymphocytes or the macrophages within the granulomas may be the source of the conversion of 25-OH D to 1,25-D. In the inflammatory state of disorders such as sarcoidosis, proinflammatory cytokines (e.g., interferon γ) can stimulate 1-α-hydroxylase activity locally. Thus, although the PTH levels are low in these conditions when hypercalcemia is present, local inflammatory mediators drive sufficient 1,25-D production from the granulomatous tissue to have systemic effects on $Ca^{2+}$ metabolism. In these cases, renal 1,25-D production is not thought to be the mediator for the hypercalcemia, and that pathway of 1,25-D synthesis is thought to be suppressed.

Other mechanisms that trigger increases in bone resorption or in intestinal $Ca^{2+}$ absorption can also cause hypercalcemia. For example, excessive levels of thyroid hormones stimulate bone resorption in hyperthyroidism, and vitamin A and its metabolites increase resorption in vitamin A intoxication states.[34] Milk-alkali syndrome results from increased $Ca^{2+}$ intake and reduced $Ca^{2+}$ excretion, usually exacerbated by alkalosis and renal failure. This syndrome has increased $Ca^{2+}$ absorption via a gastrointestinal route as one of its pathogenic mechanisms. In vitamin D intoxication, hypercalcemia and hyperphosphatemia result from increased gastrointestinal absorption of $Ca^{2+}$ and phosphate and increased bone resorption, also releasing $Ca^{2+}$ and phosphate into the circulation. Both mechanisms are mediated by VDRs in bone and gut, and the renal clearance mechanisms get overwhelmed.

## *Management of hypercalcemia*

The cornerstone of management is to address the underlying disturbance. In cases of moderate-to-severe hypercalcemia, where there is altered mental status, dehydration, hypotension, and oliguria, this is an urgent situation requiring aggressive fluid volume resuscitation and electrolyte replacement. Hypovolemia is usually addressed with intravenous normal saline solution. Once volume is restored and begins to expand, calciuresis is achieved by the use of an intravenous loop diuretic such as furosemide to promote sodium excretion via diuresis. This solution is only a temporizing solution. The etiology for the symptomatic hypercalcemia needs to be determined so that long-term management can be addressed. If the underlying process is primary HPTH, then expedited surgery can be considered once the diagnosis is established and the patient stabilized.

If the cause of the hypercalcemia is a malignancy, then the type and extent need to be established to determine what therapeutic options are available and appropriate.[34,36] Often as the diagnosis is being established, it is necessary to begin a more long-term treatment for the ongoing bone resorption that is most often the reason for the hypercalcemia. In general, once renal function is stabilized and at an acceptable level, an intravenous bisphosphonate (pamidronate in dose of 30, 60, or 90 mg or zoledronic acid ≤4 mg adjusted based on renal function) to block osteoclast-mediated bone resorption is generally the first-line pharmacotherapy. Because intravenous bisphosphonates require 48–72 h to take effect, intravenous saline and furosemide are often continued but at a less aggressive pace after the first 24–48 h. Salmon calcitonin, an agent that also blocks bone resorption, can be instituted. Salmon calcitonin (50–100 mg given by intramuscular or subcutaneous injection every 8–12 h) is often selected because of its more rapid onset of action (within 12–24 h of initial administration), compared with intravenous bisphosphonates. In addition, calcitonin is not nephrotoxic and can be given to patients with significantly reduced renal function. Because bisphosphonates are renally cleared, considerable care must be taken with their administration and dosing in patients with compromised renal function. In the most severe cases of hypercalcemia accompanied by renal failure, dialysis may be the only effective strategy, albeit temporary, for lowering the serum [$Ca^{2+}$]. Specific therapies (e.g., radiation, chemotherapy, surgery) to reduce tumor burden, if possible, are important options to explore. As noted above, generally patients with malignancy and hypercalcemia have large tumor mass, and reduction in that mass can often improve their hypercalcemia.

Glucocorticoids are an important adjunctive and at times are the primary therapy for hypercalcemia. This is the case when multiple myeloma, lymphoma, or sarcoidosis is present. In cases where 1,25-D is the mediator for the hypercalcemia, steroid therapy can reduce the inflammatory response and thereby lower 1,25-D levels. Glucocorticoids also interfere with intestinal 1,25-D actions to increase $Ca^{2+}$ uptake. In fungal infections or tuberculosis when there is associated hypercalcemia, the initial response should be to address the underlying disease with specific therapies rather than to use steroids initially to address hypercalcemia. Attention to volume status and knowing that chronic hypercalcemia promotes salt and water losses are important precepts for managing these patients.

Primary HPTH is managed in symptomatic patients with surgery as the first-line therapy. Several clinical parameters are considered in determining therapy of primary HPTH in patients who are asymptomatic. Surgery may still be offered, based on the criteria outlined in the Third International Workshop on Asymptomatic Primary HPTH (Table 11.6).[40,41,52,53] Alternatively, when patients are poor candidates for surgery, have failed it, or refuse it, oral calcimimetics can be used. A calcimimetic is a CaSR agonist that activates the receptor, bringing about an inhibition of PTH release. The calcimimetic cinacalcet was developed as a CaSR-directed therapy designed to lower serum [$Ca^{2+}$] and PTH levels in patients with uremic secondary HPTH. Cinacalcet has been shown to lower the serum [$Ca^{2+}$] into the normal range in 80%–90% of patients with mild hypercalcemia due to primary HPTH in a sustained manner.[54–57] This agent also lowers serum [$Ca^{2+}$] in patients with moderate and symptomatic primary HPTH not amenable to surgery.[58] Patients with inoperable parathyroid cancer causing symptomatic hypercalcemia can also be treated with this agent—often in higher doses than are needed to control primary or uremic secondary HPTH.[59] Oral bisphosphonates such as alendronate have also been used to improve bone mass in patients with primary HPTH who have osteoporosis.[55] Unlike the intravenous bisphosphonates that are potent enough to lower the serum [$Ca^{2+}$], oral bisphosphonates do not have a significant effect on hypercalcemia in patients with primary HPTH.

## *Hypocalcemia (see Severe hypocalcemia Chapter 24)*

Hypocalcemia should only be diagnosed when the albumin-corrected total serum [$Ca^{2+}$] or the ionized [$Ca^{2+}$] is frankly low (Table 11.3). These level(s) should be confirmed before an extensive workup is started.

### *Presentation*

It is essential for the clinician to appreciate that profound degrees of hypocalcemia may present without any significant signs or symptoms. The duration of the abnormality is the likely reason. The patient has adapted to the abnormal [$Ca^{2+}$] slowly over time. Alternatively, the presentation may be dramatic with profound neuromuscular irritability, tetany, cramping, seizures, laryngospasm, bronchospasm, and even congestive heart failure.[34,60] The full picture of how patients present with

Consider recommending parathyroid surgery for the following indications:

- Serum total [$Ca^{2+}$] ≥1.0 mg/dL (≥0.25 mmol/L) above the upper limits of normal
- Renal stones, any symptoms or complications of hypercalcemia and primary HPTH
- Estimated glomerular filtration rate <60 mL/min/1.73 $m^2$
- T score at central DXA site ≤–2.5
- Age <50 years

Monitoring recommended for patients with asymptomatic primary HPTH who do not undergo parathyroidectomy:

- Annual serum [$Ca^{2+}$] determinations
- Annual serum creatinine determinations
- Bone mineral density measurements by DXA every 1–2 years (three sites)

*Source:* Bilezikian JP et al., *J Clin Endocrinol Metab,* 94, 335–9, 2009.

***Table 11.6***
*Management of asymptomatic primary HPTH (Guidelines from the Third International Workshop).*

hypocalcemia involves those signs and symptoms due to the underlying disease plus those that are more specific to the low serum [$Ca^{2+}$] itself.

## *Symptoms and signs*

The signs and symptoms of hypocalcemia affect many different tissues in the body (Table 11.7). Neuromuscular signs and symptoms can be very troubling to the patient and include tetany, cramping of the muscles, paresthesias, numbness and tingling especially around the mouth and face and in the extremities, seizures (focal or generalized), depressed mental status, choreoathetosis, and even organic brain syndrome. Both Trousseau and Chvostek signs can be elicited in hypocalcemic patients to determine whether there is evidence of neuromuscular irritability. Trousseau sign is elicited by inflating the blood pressure cuff for at least 3 min to ~20 mm Hg over the systolic blood pressure.[34] When it is positive, painful carpal spasms involving the fingers of the tested hand occur. Chvostek sign is demonstrated by tapping the cheek over the facial nerve in front of the ear and just below the zygoma. A positive sign is twitching of the ipsilateral face. Cardiac signs include prolonged QT interval on the electrocardiography (ECG). Congestive heart failure can also occur if the abnormal serum [$Ca^{2+}$] is profoundly low, usually for a very long time, or in individuals with underlying cardiac disease.[34,60–62] Subcapsular cataracts may be seen in chronic hypocalcemia as well as papilledema. Full-blown pseudotumor cerebri can also be seen. The hair and nails are often dry and brittle.

The diverse disorders that cause hypocalcemia contribute their own clinical presentations. These disorders include pseudohypoparathyroidism, various genetic syndromes of hypoparathyroidism, hypoparathyroidism secondary to gland destruction (e.g., iron overload, autoimmune etiology, postsurgery), activating CaSR mutations, and vitamin D deficiency and resistance (Table 11.8).[7,31,32,34,46,47,60–62] The signs, symptoms, and physical findings in such an array of disorders are vast and must be looked for in a patient who does not have a clear-cut etiology for hypocalcemia after the initial history and physical examination are done. The presence of other autoimmune disorders such as adrenal insufficiency, vitiligo, and type 1 diabetes suggest autoimmune polyglandular failure type 1. The constellation of short stature, round facies, frontal bossing, mental retardation, shortened metacarpals, ectopic ossifications, and obesity is called Albright's hereditary osteodystrophy

- General
  - Weakness
  - Fatigue
- Neuromuscular manifestations
  - Tetany
  - Tingling
  - Paresthesias
  - Muscle cramps
  - Laryngospasm
  - Bronchospasm
  - Seizures (focal or generalized)
  - Altered mental status
  - Coma
- Cardiac
  - Congestive heart failure
  - Prolonged QT interval
- Ophthalmologic
  - Cataracts
  - Papilledema

***Table 11.7***
*Signs and symptoms of hypocalcemia.*

- Hypomagnesemia
  - Urinary losses due to alcoholism
  - Drug-induced renal $Mg^{2+}$ loss
  - Gastrointestinal loss of $Mg^{2+}$ due to malabsorption, diarrhea, fistula
- Hypoparathyroidism
  - Postsurgical (postthyroidectomy, parathyroidectomy, laryngectomy)
  - Metastases
  - Iron deposition (thalassemia)
  - Genetic syndromes (GATA3, GCMB mutations)
  - DiGeorge syndrome
  - Autoimmune (isolated, polyglandular)
  - Idiopathic
  - PTH gene defects
- Pseudohypoparathyroidism type 1a, 1b
- Vitamin D disorders
  - Vitamin D deficiency
  - Vitamin D–dependent rickets type 1 and 2
- Miscellaneous
  - Pancreatitis
  - Hungry bone syndrome
  - Tumor lysis syndrome

***Table 11.8***
*Disorders causing hypocalcemia.*

and is seen in pseudohypoparathyroidism type 1a, a form of resistance to the actions of PTH. There are many other findings in the syndromes associated with hypoparathyroidism, in particular, that can be helpful in arriving at the correct diagnosis and potentially ordering the correct genetic tests (Table 11.8).[61,62]

## Evaluation and differential diagnosis

An early step in the workup of hypocalcemia is the measurement of serum [$Mg^{2+}$] and intact PTH (Figure 11.6)[62]. If the serum [$Mg^{2+}$] is low, then the appropriate workup for that abnormality should be initiated and the $Mg^{2+}$ repleted. Serum intact PTH may be low or inappropriately normal in patients who have $Mg^{2+}$ depletion as a cause for their hypocalcemia. Once $Mg^{2+}$ depletion is corrected, hypocalcemia will resolve, and the PTH level may rise.

If the PTH is elevated in the presence of hypocalcemia, then vitamin D deficiency, resistance to vitamin D action, and pseudohypoparathyroidism must be considered. Physical findings are as described above for pseudohypoparathyroidism type 1a, whereas type 1b typically has no specific physical abnormalities, only the biochemical profile shown (Table 11.9). In vitamin D deficiency, 25-OH D levels are <20 ng/mL (50 nM), and phosphate levels are often low. Vitamin D deficiency should be suspected, because it is very common in patients with malabsorption, malnutrition, short gut syndrome, pancreatic insufficiency, celiac disease, and postgastric bypass surgery. In vitamin D resistance due to mutations in the 1-α-hydroxylase gene (or vitamin D–dependent rickets type 1), 1,25-D levels are low, and PTH levels are high. In vitamin D resistance due to loss of function mutations in the VDR (vitamin D–dependent rickets type 2), both 1,25-D and PTH levels are elevated. Syndromes of vitamin D resistance are extremely rare.

Hypoparathyroidism, regardless of the etiology, presents with low or inappropriately normal PTH and typically high phosphate levels. In patients with activating CaSR mutations, their hypocalcemia is usually mild and is accompanied by low normal or frankly low PTH levels. These patients, in contrast to other forms of hypoparathyroidism, excrete more $Ca^{2+}$ over 24 h when they have hypocalcemia (i.e., relative hypercalciuria) due to the concomitant renal CaSR-sensing defect.[46,61,62]

## Pathophysiology

A variety of mechanisms are involved in the pathogenesis of hypocalcemic disorders. Parathyroid tissue is either destroyed or its function impaired when there is autoimmune disease, metastatic tumor, or heavy metal deposition that affects the glands to cause hypoparathyroidism. Gland development is abnormal in patients with GATA3 or GCMB mutations, the DiGeorge syndrome, and mitochondrial disorders producing hypoparathyroidism. GATA3 mutations also affect otic vesicle and renal development so deafness and renal anomalies may also be present.

| Disorder | S-$Ca^{2\pm}$ | S-Phos | Intact PTH | 25-OH D | 1,25-D | Other lab tests |
|---|---|---|---|---|---|---|
| Hypoparathyroidism | ↓ | ↑ | ↓ or low nl | nl | nl | |
| Hypocalcemic hypercalciuria or autosomal dominant hypocalcemia | ↓ | ↑ | ↓ or low nl | nl | nl | Urinary $Ca^{2+}$ high for low serum [$Ca^{2+}$] CaSR mutation |
| Pseudohypoparathyroidism | ↓ | ↑ | ↑↑ | nl | nl | |
| Vitamin D deficiency | ↓ | ↓ | ↑↑ | ↓↓ | nl or ↓ | Urinary $Ca^{2+}$ low |
| Vitamin D resistance | | | | | | |
| Type 1 | ↓ | ↓ | ↑↑ | nl | ↓ | Urinary $Ca^{2+}$ low |
| Type 2 | ↓ | ↓ | ↑↑ | nl | ↑↑ | Urinary $Ca^{2+}$ low |
| Hypomagnesemia | sl ↓ | nl | ↓ or nl | nl | nl | Low serum [$Mg^{2+}$] |

nl, normal; sl, slight

***Table 11.9***
*Biochemical profiles of disorders causing hypocalcemia.*

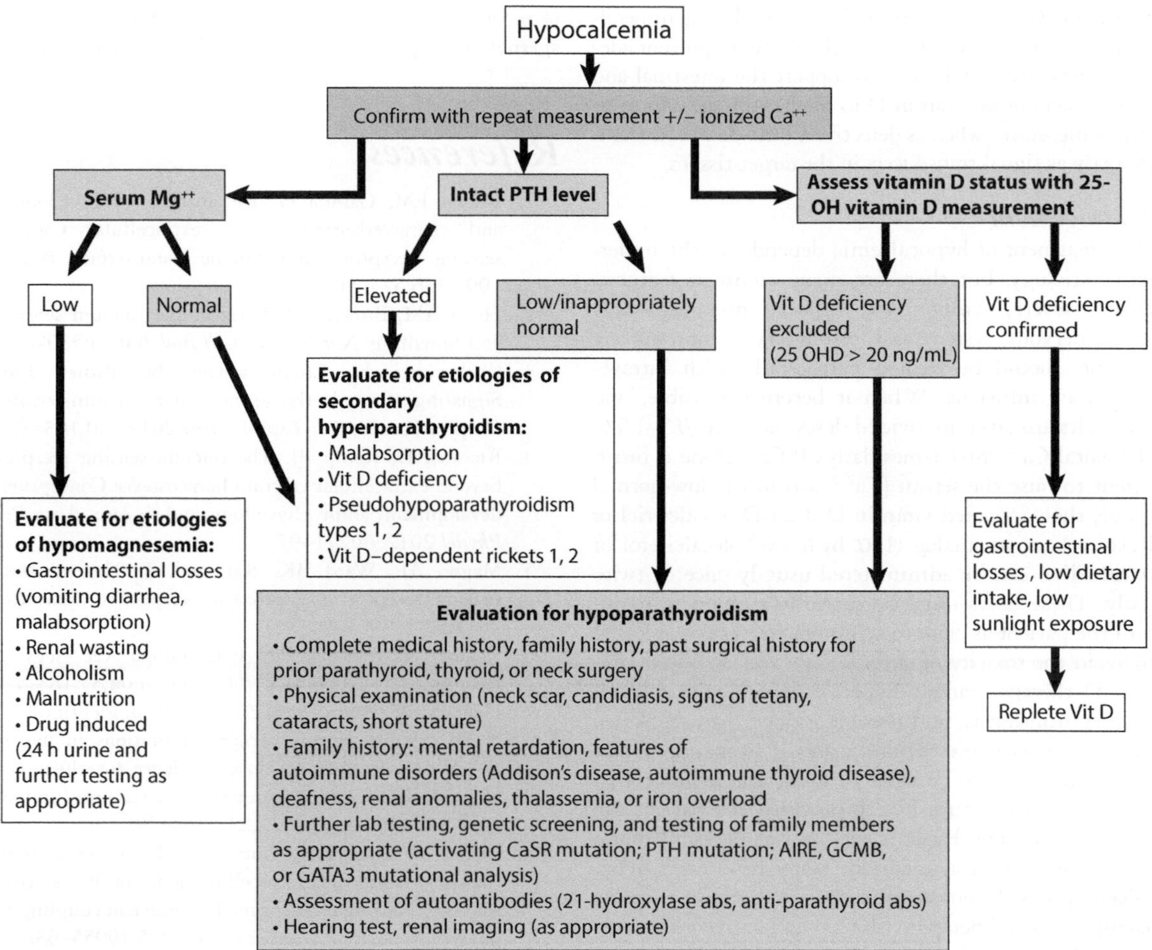


***Figure 11.6***

*Detailed algorithm for the evaluation of hypocalcemia and hypomagnesemia, including analyses that could be considered in determining the etiology for hypoparathyroidism. CaSR, Calcium-sensing receptor; PTH, Parathyroid hormone; AIRE, Autoimmune regulator gene; GCMB, Glial cell missing B;* GATA3, GATA binding protein 3. *(Modified and reproduced from Bilezikian J et al.,* J Bone Min Res, *26, 2317–37, 2011. With permission.)*

Pseudohypoparathyroidism type 1a is typically due to loss of function mutation in one allele of the stimulatory G protein α subunit coupling the PTH-R to adenylate cyclase ($G_s\alpha$). This is a heterozygous mutation, but because the $G_s\alpha$ gene is imprinted and inactivated in certain tissues such as the renal tubules, patients carrying the mutant allele may manifest the phenotypic features and the biochemical abnormalities if the mutation is maternally inherited. Resistance to PTH is most penetrant in the kidneys. There are patients with pseudohypoparathyroidism who have normal bone sensitivity to PTH and thus demineralize their bones due to their chronic secondary HPTH. They show low bone mass on DXA scanning. Some patients have even shown classic hyperparathyroid bone disease (e.g., osteitis fibrosa cystica).[34] Patients with pseudohypoparathyroidism type 1b have the same biochemical profile as type 1a patients but do not carry $G_s\alpha$ mutations. Instead the level of $G_s\alpha$ expression is altered through effects on gene transcription in many cases due to methylation defects in that gene.[34,61,62] The hypocalcemic disorders discussed above are quite uncommon, except perhaps for hypomagnesemia. Pseudohypoparathyroidism is quite rare.

The pathophysiology of the vitamin D disorders that cause hypocalcemia is straightforward. Vitamin D deficiency reflects inadequate levels of vitamin D metabolites to support $Ca^{2+}$ and phosphate balance and bone mineralization. Deficiencies in 1-hydroxylase activity prevent adequate generation of 1,25-D to support the intestinal and skeletal actions of vitamin D to maintain bone and mineral homeostasis, whereas defective VDRs do not function properly as signal transducers in the target tissues.

### Management

The treatment of hypocalcemia depends on the underlying etiology, but there are many common features. Acute, severe, symptomatic hypocalcemia, especially when nervous system and respiratory symptoms are present, should be treated parenterally with intravenous $Ca^{2+}$ infusions. When it becomes possible, oral $Ca^{2+}$ salts are given in divided doses each day (0.5–1.5 G elemental $Ca^{2+}$ three times daily). If $Ca^{2+}$ alone is insufficient to raise the serum [$Ca^{2+}$] within the low-normal range, then activated vitamin D (1,25-D or calcitriol or Rocaltrol) or its analog (1 $\alpha$ hydroxycholecalciferol or $\alpha$ calcidiol) can be administered usually once or twice daily. These doses must be carefully titrated to maintain the patient as close to symptom-free as possible and to avoid the toxicity of chronic $Ca^{2+}$ and activated vitamin D therapy, namely hypercalciuria, nephrocalcinosis, nephrolithiasis, and chronic kidney disease. When hypercalciuria is present and difficult to manage, thiazide diuretics may be used to lower the urinary $Ca^{2+}$ and elevate the serum [$Ca^{2+}$], provided the patient can tolerate this agent. Patients with activating CaSR mutations deserve special mention. Many have mild hypocalcemia and do not require therapy because they are asymptomatic. Therapy with $Ca^{2+}$ and active vitamin D metabolites or analogs has the distinct disadvantage in this group of patients of raising the urinary $Ca^{2+}$ dramatically, leading to nephrocalcinosis, renal stones, and renal insufficiency. Therapy in this group of patients should be avoided if possible.

## Acknowledgments

I thank the Research Service of the Department of Veterans Affairs Program Project Application (grant 1IP1BX001599) and the National Institutes of Health (R01 AR055588) for their funding support.

## Disclosures and Conflicts of Interest

Dr. Shoback received grant support and was a principal investigator on clinical trials to test the efficacy and safety of cinacalcet for the treatment of primary HPTH and parathyroid cancer (Amgen) and the efficacy and safety of recombinant intact human PTH (1–84) in the management of hypoparathyroidism (NPS Pharmaceuticals).

## References

*1. Brown EM, Gamba G, Riccardi D, et al. Cloning and characterization of an extracellular Ca(2+)-sensing receptor from bovine parathyroid. *Nature* 1993;366:575–80.
2. Hofer AM, Brown EM. Extracellular calcium sensing and signalling. *Nat Rev Mol Cell Biol* 2003;4:530–8.
3. Chakravarti B, Chattopadhyay N, Brown EM. Signaling through the extracellular calcium-sensing receptor (CaSR). *Adv Exp Med Biol* 2012;740:103–42.
4. Riccardi D, Kemp PJ. The calcium-sensing receptor beyond extracellular calcium homeostasis: Conception, development, adult physiology, and disease. *Annu Rev Physiol* 2012;74:271–97.
†5. Magno AL, Ward BK, Rarajczak T. The calcium-sensing receptor: A molecular perspective. *Endo Rev* 2011;32:3–30.
6. Chang W, Shoback D. Extracellular $Ca^{2+}$-sensing receptors – an overview. *Cell Calcium* 2004;35:183–96.
7. Hannan FM, Nesbit MA, Zhang C, et al. Identification of 70 calcium-sensing receptor mutations in hyper- and hypo-calcaemic patients: Evidence for clustering of extracellular domain mutations at calcium-binding sites. *Hum Mol Genet* 2012;21:2768–78.
8. Chang W, Chen T-H, Pratt S, et al. Amino acids in the second and third intracellular loops of the parathyroid $Ca^{2+}$-sensing receptor mediate efficient coupling to phospholipase C. *J Biol Chem* 2000;275:19955–63.
9. Chang W, Pratt S, Chen T-H, et al. Amino acids in the cytoplasmic carboxyterminus of the parathyroid $Ca^{2+}$-sensing receptor mediate effective cell-surface expression and phospholipase C activation. *J Biol Chem* 2001;276:44129–36.
10. Gama L, Wilt SG, Breitwieser GE. Heterodimerization of calcium sensing receptors with metabotropic glutamate receptors in neurons. *J Biol Chem* 2001;276:39053–9.
11. Margeta-Mitrovic M, Jan YN, Jan LY. Ligand-induced signal transduction within heterodimeric GABA(B) receptor. *Proc Natl Acad Sci U S A* 2001;98:14643–8.
12. Bai M, Trivedi S, Brown EM. Dimerization of the extracellular calcium-sensing receptor (CaR) on the cell surface of CaR-transfected HEK293 cells. *J Biol Chem* 1998;273:23605–10.

* Original paper reporting the cloning of the CaSR and its functional properties.
† Contemporary review of molecular properties of the CaSR and signal transduction.

13. Chang W, Tu C, Cheng Z, et al. Complex formation with type B γ-aminobutyric acid receptor affects the expression and signal transduction of the extracellular calcium-sensing receptor. *J Biol Chem* 2007;282:25030–40.
14. Cheng Z, Tu C, Rodriguez L, et al. Type B gamma-aminobutyric acid receptors modulate the function of the extracellular $Ca^{2+}$-sensing receptor and cell differentiation in murine growth plate chondrocytes. *Endocrinology* 2007;148:4984–92.
15. Riccardi D, Brown EM. Physiology and pathophysiology of the calcium-sensing receptor in the kidney. *Am J Physiol Renal Physiol* 2010;298:F485–99.
16. Kumar R, Thompson JR. The regulation of parathyroid hormone secretion and synthesis. *J Am Soc Nephrol* 2011;22:216–24.
17. Qin L, Raggatt LJ, Partridge NC. Parathyroid hormone: A double-edged sword for bone metabolism. *Trends Endocrinol Metabol* 2004;15:60–5.
*18. Silva BC, Costa AG, Cusano NE, et al. Catabolic and anabolic actions of parathyroid hormone on the skeleton. *J Endocrinol Invest* 2011;34:801–10.
19. Neer RM, Arnaud CD, Zanchetta JR, et al. Effect of parathyroid hormone (1–34) on fractures and bone mineral density in postmenopausal women with osteoporosis. *N Engl J Med* 2001;344:1434–41.
20. Orwoll ES, Scheele WH, Paul S, et al. The effect of teriparatide [human parathyroid hormone(1–34)] therapy on bone density in men with osteoporosis. *J Bone Miner Res* 2003;18:9–17.
21. Greenspan SL, Bone HG, Ettinger MP, et al. Effect of recombinant human parathyroid hormone (1–84) on vertebral fracture and bone mineral density in postmenopausal women with osteoporosis: A randomized trial. *Ann Intern Med* 2007;146:326–39.
22. Huang C, Miller RT. Regulation of renal ion transport by the calcium-sensing receptor: An update. *Curr Opin Nephrol Hypertens* 2007;16:437–43.
23. Mannstadt M, Jüppner H, Gardella TJ. Receptors for PTH and PTHrP: Their biological importance and functional properties. *Am J Physiol* 1999;277:F665–75.
24. Talmage RV, Mobley HT. Calcium homeostasis: Reassessment of the actions of parathyroid hormone. *Gen Comp Endocrinol* 2008;156:1–8.
25. Weinman EJ, Lederer ED. PTH-mediated inhibition of the renal transport of phosphate. *Exp Cell Res* 2012;318:1027–32.
†26. Haussler MR, Whitfield GK, Kaneko I, et al. The role of vitamin D in the FGF23, klotho, and phosphate bone-kidney endocrine axis. *Rev Endocrinol Metab Disord* 2012;13:57–69.
27. Perwad F, Portale AA. Vitamin D metabolism in the kidney: Regulation by phosphorus and fibroblast growth factor 23. *Mol Cell Endocrinol* 2011;347: 17–24.
28. Geibel JP, Hebert SC. The functions and roles of the extracellular $Ca^{2+}$-sensing receptor along the gastrointestinal tract. *Annu Rev Physiol* 2009;71:205–17.
29. Kos CH, Karaplis AC, Peng JB, et al. The calcium-sensing receptor is required for normal calcium homeostasis independent of parathyroid hormone. *J Clin Invest* 2003;111:1021–8.
30. Tu Q, Pi M, Karsenty G, et al. Rescue of the skeletal phenotype in CasR-deficient mice by transfer onto the Gcm2 null back ground. *J Clin Invest* 2003;111:1029–37.
31. Holick MF. Vitamin D deficiency. *N Engl J Med* 2007;357:266–81.
32. Rosen CJ. Vitamin D deficiency. *N Engl J Med* 2011;364:248–54.
33. Bikle DD. VitaminD: Newly discovered actions require reconsideration of physiologic requirements. *Trends Endocrinol Metab* 2010;21:375–84.
34. Shoback D, Sellmeyer D, Bikle D. Mineral metabolism and metabolic bone disease. In: Shoback D, Gardner D (eds), *Basic and Clinical Endocrinology*. 9th edn. Lange Medical Books/McGraw-Hill, New York; 2011, pp. 227–84.
35. Jacobs JP, Bilezikian JP. Clinical review: Rare causes of hypercalcemia. *J Clin EndocrinolMetab* 2005;90:6316–22.
36. Clines GA. Mechanism and treatment of hypercalcemia of malignancy. *Curr Opin Endocrinol Diabetes Obes* 2011;18:339–46.
‡37. Wysolmerski JJ. Parathyroid hormone-related protein: An update. *J Clin Endocrinol Metab* 2012;97:2947–56.
38. Mosekilde L. Primary hyperparathyroidism and the skeleton. *Clin Endocrinol* 2008;69:1–19.
39. Rubin MR, Bilezikian JP, McMahon DJ, et al. The natural history of primary hyperparathyroidism with or without parathyroid surgery after 15 years. *J Clin Endocrinol Metab* 2008;93:3462–70.
40. Fraser WD. Hyperparathyroidism. *Lancet* 2009; 374:145–58.
41. Silverberg SJ, Lewiecki EM, Mosekilde L, et al. Presentation of asymptomatic primary hyperparathyroidism: Proceeding of the Third International Workshop. *J Clin Endocrinol Metab* 2009;94:351–65.
42. Marcocci C, Cetani F. Clinical practice: Primary hyperparathyroidism. *N Engl J Med* 2011;365:2389–97.
43. Marcocci C, Cetani F, Rubin MR, et al. Parathyroid carcinoma. *J Bone Min Res* 2008;23:1869–80.
§44. Brown EM. Clinical lessons from the calcium-sensing receptor. *Nat Clin Pract Endocrinol Metabol* 2007;3:122–33.

* Review that describes the complex actions of PTH in bone.

† Excellent review of rapidly developing field of phosphate homeostasis and bone–kidney interactions.

‡ Recent review on the biology of the PTHrP including its functions in normal cell differentiation and function.

§ Overview of human diseases due to CaSR mutations.

45. Christensen SE, Nissen PH, Vestergaard P, et al. Familial hypocalciuric hypercalcaemia: A review. *Curr Opin Endocrinol Diabetes Obes* 2011;18:359–70.
46. Egbuna OI, Brown EM. Hypercalcaemic and hypocalcaemic conditions due to calcium-sensing receptor mutations. *Best Pract Res Clin Rheumatol* 2008;22:129–48.
47. Hannan FM, Nesbit MN, Zhang C, et al. Identification of 70 calcium-sensing receptor mutations in hyper- and hypo-calcaemic patients: Evidence for clustering of extracellular domain mutations at calcium-binding sites. *Hum Mol Genet* 2012;21:2768–78.
48. Christiansen SE, Nissen PH, Vestergaard P, et al. Discriminative power of three indices of renal calcium excretion for the distinction between familial hypocalciuric hypercalcaemia and primary hyperparathyroidism: A follow-up study on methods. *Clin Endocrinol* 2008;69:713–20.
49. Westin G, Bjorklund P, Akerstrom G. Molecular genetics of parathyroid disease. *World J Surg* 2009;33:2224–33.
50. Libutti SK, Crabtree JS, Lorang D, et al. Parathyroid gland-specific deletion of the mouse Men1 gene results in parathyroid neoplasia and hypercalcemic hyperparathyroidism. *Cancer Res* 2003;63:8022–8.
51. Imanishi Y, Hosokawa Y, Yoshimoto K, et al. Primary hyperparathyroidism caused by parathyroid-targeted overexpression of cyclin D1 in transgenic mice. *J Clin Invest* 2001;107:1093–102.
52. Udelsman R, Pasieka JL, Sturgeon C, et al. Surgery for asymptomatic primary hyperparathyroidisim: Proceedings of the Third International Workshop. *J Clin Endocrinol Metab* 2009;94:366–72.
*53. Bilezikian JP, Khan AA, Potts JT, Jr. Third International Workshop on the Management of Asymptomatic Primary Hyperparathyroidism. Guidelines for the management of asymptomatic primary hyperparathyroidism: Summary statement from Third International Workshop. *J Clin Endocrinol Metab* 2009;94:335–9.
54. Peacock M, Bilezikian JP, Klassen PS, et al. Cinacalcet hydrochloride maintains long-term normocalcemia in patients with primary hyperparathyroidism. *J Clin Endocrinol Metab* 2005;90:135–41.
55. Khan A, Grey A, Shoback D. The medical management of asymptomatic primary hyperparathyroidism. *J Clin Endocrinol Metab* 2009;94:373–81.
56. Peacock M, Bolognese MA, Borofsky M, et al. Cinacalcet treatment of primary hyperparathyroidism: Biochemical and bone densitometric outcomes in a five-year study. *J Clin Endocrinol Metab* 2009;94:4860–7.
57. Peacock M, Bilezikian JP, Bolognese MA, et al. Cinacalcet HCl reduces hypercalcemia in primary hyperparathyroidism across a wide spectrum of disease severity. *J Clin Endocrinol Metab* 2011;96:E9–18.
58. Marcocci C, Chanson P, Shoback D, et al. Cinacalcet reduces serum calcium concentrations in patients with intractable primary hyperparathyroidism. *J Clin Endocrinol Metab* 2009;94:2766–72.
59. Silverberg SJ, Rubin MR, Faiman C, et al. Cinacalcet hydrochloride reduces the serum calcium concentration in inoperable parathyroid carcinoma. *J Clin Endocrinol Metab* 2007;92:3803–8.
60. Cooper MS, Gittoes NJL. Diagnosis and management of hypocalcaemia. *BMJ* 2008;336:1298–302.
†61. Shoback D. Clinical practice: Hypoparathyroidism. *N Engl J Med* 2008;359:391–403.
62. Bilezikian J, Khan A, Potts JT, Jr., et al. Hypoparathyroidism in the adult: Epidemiology, diagnosis, pathophysiology, target organ involvement, treatment and challenges for future research. *J Bone Min Res* 2011;26:2317–37.


* International guidelines for management of primary hyperparathyroidism.

† Comprehensive review of conditions causing hypoparathyroidism.

# 12

# Metabolic bone disease

*Philip E. Harris, Pierre-Marc G. Bouloux*

## *Osteoporosis*

Osteoporosis is the most prevalent metabolic bone disease among developed countries and is characterized by compromised bone strength and increased risk of fracture.[1] An important characteristic of osteoporosis is a normal mineral/collagen ratio, which distinguishes it from osteomalacia, a disease characterized by relative deficiency of mineral in relation to collagen. Osteoporotic fractures may affect any part of the skeleton except the skull. Most commonly, fractures occur in the distal forearm (Colles fracture), thoracic and lumbar vertebrae, and proximal femur. The incidence of osteoporotic fractures increases with age, is higher in whites than in blacks, and is higher in women than in men.[2,3] The female-to-male ratio is about 1.5:1 for Colles fractures, 7:1 for vertebral fractures, and 2:1 for hip fractures. Because most osteoporotic fractures, except hip fractures, do not require admission to the hospital, it is difficult to obtain a precise knowledge on the true prevalence of this disease (Figure 12.1).

Osteoporosis in the elderly has become a major public health problem for most industrialized societies as the aging population increases.[4] The morbidity and mortality associated with osteoporosis is considerable and will impose increasing demands on health expenditures as the size of the elderly population rises.[5] Peak bone mass is higher in males and is also higher in blacks than in whites or Asians.[6] In addition, because bone loss accelerates after menopause, osteoporosis and osteoporotic fractures are much commoner among elderly women than men. There is an important genetic component to osteoporosis. Studies of twins suggest that genetic determinants are responsible for up to 85% of the variation in peak bone mass and may also determine bone turnover and fracture risk. In consequence, a family history of osteoporosis and fractures is an important part of the overall assessment of the patient.[7]

## *Bone metabolism and pathogenesis of osteoporosis*

Bone is a vascularized skeletal tissue made up of an organic matrix, a mineral phase (calcium hydroxyapatite), and bone cells (osteoclasts, osteoblasts, and osteocytes). The organic matrix is composed of fibers of collagen (chiefly type 1 collagen); elastin and other proteins, such as osteocalcin and matrix Gla proteins; the Arg-Gly-Asp (RGD)-containing proteins, such as fibronectins, thrombospondins, vitronectin, fibrillin, osteopontin, and bone sialoprotein. Other noncollagen proteins of bone include osteonectin and tetranectin. Glycosaminoglycan (GAG)–containing proteins include biglycan, decorin, fibromodulin, and osteoadherin. Apart from its ability to provide structural integrity, bone has several biochemical functions, with bone itself serving as a calcium reservoir and its marrow as a hematopoietic organ. Bone formation by osteoblasts has two phases: synthesis of the bone matrix, including the formation of a network of collagenous fibers, and mineralization of the matrix. Osteoclasts, in contrast, bring about bone resorption, which also consists of two simultaneous processes: dissolution of hydroxyapatite crystals and proteolysis of the matrix. Anatomically, bone can be divided into cortical (compact) and trabecular (spongy, cancellous) parts. In trabecular bone, the interconnecting trabecular structures increase resistance to mechanical load.

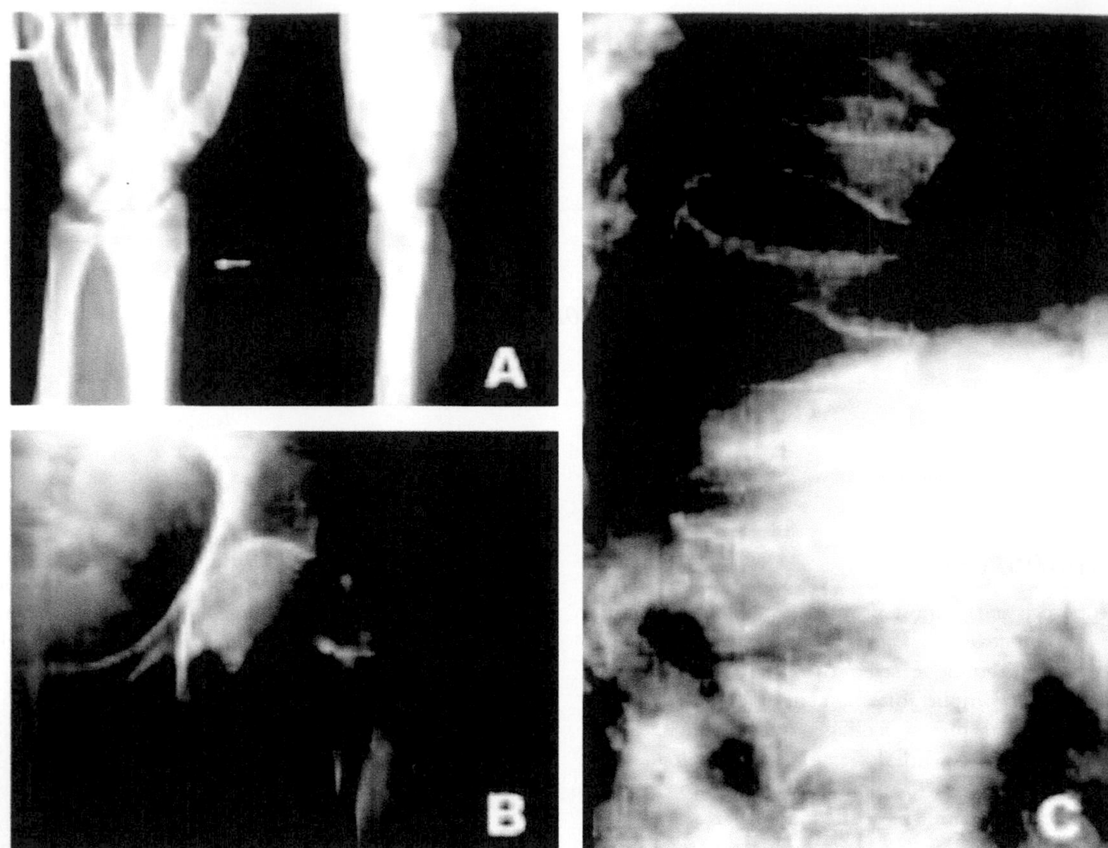


**Figure 12.1**
*Scanned images of typical osteoporotic fractures: (A) wrist, (B) hip, and (C) vertebral bodies. (From Gennari C and Avioli LV (editors),* Atlante delle malattie dell'osso, *Vol I, Chiesi Farmaceutici S.p.A., Parma, 1992. With permission.)*

Bone is constantly being remodelled, and the processes of formation and resorption of bone tissue are coupled. The cycle is initiated by resorption of old bone, recruitment of osteoblasts, deposition of new matrix, and mineralization of the newly deposited matrix. Thus, remodelling provides a mechanism for bone self-repair and adaptation to stress, by a process of renewal of old bone and replacement with new bone.[8] The annual bone turnover rate in adult women is about 2%–5% in cortical bone and 15%–25% in trabecular bone and cortical surface, with the latter two types being metabolically most active. Trabecular and cortical bones differ in their hormonal sensitivity: the vertebral spine, which is rich in trabecular bone, responds to hormonal treatments more strongly than appendicular bones with cortical bone dominance.[9]

The two most significant determinants of bone mass are the peak bone mass attained at about 30 years of age and the rate of bone loss after it. These determinants in turn are controlled by genetic, hormonal, nutritional, and environmental factors. In the lifelong process of bone turnover, formation is dominant in the growth period. Bone mass peaks at or before 30 years of age, sometimes even in late teenage years.[10,11] At peak, the activity of bone-forming cells equals that of the resorbing cells, and skeletal size remains unchanged. Soon afterward, bone mass begins to decrease, the average annual loss becoming about 0.3%–0.5% by the fifth decade of life. In women after menopause bone loss accelerates to about 2% (range, 1%–5%) for 5–10 years, stabilizing thereafter to about 1%/year, so that by age 65–70 years, bone loss is still above the premenopausal level.[12] During her lifetime, a normal woman will lose approximately half of her spinal bone and about a third from her cortical bone tissue. The increase in bone loss with age in women is made up of two components: an exponential, postmenopausal, estrogen-related component, predominantly of trabecular bone, that lasts for 5–10 years and a linear,

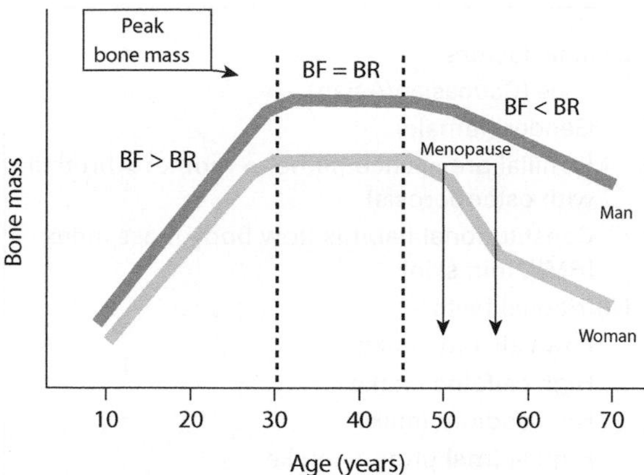


***Figure 12.2***
*Bone mass and age in male and female. BF, bone formation; BR, bone resorption.*

- Primary osteoporosis
  - Idiopathic juvenile osteoporosis
  - Idiopathic osteoporosis of the young adult
  - Involutional osteoporosis
    - Postmenopausal osteoporosis
    - Senile osteoporosis
- Secondary osteoporosis
  - Hypercortisolism (Cushing)
  - Hypogonadism
  - Hyperparathyroidism
  - Hyperthyroidism
  - Vitamin D deficiency (secondary hyperparathyroidism)
  - Malabsorption
  - Chronic renal insufficiency
  - Anorexia nervosa
  - Connective tissue diseases
    - Osteogenesis imperfecta
  - Malignancy
    - Multiple myeloma
    - Mastocytosis
  - Iatrogenic
    - Glucocorticoids Aromatase inhibitors
    - Gonadotropin-releasing hormone (GnRH) agonists/antagonists
    - Heparin
    - Anticonvulsants

***Table 12.1***
*Clinical classification of osteoporosis.*

age-related component (Figure 12.2).[11,13] This latter slower phase of bone loss affects men, starting at about age 55 years, and has been attributed to age-related factors such as reduction in renal calcium absorption as well as in intestinal calcium absorption and to a vitamin D deficiency status, mainly due to a decreased renal 1α-hydroxylase, all resulting in an increase in circulating PTH levels.[11] Estrogen-related bone loss causes type 1 osteoporosis characterized by loss of trabecular bone tissue and fractures in trabecular bones, such as crush fractures of the vertebral spine. Age-related bone loss due to declining activity of osteoblasts causes type II osteoporosis (senile osteoporosis), resulting in thinning of trabeculae and loss of cortical bone tissue which also becomes porous.

Although males do not undergo an acute loss of estrogen such as during menopause, evidence points to a key role for estrogen in the maintenance of bone mass in males. Both free testosterone and estradiol levels fall, concomitant with a rise in sex hormone binding globulin levels with age, but it is free estrogen levels that appear to be the main determinant of bone mass. There seems to be a critical threshold estradiol level, below which the fracture risk increases. Declining testosterone levels may contribute to increased fracture risk through nonskeletal effects such as muscle mass.[11]

## *Classification of osteoporosis (Table 12.1)*

Osteoporosis is commonly classified into primary or idiopathic and secondary, the latter being osteoporosis for which a clearly identifiable etiological mechanism is recognized. Primary osteoporosis is further characterized into idiopathic juvenile osteoporosis, idiopathic osteoporosis of the young adult, and involutive osteoporosis, comprising postmenopausal or type-I osteoporosis and senile or type II osteoporosis.

Depending on bone remodelling, the disease is also classified into high-turnover or low-turnover osteoporosis. It is known that the excessive bone loss that characterizes the pathogenesis of osteoporosis results from abnormality in the bone remodelling cycle. It appears that with each cycle there is a slight, imperceptible deficit in bone formation. The total bone loss is therefore a function of the number of cycles in process at any one time. Conditions that increase the rate of activation of the bone remodelling process increase the proportion of the skeleton undergoing remodelling at any one time, thus increasing the rate of bone loss. These circumstances characterize high-turnover osteoporosis. Most of the secondary causes of osteoporosis are associated with this increased rate of activation of bone remodelling cycle. In other circumstances, excessive bone loss can occur when activation of the skeleton is not increased and even when activation of the skeleton might be decreased. This loss gives rise to the concept of low-turnover osteoporosis and is typical of the normal aging process. In this case, there appears to be a progressive impairment of signaling between bone resorption and bone formation, such that with every cycle of remodelling, there is an increase in the deficit between resorption and formation, because osteoblast recruitment is inefficient.

## Diagnosis of osteoporosis

Bone loss is asymptomatic and symptoms related to fractures are often the first sign of osteoporosis. Several factors, including genetic, nutritional, lifestyle, and medical, are associated with osteoporosis (Table 12.2). It is possible that the risk of fracture could be reduced by identifying these factors in individuals and recommending appropriate lifestyle changes. Hyperthyroidism, hyperparathyroidism, and the long-term use of corticosteroids, heparin, or supraphysiological doses of thyroid hormones may also enhance bone loss. A simple clinical estimation of the risk of osteoporosis, however, is often inaccurate. Only about a third of the women at real risk for osteoporosis can be identified by the clinical indicators listed above.

Genetic factors certainly play a major role in the pathogenesis of osteoporosis. There is clear evidence of genetic modulation of bone parameters, including bone density, bone size, and bone turnover. It has been postulated that at any particular age and phase of life, genetic factors explain about 70% of the variance in bone phenotype.[7] Hormonal factors, diet, and lifestyle interact with the genetic regulators of bone, over time, to determine net bone mass.

The Endocrine Society has published guidelines on the assessment and management of osteoporosis in men.[14]

| |
|---|
| Genetic factors |
| Race (Caucasian/Asian) |
| Gender (female) |
| Familial prevalence (father > mother > brother with osteoporosis) |
| Constitutional habitus (low body mass index [BMI], thin skin) |
| Nutritional factors |
| Low calcium intake |
| High caffeine intake |
| High sodium intake |
| High animal protein intake |
| High alcohol intake |
| Lifestyle factors |
| Smoking |
| Low physical activity |
| Excessive physical activity (females) |
| Endocrine factors |
| Sex hormone status (amenorrhea/ hypogonadism) |
| Menopausal age (early menopause, ovariectomy) |

***Table 12.2***
*Risk factors for osteoporosis.*

### Bone mineral density

Bone mineral density (BMD) is closely correlated with the strength of the bone. In general, the lower the BMD, the higher the risk for fracture. Overall, 75%–85% of the variance in the ultimate strength of bone tissue is accounted by changes in BMD. Bone mass is usually assessed using dual energy X-ray absorptiometry (DXA) of the lumbar spine (L1-L4) and femoral neck/total hip. Forearm (mid-third radius) measurement may also be performed. Other techniques include quantitative computerized tomography (QCT), peripheral DXA, and heel ultrasound, although these techniques do not have the same level of predictive fracture risk data as central DXA.[15]

BMD value is compared with two standards known as the Z scores (the number of standard deviations above or below the mean population of the same gender, age, race, and weight) and T scores (the number of standard deviations above or below the mean of a young adult Caucasian population of the same gender). For postmenopausal women and men >50 years of age, T scores are classified according to the definitions of BMD set by the World Health Organization (WHO):[16]

1. Normal BMD: T-score up to 1 SD lower than the mean reference BMD
2. Osteopenia: T-score >1 SD but <2.5 SD lower than the reference mean
3. Osteoporosis: T-score ≤2.5 SD than the reference mean
4. Severe osteoporosis: T-score as in osteoporosis, plus one or more fractures

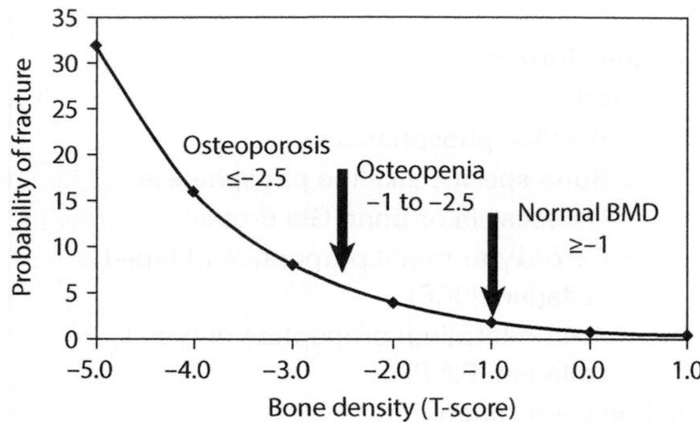


***Figure 12.3***
*Relationship between BMD and fracture probability. (From Watts NB et al.,* J Clin Endocrinol Metab, *97, 1802–22, 2012; Vokes TJ and Favus MJ,* Transl Endocrinol Metabol, *1, 9–54, 2010. With permission.)*

The T-score can also be applied to women in the perimenopausal transition. In children and young adults <50 years old, assessment of BMD should use the Z scores, with values <–2.0 being considered abnormal.[17]

Although the use of BMD measurements is an important component of the assessment of fracture risk, it is not without problems. It has high specificity but low sensitivity, the majority of postmenopausal women presenting with a fracture having T-score in the osteopenia rather than the osteoporotic range. In addition, the WHO definitions defined above are absolutes, whereas BMD is a continuous variable (Figure 12.3).[14,15]

## *Fracture Risk Assessment Tool (FRAX®)*

The importance of including factors that affect fracture risk independently of BMD has been recognized by the development of the WHO-supported FRAX risk algorithm (www.sheff.ac.uk/FRAX).[18] FRAX is a computer-driven algorithm that provides a 10-year probability of major fracture, based on risk factors (Figure 12.4). Importantly,

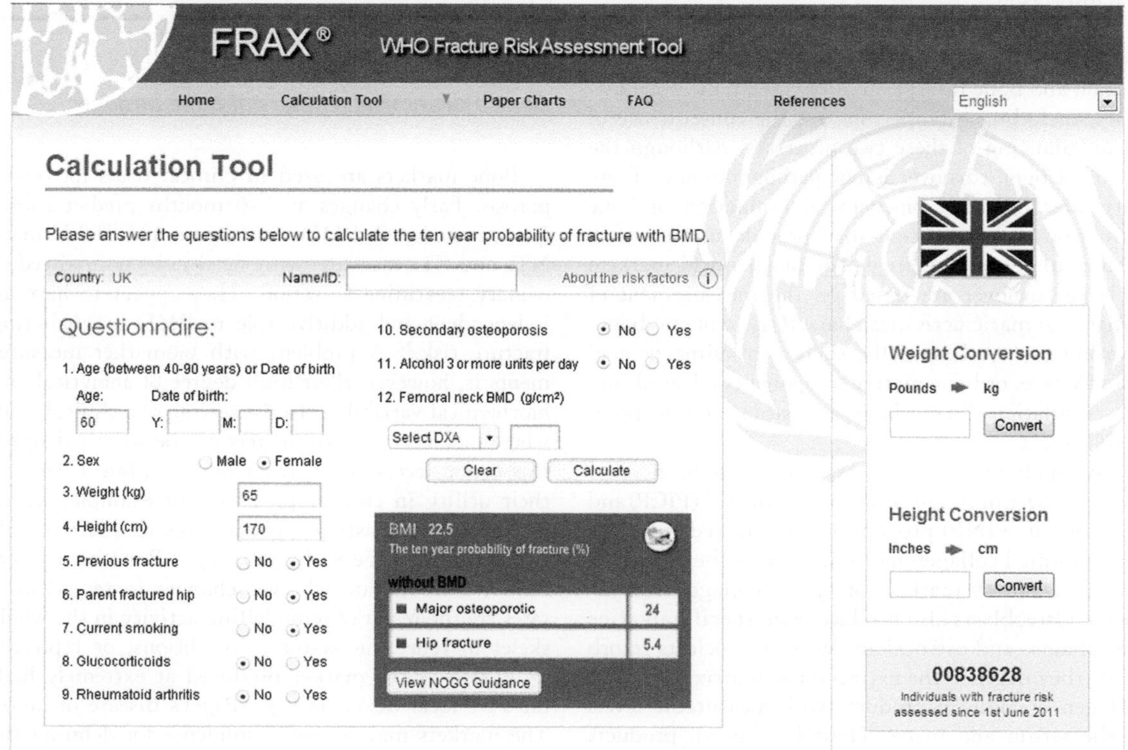


***Figure 12.4***
*WHO FRAX. Data have been entered for a 60-year-old woman who is a smoker, with a previous fracture and a positive family history. The 10-year probability of sustaining a major osteoporotic fracture is 24% and that of a hip fracture is 5.4%.*

the model provides the ability to make predictions for patients from different ethnicities, although the data are best validated for Caucasians. A limitation is that its use is limited to men and women aged ≥40 years.

## *Biochemical assessment of bone turnover*

Osteoporosis may be the only manifestation of many of the secondary causes listed in Table 12.1. It is therefore appropriate to perform simple screening analyses looking for these causes in each patient. A biochemical profile should include information about renal and hepatic function, primary hyperparathyroidism, hyperthyroidism, and possible malnutrition. A hematological profile might also provide clues to the presence of myeloma and malnutrition. A 24 h urinary collection for measurement of calcium (which should always be accompanied by the assessment of creatinine and sodium) is useful in detecting patients with hypercalciuria, the end result of excess skeletal loss. Conversely, very low levels of urinary calcium [below 50 mg (1.25 mmol) for 24 h] may be indicative of the presence of vitamin D malnutrition or malabsorption.

The bone remodelling cycle is characterized by two opposite but finely coupled processes, bone formation and bone resorption. Most metabolic bone diseases, including osteoporosis, are the consequence of an unbalancing of these two processes. Although the status of bone turnover is not pathognomonic of any particular disorder, biochemical evaluation of bone formation and resorption may provide useful information in clinical practice. The biochemical markers of bone turnover are based on the measurement of either enzymatic activities characteristic of the bone-forming or resorbing cells, such as alkaline or acid phosphatase, or bone matrix components released into the circulation during bone apposition or resorption (Table 12.3).

During bone formation, osteoblasts produce type-I collagen. Serum type-I collagen C-terminal (PICP) and N-terminal (PINP) propeptides are cleaved from the newly formed collagen molecule and can be measured in the serum as markers of type-I collagen biosynthesis. Osteoblasts also produce bone-specific alkaline phosphatase and osteocalcin. When osteoclasts resorb bone, they degrade the extracellular matrix, releasing collagen breakdown products with measurable levels in the serum and urine. These breakdown products include free pyrodinolines (PYDs) and deoxypyridinolines (DPDs), the cross-linked aminoterminal telopeptide (NTx), and cross-linked carboxyterminal-telopeptide (CTx). Osteoclasts also produce serum tartrate–resistant acid phosphatase (TRAP).[19]

A. Bone formation
- Serum
  - Alkaline phosphatase
  - Bone-specific alkaline phosphatase
  - Osteocalcin or bone Gla protein
  - Carboxy-terminal propeptide of type-I collagen (PICP)
  - Amino-terminal propeptide of type-I collagen (PINP)

B. Bone resorption
- Urine
  - Hydroxyproline
  - Free and total pyridinolines
  - Free and total deoxypyridinolines
  - N-Telopeptide of collagen cross-links (NTx)
  - C-Telopeptide of collagen cross-links (CTx)
- Serum
  - Tartrate-resistant acid phosphatase (TRAP)
  - Cross-linked C-telopeptide of type-I collagen (ICTP)

***Table 12.3***
*Bone biochemical markers of bone turnover.*

Bone markers are used in clinical trials for osteoporosis. Early changes at 3–6 months predict subsequent increases in BMD and fracture risk.[20,21] Urinary NTx and CTx measurements need to be normalized to urinary creatinine excretion. They appear to have an independent and additive role to BMD in predicting fracture risk.[22] A problem with biomarker measurements is, however, their high degree of analytical and biochemical variability. In the setting of a clinical trial, where measurement parameters can be strictly defined, this is not necessarily a major problem, but it detracts their utility in clinical practice. For example, serum osteocalcin demonstrates substantial circadian variability, peaking in the early morning.[19] Bone biomarkers cannot discriminate whether changes in remodelling rates are the result of remodelling activity in the whole skeleton, reflecting systemic conditions, or represent a dilution of the marker produced at extremely high rates by focal disorders (e.g., Paget's disease of bone). The markers may provide confidence for defining the most appropriate therapeutic intervention and for dose adjustments. Theoretically, patients with high-turnover osteoporosis, with increased levels of resorption and formation markers, should be experiencing bone loss at an accelerated rate and should respond best to therapy with drugs that inhibit bone resorption. By contrast, those with low- or normal-turnover osteoporosis should have bone markers in the physiological range, should not be losing bone at an accelerated rate, should respond less to antiresorptive therapy, and should be treated preferentially with drugs that primarily enhance bone formation.

# *Prevention and treatment of osteoporosis (Table 12.4)*

Osteoporosis is a preventable and, in its early phases, treatable disease. Maximizing peak bone mass during childhood and early adulthood is the most cost-effective way of reducing the risk of an osteoporotic fracture. An adequate intake of calcium (approximately 1000–1200 mg/day), moderate weight-bearing exercise, and the maintenance of normal body weight are important elements in building up strong bones and preserving skeletal strength lifelong. The recommended calcium intake for postmenopausal women and men >50 years old and for the treatment of osteoporosis is 1200 mg of elemental calcium per day.[14] Calcium balance is affected by dietary sodium and animal protein intake, which increase urinary calcium excretion and calcium requirements.[15] Although calcium supplementation in men and women has been shown to improve bone density, the effects on fracture risk are unclear.[14]

It is important that patients with osteoporosis are vitamin D replete. Vitamin D deficiency is defined as 25(OH)D levels ≤20 ng/mL (50 nmol/L) and insufficiency as 25(OH)D levels of 21–29 ng/mL (52.5–72.5 nmol/L).[23] Vitamin D deficiency may be associated with osteomalacia. Lesser degrees of deficiency/insufficiency may be associated with secondary hyperparathyroidism. The dose of vitamin D should be based on the clinical setting or severity of deficiency, to raise the serum level >75 nmol/L (30 ng/L).[23] Calcium and vitamin D supplementation should be included in the treatment regimen of osteoporosis, unless there is evidence of adequate calcium intake and normal vitamin D level. The recommended daily dose of vitamin D is 800 IU. Due to the high risk of vitamin D deficiency in elderly patients who are house-bound, supplementation is recommended in these patients.

Physical activity is an important component, because although the evidence for improvement in BMD is unclear, exercise improves muscle function and is associated with reduced falls and fracture risk.[14,15] Reduction in alcohol consumption and cessation of smoking are also important components of patient management.[15]

A meta-analysis of different pharmacological agents used in reducing the risk of fragility fractures has recently been reported.[24]

## *Bisphosphonates*

Bisphosphonates are analogs of inorganic pyrophosphate and are potent inhibitors of bone resorbtion. They bind to bone mineral and are then taken up by osteoclasts and rapidly inhibit resorption. They act on the mevalonate pathway by inhibiting the action of farnesyl diphosphate synthase, thereby preventing the production of prenylated proteins that are essential for osteoclast action.

They have been shown to reduce vertebral fracture rates and also hip fractures and other nonvertebral fractures in some studies. They are generally well tolerated, with good long-term safety.[14,15,25–27]

The first clinically available bisphosphonate was etidronate. Large doses or prolonged treatment may be associated with a mineralization defect in patients with Paget's disease. The newer compounds, the aminobisphosphonates, such as alendronate, risedronate, ibandronate, and zoledronic acid, are considerably more potent, and they do not appear to be associated with this problem. A small number of patients may experience severe localized bone pain, necessitating treatment with a different form of medication. Osteonecrosis of the jaw is a rare association with bisphosphonate therapy and is particularly associated with patients receiving high-dose intravenous bisphosphonates such as zoledronic acid for the treatment of malignant hypercalcemia. There is also a concern that long-term suppression of bone turnover might have adverse effects on bone strength, with reports of mid-shaft or subtrochanteric fractures of the femur. Overall, however, the beneficial effects of bisphosphonates on fracture risk are far greater than these rare potential side effects.[15]

The oral bisphosphonates should be taken with a glass of water after an overnight fast, 30–60 min before eating or drinking, or before taking other medicinal products. The patient should remain in the upright position for 30–60 min. Compliance with this treatment regimen minimizes upper gastrointestinal symptoms such as reflux and facilitates absorption. They are contraindicated in the presence of clinically significant esophageal disease. Intravenous preparations may be associated with transient flu-like symptoms (acute phase response) that may be ameliorated by taking paracetamol/acetaminophen. Oral bisphosphonates should be considered for first-line therapy for women with postmenopausal osteoporosis, men with osteoporosis, and both men and women with glucocorticoid-induced osteoporosis.

| Drug | Dosing | Comments |
|---|---|---|
| | **Inhibitors of bone resorption** | |
| *Bisphosphonates* | | |
| Etidronate | 400 mg for 14 days, then calcium carbonate 1.25 g for 76 days (oral) | Consider for first-line therapy<br>Risk of esophageal reactions reported with oral bisphosphonates. Take with glass of water after overnight fast, 30–60 min before eating, drinking, or taking other medications<br>Caution in patients with renal impairment<br>Rare association with osteonecrosis of jaw, particularly with intravenous formulations |
| Alendronate | 10 mg daily or 70 mg weekly (oral) | |
| Risedronate | 35 mg weekly or 150 mg monthly (oral) | |
| Ibandronate | 150 mg/month (oral) or 3 mg 3 monthly (intravenous injection) | |
| Zoledronic acid | 5 mg yearly (intravenous infusion over at least 15 min) | |
| | **Estrogens and SERMs** | |
| HRT | According to preparation | Increased risk of breast cancer<br>Thromboembolism |
| Raloxifene | 60 mg daily (oral) | Thromboembolism<br>Hot flushes<br>Reduced risk of breast cancer |
| RANK ligand inhibitor | | |
| Denosumab | 60 mg 6 monthly (subcutaneous injection) | Good tolerability |
| | **Calcitonin** | |
| Salmon calcitonin | 200 units daily (intranasal spray) | Modest efficacy. Use in patients unable to tolerate other forms of treatment<br>Maybe transient facial flushing and nausea<br>Additional analgesic effect |
| | **Stimulators of bone formation** | |
| Parathyroid hormone | 100 μg daily (subcutaneous injection) | Consider in severe osteoporosis if other agents not tolerated or failed<br>Hypercalcemia, hypercalciuria particularly with PTH<br>Nausea |
| Teriparatide (PTH 1-34) | 20 μg daily (subcutaneous injection) | |
| | **Dual activity** | |
| Strontium ranelate | 2 g daily in water, preferably at bedtime | Consider for patients in whom bisphosphonates are contraindicated or not tolerated<br>Efficacy demonstrated in elderly patients<br>Hypersensitivity reactions; stop if skin rash develops (DRESS)<br>Small increased risk of thromboembolism |

***Table 12.4***
*Pharmacological treatments of osteoporosis.*

### *Estrogens (hormone replacement therapy [HRT]) and selective estrogen receptor modulators (SERMs)*

HRT is an option where other therapies are contraindicated, cannot be tolerated, or are ineffective. HRT is most beneficial, however, as a prophylaxis for osteoporosis if started at early menopause and continued up to 5 years. Long-term treatment is not recommended because of the risk of breast cancer, but some patients prefer to continue treatment for symptomatic benefits. Estrogen and alendronate produce similar increase in BMD, but unlike bisphosphonates, cessation of estrogen therapy is associated with resumption of bone loss.[28] Consideration should therefore be given to continuation with an alternative therapy such as bisphosphonates, when HRT is stopped.

Raloxifene is a nonsteroidal benzothiophene compound with a high affinity for estrogen receptor (ER)–α and ERβ. It is a partial agonist in bone, reducing vertebral fractures but not nonvertebral fractures.[29] In a study of the effects of alendronate and raloxifene in postmenopausal women with osteoporosis, raloxifene and alendronate increased BMD in the lumbar spine and femoral neck, with an additive effect. The effects on BMD and bone markers with alendronate alone, however, were approximately twice those of raloxifene alone, supporting the positioning of bisphosphonates as first-line therapy for osteoporosis.[30] Raloxifene may cause or accentuate hot flushes in postmenopausal women and is also associated with an increased risk of thromboembolism, although the risk of breast cancer is decreased.[31] It reduces low-density lipoprotein levels, but does not increase high-density lipoprotein levels.[32]

### *Strontium ranelate*

Strontium ranelate is a salt consisting of two atoms of strontium linked to ranelic acid. It is gradually incorporated into the skeleton, replacing calcium ions in the hydroxyapatite lattice. In animal models, strontium has a dual effect, stimulating bone formation and inhibiting resorption, effects that are mirrored by changes in the respective bone markers in clinical studies. In addition, strontium has effects on osteoblast differentiation and proliferation.[33]

Strontium ranelate reduces both vertebral and nonvertebral fracture risk in postmenopausal women with osteoporosis and osteopenia.[34,35] Post hoc analysis of the phase III data demonstrate efficacy in patients >80 years of age.

Strontium ranelate is taken as 2 g granules in water, preferably at bedtime, avoiding food for 2 h before or after taking the medication. The main side effects are nausea and diarrhea. It is not associated with upper gastrointestinal side effects and is therefore an alternative for patients who are unable to tolerate oral bisphosphonates. A small increased risk of venous thromboembolism was seen in the clinical trials. Hypersensitivity reactions may occur and may be severe (drug reaction eosinophilia and systemic symptoms [DRESS]). If a patient develops a skin rash taking strontium ranelate, treatment should be stopped immediately, and the patient should not be retreated with the drug in the future.

### *Denosumab*

Denosumab is a human monoclonal antibody directed against receptor activator of nuclear factor (NF)-κB (RANK) ligand (RANKL). RANKL stimulates the recruitment and differentiation of osteoclast precursors. Its effects are inhibited by osteoprotegerin, a soluble decoy RANKL receptor that is secreted by osteoblasts and osteoclast precursors (Figure 12.5). Denosumab mimics the effects of osteoprotegerin on osteoclast function.[36,37]

The pivotal 3-year placebo-controlled FREEDOM trial involved the administration of denosumab 60 mg ($n$ = 3902) or placebo ($n$ = 3906) subcutaneously six monthly to postmenopausal women with osteoporosis. Treatment resulted in increased BMD and reduced new vertebrai (68%), hip (40%), and nonvertebral fractures (20%).[38] This was associated with significant increases in BMD at the lumbar spine, femoral neck, total hip, and distal one-third radius. In a subsequent extension study to FREEDOM, study participants ($n$ = 4550, 58% of those enrolled into the original FREEDOM study) all received denosumab an open label design for 7 years.[39] Results from the first 2 years of the extension study have demonstrated maintenance of the reduction in bone turnover markers (P1NP and CTx) and continued significant increases in BMD measurement in those patients who had previously received denosumab in the pivotal study. Fracture rates remained low and below those observed in the pivotal study. The patients from the placebo group, who switched to denosumab, demonstrated comparable rapid and marked falls in bone turnover markers and significant increases in BMD to the denosumab group in the pivotal study. The yearly incidence of vertebral and nonvertebral fractures was similar to those in the denosumab group of the pivotal study.

Safety data did not demonstrate any differences in incidences of adverse or serious adverse events between the placebo and treatment groups in the FREEDOM study. Comparable incidences of adverse events were seen

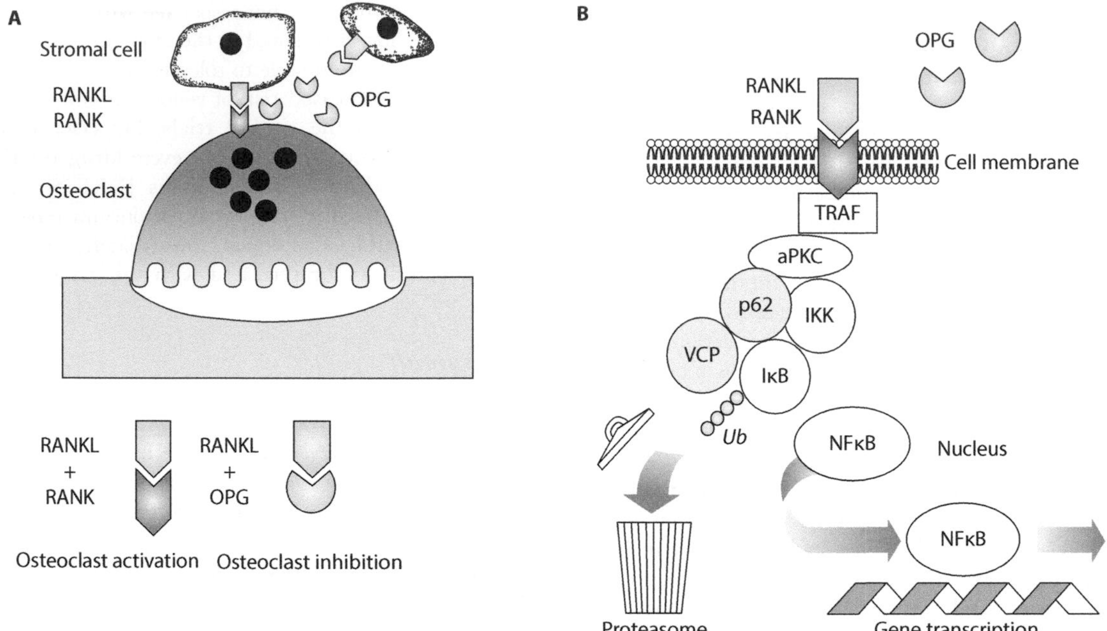


**Figure 12.5**
*Regulation of osteoblast activity by the RANK–NF-κB signaling pathway. (a) Engagement of RANK and RANKL results in osteoclast activation and inhibition of osteoclast apoptosis, and these actions are prevented by osteoprotegerin (OPG), which acts as a decoy receptor for RANKL. (b) The NF-κB signaling pathway lies downstream of the RANK receptor. Binding of RANKL to RANK results in recruitment of tumor necrosis factor (TNF)–receptor associated factors (TRAF) to the receptor complex, along with other molecules, including the* SQSTM1 *gene product p62 and atypical protein kinase C (aPKC). This binding results in phosphorylation of inhibitor of κB kinase (IKK) that, in turn, phosphorylates inhibitor of κB (IκB). The phosphorylated IκB becomes ubiquinated (Ub) and targeted for degradation by the proteasome, releasing the p65 component of NF-κB that translocates to the nucleus and activates expression of genes that stimulate osteoclast formation and function. The VCP protein that is mutated in the syndrome of inclusion body myopathy, Paget's disease, and frontotemporal dementia (IBMPFD) has also been shown to affect NF-κB signaling and is involved in regulating degradation of IκB by the proteasome. (From Ralston SH et al.,* Lancet, *372, 155–63, 2008.)*

in the extension study. There were two adverse events classified as osteonecrosis of the jaw, both of which healed, with one patient continuing with treatment.

Denosumab should be administered by subcutaneous injection six monthly. Patients should also receive calcium and vitamin D supplementation as appropriate.

### *Parathyroid hormone peptides*

Parathyroid hormone (PTH), when administered intermittently, has anabolic skeletal effects, stimulating osteoblastic new bone formation. The effect is most marked in trabecular bone.[40]

In an 18-month study in postmenopausal women with osteoporosis receiving calcium and vitamin D supplementation, human recombinant PTH 1-84 (100 µg by daily subcutaneous injection) versus placebo (daily subcutaneous injection) prevented new or worsened vertebral fracture and improved lumbar spine and hip density, although there was a reduction in forearm bone density. There was a high incidence of hypercalcemia (23%), hypercalciuria (24%), and nausea (14%) in the PTH-treated patients.[41] PTH is administered subcutaneously 100 µg by daily subcutaneous injection. Treatment is limited to a maximum of 24 months.

Teriparatide (hPTH 1-34) has a similar anabolic effect to PTH 1-84. In a study of postmenopausal women with prior vertebral fractures, daily injections of teriparatide at doses of 20 and 40 µg/day increased BMD of the spine by 9% and 13%, respectively, reducing the risk of new vertebral fractures by 65% and 69%, respectively, compared with placebo. There were also reductions in risk for nonvertebral fractures: 20 µg/day, 35%, and 40 µg/day, 40%. Adverse events were higher in the 40 µg/day group. Nausea occurred in 18% of patients. Hypercalcemia was particularly associated with this treatment group. Although urinary calcium excretion increased slightly, hypercalciuria did not occur.[42] Teriparatide, but not PTH, is approved in the United States for the treatment of osteoporosis. The dose is 20 µg/day for a maximum of 18 months. These anabolic agents are generally used in patients with severe osteoporosis, usually if they have failed other treatments such as antiresorptive agents.[15] Prior or concomitant therapy with bisphosphonates may blunt or delay the anabolic response to PTH.[43]

### Calcitonin

Calcitonin regulates calcium homeostasis by binding to osteoclasts and inhibiting bone resorption. It has mild antiresorbative activity, demonstrates modest increases in BMD,[44] and has been shown to reduce vertebral fracture risk in postmenopausal women with osteoporosis.[45] It is available as salmon calcitonin and can be administered intranasally, 200 units (1 spray), into one nostril daily. Patients sometimes experience transient facial flushing and nausea. Calcitonin has an additional variable analgesic effect. Its efficacy may wane with prolonged treatment. It may be used in patients who are unable to take other forms of treatment.

# Paget's disease of bone

Paget's disease of bone is a chronic disorder that typically results in enlarged and deformed bones in one or more regions of the skeleton. Excessive bone breakdown and formation can cause the bone to weaken. As a result, bone pain, arthritis, noticeable deformities, and fractures can occur. Paget's disease is most common in Caucasian people of European descent, but it also occurs in African Americans. It is rare in people of Asian descent. Paget's disease is rarely diagnosed in people under age 40. It affects 1%–2% of Caucasians older than 55 years, and about 8% of men and 5% of women by the eighth decade.[46]

It is important to emphasize the localized nature of Paget's disease. It may be monostotic, affecting only a single bone or a proportion of a bone, or may be polyostotic, involving two or more bones. Sites of disease are often asymmetric. In most instances, sites affected with Paget's disease at the time of diagnosis are the only ones that will show pagetic change over time. Although progression of disease within a given bone may occur, the sudden appearance of new sites of involvement some years after the initial diagnosis is not common.

## Etiology

For the majority of cases, the etiology of Paget's disease remains unclear. There is, however, an important hereditary component, with approximately 15%–40% of patients having a positive family history.[47,48]

Genome-wide linkage studies have identified several susceptibility loci for Paget's disease. Mutations have been identified in four genes that are all involved in the RANK–NF-κB pathway.[49,50] The most important gene identified so far is *sequestome 1 (SQSTM1)*, located at 5q35, a scaffold protein encoding p62 (Figure 12.5). Heterozygous mutations affecting the ubiquitin-associated domain, causing loss of ubiquitin binding, account for approximately 40% of cases of familial disease and a smaller proportion of patients with sporadic disease.[50] Other rare genetic causes have also been identified. Familial expansile osteolysis, early-onset familial Paget's disease, and expansile skeletal hyperphosphatasia are autosomal dominant disorders caused by insertion mutations in exon 1 of the *TNFRSF1A* gene that encodes the RANK receptor. Juvenile Paget's disease is an autosomal recessive disorder, caused by inactivating mutations of *TNFRSF11B* that encodes osteoprotegerin. Hereditary inclusion body myopathy, Paget's disease, and frontotemporal dementia (IBMPFD) is a dominant progressive disorder, caused by mutations in the valosin-containing protein *VCP* gene, clustered around a domain involved in ubiquitin binding.[49,50]

Viral infection has long been suggested to have a role in the pathogenesis of Paget's disease. Particles resembling paramyxovirus, as well as viral transcripts, including respiratory syncytial, measles, and canine distemper, have been reported in the nuclei and cytoplasm of osteoclasts at pagetic sites, but definitive proof has not been forthcoming.[51]

## Pathophysiology

The characteristic feature of the disease is an increased resorption followed by an increase in bone formation. It is generally believed that the primary cellular abnormality in Paget's disease is in the osteoclasts.[52] Emerging evidence suggests that osteoblasts may also have a role in disease pathogenesis.[53] Pagetic osteoclasts are markedly increased in number as well in size and contain up to 100 nuclei per cell.[54] Moreover, pagetic osteoclast precursors are hyperresponsive to $1,25(OH)_2D_3$ (calcitriol) and RANKL.[55] The marrow microenvironment also appears to be abnormal and has an enhanced capacity to induce osteoclast formation compared with the normal marrow microenvironment.[56]

Generally, the evolution of the disease follows three major phases. In the early phase, or osteolytic phase, bone resorption predominates and there is a concomitant increased vascularity of involved bones. In this phase, body calcium balance may be negative and the typical radiological picture is represented by an advancing osteolytic wedge or "blade of grass" lesion (Figure 12.6) in a long bone (i.e., femur or tibia) or by osteoporosis circumscripta, as seen in the skull ("salt and pepper") (Figure 12.7). Commonly, the excessive resorption of pagetic bone is followed closely by formation of new bone. During this second phase of the disease, the new bone that is made is structurally abnormal, presumably because of the accelerated nature of the remodelling process. Newly deposed collagen fibers are laid down in a disorganized rather than a linear manner, creating the so-called "woven bone," a reflection of high bone turnover. With time, the hypercellularity at the affected bone may diminish, leading to the development of a sclerotic, less vascular pagetic mosaic, without evidence

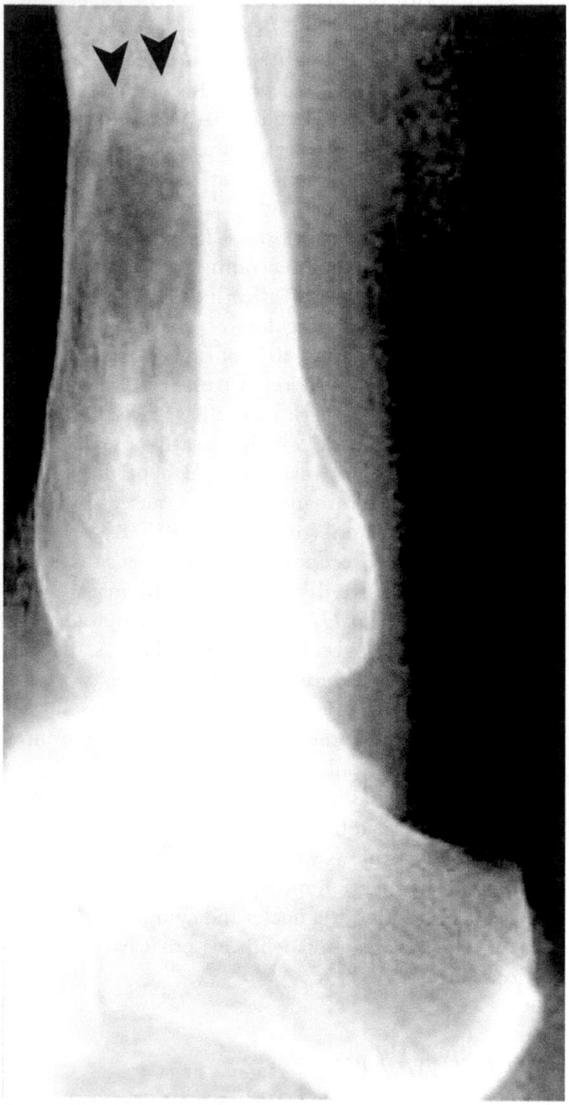

**Figure 12.6**
*Typical radiological picture of the advancing lytic wedge [arrow heads (blade of grass)] of the osteolytic phase of Paget's disease. (From Gennari C and Avioli LV (editors),* Atlante delle malattie dell'osso, *Vol II, Chiesi Farmaceutici S.p.A., Parma, 1992. With permission.)*

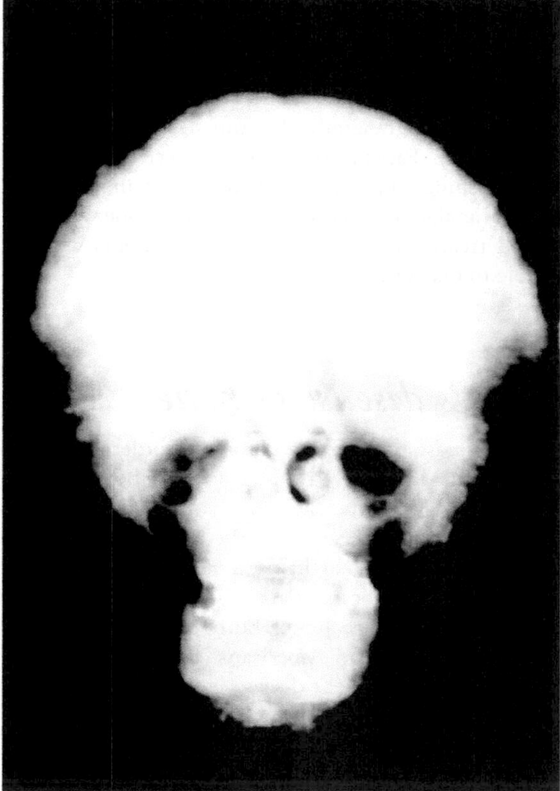

**Figure 12.7**
*Radiological picture of Pagetic lesion of the skull. (From Gennari C and Avioli LV (editors),* Atlante delle malattie dell'osso, *Vol II, Chiesi Farmaceutici S.p.A., Parma, 1992. With permission.)*

of active bone turnover. This is the so-called sclerotic or "burned-out" phase of Paget's disease. Typically, all these three phases of the disease can be seen at the same time at different sites in a single pagetic patient.

## Clinical features

In many patients, Paget's is asymptomatic. Localized bone pain is the most common presenting symptom that brings a patient with Paget's disease to a physician, sometimes associated with obvious deformity and increased local skin warmth due to increased bone microvasculature. The pain associated with Paget's disease can take many forms. It may arise from increased vascularity, from distortion of the periosteum due to disorganized remodelling, or from a focus of mechanical stress. The first phase of Paget's disease involves thinning of the bone and may be associated with painful microfractures, particularly in weight-bearing bones. Patients usually describe this pain as a deep pain that is most symptomatic at night and may lessen during the day.

Bowing of weight-bearing bones is a characteristic feature of Paget's disease. It occurs most frequently in the femur, tibia, and forearm. Because bone deformity is usually acquired later in life and is often asymmetrical, it has relatively good diagnostic specificity. This type of deformity in the femur or tibia is often associated with stress fractures on the convex surface of the bowed bone. These may present as localized areas of bone pain or tenderness and may also extend to produce a complete transverse fracture. The radiographic appearances are diagnostic and are easily distinguished from other types of stress fracture such as those typical of osteomalacia.

When Paget's disease reaches the end of a long bone, the cartilage may degenerate. When deformed, pagetic bones also damage the adjacent joints. Both of these situations result in osteoarthritis. Osteoarthritis is common among patients with Paget's disease and can be quite painful. Periarticular pain may be the presenting feature in 50% of cases.[57]

A variety of abnormalities can be associated with Paget's disease of the skull and spinal column. Skull deformity may result in enlargement of the vault, with a characteristic appearance particularly of the forehead (frontal bossing) or of the maxilla (leontiasis ossea).

## Biochemistry

Paget's disease is characteristically associated with an increase in bone turnover but normal concentrations of serum calcium, phosphate, PTH, and vitamin D metabolites. Most patients have elevated total serum alkaline phosphatase levels, reflecting the extent and activity of the disease.[58] A level of more than twice the normal range, in the absence of other potential confounding factors, is highly suggestive of Paget's disease. A normal level may occur, however, in monostotic or localized disease, in which case bone-specific alkaline phosphatase may be elevated and can be used as a biomarker. In patients with liver disease, bone-specific alkaline phosphatase should be used. Measurement of total or bone-specific alkaline phosphatase may be used to monitor disease evolution and response to treatment. Other biochemical markers of bone turnover are elevated in Paget's disease, but their measurement does not appear to offer any advantages over alkaline phosphatase.

## Radiography and scintigraphy

Radiographs of painful or deformed bones are usually diagnostic, showing the characteristic mixed appearance of areas of lysis due to increased osteoclastic resorption with sclerosis (Figure 12.8) from excessive osteoblastic bone formation. In the early stages of the disease, the changes may be predominantly lytic with flame shaped resorption fronts in the long bones or osteoporosis circumscripta in the skull. A characteristic appearance that distinguishes Paget's disease from other conditions is the increased diameter of affected bones, particularly those of the spine or the shafts of long bones.

Scintigraphy (Figure 12.9) is a sensitive but nonspecific method of detecting areas of skeletal abnormality and is the best way of assessing the skeletal distribution of Paget's disease. Although some sites may be asymptomatic, it is important that they are identified because they may be susceptible to complications, such as fracture. Biopsy of the affected lesion may be needed when the clinical features are equivocal.

## Complications of Paget's disease

Blood flow may be markedly increased in extremities involved with Paget's disease. When the disease is widespread and involves several bones, the increased blood flow may be associated with increased cardiac output and rarely with high-output heart failure. Pathologic fractures may occur at any stage even though are more common in the osteolytic phase of the disease. They particularly involve long bones with active area of advancing lytic disease (i.e., the femoral shaft or the subtrochanteric area) and may occur spontaneously or

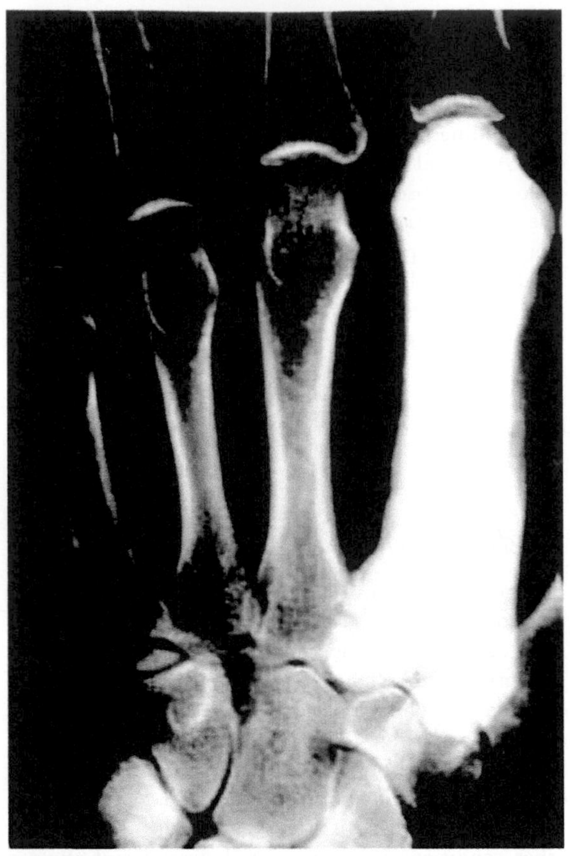

**Figure 12.8**
*Increased diameter and density at metacarpal level in monostotic Paget's disease. (From Gennari C and Avioli LV (editors),* Atlante delle malattie dell'osso, *Vol II, Chiesi Farmaceutici S.p.A., Parma, 1992. With permission.)*

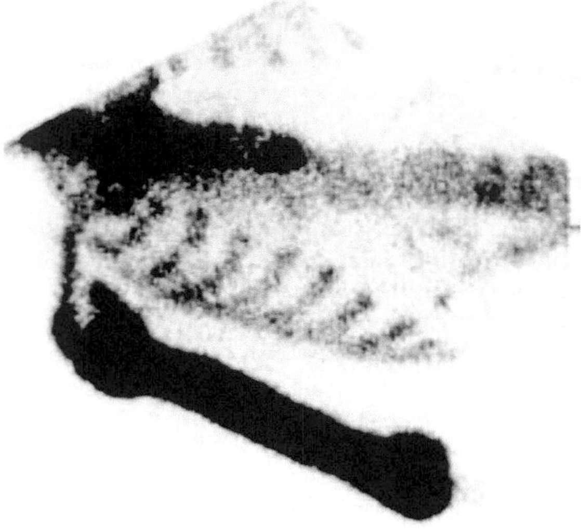

**Figure 12.9**
*Typical $^{99m}$Tc-methilene bisphosphonate scan of a patient affected with polyostotic Paget's disease. (From Gennari C and Avioli LV (editors),* Atlante delle malattie dell'osso, *Vol II, Chiesi Farmaceutici S.p.A., Parma, 1992. With permission.)*

follow slight trauma. They are estimated to occur in 6%–7% of patients.

Deafness occurs in about 13% of patients due to compression of the auditory nerve, ossicular and cochlear involvement.[57] Involvement of other cranial nerves is rare. Basilar impression (deformity of the craniocervical region) does not result in outwardly visible changes but is apparent radiologically and may cause symptoms due to internal hydrocephalus or long tract signs from brain stem compression. Pain radiating from the lower back into the legs (sciatica), can also occur because of the overgrowth of bone or the compression of discs. One of the most serious complications of Paget's disease is neoplastic degeneration of pagetic bone with an increased incidence of sarcomas, especially in polyostotic cases of the disease. The majority of these tumors are classified as osteosarcomas, although fibrosarcomas and chondrosarcomas may also be also seen. Approximately 1% of pagetic patients develop osteosarcoma, an increase in the risk that is several thousand-fold higher than in the general population. It has been estimated that 20% of the patients with osteosarcoma over the age of 60 years have Paget's disease as a predisposing condition.[59] This significantly contributes to the mortality and morbidity of Paget's disease patients. The sarcomas most frequently arise in the femur, tibia, humerus, skull, mandible, and pelvis, and they rarely occur in vertebrae. Typically, pagetic osteosarcomas are osteolytic, in contrast to the sclerotic appearance of radiation-induced osteosarcomas. Benign giant-cell tumor also may occur in pagetic bone. Radiographic evaluation of lesion as well as bone biopsy may be useful in the diagnosis. These tumors may show a great sensitivity to glucocorticoids, and in many instances, the mass may shrink or even disappear after treatment with dexamethasone or prednisone.[60]

## Medical therapy

Most pagetic patients do not have symptoms, because the disease is localized. However, appropriate treatment should be given not only to symptomatic patients but also to any patient with a pagetic lesion in a high-risk location, even if patient is asymptomatic. High-risk locations include the skull, spine, weight-bearing bones, pelvis, and areas near major joints. The treatment objective is to control symptoms and reduce the risk of long-term complications, although the evidence for this at the present time is lacking. Indications for therapy are listed in Table 12.5.

Any symptomatic pagetic lesion
- Pain
- Nerve compression
- Rapidly progressive deformity
- Repeated fractures

Asymptomatic lesions in high-risk locations
- Weight-bearing bone lesions
- Lesions affecting the skull and/or the spine
- Periarticular bone lesions

Before surgical intervention in pagetic bone
Immobilization with hypercalcemia
High-output cardiac failure

***Table 12.5***
*Indications for treatment of Paget's disease of bone.*

Two major classes of drugs, calcitonin and bisphosphonates, are available for the treatment of Paget's disease. Both classes of drugs suppress the abnormal bone cell activity that is associated with Paget's disease (Table 12.6).

### *Salmon calcitonin*

Salmon calcitonin has comparatively weak antiresorptive effects and a shorter duration of remission compared with bisphosphonates. It also has a short duration of action. It does, however, have analgesic properties and can be effective in controlling bone pain. It may be associated with nausea and flushing. The recommended dose is 50 units 3 times weekly to 100 units daily by subcutaneous or intramuscular injection, according to response. It may be useful in patients who are unable to take bisphosphonates.

### *Bisphosphonates (see "Osteoporosis")*

The introduction of these potent antiresorptive drugs has led to a dramatic improvement in the treatment of Paget's disease. An adequate dietary calcium intake (1000–1500 mg daily) and vitamin D intake (400 units) are recommended during bisphosphonate use, unless there is a history of nephrocalcinosis. Oral bisphosphonates and intravenous bisphosphonates are both effective (Table 12.6).

| *Drug* | *Dosing* | *Comments* |
|---|---|---|
| Calcitonin | 5–100 units daily (subcutaneous or intramuscular injection) | Modest efficacy. Use in patients unable to tolerate bisphosphonates<br>Maybe transient facial flushing and nausea<br>Analgesic effect may be helpful |
| Bisphosphonates | | |
| Etidronate | 5 mg/kg/day (oral) for up to 6 months—recommended dose<br>10 mg/kg/day (oral) for 3–6 months<br>11–20 mg/kg/day (oral) not to exceed 3 months | Etidronate may be associated with mineralization defect—avoid in patients with severe Paget's disease and osteolytic fronts affecting weight-bearing bone.<br>Risk of esophageal reactions with oral bisphosphonates. Take with glass of water after overnight fast 30–60 min before eating, drinking, or taking other medications.<br>Caution in patients with renal impairment.<br>Rare association with osteonecrosis of jaw, particularly with intravenous formulations |
| Tiludronate | 400 mg/day (oral) 3 months | |
| Alendronate | 40 mg/day (oral) 6 months | |
| Risedronate | 30 mg/day (oral) 2 months | |
| Pamidronate | Intravenous infusion; see dosing instructions | |
| Zoledronic acid | 5 mg intravenous infusion over at least 15 min as a single dose | |

***Table 12.6***
*Pharmacological treatments for Paget's disease of bone.*

Etidronate is moderately effective in reducing bone turnover by about 40%–60% and producing clinical improvement, but in many patients responses are incomplete. It may be associated with the development of localized osteomalacia that appears to be due to a direct effect on bone mineralization and is not correctable with vitamin D.[61] In consequence, it should be avoided in patients with severe Paget's disease and in the presence of advancing osteolytic changes in weight-bearing bone. Tiludronate usually leads to a normalization of serum alkaline phosphatase after 3 months of treatment in 30%–40% of moderately affected subjects.[62] It is generally well tolerated with a minority of patients experiencing mild upper gastrointestinal disturbances. In clinical trials with tiludronate, bone biopsy showed no evidence of defective mineralization. This drug may represent an attractive choice in patients with mild disease.

Alendronate is not associated with mineralization problems at therapeutically effective doses. In clinical trials, 6-month treatment with alendronate led to a normalized serum alkaline phosphatase in >63% of patients, compared with 17% for etidronate.[63] A similar response with normalization of serum alkaline phosphatase occurred in 54% of patients over two treatment cycles with risedronate.[64]

Intravenous bisphosphonates ensure compliance and may be used where rapid control is required, such as before surgery. They are also useful for patients who are unable to tolerate oral bisphosphonates. In a comparative study of risedronate with intravenous pamidronate in patients who had not previously received bisphosphonate therapy, similar degrees of efficacy were achieved.[65] Zoledronic acid is a highly potent bisphosphonate that can achieve long-term control over a 6–24 month period after a single intravenous infusion.[66,67] Intravenous bisphosphonates are associated with a transient fever and increase in bone pain in 10%–25% of patients.[49] This extended period of efficacy compared with other bisphosphonates offers the prospect of long-term symptomatic and biochemical control. There is, however, no evidence at the present time that this results in a reduction in long-term complications.

Most clinicians aim to control disease by means of normalizing serum alkaline phosphatase levels. The effects of this on long-term outcome are questionable. The PRISM trial compared "intensive" versus "symptomatic" treatment in 1324 patients over 5 years. The symptomatic group received treatment for bone pain, initially analgesics or anti-inflammatory drugs, followed by bisphosphonates if they did not respond. The intensive group received bisphosphonate treatment irrespective of symptoms, with the aim of maintaining serum alkaline phosphatase levels within the normal range. The trial concluded that there was no clinical difference between symptomatic treatment and intensive biochemical control.[68]

The genetic abnormalities associated with Paget's disease, in particular *SQSTM1* mutations, suggest that drugs targeting the RANK–NF-κB pathway may be effective in the treatment of Paget's disease.[69] There is also the possibility of personalized medicine with targeted intervention.

## Rickets and osteomalacia

Rickets and osteomalacia are disorders of bone mineralization of newly synthetized organic matrix (osteoid). In osteomalacia, this occurs after cessation of growth, whereas in rickets, it also affects the growth plate. Ultimately, virtually all causes of osteomalacia are caused by defects in the production of vitamin D, or the action of vitamin D (Table 12.7).

### Vitamin D and calcium deficiency (see "Osteoporosis" and Chapter 11)

Deficiencies of vitamin D, calcium, or phosphate due to inadequate nutritional intake or malabsorption may result in a defective bone mineralization. The main natural sources of vitamin D in foods are oily fish (herring, mackerel) liver, whereas the main natural sources of calcium and phosphate occur in milk and dairy products. Vitamin D is a prohormone that is also

| Causes of osteomalacia |
|---|
| Insufficient quantities or faulty metabolism of vitamin D or phosphorus |
| Renal tubular acidosis |
| Malnutrition during pregnancy |
| Malabsorption syndromes, including coeliac disease |
| Hypophosphatemia |
| Chronic renal failure |
| Tumor-induced osteomalacia |
| Drugs (see Table 12.8) |
| Cadmium poisoning (Itai-itai disease) |

**Table 12.7**
*Causes of osteomalacia.*

synthesized in the skin under the influence of ultraviolet light. Adequate synthesis occurs with 20–30 min of daily sunlight exposure to arms and legs. The most biologically active vitamin D metabolite is $1,25(OH)_2D_3$, synthesized in the kidney by hydroxylation of 25(OH) D that is produced by the liver. Calcitriol enhances calcium and phosphate absorption from the small intestine. In the presence of vitamin D deficiency, intestinal calcium and phosphate absorption are reduced, causing hypocalcaemia resulting in a (secondary) hyperparathyroid state and low plasma phosphate. Consumption of cereals and other grain products high in phytate can result in intraluminal calcium phytate formation and calcium malabsorption.[70]

### *Clinical features*

Diffuse bone pain is the most common manifestation of osteomalacia, especially in the hip area. Other clinical manifestations of osteomalacia are mainly represented by hypotonia, muscle weakness, and in severe cases tetany. Deformity of the back, including kyphosis and lordosis, may be present as also an increased risk for bone fractures (Figure 12.10). Radiologically, the long bones exhibit thin cortical radiolucent lines (stress fractures). The pelvis and ribs are the most frequently affected areas.[71] A decreased BMD is also observed. Biochemical findings include low or normal serum calcium and phosphate and elevated serum alkaline phosphatase. Serum levels of 25(OH)D are low, and PTH levels are elevated in presence of hypocalcaemia (secondary hyperparathyroidism). Chronic hypophosphatasemia exhibits similar radiological manifestations to those seen in both calcium and vitamin D deficiency. Because the serum calcium levels are in the normal range, secondary hyperparathyroidism is not an accompanying clinical feature. Consequently, bone mass is not decreased.

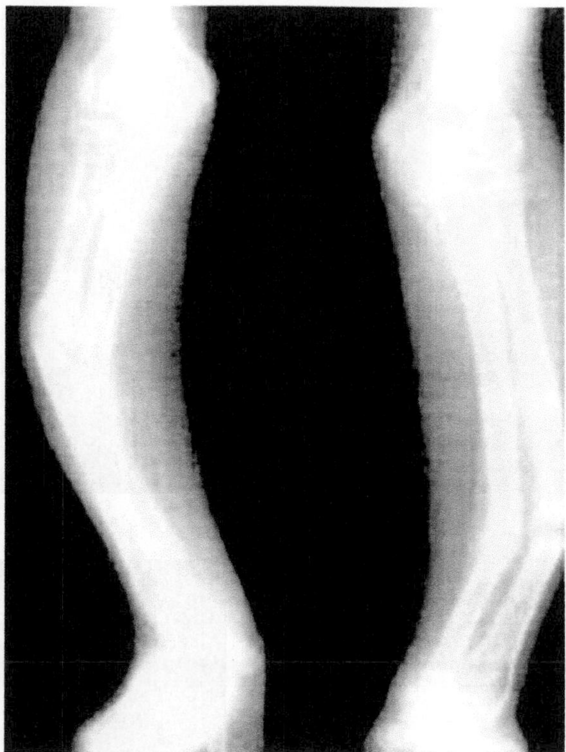

***Figure 12.10***
*Pathological fractures of radius and ulna in a patient affected by intestinal malabsorption. (From Gennari C, Avioli LV (editors),* Atlante delle malattie dell'osso, *Vol II, Chiesi Farmaceutici S.p.A., Parma, 1992. With permission.)*

## *Oncogenic osteomalacia*

In most cases, a tumor has been documented as the cause of the osteomalacia, because the metabolic disturbances improve or completely disappear on removal of the tumor. Patients usually present with vague symptoms including bone and muscle pain and muscle weakness. Fractures of long bone are occasionally reported. In younger patients, fatigue, gait disturbances, slow growth, and skeletal abnormalities occur. The biochemical findings characterizing this disorder include hypophosphatasemia, together with an abnormally low renal tubular maximum for the reabsorption of phosphate, which is caused by an excessive secretion of a phosphatonin. The serum levels of 25(OH)D are normal, and $1,25(OH)_2D_3$ are generally inappropriately normal relative to the hypophosphatasemia. Serum alkaline phosphatase is high. X-ray abnormities include osteopenia, pseudofractures [Looser's zones (Figure 12.11)], and coarsened trabeculae.

The responsible tumors are mainly represented by neoplasms of mesenchymal origin and fibrous tumors. They are often small and difficult to detect, but their successful removal is usually accompanied by rapid reversal of the osteomalacia. Fibroblast growth factor (FGF) 23 is the most likely etiological phosphatonin, but FGF7 and matrix extracellular phosphoglycoprotein (MEPE) may also be involved.[72]

## *Drug-induced osteomalacia*

Numerous drugs can cause osteomalacia by several mechanisms as summarized in Table 12.8. They include high-dose fluoride and first-generation bisphosphonates, such as disodium etidronate, as well as phenytoin.

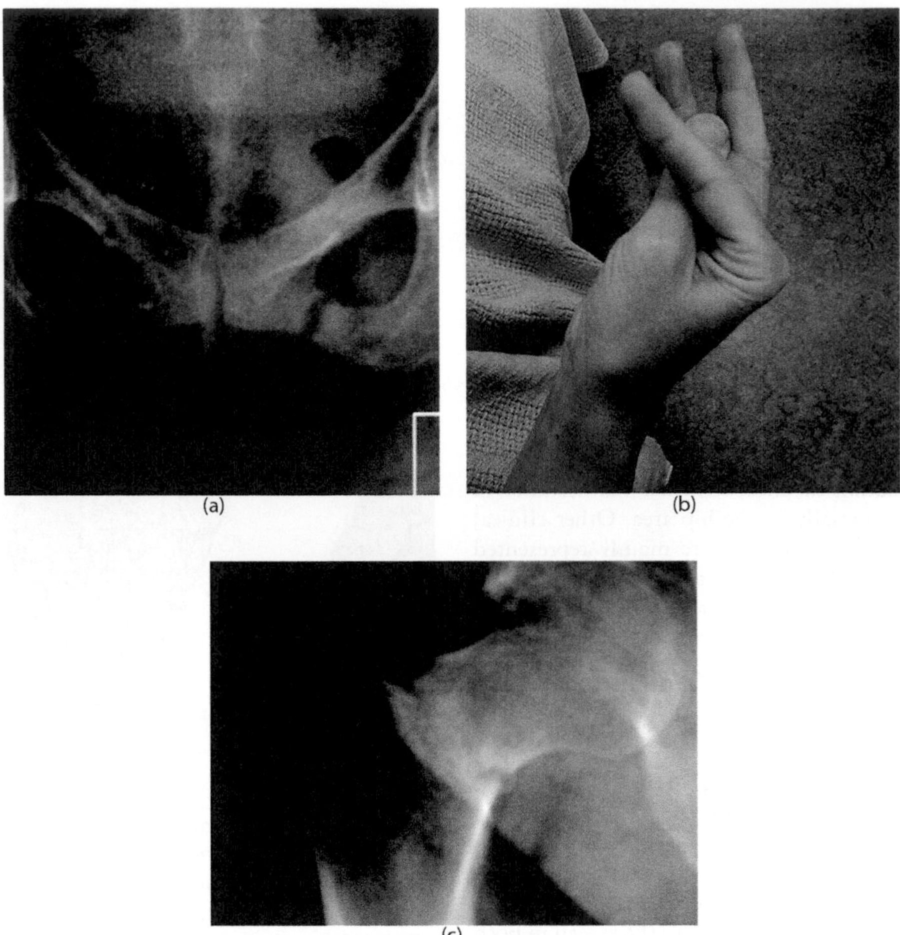

**Figure 12.11**
*(a and b) Looser's zones and carpopedal spasm in severe osteomalacia ($Ca^{2+}$ 1.25 mmol/L). (c) Pseudofracture of femoral neck in osteomalacia.*

## Disorders of vitamin D metabolism or vitamin D action and osteomalacia

Renal tubular disorders such as the Fanconi syndrome can lead to impaired 1-α-hydroxylase action. A hereditary deficiency of 1-α-hydroxylase can also occur as a rare autosomal recessive disorder causing the appearance of rickets usually in the first year of life. It is responsive to the use of calcitriol. Homozygous mutations in the vitamin D receptor cause vitamin D–resistant rickets. Affected children have alopecia, and improvements in bone disease occur in response to high-dose calcium and phosphorus.

In familial X-linked hypophosphatemia, there is a defect in renal phosphate transport leading to inappropriate hyperphosphaturia, as well as to phosphate transport in osteoblasts. The disorder is caused by inactivating mutations in the *PHEX* gene that encodes a protein of the MMP13 membrane-bound metalloproteinases that are involved in the regulation of phosphatonins and MEPE.[73] In addition, both FGF23 and secreted frizzled-related protein (SFRP) 4 inhibit the synthesis of $1,25(OH)_2D_3$ by reducing the activity of 1-α-hydroxylase. Treatment involves the lifelong use of calcitriol and phosphate.

## Renal osteodystrophy

Chronic and end stage renal disease can lead to bone disease known as renal osteodystrophy that is most

| Drugs disrupting the vitamin D endocrine system | |
|---|---|
| Cholestyramine | Inhibition of vitamin D absorption |
| Phenytoin | Alteration of vitamin D metabolism |
| Phenobarbital | |
| Rifampicin | |
| Cadmium | |
| Glucocorticoids | |
| *Drugs disrupting the phosphate homeostasis* | |
| Aluminum-containing antacid | Inhibition of phosphate absorption |
| Cadmium | Induction of renal phosphate wasting |
| Lead | |
| *Drugs disrupting bone mineralization* | |
| Aluminum | |
| Fluoride | |
| Bisphosphonates | |

***Table 12.8***
*Drug-induced osteomalacia.*

commonly caused by the decrease in the synthesis of $1,25(OH)_2D_3$, as well as phosphate retention, which further reduces calcium resorption from the gut. This results in secondary hyperparathyroidism that is sometimes sufficiently severe as to cause osteitis fibrosa cystica. In chronic kidney disease, hyperphosphatemia will stimulate production of the phosphatonin FGF23, further compromising the ability of the kidney to manufacture $1,25(OH)_2D_3$. A high bone turnover state occurs in osteitis fibrosa cystica, frequently associated with very high PTH levels. Adynamic bone disease, with a low bone turnover state can also occur, usually associated with lower PTH levels. In the high-turnover situation, very wide osteoid seams are typically observed, with particularly severe mineralization defects.[74]

It is possible to slow down the progression of bone disease by treatments aimed at reducing phosphate levels, usually by use of phosphate binders and the use of calcitriol, or analogs of calcitriol less prone to causing hypercalcemia.[75] The development of calcimimetic drugs has heralded in a new therapeutic era for reducing PTH levels. In secondary hyperparathyroidism in patients with end stage renal disease on dialysis, cinacalcet is started at a dose of 30 mg daily and adjusted every 2–4 weeks to a maximum dose of 180 mg/day. Aluminum hydroxide is now rarely used as a phosphate binder because of its propensity to cause adynamic bone disease. Rather, calcium salts, sevelamer hydrochloride, or carbonate (2.4–4.8 g daily in divided doses with meals, or lanthanum carbonate hydrate, 1.5–3 g daily) are used as phosphate-binding agents. Adynamic bone disease can occur in patients in whom secondary hyperparathyroidism has been reversed. The relationship of adynamic bone disease to PTH level, however, is variable, and an iliac crest bone biopsy may be necessary to establish the diagnosis.[76]

### Clinical features

Adults with renal osteodystrophy have bone pain and muscle weakness; in children, the condition causes growth retardation and skeletal deformities. The increased calcium-phosphate product gives a propensity to soft tissue calcification that poses a particular threat when it occurs in blood vessels, resulting in vascular insufficiency.

### Treatment

The goal is to maintain calcium and phosphate in the normal range and to minimize exposure to aluminum. Diets low in phosphate are difficult to institute but should be recommended early in the course of disease. Phosphate binders become necessary when the estimated glomerular filtration rate (eGFR) falls to <25 ml/min. Systemic acidosis should be minimized by the use of sodium bicarbonate, because acidosis can accelerate bone disease. Calcitriol is given initially as a low dose, gradually increasing to a dose of 0.25–0.5 μg/day, care being taken to avoid hypercalcemia and hypercalciuria.

Parathyroidectomy may be necessary in some cases when hypercalcemia supervenes (tertiary hyperparathyroidism). Such patients suffer from severe pruritus, extracellular calcification, and severe skeletal disease. The indication for parathyroidectomy, however, must be balanced against the risk of precipitating adynamic bone disease. Renal transplantation, although correcting many of the underlying drivers to renal osteodystrophy, may lead to progression of bone disease. Bisphosphonates and vitamin D analogs may slow the progression of bone loss after transplantation.[77]

## References


1. NIH, Consensus Panel. Osteoporosis prevention, diagnosis and therapy. *JAMA* 2001; 285: 785–95.
2. Johnell O, Kanis J. Epidemiology of osteoporotic fractures. *Osteoporos Int* 2005; 16(Suppl 2): S3–7.
3. Mackey DC, Lui LY, Ccawthon PM, et al. High-trauma fractures and low bone mineral density in older women and men. *JAMA* 2007; 298: 2381–8.
4. NOF (National Osteoporosis Foundation). *Facts on Osteoporosis*. 2008. Available from: http://www.nof.org/osteoporosis/diseasefacts.htm
5. Burge R, Dawson-Hughes B, Solomon DH, et al. Incidence and economic burden of osteoporosis-related fractures in the United States 2005–2025. *J Bone Miner Res* 2007; 22: 465–75.
6. Bonjour J, Chevalley T. Pubertal timing, peak bone mass and fragility fracture risk. *BoneKey-Osteovision* 2007; 4: 30–48.
7. Farber CR, Rosen CJ. Genetics of osteoporosis. *Transl Endocrinol Metabol* 2010; 1: 87–116.
8. Seerman E, Delmas PD. Bone quality – the material and structural basis of bone strength and fragility. *N Engl J Med* 2006; 354: 2250–61.
9. Henriksen K, Bollerslev J, Everts V, et al. Osteoclast activity and subtypes as a function of physiology and pathology – implications for future treatments of osteoporosis. *Endo Rev* 2011; 32: 31–63.
10. Theintz G, Busch B, Rizzoli R, et al. Longitudinal monitoring of bone mass accumulation in healthy adolescents; evidence for a marked reduction after 16 years of age at the level of lumbar spine and femoral neck in female subjects. *J Clin Endocrinol Metab* 1992; 75: 1060–5.
11. Khosla S. Pathogenesis of osteoporosis. *Transl Endocrinol Metabol* 2010; 1: 55–86.
12. Heaney RP. Estrogen-calcium interactions in the postmenopause: A quantitative description. *Bone Mineral* 1990; 11: 67–84.
13. Nordin BEC, Need AG, Chatterton BE, et al. The relative contributions of age and years since menopause to postmenopausal bone loss. *J Clin Endocrinol Metab* 1990; 70: 83–8.
14. Watts NB, Adler RA, Bilezikian JP, et al. Osteoporosis in men. An Endocrine Society clinical practice guideline. *J Clin Endocrinol Metab* 2012; 97: 1802–22.
15. Vokes TJ, Favus MJ. Clinical management of the patient with osteoporosis. *Transl Endocrinol Metabol* 2010; 1: 9–54.
16. World Health Organization. Assessment of fracture risk and its application to screening for postmenopausal osteoporosis. Report of a WHO study group. *World Health Organ Tech Rep Ser* 1994; 843: 1–129.
17. Baim S, Binkley N, Bilezikian JP, et al. Official Positions of the International Society for Clinical Densitometry and executive summary of the 2007 ISCD Position Development Conference. *J Clin Densitom* 2008; 11: 75–91.
18. Kanis JA. On behalf of the World Health Organization Scientific Group. Assessment of osteoporosis at the primary health care level. 2007 Technical Report. WHO Collaborating Center, University of Sheffield, UK; 2008.
19. Unnanuntana A, Gladnick BP, Donnelly E, et al. The assessment of fracture risk. *J Bone Joint Surg Am* 2010; 92: 743–53.
20. Brown JP, Albert C, Nassar BA, et al. Bone turnover markers in the management of postmenopausal osteoporosis. *Clin Biochem* 2009; 42: 929–42.
21. Reginster JY, Collette J, Neuprez A, et al. Role of biochemical markers of bone turnover as prognostic indicator of successful osteoporosis therapy. *Bone* 2008; 42: 832–6.
22. Johnell O, Oden A, De Laet C, et al. Biochemical indices of bone turnover and the assessment of fracture probability. *Osteoporos Int* 2002; 13: 523–6.
23. Holick MF, Binkley NC, Heike A, et al. Evaluation, treatment, and prevention of vitamin D deficiency. An Endocrine Society clinical practice guideline. *J Clin Endocrinol Metab* 2011; 96: 1911–30.
24. Murad MH, Mullan R, Drake M, et al. Comparative effectiveness of drug treatments to prevent fragility fractures: A systemic review and network meta-analysis. *J Clin Endocrinol Metab* 2012; 97: 1871–80.
25. Russell RG, Watts NB, Ebetino FH, et al. Mechanisms of action of bisphosphonates: Similarities and differences and their potential influence on clinical efficacy. *Osteoporos Int* 2008; 19: 733–59.
26. Black DM, Schwartz AV, Enstrud KE, et al. Effects of continuing or stopping alendronate after 5 years of treatment: The Fracture Intervention Trial Long-term

Extension (FLEX): A randomized trial. *JAMA* 2006; 296: 2927–38.

27. Bone HG, Hosking G, Devogelaer JP, et al. Ten years experience with alendronate for osteoporosis in postmenopausal women. *N Eng J Med* 2004; 350: 1189–99.
28. Greenspan SL, Emkey RD, Bone HG, et al. Significant differential effects of alendronate, estrogen, or combination therapy on the rate of bone loss after discontinuation of treatment of postmenopausal osteoporosis. A randomized, double-blind, placebo-controlled trial. *Ann Intern Med* 2002; 137: 875–83.
29. Ettinger B, Black DM, Mitlak BH, et al. Reduction of vertebral fracture risk in postmenopausal women with osteoporosis treated with raloxifene: Results from a 3-year randomized clinical trial. Multiple Outcomes of Raloxifene Evaluation (MORE) Investigators. *JAMA* 1999; 282: 637–45.
30. Johnell O, Scheele WH, Lu Y, et al. Additive effects of raloxifene and alendronate on bone density and biochemical markers of bone remodelling in postmenopausal women with osteoporosis. *J Clin Endocrinol Metab* 2002; 87: 985–92.
31. Barrett-Connor E, Mosca L, Collins P, et al. Effects of raloxifene on cardiovascular events and breast cancer in postmenopausal women. *N Engl J Med* 2006; 355: 125–37.
32. Johnston CC, Jr., Bjarnason NH, Cohen FJ, et al. Long term effects of raloxifene on bone mineral density, bone turnover and serum lipid levels in early postmenopausal women: Three year data from 2 double blind, randomised, placebo controlled trials. *Arch Intern Med* 2000; 160: 3444–50.
33. Fonseca JE, Brandi ML. Mechanism of action of strontium ranelate: What are the facts? *Clin Cases Miner Bone Metab* 2010; 7: 17–18.
34. Meunier PJ, Roux C, Seeman E, et al. The effects of strontium ranelate on the risk of vertebral fracture in women with postmenopausal osteoporosis. *N Engl J Med* 2004; 350: 459–68.
35. Reginster JY, Seeman E, De Vernejoul MC, et al. Strontium ranelate reduces the risk of nonvertebral fractures in postmenopausal women with osteoporosis. Treatment of Peripheral Osteoporosis (TROPOS) study. *J Clin Endocrinol Metab* 2005; 90: 2816–22.
36. Kostenuik PJ. Osteoprotegerin and RANKL regulate bone resorbtion, geometry and strength. *Curr Opin Pharmacol* 2005; 5: 618–25.
37. Boyle WJ, Simonet WS, Llacey DL. Osteoclast differentiation and activation. *Nature* 2003; 423: 337–42.
38. Cummings SR, San Martin J, McClung MR, et al. Denosumab for prevention of fractures in postmenopausal women with osteoporosis. *N Engl J Med* 2009; 361: 756–65.
39. Papapoulos S, Chapurlat R, Libanati C, et al. Five years of denosumab exposure in women with postmenopausal osteoporosis: Results from the first two years of the FREEDOM extension. *J Bone Miner Res* 2012; 27: 694–701.
40. Compston JE. Skeletal actions of intermittent parathyroid hormone: Effects on bone remodelling and structure. *Bone* 2007; 40: 1447–52.
41. Greenspan SL, Bone HG, Ettinger MP, et al. Effect of recombinant parathyroid hormone (1–84) on vertebral fracture and bone mineral density in postmenopausal women with osteoporosis. *Ann Int Med* 2007; 146: 326–39.
42. Neer RM, Arnaud CD, Zanchetta JR, et al. Effect of parathyroid hormone (1–34) on fractures and bone mineral density in postmenopausal women with osteoporosis. *N Engl J Med* 2001; 344: 1434–41.
43. Boonen S, Marin F, Obermayer-Pietsch B, et al. Effects of previous antiresorptive therapy on the bone mineral density response to two years of teriparatide treatment in postmenopausal women with osteoporosis. *J Clin Endocrinol Metab* 2008; 93: 852–60.
44. Downs RW, Jr., Bell NH, Ettinger MP, et al. Comparison of alendronate and intranasal calcitonin for treatment of osteoporosis in postmenopausal women. *J Clin Endocrinol Metab* 2000; 85: 1783–8.
45. Chesnut CH 3rd, Silverman S, Andriano K, et al. A randomized trial of nasal spray salmon calcitonin in postmenopausal women with established osteoporosis: The prevent recurrence of osteoporotic fractures study. PROOF Study Group. *Am J Med* 2000; 109: 267–76.
46. van Staa TP, Selby P, Leufkens HG, et al. Incidence and natural history of Paget's disease of bone in England and Wales. *J Bone Miner Res* 2002; 17: 465–71.
47. Siris ES, Canfield RE, Jacobs TP. Paget's disease of bone. *Bull New York Acad Med* 1980; 56: 285–304.
48. Morales-Piga AA, Rey-Rey JS, Corres-Gonzalez J, et al. Frequency and characteristics of familial aggregation of Paget's disease of bone. *J Bone Miner Res* 1995; 10: 663–70.
49. Ralston SH, Langston AL, Reid IR. Pathogenesis and management of Paget's disease of bone. *Lancet* 2008; 372: 155–63.
50. Lucas GJA, Daroszewska A, Ralston SH. Contribution of genetic factors to the pathogenesis of Paget's disease of bone and related disorders. *J Bone Miner Res* 2006; 21(Suppl 2): P31–7.
51. Helfrich MH, Hobson RP, Grabowski PS, et al. A negative search for paramyxoviral etiology of Paget's disease of bone; molecular, immunological, and ultrastructural studies in UK patients. *J Bone Miner Res* 2000; 15: 2315–29.
52. Robey PG, Bianco P. The role of osteogenic cells in the pathophysiology of Paget's disease. *J Bone Miner Res* 1999; 14(Suppl 2): 9–16.

53. Naot D, Bava U, Matthews B, et al. Differential gene expression in cultured osteoblasts and bone marrow stromal cells from patients with Paget's disease of bone. *J Bone Miner Res* 2007; 22: 298–309.
54. Reddy SV, Menaa C, Singer FR, et al. Cell biology of Paget's disease. *J Bone Miner Res* 1999; 14(Suppl 2): 3–8.
55. Neale SD, Smith R, Wass JA, et al. Osteoclast differentiation from circulating mononuclear precursors in Paget's disease is sensitive to 1, 25–dihydroxyvitamin D1 and RANKL. *Bone* 2000; 27: 409–16.
56. Menaa C, Reddy SV, Kurihara N, et al. Enhanced RANK ligand expression and responsivity of bone marrow cells in Paget's disease of bone. *J Clin Invest* 2000; 105: 1833–8.
57. Meunier PJ, Salson C, Mathieu L, et al. Skeletal distribution and biochemical parameters of Paget's disease. *Clin Orthop* 1987; 217: 37–44.
58. Ooi CG, Fraser WD. Paget's disease of bone. *Postgrad Med J* 1997; 73: 69–74.
59. Huvos AG. Osteogenic sarcoma of bones and soft tissues in older persons. A clinicopathologic analysis of 117 patients older than 60 years. *Cancer* 1986; 57: 1442–9.
60. Jacobs TP, Michelsen J, Polay J, et al. Giant cell tumor in Paget's disease of bone: Familial and geographic clustering. *Cancer* 1979; 44: 742–7.
61. MacGowan JR, Pringle J, Morris VH, et al. Gross vertebral collapse associated with long-term disodium etidronate treatment for Paget's disease. *Skeletal Radiol* 2000; 29: 279–82.
62. McClung MR, Tou CPK, Goldstein NH, et al. Tiludronate therapy for Paget's disease of bone. *Bone* 1995; 17: 493S–6S.
63. Siris E, Weinstein RS, Altman R, et al. Comparative study of alendronate vs. etidronate for the treatment of Paget's disease of bone. *J Clin Endocrinol Metab* 1996; 81: 961–7.
64. Siris ES, Chines AA, Altman RD, et al. Risedronate in the treatment of Paget's disease of bone: An open label, multicenter study. *J Bone Miner Res* 1998; 13: 1032–8.
65. Walsh JP, Ward LC, Stewart GO, et al. A randomized clinical trial comparing oral alendronate and intravenous pamidronate for the treatment of Paget's disease of bone. *Bone* 2004; 34: 747–54.
66. Reid IR, Miller P, Lyles K, et al. Comparison of a single infusion of zolendronic acid with risedronate for Paget's disease. *N Engl J Med* 2005; 353: 898–908.
67. Hosking D, Lyles K, Brown JP, et al. Long-term control of bone turnover in Paget's disease with zolendronic acid and risedronate. *J Bone Miner Res* 2007; 22: 142–8.
68. Langston AL, Campbell MK, Fraser WD, et al. Clinical determinants of quality of life in Paget's disease of bone. *Calcif Tissue Int* 2007; 80: 1–9.
69. Schwartz P, Rasmussen AQ, Kvist TM, et al. Paget's disease of the bone after treatment with denosumab: A case report. *Bone* 2012; 50: 1023–5.
70. Stamp TCB. Factors in human vitamin D nutrition and in the production and cure of classical rickets. *Proc Nutr Soc* 1975; 34: 119–30.
71. Sandstead HH. Clinical manifestations of certain classical deficiency diseases. In: Goodhart RS, Shils ME, eds. *Modern Nutrition in Health and Disease.* 6th ed. Philadelphia: Lea & Febiger; 1980, pp. 693–6.
72. Jonsson KB, Zahradnik R, Larsson T, et al. Fibroblast growth factor 23 in oncogenic osteomalacia and X-linked hypophosphataemia. *N Eng J Med* 2003; 348: 1656–63.
73. Berndt TJ, Schiavi S, Kumar R. "Phosphatonins' and the regulation of phosphate homeostasis. *Am J Physiol Renal Physiol* 2005; 289: F1170–82.
74. Hruska KA, Mathew S, Lund R, et al. Hyperphosphataemia of chronic kidney disease. *Kidney Int* 2008; 74: 148–57.
75. Palmer S, McGregor DO, Strippoli GF. Interventions for preventing bone disease in kidney transplant recipients. *Cochrane Database Syst Rev* 2007; 3: CD 005015.
76. Gal-Moscovici A, Popovtzer MM. New worldwide trends in presentation of renal osteodystrophy and its relationship to parathyroid hormone levels. *Clin Nephrol* 2005; 63: 284–9.
77. Cunningham J, Sprague SM, Cannata-Andia J, et al. Osteoporosis in chronic kidney disease. *Am J Kid Dis* 2004; 43: 566–71.

# 13

# Autoimmune endocrine disease

*Terry J. Smith, Laszlo Hegedüs*

## *Introduction and basic disease mechanisms*

Autoimmunity continues to represent a poorly understood set of processes where "self" is misrecognized as foreign. When left unchecked, this misidentification can activate host defense systems that, in turn, result in tissue dysfunction and disruption.[1] Thyroid immunity in many respects resembles analogous, fundamental events occurring in other tissues. Although immune surveillance is critical to organism survival, its overzealous activity can result in devastating diseases as these play themselves out in the thyroid. To regulate the intensity and specificity of immune reactivity, the body has several safeguards in place. Within the thymus, central tolerance is imposed by positive and negative B- and T-cell selection. Thymic epithelial cells express many of the so-called "tissue-specific" proteins that are known to behave as autoantigens. In the periphery, the vast array of cytokines generated by immune cells leads to polarization of T cells and can down regulate autoreactivity. In addition, the discovery of cell types that can down regulate immune reactivity, such as $CD4^+CD25^+FOXp3^+$ regulatory T cells, has provided a partial explanation for how local reactivity can be controlled.[2] These regulatory T cells are in turn influenced by multiple cytokines, such as interleukin (IL)-27, and other molecular and cellular factors. Better understanding of the defects underlying autoimmune thyroid diseases should allow the development of better treatments, such as those that are antigen specific.

Chronic inflammatory diseases of the thyroid represent the most common forms of autoimmunity. The prevalence of autoimmune thyroid disease might be as high as 2%–3% of the general population. The prevalence of the disease varies geographically, however. It is also more common amongst women. When considered in aggregate, these diseases are responsible for substantial morbidity. Two common examples of autoimmune thyroid disease that are focused upon in this chapter are Graves' disease (GD) and Hashimoto's thyroiditis. They are typically associated with very different clinical presentations but may represent common immunologic processes that diverge into distinct entities within a single disease spectrum.[3,4] In both, key components of immune dysfunction include the generation of autoreactive T lymphocytes directed against one of the thyroid autoantigens and the production of autoantibodies. GD appears to result, at least in part, from the loss of peripheral immune tolerance to the thyroid-stimulating hormone (TSH) also known as thyrotropin receptor (TSHR)[5] (Figure 13.1). Once tolerance is lost, antibodies are generated against specific epitopes of TSHR.[6] Stimulatory antibodies drive the overproduction of thyroid hormones in GD. These antibodies have been characterized extensively.[7,8] They appear restricted to the immunoglobulin (Ig) G1 subclass. Many of the actions of TSH and thyroid-stimulating antibodies (TSIs) are mediated through the generation of cAMP. The impact of TSH on cell signaling in thyroid epithelium appears to differ from that of the stimulatory antibodies (Abs). In contrast, should the antibodies be generated against epitopes that interfere with the normal binding and activity of TSH, hypothyroidism might result. These antibodies, known as TSHR-blocking antibodies, may dominate the array of IgGs in patients with GD presenting with hypothyroidism and after therapy.

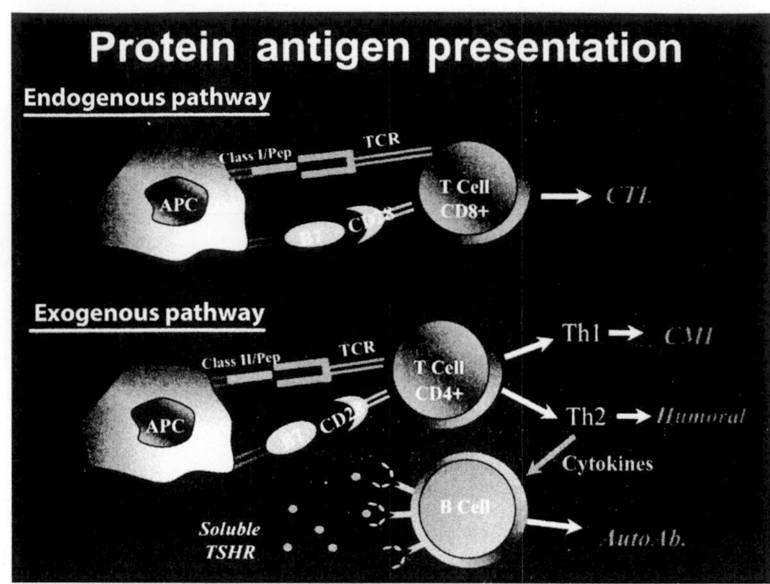


**Figure 13.1**
*Antigen-processing pathway that might be required for autoantibody production against the TSHR. Note the consequence of antigen processing by both the endogenous and exogenous pathways. Even when the antigen is exogenously processed, activation of the T-helper 2 cells might be required for an optimal antibody production. APC, antigen-presenting cell; TCR, T cell receptor; CTL, CMI, cell-mediated immunity. (From Prabhakar B et al.,* Endocr Rev, *24, 802–35, 2003. With permission. Copyright 2003, The Endocrine Society.)*

Unlike the stimulatory antibodies, blocking antibodies are not subclass restricted. The most common presentation for GD is hyperthyroidism. But GD appears to be a far more complex disease process than merely the generation of functionally active anti-TSHR antibodies. Typically, the thyroid becomes infiltrated with T cells, and ultimately the gland can become fibrotic. But in most cases, the thyroid tissue reaction observed in GD is considerably less dramatic than that seen in Hashimoto's thyroiditis.

Conversely, in Hashimoto's thyroiditis, large numbers of T lymphocytes infiltrate the gland, often are found in sheets, and ultimately the processes they drive result in glandular enlargement and failure.[3] Thyroid-infiltrating lymphocytes in Hashimoto's thyroiditis express very low levels of Fas but high levels of Bcl-2. In contrast, thyrocytes express low levels of Bcl-2 but high levels of Fas and Fas ligand. In theory, this could lead to enhanced apoptosis of these epithelial cells and thyroid failure. The long-term consequences of an often dramatic remodelling of the thyroid include autoimmune hypothyroidism (AIH) and its attendant signs and symptoms.

## Genetic and environmental factors underlying autoimmune thyroid disease

The etiologies of Hashimoto's thyroiditis and GD remain uncertain, but they are likely the result of both genetic and acquired factors.[3] Perhaps our best clues about the relative importance of each derive from twin studies in which GD affects either one or both monozygotic twins.[9] Those studies point to about a 30% genetic contribution. Frequently, the HLA-DR3 genotype is found in these patients. Several candidate susceptibility genes have been proposed as being associated with thyroid autoimmunity. Among these genes are *CTLA-4*, *CD40*, *PTPN22*, and *FCRL3*.[10] The evidence for each being involved in the pathogenesis of disease has been reviewed extensively elsewhere. Importantly, no convincing evidence yet exists for any of these candidates targeting individuals for disease-specific manifestations associated with either GD or Hashimoto's thyroiditis. Thus, factors other than those arising from genetic makeup might provide disease-specific susceptibility. With regard to the nongenetic factors, stress, diet, pollutants, and infectious agents have all been mentioned, but the successful identification of specific factors as causative in GD remains an unmet objective. Nonetheless, tobacco smoking has been identified as a major risk factor for developing GD.[11] In a study of monozygotic twins both of whom smoked, the twin with the greater exposure to cigarettes was more likely to manifest GD.

Another important void in our understanding concerns the connectivity between the thyroid, periocular structures, and regional skin involvement in GD. Why do some individuals with GD manifest severe thyroid-associated ophthalmopathy (TAO) and regional dermopathy, whereas others do not? Is it likely that different factors underlie susceptibility to the thyroidal and orbital manifestations of GD? Many leading experts in the field of thyroid autoimmunity believe that all patients with *bona fide* GD manifest all three of these maladies. Certainly, many isolated reports of subclinical disease have found their way into the literature. For instance, biopsy of innocent-appearing pretibial skin in patients with GD has revealed evidence of disease involvement.

Symptoms
- Fatigue, lethargy, decreased awareness
- Cold intolerance
- Dry skin, complaints of brittle hair
- Weight gain
- Constipation and abdominal pain
- Slowed mentation
- Decreased libido, impotence
- Increased menstrual bleeding
- Arthralgia, myalgia

Signs
- Facial edema; ankle edema
- Dry pale or yellowish skin (retinoids); cool palms
- Dry hair and diffuse hair loss
- Mental status changes, slow speech and mentation
- Bradycardia
- Diminished reflexes

Effusions (gold paint sign), ascites
Hoarse voice
Hypothermia
Breast discharge

***Table 13.1***
*In clinical findings associated with hypothyroidism, the severity of each depends on the duration and magnitude of the thyroid hormone privacy.*

## *Clinical manifestations of autoimmune diseases: Contrasts between GD and Hashimoto's thyroiditis*

The optimal approach to patients with either thyrotoxicosis or hypothyroidism should be sufficiently broad-based and comprehensive to allow discovery of the multisystemic nature of these metabolic derangements. The clinical course of hyperthyroidism associated with GD and the hypothyroidism associated with Hashimoto's thyroiditis is variable. Almost every human tissue is normally impacted by the activity of thyroid hormone and suffers as a consequence of its excesses and deficits. Hashimoto's thyroiditis represents the most common form of primary AIH, the result of substantial thyroid destruction. As the gland fails and produces an inadequate amount of thyroid hormone, characteristic symptoms dominate the clinical presentation. These symptoms include fatigue, coarsening of the hair, dry skin, cold intolerance, constipation, depression, and menorrhagia (Table 13.1). A strong family history should suggest increased suspicion in patients with these symptoms. Thyroid enlargement is common in GD but is not inevitable, and when present, it is typically symmetrical. The Hashimoto gland can be enlarged, normal-sized, or atrophic, depending on several factors such as iodine intake and the duration of the disease. It is usually firm, can present with nodularity, and in some cases is extremely firm to stony hard, depending on the duration of disease. Some of the irregularities can result from small bleeds that subsequently become calcified. The appearance of hypothyroid individuals can change dramatically as soft tissues become infiltrated with glycosaminoglycans that trap water and lead to edema (Figure 13.2)[12]. In GD, examination of the thyroid is usually dominated by a diffusely and symmetrically enlarged, firm nontender gland that may be surrounded by a mild degree of lymphadenopathy. The texture of the gland is often bosselated. The surface may be smooth. Depending on clinical circumstances, a thrill may be palpable over the thyroid

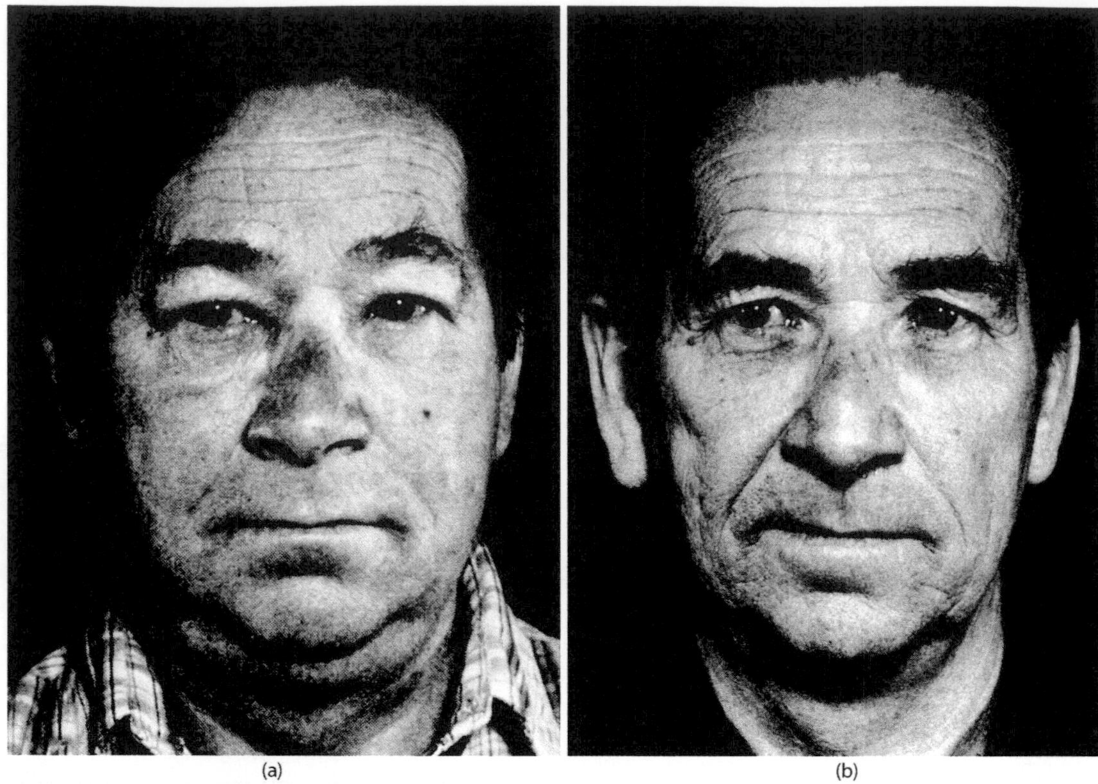


***Figure 13.2***
*Thyroprivic myxedema before (a) and after (b) treatment. (From Smith TJ et al.,* Endocr Rev, *10, 366–91, 1989. Copyright 1989, The Endocrine Society.)*

and a bruit might be audible. The gland should not be fixed but should move well with deglutition. A thyroid fixed to surrounding tissues might suggest underlying malignancy or a sclerosing, inflammatory process such as Riedel's thyroiditis causing substantial fibrosis and adherence to adjacent structures. Malignant thyroid tumors often act more aggressively in those with GD. This might result from the trophic actions of TSI.[13] In our view, finding a small, atrophic thyroid gland in a hypothyroid patient should raise the possibility of hypothalamic/pituitary gland failure. Suspicion should provoke further questioning of the patient with regard to symptoms of adrenal and gonadal failure. A more extensive examination of the patient for signs of these, such as postural hypotension and loss of secondary sex characteristics, should also be undertaken. Absence of elevations in serum TSH and abnormalities in other pituitary hormones in a hypothyroid patient will likely confirm the diagnosis. Ultimately, any anatomical abnormality, such as glandular enlargement associated with GD, must be distinguished from other causes: malignancy, infections, and inflammation can all present as thyroid enlargement. Although GD can also present as hypothyroidism, the far more common scenario is one of variably overactive thyroid function and a suppressed serum TSH. The metabolic consequences of hyperthyroidism associated with GD resemble those of any other cause of thyrotoxicosis, namely toxic nodular goiter, solitary toxic nodule, TSH-secreting pituitary adenoma, excessive exogenous thyroid hormone ingestion, and struma ovarii. The most common signs and symptoms of thyrotoxicosis are presented in Table 13.2. Tachycardia, often experienced as symptomatic palpitations, is among the most common. Increased anxiety, emotional liability, and nervousness, heat intolerance, and weight loss with increased appetite are also very frequently encountered in the untreated patient. Quality of sleep is often disturbed. The menses are generally diminished or absent in women, whereas men often experience loss of libido. Not uncommonly, thyrotoxic patients present with diaphoresis and warm moist palms. They are fidgety and restless, irritable, and often complain of diminished

| *Symptoms and signs* |
|---|
| Tachycardia and palpitations, sinus arrhythmias, atrial fibrillation |
| Tremor |
| Heat intolerance; warm moist palms, sweating |
| Irritability and nervousness, fidgeting |
| Weight loss, often despite hyperphagia, increased appetite |
| Fatigue |
| Anxiety |
| Dysphoria |
| Muscle wasting and weakness |
| Increased bowel motility, abdominal pains and cramping, diarrhea |
| Anorexia |
| Dyspnea |

***Table 13.2***
*Prevalent signs and symptoms associated with thyrotoxicosis and frequently found in GD and other forms of thyrotoxicosis.*

attention span. Often, a fine tremor can be demonstrated in these patients. The reflexes might become more brisk and the proximal muscles might exhibit diminished strength and in severe, long-standing disease might exhibit wasting. When fully expressed, GD also affects the orbital tissues surrounding the eye and is referred to as TAO. It also results in a dermal process known as pretibial myxedema or dermopathy.[14,15] This should not be confused with generalized myxedema that is associated with severe and sustained hypothyroidism.

## Laboratory testing in autoimmune thyroid disease remains an important component of patient evaluation

Laboratory examination of patients suspected of having hyperthyroidism resulting from GD should include assessment of serum TSH levels. These levels will reflect substantial suppression of the hypothalamic–pituitary axis that occurs with primary hyperthyroidism from any etiology. Wide availability of assays measuring "free" levels of thyroxine (T4) and triiodothyronine (T3) now allow uncomplicated direct assessment of the biologically available fractions of each. These determinations eliminate the potentially confounding impact of changes in thyroid hormone binding globulin, such as seen during pregnancy or oral contraceptive use. We routinely measure the titer of TSI, especially in the absence of clinically obvious TAO and when the diagnosis of GD might be in doubt. Although not disease specific, antibodies against thyroid peroxidase and thyroglobulin are often detectable in GD and fortify the diagnosis that the patient has an autoimmune thyroid disorder. Repeated assessment of TSH, T4, and T3 provides guidance regarding the adequacy of antithyroid therapy and indicates whether remission has been achieved. This may prove useful because some patients, especially the very old, can mask clinical manifestations of elevated thyroid function. Some practitioners advocate repeating antibody measurements as a guide to management, whereas others view it only as a diagnostic tool. Should additional evidence be required, 99mTc of radioiodine uptake is often an easily performed diagnostic maneuver. It offers the advantage of rendering a rapid result confirming increased thyroid uptake that is typical of the hyperthyroidism of GD.

## Management of the hyperthyroidism associated with GD

Spontaneous remission of hyperthyroidism occurs occasionally in GD but this is not the rule. When treatment is required, antithyroid drugs (ATDs), radioiodine (RAI), and surgical thyroidectomy represent the options currently available (Table 13.3). Little has changed in our understanding of the advantages and disadvantages of the various management strategies during the past 50 years.[16] It is obvious that one therapy does not serve the needs of all patients and that the final decision is based on a dialog between the patient and his or her treating physician. Twenty years ago, questionnaire studies suggested that there are geographical differences in the initial use of ATDs in Europe and Asia, compared with a propensity for using RAI in North America.[17] Whether this still holds is unknown. But the following should be considered: (1) 40%–50% of patients achieve long-term remission after use of ATD; (2) we are unable to calculate confidently the dose of RAI required to achieve and maintain a euthyroid state; and (3) the current manner in which thyroid hormone replacement is undertaken is nonphysiological, and in some patients not satisfactory in restoring premorbid sense of well-being. The many aspects of decision making have been covered in published guidelines.[18]

| Treatment | Advantages | Disadvantages |
|---|---|---|
| Thioamides | • No radiation hazard<br>• No surgical or anesthesia risk<br>• No permanent hypothyroidism<br>• Outpatient therapy | • Recurrence rate, 50%–60%<br>• Frequent thyroid function testing required<br>• Common mild adverse effects<br>• Rare but potentially lethal adverse effects |
| Radioactive iodine | • Definitive treatment of hyperthyroidism<br>• No surgical risk or risk from anesthesia<br>• Out-patient therapy<br>• Rapid control of hyperthyroidism in most<br>• Low cost<br>• Side effects: mild, rare, and transient<br>• Normalizes thyroid size within 1 year | • Potential radiation hazards<br>• Potential provocation/worsening of TAO<br>• Adherence with radiation regulations<br>• Decreasing efficacy with increasing goiter size<br>• May need to be repeated<br>• Eventually hypothyroidism in most cases<br>• Radiation thyroiditis |
| Surgical thyroidectomy | • Definitive treatment of hyperthyroidism<br>• No radiation hazard<br>• Rapid normalization of thyroid dysfunction<br>• Definitive histology<br>• Relief of compressive symptoms | • High cost<br>• Requires hospitalization<br>• Anesthesia risk[a]<br>• Hypoparathyroidism (1%–2%)[b]<br>• Recurrent laryngeal nerve damage (1%–2%)[b]<br>• Risk of bleeding, infection, scarring[b]<br>• Hypothyroidism in most[b] |

[a] The risk from anesthesia is reduced in euthyroid patients compared with those who remain hyperthyroid at time of surgery.
[b] The surgical risk is generally higher in case of total than in case of subtotal thyroidectomy. The risk of hypothyroidism and the risk of recurrence are inversely related and depend on amount of thyroid tissue removed.

***Table 13.3***
*Advantages and disadvantages of therapeutic options in GD.*

## *Antithyroid drugs*

Thioamides have been used since the early 1940s. Propylthiouracil (PTU) and methimazole (MMI) were previously preferred in Europe, Asia, and North America. However, increasing focus on PTU-related adverse effects, especially in childhood GD, has resulted in the recommendation of replacing PTU as a first-line drug, with the exception of the first trimester of pregnancy.[18–20] Carbimazole (CBZ), a precursor of MMI, is preferred in the United Kingdom. The major action of ATDs is to inhibit thyroid hormone synthesis by interfering with thyroid peroxidase–mediated iodination of tyrosine residues in thyroglobulin. PTU inhibits the type 1 deiodinase enzyme that converts T4 to T3. Therefore, T3 levels usually fall more rapidly with PTU than with MMI/CBZ, but this is only of importance in severe thyrotoxicosis. The drugs also influence intrathyroidal immune responses, leading to a decrease in TSI generation. Whether remission in GD results from the effects on immune response or is the consequence of thyroid activity normalization is still debated.[21,22] Table 13.4 describes the properties of MMI and PTU.

The decision to use a particular ATD is based on custom, personal preference, and consideration of side effects, because few large, randomized trials have been performed.[23] MMI carries the advantage of 1–2 times daily dosing compared with 2–3 times with PTU. There is no significant difference in cost of the drugs or

| Characteristic | MMI | PTU |
|---|---|---|
| Relative potency | 10–50 | 1 |
| Administration | Oral | Oral |
| Absorption | Nearly complete | Nearly complete |
| Binding to serum proteins (%) | Negligible | 80–90 |
| Serum half-life (h) | 4–6 | 1–2 |
| Volume of distribution (L) | 40 | 20 |
| Duration of action (h) | >24 | 12–24 |
| Metabolism during liver disease | Decreased | Normal |
| Metabolism during kidney disease | Normal | Normal |
| Transplacental passage | Low | Even lower |
| Effect on neonatal thyroid function[a] | Negligible | Negligible |
| Level in breast milk | Low | Even lower |
| Inhibition ofT4/T3 conversion | No | Yes |
| Dosing[a] | 1–2 times daily | 2–3 times daily |

[a] At initial therapy. During titrated ATD therapy, when reaching doses of 5 mg MMI or 100 PTU, once daily dosing is thought to be prudent and probably secures a higher compliance than if divided doses are given; in case of MMI doses of no >20 mg daily, or PTU doses of no >250 mg daily.[16,21]

***Table 13.4***
*Characteristics of MMI and PTU.*

their ability to provoke remission. Higher initial dosing of MMI does not result in more rapid normalization of thyroid function or higher remission rates.[24] The usual starting dose for MMI/CBZ is 10–40 mg daily, increasing with larger glands and greater iodine intake. The initial dose of PTU is usually 300–600 mg per day in 2–3 daily doses. Thyroid function should be evaluated monthly. Within 1–3 months of therapy, ATDs can often be tapered to 5–10 mg of MMI/CBZ or 100–200 mg of PTU. An alternative to the dose–titration regimen is the block-and-replace regimen, the objective of which is normalization of thyroid function by administering high dose ATD in combination with levothyroxine (LT4). This regimen confers more stable thyroid function, necessitates less frequent monitoring, and probably leads to greater patient compliance. However, no evidence exists for increased remission rates.[25,26] The maximal remission rate may occur more rapidly with the block–replace regimen compared to the titration regimen.[27]

After stopping treatment, patients should be monitored frequently because of the high rate of relapse. Two out of three patients who relapse (50%–60% overall) do so within the first year. Thereafter, annual testing is advised because relapses and hypothyroidism can occur decades later, in up to 20%.[28] TSH levels may remain subnormal, despite depressed thyroid hormone levels, for some time after clinical euthyroidism is achieved. Therefore, free T4 and or T3 levels are needed to evaluate thyroid status. Continuing T4 treatment after withdrawal of the block–replace regimen is not recommended, because remission rates are unaffected.[26,29]

Retrospective studies have suggested that several factors are associated with relapse after a course of ATD[14] (Table 13.5). Unfortunately, the associations with these factors and known genetic markers lack sufficient sensitivity[30] and specificity to allow risk stratification and robust guidance for therapy.[31] In our opinion, a combination of patient characteristics, including goiter size, high T3/T4 ratio, and elevated TSI, suggest a high risk of recurrence.

The side effects of ATDs (Table 13.6) are underreported. Drug comparisons are hampered because of the scarcity of randomized controlled studies (RTCs).[23] Side effects occur in approximately 5% of exposed patients. These side effects are most frequently mild, with the most common being skin rash. No convincing differences exist between drugs,[21,32] although some report a higher frequency with PTU.[21,23] Side effects of MMI are dose related and most occur within the first 3 months of

- Recurrence after a previous course of ATD therapy
- Long duration of symptoms pretreatment
- Young age and male sex
- Family history of autoimmune thyroid disease
- Certain genetic markers
- Cigarette smoking
- Presence of thyroid-associated ophthalmopathy
- Pronounced hyperthyroidism at presentation
- High serum T3/T4 ratio
- High ATD dose at end of therapy
- High-level TSHRAbs initially and/or after ATD therapy
- Large goiter size initially and/or after ATD therapy[a]
- Increasing goiter size during therapy[a]
- Nodularity, and/or hypoechogenicity, and/or high intrathyroidal flow (Doppler ultrasound) initially or after ATD therapy[a]

[a] Denotes determination of size, morphology, and echogenicity by high-frequency ultrasound and flow using Doppler ultrasound.
ATD; antithyroid drugs (thioamides); TSHRAb; thyrotropin receptor antibodies.
*Note:* Certain genetic markers are associated with an increased risk of developing GD. However, in the individual patient sensitivity and specificity is too low for clinical use.

**Table 13.5**
*Factors thought to be associated with higher recurrence rate after ATD in GD.*

therapy. The side effects of PTU are less clearly associated with dose and occur more idiosyncratically.[21] Most side effects resolve, either spontaneously or after dose adjustment or after antihistamine treatment. Cross-reactivity occurs in half those patients experiencing side effects. Serious side effects occur in about 0.3% of users per year. The most serious of these is agranulocytosis. Should fever, sore throat, or urinary tract infection develop, treatment should be curtailed, and a white blood cell count should be obtained. Granulocytes usually recover spontaneously, but broad-spectrum antibiotics may be necessary. There is no consensus on the use of colony-stimulating factor that, in a randomized study, did not improve recovery time.[33] Hepatotoxicity is an even rarer side effect (0.1%–0.2%) as is vasculitis. These side effects are more common with PTU than

| *Common (5%–10% of treated individuals)* | *Uncommon or rare (in general <1%)* |
|---|---|
| • Rash | • Agranulocytosis, thrombocytopenia, aplastic anemia |
| • Arthralgias | • Jaundice, hepatic failure |
| • Fever | • Vasculitis, SLE-like syndrome, lymphadenopathy |
| • Pruritus | • Rhinitis, conjunctivitis |
| • Urticaria | • Enlargement or inflammation of salivary glands |
| • Nausea | • Loss of taste |
| • Headache | • Alopecia |
| | • Edema |
| | • Diarrhea |

**Table 13.6**
*Side effects associated with antithyroid drugs.*

with MMI/CBZ.[21,32] We advocate routine monitoring of white cell counts and hepatic function tests routinely during therapy.

## *Other drugs*

Beta blockers such as propranolol, or calcium channel blockers, are often used to ameliorate symptoms of increased sympathetic nervous system activity, including sweating, palpitations, and restlessness. Beta blockade is particularly useful while the antithyroid therapy takes effect and the euthyroid state is achieved.

Lithium carbonate is rarely used in the therapy of GD. It can block iodine release and is sometimes prescribed to enhance the effectiveness of RAI therapy. If used, serum lithium levels must be monitored.[34]

Potassium perchlorate reduces iodine stores within the thyroid and can induce remission in GD. It is more commonly used in combination with ATDs and steroids to control amiodarone-induced thyrotoxicosis. Agranulocytosis and aplastic anemia can occur at a higher rate than that associated with ATD use and therefore is rarely used.[35]

Nonradioactive iodine, in the form of Lugol's iodine (5% iodine, 10% potassium iodide), or potassium iodide is useful for preparing patients for surgery because they decrease blood flow and thyroid mass.

The blocking effects of iodine are sometimes transient, and the thyroid can escape inhibition and thyrotoxicosis can recur.[36]

## *Radioactive iodine (see Chapter 7)*

Radioactive iodine (RAI) has been used since the mid-1940s for treatment of thyroid maladies. Today, it is considered safe, effective, and inexpensive compared with long-term ATD or surgical thyroidectomy.[37] Neither cost nor quality of life, which is negatively impacted,[38] differs significantly among the three treatment options.[39–41] The isotope of choice is $^{131}$I. It is given orally, usually as a capsule. It emits beta radiation that causes that causes inflammation and vascular occlusion followed by thyroid fibrosis, the consequence of which is decreased thyroid size and eventually hypothyroidism. It is contraindicated in pregnant and lactating patients and those who cannot comply with safety regulations. We rarely use RAI in adolescents below the age of 20 years because the long-term impact of radiation is yet to be definitively established. Nonetheless, RAI is becoming more commonly used in young patients above the age of 10 years. This is justified by the lack of definitive evidence of increased risks of malignancy.[37,42] Pregnancy should be avoided for at least 4 months after RAI therapy, although many in North America advise waiting 1 year before initiating pregnancy. There remains a theoretical risk for genetic damage in germ cells. Patients should be reassured in relation to risk of malformations and infertility. Post-RAI radiation regulations, which vary between countries, need to be followed. They mainly focus on minimizing close contact with children and pregnant women.

Ideally, the therapy should rapidly render the patient euthyroid without causing hypothyroidism. However, this is an elusive goal.[16,37] A positive relationship has been established between the $^{131}$I dose and the risk of hypothyroidism within the first year. The incidence of hypothyroidism after 1 year (2%–3% yearly) seems independent of dose.[37,43] RAI activity is often determined by the following algorithm: Activity (mCi) = 80–200 μCi $^{131}$I/g thyroid × estimated thyroid gland weight (g)/24 h radioiodine uptake.

Typical activities are in the range of 5–15 mCi (185–555 MBq), corresponding to absorbed doses of 50–100 Gy. This algorithm is typically associated with a hypothyroidism rate of 10% during the first year and necessitates retreatment in 20%. However, because the ideal dose is yet to be established, many administer fixed activities based on clinical features such as thyroid size.[44] Failure to obtain euthyroidism is related to young age, a large thyroid, more severe hyperthyroidism, prior exposure to ATD, and a high RAI uptake.[45] In such cases, aiming for a higher dose seems prudent. This also concerns the elderly and patients with recurrent disease. Using this deliberate ablation regimen, the 1-year relapse rate is about 5% at the expense of a hypothyroidism rate of about 65%.[16] An account of complications of RAI, other than hypothyroidism, is given in Table 13.3. Many prepare their patients with propranolol alone. Due to a small risk of thyroid storm and the slow onset of RAI effects, many treat with ATDs before RAI, especially in patients with severe hyperthyroidism, atrial fibrillation, and cardiac failure. Importantly, ATDs potentially increase rates of failure and reduce rates of hypothyroidism if they are given during the weeks before or after RAI treatment, respectively.[46] In North America, many practitioners aim for complete ablation of thyroid function and routinely prepare the patient for the early and predictable need for life-long thyroid hormone replacement.

Thyroid function gradually declines and is normalized in 50%–80% within 6–8 weeks.[43] Concomitantly, thyroid size decreases and becomes normal in virtually all, independent of pretreatment size.[43] Our policy is to review thyroid function at 4- to 6-week intervals until a steady state is reached and annually thereafter. Importantly, hypothyroidism occurring up to 3–6 months after RAI can be transient. In case of persistent or recurrent hyperthyroidism, a second RAI dose should be given >6 months after the initial treatment.

## *Surgery*

Surgery is the oldest but may represent the least used treatment option.[17] The advantages and disadvantages of surgery are listed in Table 13.3.[39,47,48] Besides patient preference, there are few absolute indications for surgery. However, we favor surgery in case of (1) inconclusive fine needle aspiration from a thyroid nodule; (2) a very large goiter with pressure symptoms; (3) severe, active TAO, especially in individuals who cannot tolerate steroid therapy; and (4) during pregnancy, childhood, and adolescence in those who prove intolerant to ATDs.

In Europe, most surgeons recommend lobectomy and subtotal/total contralateral lobectomy to minimize recurrence, the risk of which is substantial if >5 g remains. In contrast, North American thyroid surgeons often recommend total thyroidectomy. The risk of general anesthesia is very low, and mortality is extremely rare, especially if the patients are rendered euthyroid before surgery. There is an inverse relation between the postoperative thyroid remnant and risk of hypothyroidism, the latter being the aim if surgery is used. Risk of complications is inversely related to the experience of the surgeon and increases with patient age, size of the goiter, and degree of hyperthyroidism.[48] If hyperthyroidism recurs after surgery, RAI is the therapy of choice. Many use preoperative inorganic iodine for 10 days to decrease thyroid blood flow, but blood loss is not affected. In combination with a beta blocker, inorganic iodine or oral cholecystographic agents can be used to rapidly normalize thyroid function before surgery, in patients intolerant to ATDs.[49]

## Thyroid-associated ophthalmopathy

Besides the manifestations of GD occurring within the thyroid, connective tissues in the orbit and surrounding the eye are also involved.[50] Tissue reactivity and remodeling around the eye are referred to as TAO, Graves' orbitopathy, or thyroid eye disease. The etiology of TAO remains uncertain as does its relationship to the overactivity and abnormal enlargement of the thyroid. Orbital tissues, including fat and the extraocular muscles, become enlarged and inflamed.[51] The classic appearance of individuals with TAO can be seen in Figure 13.3. TAO runs a characteristic course that can be divided into two phases.[52] First, there is active TAO, the hallmarks of which are tissue reactivity and change over time. This early phase usually lasts 24–36 months. It gives way to stable TAO where the characteristic signs of inflammation and swelling are diminished. The histology of TAO has been described in some detail. Orbital tissues are infiltrated with lymphocytes and other mononuclear cells, such as mast cells.[53] This infiltrate can involve the fatty connective tissue and the extraocular muscles. Typically, the muscles themselves remain intact and the motor fibers are intercalated with

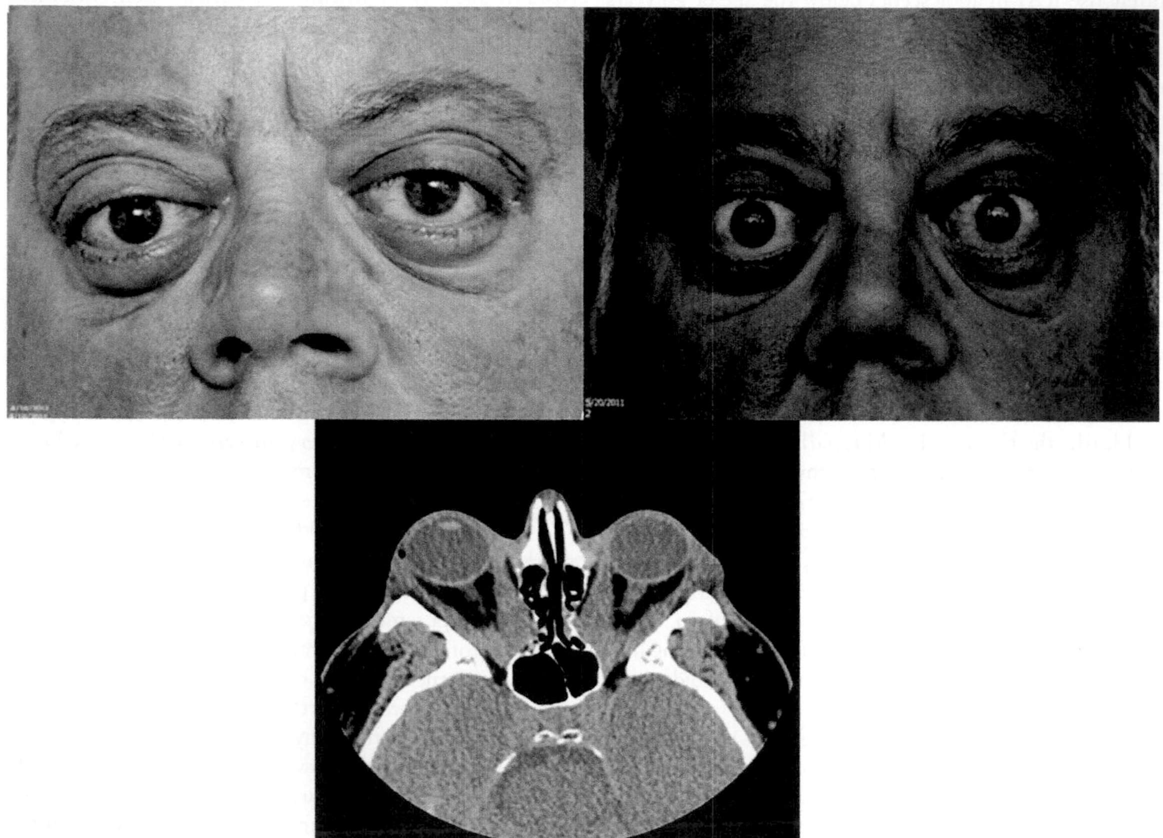

**Figure 13.3**
*Patient with active severe TAO (left) and 1 month later (right). Note the proptosis and inflammatory signs around the orbit, eyelids, and upper face. There is a remarkable progression of lid retraction and proptosis 1 month later. The CT demonstrates enlargement of the extraocular muscles, including the medial rectus, crowding of the apex, and medial wall bone remodeling in the same patient.*

inflammatory cells until very late in the process when irregularities in eye motility might prove problematic. These most often culminate in restricted eye movements and diplopia. In most individuals, both extraocular muscles and orbital fat expand (Figure 13.2). Either tissue can dominate the clinical picture. $CD34^+$ monocyte lineage progenitor cells have been found to accumulate in the orbit in TAO.[54] These fibrocytes express relatively high levels of TSHR, potentially identifying a mechanism by which the thyroid and orbit could be connected in GD. In fact, these $CD34^+$ fibrocytes also accumulate in the thyroid in GD.[55] Perhaps they could ultimately explain how high levels of TSI might influence the clinical evolution of TAO. Fibrocytes have been shown to differentiate into fat cells and myofibroblasts.[56] Thus, they might play important roles, once recruited to the orbit in TAO, in the expansion of fat volume and fibrosis seen in end stage disease. Any patient with diffuse thyroid enlargement and thyrotoxicosis should arouse suspicion of TAO. Several symptoms and signs are often associated with orbital GD, including proptosis, diplopia, strabismus, eye lid edema, redness, lagophthalmos, and ocular dryness. Patients will often complain of eye pain, gritty sensations, and dry eye, especially when exposed to wind.

## Eye evaluation in GD

The evaluation of anyone suspected of having GD should include a thorough eye exam. In our practice, we often refer such patients to the ophthalmologist for a baseline assessment. This occurs even in patients without any outward manifestations of the disease. In early TAO, only very subtle symptoms can be identified, such as increased sensitivity to the desiccating effects of sun and wind. The components of a baseline ophthalmic exam are enumerated in Table 13.7. Should clear-cut signs of TAO exist, orbital imaging is often obtained in the form of computed tomography (CT) or magnetic resonance imaging (MRI). Visual acuity should be assessed, including visual fields, and photographs should be taken, including detailed views of eye movements. Proptosis can be easily evaluated with an exophthalmometer. Multiple varieties are commercially available. Exophthalmometry involves measuring the distance between the tangent to the corneal apex with the line of the lateral orbital margin. The Hertel instrument is the most commonly used. The Luedde exophthalmometer is extremely simple and in some hands has proven more reliable. Interobserver variation often confounds detection of subtle interval changes, and thus reliance on a single operator is preferable.

*Clinical exam*

- Visual acuity and refraction
- Pupil exam
- Schirmer basal tear secretion test
- Color vision testing
- Visual field testing (Humphrey visual field SITA standard)
- Ductions and versions
- Alignment testing
- Exophthalmometry
- Slit lamp exam
- Fundus exam

**Table 13.7**
*Baseline eye exam undertaken in all newly diagnosed patients with GD.*

| *Class* | *Signs and symptoms* |
|---|---|
| 0 | No physical signs or symptoms |
| 1 | Only signs, no symptoms (lid lag, stare, etc.) |
| 2 | Soft tissue involvement |
| 3 | Proptosis |
| 4 | Extraocular muscle involvement (eye motility deficits) |
| 5 | Corneal involvement (such as ulceration) |
| 6 | Sight loss (secondary to optic nerve compression) |

*Source:* Pinchera A et al., *Thyroid*, 2, 235–6, 1992. With permission.

**Table 13.8**
*NOSPECS classification scheme and the derivative indices are not particularly useful as objective measurements for interval change; they do contain important elements of assessment for these patients.*

Unfortunately, no reliable biomarkers that accurately reflect either the severity or activity have yet been validated. Multiple classification systems have been developed. The NOSPECS scheme is depicted in Table 13.8.[57] The clinical activity score (CAS) was developed to identify active TAO and to predict the likely impact of corticosteroid therapy. It relies heavily on subjective assessment. The CAS system is based on four signs of inflammation, including pain, redness, swelling, and functional impairment.[58] It is imprecise and thus methods of assessment with greater objectivity and precision are necessary for the implementation of robust clinical trials. Efforts to develop better markers for the disease and its response to therapy are under development on both sides of the Atlantic.

## *Therapy for TAO*

Management of TAO very much depends on the severity and activity of the disease. The majority of patients with GD present with mild eye disease. This most often requires only conservative management. Maintaining adequate ocular hydration with artificial tears or plugging the punctum can provide substantial symptomatic relief. Punctal plugs are useful but are frequently displaced. Cautery of the punctum can offer more permanent improvement of dry eye symptoms. If substantial lagophthalmos develops, maintaining proper nighttime eye coverage might become challenging. Patients should be instructed in covering their eyes with saran wrap and petroleum to retard ocular desiccation. Use of irritating eye cosmetics and harsh soaps should be avoided. When diplopia complicates the presentation, the use of Fresnel prisms can greatly improve the daily functional status of patients. Congruent with their deleterious impact on GD, cigarettes appear to increase the incidence and severity of TAO in patients with GD. Moreover, the benefits of corticosteroids and orbital radiotherapy are minimized by tobacco use. Controlling the excursions in thyroid function that accompany suboptimally treated hyperthyroidism is associated with reduced incidence and severity of TAO. Initiating thyroid hormone replacement in a timely manner after RAI thyroid ablation avoids the untoward effects of elevated serum TSH levels and has been shown to reduce the risk of worsening eye disease.[59]

Moderate-to-severe TAO during the active phase of the disease is usually treated conservatively. But these patients can experience substantially diminished quality of life.[60–64] Thus, appropriate measure of supportive care and anti-inflammatory therapies are sometimes implemented, such as systemic corticosteroids. These agents are not thought to alter the natural course of disease but rather to reduce the inflammation associated with it. In severe disease or when concern exists about the impending development of optic neuropathy, the decision to treat with steroids is usually made by the ophthalmologist in collaboration with the endocrinologist. Current use of high-dose pulse intravenous steroids rather than orally administered prednisone derives in large part from reports that the former might be associated with fewer and less severe side effects.[65–67] Rarely, intravenous administration has resulted in liver failure and a few deaths. The most extensive use of parenteral corticosteroids comes from Europe, but its popularity is growing in North America.

Although corticosteroids are useful for dampening the inflammation associated with active phase TAO, these agents do not appear to alter the ultimate outcome of the disease process. Thus, a continuing quest is currently underway for identifying therapies that will modify the course of the disease and spare the patient from surgeries. Several of the drugs that have found utility in the treatment of rheumatoid arthritis and other collagen vascular diseases are currently under examination for their potential benefit in TAO. Most notable of these is the B-cell–depleting drug rituximab.[68] Rituximab is a fully humanized monoclonal antibody that targets the cell surface protein determinant CD20 present on B lymphocytes. This interaction results in the elimination of these cells. Several studies have suggested that rituximab can substantially reduce the clinical activity of TAO and might be useful in patients with impending optic neuropathy who have failed to improve sufficiently with corticosteroids, thus sparing them from surgery.[69–75] Besides rituximab, several anticytokine monoclonal antibodies such as those directed against tumor necrosis factor (TNF)-$\alpha$, IL-1$\beta$, and IL-6 are being evaluated because these agents have also found utility in the treatment of rheumatoid arthritis and its allied diseases.

Dietary supplementation of selenium is another potentially useful therapy that should be well tolerated.[76] A recent study involving 159 subjects demonstrates an improved quality of life score and decreased eyelid aperture, reduced soft tissue signs, and a slowed progression of TAO.[77] Although additional studies are warranted, including additional controls such as assessment of baseline selenium dietary content,[78] this study breaks new ground and focuses on relatively mild TAO.

Surgical rehabilitation of the eye in TAO can be broken down into broad categories depending on the clinical circumstances. As a general principle, most elective surgeries are withheld until the disease has entered the stable phase and no signs of inflammation and change remain. If the volume of orbital contents has expanded and resulted in compromised ocular motility and proptosis that causes cosmetic concerns or compromised ocular surface, orbital decompression becomes appropriate. Several surgical approaches have been refined over the past few decades for decompressing the orbit in TAO. These can target removal of the boney walls or attempt to reduce the volume of fat. Whichever approach is taken, the main objective is to reduce the overcrowding of the orbital contents, either by reducing its volume or increasing the orbital space. The relatively rare exception from delaying surgery until TAO stabilizes can occur with impending optic neuropathy where the threat of permanent loss of vision is greatest. In this case, emergent orbital decompression can be undertaken by a skilled oculoplastic surgeon or neuro-ophthalmologist. The objective in this case is to provide immediate relief of mechanical embarrassment of the optic nerve. In addition to orbital decompression, eyelid repair and strabismus surgeries are often required to restore eye function. Each can be approached in several ways depending on the particulars of each case and the preferences of the surgeon. The ultimate goal of these procedures is to restore the orbit, its contents, and the structures of the upper face to their premorbid function and appearance.

## Dermopathy in GD

The third component of fully expressed GD is an infiltrative process confined to the skin, called pretibial or regional dermopathy or sometimes localized myxedema.[79] The lesions result from the accumulation of glycosaminoglycans.[80] Some evidence points to antibodies driving its pathogenesis,[81] but definitive evidence for a disease mechanism does not yet exist. This manifestation, the rarest of the three, usually involves the skin of the anterior shin, but rarely can be detected in other body regions, especially after trauma. It can present in one of three forms: (1) diffuse dermopathy with characteristic, nonpitting lesions; (2) nodular lesions that are sharply circumscribed; and (3) the elephantiasis form. Representative appearances are shown in Figure 13.4. Histologically, the skin takes on an appearance that is remarkably similar to that seen in hypothyroid myxedema. The subcutaneous tissue is infiltrated with hyaluronidase-digestible material that stains metachromatically. Most lesions are relatively devoid of infiltrating mononuclear cells with inflammatory phenotypes; in this regard, the process seems distinct from that occurring in the orbit in TAO.

Treatment of dermopathy usually results in disappointing responses. Corticosteroids have been administered either systemically, by intralesional injection, or through topical application. The side effects of these agents and the frequently mild clinical course taken by

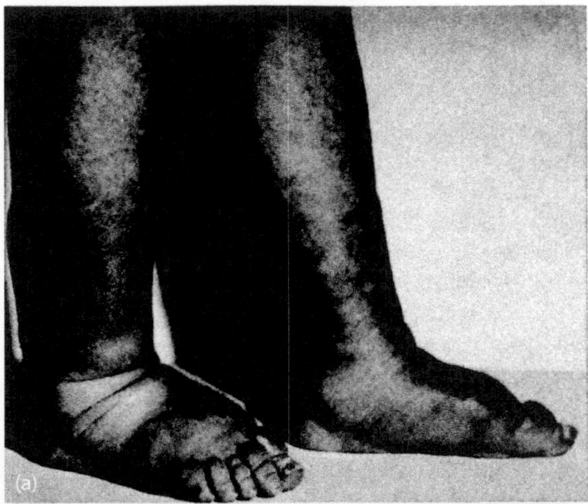


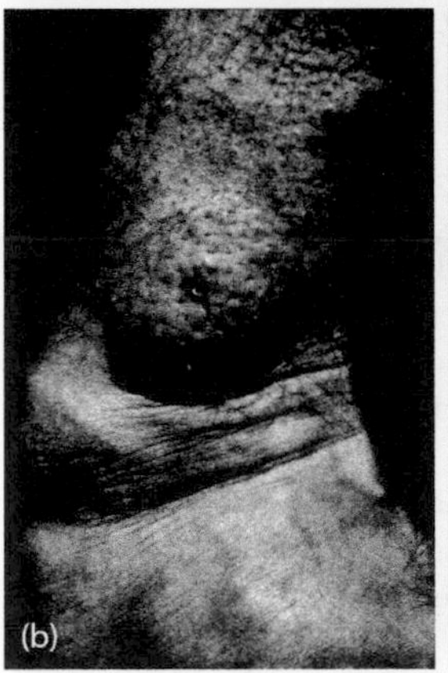


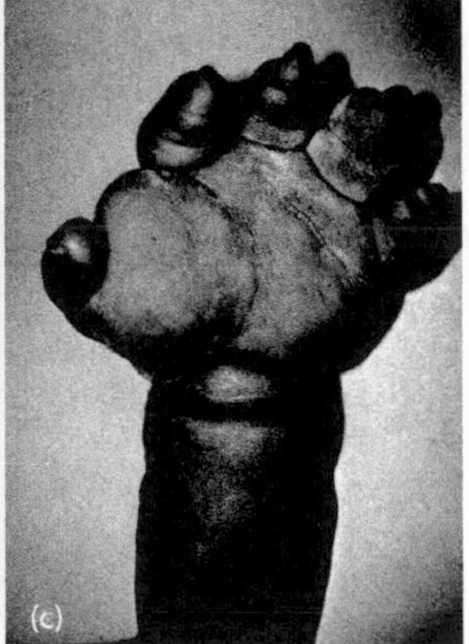


***Figure 13.4***
*Types of thyroid dermopathy. (a) Elephantiasic form. (b) Nodular form. Note the thickened "orange-peel" appearance of the skin. Prominence of hair follicles is caused by interfollicular edema. (c) Severe thyroid dermopathy of upper extremity in patient who had self-administered many intravenous injections. (From Smith TJ et al.,* Endocr Rev, *10, 366–91, 1989. Copyright 1989, The Endocrine Society.)*

dermopathy make the use of steroids unattractive in the majority of cases. Some experts advocate the use of topical agents such as fluocinolone acetonide applied under occlusive film. This can be repeated several times each week until the process seems to abate. The frequency of application can then be reduced to a few times each month. Elastic stockings are said to slow the rate of lesion recurrence. Surgical remediation in the form of skin grafts and excisional biopsies are usually futile because the disease can return.

## Thyroid acropachy

A process literally named "thickening of the extremities," acropachy is extremely rare and occurs exclusively in patients with GD and severe TAO.[82] It involves soft tissue swelling associated with clubbing of the fingers (Figure 13.5). There can be hyperpigmentation of the overlying skin. Underlying this process is the accumulation of glycosaminoglycans that intercalate collagen bundles, nodular fibrosis of the periosteum, and subperiosteal bone formation.[83,84] The affected tissues are not painful but have a striking appearance. No treatments appear to be beneficial and surgical intervention should be avoided because the affected tissues are characteristically slow to heal.

## GD during pregnancy and breastfeeding

GD occurs in up to 0.2%–0.3% of all pregnancies, mostly in females with on going or previously treated GD, and it should ideally be dealt with before pregnancy. It can be associated with infertility, intrauterine growth retardation, pre eclampsia, low birth weight, and miscarriage.[85] Fetal hyperthyroidism occurs in about 1% of neonates from mothers with GD and should always be considered in these pregnancies. It is characterized by fetal goiter, tachycardia, hydrops, and small fontanelles and is the consequence of transplacental passage of TSI.

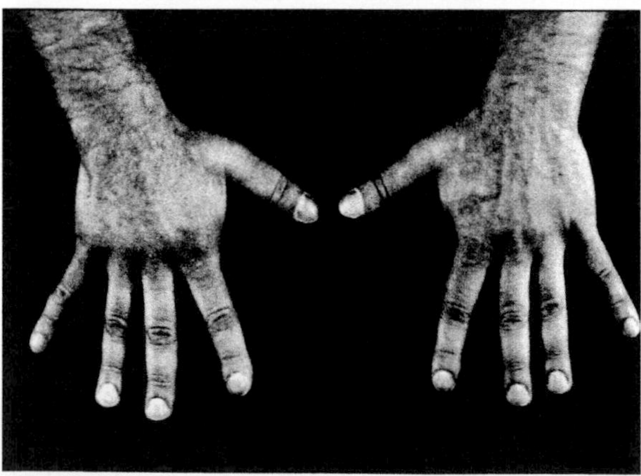

**Figure 13.5**
*Thyroid acropachy. Note that disease is most apparent on index fingers and thumbs of both hands; these digits are slightly clubbed with soft tissue thickening adjacent to the nail beds. (From Smith TJ et al.,* Endocr Rev*, 10, 366–91, 1989. Copyright 1989, The Endocrine Society.)*

Therefore, patients previously treated with surgery or RAI for GD should be evaluated in early pregnancy for TSI that may persist independently of thyroid status. If these are >40 U/L in the third trimester, the risk of neonatal hyperthyroidism is considerable.[86]

Medical management is the preferred therapeutic option for hyperthyroidism in pregnancy. Surgery is an alternative during the second trimester. Key elements of care are enumerated in Table 13.9. MMI and PTU cross the placenta to the same degree and have similar effects on fetal and neonatal thyroid function. Although the evidence is limited and not based on RCTs, PTU is recommended in the first trimester of pregnancy. This is largely based on a lower risk of congenital abnormalities, including aplasia cutis and choanal and esophageal atresia. MMI is recommended in the second and third trimesters.[18] Thyroid function should be monitored every 4–6 weeks, with a target in the high reference range. The block–replace regimen should not be used. Typically, 30% of women are able to discontinue ATD during the second half of pregnancy.

The fractional excretion of MMI into breast milk is much higher than that for PTU. However, studies have demonstrated that MMI doses <20 mg/day and PTU

*Essential points*

- Share care with obstetrician and consult with pediatrician
- Evaluate TSHRAb early in pregnancy and, if elevated, also in third trimester
- PTU recommended in first trimester and MMI in the rest of the pregnancy, but both may be used
- Use smallest possible dose aiming at free T4 in the high-normal nonpregnant reference range
- Evaluate thyroid function every 4–6 weeks throughout pregnancy
- About 30% may be taken off ATD treatment; postpartum recurrence common
- PTU (up to 250 mg daily) and MMI (up to 20 mg daily) do not affect neonatal thyroid function, which does not need to be monitored
- Both PTU and MMI may be given during lactation without monitoring of infant thyroid function

**Table 13.9**
*Important aspects of medical management of GD in pregnancy.*

doses <250 mg/day do not affect infant thyroid function. Women on ATD should thus not be advised against breastfeeding.[85]

## Autoimmune hypothyroidism

Hashimoto's thyroiditis represents the most common cause of hypothyroidism in iodine-replete regions of the world. It results from complex interactions between genetic and environmental factors, such as iodine intake and tobacco use.[85,86] Both MHC and non-MHC genes appear to confer disease susceptibility. Those unrelated to MHC can be divided into two groups: those involved in immunoregulation, such as CD40, CTLA-4, and PTPN22, and those traditionally thought to be "thyroid-specific," including thyroglobulin and TSH-receptor. The life-time risk of AIH is about 5%, with an approximately 5:1 female preponderance.[89] Despite adequate treatment, AIH negatively impacts quality of life,[38] whereas overall mortality seems only marginally affected.[90]

The autoimmune process leads to destruction of thyroid follicular cells and hypothyroidism. Antibodies against thyroid peroxidase (TPO Ab) and thyroglobulin (Tg Ab) are markers of the disease but do not appear pathogenic, because transplacental transfer fails to elicit neonatal thyroid dysfunction. In contrast, TSHR-blocking antibodies can promote transient neonatal hypothyroidism.[91]

## Work-up and clinical manifestations associated with AIH

Signs and symptoms of hypothyroidism appear in Table 13.2. Most patients manifest nonspecific symptoms and are diagnosed relatively early in the course of disease. Depression may dominate the clinical picture in the elderly. Some patients do not have thyroid enlargement, whereas goiter may prompt others to seek medical attention.[89] Typically, thyroxine therapy reduces glandular size and eventually thyroid autoantibody levels drop.[92] Lymphoma of the thyroid, although rare, occurs almost exclusively in patients with Hashimoto's thyroiditis. Large needle or open biopsy is needed to make the diagnosis and to determine the response to therapy.[93] Pain associated with thyroiditis usually disappears with thyroxine treatment and mild analgesics, but it may require corticosteroids or surgical intervention.[94]

Several drugs such as amiodarone, iodine, lithium, interferon-α, and IL-2 can precipitate AIH. Sometimes cessation of these drugs can lead to remission.

The diagnosis of AIH is confirmed by an elevated TSH. The degree of hypothyroidism is evaluated by assessing free T4 which if subnormal indicates overt hypothyroidism. If free T4 remains in the reference range, the condition is referred to as mild, subclinical, or compensated hypothyroidism. Free T3 is unreliable for this purpose because the body defends maintaining its levels in the normal range. Autoimmunity is confirmed by demonstrating the presence of high titer anti-TPO and/or anti-Tg Abs. These are detectable in >95% of individuals. A relationship can usually be demonstrated between TSH levels and symptoms. Other autoimmune conditions such as pernicious anemia and Addison's disease, should be considered in these patients because of their increased incidence.

Screening for hypothyroidism is indicated in several clinical situations; patients presenting with typical symptoms and physical signs, those treated with amiodarone or lithium, those diagnosed with Addison's disease or autoimmune polyglandular syndrome (APS) type 2, those with unexplained infertility, as a follow-up of postpartum thyroiditis, and those with Down's and Turner's syndromes all deserve assessment. Consideration of the diagnosis of AIH seems warranted in dementia, those with strong family history of thyroid autoimmunity, obesity, and breast disease. Screening should be delayed in acutely ill patients.[95] Approximately, 10% of those will be diagnosed with subclinical hypothyroidism, a similar number of females will be found to have anti-thyroid Abs, and these numbers increase with advancing age.[96] The annual risk of progression to overt hypothyroidism is 2%–3% in those with either elevated TSH or Abs and 4%–5% with both.[96] Higher serum TSH is associated with greater risk.[97]

## Management of hypothyroidism

Treatment can be initiated with 50–100 μg of LT4 daily in individuals without cardiovascular disease. The effects on appearance can be rapid and dramatic (Figure 13.2). In those with cardiac issues, starting at a lower dose is advisable, such as 25 μg daily. Dose adjustments are typically made after 6 weeks at a given dosage, when new steady-state levels are achieved. Symptomatic improvement usually lags behind normalization of thyroid function tests. Normalization of TSH level is generally reached with LT4 doses of 75–150 μg daily, depending on residual thyroid function and body weight. Requirements of >200 μg daily may indicate poor compliance or malabsorption, as does an elevated free T4 associated with high TSH levels. Because the serum half-life of T4 is 7 days in individuals with normal thyroxine-binding globulin levels, the weekly dose can be safely ingested as a single dose.[98] Neglecting concomitant adrenal insufficiency as thyroid hormone replacement is initiated can precipitate Addison crisis. Thyroxine requirements may decline with loss of body weight or increase as the thyroid gland continues to fail.[99]

Evidence suggests that small adjustments of serum TSH within the normal reference range do not improve quality of life. Although a meta-analysis[100] concluded that this was not the case, a subgroup of patients with deiodinase 2 gene polymorphisms exhibited improved well-being on a combination of T4/T3 compared with T4 alone.[101] Our policy is to institute therapy with LT4 in patients with elevated TSH and thyroid antibodies, targeting TSH levels in the lower half of the reference range.

## Hypothyroidism in pregnancy

Both overt (0.3%–0.5%) and subclinical hypothyroidism (2%–3%) are common in pregnancy. These conditions are frequently overlooked.[85,102] Untreated maternal hypothyroidism is associated with adverse fetal and obstetric outcomes, including miscarriage, pre-eclampsia, abruptio placenta, and postpartum hemorrhage. In addition, it is associated with low birth weight and increased respiratory distress in the newborn. These adverse events are also found in mothers with subclinical hypothyroidism and may also result from underlying thyroid autoimmunity, independent of thyroid function.[85] Treatment with LT4 in all these groups reduces adverse outcomes.[85,103]

Serum TSH level should be maintained <2.5 mU/L in the first trimester and <3.0 mU/L thereafter. Early in pregnancy, the LT4 requirements tend to increase by 30%–50%. Thus, thyroid function should be monitored at 6-week intervals. Postpartum LT4 requirements return rapidly to prepregnancy levels.[85]

## Postpartum thyroiditis (see Chapter 14)

Postpartum thyroid dysfunction (PPTD) represents thyroid dysfunction within the year after delivery. It results from the resetting of immune function after pregnancy. It is usually transient, with hyperthyroidism occurring around post-partum week 13, followed by transient hypothyroidism at week 19.[85,104] However, many variations of thyroid dysfunction have been reported. PPTD can recur in 70% of women not developing permanent hypothyroidism.[104] It occurs in half of those patients in whom TPO Abs can be detected and has an overall incidence of 1%–21%.[105] Its severity may be positively related to the level of TPO Ab in early pregnancy.[106] Permanent hypothyroidism is reported in about half of those developing postpartum hypothyroidism within 10 years.[104,106]

PPTD can be distinguished from GD by the lack of TSHR Abs, TAO, and dermopathy. In addition, absent or low iodine uptake is characteristic. Breastfeeding needs to be discontinued for 24 h for this test. The hyperthyroid phase is often transient and short-lived. Propranolol may be given at low doses (20–40 mg/day) for several weeks without adverse effects. Hypothyroidism in this condition is treated with LT4 but usually can be stopped several months after delivery. The risk of developing permanent hypothyroidism is life long.[102,104,108] In general, screening of pregnant woman is reserved for those at high risk.[107] The impact of screening and treating individuals found to have subclinical thyroid dysfunction associated with pregnancy is currently under investigation.[107]

## Addison's disease (see Secondary adrenal insufficiency, Chapter 5; Addisonian crisis/acute adrenal insufficiency, Chapter 24)

Primary adrenal failure is most frequently caused by autoimmune destruction of the gland.[109] Historically, tuberculosis and other infectious processes accounted for a large fraction of the disease. Autoimmunity now accounts for 80%–90% of cases in the United Kingdom[110] (Table 13.10). Evidence suggests that both cellular and humoral immunity play parts in its pathogenesis. A variety of autoantibodies have been described that fall into two classes: adrenal specific, directed against cytochrome P450 21-hydroxylase enzyme, and those reacting with any steroid-producing tissue, directed against P450 17α-hydroxylase and side chain–cleaving enzymes.[110] They are valuable diagnostic tools and can be identified in 80%–90% of patients with autoimmune Addison's disease. They and are absent in nonautoimmune cases.[111]

| |
|---|
| Autoimmune destruction |
| Infection |
| Tuberculosis |
| Fungal infection |
| AIDS |
| Cytomegalovirus |
| Congenital |
| Adrenoleukodystrophy |
| Adrenal hyperplasia or hypoplasia |
| Inactivating ACTH receptor mutation |
| Drugs (metyrapone, ketoconazole, mitotane, suramin, etomidate) |
| Hemorrhage |
| Waterhouse–Friedrichsen syndrome after infection, especially meningococcal |
| Antiphospholipid syndrome |
| Warfarin |
| Infiltration |
| Metastases |
| Amyloidosis |
| Sarcoidosis |
| Hemochromatosis |
| ACTH, adrenocorticotropic hormone. |

***Table 13.10***
*Causes of primary adrenal failure (Addison's disease).*

The clinical presentation of Addison's disease is variable as is the clinical context, ranging from a slow, progressive process to an acute medical emergency. Primary adrenal failure is frequently accompanied by a darkening of the skin and such an occurrence should arouse suspicion (Table 13.11). The possible occurrence of Addison's disease as part of APS types 1 and 2 should always be considered.

Recognizing its presence, especially in the setting of acutely stressful events (e.g., trauma, thermal burns, myocardial infarction), can be critical to survival. Our approach in the emergency room is to treat with exogenous corticosteroids immediately, before confirmatory laboratory testing and then document steroid deficiency later. Typical physical signs and symptomatology include nausea and vomiting, hypoglycemia, hypotension (especially that proving to be refractory to treatment), abdominal pain, and mental confusion lapsing into frank coma.

Clues to the diagnosis are the presence of hyponatremia; hyperkalemia; raised urea and creatinine; hypoglycemia; hypercalcemia; a normochromic; normocytic anemia; eosinophilia; and neutropenia. Definitive diagnosis depends on demonstrating a low cortisol, excluding secondary adrenal failure due to pituitary disease and determining the etiology. Random cortisols are not particularly helpful, but in the setting of an acutely ill patient, a value <200 nmol/L, together with an adrenocorticotropic hormone (ACTH) level of >80 ng/L, is diagnostic, whereas a cortisol level of >550 nmol/L excludes Addison's disease. Blood should be stored for retrospective analysis and the treatment commenced immediately in this setting. Cortisol levels <100 nmol/L and >525 nmol/L at 0800–0900 h are also sometimes used to demonstrate or exclude Addison's disease[112] If cortisol levels are between these extremes, a short Synacthen test should be performed that involves giving 250 μg of synthetic ACTH intramuscularly or intravenously at 0800–1000 h and measuring cortisol at 0, 30, and 60 min. Failure to achieve levels of ≥550 nmol/L confirms hypoadrenalism. The measurement of ACTH levels enables the differentiation of primary from secondary adrenal failure.

| |
|---|
| Increased pigmentation, especially skin creases, recent scars, and inside cheeks |
| Fatigue, weakness |
| Depression |
| Nausea and weight loss |
| Postural hypotension |
| Salt craving |
| Abdominal pain, vomiting, diarrhea |
| Confusion leading to coma |
| Amenorrhea, decreased libido |
| Loss of axillary and pubic hair in postmenopausal women |
| Associated autoimmune disorders: vitiligo, alopecia, thyroid disease, type 1 diabetes mellitus (25%–50% of patients) |

***Table 13.11***
*Clinical manifestations of Addison's disease.*

Adrenal antibodies to 21-hydroxylase can be demonstrated in >75% of patients with autoimmune Addison's disease, with high specificity. Antibody-positive individuals with normal cortisol levels are at risk of developing adrenal failure and must be followed up.[113] In the absence of adrenal autoantibodies or other evidence suggesting APS type 1 or 2, other causes of adrenal failure must be considered (Table 13.10). These are usually apparent from the clinical history. Tuberculosis in particular must be excluded. CT scan of the adrenal is the best investigation, because the adrenals are atrophic with autoimmune Addison's disease but are usually enlarged with tuberculosis and other infiltrative conditions.

The emergency management of an Addisonian crisis consists of an intravenous. Treatment consists of an intravenous or intramuscular injection of 100 mg of hydrocortisone, followed by an intravenous infusion of 4 mg/h or 6 hourly intramuscular injections of 50–100 mg. Patients are usually severely dehydrated and require rapid fluid replacement with normal saline. Electrolytes need to be closely monitored because the potassium levels usually fall rapidly and require supplementation in the saline infusion. Fluid replacement needs to be closely monitored by urine output and blood pressure. Particular care needs to be taken with elderly patients and patients with underlying cardiac disease.

The usual replacement dose of hydrocortisone 20–30 mg/day is given in divided doses, with the highest dose taken in the morning immediately on waking. At minimum, there should be a second dose early evening, but many patients benefit from a third dose at lunchtime. Anticonvulsant drugs and rifampicin increase hydrocortisone clearance, and patients taking these medications may require higher doses of replacement therapy.

In addition, fludrocortisone is required to provide mineralocorticoid replacement. The usual dose is 50–200 μg/day as a single dose. The dose is adjusted to ensure a normal blood pressure with the absence of edema, together with measurement of electrolytes and plasma renin, which should be in the upper half of the reference range.[114] The benefits of dehydroepiandrosterone replacement therapy are unclear, and there are no approved formulations available for prescription.[115]

All patients require a careful explanation of the principles of their treatment, and clear instructions should be given about the need to double the dose of hydrocortisone during intercurrent illness and the need to urgently seek medical attention if the medication cannot be taken because of vomiting. Diarrhea and vomiting in particular are associated with the risk of adrenal crisis. It is important that close members of the family and friends should also be aware of these instructions. A steroid card must be issued, detailing the use of hydrocortisone, and the patient should also wear a medical bracelet or necklace stating that the patient is taking glucocorticoid replacement therapy. Patients who are traveling abroad or who live in remote locations should be issued with hydrocortisone for injection for use in an emergency (100-mg vial, water for injection, syringe and needle). They and their companions should be instructed on its administration by intramuscular injection.

Pregnancy does not usually cause problems in patients with Addison's disease, and the medication does not usually require adjustment. During labor, the dose of replacement therapy should be doubled.

Patients should undergo routine annual review to ensure optimum replacement therapy and to check for other autoimmune conditions. A minimum check should enquire about general health, periods in women of reproductive age, TSH, glucose, full blood count, and/or vitamin $B_{12}$ levels and antibody testing for pernicious anemia.

## *Autoimmune polyglandular syndrome type 1*

APS-1 represents an autosomal recessive disorder caused by mutations in the *AIRE* (autoimmune regulator) gene on chromosome 21q22.3.[116] AIRE appears to drive the expression of tissue-restricted antigens (TRAs) in the epithelial cells of the adrenal medulla, resulting in the negative selection of TRA-reactive thymocytes and preventing autoimmune disease.[117] The diagnosis is based on distinctive features (Table 13.12),

| | Approximate frequency (%) |
|---|---|
| Major components | |
| Chronic mucocutaneous candidiasis | 80–100 |
| Hypoparathyroidism | 80 |
| Addison's disease | 70 |
| Other features | |
| Enamel hypoplasia | 80 |
| Gonadal failure | 10 men; 60 women |
| Nail dystrophy | 50 |
| Keratopathy | 40 |
| Tympanic membrane calcification | 30 |
| Vitiligo | 30 |
| Alopecia | 30 |
| Malabsorption | 20 |
| Insulin-dependent diabetes mellitus | 10 |
| Hypothyroidism | 10 |
| Pernicious anemia | 10 |
| Chronic active hepatitis | 10 |

**Table 13.12**
*Clinical features of APS-1.*

including the presence of at least two of the three major components, that is, chronic mucocutaneous candidiasis, hypoparathyroidism, and Addison's disease,[118–120] appearing in this order in childhood, or occasionally in later life.

The presentation and management of Addison's disease in APS-1 are as for the isolated type. Chronic mucocutaneous candidiasis affects the nails (70%), skin (10%), and oropharynx and esophagus (20%). It responds well to ketoconazole, but this often needs to be prolonged and repeated. Hypoparathyroidism presents with circumoral paresthesiae, tetany (including carpopedal spasms), or seizures; depression and other mental changes may be prominent. Cataracts, calcification of the basal ganglia, and prolonged Q-T interval may also occur. Diagnosis depends on demonstrating hypocalcemia and low parathyroid hormone levels, with the exclusion of other causes of hypoparathyroidism. Treatment is with vitamin D analogs such as alphacalcidol with a usual adult dose of 1–2 μg/day. Calcium levels need to be regularly monitored and the dose of vitamin D analog adjusted to maintain the serum calcium within the normal range.

Once a patient has been diagnosed, family members will require screening.

Major endocrinopathies
- Autoimmune thyroid disease (Graves' disease, primary myxedema, Hashimoto's thyroiditis, postpartum thyroiditis)
- Type 1 diabetes mellitus
- Addison's disease
- Premature ovarian failure

Other endocrinopathies
- Lymphocytic hypophysitis
- Lymphocytic infundibuloneurohypophysitis

Other features
- Vitiligo
- Alopecia or leukotrichia
- Pernicious anemia
- Celiac disease/dermatitis herpetiformis
- Myasthenia gravis
- Serositis

***Table 13.13***
*Clinical features of APS-2.*

## Autoimmune polyglandular syndrome type 2

APS-2 is the most common autoimmune polyglandular syndrome. The key features of APS-2 are detailed in Table 13.13. The presence of two or more of the major endocrinopathies can be regarded as diagnostic, whereas one major endocrinopathy and one or more associated features are suggestive of APS-2 and the need for follow-up.[118] APS-2 is an autosomal dominant disorder, strongly associated with HLA-A1, -B8, -DR3 haplotypes and polymorphisms of the CTLA-4 gene.[121]

The assessment, diagnosis, and management of each individual component follows the standard lines for the isolated disorder. The recognition of the syndrome is important, because the patient and family need to be screened clinically and biochemically on an annual basis, to ensure that each of the individual components is recognized.

## References


1. Cheng MH, Anderson MS. Monogenic autoimmunity. *Annu Rev Immunol* 2012;30:393–427.
2. Shen S, Ding Y, Tadokoro CE, et al. Control of homoeostatic proliferation by regulatory T cells. *J Clin Invest* 2005;115:3517–26.
3. Dayan CM, Daniels GH. Chronic autoimmune thyroiditis. *N Eng J Med* 1996;335:99–107.
4. Brent GA. Graves' disease. *N Eng J Med* 2008;358:2594–605.
5. Vassart G, Dumont JE. The thyrotropin receptor and the regulation of thyrocyte function and growth. *Endocrine Rev* 1992;13:596–611.
6. Costagliol S, Bonomi M, Morgenthaler NG, et al. Delineation of the discontinuous-conformational epitope of a monoclonal antibody displaying full in vitro and in vivo thyrotropin activity. *Mol Endocrinol* 2004;18:3020–34.
7. Zakarija MJ. Immunochemical characterization of the thyroid-stimulating antibody (TSab) of Graves' disease: Evidence for restricted heterogeneity. *J Clin Lab Immunol* 1983;10:77–85.
8. Weetman AP, Yateman ME, Ealey PA, et al. Thyroid-stimulating antibody activity between different immunoglobulin G subclasses. *J Clin Invest* 1990;86:723–7.
9. Brix TH, Kyvik KO, Christensen K. Evidence for a major role in heredity in Graves' disease; a population-based study of two Danish twin cohorts. *J Clin Endocrinol Metab* 2001;86:930–4.

10. Brand OJ, Gough SCL. Genetics of thyroid autoimmunity and the role of the TSHR. *Mol Cell Endocrinol* 2010;322:135–43.
11. Brix TH, Hansen PS, Kyvik KO, et al. Cigarette smoking and the risk of clinically overt thyroid disease: A population-based twin case-control study. *Arch Intern Med* 2000;160:661–6.
12. Smith TJ, Bahn RS, and Gorman CA. Connective tissue, glycosaminoglycans, and diseases of the thyroid. *Endocr Rev* 1989;10:366–91.
13. Pellegriti G, Belfiore A, Guiffrida D, et al. Outcome of differentiated thyroid cancer in Graves' disease. *J Clin Endocrinol Metab* 1998;83:2805–9.
14. Kazim M, Goldberg RA, Smith TJ. Insights into the pathogenesis of thyroid-associated orbitopathy: Evolving rationale for therapy. *Arch Ophthalmol* 2002;120:380–6.
15. Fatourechi V. Pretibial myxedema: Pathophysiology and treatment options. *Am J Clin Dermatol* 2005;6(5):295–309.
16. Hegedüs L. Treatment of Graves' hyperthyroidism: Evidence-based and emerging modalities. *Endocrinol Metabolism Clin N Am* 2009;38:355–71.
17. Wartofsky L, Glinoer D, Solomon B, et al. Differences and similarities in the diagnosis and treatment of Graves' disease in Europe, Japan, and the United States. *Thyroid* 1991;1:129–35.
18. Bahn RS, Burch HB, Cooper DS, et al. Hyperthyroidism and other causes of thyrotoxicosis: Management guidelines of the American Thyroid Association and American Association of Clinical Endocrinologists. *Thyroid* 2011;21:593–646. Erratum: *Thyroid* 2011;21:1169.
19. Rivkees SA, Szarfman A. Dissimilar hepatotoxicity profiles of propylthiouracil and methimazole in children. *J Clin Endocrinol Metab* 2010;95:3260–6.
20. Kahaly GJ, Bartalena L, Hegedus L. The American Thyroid Association/American Association of Clinical Endocrinologists guidelines for hyperthyroidism and other causes of thyrotoxicosis: A European perspective. *Thyroid* 2011;21:585–91.
21. Cooper DS. Antithyroid drugs. *N Engl J Med* 2005;352:905–17.
22. Laurberg P. Remission of Graves' disease during antithyroid drug therapy. Time to reconsider the mechanism? *Eur J Endocrinol* 2006;155:783–6.
23. Nakamura H, Noh JY, Itoh K, et al. Comparison of methimazole and propylthiouracil in patients with hyperthyroidism caused by Graves' disease. *J Clin Endocrinol Metab* 2007;92:2157–62.
24. Reinwein D, Benker G, Lazarus JH, et al. A prospective randomized trial of antithyroid drug dose in Graves' disease therapy. European Multicenter Study Group on Antithyroid Drug Treatment. *J Clin Endocrinol Metab* 1993;76:1516–21.
25. Benker G, Reinwein D, Kahaly G, et al. Is there a methimazole dose effect on remission rate in Graves' disease? Results from a long-term prospective study. The European Multicenter Trial Group of the Treatment of Hyperthyroidism with Antithyroid Drugs. *Clin Endocrinol (Oxf)* 1998;49:451–7.
26. Abraham P, Avenell A, Watson WA, et al. Antithyroid drug regimen for treating Graves' hyperthyroidism. *Cochrane Database Syst Rev* 2004;(2):CD003420.
27. Weetman AP, Pickerill AP, Watson P, et al. Treatment of Graves' disease with the block-replace regimen of antithyroid drugs: The effect of treatment duration and immunogenetic susceptibility on relapse. *Q J Med* 1994;87:337–41.
28. Tamai H, Kasagi K, Takaichi Y, et al. Development of spontaneous hypothyroidism in patients with Graves' disease treated with antithyroidal drug: Clinical, immunological, and histological findings in 26 patients. *J Clin Endocrinol Metab* 1989;69:49–53.
29. McIver B, Rae P, Beckett G, et al. Lack of effect of thyroxine in patients with Graves' hyperthyroidism who are treated with an antithyroid drug. *N Engl J Med* 1996;334:220–4.
30. Pearce SH, Meeriman TR. Genetics of type 1 diabetes and autoimmune thyroid disease. *Endocrinol Metabolism Clin N Am* 2009;38:289–301.
31. Vitti P, Rago T, Chiovato L, et al. Clinical features of patients with Graves' disease undergoing remission after antithyroid drug treatment. *Thyroid* 1997;7(3):369–75.
32. Pearce SH. Spontaneous reporting of adverse reactions to carbimazole and propylthiouracil in the UK. *Clin Endocrinol (Oxf)* 2004;61:589–94.
33. Fukata S, Kuma K, Sugawara M, et al. Granulocyte colony-stimulating factor (G-CSF) does not improve recovery from antithyroid drug-induced agranulocytosis: A prospective study. *Thyroid* 1999;9:29–31.
34. Bogazzi F, Bartalena L, Brogioni S, et al. Comparison of radioiodine with radioiodine plus lithium in the treatment of Graves' hyperthyroidism. *J Clin Endocrinol Metab* 1999;84:499–503.
35. Bogazzi F, Bartalen L, Martino E. Approach to the patient with amiodarone-induced thyrotoxicosis. *J Clin Endocrinol Metab* 2010;95:2529–35.
36. Nayak B, Burman K. Thyrotoxicosis and thyroid storm. *Endocrinol Metab Clin North Am* 2006;35:663–86.
37. Ross DS. Radioiodine therapy for hyperthyroidism. *N Engl J Med* 2011;364:542–50.
38. Watt T, Groenvold M, Rasmussen AK, et al. Quality of life in patients with benign thyroid disorders. A review. *Eur J Endocrinol* 2006;154:501–10.
39. Stålberg P, Svensson A, Hessman O, et al. Surgical treatment of Graves' disease: Evidence-based approach. *World J Surg* 2008;32:1269–77.
40. Ljunggren JG, Törring O, Wallin G, et al. Quality of life aspects and costs in treatment of Graves'

hyperthyroidism with antithyroid drugs, surgery, or radioiodine: Results from a prospective, randomized study. *Thyroid* 1998;8:653–9.
41. Abraham-Nordling M, Törring O, Hamberger B, et al. Graves' disease: A long-term quality-of-life follow up of patients randomized to treatment with antithyroid drugs, radioiodine, or surgery. *Thyroid* 2005;15:1279–86.
42. Franklyn JA, Maisonneuve P, Sheppard MC, et al. Mortality after the treatment of hyperthyroidism with radioactive iodine. *New Engl J Med* 1998;338:712–18.
43. Nygaard B, Hegedüs L, Gervil M, et al. Influence of compensated radioiodine therapy on thyroid volume and incidence of hypothyroidism in Graves' disease. *J Intern Med* 1995;238:491–7.
44. Jarløv AE, Hegedüs L, Kristensen LØ, et al. Is calculation of the dose in radioiodine therapy of hyperthyroidism worthwhile? *Clin Endocrinol (Oxf)* 1995;43:325–9.
45. Allahabadia A, Daykin J, Sheppard MC, et al. Radioiodine treatment of hyperthyroidism – prognostic factors for outcome. *J Clin Endocrinol Metab* 2001;86:3611–17.
46. Walter MA, Briel M, Christ-Crain M, et al. Effects of antithyroid drugs on radioiodine treatment: Systematic review and meta-analysis of randomised controlled trials. *Br Med J* 2007;334:514.
47. Palit TK, Miller CC III, Miltenburg DM, et al. The efficacy of thyroidectomy for Graves' disease: A meta-analysis. *J Surg Res* 2000;90:161–5.
48. Sosa JA, Bowman HM, Tielsch JM, et al. The importance of surgeon experience for clinical and economic outcomes from thyroidectomy. *Ann Surg* 1998;228:320–30.
49. Baeza A, Aguayo J, Barria M, et al. Rapid preoperative preparation in hyperthyroidism. *Clin Endocrinol (Oxf)* 1991;35:439–42.
50. Bahn RS. Mechanisms of disease: Graves' ophthalmopathy. *N Engl J Med* 2010;362:726–38.
51. Cockerham KP, Chan SS. Thyroid eye disease. *Neurol Clin* 2010;28:729–55.
52. Rundle FF, Wilson CW. Ophthalmoplegia in Graves' disease. *Clin Sci* 1944;5:17–29.
53. Hufnagel TJ, Hickey WF, Cobbs WH, et al. Immunohistochemical and ultrastructural studies on the exenterated orbital tissues of a patient with Graves' disease. *Ophthalmol* 1984;91:1411–19.
54. Douglas RS, Afifiyan NF, Hwang CJ, et al. Increased generation of fibrocytes in thyroid-associated ophthalmopathy. *J Clin Endrocrinol Metab* 2010;95:430–8.
55. Smith TJ, Padovani-Claudio DA, Lu Y, et al. Fibroblasts expressing the thyrotropin receptor overarch thyroid and orbit in Graves' disease. *J Clin Endocrinol Metab* 2011;96:3827–37.
56. Herzog EL, Bacula R. Fibrocytes in health and disease. *Exp Hematol* 2010;38:548–56.
57. Multiple authors. Classification of eye changes of Graves' disease. *Thyroid* 1992;2:235–6.
58. Mourits MP, Prummel MF, Wiersinga WM, et al. Clinical activity score as a guide in the management of patients with Graves' ophthalmopathy. *Clin Endocrinol (Oxf)* 1997;47:9–15.
59. Stan MN, Bahn RS. Risk factors for development of deterioration of Graves' ophthalmopathy. *Thyroid* 2010;20(7):777–83.
60. Yeatts RP. Quality of life in patients with Graves' ophthalmopathy. *Trans Am Ophthalmol Soc* 2005;103:368–441.
61. Bradley EA, Sloan JA, Novotny PJ, et al. Evaluation of the National Eye Institute Visual Function questionnaire in Graves' ophthalmopathy. *Ophthalmol* 2006;113:1450–4.
62. Elberling TV, Rasmussen AK, Feldt-Rasmussen U, et al. Impaired health-related quality of life in Graves' disease. A prospective study. *Eur J Endocrinol* 2004;151:549–55.
63. Terwee CB, Gerding MN, Dekker FW, et al. Development of a disease specific quality of life questionnaire for patients with Graves' ophthalmopathy: The GO-QOL. *Br J Ophthalmol* 1998;82:773–9.
64. Terwee C, Wakelkamp I, Tan S, et al. Long-term effects of Graves' ophthalmopathy on health-related quality of life. *Eur J Endocrinol* 2002;146:751–7.
65. Stiebel-Kalish H, Robenshtok E, Hasanreisoglu M, et al. Treatment modalities for Graves' ophthalmopathy: Sytematic review and metaanalysis. *J Cin Endocrinol Metab* 2010;94:2708–16.
66. Kahaly GJ, Pitz S, Hommel G, et al. Randomized, single blind trial of intravenous versus oral steroid monotherapy in Graves' orbitopathy. *J Clin Endocrinol Metab* 2005;90:5234–40.
67. Zang S, Ponto KA, Kahaly GJ. Intravenous glucocorticoids for Graves' orbitopathy: Efficacy and morbidity. *J Clin Endocrinol Metab* 2011;96:320–32.
68. Sacchi S, Federico M, Dastoli G, et al. Treatment of B-cell non-Hodgkin's lymphoma with anti CD 20 monoclonal antibody Rituximab. *Clin Rev Onc Hematol* 2001;37:13–25.
69. El Fassi D, Banga JP, Gilbert JA, et al. Treatment of Graves' disease with rituximab specifically reduces the production of thyroid stimulating autoantibodies. *Clin Immunol* 2009;130:252–8.
70. El Fassi D, Nielsen CH, Bonnema SJ, et al. B lymphocyte depletion with the monoclonal antibody Rituximab in Graves' disease: A controlled pilot study. *J Clin Endocrinol Metab* 2007;92(5):1769–72.
71. Silkiss RZ, Reier A, Coleman M, et al. Rituximab for thyroid eye disease. *Ophthalmic Plast Rec* 2010;26:310–14.
72. Wang SH, Baker JR. Targeting B cells in Graves' disease. *Endocrinol* 2006;147:4559–60.

73. Vannucchi G, Campi I, Bonomi M, et al. Rituximab treatment in patients with active Graves' orbitopathy: Effects on proinflammatory and humoral immune reactions. *Clin Exp Immonol* 2010;161:436–43.
74. Salvi M, Vannucchi G, Campi I, et al. Rituximab treatment in a patient with severe thyroid-associated ophthalmology: Effects on the orbital lymphocytic infiltrates. *Clin Immunol* 2009;131:360–5.
75. Khanna D, Chong KKL, Afifiyan NF, et al. Rituximab treatment of patients with severe, corticosteroid-resistant thyroid-associated ophthalmopathy. *Ophthalmol* 2010;117:133–9.
76. Stoedter M, Renko K, Hog A, et al. Selenium controls the sex-specific immune response and selenoprotein expression during the acute-phase response in mice. *Biochem J* 2010;429:43–50.
77. Marcocci C, Kahaly GJ, Drassas GE, et al. Selenium and the course of mild Graves' orbitopathy. *N Engl J Med* 2011;365:1920–31.
78. Smith TJ, Douglas RD. Does selenium supplementation improve Graves' ophthalmology? *Nat Rev Endocrinol* 2011;7:505–6.
79. Niepomniszcze H, Amad RH. Skin disorders and thyroid diseases. *J Endocrinol Invest* 2001;24:628–38.
80. Fatourechi V, Pajouhi M, Fransway AF. Dermopathy of Graves' disease (pretibial myxedema). *Medicine* 1994;73:1–7.
81. Tao TW, Leu SL, Kriss JP. Biological activity of autoantibodies associated with Graves' dermopathy. *J Clin Endocrinol Metab* 1989;69:90–9.
82. Nixon DW, Samols E. Acral changes associated with thyroid diseases. *JAMA* 1970;212:1175–80.
83. Vanhoenacker FM, Pelckmans MC, DeBeuckeleer LH, et al. Thyroid acropachy: Correlation of imaging and pathology. *Eur Radiol* 2001;11:1058–62.
84. Torres-Reyes E, Staple TW. Roentgenographic appearance of the thyroid acropachy. *Clin Radiol* 1970;21:95–100.
85. Okosieme OE, Marx H, Lazarus JH. Medical management of thyroid dysfunction in pregnancy and the postpartum. *Expert Opin Pharmacother* 2008;9:2281–93.
86. Laurberg P, Nygaard B, Glinoer D, et al. Guidelines for TSH-receptor antibody measurements in pregnancy: Results of an evidence-based symposium organized by the European Thyroid Association. *Eur J Endocrinol* 1998;139:584–6.
87. Brix TH, Hegedüs L. Twin studies as a model for exploring the aetiology of autoimmune thyroid disease. *Clin Endocrinol (Oxf)* 2012;76:457–64.
88. Eschler DC, Hasham A, Tomer Y. Cutting edge: The etiology of autoimmune thyroid diseases. *Clin Rev Allergy Immunol* 2011;41:190–7.
89. Calé A, Pedersen IB, Knudsen N, et al. Thyroid volume in hypothyroidism due to autoimmune disease follows a unimodal distribution: Evidence against primary thyroid atrophy and autoimmune thyroiditis being distinct diseases. *J Clin Endocrinol Metab* 2009;94:833–9.
90. Thvilum M, Brandt F, Brix TH, et al. A review for and against increased mortality in hypothyroidism. *Nature Rev Endocrinol* 2012;8:417–24.
91. Evans C, Gregory JW, Barton J, et al. Transient congenital hypothyroidism due to thyroid-stimulating hormone receptor blocking antibodies: A case series. *Ann Clin Biochem* 2011;48:386–90.
92. Hegedüs L, Hansen JM, Feldt-Rasmussen U, et al. Influence of thyroxine treatment on thyroid size and anti-thyroid peroxidise antibodies in Hashimoto's thyroiditis. *Clin Endocrinol (Oxf)* 1991;35:235–8.
93. Penney SE, Homer JJ. Thyroid lymphoma: Acute presentation and long-term outcome. *J Laryngol Otol* 2011;125:1256–62.
94. Zimmerman RS, Brennan MD, McConahey WM, et al. Hashimoto's thyroiditis. An uncommon cause of painful thyroid unresponsive to corticosteroid therapy. *Ann Intern Med* 1986;104:355–7.
95. Weetman AP. Hypothyroidism: Screening and subclinical disease. *BMJ* 1997;314:1175–8.
96. Vanderpump MPJ, Tunbridge WMG, French JM, et al. The incidence of thyroid disorders in the community: A twenty-year follow-up of the Whickham survey. *Clin Endocrinol* 1995;43:55–68.
97. Åsvold BO, Vatten LJ, Midthjell K, et al. Serum TSH within the reference range as a predictor of future hypothyroidism and hyperthyroidism: 11-year follow-up of the HUNT study in Norway. *J Clin Endocrinol Metab* 2012;97:93–9.
98. Grebe SKG, Cooke RR, Ford HC, et al. Treatment of hypothyroidism with once weekly thyroxine. *J Clin Endocrinol Metab* 1997;82:870–5.
99. Devdhar M, Drooger R, Pehlivanova M, et al. Levothyroxine replacement doses are affected by gender and weight, but not age. *Thyroid* 2011;21:821–7.
100. Grozinsky-Glasberg S, Fraser A, Nahshoni E, et al. Thyroxine-triiodothyronine combination therapy versus thyroxine monotherapy for clinical hypothyroidism: Meta-analysis of randomized controlled trials. *J Clin Endocrinol Metab* 2006;91:2592–9.
101. Panicker V, Saravanan P, Vaidya B, et al. Common variation in the DIO2 gene predicts baseline psychological well-being and response to combination thyroxine plus triiodothyronine therapy in hypothyroid patients. *J Clin Endocrinol Metab* 2009;94:1623–9.
102. Klein RZ, Haddow JE, Faix JD, et al. Prevalence of thyroid deficiency in pregnant women. *Clin Endocrinol (Oxf)* 1991;35:41–6.
103. Negro R, Formoso G, Mangieri T, et al. Levothyroxine treatment in euthyroid pregnant women with autoimmune thyroid disease:effects on obstetrical complications. *J Clin Endocrinol Metab* 2006;91:2587–91.

104. Muller AF, Drexhage HA, Berghout A. Postpartum thyroiditis and autoimmune thyroiditis in women of childbearing age: Recent insights and consequences for antenatal and postnatal care. *Endocrine Rev* 2001;22:605–30.
105. Lazarus JH. The continuing saga of postpartum thyroiditis. *J Clin Endocrinol Metab* 2011;96:614–16.
106. Premawardhana LD, Parkes AB, Ammari F, et al. Postpartum thyroiditis and long-term thyroid status: Prognostic influence of thyroid peroxidise antibodies and ultrasound echogenicity. *J Clin Endocrinol Metab* 2000;85:71–5.
107. Abalovich M, Amino N, Barbour LA, et al. Management of thyroid dysfunction during pregnancy and postpartum: An Endocrine Society clinical practice guideline. *J Clin Endocrinol Metab* 2007;92(8 Suppl):S1–47.
108. Lazarus JH, Bestwick JP, Channon S, et al. Antenatal thyroid screening and childhood cognitive function. *N Engl J Med* 2012;366:493–501.
109. Irvine WJ, Barnes EW. Addison's disease, ovarian failure and hypoparathyroidism. *Clin Endocrinol Metab* 1975;4:379–434.
110. Weetman AP. Autoantigens in Addison's disease and associated syndromes. *Clin Exp Immunol* 1997;107:227–9.
111. Betterle C, Volpato M, Pedini B, et al. Adrenal-cortex autoantibodies and steroid-producing cells autoantibodies in Addison's disease: Comparison of immunofluorescence and immunoprecipitation assays. *J Clin Endocrinol Metab* 1999;84:618–22.
112. Grinspoon SK, Biller BMK. Laboratory assessment of adrenal insufficiency. *J Clin Endocrinol Metab* 1994;79:923–31.
113. De Bellis A, Bizzarro A, Rossi R, et al. Remission of subclinical adrenocortical failure in subjects with adrenal autoantibodies. *J Clin Endocrinol Metab* 1993;76:1002–7.
114. Oelkers W, Diederich S, Bahr V. Diagnosis and therapy surveillance in Addison's disease: Rapid adrenocorticotropin (ACTH) test and measurement of plasma renin activity and aldosterone. *J Clin Endocrinol Metab* 1992;72:259–64.
115. Alkatib AA, Cosma M, Elamin MB, et al. A systematic review and meta-analysis of randomized placebo-controlled trials of DHEA treatment effects on quality of life in women with adrenal insufficiency. *J Clin Endocrinol Metab* 2009;94:3676–81.
116. Peterson P, Nagamine K, Scott H, et al. APECED: A monogenic autoimmune disease providing new clues to self-tolerance. *Immunol Today* 1998;19:384–6.
117. Danso-Abeam D, Humblet-Baron S, Dooley J, et al. Models of AIRE-dependent gene regulation for thymic negative selection. *Front Immunol* 2011;2:14.
118. Neufeld M, Maclaren NK, Blizzard RM. Two types of autoimmune Addison's disease associated with different polyglandular autoimmune (PGA) syndromes. *Medicine* 1981;60:355–62.
119. Betterle C, Greggio NA, Volpato M. Autoimmune polyglandular syndrome type 1. *J Clin Endocrinol Metab* 1998;83:1049–55.
120. Ahonen P, Myllärniemi S, Sipilä I, et al. Clinical variation of autoimmune polyendocrinopathy-candidiasis-ectodermal dystrophy (APECED) in a series of 68 patients. *New Engl J Med* 1990;322:1829–36.
121. Vaidya B, Imrie H, Greatch DR, et al. Association analysis of the cytotoxic T lymphocyte antigen-4 (CTLA-4) and autoimmune regulator-1 (AIRE-1) genes in sporadic autoimmune Addison's disease. *J Clin Endocrinol Metab* 2000;85:688–91.
122. Prabhakar BS, Bahn RS, Smith TJ. Current perspective on the pathogenesis of Graves' disease and ophthalmopathy. *Endocr Rev*. 2003;24(6):802–35.

# 14

# Nonautoimmune thyroid disease

*Arie Berghout, Alex F. Muller, Philip E. Harris*

## Multinodular goiter

Multinodular goiter is an enlargement of the thyroid gland consisting of multiple nodules. Sometimes, only a single nodule is found in a thyroid, often the prelude to more nodules. If a single nodule is hyperactive, it is called toxic adenoma.

Multinodular goiter is quite prevalent: In the Framingham study (United States), it was observed in 6.4% of females and in 1.5% of males[1]; Whickham Survey (United Kingdom) found that 10% of females and 2% of males had multinodular goiter.[2] Even a higher prevalence is documented in ultrasound studies and at necropsy, notably in higher age groups. Iodine deficiency can increase the prevalence to up to 30%; cigarette smoking is also an environmental risk factor.[3] Moreover, family and twin studies suggest a strong genetic predisposition.

## Pathogenesis

Most goiters consist of nodules, cysts, and areas of hemorrhage and calcification. Single nodules and adenomas, as well as most nodules in multinodular goiters, are monoclonal in origin. The early literature suggests that diffuse goiters precede nodular goiters and that thyroid-stimulating hormone (TSH) is involved in the earlier phases of growth. Evidence for this hypothesis is lacking. Current opinion favors a continuous pathophysiological process operating on the background of the natural heterogeneity and polyclonality of human thyroid cells, where, in addition to TSH and iodine, growth factors and goitrogens are also involved in the evolution of thyroid nodules.[4,5] In contrast, genetic alterations can explain thyroid growth. In autonomously functioning thyroid adenomas, activating mutations of the TSH receptor and $G_s$ $\alpha$ genes have been demonstrated. Multinodular goiters are functionally heterogeneous and thus appear polyclonal. However, most nodules are monoclonal in origin.[6] Because the family history in patients with multinodular goiter is often positive, genetic research could be of clinical benefit in the future. Indeed, a germline polymorphism of codon 727 of the human TSH receptor was found to be associated with toxic multinodular goiter, and a familial form of goiter has been found with a link to markers on chromosome 14q.[7,8] Recent studies found new susceptibility loci on 2q, 3p, 7q, and 8p for familial euthyroid goiter, confirming the genetic heterogeneity.[9] In selected cases of toxic adenoma, gain-of-function somatic mutations and mutations in the gene coding for G proteins have been demonstrated.[10] However, these findings are not universal, and other studies have failed to confirm the presence of these nonfunctional mutations. Furthermore, these mutations may be secondary phenomena and thus not etiologically related to adenoma or goiter formation.

## Clinical presentation

In about 50% of cases, the goiter is detected by the patients; in the remaining cases, it is detected by relatives or a physician. Complaints are neck discomfort (61%), cosmetics (17%), and dyspnea (17%). Fear of malignancy is expressed spontaneously by a minority of patients but by most when asked directly.[11]

## Diagnosis

Ultrasonography is nowadays the preferred investigative tool for thyroid and is used by many endocrinologists worldwide. Ultrasonography has replaced diagnosis of goiter by inspection and palpation.[12] This approach has also led to frequent coincidental detection of thyroid nodules and cysts. Ultrasound can be applied to measure the volume of goiters and the size of nodules and is also indispensable for fine-needle aspiration (FNA).[13] In cases of substernal extension of the goiter, magnetic resonance imaging (MRI) should be used. Computed tomography (CT) scanning should be avoided because it requires iodine-containing contrast agents.

It is important to exclude thyroid malignancy. The risk of malignancy is higher in solitary, rapidly growing nodules; in children or in the elderly; in males; and in subjects with a history of neck irradiation, particularly in childhood.

In goiters removed at surgery, carcinoma is found in 10%–15%, the majority being occult. In general, the risk of clinically important carcinoma in multinodular goiter is considered to be low, and, therefore, more aggressive therapy for nontoxic goiter is not justified.

Ultrasound-guided FNA is now the diagnostic procedure of first choice in the evaluation of solitary or dominant nodules.[16,17] Since its introduction, the numbers of thyroidectomies have declined dramatically.[18] Certain ultrasonographic features are associated with an increased risk of malignancy: nodule hypoechogenicity, microcalcifications, increased vascular flow, irregular borders, and the absence of a halo.[19,20] Applying these criteria can also be helpful in selecting the nodules within a multinodular goiter for aspiration. FNA cytology is a simple outpatient procedure. The test result can be benign, suspicious, malignant, or nondiagnostic. Repeat aspiration can augment the diagnostic accuracy and is indicated in case of increase of nodular size. Surgery is indicated in case of suspicion of malignancy or of a repeated nondiagnostic FNA test result. The number of diagnostic surgeries could possibly be further reduced by the application of molecular diagnosis by testing for common somatic mutations, BRAF, RAS, RET/PTC, and PAX8/PPARg, notably in case of nondiagnostic test results.[21]

In all patients, TSH should be measured. Subclinical hyperthyroidism is more prevalent in patients with multinodular goiter and is a risk for cardiovascular morbidity and mortality. TSH can also be helpful as an adjunct to FNA. It was found that the risk of malignancy increased with the TSH level. This is explained by the trophic effect of TSH on thyroid malignant cells.[22]

## Natural history and prognosis

The natural history of multinodular goiter is characterized by the increase of thyroid volume at a rate of about 4% per year. Concomitant with the increase in size, TSH values decline, followed by a rise of T3 and T4 levels, respectively.[11] This is called the evolution of "autonomy" of thyroid function, and eventually hyperthyroidism can follow.[23] Toxic multinodular goiter is often complicated by atrial fibrillation.[24] Furthermore, epidemiologic studies found a relation of increased vascular morbidity and mortality in elderly people with a low TSH.[25,26] Cardiac abnormalities have been demonstrated not only in epidemiologic studies but also in series of patients with "endogenous" subclinical hyperthyroidism.[27] Also, increased heart rate, left ventricular mass, and impaired diastolic function have been found in patients on thyroxine therapy in doses that suppress TSH levels.[28] Data about the significance of subclinical hyperthyroidism on other parameters vary. Cholesterol levels have been found to be lower; in other studies, bone gla protein, osteocalcin, and sex hormone–binding globulin (SHBG) levels were found to be higher in patients compared with controls.[29–31] Of theoretical interest is the difference between endogenous subclinical hyperthyroidism in patients with goiter with an initial rise in T3 levels and patients with exogenous subclinical hyperthyroidism due to thyroxine therapy, in whom T4 levels are elevated. Large multicenter studies are needed to investigate the preventive effect of low-dose radioactive iodine on the development of atrial fibrillation, the most serious long-standing consequence of multinodular goiter.

## Treatment (see Chapter 7)

The aim of treatment of a patient with a multinodular goiter is the reduction of goiter size and the prevention of thyrotoxicosis. Given that the goiter is an incidental finding in the majority of cases, general advice in euthyroid patients is to refrain from treatment and to advise follow-up. In case of obstruction, the choice is between surgery and radioactive iodine. Treatment with thyroxine to suppress the endogenous TSH secretion is only partially and temporarily effective and therefore no longer advised.[11]

Radioactive iodine is nowadays the treatment of choice, particularly in elderly subjects who represent the majority of the patients with a multinodular goiter. The efficacy of this treatment as evaluated by MRI is excellent. Both obstructive symptoms and thyroid volume decrease significantly in nearly all patients.[32,33] Most patients are treated with doses of 3–15 MBq/g tissue. The efficacy of treatment is enhanced by the administration of recombinant TSH.[34] Moreover, in the long-term, tracheal compression is diminished and inspiratory capacity is improved.[35] The treatment with radioactive iodine is complicated by mild and transient hyperthyroidism in the majority of patients. This treatment is generally well tolerated. Between 3 and 6 months, the majority of patients will have regained euthyroidism; only a minority has become hypothyroid.[36] However, sometimes hyperthyroidism is caused by the formation of TSH receptor autoantibodies, probably as a result of a toxic effect of the radioactive iodine on thyroid tissue. The onset of this form of thyrotoxicosis is insidious, can cause tachycardia and atrial fibrillation, and can occur even after several months.[37]

Surgery is performed in case of very large goiter, on patient's preference, and it can be a good option for a one-sided multinodular goiter.

# Toxic adenoma (see Chapter 7)

A toxic adenoma is a single hyperfunctioning thyroid nodule in an otherwise normal thyroid gland. A hyperfunctioning nodule can also be found in a multinodular goiter. From all patients presenting with hyperthyroidism, about 5% has a single hyperfunctioning nodule, and this rate is somewhat higher in iodine-deficient areas. Patients are mostly female and of middle age as in most thyroid disorders. The diagnosis is made by scintigraphy—one of the rare reasons nowadays to perform this diagnostic test—where uptake of the iodine is shown in the nodule and virtually no uptake in the other thyroid tissue. In case of incomplete suppression of uptake in surrounding thyroid tissue, the term *warm nodule* is used. In a toxic multinodular goiter, different areas can show enhanced uptake and result in a patchy distribution of the radiofarmacon.

Radioactive iodine is the treatment of choice. In most cases, the nodule reduces in size after therapy.[38] It is highly efficacious. Unlike Graves' disease, there is a much lower risk of developing hypothyroidism. Alternatively, surgery can be a good option as the excision of a single nodule is relatively simple, has a low risk, and offers immediate cure.

# Thyroiditis

The hallmark of thyroiditis is thyroid inflammation. Thyroid inflammation can be due to different causes: physical factors (palpation, radiation), pharmacotherapeutic agents, microorganisms, and autoimmunity. In this section, we focus on subacute granulomatous thyroiditis, subacute lymphocytic thyroiditis, and postpartum thyroiditis. Riedel's thyroiditis and infectious thyroiditis are discussed only briefly.

## Subacute granulomatous thyroiditis

Subacute granulomatous thyroiditis goes by several names: subacute (Quervain's) thyroiditis, subacute nonsuppurative thyroiditis, pseudo tuberculous thyroiditis, giant cell thyroiditis, pseudo-giant-cell thyroiditis, or struma granulomatosa.

### Prevalence

The incidence of subacute granulomatous thyroiditis is reported to be 4.9 cases per 100,000 per year.[39] Subacute granulomatous thyroiditis develops most frequently between the third and sixth decades.[39] The male-to-female ratio is reported to be in the range of 1 to 4–5.[39] Given the presumed etiology (see below), it is not surprising that in the majority of patients the disease is diagnosed in the summer. Also, some disease clusters have been described below.

### Pathogenesis

Several studies have investigated the etiology of subacute granulomatous thyroiditis. These studies support the notion that subacute granulomatous thyroiditis is caused by a viral infection or a postviral inflammatory process.[40]

Indirect evidence from case series for a viral origin has emerged from studies in which viral antibodies were measured in case of subacute granulomatous thyroiditis.[41,42] Associations between mumps, measles, coxsackie, and other viral pathogens and the occurrence of subacute granulomatous thyroiditis have been found.[41,42]

In the course of subacute granulomatous thyroiditis, autoimmune phenomena have also been described. Approximately 50% of patients with subacute granulomatous thyroiditis have thyroid autoantibodies; however, they are generally transient and their titer is low.[43] Moreover, circulating and intrathyroidal antigen-binding T cells are also observed in subacute granulomatous thyroiditis.[43] Because these phenomena are transient, they are unlikely to be the primary disruptive events in the pathogenesis of subacute granulomatous thyroiditis.[43]

Genetic associations have also been described in subacute granulomatous thyroiditis. Most important are the genes of the major histocompatibility complex (MHC) region located on the short arm of chromosome 6. MHC comprises the antigen-presenting molecules located on the cell membranes of antigen-presenting cells. HLA-B35 and HLA-B67 have been reported to be strongly associated with subacute granulomatous thyroiditis.[44] Collectively, the evidence supports a viral etiology, either direct or indirect, for subacute granulomatous thyroiditis and is consistent with subacute granulomatous thyroiditis being the result of a "final common pathway" occurring after a viral infection in genetically susceptible individuals.

## Clinical presentation

Biochemically, subacute granulomatous thyroiditis is characterized by a transient thyrotoxicosis occurring in about 75% of cases during which symptoms are usually mild compared with Graves' disease.[45,46] Nevertheless, thyrotoxic symptoms such as heat intolerance, palpitations, nervousness, and increased sweating can occur. The thyrotoxic phase of subacute granulomatous thyroiditis is due to leakage of thyroid hormones from destroyed thyrocytes and is therefore self-limiting, usually lasting 2–10 weeks.[45,46] In a minority of cases, the thyrotoxic phase is followed by a transient hypothyroid phase[45,46] (Figure 14.1).

Subsequent permanent hypothyroidism seems to be a rare event. Nikolai et al.[47] could find no cases of hypothyroidism in their 1–15 years of follow-up of 124 patients who had suffered an episode of subacute granulomatous thyroiditis.[47] Although considered to be a rare event, in another study, 15% of the patients are receiving T4 therapy after 28 years of follow-up.[46]

Iitaka et al.[48] have specifically addressed the question of recurrence of subacute granulomatous thyroiditis after complete recovery. They surveyed their database of 3344 patients who experienced an episode of subacute granulomatous thyroiditis between 1970 and 1993. They concluded that late recurrences arise in at least 2% of cases. The mean latency period (±SD) between the first and second episodes of subacute granulomatous thyroiditis was 14.5 ± 4.5 years.

## Diagnosis

The diagnosis of subacute granulomatous thyroiditis is fairly straightforward and is primarily clinical. The most prominent symptom of subacute granulomatous thyroiditis is pain in the region of the thyroid, frequently described as a sore throat. Indeed, most authors consider it a *conditio sine qua non* for the diagnosis to be made.[45] Frequently, this pain radiates to the jaw and ear. Other reported symptoms are malaise, fatigue, myalgia, and arthralgia.[42] Physical signs include fever and a small- to medium-sized diffuse goiter that is nearly always painful on palpation.[42,45] Further diagnostic confirmation can be obtained by finding a raised erythrocyte sedimentation rate, >40 mm/h in 97%

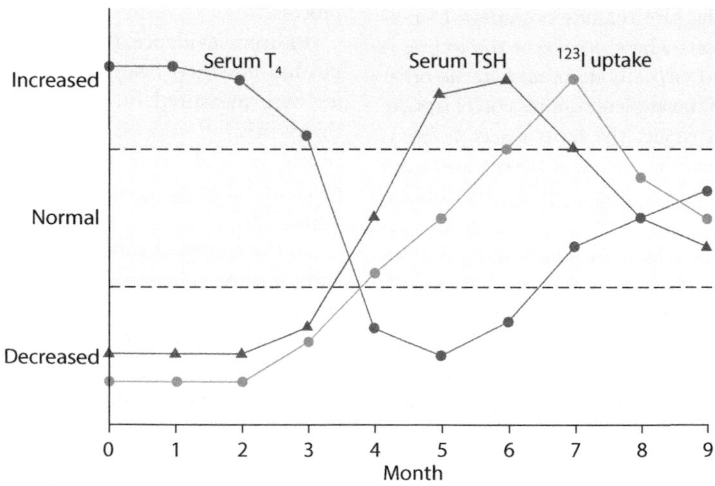


***Figure 14.1***
*Clinical course of subacute granulomatous thyroiditis, subacute lymphocytic thyroiditis, and postpartum thyroiditis. Measurements of serum TSH and $^{123}$I uptake show thyrotoxicosis during the first 3 months, followed by hypothyroidism for 3 months and then by euthyroidism. T4 denotes thyroxine. (Reproduced from Pearce EN et al.,* N Engl J Med, *348, 2646–55, 2003. With permission.)*

of patients, and a reduced or absent radioactive iodine uptake (usually <2%).[48] Other reported findings are mild anemia and leucocytosis.[48]

With respect to late recurrences, it should be noted that although the biochemical severity of thyrotoxicosis is similar to that of the previous event, erythrocyte sedimentation rate is lower and the radioactive iodine uptake higher, indicating a less severe inflammatory response.[48]

The differential diagnosis of pain in the thyroid region comprises primarily acute pharyngitis and, within the spectrum of thyroid disorders, acute infectious thyroiditis and hemorrhage into a preexistent thyroid nodule or cyst. Because the treatment of subacute granulomatous thyroiditis and acute infectious thyroiditis differ considerably, it is of paramount importance to establish a causal diagnosis. Symptoms can be localized to the thyroid by finding a painful goiter. Thyroid function testing should be performed because thyrotoxicosis is the rule in subacute granulomatous thyroiditis, whereas acute infectious thyroiditis and hemorrhage in a preexistent thyroid nodule do not present with thyroid dysfunction. Moreover, acute infectious thyroiditis, but not hemorrhage into a preexistent thyroid nodule, is generally accompanied by more prominent systemic manifestations, including a markedly elevated erythrocyte sedimentation rate (ESR). In cases of doubt, a needle aspiration under ultrasound guidance can be of diagnostic value.

Measurement of radioactive iodine uptake will confirm the destructive nature of the thyrotoxicosis, but it is usually not indicated. In exceptional cases where the cervical pain is not a prominent feature and Graves' disease is being considered as a plausible diagnosis, thyroid scintigraphy is valuable in distinguishing between these conditions.

### *Treatment*

Treatment of subacute granulomatous thyroiditis consists of relief of pain and symptomatic treatment of thyrotoxic symptoms. It has not been shown that subsequent permanent hypothyroidism can be prevented. If treatment is considered, nonsteroidal anti-inflammatory drugs or corticosteroids are the drugs of choice.[45,46,48] Generally, a nonsteroidal anti-inflammatory drug (e.g., aspirin 600 mg, 3–6 times daily) is given, followed by corticosteroids in case of insufficient pain relief within 3 days. A typical dose regimen consists of a starting dose of prednisone (40 mg/day, single dose) that should lead to a significant reduction in pain within 48 h. The dose is reduced to 30 mg after 4 days, followed by a dose reduction of 5 mg each week. With respect to thyrotoxicosis, 4–6 weeks of treatment with a beta blocker (e.g., 40–120 mg of propranolol or 25–50 mg of atenolol daily) is usually beneficial in symptomatic cases. Antithyroid drug therapy is ineffective and should not be given, because there is no increased thyroid hormone synthesis. After weeks to months, the thyroid dysfunction returns to normal.

Symptomatic hypothyroidism is temporarily treated with L-thyroxine replacement therapy.

Regarding follow-up, permanent hypothyroidism is the most important sequel of subacute granulomatous thyroiditis. Permanent hypothyroidism develops in <15% of patients after an episode of subacute granulomatous thyroiditis.

## *Lymphocytic thyroiditis: Subacute lymphocytic thyroiditis and postpartum thyroiditis (see Chapter 13)*

Subacute lymphocytic thyroiditis and postpartum thyroiditis are variants of chronic autoimmune (Hashimoto's) thyroiditis. If subacute lymphocytic thyroiditis manifests itself in the first year after delivery, the term postpartum thyroiditis is more appropriate. Synonyms are silent thyroiditis, hyperthyroiditis, atypical thyroiditis, and lymphocytic thyroiditis with spontaneously resolving hyperthyroidism.

### *Prevalence*

The prevalence of subacute lymphocytic thyroiditis varies widely.[49] In various studies, subacute lymphocytic thyroiditis accounts for 0%–23% of all cases of thyrotoxicosis. Because of the close temporal association with parturition, which facilitates prospective studies, more data are available on the epidemiology of postpartum thyroiditis than for other variants. The reported prevalence of postpartum thyroiditis varies widely, from 1.1% to 21.1%[50] (Table 14.1). A critical appraisal of the available literature concluded that the prevalence of postpartum thyroiditis in iodine-sufficient areas ranges between 5% and 7%.[50]

Subacute lymphocytic thyroiditis can occur at virtually any age. It has been described in 5–93-year-olds.[49,51] There is a slight female preponderance, with a female: male ratio of 2:1.[49,51]

Postpartum thyroiditis occurs more frequently in patients with type I diabetes mellitus. The incidence of PPTD in patients with type I diabetes mellitus is at least 15%.[52]

| First author | Year | Country | No. in source population | Inclusion criteria | No. included | Time of inclusion & last fu | No. of source population included (%)/ last fu (%) | Prevalence of TD (n) |
|---|---|---|---|---|---|---|---|---|
| Amino | 1982 | Japan | 507 consecutive F who delivered | TD, Tab+ or G | 63 | 3 mo pp/6 mo pp | 63 (12)/63 (12) | 5.5 (28/507) |
| Jansson | 1984 | Sweden | 644 consecutive F who delivered | Informed consent | 460 | 2 mo pp/5 mo pp | 460 (71)/460 (71) | 6.5 (30/460) |
| Freeman | 1986 | United States | 216 F at routine pp visits | Informed consent | 212 | 4–8 weeks pp/8–12 weeks pp | 212 (98)/44 (21) | 1.9 (4/212) |
| Lervang | 1987 | Denmark | 694 F who delivered | Informed consent | 591 | 3 mo pp/12 mo pp | 591 (85)/23 (4) | 3.9 (23/591) |
| Nicolai | 1987 | United States | 238 F who delivered | Informed consent | 238 | delivery/3 mo pp | 238 (100)/154 (65) | 6.7 (16/238) |
| Hayslip | 1988 | United States | 1034 F who delivered | Tab+ | 63 | 2nd day pp/6 mo pp | 63 (6)/51 (5) | 3.3 (34/1034) |
| Vargas | 1988 | United States | 261 F completing 1 year fu | Informed consent | 261 | delivery/12 mo pp | 261 (100)/261 (100) | 21.1 (55/261) |
| Fung | 1988 | United Kingdom | 901 F attending an antenatal clinic | Tab+ (tab-co's) | 100 (132) | 1st trimester/12 mo pp | 220 (24)/82 (9) | 16.7 (49/220)[a] |
| Rajatanavin | 1990 | Thailand | 812 F who delivered | Tab+ | 812 | 6 weeks pp/12 mo pp | 812 (100)/67 (8) | 1.1 (9/812) |
| Rasmussen | 1990 | Denmark | 1163 F in the 1st trimester | Tab+ (tab-co's) | 36 (20) | 1st trimester/12 mo pp | 56 (5)/56 (5) | 3.3 (33% of 10% TAb) |
| Roti | 1991 | Italy | 372 F who delivered | Informed consent | 219 | 1 mo pp/12 mo pp | 219 (59)/42 (11) | 8.7 (19/219) |
| Walfish | 1992 | Canada | 1376 F who delivered | Informed consent | 1376 | delivery/12 mo pp | 1376 (100)/ 300 (22) | 5.9 (81/1376) |

| | | | | | | | | |
|---|---|---|---|---|---|---|---|---|
| Stagnaro-Green | 1992 | United States | 552 F in the 1st trimester | Tab+ (tab-co's) | 38 (32) | 1st trimester/6 mo pp | 60 (11) /60 (11) | 8.8[a,b] |
| Harris | 1992 | United Kingdom | 1248 F attending an antenatal clinic | Tab+ (tab-co's) | 145 (229) | 2nd trimester/8 mo pp | 374 (30) /374 (30) | 5.0 (62/1248)[a,c] |
| Pop | 1993 | Netherlands | 382 pregnant F | Informed consent | 303 | 3rd trimester/8 mo pp | 303 (79) /293 (77) | 7.2 (21/293) |
| Kuijpens | 1998 | Netherlands | 448 pregnant F | Informed consent | 310 | 1st trimester/9 mo pp | 310 (69) /291 (65) | 5.2 (15/291) |
| Kent | 1999 | Australia | 1816 F who delivered | Informed consent | 748 | 6 mo pp/6 mo pp | 748 (41) /748 (41) | 10.3 (76/739) |
| Lucas | 2000 | Spain | 757 pregnant F | Informed consent | 605 | delivery/12 mo pp | 605 (80) /444 (59) | 7.4 (45/605) |
| Barca | 2000 | Brazil | 830 pregnant F with no TD, no G/C/N, Tab– | Informed consent | 800 | 1st trimester/12 mo pp | 800 (96) /335 (40) | 14.6 (49/335) |
| Sakaihara | 2000 | Japan | 4072 pregnant F in a screen program | — | 4072 | 1st trimester/3 mo pp | 1161/4072 | 6.5 (76/1161) |

fu, follow-up Tab, thyroid antibodies; TD, thyroid dysfunction; TF, thyroid function; F, females; pp, postpartum; G/C/N, goiter, cysts, or nodules.
(Reproduced from Muller AF et al., *Endocr Rev*, 22, 605–30, 2001. With permission.)

[a] Estimated prevalence.
[b] 33% of 18% Tab+ and 3% of 82% Tab–.
[c] 43% of 12% Tab+ and 0% of 78% Tab–.

***Table 14.1***
*Epidemiological data on postpartum thyroiditis.*

## Pathogenesis

Subacute lymphocytic thyroiditis and postpartum thyroiditis are acute phases of autoimmune destruction in the context of an existing and ongoing process of thyroid autosensitization[50] (Figure 14.2). This is suggested by the presence of thyroid autoantibodies, the histology of both focal organized and diffuse destructive lymphocytic thyroiditis with folliculolysis and disruption, the presence of circulating activated T cells, and the association between specific MHC haplotypes.[50]

At present, the initiating events in subacute lymphocytic thyroiditis and postpartum thyroiditis remain unknown. Immunotherapy with interferon-α and interleukin-2 can induce thyroid autoantibodies and a clinical picture similar to that of lymphocytic thyroiditis.[51] In postpartum thyroiditis, it is clear that, after the profound pregnancy-associated immunomodulation, there is a rebound effect leading to aggravation of thyroid autoimmunity during the puerperal period that plays an important in the pathogenesis of this condition.[50] These observations indicate that a sudden change in "immunohomeostasis" plays an important role in the initiation of the disorder.

Iodine has been implicated in several ways. Most important is iodine excess in autoimmune-prone individuals. After the introduction of iodine supplementation to a population, a rise in thyroid autoantibodies and a higher incidence of lymphocytic thyroiditis have been observed.[50] Besides iodine, other environmental factors such as toxins and cigarette smoking have been implicated as pathogenetic factors in the development of thyroid autoimmunity.[51]

## Presentation

Subacute lymphocytic thyroiditis and postpartum thyroiditis classically run a biphasic course: a thyrotoxic phase is followed by a hypothyroid phase.[50,51]

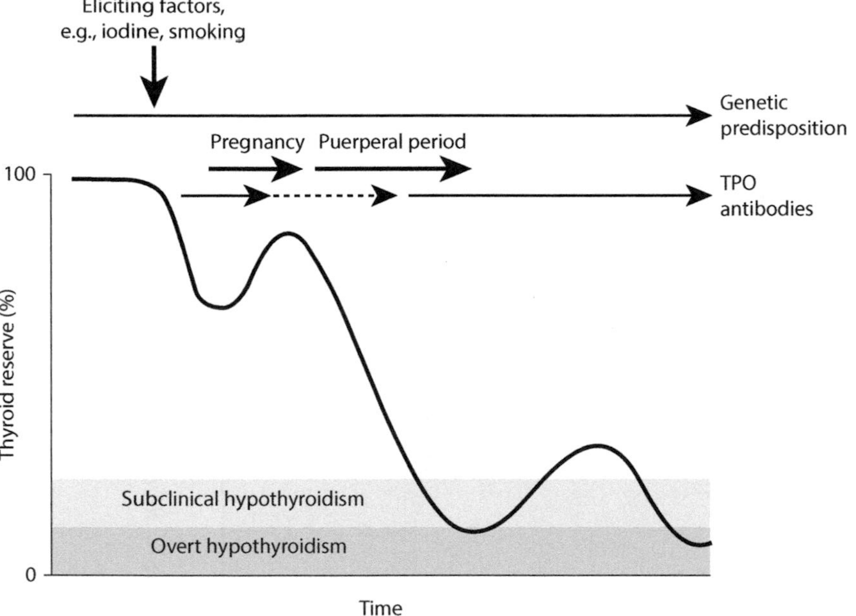


***Figure 14.2***
*A scheme depicting the gradual loss of thyroid reserve over time (often years) due to thyroid autoimmune mechanisms. On the basis of a genetic predisposition for endocrine and thyroid autoreactivity, an insult on the level of the thyroid (leading to the attraction of antigen-presenting cells [APCs]), and various other eliciting factors (e.g., iodine, smoking), a thyroid autoimmune reaction is initiated. TPO antibodies are markers of the ongoing thyroid autosensitization process. Pregnancy ameliorates the process, whereas the puerperal period aggravates thyroid autoimmunity. If thyroid reserve was already considerably compromised before pregnancy, or if the transient autoimmune attack in the puerperal period is severe enough, subclinical hypothyroidism and even overt hypothyroidism will develop (PPTD). (Reproduced from Muller AF et al.,* Endocr Rev, *22, 605–30, 2001. With permission.)*

The disease can also present as either transient thyrotoxicosis or hypothyroidism[50,51] (Figure 14.1). The duration of thyrotoxicosis is variable and can be 1–2 months.[50,51] The onset of thyrotoxicosis in postpartum thyroiditis is variable, ranging from the first to the sixth month postpartum.[50] During the thyrotoxic phase, the physical symptoms are usually mild compared to Graves' thyrotoxicosis and toxic multinodular goiter.[50,51] The thyrotoxic phase is due to leakage of thyroid hormones from destroyed thyrocytes and is therefore self-limiting.[50,51] Permanent hypothyroidism is the most important sequel of subacute lymphocytic thyroiditis and postpartum thyroiditis and occurs in about 6% and 12%–61% of patients, respectively.[50,51]

### Treatment

Because management and follow-up of postpartum destructive thyrotoxicosis and Graves' disease differ, it is important to establish a causal diagnosis. The presence of ophthalmopathy and TSH receptor antibodies points to a diagnosis of Graves' disease. In cases of doubt, thyroid scintigraphy should be performed, with a diffusely elevated uptake in Graves' disease and a suppressed uptake in cases of subacute lymphocytic thyroiditis and postpartum thyroiditis.[50,51]

It is important to be aware that thyrotoxicosis in patients with a previous episode of Graves' disease does not necessarily represent a relapse; postpartum thyroiditis can be superimposed on Graves' disease, emphasizing the role of thyroid scintigraphy in establishing a correct diagnosis.[53] During breastfeeding, however, the administration of $^{131}I$ is contraindicated.[54] When $^{123}I$ is used, breastfeeding should be stopped for 3 days, followed by measurement of radioactivity in the milk to assess safety of resuming breastfeeding.[54]

Due to the nature of the thyrotoxicosis—destruction mediated—antithyroid drug therapy should not be given. In symptomatic cases, a short course of beta blockade may be beneficial, for example, 40–120 mg of propranolol or 25–50 mg of atenolol daily until serum-free T4 is normal. In cases of hypothyroidism, treatment with L-thyroxine is given. Spontaneous recovery of thyroid function should not be awaited. Instead, it is reasonable to stop thyroxine after 2–6 months to see whether remission has occurred. If so, yearly assessment of thyroid function is advised. The risk of recurrence of thyroiditis after another pregnancy is 25%–50%. A pragmatic approach is to maintain the thyroxine replacement therapy and postpone the cessation of therapy until completion of the family.

The prevalence of permanent, clinically overt hypothyroidism after an episode of subacute lymphocytic thyroiditis or postpartum thyroiditis is sufficiently high to warrant yearly determination of TSH levels.[47]

## Riedel's thyroiditis

Riedel's thyroiditis is also known as Riedel's struma, fibrous thyroiditis, or invasive thyroiditis. It is a rare disorder of unknown cause.[51]

Because Riedel's thyroiditis is sometimes associated with fibrosis in other areas (retroperitoneal, mediastinal, orbital) and organs (lung, heart, bile ducts, parotids, and lacrimal glands), it is considered a rare manifestation of systemic collagenosis.[55] Indeed, on histology, the thyroid is densely infiltrated with connective tissue, with the presence inflammatory cells, especially lymphocytes and plasma cells.[56]

The clinical hallmark is an unusually hard thyroid gland that is often diffusely enlarged and attached to adjacent muscles, nerves, blood vessels, and trachea.[51] Other symptoms include anterior neck pain, dysphagia, and tracheal compression, with dyspnea and hoarseness.[51] As thyroid infiltration progresses, hypothyroidism occurs in about 25% of cases.[55] In exceptional cases, even hypoparathyroidism can ensue. Carcinomas and sclerosing lymphomas should be ruled out; this is best achieved by surgical biopsy. Systemic steroids and tamoxifen can stabilize the fibrosis and alleviate symptoms.[57,58] Hypothyroidism should be treated with thyroxin replacement therapy. Long-term follow-up with yearly check of thyroid function is warranted.

## Infectious thyroiditis

Infection of the thyroid is a rare event. Most thyroid infections involve pyogenic bacteria, although other microorganisms can also be involved.[59]

Infectious thyroiditis is often observed in two age groups: in children under age 10 years, when the infection frequently reaches the thyroid via a fistula from the left pyriform sinus, and in young middle-aged adults, in whom underlying thyroid disease—goiter, thyroiditis, adenoma, or carcinoma—seems to be a predisposing factor.[60]

Infectious thyroiditis should be considered whenever there are signs of infection accompanied by neck pain. Signs often include a uni- or bilateral tenderness to palpation, local erythema and warmth, dysphagia, and dysphonia. Thyroid function is usually normal. The differential diagnosis comprises infection of neck cysts (thyroglossal duct cyst, cystic hygroma, bronchial cleft cyst); subacute granulomatous thyroiditis; hemorrhage in a nodule; and, in case of slowly growing infectious agents, diffuse goiter or carcinoma. If infectious thyroiditis is suspected, a causal diagnosis is best established by FNA or surgical excision of the involved thyroid lobe. This will enable drainage as well as initiation of antibiotic therapy based on direct staining and culture results. In children, and in adults with recurrent episodes of suppurative thyroiditis, antibiotic cover should be directed against oropharyngeal flora, because in these groups infection is most likely caused by a fistula from the pyriform sinus. In these cases, barium swallow or CT scanning should be performed after recovery. In cases of pyriform fistula, fistulectomy should then be considered. There is no reason to advocate long-term follow-up after appropriate treatment for infectious thyroiditis.

## TSH receptor mutations and thyroid disease

The TSH receptor (TSHR) is a G protein–coupled receptor with the typical serpentine seven-transmembrane domains. It is preferentially coupled to $G_s$ that activates adenylyl cyclase, generating cyclic adenosine monophosphate (cAMP), when TSH binds to the receptor.[61] At higher levels of TSH, the TSHR also binds to $G_q$ with activation of phospholipase C and the production of inositol phosphate.[62] The cAMP pathway regulates expression of the thyroglobulin and thyroperoxidase genes, thyrocyte growth, and thyroid hormone secretion, whereas the inositol phosphate pathway is primarily involved in the control of organification of iodine and hormone synthesis.

Activating mutations of the TSHR have been described in familial nonautoimmune hyperthyroidism, sporadic congenital nonautoimmune hyperthyroidism, and autonomously functioning adenomas (toxic adenomas). Activating mutations have been described in the extracellular domains and N terminus and intracellular domains and C terminus and transmembrane domains. The majority of mutations are localized in the transmembrane domains, in particular the sixth transmembrane domain[63] (Figure 14.3).

### Somatic activating mutations of the TSHR in toxic adenomas

Somatic mutations of the TSHR were first described in toxic adenomas.[64] Activating somatic mutations were identified in the carboxyl-terminal portion of the third cytoplasmic loop in 3/11 toxic adenomas. The mutations were only found in the tumor tissue, involving B619G in two cases and A623I in one case. Activating mutations have since been reported in up to 80% of toxic adenomas and in a proportion of hyperfunctioning nodules in toxic multinodular goiters. Activating mutations of $G_s$ (*gsp*) have also been detected in ~10% of toxic adenomas.[65–67]

The treatment for toxic adenomas is the same, whether or not there is a TSHR or $G_s$ mutation present. The situation for germline mutations, however, is quite different.

### Germline activating mutations of the TSHR

Autosomal dominant nonautoimmune hyperthyroidism is defined clinically by the familial occurrence of thyroid autonomy in two or more generations. The demographic prevalence is difficult to estimate. The reported prevalence is increasing as awareness of the disease grows. The onset of thyrotoxicosis varies from fetal/neonatal presentation, through to adulthood. Neonatal sporadic or nonautoimmune hyperthyroidism, unlike Graves' disease, is characterized by the absence of TSH-binding inhibitory immunoglobulins and the persistence of thyrotoxicosis beyond 3 months of age. It is associated with intrauterine growth retardation, low birth weight, and tachycardia. The presence of goiter at presentation is variable. There may be other associated features such as microcephaly and developmental delay. Characteristically, the patients have severe disease that is difficult to control and relapses after medical therapy.[63,68] Goiters tend to enlarge and become multinodular in later life.

Two heterozygous activating germline mutations of the TSHR, associated with familial nonautoimmune hyperthyroidism, were first described in two families with autosomal dominant hyperthyroidism involving residues in the third (V509A) and seventh (C672T) transmembrane domains.[69] Since then, numerous different mutations have been described in many families. Some of the mutations have also been found in toxic adenomas (Figure 14.3). Most of the mutations activate cAMP, but a subset also activates phospholipase C.[63]

Graves' disease is the main differential diagnosis of familial nonautoimmune hyperthyroidism. Unlike Graves' disease, nonautoimmune hyperthyroidism is not associated with a high female preponderance. It also lacks the autoimmune features characteristic of Graves' disease. Interestingly, however, some patients present with associated ocular symptoms, in particular proptosis. They have been particularly described in spontaneous congenital nonautoimmune hyperthyroidism. Unlike autoimmune thyroid disease, however, there are no inflammatory components.[63]

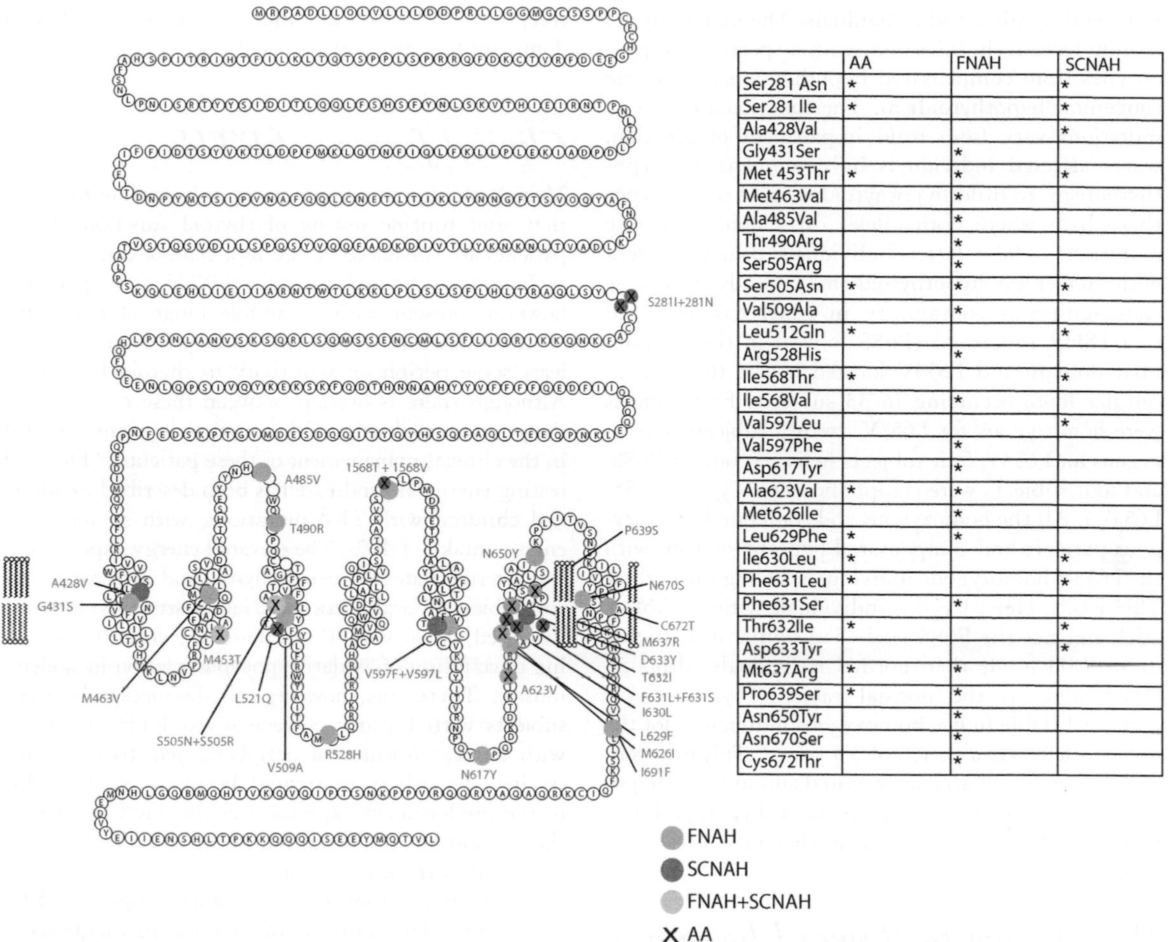

| | AA | FNAH | SCNAH |
|---|---|---|---|
| Ser281 Asn | * | | * |
| Ser281 Ile | * | | * |
| Ala428Val | | | * |
| Gly431Ser | | * | |
| Met 453Thr | * | * | * |
| Met463Val | | * | |
| Ala485Val | | * | |
| Thr490Arg | | * | |
| Ser505Arg | | * | |
| Ser505Asn | * | * | * |
| Val509Ala | | * | |
| Leu512Gln | * | | * |
| Arg528His | | * | |
| Ile568Thr | * | | * |
| Ile568Val | | * | |
| Val597Leu | | | * |
| Val597Phe | | * | |
| Asp617Tyr | | * | |
| Ala623Val | * | * | |
| Met626Ile | | * | |
| Leu629Phe | * | * | |
| Ile630Leu | * | | * |
| Phe631Leu | * | | * |
| Phe631Ser | | * | |
| Thr632Ile | * | | * |
| Asp633Tyr | | | * |
| Mt637Arg | * | * | |
| Pro639Ser | * | * | |
| Asn650Tyr | | * | |
| Asn670Ser | | * | |
| Cys672Thr | | * | |



**Figure 14.3**

*Activating mutations of the* TSHR *gene in the various genetic hyperthyroidism syndromes. Comparison of amino acid structure of the TSHR and locations of gain-of-function mutations found in familial non autoimmune hyperthyroidism (FNAH) (green), sporadic congenital nonautoimmune hyperthyroidism (SCNAH) (red), or in FNAH and SCNAH (yellow); autonomous adenomas (AA) X. (From Hébrant A et al.,* Eur J Endocrinol, *164, 1–9, 2011.)*

In contrast to Graves' disease, although patients may respond to antithyroid medical therapy, they inevitably relapse when treatment is withdrawn. Definitive treatment is required in the form of total thyroidectomy and/or radioiodine.

## Germline inactivating mutations of the TSHR

Resistance to TSH is characterized by elevated TSH levels, normal or low levels of T3 and T4, and the absence of a goiter (normal or hypoplastic thyroid gland). The first mutation responsible for the inactivation of the TSHR was described in the *hyt/hyt* mouse. Homozygous *hyt/hyt* mice have thyroid hypoplasia and are hypothyroid.[70] Loss-of-function mutations were first described in a family with compensated hypothyroidism, that is, clinically euthyroid with elevated serum TSH but normal T3 and T4 levels.[71] The trait appeared in three sisters from parents who were clinically and biochemically euthyroid. The sisters were found to be compound heterozygotes, with two different mutations in the extracellular domain of TSHR (maternal allele, P162A; paternal allele, I167N). Since then, loss-of-function mutations have been described in several families and individuals. The mutations are mainly recessively inherited, with a spectrum of phenotypes from compensated hypothyroidism to severe congenital hypothyroidism. The functional effects of mutations vary from mild impairment of function, where affected individuals have compensated hypothyroidism, to mild hypothyroidism and severe hypothyroidism where both alleles carry nonfunctioning mutations. These latter individuals usually present with congenital hypothyroidism. A study of a large consanguineous community in Israel has identified two TSHR mutations (P68S located in the extracellular domain and L653V located in the third extracellular loop) occurring in 33 subjects. Five subjects were homozygous for L653V, twenty subjects heterozygous for L653V, four subjects heterozygous for P68S, and four subjects were compound heterozygous P68S/L653V4. All the homozygous and compound heterozygous patients had compensated hypothyroidism, with the L653V homozygous individuals having the highest TSH levels. Heterozygous individuals with the L653V allele but not the P68S allele had significantly higher mean TSH levels than normal individuals, although many were in the normal range. Thyroid status remained stable in five homozygous individuals for the L653V allele over a period of 3.5 years.[72] This is in contrast to patients with compensated autoimmune hypothyroidism who may develop frank hypothyroidism requiring thyroxine replacement therapy.

## Resistance to thyroid hormone

Thyroid hormone action is encoded by two highly homologous receptors, TRα and TRβ, encoded by genes on chromosomes 17 and 3, respectively. Alternate splicing generates three highly homologous nuclear receptor isoforms (TRα1, TRβ1, and TRβ2) that have differing tissue distributions.[73] TRα1is most abundant in the central nervous system, myocardium, and skeletal muscle; TRβ1 in liver and kidney; and TRβ2 in the pituitary and hypothalamus.

RTH is rare and is characterized by elevated thyroid hormone levels, together with an unsuppressed TSH level, reflecting RTH in the hypothalamic–pituitary–thyroid axis. Peripheral RTH appears to be variable, resulting in variable clinical manifestations of the abnormality.[74] The condition is inherited in an autosomal dominant manner, associated with diverse, heterozygous *TRβ* gene mutations that occur *de novo* in approximately 10% of sporadic cases. A large number of mutations have been identified that impair binding to thyroid hormones and/or transcriptional activity of the receptors.[75–77] In addition, mutant receptors also have a dominant negative action on wild-type receptors.[78,79]

## Clinical features of RTHs

Many patients are asymptomatic, only coming to attention after routine testing of thyroid function. These patients are considered to be in a state of compensated euthyroidism, termed generalized RTH. Some patients, however, present with a variable range of symptoms of thyrotoxicosis, consistent with preservation of at least some peripheral sensitivity to thyroid hormones. Although there is overlap between these two entities, the presence or absence of thyrotoxic symptoms is useful in the clinical management of these patients.[80] Elevated resting energy expenditure has been described in adults and children with TRβ mutations, with an increased energy intake of 40%. The elevated energy expenditure was intermediate between euthyroid and thyrotoxic control subjects. Basal mitochondrial substrate oxidation is increased, whereas ATP synthesis is decreased, indicating uncoupling of oxidative phosphorylation in skeletal muscle. There was, however, no distinction between subjects with features of generalized RTH and those with clinical features of peripheral sensitivity.[81] This retained sensitivity to thyroid hormone is likely due to the predominant expression of the TRα isoform in skeletal muscle. A similar retained sensitivity has been described in the myocardium.[82]

Goiter is the commonest presenting sign in >50% of patients. The most common error in diagnosis is Graves' disease. If a patient undergoes a thyroidectomy, the goiter will usually recur, often with multinodular features. The main differential diagnosis in patients with elevated TSH and thyroid hormone levels is a thyrotropin-secreting pituitary tumor. These patients are clinically thyrotoxic and may have other features indicative of a pituitary tumor. Other causes of a raised serum T4 and TSH that need to be considered are listed in Table 14.2. Assay artifacts due to interfering protein binding or antibodies can usually be excluded using a two-step assay or equilibrium dialysis for fT4, and serial dilutions for TSH.

Recently, patients with heterozygous inactivating mutations in TRα1 have been identified.[83–85] The phenotype of these patients includes growth retardation, delayed skeletal development mildly delayed motor and cognitive development and constipation. Thyroid function tests demonstrate low free T4, high T3, low rT3 and normal TSH levels.

There may be associated low growth hormone and IGF-I levels and dyslipidaemia.

| |
|---|
| Raised serum-binding proteins |
| Familial dysalbuminemic hyperthyroxinemia |
| Anti-iodothyronine/anti-TSH antibodies |
| Nonthyroidal illness |
| Acute psychiatric illness |
| Drugs, e.g., amiodarone, heparin |
| Intermittent T4 therapy or T4 overdose |
| Thyrotropin-secreting pituitary tumor |
| RTH |

***Table 14.2***
*Causes of raised serum T4 with nonsuppressed TSH.*

## Management of RTHs

The need for therapy is guided by the presence or absence of features of thyrotoxicosis or hypothyroidism. Most patients are clinically euthyroid and do not require treatment, unless they have a large goiter. Surgery or radioiodine should be avoided, because the goiter will often recur. Supraphysiological doses of thyroxine may be considered in this situation and also in patients who have features of hypothyroidism. In this situation, careful clinical monitoring is required, particularly of basal metabolic rate, cardiac function, and bone (biomarkers of turnover, bone density). Ideally, TSH should be normalized. Additional useful biomarkers are SHBG, ferritin, cholesterol, and angiotensin-converting enzyme. Tachycardia may be managed with cardioselective beta blockers.

Although antithyroid drugs may be considered for patients with features of thyrotoxicosis, they may be associated with a further rise in TSH levels, overriding their effects, with an increase in the size of a goiter. Thyroid hormone analogues such as TRIAC (3,3,5-triiodothyroacetic acid) may be used. TRIAC has has predominantly pituitary and hepatic thyromimetic effects—tissues that are relatively refractory to thyroid hormones in RTH, and it has a preferential affinity for TRβ *in vitro*.[86] The Food and Drug Administration (FDA) has issued several health warnings referring to the use of TRIAC for nonmedical reasons, such as weight loss and reduction in body fat in body builders. Patients who cannot be controlled with TRIAC alone may respond to combined therapy with an antithyroid drugs such as carbimazole/methimazole.[87] An alternative therapy that may be considered is with dextrothyroxine (D-T4).

Patients with TRα1 mutations have been reported to demonstrate partial responses to treatment with thyroxine, although cognitive and motor functions have been unaffected.[83–85]

# *Thyrotropin-secreting pituitary adenomas (see Chapter 1)*

Thyrotropin-secreting pituitary adenomas (TSH-omas) are rare. An observational study in Sweden has estimated an age-standardized incidence of 0.26 per million between 2005 and 2009, with a prevalence of 2.8 per million in 2010. The peak age-specific incidence was 55–69 years.[88] There is no clear gender predominance. In a Franco-Belgian study of 43 patients presenting between 1976 and 2001, the mean age of diagnosis was 44 ± 13 years.[89]

## Clinical features of TSH-omas

Patients may present with symptoms and signs of thyrotoxicosis, although this may be mild or subclinical. Some patients present with symptoms of a pituitary adenoma. The tumors are most frequently macroadenomas; they may be invasive and are often associated with chiasmal compression. Rarely, TSH-omas are malignant.[90]

Macroadenomas occurred in 16.28 (57%) of patients in the Swedish study.[88] In contrast, in the Franco-Belgian study, 34/43 (79%) had a macroadenoma that was invasive in 31(72%). Three tumors were giant macroadenomas. Two patients did not have demonstrable tumors on pituitary imaging, indicating that a normal MRI scan cannot unequivocally exclude a TSH-oma.[89] Similarly, a pituitary abnormality on an MRI scan in a patient with elevated TSH and thyroid hormone levels does not necessarily exclude a diagnosis of thyroid hormone resistance.[91] In questionable cases, inferior petrosal sinus sampling with central and peripheral measurement of TSH, $^{111}$In-pentetreotide scintigraphy, and positron emission tomography may be helpful.[89]

There is often concomitant evidence of pituitary disease. In the Swedish study, 5/27(18.5%) of patients had some degree of hypopituitarism. Cosecretion of prolactin is the most frequent additional endocrine secretory abnormality, occurring in 9/27 (33%) of patients in the Swedish study, 9/43 (21%) in the Franco-Belgian study, and 3/25 (12%) in a U.S. study.[90] Growth hormone secretion, sometimes with features of acromegaly, may also occur, ranging from 4%[90] to 14%[88] to 19%.[89]

## Investigation of TSH-omas

The differential diagnosis of a TSH-oma from RTH is summarized in Figure 14.4.

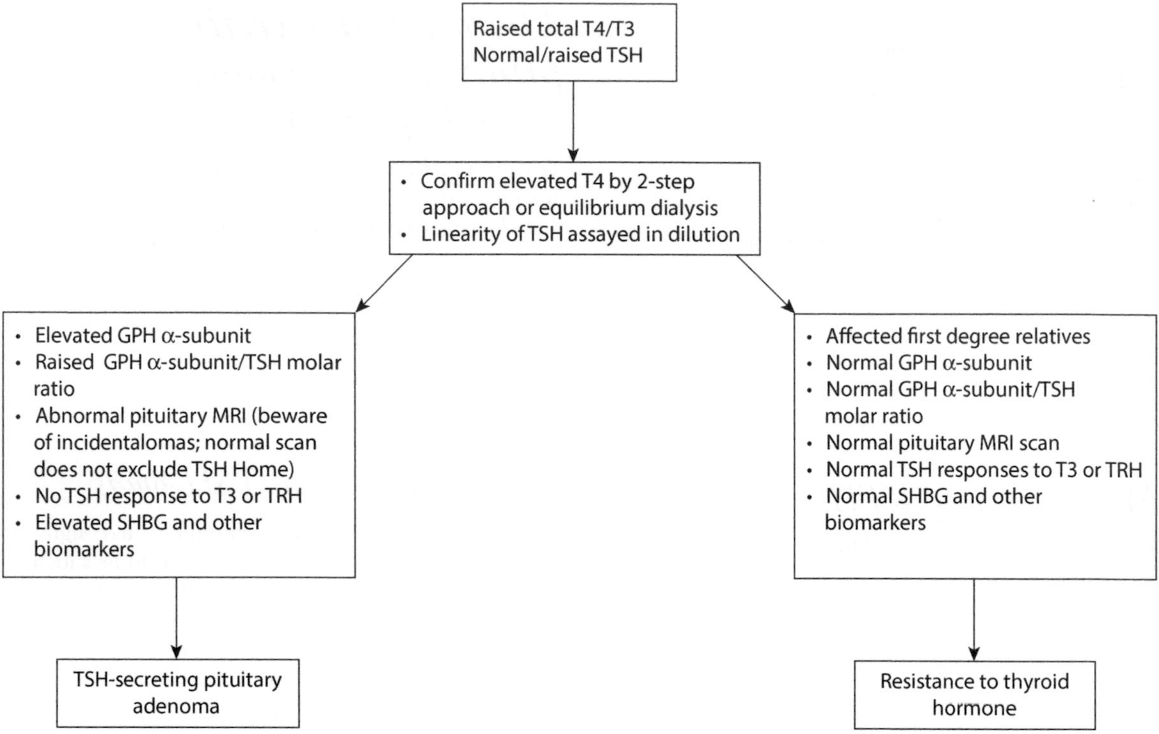


***Figure 14.4***
*Differential diagnosis of thyrotroph-secreting pituitary adenoma from resistance to thyroid hormone.*

Thyrotropin-secreting adenomas characteristically secrete glycoprotein hormone α-subunit (GPH α-subunit), with elevated basal levels in the majority of patients. Glycoprotein hormone α-subunit levels can, however, be misleading in patients with elevated gonadotropin levels, such as postmenopausal women and in patients who have had previous thyroid treatment associated with elevated TSH levels. Additional sensitivity is achieved by measuring the GPH α-subunit/TSH molar ratio TSH molar ratio which is usually >1.0. Thyrotroph-secreting adenomas usually fail to suppress TSH secretion with the pharmacological doses of T3 (80–100 μg/day for 8–10 days). They may also demonstrate a lack of TSH response to thyrotropin-releasing hormone (TRH).[90] The majority of TSH-omas express somatostatin receptors (SSTs) 2 and 5, demonstrating TSH suppression in response to acute octreotide challenge (octreotide 100 μg s.c.),[89,90] although responsivity does not necessarily predict efficacy with long-term treatment with somatostatin analogs.

## Management of TSH-omas

Surgery is the treatment of choice. Due to the size and invasiveness of many tumors, however, surgical cure may not be achieved. In addition, these tumors often have a fibrotic consistency, rendering surgery difficult. In patients selected for first-line surgery, long-term remission/cure has been achieved in 16/22 (73%),[88] 19/36 (53%),[89] and 8/25 (32%)[90] of patients. Patients with invasive residual disease should be considered for radiotherapy. Adjuvant medical therapy with octreotide or lanreotide may achieve medical control in these patients. Patients may be treated with somatostatin analogs presurgically, although there is no evidence that this improves surgical outcome and, unlike somatotroph adenomas, tumor shrinkage is seen less frequently.[89,90] Nonetheless, consideration can be given to somatostatin analogs as primary medical therapy in selected patients. Dopamine (D2) receptors are expressed by TSH-omas.[92] Occasionally, tumors may respond to DA agonist therapy.[89,90] The coexpression of SST2 and 5 and DA2 on

TSH-omas may render them amenable to treatment with somatostatin–dopamine analog chimeric molecules in the future.[92]

# References


1. Vander JB, Gaston EA, Dawber TR. The significance of nontoxic thyroid nodules. Final report of a 15-year study of the incidence of thyroid malignancy. *Ann Intern Med*. 1968;69(3):537–40.
2. Vanderpump MP, Tunbridge WM, French JM, et al. The incidence of thyroid disorders in the community: A twenty-year follow-up of the Whickham Survey. *Clin Endocrinol (Oxf)*. 1995;43(1):55–68.
3. Berghout A, Wiersinga WM, Smits NJ, et al. Determinants of thyroid volume as measured by ultrasonography in healthy adults in a non-iodine deficient area. *Clin Endocrinol (Oxf)*. 1987;26(3):273–80.
4. Derwahl M, Studer H. Nodular goiter and goiter nodules: Where iodine deficiency falls short of explaining the facts. *Exp Clin Endocrinol Diabetes*. 2001;109(5):250–60.
5. Studer H, Ramelli F. Simple goiter and its variants: Euthyroid and hyperthyroid multinodular goiters. *Endocr Rev*. 1982;3(1):40–61.
6. Aeschimann S, Kopp PA, Kimura ET, et al. Morphological and functional polymorphism within clonal thyroid nodules. *J Clin Endocrinol Metab*. 1993;77(3):846–51.
7. Bignell GR, Canzian F, Shayeghi M, et al. Familial nontoxic multinodular thyroid goiter locus maps to chromosome 14q but does not account for familial nonmedullary thyroid cancer. *Am J Hum Genet*. 1997;61(5):1123–30.
8. Gabriel EM, Bergert ER, Grant CS, et al. Germline polymorphism of codon 727 of human thyroid-stimulating hormone receptor is associated with toxic multinodular goiter. *J Clin Endocrinol Metab*. 1999;84(9):3328–35.
9. Bayer Y, Neumann S, Meyer B, et al. Genome-wide linkage analysis reveals evidence for four new susceptibility loci for familial euthyroid goiter. *J Clin Endocrinol Metab*. 2004;89(8):4044–52.
10. Parma J, Duprez L, Van Sande J, et al. Diversity and prevalence of somatic mutations in the thyrotropin receptor and Gs alpha genes as a cause of toxic thyroid adenomas. *J Clin Endocrinol Metab*. 1997;82(8):2695–701.
11. Berghout A, Wiersinga WM, Smits NJ, et al. Interrelationships between age, thyroid volume, thyroid nodularity, and thyroid function in patients with sporadic nontoxic goiter. *Am J Med*. 1990;89(5):602–8.
12. Bahn RS, Castro MR. Approach to the patient with nontoxic multinodular goiter. *J Clin Endocrinol Metab*. 2011;96(5):1202–12.
13. Berghout A, Wiersinga WM, Smits NJ, et al. The value of thyroid volume measured by ultrasonography in the diagnosis of goitre. *Clin Endocrinol (Oxf)*. 1988;28(4):409–14.
14. Harach HR, Franssila KO, Wasenius VM. Occult papillary carcinoma of the thyroid. A "normal" finding in Finland. A systematic autopsy study. *Cancer*. 1985;56(3):531–8.
15. Sampson RJ, Woolner LB, Bahn RC, et al. Occult thyroid carcinoma in Olmsted County, Minnesota: Prevalence at autopsy compared with that in Hiroshima and Nagasaki, Japan. *Cancer*. 1974;34(6):2072–6.
16. Danese D, Sciacchitano S, Farsetti A, et al. Diagnostic accuracy of conventional versus sonography-guided fine-needle aspiration biopsy of thyroid nodules. *Thyroid*. 1998;8(1):15–21.
17. Gharib H. Fine-needle aspiration biopsy of thyroid nodules: Advantages, limitations, and effect. *Mayo Clin Proc*. 1994;69(1):44–9.
18. Berghout A, Hoogendoorn D, Wiersinga WM. [A diminishing number of thyroid operations in The Netherlands in 1972–1986]. *Ned Tijdschr Geneeskd*. 1989;133(26):1313–17.
19. Fish SA, Langer JE, Mandel SJ. Sonographic imaging of thyroid nodules and cervical lymph nodes. *Endocrinol Metab Clin North Am*. 2008;37(2):401–17, ix.
20. Papini E, Guglielmi R, Bianchini A, et al. Risk of malignancy in nonpalpable thyroid nodules: Predictive value of ultrasound and color-Doppler features. *J Clin Endocrinol Metab*. 2002;87(5):1941–6.
21. Ferraz C, Eszlinger M, Paschke R. Current state and future perspective of molecular diagnosis of fine-needle aspiration biopsy of thyroid nodules. *J Clin Endocrinol Metab*. 2011;96(7):2016–26.
22. Boelaert K, Horacek J, Holder RL, et al. Serum thyrotropin concentration as a novel predictor of malignancy in thyroid nodules investigated by fine-needle aspiration. *J Clin Endocrinol Metab*. 2006;91(11):4295–301.
23. Elte JW, Bussemaker JK, Haak A. The natural history of euthyroid multinodular goitre. *Postgrad Med J*. 1990;66(773):186–90.
24. Sawin CT, Geller A, Wolf PA, et al. Low serum thyrotropin concentrations as a risk factor for atrial fibrillation in older persons. *N Engl J Med*. 1994;331(19):1249–52.
25. Cappola AR, Fried LP, Arnold AM, et al. Thyroid status, cardiovascular risk, and mortality in older adults. *JAMA*. 2006;295(9):1033–41.
26. Parle JV, Maisonneuve P, Sheppard MC, et al. Prediction of all-cause and cardiovascular mortality in

elderly people from one low serum thyrotropin result: A 10-year cohort study. *Lancet*. 2001;358(9285):861–5.
27. Biondi B, Cooper DS. The clinical significance of subclinical thyroid dysfunction. *Endocr Rev*. 2008;29(1): 76–131.
28. Smit JW, Eustatia-Rutten CF, Corssmit EP, et al. Reversible diastolic dysfunction after long-term exogenous subclinical hyperthyroidism: A randomized, placebo-controlled study. *J Clin Endocrinol Metab*. 2005;90(11):6041–7.
29. Parle JV, Franklyn JA, Cross KW, et al. Circulating lipids and minor abnormalities of thyroid function. *Clin Endocrinol (Oxf)*. 1992;37(5):411–14.
30. Faber J, Perrild H, Johansen JS. Bone Gla protein and sex hormone-binding globulin in nontoxic wgoiter: Parameters for metabolic status at the tissue level. *J Clin Endocrinol Metab*. 1990;70(1):49–55.
31. Berghout A, van de Wetering J, Klootwijk P. Cardiac and metabolic effects in patients who present with a multinodular goitre. *Neth J Med*. 2003;61(10):318–22.
32. Hegedus L, Hansen BM, Knudsen N, et al. Reduction of size of thyroid with radioactive iodine in multinodular non-toxic goitre. *BMJ*. 1988;297(6649):661–2.
33. Huysmans DA, Hermus AR, Corstens FH, et al. Large, compressive goiters treated with radioiodine. *Ann Intern Med*. 1994;121(10):757–62.
34. Fast S, Hegedus L, Grupe P, et al. Recombinant human thyrotropin-stimulated radioiodine therapy of nodular goiter allows major reduction of the radiation burden with retained efficacy. *J Clin Endocrinol Metab*. 2010;95(8):3719–25.
35. Bonnema SJ, Nielsen VE, Boel-Jorgensen H, et al. Recombinant human thyrotropin-stimulated radioiodine therapy of large nodular goiters facilitates tracheal decompression and improves inspiration. *J Clin Endocrinol Metab*. 2008;93(10):3981–4.
36. Graf H, Fast S, Pacini F, et al. Modified-release recombinant human TSH (MRrhTSH) augments the effect of (131)I therapy in benign multinodular goiter: Results from a multicenter international, randomized, placebo-controlled study. *J Clin Endocrinol Metab*. 2011;96(5):1368–76.
37. Nygaard B, Faber J, Veje A, et al. Appearance of Graves'-like disease after radioiodine therapy for toxic as well as non-toxic multinodular goitre. *Clin Endocrinol (Oxf)*. 1995;43(1):129–30.
38. Nygaard B, Hegedus L, Nielsen KG, et al. Long-term effect of radioactive iodine on thyroid function and size in patients with solitary autonomously functioning toxic thyroid nodules. *Clin Endocrinol (Oxf)*. 1999;50(2):197–202.
39. Golden SH, Robinson KA, Saldanha I, et al. Clinical review: Prevalence and incidence of endocrine and metabolic disorders in the United States: A comprehensive review. *J Clin Endocrinol Metab*. 2009;94(6):1853–78.
40. Desailloud R, Hober D. Viruses and thyroiditis: An update. *Virol J*. 2009;6:5.
41. Hung W. Mumps thyroiditis and hypothyroidism. *J Pediatr*. 1969;74(4):611–13.
42. Volpe R, Row VV, Ezrin C. Circulating viral and thyroid antibodies in subacute thyroiditis. *J Clin Endocrinol Metab*. 1967;27(9):1275–84.
43. Tomer Y, Davies TF. Infection, thyroid disease, and autoimmunity. *Endocr Rev*. 1993;14(1):107–20.
44. Ohsako N, Tamai H, Sudo T, et al. Clinical characteristics of subacute thyroiditis classified according to human leukocyte antigen typing. *J Clin Endocrinol Metab*. 1995;80(12):3653–6.
45. Erdem N, Erdogan M, Ozbek M, et al. Demographic and clinical features of patients with subacute thyroiditis: Results of 169 patients from a single university center in Turkey. *J Endocrinol Invest*. 2007;30(7):546–50.
46. Fatourechi V, Aniszewski JP, Fatourechi GZ, et al. Clinical features and outcome of subacute thyroiditis in an incidence cohort: Olmsted County, Minnesota, study. *J Clin Endocrinol Metab*. 2003;88(5):2100–5.
47. Nikolai TF, Coombs GJ, McKenzie AK. Lymphocytic thyroiditis with spontaneously resolving hyperthyroidism and subacute thyroiditis. Long-term follow-up. *Arch Intern Med*. 1981;141(11):1455–8.
48. Iitaka M, Momotani N, Ishii J, et al. Incidence of subacute thyroiditis recurrences after a prolonged latency: 24-year survey. *J Clin Endocrinol Metab*. 1996;81(2):466–9.
49. Lazarus JH. *Sporadic and Postpartum Thyroiditis. Werner & Ingbar's The thyroid A Fundamental and Clinical Text*. 9th edn. Philadelphia: Lippincott Williams & Wilkins; 2005. pp. 524–35.
50. Muller AF, Drexhage HA, Berghout A. Postpartum thyroiditis and autoimmune thyroiditis in women of childbearing age: Recent insights and consequences for antenatal and postnatal care. *Endocr Rev*. 2001;22(5):605–30.
51. Pearce EN, Farwell AP, Braverman LE. Thyroiditis. *N Engl J Med*. 2003;348(26):2646–55.
52. Gallas PR, Stolk RP, Bakker K, et al. Thyroid dysfunction during pregnancy and in the first postpartum year in women with diabetes mellitus type 1. *Eur J Endocrinol*. 2002;147(4):443–51.
53. Momotani N, Noh J, Ishikawa N, et al. Relationship between silent thyroiditis and recurrent Graves' disease in the postpartum period. *J Clin Endocrinol Metab*. 1994;79(1):285–9.
54. McDougall IR. In vivo radionuclide tests and imaging. In: Braverman LE, Utiger RD, eds. *Werner & Ingbar's The thyroid A Fundamental and Clinical Text*. 9th ed. Philadelphia: Lippincott Williams & Wilkins; 2005. pp. 309–28.
55. de Lange WE, Freling NJ, Molenaar WM, et al. Invasive fibrous thyroiditis (Riedel's struma): A manifestation

of multifocal fibrosclerosis? A case report with review of the literature. *Q J Med*. 1989;72(268):709–17.

56. Baloch ZW, LiVolsi VA. Pathology. In: Braverman LE, Utiger RD eds. *Werner & Ingbar's The thyroid A Fundamental and Clinical Text*. 9th ed. Philadelphia: Lippincott Williams & Wilkins; 2005. pp. 427.
57. Vaidya B, Harris PE, Barrett P, et al. Corticosteroid therapy in Riedel's thyroiditis. *Postgrad Med J*. 1997;73(866):817–19.
58. Jung YJ, Schaub CR, Rhodes R, et al. A case of Riedel's thyroiditis treated with tamoxifen: Another successful outcome. *Endocr Pract*. 2004;10(6):483–6.
59. Paes JE, Burman KD, Cohen J, et al. Acute bacterial suppurative thyroiditis: A clinical review and expert opinion. *Thyroid*. 2010;20(3):247–55.
60. Berger SA, Zonszein J, Villamena P, et al. Infectious diseases of the thyroid gland. *Rev Infect Dis*. 1983;5(1):108–22.
61. Vassart G, Dumont JE. The thyrotropin receptor and the regulation of thyrocyte function and growth. *Endocrine Rev*. 1992;13:596–611.
62. Van Sande J, Raspe E, Perret J, et al. Thyrotropin activates both the cyclic AMP and PIP2 cascades in CHO cells expressing the human cDNA of TSH receptor. *Mol Cell Endocrinol*. 1990;74:R1–6.
63. Hébrant A, van Staveren WCG, Maenhaut C, et al. Genetic hyperthyroidism: Hyperthyroidism due to activating TSHR mutations. *Eur J Endocrinol*. 2011;164:1–9.
64, Parma J, Duprez L, van Sande J, et al. Somatic mutations of the thyrotropin receptor gene cause hyperfunctioning thyroid adenomas. *Nature*. 1993;365:649–51.
65. Krohn K, Paschke R. Somatic mutations in thyroid nodular disease. *Mol Genet Metab*. 2002;75:202–8.
66. Palos-Paz F, Perez-Guerra O, Cameselle-Teijeiro J, et al. Prevalence of mutations in TSHR, GNAS, PRKAR1A and RAS genes in a large series of toxic thyroid adenomas from Galacia, an iodine-deficient area in Northern Spain. *Eur J Endocrinol*. 2008;159:623–31.
67. Nishihara E, Amino N, Maekawa K, et al. Prevalence of TSH receptor and Gsα mutations in 45 autonomously functioning thyroid nodules in Japan. *Endocr J*. 2009;56:791–8.
68. Esapa CT, Duprez L, Ludgate M, et al. A novel thyrotropin receptor mutation in an infant with severe thyrotoxicosis. *Thyroid*. 1999;9:1005–10.
69. Duprez L, Parma J, Van Sande J, et al. Germline mutations in the thyrotropin receptor gene cause nonautoimmune autosomal dominant hyperthyroidism. *Nat Genet*. 1994;7:396–401.
70. Stein SA, Oates EL, Hall CR, et al. Identification of a point mutation in the thyrotropin receptor of the hyt/hyt hypothyroid mouse. *Mol Endocrinol*. 1994;8:129–38.
71. Sunthornthepvarakui T, Gottschalk ME, Hayashi Y, et al. Brief report: Resistance to thyrotropin caused by mutations in the thyrotropin-receptor gene. *N Engl J Med*. 1995;332:155–60.
72. Tenenbaum-Rakover Y, Grasberger H, Mamanasiri S, et al. Loss-of-function mutations in the thyrotropin receptor gene as a major determinant of hyperthyrotropinemia in a consanguineous community. *J Clin Endocrinol Metab*. 2009;94:1706–12.
73. Mazar MA. Thyroid hormone receptors: Multiple forms, multiple possibilities. *Endocr Rev*. 1993;14:184–93.
74. Refetoff S, Weiss RE, Usala SJ. The syndromes of resistance to thyroid hormone. *Endocr Rev*. 1993;14:348–99.
75. Parrilla R, Mixson AJ, McPherson JA, et al. Characterization of seven novel mutations of the c-erbAb gene in unrelated kindreds with generalized thyroid hormone resistance: Evidence for two 'hot spot' regions of the ligand binding domain. *J Clin Invest*. 1991;88:2123–30.
76. Weiss RE, Weinberg M, Refetoff S. Identical mutations in unrelated families with generalized resistance to thyroid hormone occur in cytosine-guanine-rich areas of the thyroid hormone receptor beta gene. Analysis of 15 families. *J Clin Invest*. 1993;91:2408–15.
77. Adams M, Matthews C, Collingwood TN, et al. Genetic analysis of 29 kindreds with generalized and pituitary resistance to thyroid hormone. Identification of thirteen novel mutations in the thyroid hormone receptor beta gene. *J Clin Invest*. 1994;94:506–15.
78. Sakurai A, Miyamoto T, Refetoff S, et al. Dominant negative transcriptional regulation by a mutant thyroid hormone receptor-β in a family with generalized resistance to thyroid hormone. *Mol Endocrinol*. 1990;4:1988–94.
79. Chatterjee VKK, Nagaya T, Madison LD, et al. Thyroid hormone resistance syndrome. Inhibition of normal receptor function by mutant thyroid hormone receptors. *J Clin Invest*. 1991;87:1977–84.
80. Beck-Peccoz P, Chatterjee VK. The variable clinical phenotype in thyroid hormone resistance syndrome. *Thyroid*. 1994;4:225–32.
81. Mitchell CS, Savage DB, Dufour S, et al. Resistance to thyroid hormone is associated with raised energy expenditure, muscle mitochondrial uncoupling and hyperphagia. *J Clin Invest*. 2010;120:1345–54.
82. Kahaly GJ, Matthews CH, Mohr-Kahaly S, et al. Cardiac involvement in thyroid hormone resistance. *J Clin Endocrinol Metab*. 2002;87:204–12.
83. Bochukova E, Schoenmakers N, Agostini M et al. A mutation in the thyroid hormone receptor alpha gene. *N Engl J Med*. 2012;366:243–49.
84. van Mullem A, van Heerebeek R, Chrysis D et al. Clinical phenotype and mutant TRalpha1. *N Engl J Med*. 2012;366:1451–53.
85. van Mullem A, Chrysis D, Eythimiadou A et al. Clinical phenotype of a new thyroid hormone resistance caused by a mutation of the TRα1 receptor: Consequences of LT4 treatment. *J Clin Endocrinol Metab*. 2013;98:3029–38.

86. Messier N, Laflamme L, Hamann G, et al. In vitro effect of TRIAC on resistance to thyroid hormone receptor mutants; potential basis for therapy. *Mol Cell Endocrinol*. 2001;174:59–69.
87. Ali K, Culley V, Morovar R, et al. TRIAC and carbimazole combination therapy in pituitary thyroid hormone resistance. *Endocr Abstr*. 2008;17:P32.
88. Önnestam L, Berinder K, Burman P, et al. National incidence of TSH-secreting pituitary adenomas in Sweden. *J Clin Endocrinol Metab*. 2013;98:626–35.
89. Socin HV, Chanson P, Delemer B, et al. The changing spectrum of TSH-secreting pituitary adenomas: Diagnosis and management in 43 patients. *Eur J Endocrinol*. 2003;148:433–42.
90. Brucker-Davis F, Oldfield EH, Skarulis MC, et al. Thyrotropin-secreting pituitary tumors: Diagnostic criteria, thyroid hormone sensitivity and treatment outcome in 25 patients followed at the National Institutes of Health. *J Clin Endocrinol Metab*. 1999;84:476–86.
91. Freda PU, Backers AM, Katznelson L, et al. Pituitary incidentaloma: An Endocrine Society clinical practice guideline. *J Clin Endocrinol Metab*. 2011;94:894–904.
92. Gatto F, Barbieri F, Gatti M, et al. Balance between somatostatin and D2 receptor expression drives TSH-secreting adenoma response to somatostatin analogues and dopastatins. *Clin Endocrinol*. 2012;76:407–14.

# 15

# Differentiated and undifferentiated thyroid cancer

*Michael J. Stechman, David Scott-Coombes*

## *Introduction*

Thyroid cancer is the commonest endocrine malignancy, but itself is rare, accounting for <1% of all cancers. Thyroid cancer includes a wide spectrum of diseases of which there are four distinct subtypes. Differentiated thyroid cancer (DTC) accounts for most malignancies (85%) and arises from the follicular cell. Anaplastic thyroid cancer (ATC) (1%–3%) is undifferentiated and may arise from preexisting differentiated tumor or *de novo.* Medullary thyroid cancer (10%) is a tumor of the parafollicular C cells. It may occur sporadically, as an isolated familial condition or in association with multiple endocrine neoplasia type 2 (MEN2) (see Chapters 7, 9). Thyroid lymphoma (3%) is usually of the non-Hodgkin's B-cell type arising on a background of Hashimoto's thyroiditis and is best managed by hemato-oncologists.

## *Differentiated thyroid cancer*

### *Epidemiology*

The incidence of DTC has a geographical variation and is more common in women (2.4/100,000 in the United Kingdom; 5.2/100,000 in the United States) compared with men (0.9/100,000 in the United Kingdom; 2.1/100,000 in the United States).[1] Between 1973 and 2002, there has been a 2.4-fold increase in its incidence in the United States, but the mortality has not altered, suggesting that this phenomenon may simply be increased detection of smaller tumors.[2] The principle subtypes of DTC are papillary and follicular. Their prevalence is partly dependent upon iodine intake in a particular geographic area. In iodine-sufficient areas, papillary carcinomas account for about 80% of tumors, whereas in areas of iodine deficiency, as the prevalence of follicular carcinoma rises, the prevalence of papillary carcinoma falls to 35%–55%.[3]

### *Pathology*

#### *Papillary thyroid carcinoma*

Papillary thyroid carcinoma (PTC) tumors present in the third and fourth decades, predominantly in women. The tumor is unencapsulated with both papillary and follicular structures. The papillae have a fibrovascular core covered by a single layer of tumor cells (Figure 15.1). The nuclei are typically pale-staining "glass-ground" in appearance with longitudinal grooves and cytoplasmic inclusion vacuoles, producing the "Orphan Annie" appearance. Psammoma bodies are calcified degenerative changes that occur in the papillae and are characteristic of papillary carcinomas, occurring in 40%–50% of tumors. Multifocality is present in 20%–80% of cases, with 30% being bilateral.[4] Several subtypes or variants of papillary carcinoma have been identified[4] (Table 15.1). The main variant that seems to be clinically significant is the tall cell variant (height of cell greater than twice its width). This variant is more likely to present at an older age, and these tumors have a higher recurrence rate, mortality, and rate of progression to more poorly differentiated subtypes such as ATC.[5] Papillary carcinomas frequently spread to local lymph nodes,[6] more commonly in children than adults, being seen in 50%–89% of cases.[4] Microscopic nodal disease has minimal impact on overall survival, although local recurrence rates may be higher. In contrast, bulky nodal disease in high-risk patients affects survival and

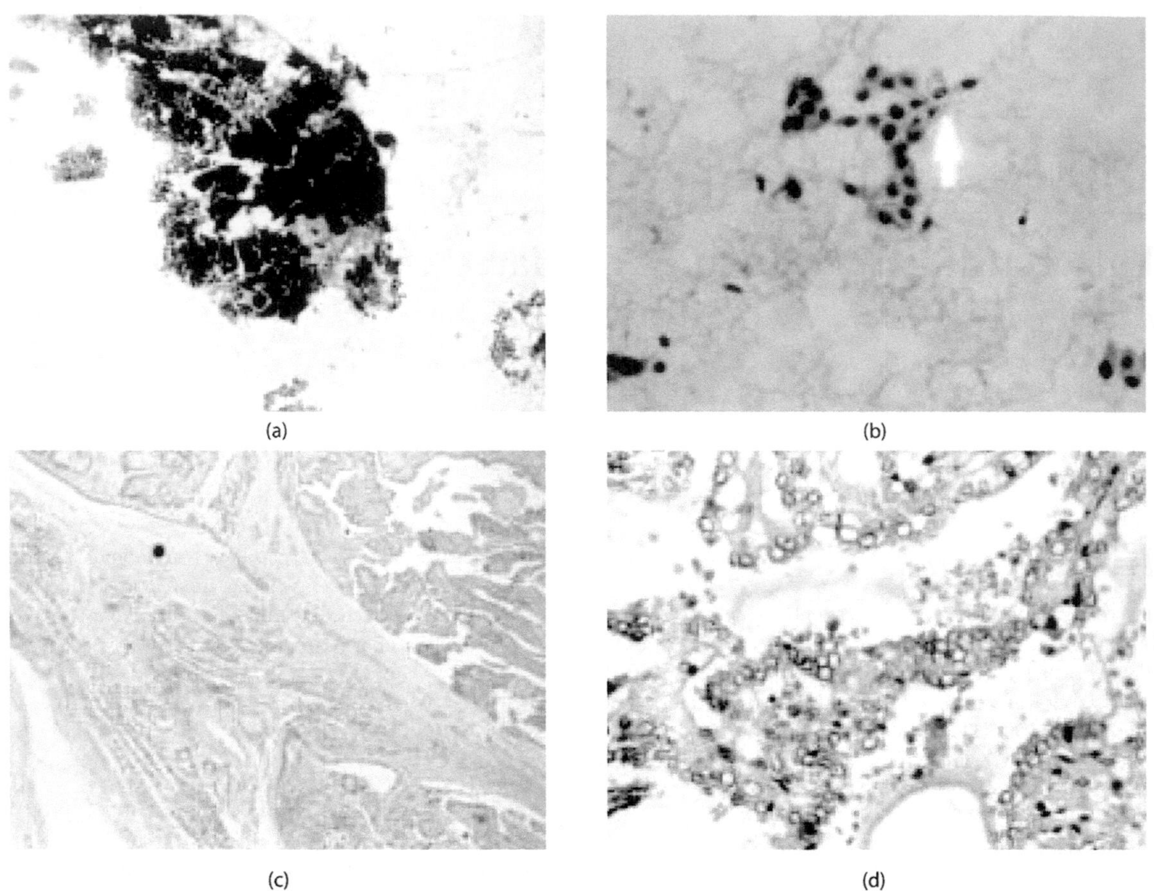


**Figure 15.1**
*Histopathology of PTC. (a) Low-power (×40) FNA demonstrating papillary structures. (b) High-power (×400) FNA demonstrating intranuclear cytoplasmic inclusion (arrow). (c) Low-power (×40) demonstrating papillary tumor surrounded by normal, compressed thyroid tissue. (d) High-power (×400) demonstrating ground glass nuclei.*

| *Histological type* | *Relative proportion (%)* | *Prognosis compared with classical type* |
|---|---|---|
| Classical | 50 | |
| Follicular variant | 25–30 | Similar |
| Encapsulated | 10 | Better |
| Tall cell | 10 | Less favorable |
| Diffuse sclerosing | 4 | Less favorable |
| Columnar cell | <1 | Poor |

***Table 15.1***
*Subtypes of papillary carcinoma.*

loco regional recurrence rates.[7] Distant metastatic spread is uncommon, occurring in <10% of patients.

## *Follicular neoplasm*

Unlike PTC, follicular tumors can either be benign (adenoma) or malignant (carcinoma). Follicular thyroid carcinomas (FTCs) present at a later age, peaking in the fourth and fifth decades. They are encapsulated tumors with follicular differentiation but without the characteristic nuclear changes of PTC. Capsular invasion is the key feature that distinguishes follicular carcinomas from follicular adenomas.[8] It is for this reason that follicular carcinomas *cannot* be differentiated from benign follicular adenomas using cytology. Two main types are recognized: minimally invasive, infiltrating the tumor capsule, and widely invasive, with involvement of surrounding blood vessels (Figure 15.2). Follicular tumors,

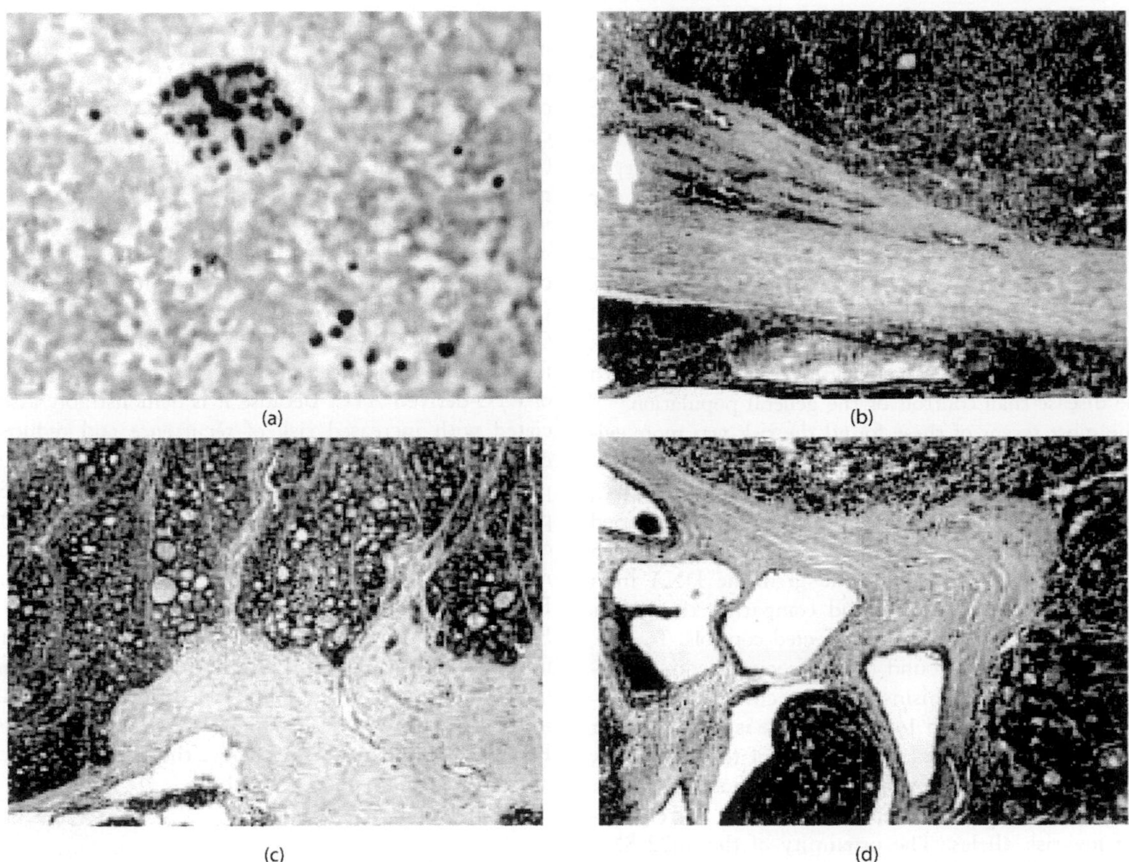


***Figure 15.2***
*Histopathology of FTC. (a) FNA (×200) demonstrating microfollicles, follicular neoplasm. (b) Follicular carcinoma demonstrating minimal invasion of the tumor capsule (arrow) (×100). (c) Follicular carcinoma demonstrating capsular invasion (×100). (d) Follicular carcinoma demonstrating vascular invasion (×100).*

unlike PTCs, characteristically metastasize by hematogenous spread, most commonly to lung and bone. Hürthle cell carcinomas (oncocytic variant) are uncommon and are more often multifocal, frequently involving regional nodes. However, only 10% of these tumors take up radioiodine, and they have a greater tendency for tumor recurrence and increased mortality.[9] Insular carcinoma is a morphologically distinct tumor (neither PTC nor FTC) derived from the follicular cell that has an aggressive biological course. These tumors affect elderly patients and have a poor prognosis.

# Etiology and molecular pathogenesis

The exact etiology of DTC remains largely unknown; however, the two most significant risk factors associated with its development are exposure to ionizing radiation and a positive family history for the disease.

### Exposure to radiation

Pooled analysis of atomic bomb survivors, children exposed to therapeutic external radiotherapy, and children exposed to the Chernobyl nuclear accident[10,11] have demonstrated that childhood exposure to radiation is associated with the development of both benign and malignant thyroid tumors. The risk is inversely proportional to age and the dose–response curve is linear, reaching its maximum at doses of 20–30 Gy, but tapering off at doses >30 Gy.[12] Nodules found in radiation-exposed individuals should be investigated in the same manner as nonexposed individuals, but if found to be suspicious or malignant, surgical treatment should be more aggressive because more than half of these tumors are multicentric.[13] Once exposed, the risk persists for up to 40 years and may lead to other head-and-neck tumors, including those of the salivary[14] and parathyroid glands.[15]

### Family history and genetic epidemiology

In common with some other solid tumors, patients with DTC are more likely than the general population to have a relative affected by the disease. A study of 9.6 million individuals on the Swedish Family-Cancer database estimated the genetic component, or heritability of thyroid cancer, to be 53%.[16] This was higher than any other tumor studied but may be skewed by the inclusion of medullary thyroid cancer. Other studies comparing hospital and population-based samples of patients with DTC with unaffected controls have determined that those with DTC are between 4.1 and 8.6 times more likely to have a first-degree relative (FDR) with the disease than controls or the general population.[17–19] The most recent of these found the risk was more evident in those with a sibling FDR.[19] To determine the underlying genetic cause for apparently sporadic DTC, genome-wide association studies have been performed in U.S., European, and U.K. populations.[20–24] Such studies involve genotyping the germline DNA from patients affected by DTC and comparing the results with those obtained from unaffected controls. To date, DTC risk has been found to be associated with single-nucleotide polymorphisms (SNPs) at chromosomal locations 8q24, 9q22, and 14q13; evidence is conflicting for a further SNP at 5q24. Inheritance of these high-risk alleles appears to confer up to a 10-fold increase in risk of developing DTC compared with the corresponding low-risk alleles. The proximity of the 9q22 SNP to the FOXE1 (TTF2) gene and the 14q13 SNP to the NKX2-1 (TTF1) gene suggests that they may have a role in the etiology of sporadic DTC.

### Familial DTC

Despite evidence supporting a genetic or heritable cause for DTC, <5% of cancers have a clear, genetic origin. They may occur as Mendelian tumor syndromes (phosphatase and tensin [PTEN]-hamartoma tumor syndrome/Cowden syndrome, familial adenomatous polyposis/Gardner syndrome, Carney complex type 1, Werner syndrome, and Pendred syndrome) or as familial syndromes in which PTC is the predominant feature, such as pure familial PTC, familial PTC associated with papillary renal cell carcinoma, and familial PTC with multinodular goiter. Details on these rare disorders are provided in Table 15.2.

### Molecular pathogenesis of DTC

Somatic alterations in genes affecting several signal transduction pathways have been demonstrated in thyroid cancer and can be broadly classified into point mutations and chromosomal rearrangements.[25] It is proposed that point mutations arise due to chemical mutagenesis, whereas chromosomal rearrangements occur with exposure to ionizing radiation.[25] Mutations of the B-type Raf kinase (BRAF) and RAS oncogenes cause activation of the mitogen-activated protein kinase (MAPK) and the phosphatidylinositol 3-kinase/v-Akt murine thymoma viral oncogene (PI3K/AKT1) signaling pathways, and lead to downstream effects on the nuclear expression of genes involved in cell proliferation, cell differentiation, cell survival, and tumorigenesis. In particular, the T1799A missense mutation in BRAF (leading to V600E amino acid change) appears specific for PTC and is observed in up to 69% of PTC and 24% of PTC-derived ATC. Because it is demonstrably associated with increased risk of recurrence and reduced disease-specific survival,[26] it may become a useful prognostic marker in PTC. The RET/PTC and PAX8/peroxisome proliferator-activated receptor (PPAR)γ chromosomal arrangements are seen in PTC and FTC, respectively. The recombinant protein product of the RET/PTC fusion gene leads to a constitutively active RET tyrosine kinase that activates the MAPK pathway upstream of BRAF.[27] PAX8 is a thyroid transcription factor and PPARγ promotes cell differentiation and inhibits cell growth. The likely effect of the PAX8/PPARγ rearrangement is to remove the inhibitory effect of PPARγ gene upon cell growth.[28]

## Clinical presentation

Most cancers present with a goiter. Thyroid nodules occur in about 5%–10% of adults of which the overwhelming majority (95%) are benign. Features in the history that alert the physician to a cancer and warrant an urgent referral are listed in Table 15.3. Every patient should undergo a thorough clinical examination and particular attention should be paid to the size and consistency of the goiter as well as presence–absence of cervical lymphadenopathy. Increasingly thyroid nodules are incidentally identified during radiological imaging for indications other than the thyroid (thyroid incidentalomas), for example, carotid artery duplex (9%), cross-sectional scans (15%), and positron emission tomography (PET) scans (3%).[29]

## Investigation of thyroid nodule and staging

Thyroid function tests should be requested in all patients. Thyroid scintiscan and serology should be considered when thyroid-stimulating hormone (TSH) is suppressed. Any new thyroid nodule should undergo fine needle

| Syndrome | Features | Inheritance | Chromosome | Gene |
|---|---|---|---|---|
| Cowden syndrome | Hamartomas, breast cancer, FTC, and rarely PTC | A-D | 10q23.31 | PTEN |
| Familial adenomatous polyposis | Gastrointestinal polyps, osteomas, retinal hypertrophy, desmoid tumors, cribriform PTC | A-D | 5q22.2 | APC |
| Carney complex | Adrenal, pituitary, and gonadal cancers, PTC, FTC | A-D | 17q23-24 | PRKAR1a |
| Werner syndrome | Premature aging, sarcomas, osteosarcomas, FTC/PTC | A-R | 8p11-12 | WRN |
| Pendred syndrome | Deafness, diffuse goiter, PTC | A-R | 7q22.3 | SLC26A4 |
| Familial PTC | PTC | — | 2q21 | ? |
| Familial PTC and papillary renal neoplasia | PTC and renal tumors | — | 1q21 | ? |
| Familial PTC and multinodular goiter | PTC and goiter | — | 14q32 | ? |

A-D, autosomal dominant; A-R, autosomal recessive; ?, unknown.

***Table 15.2***
*Familial syndromes associated with DTC.*

| |
|---|
| Extremes of age (<20 years, >70 years) |
| Family history of thyroid cancer |
| History of exposure to radiation |
| Hoarseness |
| Rapid enlargement of goiter (over 4–6 weeks) |
| Presence of cervical lymphadenopathy |

***Table 15.3***
*"Red flag" features and symptoms for thyroid cancer.*

aspiration biopsy (FNAB) that can be undertaken by the clinician in the outpatient clinic or under ultrasound control. The FNAB report should be reported according to British Thyroid Association (BTA)/American Thyroid Association (ATA) guidelines[30] (Table 15.4). Cases of thyroid incidentalomas should undergo an ultrasound scan, and those with suspicious sonographic features (calcification, irregularity, solid lesion, hypervascularity) should undergo ultrasound-guided FNAB.[31] When a diagnosis of PTC is made, patients should undergo an ultrasound staging of the neck (Figure 15.3). Computed tomography (CT) scanning is avoided because it is less sensitive than ultrasound for lymph node staging, and administration

| Classification | Definition |
|---|---|
| Thy 1a | Insufficient cellular material |
| Thy 1c | Consistent with benign cyst contents |
| Thy 2 | Benign |
| Thy 3a | Some features of PTC |
| Thy 3f | Suspicious for follicular neoplasm |
| Thy 4 | Suspicious for PTC |
| Thy 5 | Malignant |

**Table 15.4**
*Classification of thyroid cytology results.*

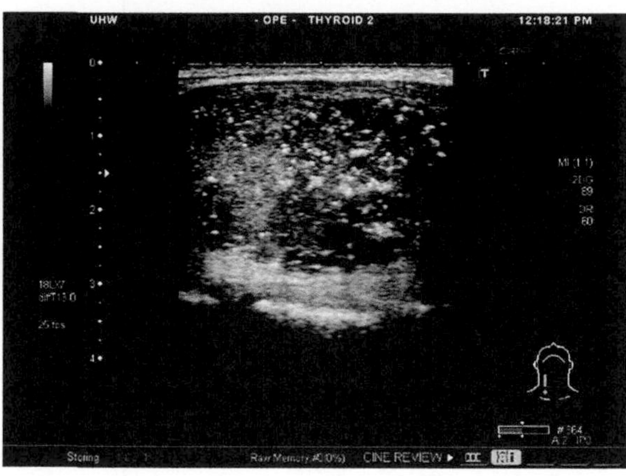


**Figure 15.3**
*Ultrasound of a malignant lateral cervical node showing the characteristic punctuate microcalcification of psammoma bodies within a metastatic node.*

of intravenous contrast can saturate iodine-avid tissue and significantly delay radioiodine treatment. However, cross-sectional imaging (ideally without contrast) is indicated when there is suspicion of local invasion or significant retrosternal extension. A suggested algorithm is presented in Figure 15.4.

# Surgery for DTC

Thyroidectomy with or without lymphadenectomy is the mainstay of treatment for DTC and should aim to gain local control of disease, preserve function, provide accurate staging, and prevent loco regional recurrence. The minimum operation for low-risk tumors should be lobectomy and isthmusectomy, whereas higher risk tumors will require total thyroidectomy. Apart from risk to the recurrent laryngeal nerve that is common to both operations, total thyroidectomy requires long-term levothyroxine replacement and may result in hypoparathyroidism. The risk of recurrent laryngeal nerve injury and hypoparathyroidism should also be taken into consideration when balancing the risk of lymph node dissection with the risk of local recurrence. Discussion and planning of treatment for patients with thyroid cancer is ideally managed in a multidisciplinary setting with appropriate audit of complications and outcomes.

# Surgery for PTC

The diagnosis of PTC is usually possible preoperatively with FNAB, allowing staging and planned treatment. Tumor size, age, and metastases at presentation will dictate the extent of thyroidectomy required. Thus, multivariate analysis has demonstrated that clinically significant tumors (>1 cm in diameter) should be treated with total thyroidectomy.[32] Those over the age of 45 years are at greater risk of recurrence, with a higher mortality and should be treated similarly.[33] Regardless of tumor size, those with metastases require total thyroidectomy for local control and also to facilitate radioactive iodine therapy. Other factors that increase the risk of contralateral disease and that should prompt total thyroidectomy in patients with tumors close to 1 cm in size are prior exposure to head-and-neck irradiation, FDR family history of DTC, and evidence of multifocality (e.g., two or more foci). Micropapillary thyroid cancer (<1 cm) with no other risk factors has a very low risk in terms of mortality and local recurrence and can be managed by thyroid lobectomy alone. Finally, despite the overwhelmingly good prognosis of most patients with PTC, a minority will present with locally advanced disease. Tumor invasion into the trachea or larynx should be treated by excision of all macroscopic tumor, including, if necessary, tracheal resection or vertical hemilaryngectomy and reconstructive surgery,[7] provided the patient has a good performance status and is free from metastatic disease. Fortunately, the necessity for such procedures is rare and macroscopic clearance is usually feasible by tracheal shave procedure. Adjuvant therapy with external beam radiotherapy as well as radioactive iodine should be considered in these patients to reduce the risk of local recurrence.

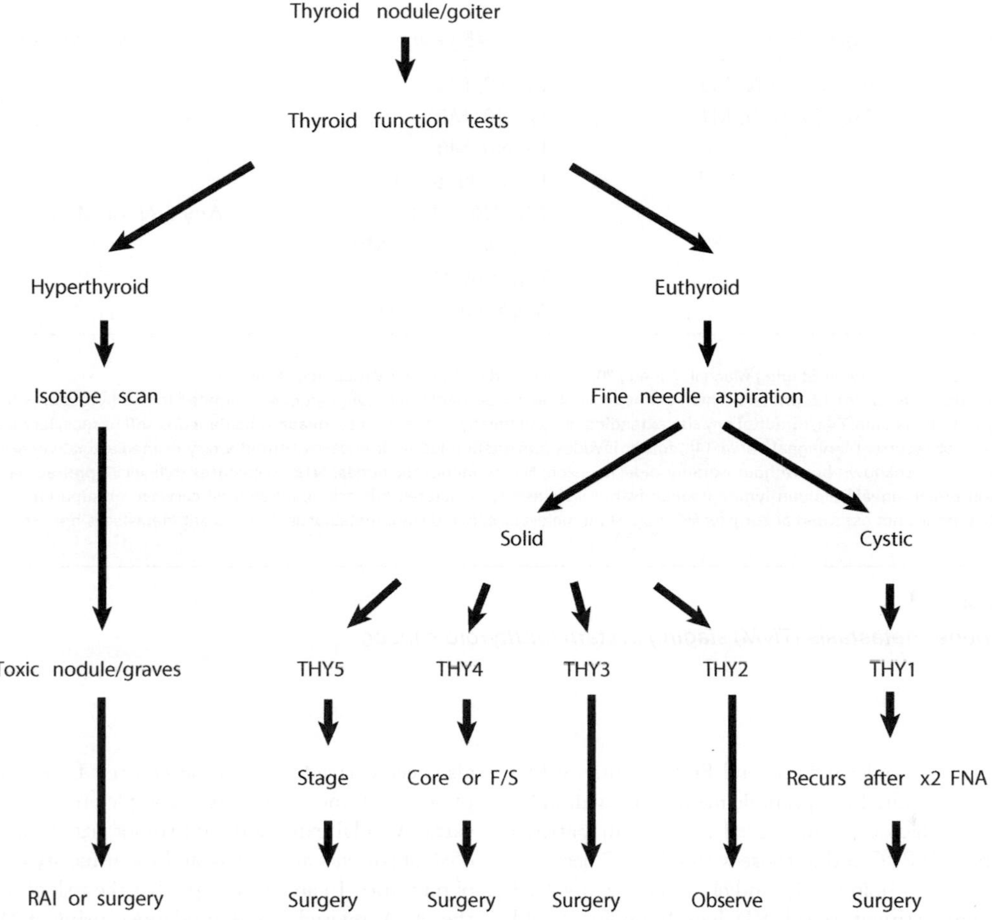


***Figure 15.4***
*Algorithm for the management of a thyroid nodule. RAI, radioactive iodine; Core, core biopsy; F/S, intraoperative frozen section; FNA, fine needle aspiration cytology.*

# *Surgery for FTC*

Approximately 15%–20% of lesions with Thy3f cytology will be invasive FTC, but definitive diagnosis requires paraffin-block histology, usually via diagnostic lobectomy. The necessity for further treatment (completion thyroidectomy and radioactive iodine) depends upon tumor size, whether the disease is minimally or widely invasive, the presence of vascular invasion, and the histological subtype. Thus, patients >45 years, tumors >4 cm, widely invasive FTC, Hürthle cell variant histology, or vascular invasion are all best treated by completion thyroidectomy and radioactive iodine (RAI) after initial lobectomy. Those with T1 tumors (<2 cm) (Table 15.5) that are minimally invasive, with no other adverse features (age >45 years, vascular invasion, aggressive histological features) can be managed with thyroid lobectomy alone. Some minimally invasive T2 tumors (2–4 cm) may also be managed with lobectomy alone, provided they are in young patients with no contralateral thyroid nodules and without any of the abovementioned adverse features.

# *Lymph node dissection*

Micro- or macroscopic regional lymph node metastases are present in up to 60% of patients with PTC but at a lower frequency in other histological subtypes.[7] Although nodal metastasis is reported to have minimal impact upon overall survival, it is likely that it does increase local recurrence rates. Furthermore,

| Stage | Age <45 years | Age >45 years | Anaplastic (any age) |
|---|---|---|---|
| I | Any T, any N, M0 | T1, N0, M0 | |
| II | Any T, any N, M1 | T2, N0, M0 | |
| III | | T3, N0, M0 | |
| | | T1/2/3, N1a, M0 | |
| IVA | | T4a, N0/1, M0 | Any T, N, or M |
| | | T1/2/3/4a, N1b, M0 | |
| IVB | | T4b, Any N, M0 | |
| IVC | | Any T, any N, M1 | |

*Source:* From AJCC Cancer Staging Manual, 7th ed., 2010, published by Springer-Verlag, Inc., New York.
T1, tumor, diameter ≤2 cm; T2, primary tumor, diameter >2–4 cm; T3, primary tumor, diameter >4 cm limited to the thyroid or with minimal extrathyroidal extension; T4a, tumor of any size extending beyond the thyroid capsule to invade subcutaneous soft tissues, larynx, trachea, esophagus, or recurrent laryngeal nerve; T4b, tumor invades prevertebral fascia or encases carotid artery or mediastinal vessels; TX, primary tumor size unknown but without extrathyroidal invasion; N0, no metastatic nodes; N1a, metastases to level VI (pretracheal, paratracheal, and prelaryngeal/Delphian lymph nodes); N1b, metastasis to unilateral, bilateral, contralateral cervical, or superior mediastinal nodes; NX, nodes not assessed at surgery; M0, no distant metastases; M1, distant metastases; MX, distant metastases not assessed.

***Table 15.5***
*Tumor-node-metastasis (TNM) staging system for thyroid cancer.*

a Surveillance, Epidemiology, and End Results (SEER) database report cited lymph node metastasis as an independent risk factor for decreased survival in patients >45 years with PTC and in those with FTC.[34] Therefore, patients with radiologically and/or clinically involved central compartment (level VI) lymph nodes should undergo therapeutic central compartment neck dissection at time of thyroidectomy. If lateral nodal involvement is present (levels II–V), a selective neck dissection of involved levels should also be performed; "berry picking" should be avoided. The evidence for lymph node dissection in those with radiological and clinically negative lymph nodes (prophylactic dissection) is less clear but is currently reserved for those patients with high-risk features such as age >45 years and locally advanced (T3 and T4) (Table 15.5) primary tumors.[35]

## *Risk stratification in the follow up of DTC*

To provide accurate information on tumor extent, patients should be staged according to the American Joint Committee on Cancer (AJCC) Tumor-node-metastasis (TNM) staging system (Table 15.5). Several scoring systems, for example, MACIS, AMES, and AGES, have also been derived and score several risk factors, including presence of metastasis, age, completeness of resection, extrathyroidal extension, and tumor size, to identify the 85% of patients at low risk and the minority at high risk of mortality. In an effort to predict the risk of recurrence, the ATA revised 2009 guidelines using a three-level stratification system (low, intermediate, and high risk)[35] (Table 15.6).

### *Low-risk patients*

This subgroup has either minimal or no benefit from RAI therapy in terms of reduced risk of recurrence or death, but remnant ablation may aid follow-up (see below); so, RAI may be used in selected cases, according to MDT discussion.

### *Intermediate- and high-risk patients*

Intermediate- and high-risk subgroups have either demonstrable benefit in terms of reduced risk of death, or reduced risk of recurrence, and RAI should be recommended.

Stratifying patients in the light of their response to therapy improves prognostic assessment and allows better planning for follow-up.[36] The ATA system has

| Low risk (all the following are present) | Intermediate risk (any of the following is present) | High risk (any of the following is present) |
|---|---|---|
| No local or distant metastasis | Microscopic invasion into the perithyroidal soft tissues | Macroscopic tumor invasion |
| All macroscopic tumors resected | Cervical lymph node metastases or $^{131}$I uptake outside the thyroid bed on the posttreatment scan, if done after remnant ablation | Incomplete tumor resection with gross residual disease |
| Tumor does not have aggressive histology (tall cell, insular, columnar cell, Hürthle cell carcinoma, FTC) | Tumor with aggressive histology or vascular invasion (tall cell, insular, columnar cell, Hürthle cell carcinoma, FTC) | Distant metastases |
| No vascular invasion | | |
| No $^{131}$I uptake outside the thyroid on posttreatment scan, if done | | |

*Source:* From ATA, *Thyroid Cancer Guidelines*, 2009; Cooper DS et al., *Thyroid*, 19, 1167–214, 2009. With permission.

***Table 15.6***
*Risk stratification for recurrent disease.*

since been validated in a large retrospective study[37] and refined by the addition of measurements of response to therapy such as postoperative imaging, TSH-suppressed thyroglobulin (Tg), and stimulated Tg.

# RAI therapy (see Chapter 7)

Most DTC cells retain the ability to trap and organify iodine, although not with the same efficiency as that of a normal follicular cell. This property paves the way for adjuvant RAI therapy whereby uptake of $^{131}$I into cancer cells leads to a targeted destruction (owing to beta-emitting properties of the isotope). This treatment has been deployed for decades, but a lack of randomized trials and national differences in practice means that there is no standardized approach to this treatment. There are three principle applications of RAI[38] (Table 15.7). Patients at high-risk of recurrence or death will be offered adjuvant therapy with RAI, and there is good evidence for a survival benefit in patients with metastatic disease.[39] Two weeks before RAI therapy, the patient is commenced on a low-iodine diet. At the time of taking the RAI, TSH must be high to stimulate radioiodine uptake. This is either achieved by thyroid hormone withdrawal (THW) or the use of recombinant human TSH (rhTSH). A prospective randomized study found that THW and rhTSH

| Application | Benefit |
|---|---|
| Remnant ablation | To facilitate follow-up by achieving undetectable serum Tg and a negative iodine whole-body scan. It will also facilitate detection of metastases by preventing iodine uptake by normal thyroid tissue |
| Adjuvant therapy | Destruction of occult cancer cells in the neck not treated by surgery |
| Treatment of persistent disease | Treatment of RAI-avid distant metastases |

*Source:* Reproduced from Tala H, Tuttle RM, *Clin Oncol (R Coll Radiol)*, 22, 419–29, 2010. Copyright 2011, with permission from Elsevier.

***Table 15.7***
*Applications of RAI.*

stimulation were equally effective in preparing patients for RAI ablation with significant improved quality of life in the rhTSH group.[40] Current advice discourages the use of a tracer scan before RAI treatment because of "thyroid stunning" that reduces the efficacy of an ablation dose.[41] At the time of treatment, the patient is resident in an isolation room and is not fit for discharge until the radiation level falls to below national guidelines. The commonest side effect is transitory sialadenitis because RAI is also taken up by salivary gland tissue. Patients receive a combination of lozenges, antiemetics, and antacids in an attempt to ameliorate side effects. Long-term side effects are remarkably few, but patients with extensive metastatic pulmonary disease may develop lung fibrosis. After RAI therapy, patients are prescribed levothyroxine.

## TSH suppression

DTC expresses TSH receptors on the cell membrane and responds to TSH stimulation by increasing rates of cell growth. Long-term suppression of TSH using supraphysiological doses of levothyroxine has been a cornerstone in the treatment of these patients in an attempt to decrease the risk of thyroid cancer recurrence and even cancer-related mortality.[42] There is emerging evidence that suppressive therapy may be beneficial in high-risk patients, but the data in low- to intermediate-risk patients are less convincing.[43,44] The benefits of TSH suppression need to be balanced against the adverse effects of TSH suppression on the heart and skeleton.[38]

## Follow up

The goal of follow-up is to detect recurrence early. Most recurrences will be in the neck (thyroid bed or lateral lymph nodes). Serum Tg is a specific tumor marker for DTC and is an excellent predictor of relapse and indicator of residual disease.[3] It should be undetectable in patients who have undergone total thyroid ablation. A measurable Tg indicates the presence of thyroid tissue or recurrent disease. Circulating anti-Tg antibodies interfere with Tg assays, making the interpretation of Tg levels difficult. However, a rising antibody titer is a surrogate marker for recurrent disease. Tg can either be measured in patients on levothyroxine (suppressed) or off-thyroxine and/or with recombinant TSH (stimulated).[45] Low-risk patients can be followed up every 9 months with a suppressed Tg, whereas high-risk patients (for death or recurrence) are followed up with stimulated Tg every 6 months and an annual neck ultrasound scan.[38]

## Recurrence

Surgery should be the first consideration in the management of recurrent disease. A compartment-oriented surgical resection of biopsy-proven loco regional metastases is recommended for metastases >1 cm. This surgery is challenging and should only be undertaken in expert surgical centers. Radiotherapy should be considered in patients with evidence of rapidly progressive disease or in whom there is no radioiodine uptake in known tumor sites. It should be considered in patients with extensive inoperable residual disease invading the aerodigestive system. Radiotherapy is particularly effective as palliation in patients with painful bone metastases. Chemotherapy has no proven role in patients with differentiated FTC or PTC. Its palliative use may be considered in patients with dedifferentiating tumors.

# Anaplastic thyroid carcinoma

Anaplastic thyroid carcinoma (ATC) has a dismal prognosis. It has an incidence of 1–2 per million, and this incidence is decreasing, whereas the incidence of differentiated cancer is increasing.[46] It is predominantly a disease of the elderly (>70 years). Up to 25% of cases have a preexisting goiter[47] presenting with a rapidly enlarging goiter (Figure 15.5). Local invasion is common (Figure 15.6) and dysphagia, hoarseness, and stridor are frequent symptoms. Metastases are found in 50% of patients at presentation.[48] The median survival is 3–5 months.[49] Similar to DTC, ATC is associated with genetic mutations, particularly involving the mitogen-activated protein (MAP) kinase PI3K pathways. The BRAF mutation is a major cause of aberrant activation of the MAP kinase pathway, and this is associated with dedifferentiation of PTC.[50] The PI3K signaling pathway plays a fundamental role in the regulation of cell growth, and proliferation and PI3K mutation are particularly common in ATC.[51]

## Management

All patients with ATC are regarded as having systemic disease. Surgery is considered as an option to achieve local control, but for many patients the disease is too advanced to make resection feasible. ATC loses its ability to take up iodine, so RAI therapy is not an option. There is little evidence that external beam radiotherapy to the primary tumor alters the course of the disease, but it may be considered on an individual basis and its benefits must be weighed against toxic side effects

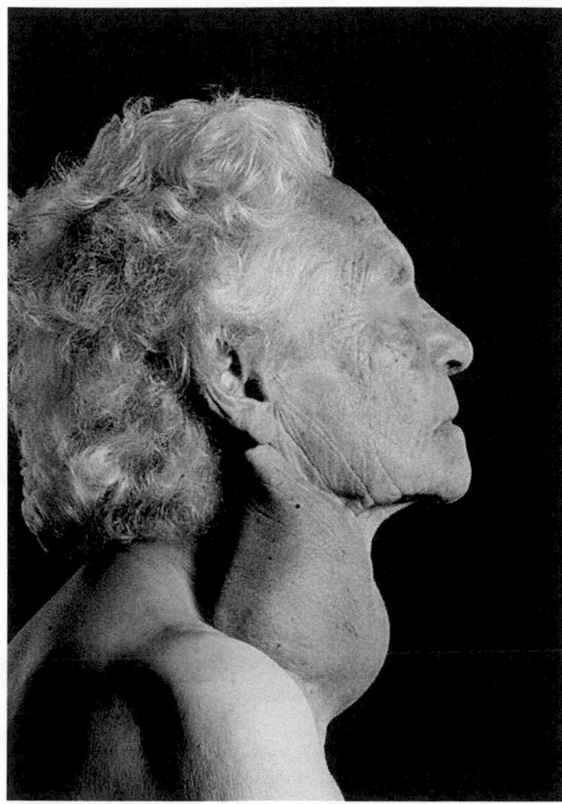

***Figure 15.5***
*Elderly woman presenting with a rapidly enlarging neck mass over the past 5 weeks.*

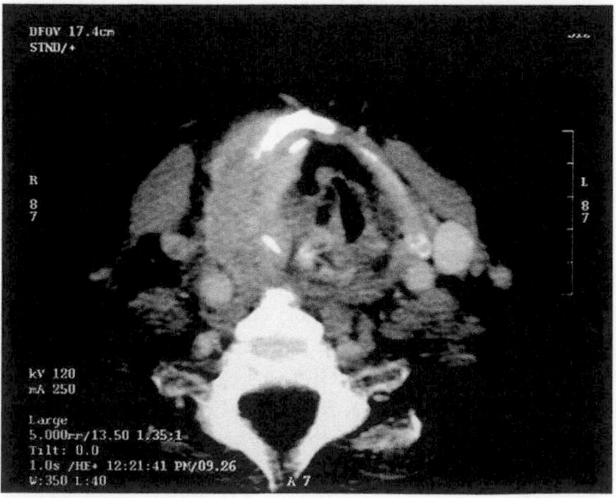


***Figure 15.6***
*CT scan demonstrating local invasion of the larynx by an ATC.*

(skin, esophagus, myelopathy).[52] The most successful results from the use of conventional chemotherapy have been achieved with doxorubicin with a response rate of about 20%.[53] Because the genetic basis of ATC tumorigenesis is better understood, targeted therapies are emerging, particularly the use of tyrosine kinase inhibitors, and their outcomes are currently under investigation. It is important that patients are considered for entry into clinical trials.

## *References*

1. Cancer Statistics Registrations for 1982, Series MB1, England and Wales. Biometry Branch Division of Cancer Cause and Prevention 1975. Third National Cancer Survey Incidence Data. In: Cutler S, Young J, eds. *Office of Population Censuses and Surveys*. NCI Monograph No.75-789. Washington, DC: DHEW Publications, 1985; pp. 25.
2. Davies L, Welch HG. Increasing incidence of thyroid cancer in the United States, 1973–2002. *JAMA* 2006; **295**(18): 2164–7.
3. Schlumberger MJ. Papillary and follicular thyroid carcinoma. *N Engl J Med* 1998; **338**(5): 297–306.
4. Ain KB. Papillary thyroid carcinoma. Etiology, assessment, and therapy. *Endocrinol Metab Clin North Am* 1995; 24(4): 711–60.
5. Leung AK, Chow SM, Law SC. Clinical features and outcome of the tall cell variant of papillary thyroid carcinoma. *Laryngoscope* 2008; 118(1): 32–8.
6. DeGroot LJ, Kaplan EL, McCormick M, Straus FH. Natural history, treatment, and course of papillary thyroid carcinoma. *J Clin Endocrinol Metab* 1990; 71(2): 414–24.
7. Iyer NG, Shaha AR. Management of thyroid nodules and surgery for differentiated thyroid cancer. *Clin Oncol (R Coll Radiol)* 2010; 22(6): 405–12.
8. Grebe SK, Hay ID. Follicular thyroid cancer. *Endocrinol Metab Clin North Am* 1995; 24(4): 761–801.
9. McLeod MK, Thompson NW. Hurthle cell neoplasms of the thyroid. *Otolaryngol Clin North Am* 1990; 23(3): 441–52.
10. Ron E, Lubin JH, Shore RE, Mabuchi K, Modan B, Pottern LM, Schneider AB, Tucker MA, Boice JD, Jr. Thyroid cancer after exposure to external radiation: A pooled analysis of seven studies. *Radiat Res* 1995; 141(3): 259–77.
11. Hancock SL, Cox RS, McDougall IR. Thyroid diseases after treatment of Hodgkin's disease. *N Engl J Med* 1991; 325(9): 599–605.
12. Sigurdson AJ, Ronckers CM, Mertens AC, Stovall M, Smith SA, Liu Y, Berkow RL, Hammond S, Neglia JP, Meadows AT, Sklar CA, Robison LL, Inskip PD.

Primary thyroid cancer after a first tumour in childhood (the Childhood Cancer Survivor Study): A nested case-control study. *Lancet* 2005; **365**(9476): 2014–23.

13. Mihailescu DV, Schneider AB. Size, number, and distribution of thyroid nodules and the risk of malignancy in radiation-exposed patients who underwent surgery. *J Clin Endocrinol Metab* 2008; **93**(6): 2188–93.
14. Schneider AB, Lubin J, Ron E, Abrahams C, Stovall M, Goel A, Shore-Freedman E, Gierlowski TC. Salivary gland tumors after childhood radiation treatment for benign conditions of the head and neck: Dose-response relationships. *Radiat Res* 1998; **149**(6): 625–30.
15. Tisell LE, Carlsson S, Fjalling M, Hansson G, Lindberg S, Lundberg LM, Oden A. Hyperparathyroidism subsequent to neck irradiation. Risk factors. *Cancer* 1985; **56**(7): 1529–33.
16. Czene K, Lichtenstein P, Hemminki K. Environmental and heritable causes of cancer among 9.6 million individuals in the Swedish Family-Cancer Database. *Int J Cancer* 2002; **99**(2): 260–6.
17. Pal T, Vogl FD, Chappuis PO, Tsang R, Brierley J, Renard H, Sanders K, Kantemiroff T, Bagha S, Goldgar DE, Narod SA, Foulkes WD. Increased risk for nonmedullary thyroid cancer in the first degree relatives of prevalent cases of nonmedullary thyroid cancer: A hospital-based study. *J Clin Endocrinol Metab* 2001; **86**(11): 5307–12.
18. Goldgar DE, Easton DF, Cannon-Albright LA, Skolnick MH. Systematic population-based assessment of cancer risk in first-degree relatives of cancer probands. *J Natl Cancer Inst* 1994; **86**(21): 1600–8.
19. Xu L, Li G, Wei Q, El-Naggar AK, Sturgis EM. Family history of cancer and risk of sporadic differentiated thyroid carcinoma. *Cancer* 2012; **118**(5): 1228–35.
20. Gudmundsson J, Sulem P, Gudbjartsson DF, Jonasson JG, Sigurdsson A, Bergthorsson JT, He H, Blondal T, Geller F, Jakobsdottir M, Magnusdottir DN, Matthiasdottir S, Stacey SN, Skarphedinsson OB, Helgadottir H, Li W, Nagy R, Aguillo E, Faure E, Prats E, Saez B, Martinez M, Eyjolfsson GI, Bjornsdottir US, Holm H, Kristjansson K, Frigge ML, Kristvinsson H, Gulcher JR, Jonsson T, Rafnar T, Hjartarsson H, Mayordomo JI, de la Chapelle A, Hrafnkelsson J, Thorsteinsdottir U, Kong A, Stefansson K. Common variants on 9q22.33 and 14q13.3 predispose to thyroid cancer in European populations. *Nat Genet* 2009; 41(4): 460–4.
21. Jazdzewski K, Liyanarachchi S, Swierniak M, Pachucki J, Ringel MD, Jarzab B, de la Chapelle A. Polymorphic mature microRNAs from passenger strand of pre-miR-146a contribute to thyroid cancer. *Proc Natl Acad Sci U S A* 2009; **106**(5): 1502–5.
22. Jones AM, Howarth KM, Martin L, Gorman M, Mihai R, Moss L, Auton A, Lemon C, Mehanna H, Mohan H, Clarke SE, Wadsley J, Macias E, Coatesworth A, Beasley M, Roques T, Martin C, Ryan P, Gerrard G, Power D, Bremmer C, Tomlinson I, Carvajal-Carmona LG. Thyroid cancer susceptibility polymorphisms: Confirmation of loci on chromosomes 9q22 and 14q13, validation of a recessive 8q24 locus and failure to replicate a locus on 5q24. *J Med Genet* 2012; 49(3): 158–63.
23. Ruiz-Llorente S, Montero-Conde C, Milne RL, Moya CM, Cebrian A, Leton R, Cascon A, Mercadillo F, Landa I, Borrego S, Perez de Nanclares G, Alvarez-Escola C, Diaz-Perez JA, Carracedo A, Urioste M, Gonzalez-Neira A, Benitez J, Santisteban P, Dopazo J, Ponder BA, Robledo M. Association study of 69 genes in the RET pathway identifies low-penetrance loci in sporadic medullary thyroid carcinoma. *Cancer Res* 2007; **67**(19): 9561–7.
24. Wokolorczyk D, Gliniewicz B, Sikorski A, Zlowocka E, Masojc B, Debniak T, Matyjasik J, Mierzejewski M, Medrek K, Oszutowska D, Suchy J, Gronwald J, Teodorczyk U, Huzarski T, Byrski T, Jakubowska A, Gorski B, van de Wetering T, Walczak S, Narod SA, Lubinski J, Cybulski C. A range of cancers is associated with the rs6983267 marker on chromosome 8. *Cancer Res* 2008; **68**(23): 9982–6.
25. Nikiforov YE, Nikiforova MN. Molecular genetics and diagnosis of thyroid cancer. *Nat Rev Endocrinol* 2011; 7(10): 569–80.
26. Elisei R, Ugolini C, Viola D, Lupi C, Biagini A, Giannini R, Romei C, Miccoli P, Pinchera A, Basolo F. BRAF(V600E) mutation and outcome of patients with papillary thyroid carcinoma: A 15-year median follow-up study. *J Clin Endocrinol Metab* 2008; **93**(10): 3943–9.
27. Ciampi R, Nikiforov YE. RET/PTC rearrangements and BRAF mutations in thyroid tumorigenesis. *Endocrinology* 2007; **148**(3): 936–41.
28. Kroll TG, Sarraf P, Pecciarini L, Chen CJ, Mueller E, Spiegelman BM, Fletcher JA. PAX8-PPARgamma1 fusion oncogene in human thyroid carcinoma [corrected]. *Science* 2000; **289**(5483): 1357–60.
29. Gough J, Scott-Coombes D, Palazzo F. Thyroid incidentaloma: An evidence-based assessment of management strategy. *World J Surg* 2008; **32**(7): 1264–8.
30. BTA. *Guidelines for the management of thyroid cancer*. 2nd ed. London: Royal College of Physicians; 2007.
31. Frates MC, Benson CB, Charboneau JW, Cibas ES, Clark OH, Coleman BG, Cronan JJ, Doubilet PM, Evans DB, Goellner JR, Hay ID, Hertzberg BS, Intenzo CM, Jeffrey RB, Langer JE, Larsen PR, Mandel SJ, Middleton WD, Reading CC, Sherman SI, Tessler FN. Management of thyroid nodules detected at US: Society of Radiologists in Ultrasound consensus conference statement. *Ultrasound Q* 2006; **22**(4): 231–8; discussion 239–40.
32. Bilimoria KY, Bentrem DJ, Ko CY, Stewart AK, Winchester DP, Talamonti MS, Sturgeon C. Extent of

surgery affects survival for papillary thyroid cancer. *Ann Surg* 2007; 246(3): 375–81; discussion 381–4.

33. Hay ID, Thompson GB, Grant CS, Bergstralh EJ, Dvorak CE, Gorman CA, Maurer MS, McIver B, Mullan BP, Oberg AL, Powell CC, van Heerden JA, Goellner JR. Papillary thyroid carcinoma managed at the Mayo Clinic during six decades (1940–1999): Temporal trends in initial therapy and long-term outcome in 2444 consecutively treated patients. *World J Surg* 2002; 26(8): 879–85.
34. Zaydfudim V, Feurer ID, Griffin MR, Phay JE. The impact of lymph node involvement on survival in patients with papillary and follicular thyroid carcinoma. *Surgery* 2008; 144(6): 1070–7; discussion 1077–8.
35. Cooper DS, Doherty GM, Haugen BR, Kloos RT, Lee SL, Mandel SJ, Mazzaferri EL, McIver B, Pacini F, Schlumberger M, Sherman SI, Steward DL, Tuttle RM. Revised American Thyroid Association management guidelines for patients with thyroid nodules and differentiated thyroid cancer. *Thyroid* 2009; **19**(11): 1167–214.
36. Tuttle RM, Leboeuf R. Follow up approaches in thyroid cancer: A risk adapted paradigm. *Endocrinol Metab Clin North Am* 2008; 37(2): 419–35, ix–x.
37. Tuttle RM, Tala H, Shah J, Leboeuf R, Ghossein R, Gonen M, Brokhin M, Omry G, Fagin JA, Shaha A. Estimating risk of recurrence in differentiated thyroid cancer after total thyroidectomy and radioactive iodine remnant ablation: Using response to therapy variables to modify the initial risk estimates predicted by the new American Thyroid Association staging system. *Thyroid* 2010; **20**(12): 1341–9.
38. Tala H, Tuttle RM. Contemporary post surgical management of differentiated thyroid carcinoma. *Clin Oncol (R Coll Radiol)* 2010; 22(6): 419–29.
39. Mazzaferri EL, Jhiang SM. Long-term impact of initial surgical and medical therapy on papillary and follicular thyroid cancer. *Am J Med* 1994; 97(5): 418–28.
40. Pacini F, Ladenson PW, Schlumberger M, Driedger A, Luster M, Kloos RT, Sherman S, Haugen B, Corone C, Molinaro E, Elisei R, Ceccarelli C, Pinchera A, Wahl RL, Leboulleux S, Ricard M, Yoo J, Busaidy NL, Delpassand E, Hanscheid H, Felbinger R, Lassmann M, Reiners C. Radioiodine ablation of thyroid remnants after preparation with recombinant human thyrotropin in differentiated thyroid carcinoma: Results of an international, randomized, controlled study. *J Clin Endocrinol Metab* 2006; **91**(3): 926–32.
41. Clarke SE. Radioiodine therapy in differentiated thyroid cancer: A nuclear medicine perspective. *Clin Oncol (R Coll Radiol)* 2010; 22(6): 430–7.
42. Mazzaferri EL, Young RL, Oertel JE, Kemmerer WT, Page CP. Papillary thyroid carcinoma: The impact of therapy in 576 patients. *Medicine (Baltimore)* 1977; 56(3): 171–96.
43. Sugitani I, Fujimoto Y. Does postoperative thyrotropin suppression therapy truly decrease recurrence in papillary thyroid carcinoma? A randomized controlled trial. *J Clin Endocrinol Metab* 2010; **95**(10): 4576–83.
44. Pujol P, Daures JP, Nsakala N, Baldet L, Bringer J, Jaffiol C. Degree of thyrotropin suppression as a prognostic determinant in differentiated thyroid cancer. *J Clin Endocrinol Metab* 1996; **81**(12): 4318–23.
45. Ladenson PW, Braverman LE, Mazzaferri EL, Brucker-Davis F, Cooper DS, Garber JR, Wondisford FE, Davies TF, DeGroot LJ, Daniels GH, Ross DS, Weintraub BD. Comparison of administration of recombinant human thyrotropin with withdrawal of thyroid hormone for radioactive iodine scanning in patients with thyroid carcinoma. *N Engl J Med* 1997; **337**(13): 888–96.
46. Burke JP, Hay ID, Dignan F, Goellner JR, Achenbach SJ, Oberg AL, Melton LJ, 3rd. Long-term trends in thyroid carcinoma: A population-based study in Olmsted County, Minnesota, 1935–1999. *Mayo Clin Proc* 2005; **80**(6): 753–8.
47. Hundahl SA, Cady B, Cunningham MP, Mazzaferri E, McKee RF, Rosai J, Shah JP, Fremgen AM, Stewart AK, Holzer S. Initial results from a prospective cohort study of 5583 cases of thyroid carcinoma treated in the United States during 1996. U.S. and German Thyroid Cancer Study Group. An American College of Surgeons Commission on Cancer Patient Care Evaluation study. *Cancer* 2000; **89**(1): 202–17.
48. Hundahl SA, Fleming ID, Fremgen AM, Menck HR. A National Cancer Data Base report on 53,856 cases of thyroid carcinoma treated in the U.S., 1985–1995 [see comments]. *Cancer* 1998; **83**(12): 2638–48.
49. McIver B, Hay ID, Giuffrida DF, Dvorak CE, Grant CS, Thompson GB, van Heerden JA, Goellner JR. Anaplastic thyroid carcinoma: A 50-year experience at a single institution. *Surgery* 2001; **130**(6): 1028–34.
50. Xing M. BRAF mutation in papillary thyroid cancer: Pathogenic role, molecular bases, and clinical implications. *Endocr Rev* 2007; **28**(7): 742–62.
51. Hou P, Liu D, Shan Y, Hu S, Studeman K, Condouris S, Wang Y, Trink A, El-Naggar AK, Tallini G, Vasko V, Xing M. Genetic alterations and their relationship in the phosphatidylinositol 3-kinase/Akt pathway in thyroid cancer. *Clin Cancer Res* 2007; 13(4): 1161–70.
52. Wong CS, Van Dyk J, Simpson WJ. Myelopathy following hyperfractionated accelerated radiotherapy for anaplastic thyroid carcinoma. *Radiother Oncol* 1991; **20**(1): 3–9.
53. Ahuja S, Ernst H. Chemotherapy of thyroid carcinoma. *J Endocrinol Invest* 1987; **10**(3): 303–10.
54. Edge SB, Byrd DR, Compton CC, Fritz AG, Greene FL, Trotti A, et al. *AJCC Cancer Staging Manual*. 7th ed. New York, NY: Springer-Verlag; 2010.

# 16

# The inherited basis of hypogonadotropic hypogonadism

*Pierre-Marc G. Bouloux*

## *Introduction*

Congenital isolated hypogonadotropic hypogonadism (CIHH) is a well-known cause of absent pubertal development in both boys and girls and results from inadequate secretion of the two pituitary gonadotropins, luteinizing hormone (LH) and follicle-stimulating hormone (FSH), with consequent impairment of normal testicular or ovarian function. With a prevalence estimation, based on a civilian and military hospital series, of 1/4000 to 1/10,000 in males,[1] CIHH is reported to be between two and five times more common in boys than in girls.[2] Patients with CIHH usually come to clinical attention during adolescence or adulthood because of incomplete or absent pubertal development; owing to progress in molecular genetics and clinical practice, the diagnosis can be made earlier in cases where the diagnosis is specifically sought.

Congenital hypogonadotropic hypogonadism is a component of several syndromes, usually managed in the pediatric setting (Table 16.1), when it may occur together with nongonadal features such as short stature due to growth hormone deficiency and other anterior pituitary hormone deficiencies,[3,4] primary adrenal failure,[5] (early onset) childhood obesity,[6,7] or in association with several neurological disorders,[8–10] when early onset of the extragonadal features may predominate.

Current understanding of the pathophysiology and origins of CIHH can be gleaned from the ontogeny of the gonadotropin-releasing hormone (GnRH) neuronal system and the rapid progress made in the molecular genetics of this condition.

## *Ontogeny of the GnRH system*

Embryological studies conducted in mammals,[11–14] birds,[15] amphibians,[16] and fish[17] have established that neuroendocrine GnRH cells originate, proliferate, and then migrate from the medial part of the olfactory pit into the brain in an axonophilic manner along the olfactory–vomeronasal nerve pathway. The stem cell population giving rise to GnRH neurons is as yet unknown because cells are only identifiable once they express GnRH. In humans, GnRH neuronal migration begins during the sixth embryonic week, at a time when axon terminals of the olfactory sensory neurons first come into contact with the rostral pole of the forebrain just before the emergence of the olfactory bulbs. On reaching the base of the telencephalon, GnRH neurons penetrate into the brain, just caudal to the olfactory bulb anlage, before making their way superficially along the medial wall of the cerebral hemisphere to their final resting location in the septopreoptic hypothalamic region.[18]

The fully developed GnRH system consists between 1500 and 2000 neurons scattered in the anterior septopreoptic area of the hypothalamus, whose axons converge onto the median eminence portal capillaries where neurosecretion occurs. This full developmental sequence, completed by the eighth to ninth week of embryonic development, can therefore be compartmentalized into several discrete but well-coordinated events, starting with (1) fate specification of GnRH neurons; (2) expansion of cell numbers (mitosis and apoptosis); (3) cell migration (a mixture of chemorepulsive and chemorepellent events); (4) coalescence of individual GnRH neurons into a responsive, secreting,

| Syndrome | Phenotype | Genetic defect |
|---|---|---|
| Prader–Willi | Mental retardation, morbid obesity, hypotonia | Deletions within paternally imprinted 15q11.2-12 region |
| | Carbohydrate intolerance | |
| | Autosomal dominant | |
| | Cryptorchidism | |
| Laurence–Moon–Bardet–Biedl | Mental retardation, obesity retinitis pigmentosa, autosomal recessive post-axial polydactyly | BBS-1-11 (multiple loci) |
| | | 20p12 |
| | | 16q21,15q22.3-23,14q32.1 |
| Biemond | Iris coloboma polydactyly, developmental delay | |
| CHARGE anomaly (see text) | Adrenohypoplasia | |
| | Primary adrenal deficiency | DAX-1 |
| | Congenita | |
| Septo-optic dysplasia | Small, dysplastic pale optic discs | HESX1 |
| | Pendular nystagmus, midline Hypothalamic defect with DI, GH, ACTH,TSH and LH/FSH deficiency, absent septum pellucidum | |
| Solitary median maxillary incisor syndrome | Prominent midpalatal ridge | SHH 7q3 |
| | Hypopituitarism | PROP1 |
| | GH,TSH, LH/FSH deficiency | PROP1 5q |
| | LH, FSH + multiple hormone deficiencies | LHX3 |
| | Severe restriction of head rotation due to rigid cervical spine | |
| | Anterior pituitary hypoplasia | SOX2 |
| | Anophthalmia, microphthalmia | |
| | Coloboma | |
| Borjeson–Forssman–Lehmann syndrome | Mental retardation | X-linked ataxia |
| Gordon Holmes | HH, ataxia, dementia | Inactivating mutations in RNF216/OTUD4 |

***Table 16.1***
*Congenital syndromes associated with HH.*

and coordinating network functioning in an integrated manner; and (5) the development of a capacity to incorporate and integrate internal and external feedback signals into the final feedback control mechanisms that modulate GnRH release. Mutations in the genes whose actions determine any one or more of these pathways could theoretically underpin congenital forms of hypogonadotropic hypogonadism. Postnatally, a further tier of regulation of these neurosecretory events involves the reversible detachment of these nerve endings onto the capillary loops of the median eminence.[19]

Over the past 22 years, steady progress has been made toward unraveling the molecular genetic abnormalities that can underpin the inherited forms of hypogonadotropic hypogonadism. What has emerged is a complex group of genes and patterns of inheritance spanning from classical monogenic to what seems progressively to have become classified an oligogenic disorder of potentially interacting genes underpinning the phenotype.

## Development of reproductive activity

In humans, the fetal GnRH pulse generator and its downstream gonadotrope and gonadal axis activation are functional in both sexes by the end of the first trimester of gestation but then become quiescent *in utero* such that by the time of parturition, serum LH and FSH are fully suppressed in cord blood, the consequence of negative feedback inhibition from placentally derived sex steroids. Shortly after birth, male infants demonstrate a brief surge of LH and testosterone that persists for about 12 h, followed by, about 1–2 weeks later (with the gradual elimination of placentally derived inhibitory hormonal influences), what is tantamount to a minipuberty, differing in its duration between the two sexes.[20] Thus, in males, LH, FSH, and testosterone peak between 4 and 10 weeks. The hypothalamo–pituitary axis then gradually becomes less active until around 6 months, after which GnRH quiescence becomes complete,[21] only to be reawakened with the onset of puberty. At the onset of puberty, Sertoli cells undergo a radical change in their morphology and function, switching from an immature proliferative state to a mature, nonproliferative state. FSH induces proliferation of immature Sertoli cells, and the number of Sertoli cells is directly associated with sperm-producing capability. In females, there is a greater persistence of GnRH secretory activation for up to 3 years, with a greater preponderance of FSH secretion throughout. The male minipuberty serves to expand the pool of Sertoli cells, with a concomitant increase in germ cells available for future fertility.[22] In macaque monkeys, exposure to superactive GnRH analogs at this critical phase leads to suppression of future fertility potential.[23] A further effect of the minipuberty is the exposure of the developing male brain to testosterone concentrations not far short of adult values, as well as those of hormone-sensitive tissues such as the penis and for completion of testicular descent. Absence of *in utero* and early postnatal sex steroid exposure may explain in part the frequency of micropenis seen in males with idiopathic hypogonadotropic hypogonadism (IHH). Gonadotropin secretion then becomes effectively silenced by an ill-understood restraint mechanism until the onset of puberty.

## Clinical presentation of hypogonadotropic hypogonadism

HH is suspected when onset of pubertal development is incomplete or absent after the age of 13 years in girls and 14 years in boys, particularly if pubertal delay is associated with cryptorchidism or micropenis or is persistent after the age of 18 years. In females, it is likely to present as failure of breast and secondary sexual hair development in association with primary amenorrhea, associated with low levels of FSH and LH and estradiol levels.

Prepubertal diagnosis in boys with CIHH is rarely made before puberty, although the presence of neonatal unilateral or bilateral cryptorchidism or micropenis or hyposmia/anosmia may suggest the diagnosis; the finding of low gonadotropins and testosterone during the expected minipuberty (within the first 6 months of postnatal life) can establish an early diagnosis if cryptorchidism, micropenis, or both are present.[24]

Constitutional short stature and pubertal delay (CSSPD) can cause diagnostic confusion: in complete forms, CIHH can be usually distinguished from CSSPD by virtue of the growth pattern, with CIHH having normal height for chronological age and CSSPD tending to be short.[25] In mild or partial forms, additional associated physical signs (e.g., cryptorchidism or micropenis) suggestive of a syndromic form can be helpful. CIHH has a normal growth pattern during childhood but lacks the usual pubertal growth spurt. The absence of long-bone epiphyseal closure results in eunuchoid proportions and relative tall stature, and an arm span exceeding height. Lack of exposure to testosterone not only leads to relative stunting of upper segment growth, and general retardation of bone maturation, but also predisposes to osteopenia, and osteoporosis in later life.[26]

Gynecomastia is occasionally seen in patients with untreated CIHH, although more usually after human chorionic gonadotropin (hCG) or supraphysiological testosterone exposure, the latter being due to aromatization into estradiol. Partial congenital gonadotropin deficiency affects only a minority of male patients and is characterized by incomplete virilization, gynecomastia, and a testicular volume >4 mL or even close to normal and with only moderate clinical and endocrine abnormalities.

## CIHH in women

In >90% of women, CIHH is characterized by primary amenorrhea, with variable breast development ranging from absent to almost normal. Pubic hair may be absent, sparse, or even normal. Partial forms may lead to an underestimation of the true prevalence of this condition in females. The mildest form, present in a minority of women, is associated with isolated chronic anovulation, with estradiol secretion adequate for endometrial development as evidenced by progestogen-induced endometrial stripping; oligomenorrhea may be present in these women. These attenuated forms have also been described in women having conceived spontaneously.

Diagnostic difficulty may arise in women with primary amenorrhea, normal olfaction, and no identified mutation where the differential diagnosis lies between CIHH and functional hypothalamic amenorrhea. In such cases, it is important to exclude other causes of HH such as those due to low body mass, eating disorders, excessive physical activity, and chronic underlying conditions. Sometimes, only after a period of observation with later reassessment of the hypothalamo–pituitary ovarian axis can the diagnosis be established. It has recently become recognized that a genetic lesion responsible for CIHH may be present in a significant number of women presenting with hypothalamic amenorrhea.[27]

## Clinical evaluation of suspected CIHH

The first step in the evaluation is a thorough anamnesis and family history followed by physical examination. Certain physical signs will increase suspicion of underlying CIHH, such as hyposmia/anosmia, cleft lip/palate, bimanual synkinesia,[28,29] and features suggesting the CHARGE syndrome[30] as well as skeletal abnormalities (Figure 16.1). Pubertal status according to Tanner staging should be established. Family history should focus on the reproductive histories of male and female family members.

The many nonreproductive phenotypes associated with CIHH therefore include the following: mirror movements of the upper limbs (bimanual synkinesis),[31–34] eye movement abnormalities,[29] congenital ptosis and abnormal visual spatial attention,[35] hearing impairment,[36] renal agenesis,[37] cleft lip or palate,[38] agenesis of one or several teeth (hypodontia),[39] obesity and digital abnormalities.[40]

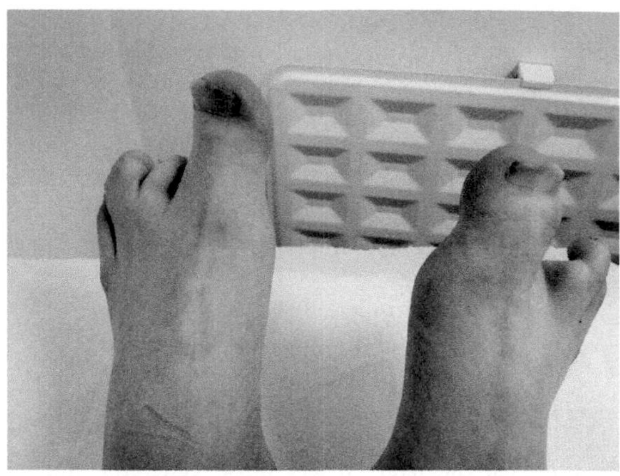

**Figure 16.1**
*Digital abnormality of the toes, with broad great toe in a male with a de novo mutation of FGFR1, anosmia, and HH. The hands were normal.*

## Kallmann syndrome

Kallmann syndrome (KS) is diagnosed when low serum gonadotropins and gonadal steroids are coupled with a compromised sense of smell (hyposmia or anosmia), with the latter being ascertainable on the anamnesis (subjective) or by means of detailed questioning or objectively by formal olfactory test, such as the Pennsylvania smell test.

Even severe CIHH in men is not associated with ambiguous external genitalia, and the penis can range from normal to micropenis proportions (Figure 16.2). Although LH and FSH will have been deficient in these cases, testosterone secretion secondary to fetal Leydig cell stimulation by placental hCG will have occurred during early development.

## Investigations

In males, the diagnosis of HH is based on low plasma total testosterone levels, usually associated with an inappropriately low or "normal" LH and FSH. Although it was thought that the use of ultrasensitive gonadotropin assays might also give an insight into the central control of gonadotropin secretions in affected individuals, with some patients showing no discernible pulsatile LH secretion, with others demonstrating reduced LH pulse frequency or amplitude, and still others an exclusively LH nocturnal secretion, it has become evident that there is no genotype–phenotype relationship between

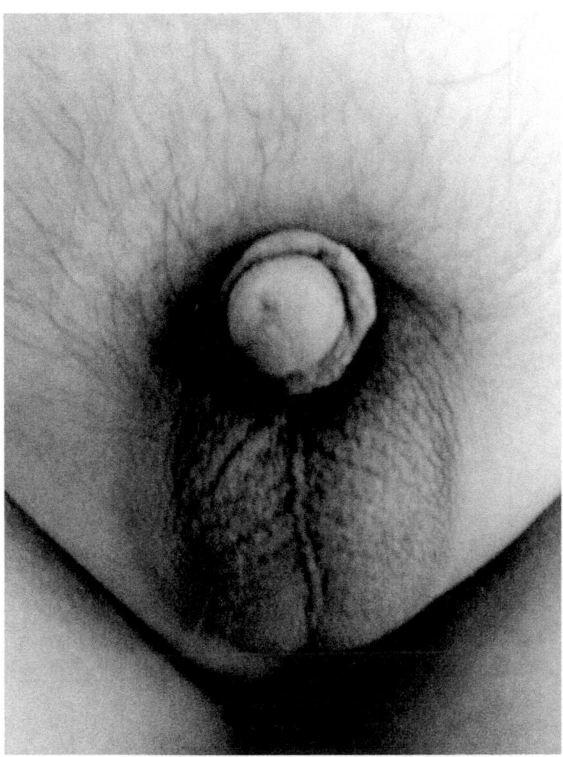

**Figure 16.2**
*Genitalia of a 21-year-old man with KS. Sparse pubic hair represents the effects of adrenarche, and the penile shaft is short and the scrotum hypoplastic. LH <0.1, FSH <0.1, testosterone <0.5 nmol/L.*

the LH secretion profile and underlying genetic abnormality (See Figure 16.3).

Patients with complete gonadotropin deficiency pose no diagnostic difficulties with prepubertal range testosterone levels and low inhibin B concentrations, a marker of FSH deficiency. Difficulties arise in partial forms of CIHH when gonadotropin and inhibin B levels can be in the reference range. Other studies have shown that patients with CIHH retain prepubertal circulating anti-Müllerian hormone concentrations indicative of absent pubertal FSH-dependent testicular maturation, induced by intratesticular testosterone.[41] Its use for diagnostic purposes is still under evaluation.

# GnRH test

It is doubtful whether the GnRH test provides any additional information to that gleaned from ultrasensitive baseline gonadotropin assays. The conventional 100-μg GnRH test does not usually discriminate between gonadotropin deficiency of hypothalamic or pituitary origin, and a partial response is usually present in partial pituitary deficiency, both in patients with CIHH and in those with acquired postpubertal HH. In congenital gonadotropin deficiencies, the response to GnRH test is highly variable; absent responses are seen when the testes are very small in men and breast development is absent in women. In complete forms with testicular volumes <2 mL, a slight or totally absent gonadotropin response is observed. In partial forms with testicular volume >6 mL, the response can be positive, or even supranormal in the case of LH.

Plasma estradiol concentrations are often near the detection limit in CIHH, paralleling the degree of breast development, whereas estradiol can range from just detectable when a little breast development is present to the levels seen in the mid-follicular phase in patients with Tanner 3–4 breast development.

Finally, before making a firm diagnosis of isolated congenital gonadotropin deficiency, all anterior pituitary functions must be investigated to exclude hyperprolactinemia, or other anterior pituitary deficiencies, or an associated endocrine disorder that may be part of syndromic forms of CHH. In all cases of IHH, the diagnostic work-up should include serum iron binding capacity and ferritin levels to rule out hemochromatosis, and the anamnesis should rule out other underlying chronic illness and opioid use.

# Ultrasound examination

Renal ultrasound examination can reveal malformation or unilateral agenesis in patients with X-linked *KAL1* but is invariably normal in other causes of CIHH (euosmic and hyposmic).[42] Ultrasound examination of the scrotum and testes is helpful in situations where there is difficulty palpating the testes, and to give objective evidence of maldescent and its level.

In women, transabdominal ultrasound can help size the uterus, an indicator of estrogenic exposure and transvaginal ultrasound, where possible can enable direct visualization of endometrial thickness, ovary volume, and the number of developing follicles and their size, which reflects the severity of gonadotropin deficiency.

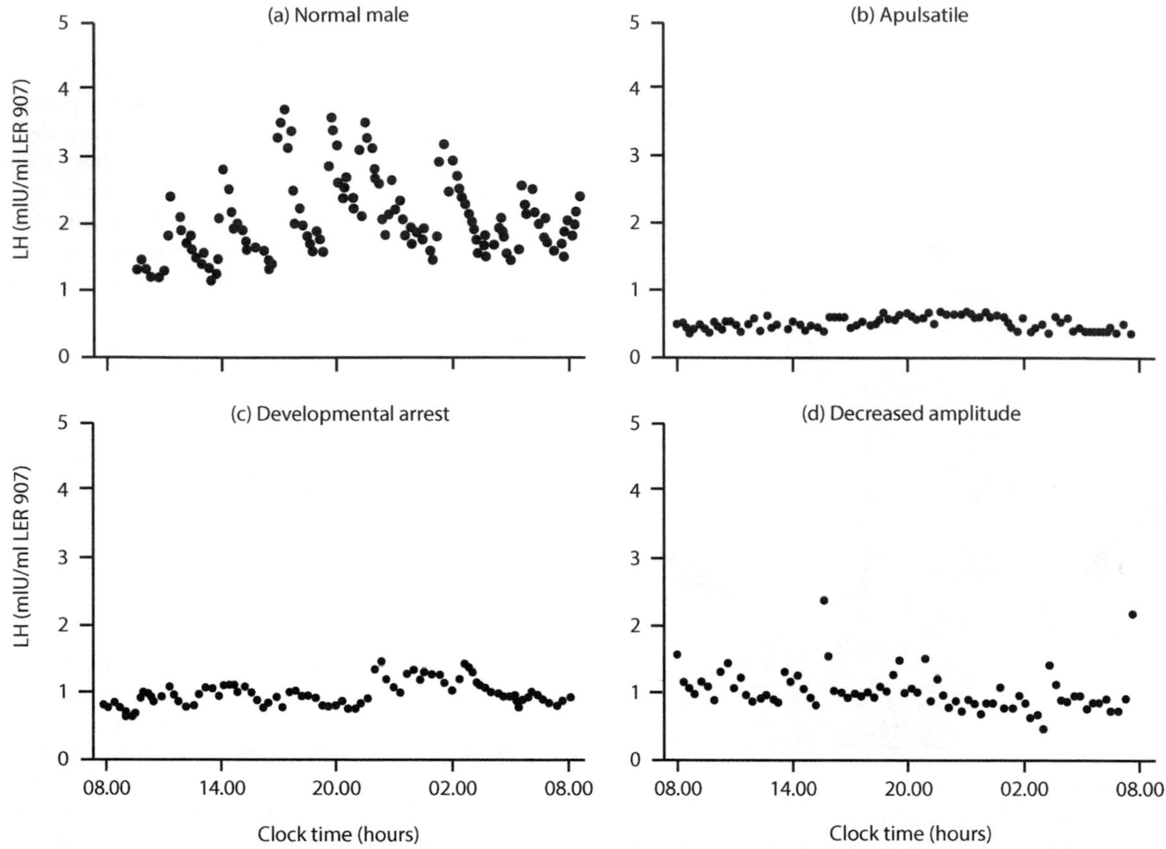


***Figure 16.3***
*Heterogeneity in the profiles of LH and follicle-stimulating hormone (FSH) secretion in patients with IHH. The pulsatile LH secretion in a healthy young man (a) is contrasted with a complete absence of LH pulses in a man with IHH (b). The patient in (c) has a few low-amplitude, nighttime LH pulses, reminiscent of early puberty, while the patient in (d) has a normal frequency of LH pulses, all of which have low amplitude. We do not know whether this clinical heterogeneity in LH pulsatile secretion is due to different degrees of gonadotropin-releasing hormone (GnRH) deficiency or whether it reflects genetic heterogeneity in the pathophysiology of this syndrome. (Adapted from Crowley WF Jr, et al.,* Recent Prog Horm Res, 41, *473–531, 1985.)*

# Hypothalamo–pituitary imaging

Magnetic resonance imaging (MRI) of the brain and olfactory bulbs is useful in CIHH and can demonstrate absent or hypoplastic olfactory bulbs and sulci in cases of KS[31,43] (Figure 16.4). MRI is also useful to exclude hypothalamic or pituitary lesions as the cause of HH. MRI is invariably normal in IHH but can occasionally show structural abnormalities such as absent corpus callosum and abnormal cerebellum.

# Classification of genetic causes of HH

Rapid progress has been made in unraveling the genetic basis of CIHH. Targeted clinical investigation, together with the catalyst provided by mapping of the human genome, has enabled the identification of several genes involved in GnRH ontogeny and whose loss of function, singly or in combination, results in the phenotype of HH.

The genes whose loss of function result in HH can broadly be classified into three groups.

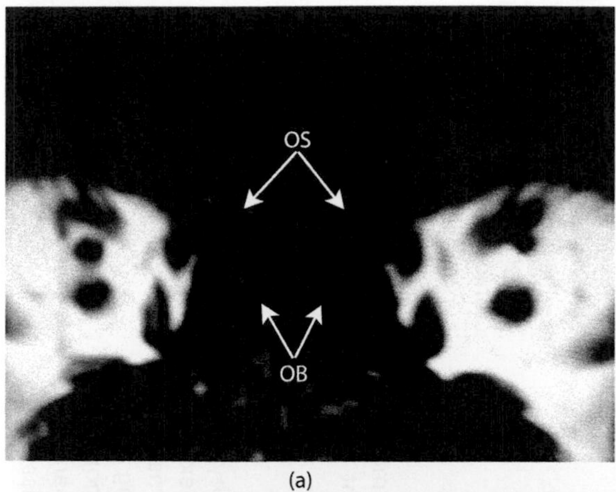


(a)

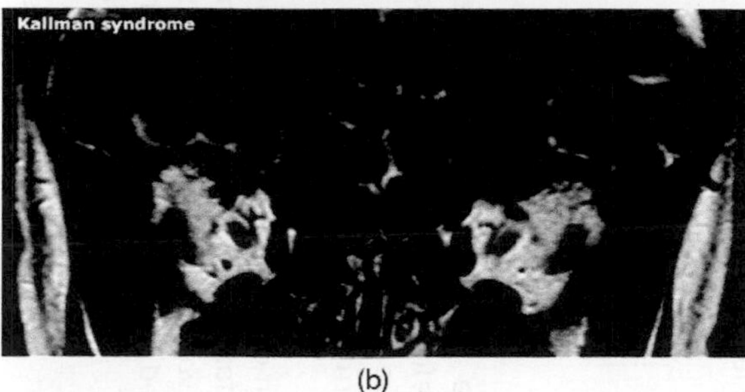


(b)

***Figure 16.4***
*Coronal MRI showing olfactory sulci and bulbs in a normal subject (a) and absent bulbs and sulci in a patient with KS (b). OS, OB.*

1. Genes that appear to represent purely neurodevelopmental genes whose loss of function affects the development and migration of GnRH neurons (KAL1, NELF, fibroblast growth factor receptor [FGFR]1, fibroblast growth factor [FGF] [and its synexpression group], PROKR2, PROK2, CHD7, SEM3A, SEM3E, HPSST 3, WDR11) into the hypothalamus
2. Genes that appear to have a purely neuroendocrine role (GnRH1, GnRHR, KISS 1, KISS1R, TAC3, TACR3)
3. Genes that appear to have a mixed role and are implicated in both development and neuroendocrine function (FGF8, FGF1,PROK2, PROKR2) (Table 16.2)

## Genes mutated in HH

Multiple genetic defects can cause KS (Table 16.2), and multiple inheritance patterns have been reported, including X-linked recessive, autosomal dominant, and autosomal recessive. Frequently, however, the condition is sporadic. For each genetic form of KS identified so far, the clinical heterogeneity of the disease within affected families clearly indicates that the manifestation of KS phenotypes is dependent on factors other than the mutated gene itself. These factors may include epigenetic factors and modifier genes effects. More recently, it has become evident that CIHH is not infrequently a digenic or oligogenic condition, a further explanation for the variable penetrance of the disease within pedigrees.[44]

A greater variability in the degree of hypogonadism has been observed in patients carrying mutations in *FGFR1*, *FGF8*, *PROKR2*, or *PROK2* than in *KAL1* patients, in which the phenotype is invariably severe.[45,46] Spontaneously fertile individuals carrying mutations in many of the autosomal KS genes account for the transmission of the disease over several generations, whereas the X-linked form of KS is usually transmitted by the female carriers of *KAL1* mutations, who are clinically unaffected. Among the variety of nonreproductive and nonolfactory disorders that affect a fraction of the KS patients, some have been reported for specific genetic forms of the disease.

Unilateral renal agenesis occurs in approximately 30% of *KAL1* patients[42] but has so far not been reported in patients with *FGFR1*, *FGF8*, *PROKR2*, or *PROK2* mutations. The loss of nasal cartilage, external ear hypoplasia, and skeletal anomalies of the hands or feet have only been reported in *KAL2* (FGFR1) patients. In contrast, hearing impairment is common to several genetic forms of KS, although it should be noted that the underlying defect (conductive, perceptive, or mixed) is likely to vary between different genetic forms. Palate defects should also be considered as one of these shared traits, even though the severity differs between *KAL1* (high arched palate) and *KAL2* (cleft palate). The cleft lip, palate, or both may occur in as many as 25%–30% of the *KAL2* cases. Finally, bimanual synkinesis is highly prevalent in *KAL1* (maybe >75% of the cases), but it seems to be much less common in *KAL2*.

## KAL1 (anosmin 1)

The *KAL1* gene, located on the X chromosome at the Xp22.3 locus, was the first gene identified to be mutated in X-linked KS.[47] It encodes an extracellular cell membrane associated glycoprotein (anosmin 1) involved in cellular adhesion, cell migration, and neurite outgrowth and is bound extracellularly to heparan sulfate glycosaminoglycans, via its FnIII domains.[48,49]

| *Gene* | *Gene product* | *Function* | *Inheritance* | *Clinical phenotype* |
|---|---|---|---|---|
| KAL1 | Anosmin 1 | Promotes neurite outgrowth, axon branching and targeting, chemoattractive on GnRH neuronal migration, cell adhesion | X-KS | KS (anosmia + HH), bimanual synkinesis, renal agenesis, cryptorchidism, neurosensorial deafness |
| FGFR1 (KAL2) | FGF receptor 1 | FGF signaling for cell proliferation, differentiation and GnRH neuronal migration | Autosomal dominant | Normosmic IHH, KS, primary amenorrhea, craniofacial defects, abnormal limb development, cleft palate, dental agenesis, digital bony abnormalities |
| FGF8 (KAL3) | Fibroblast growth factor 8 | Ligand of FGFR for the genesis of the GnRH neuronal system and olfactory bulb development, *Fgf8*-conditional-knockout mice exhibit increased levels of apoptosis in the developing olfactory epithelium | Predominantly inherited in an autosomal dominant manner | Normosmic IHH, KS, primary amenorrhea, cleft lip and palate, neurosensorial deafness, digital bony abnormalities, dental agenesis, recessive holoprosencephaly, craniofacial defects, and hypothalamo–pituitary dysfunction |
| FGF17 | Fibroblast growth factor 17 | FGF8 synexpression member, mice lacking FGF17 have cerebellar defects and selective reduction in the size of the dorsal frontal cortex, but normal OB | One allelic defect is most likely not sufficient | Congenital hypogonadotropic hypogonadism |
| HS6ST1 | Heparan-sulfate 6-*O*-sulfotransferase 1 | An enzyme involved in 6O sulfation on glycosaminoglycan heparan sulfate, regulates neural branching *in vivo* in concert with other IHH-associated genes, including *kal-1*, the *FGF receptor*, and *FGF* | Heterozygous/homozygous mutations; complex inheritance patterns not readily conforming to Mendelian definitions of autosomal dominant or recessive transmission | IHH, KS, microphallus, unilateral cryptorchidism |

| | | | | |
|---|---|---|---|---|
| IL17RD | Interleukin 17 receptor D | FGF8 synexpression member, inhibits FGF signaling by acting both at the level of the FGF receptors (FGFR1 and FGFR2) and on downstream components of the Ras—extracellular-signal-regulated kinase (ERK)1/2 pathway by capturing active mitogen-activated protein kinase (MEK) and ERK complexes at the Golgi apparatus and inhibiting their dissociation | One allelic defect is most likely not sufficient | KS individuals and strongly linked to hearing loss |
| DUSP6 | Dual-specificity phosphatase 6 | FGF8 synexpression member, inhibits MAPK pathway by dephosphorylating and thereby inactivating MAP kinases | One allelic defect is most likely not sufficient | Congenital hypogonadotropic hypogonadism |
| SPRY4 | Sprouty homolog 4 | FGF8 synexpression member, inhibits MAPK pathway | One allelic defect is most likely not sufficient | Congenital hypogonadotropic hypogonadism |
| FLRT3 | Fibronectin leucine-rich transmembrane protein 3 | FGF8 synexpression member, stimulates FGFR by increasing ERK phosphorylation via intracellular domain interaction with FGFR | One allelic defect is most likely not sufficient | Congenital hypogonadotropic hypogonadism |
| NELF | Nasal embryonic LHRH factor | GnRH neuronal migration | Heterozygous mutation, mutation of one NELF allele may not be sufficient to result in disease | Normosmic IHH and KS |
| CHD7 (KAL5) | Chromodomain helicase DNA-binding protein-7 | Hydrolyze ATP to alter nucleosome structure (DNA wrapped in histones), two N-terminal chromodomains that function to bind histones, whereas SNF2/helicase domains are important in chromatin remodeling; CHD7 may function in DNA binding, transcription regulation, cell cycle regulation, apoptosis, and embryonic stem cell pluripotency | Predominantly inherited in an autosomal dominant manner | nIHH, KS + hearing loss, CHARGE syndrome: eye coloboma, heart malformations, atresia of the choanae, retardation of growth/development, genital anomalies, and ear abnormalities |

***Table 16.2***
*Genes incriminated in anosmic CIHH (KS) and normosmic CIHH.*

| *Gene* | *Gene product* | *Function* | *Inheritance* | *Clinical phenotype* |
|---|---|---|---|---|
| PROK2 | Ligand for G protein–coupled prokineticin receptor-2 | Effects on neuronal survival, gastrointestinal smooth muscle contraction, circadian locomotor rhythm, survival and migration of adrenal cortical capillary endothelial cells; in appetite regulation its anorectic effect is mediated partly by the melanocortin system; *PROK2* deficiency in mice leads to a loss of normal olfactory bulb architecture and accumulation of neuronal progenitors in the rostral migratory stream; PROK2 is a clock-controlled gene; PROK2-null mice show accelerated acquisition of food anticipatory activity during a daytime food restriction, exhibit reduced total sleep time predominantly during the light period, and also have an impaired response to sleep disturbance | Heterozygous mutations in most cases and homozygous in minority (or compound heterozygous) indicating a digenic or oligogenic mode of inheritance in heterozygous patients | IHH, KS, but not associated with hypopituitarism and septo-optic dysplasia |
| PROKR2 | G protein–coupled prokineticin receptor-2 | *Prokr2–/–* knockout mice exhibit early hypoplasia of the olfactory bulbs and severe atrophy of the reproductive organs in both sexes | Heterozygous mutations in most cases and homozygous in minority (or compound heterozygous), indicating a digenic or oligogenic mode of inheritance in heterozygous patients | IHH, KS, hypopituitarism and septo-optic dysplasia |
| WRD11 | WD repeat –containing protein 11 and also known as bromodomain and WD repeat –containing protein 2 (BRWD2) | Expressed in the developing olfactory and GnRH migratory pathway, as well as in the hypothalamus in adults; in addition, WDR11 protein was found to colocalize with EMX1 *in vivo* and *in vitro,* and three of the human mutations failed to bind EMX1 | Heterozygous missense mutations | nIHH, KS |

| | | | | |
|---|---|---|---|---|
| GPR54 | KISS1-derived peptide receptor/ kisspeptin receptor | G protein–coupled receptor for kisspeptin to stimulate GnRH release | Homozygous mutation in affected patients | nIHH |
| KISS1 | Metastin or kisspeptin | Ligand for GPR54 to stimulate gonadotropin release in several species by inducing GnRH secretion from hypothalamic GnRH neurons expressing GPR54 | Homozygous mutation in all affected family members as an autosomal recessive trait | nIHH |
| TACR3 | Neurokinin B receptor/NK3R | Coordinated activity with kisspeptin to regulate GnRH secretion | Most affected individuals are homozygous for loss-of-function mutations | nIHH |
| TAC3 | Neurokinin B | Substance P–related tachykinin family, coordinated activity with kisspeptin to regulate GnRH secretion | Most affected individuals are homozygous for loss-of-function mutations | nIHH |
| LEP | Leptin | Regulation of kisspeptin expression and involved in coordinating metabolic status with the reproductive axis | Homozygous mutations | Severe early-onset obesity with major hyperphagia associated with HH |
| LEPR | Leptin receptor | Regulation of kisspeptin expression and involved in coordinating metabolic status with the reproductive axis | Homozygous mutations | Severe early-onset obesity with major hyperphagia associated with HH |
| GnRH | Gonadotropin-releasing hormone | Ligand for GnRH receptor to induce signal transduction; GnRH is released from the hypothalamus and stimulates cells in the anterior pituitary to release LH and FSH | Homozygous frameshift mutation and heterozygous variants | nIHH |
| GnRHR | Gonadotropin-releasing hormone receptor | Secretion of LH and FSH in anterior pituitary | As the first gene involved in autosomal recessive normosmic IHH | nIHH |
| LHβ | Luteinizing hormone β | Triggers ovulation and development of the corpus luteum and stimulates production of testosterone | Compound heterozygous state | HH |

***Table 16.2* (Continued)**
*Genes incriminated in anosmic CIHH (KS) and normosmic CIHH.*

| *Gene* | *Gene product* | *Function* | *Inheritance* | *Clinical phenotype* |
|---|---|---|---|---|
| FSHβ | Follicle-stimulating hormone β | Regulates the development, growth, pubertal maturation, and reproductive processes of the body | homozygous mutations | HH |
| SEMA3A | Semaphorin-3A | A secreted guidance protein acting on neuropilin-1 with repulsive effects on primary olfactory axons and GnRH neurons | Autosomal dominant | KS |
| SOX10 | SOX10 | Transcription factor, maintenance of progenitor cell multipotency, lineage specification, cell differentiation, OEC development | *SOX10* mutations in the heterozygous state in both KS and WS individuals | KS individuals and strongly linked to hearing loss, pigmentation defects, intellectual disability, psychomotor delay |
| NR0B1 | DAX-1 | Act on both the hypothalamus and pituitary | X-linked | X-linked adrenal hypoplasia congenita and HH |

***Table 16.2*** **(Continued)**
*Genes incriminated in anosmic CIHH (KS) and normosmic CIHH.*

Structurally, *KAL1* is a modular protein comprising a large cysteine-rich N-terminal domain, a whey acidic protein (WAP)–like domain, four contiguous fibronectin-like type III (FnIII) repeats, and a small C-terminal domain rich in basic residues. The WAP domain is structurally similar to those of many serine protease inhibitors, whereas the FnIII repeats are structurally related to some cell adhesion molecules. Early indicators, gleaned from a human fetus carrying a chromosomal deletion at Xp22.3 that included *KAL1*, showed that GnRH cellular migration was abnormal, with GnRH neurons accumulating in the upper nasal region[50]; the olfactory bulbs were also absent. It was inferred that *KAL1* gene mutations led to the failure of the later phases of GnRH neuronal migration (GnRH neuronal arrest in the subcribriform plate area) coupled with failed olfactory bulb development.

Mutations in *KAL1* are mainly nonsense or frameshift mutations, or large gene deletions. They tend to be associated with a more severe KS phenotype, with anosmia and HH, a high frequency of cryptorchidism, microphallus, and small testes in males. All reported families with *KAL1* mutations and HH have exclusively anosmic HH. Indeed, in a patient with KS, a family history of normosmic HH makes an underlying *KAL1* mutation unlikely.

In the embryo, anosmin 1 is expressed in the interstitial matrix of the presumptive olfactory bulbs during the sixth embryonic week,[51] although it is also present in the olfactory pit epithelium. Such a distribution is consistent with a role of anosmin 1 in the initial stage of olfactory bulb morphogenesis, which occurs at the end of the sixth embryonic week. Evidence has accrued that anosmin 1 is a modulator of FGFR1 signaling,[52] with FGFR1 having an important role in the evagination of the olfactory bulbs from the neuroepithelial wall.[53]

# FGFR1 (KAL2) mutations

FGFR1, a member of the receptor tyrosine kinase superfamily located on chromosome 8, is also implicated in cell migration and has an obligatory requirement for heparin sulfate (as does anosmin 1) for its signaling. In the presence of heparan sulfate proteoglycans (HSPGs), FGF binds with high affinity to FGFR and induces receptor dimerization, thereby triggering transautophosphorylation of tyrosine residues in the intracellular domain. FGF signaling also controls cell proliferation, differentiation, and survival and thus plays essential roles in various processes of embryonic development. Several signaling proteins are phosphorylated in response to FGF stimulation (Shc, phospholipase Cγ, STAT1, Gabl, FRS2α), leading to activation of downstream signaling pathways that include Ras/mitogen-activated protein kinase (MAPK) and phosphatidylinositol-3 kinase/Akt pathways. FGF8 can activate the FGFR1c splice form of FGFR1.[54]

Both FGFR1 and anosmin 1 represent separate though interacting genes involved in GnRH neuronal migration to the hypothalamus. Although loss-of-function mutations in FGFR1 and *KAL1* can present with very similar phenotypes, FGFR1-related phenotypes are highly variable, with patients having both normosmic or anosmic forms of HH; indeed females with anosmia and normal reproductive function have been described with FGFR1 mutations.[55,56] Moreover, reversal of GnRH deficiency has even been reported in some male patients with FGFR1 mutations after therapy with testosterone.

# FGF8 mutations

Fibroblast growth factor 8 (FGF8) is one of the ligands for FGFR1. Mutations in FGF8 have been associated with KS in humans; in mice, homozygous mutation in FGF8 leads to absent hypothalamic GnRH neurons, whereas heterozygous mice had markedly fewer hypothalamic GnRH neurons.[57] As with FGFR1 mutations, humans with FGF8 mutations have a range of phenotypes, including adult onset HH.[58] In common with FGFR1 mutations, patients with FGF8 mutations have a cleft palate in 30% of cases and may also display ear, cartilage, and digital abnormalities (Table 16.3). The presence of these abnormalities in a patient with HH should raise suspicion for FGFR1/FGF8 mutation.

# PROKR2/PROK2

The clinical phenotypes of PROKR2/PROK2 mutations, encoding prokineticin receptor-2 and prokineticin-2, respectively, range from both classical KS to normosmic hypogonadotropic hypogonadism.[59] Nonreproductive phenotypes include fibrous dysplasia, bimanual synkinesia, and epilepsy. Patients with the more severe reproductive dysfunction tend to have biallelic mutations in PROK2/PROKR2 and fewer associated nonreproductive abnormalities. Patients with monoallelic mutations have less severe reproductive dysfunction and more nonreproductive abnormalities. The PROKR2 is a G protein–coupled receptor that binds to the ligand PROK2. Mouse *prok2* knockout models have small, abnormally shaped olfactory bulbs with an accumulation of neurons in the rostral migratory stream (RMS) between the subventricular zone and the olfactory bulb.[60]

| |
|---|
| Skeletal phenotypes |
| Cleft lip/palate |
| Dental agenesis |
| Absent nasal cartilage |
| External ear hypoplasia |
| Mandibular hypoplasia |
| Thoracic dystrophia |
| Asymmetry of limbs |
| Cubitus valgus |
| Syndactyly |
| Clinodactyly |
| Osteoporosis |
| Miscellaneous phenotypes |
| Synkinesia |
| Agenesis of corpus callosum |
| Frontal bossing |
| Hypertelorism |
| Iris Coloboma |
| Hearing loss |
| Epilepsy |
| Sleep disorder |
| Obesity |

***Table 16.3***
*Nonreproductive phenotypic abnormalities reported in patients with FGFR1 mutations.*

Putative loss-of-function mutations in *PROKR2* or *PROK2* have been detected in approximately 9% of the KS patients.[61–63] Most of these mutations are missense (loss-of-function) mutations, and many have also been found in apparently unaffected individuals, challenging their pathogenic role in the disease. Although the PROK2/PROKR2 system regulates various biological processes, including intestinal contraction, circadian rhythms, and vascular function, its role in GnRH neuronal migration remains unclear. It is not expressed in GnRH neurons.

## *CHARGE syndrome*

The CHARGE syndrome (Hall–Hittner syndrome) acronym stands for coloboma, heart malformations, atresia of the choanae, retardation of growth and development, genital anomalies, and ear anomalies (auditory and vestibular). In addition, HH may be present, and most if not all CHARGE patients have both olfactory bulb aplasia or hypoplasia, two KS-defining features.[64] CHARGE has an estimated birth incidence of 1 in 8500–12,000. Other infrequently occurring features include characteristic face and hand dysmorphia, hypotonia, arhinencephaly, semicircular canal agenesis or hypoplasia, hearing impairment, urinary tract anomalies, orofacial clefting, dysphagia, and tracheoesophageal anomalies. Multiple sets of diagnostic criteria for CHARGE syndrome have been proposed.[65]

The causative *CHD7* gene encodes a chromodomain (chromatin organization modifier domain) helicase DNA–binding protein expressed in the olfactory placode, which gives rise to GnRH neurons, spinal cord, nasopharynx, and eye. This protein may explain some of the organ involvement. Most patients are heterozygous for loss-of-function mutations in *CHD7*.

KS cases occurring in association with congenital heart disease or choanal atresia may represent unrecognized mild CHARGE cases. Additional traits shared between CHARGE and the *KAL2* (FGFR1) genetic form of KS include cleft lip or palate (present in 20%–35% of *KAL2* and CHARGE patients), external ear malformation (present in virtually all CHARGE patients and a few *KAL2* patients), agenesis of the corpus callosum, and coloboma. Because of the similarity between CHARGE and *KAL2* phenotypes, it is tempting to speculate that there are functional interactions between CHD7 and the FGFR1 signaling. Thus, IHH/KS may be a mild allelic form of the CHARGE syndrome; indeed, CHD7 has been designated as KAL5.

## *Kisspeptin and GPR54*

Kisspeptin, a peptide encoded by the gene KISS1, was originally described as a metastasis suppressor in melanoma and breast cancer.[66] It binds to GPR54, encoded by the gene *KISS1R*. The kisspeptin–KISS1R system is established as an important positive regulator of GnRH secretion, and in humans, intravenous kisspeptin acutely releases gonadotropins.[67] Loss-of-function mutations in GPR54/*KISS1R* in patients can cause both familial and sporadic forms of normosmic CIHH,[68,69] although they represent a rare cause of HH. Further studies in affected humans and in knockout mice have revealed that mutations in GPR54 resulted in normosmic (n)IHH with an autosomal recessive mode of inheritance. Although animal models have not conclusively demonstrated HH with loss of function in kisspeptin, a loss-of-function mutation leading to nIHH has been recently described in the kisspeptin gene *KISS1* in humans.[70]

Clinical and endocrinological evaluation of individuals with CIHH affected by mutations in GPR54 reveal low sex steroid levels and low gonadotropin levels. In males, micropenis and cryptorchidism are frequently noted, and in females primary amenorrhoea and partial breast development are evident. Exogenous gonadotropin therapy leads to testicular maturation, with the appearance of sperm in the ejaculate and subsequent fertility ruling out primary testicular dysfunction. Pulsatile GnRH therapy in affected females leads to ovulation and conception. These findings indicate that loss-of-function mutations in GPR54/*KISS1R* do not diminish the sensitivity of gonadotropic cells to GnRH nor the sensitivity of the gonads to gonadotropins. Thus, in humans as in mice, GPR54/*KISS1R* loss of function mainly appears to affect hypothalamic GnRH secretion, with no discernible direct effect on the pituitary or gonads. Patients with GPR54 defects demonstrate a markedly higher sensitivity to exogenous pulsatile GnRH than a cohort of CIHH patients receiving similar therapy; indeed, some patients retain a persistent pulsatile LH secretion with a normal frequency but a very low amplitude, suggesting that GPR54 inactivation impaired but did not prevent the neuroendocrine onset of puberty.

## GnRHR

Whereas KS genes are primarily involved in GnRH neuronal ontogeny, genes in which mutations lead to normosmic hypogonadotropic hypogonadism are involved in the regulation of the hypothalamic–pituitary–gonadal axis. GnRHR gene defects were the first identified cause of nonsyndromic CHH. Mutations in the GnRHR are responsible for roughly one fifth of the sporadic cases and about half of autosomal recessive inherited cases of nIHH, whereas mutations in the gene for GnRH have proven rare, accounting for about 1% of cases.[71] The most consistent characteristic of patients with GnRHR mutations is their pituitary resistance to pulsatile GnRH administration when the phenotype is severe and their spontaneous LH secretion is nonpulsatile. Mutations can affect GnRH binding, receptor activation, or interaction with coupled effectors, but it has also been shown that GnRHR protein misfolding with misrouting may also be caused by mutations and lead to loss of human GnRHR function. High-dose GnRH may elicit a response in partial forms, with an increase in the LH pulse amplitude, and occasional pregnancies have been reported after pulsatile GnRH administration.

## GnRH1 mutations as a cause of CIHH in humans

GnRH is crucial for regulating reproduction in mammals. It is synthesized by hypothalamic neurons and released from nerve endings into the portal circulation. After binding to the membrane GnRHR type 1 receptor, it stimulates gonadotropic cells of the anterior pituitary to synthesize and release LH and FSH, which in turn, stimulate synthesis and secretion of sex steroid hormones, and gametogenesis. Proof that GnRH mutations are involved in CIHH pathogenesis appeared in two reports in 2009.[72,73]

As would be anticipated, pulsatile GnRH administration restored the patient's ovarian function, as indicated by increased circulating estradiol and inhibin B levels and the appearance of a single dominant follicle seen on ultrasonography. Both index subjects were homozygous for the mutation, whereas their unaffected parents and sisters were heterozygous and had a normal reproductive phenotype.

## Leptin and LEPR mutations

Mutations in both leptin and leptin receptor (LEPR) are associated with HH in addition to obesity and hyperphagia.[6,7] In 300 patients studied with severe early-onset obesity and hyperphagia, 3% had a mutation in the LEPR. These subjects were characterized by altered immune systems and HH in addition to their obesity. Interestingly, they had relatively normal levels of leptin.

## DAX-1

X-linked congenital adrenal hypoplasia (CAH) is associated with normosmic HH, and the DAX-1 gene has been implicated in this relationship.[74] DAX-1 works during embryologic development to antagonize SRY and is therefore essential in sexual differentiation. It is also a transcriptional repressor of SF1.[75] DAX-1 encodes a nuclear receptor that is expressed in embryonic stem cells, steroidogenic tissues, the ventromedial hypothalamus, and the pituitary gonadotrophs. The adrenal failure reflects a developmental abnormality in the transition of the fetal to adult zone, resulting in mineralocorticoid and glucocorticoid deficiency, whereas the etiology of the HH involves a combined and variable deficiency of hypothalamic GnRH secretion and/or pituitary responsiveness to GnRH, resulting in low gonadotropins and low testosterone. Treatment with exogenous gonadotropins does not generally result in spermatogenesis. It is always the adrenal dysfunction that prompts investigation into the function of the hypothalamic–pituitary–gonadal axis as infants with CAH that are not recognized clinically are unlikely to survive until puberty.

## Neurokinin B and NKB receptor mutations

Neurokinin B (NKB/TAC3) and its receptor (NKBR/TAC3R) represent a further system whose malfunction is linked to normosmic (n)HH. NKB is highly expressed in the arcuate nucleus, a region of the brain that also expresses high levels of kisspeptin. In a study of four separate families with strong histories of nHH without known mutations in other CIHH genes, affected individuals were found to have homozygous mutations in either the TAC3 gene that encodes NKB or the TAC3R gene that encoded the NKBR.[76,77]

The anatomical and functional relationship between the GPR54/kisspeptin and NKB/NKBR has led to a greater understanding of the physiological regulation of GnRH release. Kisspeptin and NKB are directly involved in signaling between the arcuate nucleus and GnRH neurons and are found together with dynorphin 23 in these arcuate neurons. They may represent the GnRH pulse generator. Continuous kisspeptin infusion results in normal GnRH secretion in patients with loss-of-function mutations in TAC3 or TAC3R, suggesting that NKB is proximal to kisspeptin in the pathway for GnRH release possibly acting as a modulator of kisspeptin release.

NK3R is expressed on rodent GnRH-expressing neurons, and axons of neurons expressing neurokinin B are closely anatomically apposed to those of GnRH neurons within the median eminence where NKB-immunoreactive varicosities have been reported to be in direct contact with GnRH-immunoreactive axons. NKB expression is highest in the arcuate nucleus, where it colocalizes with estrogen receptor-α and dynorphin 23, both of which are involved in progesterone feedback in response to GnRH secretion.

## HS6ST1

Insights from studies of cell-specific overexpression of *kal-1* in a set of *Caenorhabditis elegans* interneurons that demonstrated a *kal-1*–dependent axonal branching phenotype prompted a genetic modifier screen that uncovered mutations in the *C. elegans* HS 6-*O*-sulfotransferase gene (*hst-6*) as suppressors of a *kal-1* gain-of-function phenotype. This finding supported earlier studies indicating that anosmin 1 required HS with specific 6-*O*-sulfate modifications for its *in vivo* action. Heparan 6-*O*-sulfation is also required for the function of FGFR1 and its ligand FGF8, with loss-of-function mutations in both genes being associated with human GnRH deficiency. The human *HS6ST1* homolog has been investigated as a candidate gene for GnRH deficiency, leading to the identification of mutations associated with reduced enzymatic activities in *in vivo* and *in vitro* HST6ST1 in 2% of IHH patients.[78]

## WDR11

By defining the chromosomal breakpoint of a balanced t(10;12) translocation from a subject with KS and scanning genes in its vicinity in unrelated hypogonadal subjects, *WDR11* has been identified as an autosomal dominant gene involved in human puberty. Six patients with a total of five different heterozygous WDR11 missense mutations, including three alterations (A435T, R448Q, and H690Q) in WD domains important for β propeller formation and protein–protein interaction, were identified.[79] WDR11 has been shown to interact with EMX1, a homeodomain transcription factor involved in the development of olfactory neurons; moreover, missense alterations in WDR11 reduce or abolish this interaction. These findings suggested that impaired pubertal development in these patients resulted from a deficiency of productive WDR11 protein interaction.

## FGF8 synexpression group

The hypothesis that mutations in genes encoding a broader range of modulators of the FGFR1 pathway might contribute to the genetics of CIHH as causal or modifier has been tested in a large group of IHH individuals and has revealed that mutations in members of the so-called FGF8 synexpression group, namely FGF17, IL17RD, DUSP6, SPRY4, and FLRT3, harbor potential loss-of-function mutations in CIHH patients.[80] On the basis of their protein–protein interaction patterns with proteins known to be altered in CIHH, FGF17 and IL17RD were predicted to be potentially important genes in IHH. Most of the FGF17 and IL17RD mutations altered protein function *in vitro*. IL17RD mutations were found only in KS individuals and were strongly linked to hearing loss (six of eight individuals). Mutations in genes encoding components of the FGF pathway were found to be associated with complex modes of CIHH inheritance acting primarily as contributors to an oligogenic genetic architecture underlying CIHH.

## SOX10

The transcription factor SOX10 plays an important role in the development of the neural crest and is involved in the maintenance of progenitor cell multipotency, lineage specification, and cell differentiation. Mutations in

SOX10 have been implicated in Waardenburg syndrome (WS), a rare disorder characterized by the association between pigmentation abnormalities and deafness. SOX10 mutations cause a variable phenotype that spreads over the initial limits of the syndrome definition. On the basis of findings of olfactory bulb agenesis in WS individuals, SOX10 was hypothesized to be also involved in KS. SOX10 loss-of-function mutations were found in approximately one third of KS individuals with deafness, indicating a substantial involvement in this clinical condition. Study of SOX10-null mutant mice revealed a developmental role of SOX10 in a subpopulation of glial cells called olfactory ensheathing cells. These mice showed an almost complete absence of these cells along the olfactory nerve pathway, as well as defasciculation and misrouting of the nerve fibers, impaired migration of GnRH cells, and disorganization of the olfactory nerve layer of the olfactory bulbs.[81]

## SEMA3A

Cosegregation between the KS phenotype and a heterozygous (i.e., autosomal dominant) SEMA3A deletion in a family with several affected members has been reported. If semaphorin 3A haploinsufficiency can be validated as causally linked to (irreversible) KS, this relationship would contrast with the situation in model mice, in which only homozygous knockout leads to a similar phenotype. Interestingly, none of the family members with KS reported had any other clinical neurological abnormalities, suggesting that the role of semaphorin 3A in neuronal migration is restricted in humans to the olfactory system development and GnRH neuron migration, despite its expression in other neuronal and non neuronal structures.[82]

## Ataxia, dementia, and HH

Whole-exome sequencing in a patient with ataxia and HH, followed by target sequencing of candidate genes in similarly affected patients, has revealed that the syndrome of ataxia, dementia, and HH can be caused by inactivating mutations in RNF216, or by a combination of mutations in RNF216 and OTUD4, linking disordered ubiquitination to neurodegeneration and reproductive dysfunction.[83]

## Reversible forms of CIHH

So-called reversible male forms of CIHH have been recognized for several decades[84,85] and have been demonstrated with several CIHH genotypes, including *KAL1*, *FGFR1*, the GnRH receptor (GnRHR) gene, and *PROKR2*.[86–88] In these patients, very late activation of pulsatile gonadotropin secretion (due to late activation of GnRH pulse generator, or gonadotroph responsiveness) occurs, such that gonadotropin secretion improves with time. This clinical variant, estimated to affect about 10% of cases, should be actively sought either by regular monitoring of testicular volumes, or periodic interruption of testosterone replacement therapy (TRT), and measurement of gonadotropins with 09.00 testosterone. It is evident that when reversible forms occur before 20 years of age in a euosmic subject with no identifiable mutations, an alternative diagnosis is severe constitutional pubertal delay.

## Oligogenic inheritance

Although normosmic CIHH and KS have long been considered as monogenic disorders with a Mendelian inheritance pattern, several cases of possible digenic/oligogenic inheritance in KS[44] have been reported. Such digenic inheritance has been shown in both KS and normosmic CIHH patients who bore mutations in both *PROKR2* and *PROK2,* in *FGFR1* and *NELF,* or in *GNRHR* as well as in *PROKR2,* and *GnRH1*, *GNRHR*, or *KISS1R*.[89] Defects in different genes could act synergistically to induce the CIHH or the KS phenotype, or to modify the severity of the GnRH deficiency, partially explaining the phenotypic variability observed within and across families with CHH and KS.

## When should clinical genetic testing be undertaken in KS?

Given the large array of genetic defects that may be causally linked to both normosmic CIHH and KS, what should be the clinician's approach to genetic testing in any one individual? The mode of inheritance is clearly of relevance and needs to be discussed with patients. In a study of eight KS genes in six pathways (KAL1, FGF8/FGFR1, PROK2/PROKR2, HS6ST1, NELF, and CHD7) conducted in 219 male and female patients with KS (not nHH), it was hypothesized that mutations in these six pathways would exhibit specific phenotypes that could be used to direct genetic testing.[90] Of 219 KS patients, 151 had rare sequence variants (RSVs) in at least one of these genes, and none was found in 68 patients. Several phenotypes were examined: reproductive phenotype, presence of unilateral renal agenesis, bimanual synkinesis, hearing loss, presence of cleft palate, dental agenesis, and skeletal anomalies. A severe reproductive phenotype was seen most commonly in *KAL1*, and renal agenesis in *KAL1* but also in the RSV-negative group. Synkinesia was seen in *KAL1* and *FGFR1* genotypes but also in other groups, including the RSV-negative groups, but not *HS6ST1*. Hearing loss was more common in the CHD7 versus non-CHD7 groups but was also seen in all other groups except *HS6ST1*. Cleft lip/palate was seen in all groups except KAL1 and PROK2/PROKR2. Dental agenesis was seen most commonly in the FGFR1/FGF8 group but also identified in the CHD7/RSV-negative group. Syndactyly, polydactyly, or camptodactyly were seen exclusively in the FGFR1/FGF8 group (Figure 16.3); scoliosis, kyphosis, excessive joint mobility, short fourth metacarpal bones, clinodactyly, foreshortened limb bones, and flat feet were seen in all groups.

# Treatment for CIHH

The treatment for both normosmic CIHH and KS is that of the resulting hypogonadism. Treatment is first to initiate virilization or breast development and second to develop fertility. Hormone replacement therapy, with testosterone for males and combined estrogen and progesterone for females, is required to stimulate the development of secondary sexual characteristics. When fertility is desired, either gonadotropins or pulsatile GnRH is used to obtain testicular growth and sperm production in males or ovulation in females, although less successfully in males who have a history of cryptorchidism. Both treatments restore fertility in the majority of affected individuals. It is still unknown whether transient hormone replacement therapy in affected male infants to simulate the postnatal surge in gonadotropins could have later salutary impact on their sexual life and reproductive prognosis.

# Treatment of HH in the male patient

## Testosterone replacement therapy

TRT is available in a variety of formulations for clinical use, including oral, injectable esters, transdermal patch, and gel preparations, each with its own unique pharmacokinetic profile. This topic is covered in Chapter 17. Treatment is commenced at a low dose initially and gradually increased at 6-month intervals to respect the normal cadence of puberty in the male. Tostran gel and Testim gel are particularly useful, allowing upward titration of the administered dose. Injectables (e.g., testosterone enanthate, 50 mg every month) are given for 9 months, and the dose is gradually escalated to the adult dose of 200 mg every 2–3 weeks over the course of 3–4 years.

## Induction of spermatogenesis

In men desirous of fertility, options for spermatogenesis induction include exogenous gonadotropins or pulsatile GnRH. GnRH substitution is more effective for hypothalamic than pituitary disorders, whereas administration of exogenous gonadotropins is suitable for patients with both pituitary and hypothalamic disorders. hCG, with its longer biological half-life, is used as an LH substitute, in conjunction with FSH in the form of either human menopausal gonadotropins, highly purified urinary FSH preparations, or recombinant FSH formulations (Gonal F, Puregon).

FSH is necessary for the maintenance of spermatogenesis, as evidenced by the findings in contraceptive trials using testosterone esters, where azoospermia was only attained in patients in whom serum FSH levels were fully suppressed.[91] In a subset of patients with HH and larger testicular size, spermatogenesis can be stimulated with hCG alone,[92] although it is likely that men with the fertile eunuch syndrome and sufficient endogenous FSH secretion to sustain normal spermatogenesis with hCG alone are well represented in this subgroup.

High intratesticular testosterone concentrations are essential for normal spermatogenesis. Thus, spermatogenesis can be induced by a combination of hCG and human menopausal gonadotropin (hMG), though not by a regimen of purified FSH and testosterone alone.[93]

## Exogenous gonadotropin therapy

Traditionally, FSH has been administered using hMG derived from the urine of postmenopausal women. In this preparation, FSH activity predominates and LH activity is low, necessitating combined administration with hCG to achieve fertility.[94] Highly purified urinary FSH preparations give enhanced specific activity in comparison to hMG (10,000 vs. 150 U/mg protein for hMG); however, these preparations have been superseded by recombinant human FSH (r-hFSH) formulations made in Chinese hamster ovary cells with a 48 ± 5 h half-life and devoid of intrinsic LH activity (Puregon, Gonal F).

Recombinant gonadotropins can be administered subcutaneously, a route that is as effective a mode of delivery as the intramuscular route, and is conducive to good compliance. hCG alone at a dose of 1000 U on alternate days, or 1500U twice weekly (with dosage titration based on trough testosterone levels), is given initially. With larger initial testicular volume, spermatogenesis can be initiated with hCG alone, most likely due to residual FSH secretion.[95,96]

Once there is a plateau in the response to hCG, and assuming no spermatozoa are seen in the ejaculate after 3–4 months of treatment, therapy with FSH (in one of the three forms described above) is added at a dose of 75 U on alternate days initially, increasing to daily, if necessary.[97,98] Continuation of this combined regimen for 12–24 months induces testicular growth in almost all patients, with spermatogenesis in a large proportion and pregnancy rates in the range of 50%–80%.[97,98] Better outcome can be expected with larger baseline testicular size, and absence of previous cryptorchidism gynecomastia is seen in up to 33% of patients on gonadotropin therapy, the consequence of excessive secretion of estrogen by Leydig cells in response to hCG, and is avoidable by using the lowest dose of hCG capable of maintaining serum testosterone levels toward the lower end of the normal range.[99,100]

Gonadotropin therapy of HH patients rarely generates sperm concentration in the World Health Organization (WHO) reference range. This result may be because initial "priming" of testes did not occur during the minipuberty and also because of the high incidence of undescended testes. Failure to achieve normal sperm counts does not preclude fertility, however, and in one study the median sperm concentration achieved at conception was reported to be 5 million/mL. The smaller the initial testicular volume, the longer the duration of treatment required, and it may take up to 24 months for spermatogenesis to be induced.

Given the aforementioned findings, it is sensible to start treatment 6–12 months before the time at which fertility is desired. Once pregnancy is achieved, therapy should be continued until at least the second trimester, and if a further conception is planned shortly thereafter, therapy with hCG alone should be continued. In contrast, if a longer interval is anticipated, testosterone therapy can be recommenced. The option of storing sperm for subsequent use in intrauterine insemination or intracytoplasmic sperm injection should also be discussed. In patients in whom the combination of hCG and FSH is required to induce spermatogenesis initially, treatment with hCG alone may be sufficient for subsequent pregnancies due to larger starting testicular size.

## Pulsatile GnRH therapy

The alternative to gonadotropin therapy is pulsatile administration of GnRH administered by a programmable, portable mini-infusion pump. Although intravenous administration produces the most physiologic GnRH pulse contour and ensuing LH response, the subcutaneous route is clearly more practical for the long-term treatment required to stimulate spermatogenesis. The frequency of GnRH administration recommended is every 2 h at a dose of 25–600 ng/kg/bolus, with the GnRH dose being titrated for each individual to ensure normalization of testosterone, LH, and FSH. Serum testosterone and gonadotropin levels should be monitored monthly, and once testicular volume reaches 8 mL, regular semen analyses are obtained.

The majority of patients require treatment for at least 2 years to maximize testicular growth and achieve spermatogenesis, although, similar to the response to gonadotropin therapy, the time taken to reach these endpoints tends to be shorter in patients with a larger initial gonadal size, and a poorer response is expected in patients with a history of bilateral cryptorchidism.

## Effect of postnatal gonadotropin therapy in males with HH

Because patients with HH may be diagnosed shortly after birth because of micropenis and cryptorchidism, combined with subnormal LH and FSH concentrations during the postnatal period, treating these patients with gonadotropins postnatally, to mimic physiological development, could improve testicular growth and fertility potential later in life. There has been one report of an HH male being treated by recombinant human LH and FSH in doses of 20 and 21.3 U s.c. twice weekly, respectively, from 7.9 to 13.7 months of age. During treatment, concentrations of LH, FSH, inhibin B, and estradiol increased to values within normal limits, whereas serum testosterone remained undetectable. Penile length increased from 1.6 to 2.4 cm and testicular volume, assessed by ultrasound, increased by 170%.[101]

# Management of HH in females

## Estrogen replacement therapy

Initial therapy is with ethinylestradiol 5 μg orally, for at least 6 months. A transdermal twice weekly estradiol patch may be used as an alternative. Treatment is continued until breakthrough bleeding occurs, after which cyclical therapy with medroxyprogesterone acetate 5 mg daily for 2 weeks is introduced. The dose of ethinyl estradiol is gradually increased over a 2- to 3-year period to a final dose of 20–30 μg daily.

## Gonadotropin therapy

Originally introduced more than 50 years ago, purified human urinary postmenopausalgonadotropins (HMGs) containing LH to FSH bioactivity of 1:1 have been successfully used to induce ovulation in hypogonadotropic hypogonadal states. The availability of purified and highly purified urinary FSH, and recombinant human FSH (rFSH, >99% purity), has largely superseded HMG and can be given subcutaneously with none of the batch-to-batch variability observed with HMG. The aim of ovulation induction with gonadotropins is the generation of a single dominant follicle.

## Step-up and step-down protocols

A conventional step-up gonadotropin protocol would involve a starting FSH dose of 37.5–75 U/day designed to allow the FSH threshold to be reached gradually, minimizing excessive stimulation and thereby reducing the risk of development of multiple follicles. The dose is increased only if, after 7 days, no response is documented on ultrasonography and serum estradiol monitoring. The dose is incrementally increased at weekly intervals by 37.5–75 U to a maximum of 225 U/day, and the response is then monitored by ultrasonic cycle tracking with measurement of endometrial thickness and follicular diameter.

In the step-down protocol, therapy with 150 U FSH/day is started until a dominant follicle (>10 mm) is seen on transvaginal ultrasonography, with the dose then being decreased to 112.5 U/day, followed by a further decrease to 75 U/day 3 days later, a dose that is continued until hCG is administered to induce ovulation.

Purified urinary FSH has some LH activity but rFSH does not. The experience with rFSH in hypogonadotropic hypogonadal women (WHO class 1) indicates that women who have very low serum LH concentrations (<0.5 U/L) need exogenous hCG (or 75 U/day s.c. recombinant LH) to maintain adequate estradiol biosynthesis and follicle development.

hCG at 5000–10,000 U i.m. is used to trigger ovulation when ovarian follicles >20 mm are achieved and the endometrium is >10 mm thick.[102]

## Cycle tracking

Transvaginal ultrasonography is used to measure follicular diameter and endometrial thickness, with an optimal scanning frequency of every 2 or 3 days in the late follicular phase. The criteria for follicle maturity are a follicle diameter of 18–20 mm and/or a serum estradiol >734 pmol/L/dominant follicle.

hCG is given on the day that at least one follicle appears to be mature. If three or more follicles >15 mm are present, stimulation is stopped, hCG is withheld, and a barrier contraceptive is advised to prevent multiple pregnancies and ovarian hyperstimulation. Preovulatory concentrations of estradiol above the normal range may predict ovarian hyperstimulation.

## Pulsatile GnRH therapy

Pulsatile administration of GnRH using an infusion pump stimulates the production of endogenous FSH and LH and can be used in patients whose HH is not caused by GnRHR loss-of-function mutations. The resulting serum FSH and LH concentrations remain within the normal range, so the chances of multifollicular development and ovarian hyperstimulation are low. The subcutaneous route can be used, and to mimic normal pulsatile GnRH release, the pulse interval is 60–90 min and the dose is 2.5–10 μg/pulse.[103–106] The lower dose should be used initially to minimize the likelihood of multiple pregnancies; the dose should then be increased to the minimum dose required to induce ovulation. Pulsatile GnRH administration may be discontinued after ovulation, and the corpus luteum supported by hCG.

## Outcomes

Ovulation rates of 90% and pregnancy rates of 80% have been reported in women treated with pulsatile GnRH. Local complications such as phlebitis may occasionally occur.

## References


1. Fromantin M, Gineste J, Didier A, et al. Impuberism and hypogonadism at induction into military service. Statistical study. *Probl Actuels Endocrinol Nutr* 1973; 16: 179–99.
2. Seminara SB, Hayes FJ, Crowley WF, Jr. Gonadotropin-releasing hormone deficiency in the human (idiopathic hypogonadotropic hypogonadism and Kallmann's syndrome): Pathophysiological and genetic considerations. *Endocr Rev* 1998; 19: 521–39.
3. Reynaud R, Barlier A, Vallette-Kasic S, et al. An uncommon phenotype with familial central hypogonadism caused by a novel PROP1 gene mutant truncated in the transactivation domain. *J Clin Endocrinol Metab* 2005; 90: 4880–7.
4. Netchine I, Sobrier ML, Krude H, et al. Mutations in LHX3 result in a new syndrome revealed by combined pituitary hormone deficiency. *Nat Genet* 2000; 25: 182–6.
5. Lin L, Gu WX, Ozisik G, et al. Analysis of DAX1 (NR0B1) and steroidogenic factor-1 (NR5A1) in children and adults with primary adrenal failure: Ten years' experience. *J Clin Endocrinol Metab* 2006; 91: 3048–54.
6. Clement K, Vaisse C, Lahlou N, et al. A mutation in the human leptin receptor gene causes obesity and pituitary dysfunction. *Nature* 1998; 392: 398–401.
7. Strobel A, Issad T, Camoin L, et al. A leptin missense mutation associated with hypogonadism and morbid obesity. *Nat Genet* 1998; 18: 213–15.
8. Goldstone AP, Holland AJ, Hauffa BP, et al. Recommendations for the diagnosis and management of Prader–Willi syndrome. *J Clin Endocrinol Metab* 2008; 93: 4183–97.
9. Dollfus H, Verloes A, Bonneau D, et al. Update on Bardet–Biedl syndrome. *J Fr Ophtalmol* 2005; 28: 106–12.
10. Quinton R, Barnett P, Coskeran P, et al. Gordon Holmes spinocerebellar ataxia: A gonadotropin deficiency syndrome resistant to treatment with pulsatile gonadotropin-releasing hormone. *Clin Endocrinol* 1999; 51: 525–9.
11. Schwanzel-Fukuda M. Origin and migration of luteinizing hormone-releasing hormone neurons in mammals. *Microsc Res Tech* 1999; 44: 2–10.
12. Schwanzel-Fukuda M, Pfaff DW. Origin of luteinizing hormone-releasing hormone neurons. *Nature* 1989; 338: 161–4.
13. Wray S. Development of luteinizing hormone releasing hormone neurones. *J Neuroendocrinol* 2001; 13: 3–11.
14. Wray S, Grant P, Gainer H. Evidence that cells expressing luteinizing hormone-releasing hormone mRNA in the mouse are derived from progenitor cells in the olfactory placode. *Proc Natl Acad Sci U S A* 1989; 86: 8132–6.
15. Murakami S, Seki T, Arai Y. Structural and chemical guidance cues for the migration of GnRH neurons in the chick embryo. *Prog Brain Res* 2002; 141: 31–44.
16. Muske L, Moore FL. Ontogeny of gonadotropin-releasing hormone neuronal systems in amphibians. *Brain Res* 1990; 534: 177–87.
17. Parhar IS. Cell migration and evolutionary significance of GnRH subtypes. *Prog Brain Res* 2002; 141: 3–17.
18. Muller F, O'Rahilly R. The human brain at stage 17, including the appearance of the future olfactory bulb and the first amygdaloid nuclei. *Anat Embryol* 1989; 180: 353–69.
19. Prevot V, Bellefontaine N, Baroncini M, et al. Gonadotropin-releasing hormone nerve terminals, tanycytes and neurohaemal junction remodelling in the adult median eminence: Functional consequences for reproduction and dynamic role of vascular endothelial cells. *J Neuroendocrinol* 2010; 22(7): 639–49.
20. Massa G, de Zegher F, Vanderschueren-Lodeweyckx M. Serum levels of immunoreactive inhibin, FSH, and LH in human infants at preterm and term birth. *Biol Neonate* 1992; 61(3): 150–5.
21. Andersson AM, Toppari J, Haavisto AM, et al. Longitudinal reproductive hormonal profiles in infants: Peak of inhibin B levels in infant boys exceeds levels in adult men. *J Clin Endoc Metab* 1998; 83(2): 675–81.
22. Sharpe RM, Fraser HM, Brougham MF, et al. Role of the neonatal period of pituitary-testicular activity in germ cell proliferation and differentiation in the primate testes. *Hum Reprod* 2003; 18(10): 2110–17.
23. Mann DR, Smith MM, Gould KG, et al. Effects of a gonadotropin-releasing hormone agonist on luteinizing hormone and testosterone secretion and testicular histology in male rhesus monkeys, Macaca fascicularis. *Fertil Steril* 1985; 43: 115–21.
24. Grumbach MM. A window of opportunity: The diagnosis of gonadotropin deficiency in the male infant. *J Clin Endocrinol Metab* 2005; 90: 3122–7.
25. Uriarte MM, Baron J, Garcia HB, et al. The effect of pubertal delay on adult height in men with isolated hypogonadotrophic hypogonadism. *J Clin Endo Metab* 1992; 74: 436–40.
26. Finkelstein JS, Klibanski A, Neer RM, et al. Osteoporoais in men with idiopathic hypogonadotrophic hypogonadism. *Ann Intern Med* 1987; 106: 354–61.
27. Caronia LM, Martin C, Welt CK, et al. A genetic basis for functional hypothalamic amenorrhea. *N Engl J Med* 2011; 364(3): 215–25.
28. Conrad B, Kriebel J, Hetzel WD. Hereditary bimanual synkinesis combined with hypogonadotropic hypogonadism and anosmia in four brothers. *J Neurol* 1978; 218: 263–74.

29. Schwankhaus JD, Currie J, Jaffe MJ, et al. Neurologic findings in men with isolated hypogonadotropic hypogonadism. *Neurology* 1989; 39: 223–6.
30. Pinto G, Abadie V, Mesnage R, et al. CHARGE syndrome includes hypogonadotropic hypogonadism and abnormal olfactory bulb development. *J Clin Endocrinol Metab* 2005; 90: 5621–6.
31. Quinton R, Duke V, de Zoysa P, et al. The neuroradiology of Kallmann's syndrome: A genotypic and phenotypic analysis. *J Clin Endocrinol Metab* 1996; 81: 3010–17.
32. Quinton R, Duke VM, Robertson A, et al. Idiopathic gonadotropin deficiency: Genetic questions addressed through phenotypic characterization. *Clin Endocrinol* 2001; 55: 163–74.
33. Mayston MJ, Harrison LM, Quinton R, et al. Mirror movements in X-linked Kallmann's syndrome. I. A neurophysiological study. *Brain* 1997; 120: 1199–216.
34. Krams M, Quinton R, Ashburner J, et al. Kallmann's syndrome: Mirror movements associated with bilateral corticospinal tract hypertrophy. *Neurology* 1999; 52: 816–22.
35. Kertzman C, Robinson DL, Sherins RJ, et al. Abnormalities in visual spatial attention in men with mirror movements associated with isolated hypogonadotropic hypogonadism. *Neurology* 1990; 40: 1057–63.
36. Santen RJ, Paulsen CA. Hypogonadotropic eunuchoidism. I. Clinical study of the mode of inheritance. *J Clin Endocrinol Metab* 1972; 36: 47–54.
37. Wegenke JD, Uehling DT, Wear JBJ, et al. Familial Kallmann syndrome with unilateral renal aplasia. *Clin Genet* 1975; 7: 368–81.
38. Murray J, Schutte B. Cleft palate: Players, pathways, and pursuits. *J Clin Invest* 2004; 113: 1676–8.
39. Molsted K, Kjaer I, Giwercman A, et al. Craniofacial morphology in patients with Kallmann's syndrome with and without cleft lip and palate. *Cleft Palate Craniofac J* 1997; 34: 417–24.
40. Lieblich JM, Rogol AD, White BJ, et al. Syndrome of anosmia with hypogonadotropic hypogonadism (Kallmann syndrome). *Am J Med* 1982; 73: 506–19.
41. Young J, Rey R, Couzinet B, et al. Antimüllerian hormone in patients with hypogonadotropic hypogonadism. *J Clin Endo Metab* 1999; 84(8): 2696.
42. Kirk J, Grant D, Besser G, et al. Unilateral renal aplasia in X-linked Kallmann's syndrome. *Clin Genet* 1994; 46: 260–2.
43. Klingmüller D, Duwes W, Krahe T, et al. Magnetic resonance imaging of the brain in patients with anosmia and hypothalamic hypogonadism (Kallmann's syndrome). *J Clin Endocrinol Metab* 1987; 65: 581–4.
44. Pitteloud N, Quinton R, Pearce S, et al. Digenic mutations account for variable phenotypes in idiopathic hypogonadotropic hypogonadism. *J Clin Invest* 2007; 117: 457–63.
45. Hardelin J-P, Dodé C. The complex genetics of Kallmann syndrome: KAL1, FGFR1, FGF8, PROKR2, PROK2, et al. *Sex Dev* 2008; 2: 181–93.
46. Salenave S, Chanson P, Bry H, et al. Kallmann's syndrome: A comparison of the reproductive phenotypes in men carrying *KAL1* and *FGFR1/KAL2* mutations. *J Clin Endocrinol Metab* 2008; 93(3): 758–6.
47. Legouis R, Hardelin JP, Levilliers J, et al. The candidate gene for the X-linked Kallmann syndrome encodes a protein related to adhesion molecules. *Cell* 1991; 67: 423–35.
48. Soussi-Yanicostas N, Hardelin J-P, Arroyo-Jimenez M, et al. Initial characterization of anosmin-1, a putative extracellular matrix protein synthesized by definite neuronal cell populations in the central nervous system. *J Cell Sci* 1996; 109: 1749–57.
49. Hu Y, Gonzalez-Martinez D, Kim S, et al. Cross-talk of anosmin-1, the protein implicated in X-linked Kallmann's syndrome, with heparan sulphate and urokinase-type plasminogen activator. *Biochem J* 2004; 384: 495–505.
50. Schwanzel-Fukuda M, Bick D, Pfaff DW. Luteinizing hormone-releasing hormone (LHRH)-expressing cells do not migrate normally in an inherited hypogonadal (Kallmann) syndrome. *Mol Brain Res* 1989; 6(4): 311–26.
51. Hardelin J-P, Julliard AK, Moniot B, et al. Anosmin-1 is a regionally restricted component of basement membranes and interstitial matrices during organogenesis: Implications for the developmental anomalies of X chromosome-linked Kallmann syndrome. *Dev Dyn* 1999; 215: 26–44.
52. Gonzalez-Martinez D, Kim S, Hu Y, et al. Anosmin-1 modulates fibroblast growth factor receptor 1 signaling in human gonadotropin-releasing hormone olfactory neuroblasts through a heparan sulfate-dependent mechanism. *J Neurosci* 2004; 24: 10384–92.
53. Hébert JM, Partanen J, Rossant J, et al. FGF signaling through FGFR1 is required for olfactory bulb morphogenesis. *Development* 2003; 130: 1101–11.
54. Zhang X, Ibrahimi OA, Olsen SK, et al. Receptor specificity of the fibroblast growth factor family. The complete mammalian FGF family. *J Biol Chem* 2006; 281: 15694–700.
55. Pitteloud N, Meysing A, Quinton R, et al. Mutations in fibroblast growth factor receptor 1 cause Kallmann syndrome with a wide spectrum of reproductive phenotypes. *Mol Cell Endocrinol* 2006; 254–255: 60–9.
56. Trarbach EB, Costa EM, Versiani B, et al. Novel fibroblast growth factor receptor 1 mutations in patients with congenital hypogonadotropic hypogonadism with and without anosmia. *J Clin Endocrinol Metab* 2006; 91: 4006–12.
57. Chung WC, Moyle SS, Tsai PS. Fibroblast growth factor 8 signaling through Fgf receptor 1 is required

for the emergence of gonadotropin-releasing hormone neurons. *Endocrinology* 2008; 149: 4997–5003.

58. Falardeau J, Chung WC, Beenken A, et al. Decreased FGF8 signaling causes deficiency of gonadotropin-releasing hormone in humans and mice. *J Clin Invest* 2008; 118: 2822–31.
59. Pitteloud N, Zhang C, Pignatelli D, et al. Loss-of-function mutation in the prokineticin 2 gene causes Kallmann syndrome and normosmic idiopathic hypogonadotropic hypogonadism. *Proc Natl Acad Sci U S A* 2007; 104: 17447–52.
60. Matsumoto S, Yamazaki C, Masumoto KH, et al. Abnormal development of the olfactory bulb and reproductive system in mice lacking prokineticin receptor PKR2. *Proc Natl Acad Sci U S A* 2006; 103: 4140–5.
61. Cole LW, Sidis Y, Zhang C, et al. Mutations in prokineticin 2 (PROK2) and PROK2 receptor 2 (PROKR2) in human gonadotropin-releasing hormone deficiency: Molecular genetics and clinical spectrum. *J Clin Endocrinol Metab* 2008; 93: 3551–9.
62. Monnier C, Dodé C, Fabre L, et al. *PROKR2* missense mutations associated with Kallmann syndrome impair receptor signalling-activity. *Hum Mol Genet* 2008; 18(1): 75–81.
63. Leroy C, Fouveaut C, Leclercq S, et al. Biallelic mutations in the prokineticin-2 gene in two sporadic cases of Kallmann syndrome. *Eur J Hum Genet* 2008; 16: 865–8.
64. Topaloglu AK, Kotan LD. Molecular causes of hypogonadotropic hypogonadism. *Curr Opin Obstet Gynecol* 2010; 22: 264–70.
65. Kim HG, Layman LC. The role of CHD7 and the newly identified WDR11 gene in patients with idiopathic hypogonadotropic hypogonadism and Kallmann syndrome. *Mol Cell Endocrinol* 2011; 346: 74–83.
66. Ohtaki T, Shintani Y, Honda S, et al. Metastasis suppressor gene KiSS-1 encodes peptide ligand of a G-protein-coupled receptor. *Nature* 2001; 411: 613–17.
67. Roa J, Aguilar E, Dieguez C, et al. New frontiers in kisspeptin/GPR54 physiology as fundamental gatekeepers of reproductive function. *Front Neuroendocrinol* 2008; 29: 48–69.
68. Seminara SB, Messager S, Chatzidaki EE, et al. The GPR54 gene as a regulator of puberty. *New Engl J Med* 2003; 349: 1614–27.
69. de Roux N, Genin E, Carel JC, et al. Hypogonadotropic hypogonadism due to loss of function of the KiSS1-derived peptide receptor GPR54. *Proc Natl Acad Sci U S A* 2003; 100: 10972–6.
70. Topaloglu AK, Tello JA, Kotan LD, et al. Inactivating KISS1 mutation and hypogonadotropic hypogonadism. *New Engl J Med* 2012; 366: 629–35.
71. Bianco SD, Kaiser UB. The genetic and molecular basis of idiopathic hypogonadotropic hypogonadism. *Nat Rev Endocrinol* 2009; 5: 569–76.
72. Bouligand J, Ghervan C, Tello JA, et al. Isolated familial hypogonadotropic hypogonadism and a GNRH1 mutation. *New Engl J Med* 2009; 360: 2742–8.
73. Chan YM, de Guillebon A, Lang-Muritano M, et al. GNRH1 mutations in patients with idiopathic hypogonadotropic hypogonadism. *Proc Natl Acad Sci U S A* 2009; 106: 11703–8.
74. Muscatelli F, Strom TM, Walker AP, et al. Mutations in the DAX-1 gene give rise to both X-linked adrenal hypoplasia congenita and hypogonadotrophic hypogonadism. *Nature* 1994; 372: 672–6.
75. Ito M, Yu R, Jameson JL. DAX-1 inhibits SF-1 mediated transactivation via a carboxy terminal domain that is deleted in adrenal hypoplasia congenital. *Mol Cell Biol* 1997; 17: 1476–83.
76. Topaloglu AK, Reimann F, Guclu M, et al. TAC3 and TACR3 mutations in familial hypogonadotropic hypogonadism reveal a key role for Neurokinin B in the central control of reproduction. *Nat Genet* 2009; 41: 354–8.
77. Guran T, Tolhurst G, Bereket A, et al. Hypogonadotropic hypogonadism due to a novel missense mutation in the first extracellular loop of the neurokinin B receptor. *J Clin Endocrinol Metab* 2009; 94: 3633–9.
78. Tornberga J, Sykiotisb GP, Keefe K, et al. Heparan sulfate 6-O-sulfotransferase 1, a gene involved in extracellular sugar modifications, is mutated in patients with idiopathic hypogonadotrophic hypogonadism. *Proc Nat Acad Sci U S A* 2011; 108(28): 11524–9.
79. Kim H, Ahn JW, Kurth I, et al. WDR11, a WD Protein that interacts with transcription factor EMX1, is mutated in idiopathic hypogonadotropic hypogonadism and Kallmann syndrome. *Am J Hum Genet* 2010; 87(4): 465–79.
80. Miraoi H, Dwyer AA, Sykiotis GP, et al. Mutations in FGF17, IL17RD, DUSP6, SPRY4, and FLRT3 are identified in individuals with congenital hypogonadotropic hypogonadism. *Am J Hum Genet* 2013; 92(5): 725–43.
81. Pingault V, Bodereau V, Baral V, et al. Loss-of-function mutations in SOX10 cause Kallmann syndrome with deafness. *Am J Hum Genet* 92(5): 707–24.
82. Young J, Metay C, Bouligand J, et al. SEMA3A deletion in a family with Kallmann syndrome validates the role of semaphorin 3A in human puberty and olfactory system development. *Hum Reprod* 2012; 27(5): 1460–5.
83. Margolin DH, Kousi M, Chan Y-M, et al. Ataxia, dementia and hypogonadotrophic hypogonadism caused by disordered ubiquitination. *N Eng J Med* 2013; 368: 1992–2003.
84. Quinton R, Cheow HK, Tymms DJ, et al. Kallmann's syndrome: Is it always for life? *Clin Endocrinol* 1999; 50: 481–5.
85. Raivio T, Falardeau J, Dwyer A, et al. Reversal of idiopathic hypogonadotrophic hypogonadism. *New Engl J Med* 2007; 357: 863–73.

86. Ribeiro RS, Vieira TC, Abucham J. Reversible Kallmann syndrome: Report of the first case with a Kal 1 mutation and literature review. *Eur J Endocrinol* 2007; 156: 285–90.
87. Pitteloud N, Acierno JS, Jr., Meysing AU, et al. Reversible Kallmann syndrome, delayed puberty, and isolated anosmia occurring in a single family with a mutation in the fibroblast growth factor receptor 1 gene. *J Clin Endocrinol Metab* 2005; 90: 1317–22.
88. Sinisi AA, Asci R, Bellastella G, et al. Homozygous mutation in the prokineticin-receptor 2 gene (Val274Asp) presenting as reversible Kallmann syndrome and persistent oligozoospermia: Case report. *Hum Reprod* 2008; 23: 2380–4.
89. Sykiotis GP, Plummer L, Hughes VA, et al. Oligogenic basis of isolated gonadotropin-releasing hormone deficiency. *Proc Natl Acad Sci U S A* 2010; 107: 15140–4.
90. Costa-Barbosa F, Balasubramanian R, Keefe KW, et al. Prioritizing genetic testing in patients with Kallmann syndrome using clinical phenotype. *J Clin Endo Metab* 2013; 98: E943–53.
91. Behre HM, Baus S, Kliesch S, et al. Potential of testosterone buciclate for male contraception: Endocrine differences between responders and nonresponders. *J Clin Endocrinol Metab* 1995; 80: 2394–403.
92. Burris AS, Rodbard HW, Winters SJ, et al. Gonadotropin therapy in men with isolated hypogonadotropic hypogonadism: The response to human chorionic gonadotropin is predicted by initial testicular size. *J Clin Endocrinol Metab* 1988; 66: 1144–51.
93. Schaison G, Young J, Pholsena M, et al. Failure of combined follicle-stimulating hormone-testosterone administration to initiate and/or maintain spermatogenesis in men with hypogonadotropic hypogonadism. *J Clin Endocrinol Metab* 1993; 77: 1545–9.
94. Buchter D, Behre HM, Kliesch S, et al. Pulsatile GnRH or human chorionic gonadotropin/human menopausal gonadotropin as effective treatment for men with hypogonadotropic hypogonadism: A review of 42 cases. *Eur J Endocrinol* 1998; 139: 298–303.
95. Finkel DM, Phillips JL, Snyder PJ. Stimulation of spermatogenesis by gonadotropins in men with hypogonadotropic hypogonadism. *N Engl J Med* 1985; 313: 651–5.
96. Vicari E, Mongioi A, Calogero AE, et al. Therapy with human chorionic gonadotropin alone induces spermatogenesis in men with isolated hypogonadotrophic hypogonadism—long-term follow-up. *Int J Androl* 1992; 15: 320–9.
97. Mannaerts B, Fauser B, Lahlou N, et al. Serum hormone concentrations during treatment with multiple rising doses of recombinant follicle stimulating hormone (Puregon) in men with hypogonadotropic hypogonadism. *Fertil Steril* 1996; 65: 406–10.
98. European Metrodin HP Study Group. Efficacy and safety of highly purified urinary follicle-stimulating hormone with human chorionic gonadotropin for treating men with isolated hypogonadotropic hypogonadism. *Fertil Steril* 1998; 70: 256–62.
99. Liu PY, Turner L, Rushford D, et al. Efficacy and safety of recombinant human follicle stimulating hormone (Gonal-F) with urinary human chorionic gonadotropin for induction of spermatogenesis and fertility in gonadotropin-deficient men. *Hum Reprod* 1999; 14: 1540–5.
100. Liu L, Banks SM, Barnes KM, et al. Two-year comparison of testicular responses to pulsatile gonadotropin-releasing hormone and exogenous gonadotropins from the inception of therapy in men with isolated hypogonadotropic hypogonadism. *J Clin Endocrinol Metab* 1988; 67: 1140–5.
101. Main KM, Schmidt IM, Toppari J, et al. Early postnatal treatment of hypogonadotropic hypogonadism with recombinant human FSH and LH. *Eur J Endocrinol* 2002; 146(1): 75–9.
102. Ludwig M, Doody KJ, Doody KM. Use of recombinant human chorionic gonadotropin in ovulation induction. *Fertil Steril* 2003; 79: 1051.
103. Martin KA, Hall JE, Adams JM, Crowley WF Jr. Comparison of exogenous gonadotropins and pulsatile gonadotropin-releasing hormone for induction of ovulation in hypogonadotropic amenorrhea. *J Clin Endocrinol Metab* 1993; 77: 125.
104. Jansen RP. Pulsatile intravenous gonadotropin releasing hormone for ovulation induction: Determinants of follicular and luteal phase responses. *Hum Reprod* 1993; 8(Suppl 2): 193.
105. Martin K, Santoro N, Hall J, et al. Clinical review 15: Management of ovulatory disorders with pulsatile gonadotropin-releasing hormone. *J Clin Endocrinol Metab* 1990; 71: 1081A.
106. Filicori M, Flamigni C, Dellai P, et al. Treatment of an ovulation with pulsatile gonadotropin-releasing hormone: Prognostic factors and clinical results in 600 cycles. *J Clin Endocrinol Metab* 1994; 79: 1215.

# 17

# Hypogonadism, erectile dysfunction, and infertility in men

*Pierre-Marc G. Bouloux, Shalender Bhasin*

## *Hypogonadism in men*

Hypogonadism is a multisystem syndrome associated with impaired androgen production or action. Androgen deficiency can result from abnormalities of testicular function (primary hypogonadism), hypothalamic or pituitary regulation of testicular function (secondary hypogonadism), or impairment of androgen action at the target tissue (androgen resistance).

Failure to diagnose and treat androgen deficiency can have potentially serious health consequences. It is important to screen for androgen deficiency, because hypogonadism may be a manifestation of a serious underlying disease such as a pituitary tumor or some other systemic illness such as human immunodeficiency virus (HIV) infection. Left untreated, severe androgen deficiency may result in osteoporosis and increased risk of fracture,[1–6] loss of muscle mass (sarcopenia) and function,[2,7–9] impaired sexual function,[10–15] lowered mood and energy level,[7] increased fat mass (particularly in the visceral fat compartment),[16–20] and insulin resistance.[16–20]

## *Frequency of androgen deficiency*

Androgen deficiency is a common disorder that frequently remains undetected because the symptoms of androgen deficiency in adult men are often nonspecific.[21,22] For instance, in the Massachusetts Male Aging Study,[21,22] 4% of men, aged 40–70 years, who were asymptomatic had serum testosterone levels less than 150 ng/dL (4.5 nmol/L) in association with increased luteinizing hormone (LH) levels (indicative of primary gonadal malfunction). The symptoms commonly attributed to androgen deficiency, such as decreased sexual desire and activity and low energy, did not demonstrate a high correlation with low testosterone levels.[21,22]

In the European Male Aging Study (EMAS), a random population of 3369 men aged between 40 and 79 years were surveyed, with data collected for subjects' general, sexual, physical, and psychological health.[23] Levels of total testosterone were measured in morning samples by mass spectroscopy, and free testosterone was computed using the Vermeulen formula. Symptoms of poor morning erections, low sexual desire, erectile dysfunction, inability to perform vigorous physical activity, depression, and fatigue were significantly related to the testosterone level. Increased probabilities of the three sexual symptoms and reduced physical vigor were discernible with total testosterone levels of 8–13 nmol/L (2.3–3.7 ng/mL) and free testosterone levels of 160–280 pmol/L (46–81 pg/mL). Using these data, Wu et al. proposed that late-onset hypogonadism (LOH) could be defined by the presence of at least three sexual symptoms, associated with a total testosterone level of less than 11 nmol/L (3.2 ng/mL) and a free testosterone level of less than 220 pmol/L (64 pg/mL). Using these criteria, it was found that only 2.1% of men in the population studied could be classified as having LOH.[24]

A high index of suspicion is therefore the key to diagnosis. It is important to recognize that while men presenting with loss of sexual desire and function and diminished secondary sex characteristics should undoubtedly be screened for androgen deficiency, the Massachusetts Male Aging Study[21,22] demonstrated that these symptoms are uncommon in middle-aged men with androgen deficiency. If screening was triggered only by the presence of these symptoms, a significant

| The following groups of men have high prevalence of androgen deficiency and warrant measurement of serum testosterone levels: |
|---|
| 1. Men with loss of sexual desire and function |
| 2. Men with loss of secondary sex characteristics |
| 3. Men with delayed pubertal development |
| 4. Men being evaluated for infertility |
| 5. Men with erectile dysfunction |
| 6. Men presenting with minimal trauma fracture before the age of 50 |
| 7. Men with chronic illness such as that associated with HIV infection, chronic obstructive lung disease, and end-stage renal disease |
| 8. Men being treated with medications that impair testosterone production or action |
| 9. Men over the age of 60 |

***Table 17.1***
*Clinical states that are associated with a high prevalence of androgen deficiency and warrant screening.*

number of hypogonadal men would remain undiagnosed. Since the following patient groups have a high prevalence of low testosterone levels, they should be screened for androgen deficiency (Table 17.1):

1. Patients presenting with delayed sexual development may have constitutional delay of puberty, primary or secondary hypogonadism, or one of a variety of other causes; testosterone levels should be measured in all such patients.
2. Men presenting with infertility. Approximately 10% of men presenting with infertility have Klinefelter's syndrome,[25,26] and an additional 1%–3% have hypogonadotropic hypogonadism.
3. Men younger than the age of 50 presenting with minimal trauma fractures. Minimal trauma fractures are uncommon in men younger than age 50,[6,7] but when they do occur in younger men, impaired androgen secretion or action is often a contributory cause.
4. Men with chronic illness. There is a high prevalence of low testosterone levels in men with chronic illness,[27–36] such as that associated with HIV infection,[27–32] end-stage renal disease,[33–35] and chronic obstructive pulmonary disease (COPD).[36] Testosterone replacement increases lean body mass and muscle strength in HIV-infected men with weight loss and low testosterone levels.[37–39]
5. Men being treated with medications that impair testosterone secretion, alter its metabolism, or attenuate its action. Particular attention should be paid to the use of glucocorticoids,[40,41] ketoconazole,[42,43] megestrol acetate,[44,45] gonadotropin-releasing hormone agonists,[46,47] neuropsychiatric drugs,[48–50] cancer chemotherapeutic drugs, and long-term opiate use.
6. Men over the age of 60. Serum testosterone levels progressively decrease with advancing age,[1,51–57] so that by age 60, approximately 25% of men have serum testosterone levels in the hypogonadal range. Testosterone replacement therapy in older men with low-normal testosterone levels is associated with gains in lean body mass, reduction in fat mass, and increased muscle strength and bone mineral density.[56–63]
7. Men presenting with erectile dysfunction. Eight percent of men presenting with erectile dysfunction have low testosterone levels.[53,64–71] Androgen deficiency and erectile dysfunction are two common, but independently distributed, clinical disorders in middle-aged and older men.[53,64–71]

Although attempts have been made to generate disease-specific questionnaires to detect older male candidates for testosterone testing[72,73] (e.g., Morley developed and validated a 10-question Androgen Deficiency in Aging Males [ADAM] scale; see Table 17.2), in practice they tend to lack specificity, although many have considerable sensitivity.

## *Evaluation*

### *History*

The diagnostic workup of androgen deficiency is initiated by an assessment of the general health of the patient, because systemic illness is frequently associated with low testosterone levels (Figure 17.1). Twenty to thirty percent of men infected with HIV have previously been

| Questions Used as Part of the Saint Louis University ADAM Questionnaire |
|---|
| 1. Do you have a decrease in libido (sex drive)? |
| 2. Do you have a lack of energy? |
| 3. Do you have a decrease in strength and/or endurance? |
| 4. Have you lost height? |
| 5. Have you noticed a decreased "enjoyment of life"? |
| 6. Are you sad and/or grumpy? |
| 7. Are your erections less strong? |
| 8. Have you noticed a recent deterioration in your ability to play sports? |
| 9. Are you falling asleep after dinner? |
| 10. Has there been a recent deterioration in your work performance? |

*Source:* Table reprinted with permission from Morley JE, et al., Validation of a screening questionnaire for androgen deficiency in aging males. *Metabolism* 49(9): 1239–42, 2000.
*Note:* A positive questionnaire result is defined as a "yes" answer to questions 1 or 7 or any three other questions.

***Table 17.2***
*A 10-question Androgen Deficiency in Aging Males (ADAM) questionnaire, developed and validated by Morley.*

reported to have low testosterone levels,[27–32] although with more effective antiretroviral therapy, the prevalence is probably lower nowadays.

Similarly, a substantial proportion of patients with COPD,[36] diabetes mellitus (type 2 diabetes), end-stage renal disease,[33–35] and many types of cancer have low testosterone levels.

It is important to evaluate lifestyle factors and substance abuse, because they can be associated with androgen deficiency. Eating disorders, excessive exercise, and recreational drug abuse (e.g., opiates) are often associated with both delayed pubertal development and hypogonadism in adults.[74–76]

The energy balance and the hypothalamic control of the reproductive axis are intimately linked. Excessive exercise is associated with hypogonadotropic hypogonadism, probably as a consequence of increased central corticotropin-releasing hormone tone, the degree of gonadotropin deficiency being correlated with the magnitude of energy drain.[75]

Weight loss in patients with anorexia nervosa is associated with functional gonadotropin-releasing hormone (GnRH) deficiency, hypogonadotropic hypogonadism, and slow GnRH pulse frequency.[75,76] Leptin is believed to be one of the biochemical links between energy stores and the central regulation of reproduction.[77]

Use of recreational drugs such as alcohol, marijuana, opiates, and cocaine can be associated with hypogonadotropic hypogonadism.[78,79] Alcohol has inhibitory effects at all levels of the hypothalamic–pituitary–testicular axis. The physician should inquire about the use of glucocorticoids,[40,41] ketoconazole,[42,43] cancer chemotherapeutic agents, GnRH agonists and antagonists,[46,47] and neuroleptic agents,[49,50] or a previous history of pelvic irradiation. Pharmacological doses of glucocorticoids inhibit LH and follicle-stimulating hormone (FSH) secretion by multiple mechanisms and also directly inhibit testicular synthesis of testosterone.[40,41] Ketoconazole is an inhibitor of several P450-linked steroidogenic enzymes in the testosterone biosynthetic pathway, including CyP450scc.[42,43] Androgen deficiency and subfertility are well-known, frequent, long-term complications of cancer chemotherapy. Many antipsychotic and antidepressant drugs are associated with hyperprolactinemia that can cause hypogonadotropic hypogonadism.[49,50]

The physician should inquire about early-morning erections, frequency of sexual thoughts, intensity of sexual feelings, and frequency of sexual acts such as masturbation and intercourse. Overall frequency of sexual acts and libido are decreased in androgen-deficient men.[7,10–15] However, young, hypogonadal men retain the ability to achieve erections in response to visual erotic stimuli.[13] Mood and energy level should be ascertained; men with acquired androgen deficiency often report decreased energy and increased irritability ("grumpiness").[80] Androgen replacement improves positive aspects of mood and reduces irritability in androgen-deficient men.[80]

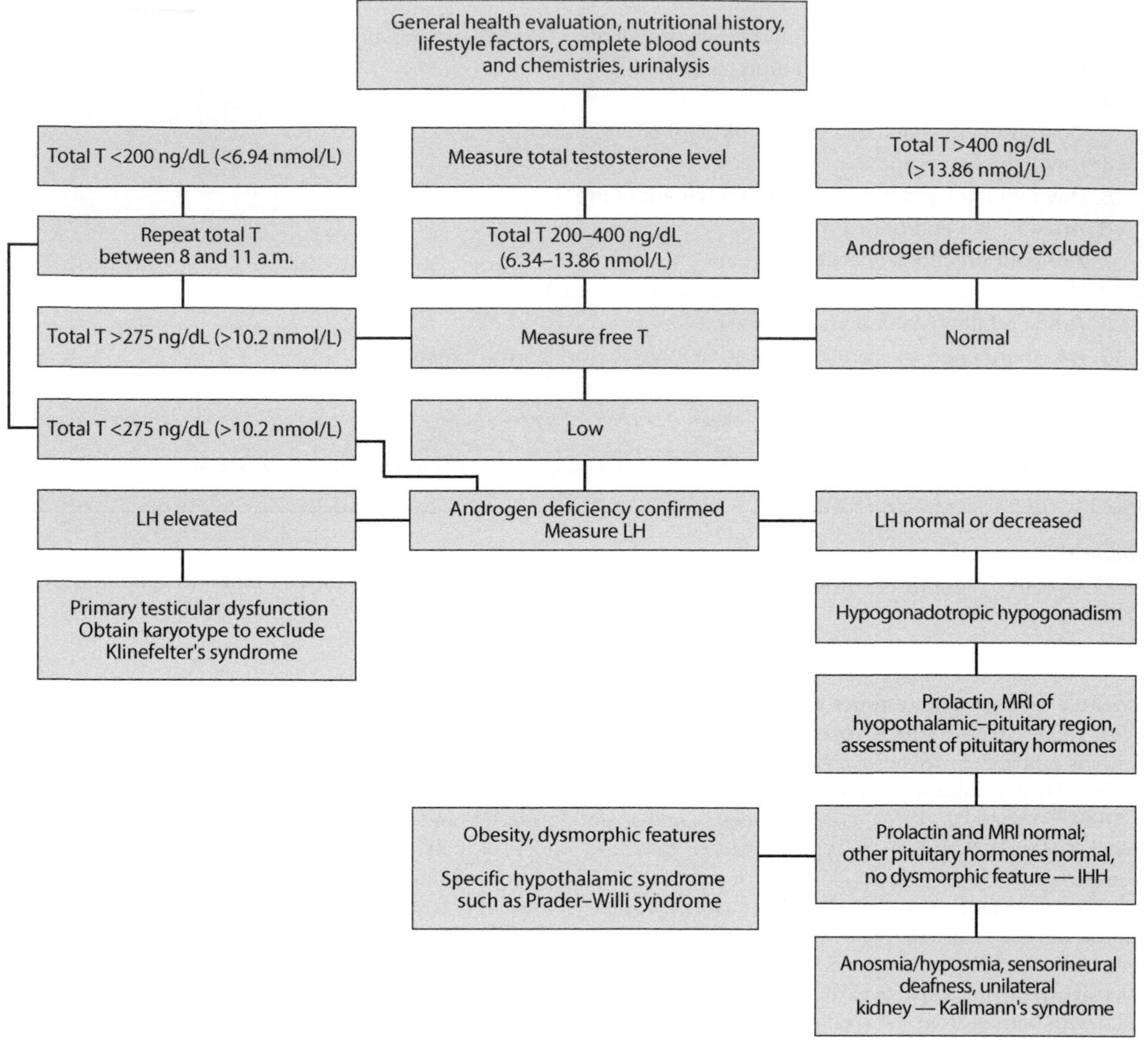


***Figure 17.1***
*An algorithmic approach to the diagnosis of androgen deficiency. T, testosterone; IHH, idiopathic hypogonadotropic hypogonadism.*

## *Physical examination*

In addition to the general physical examination, attention should be focused on assessing secondary sex characteristics such as hair growth, testicular volume, breast enlargement, prostate size and consistency, height, and span and body proportions (to look for eunuchoidism, where span exceeds height and lower segment length exceeds upper segment length). Hair growth in the beard, chest, and pubic regions is androgen dependent. There are ethnic differences in the intensity of hair growth (e.g., a paucity of facial and body hair in the Chinese).

Testicular volume can be measured by using a Prader orchidometer and taking note of testicular consistency and any inguinal scars pertaining to previous orchidopexy operations for cryptorchidism. Patients with Klinefelter's syndrome have markedly reduced testicular volumes (1–2 mL).[25,26]

In men with congenital hypogonadotropic hypogonadism, testicular volume is a good marker of the degree of gonadotropin deficiency and the likelihood of response to therapy.[81,82] In general, men with idiopathic hypogonadotropic hypogonadism (IHH) whose testicular volume is less than 4 mL have more severe gonadotropin deficiency and are less likely to respond to human chorionic gonadotropin (hCG) alone than those with testicular volumes greater than 8 mL.

Androgen deficiency can be associated with breast enlargement in men, although gynecomastia is more often due to other causes such as liver and kidney disease, medication, or physiological hormonal changes during the neonatal period, puberty, and old age. Breast enlargement may also occur after both institution of androgen replacement therapy and pharmacological administration such as in body building. The propensity to gynecomastia reflects underlying aromatase activity.

### Inactivating mutations of the LH receptor gene

Inactivating mutations of the LH receptor gene are associated with hypogonadism and Leydig cell hypoplasia.[92,93] Several families with resistance to LH action due to inactivating mutations of the LH receptor have been reported. Men with LH receptor mutations present with a spectrum of phenotypic abnormalities ranging from feminization of external genitalia in 46,XY males to Leydig cell hypoplasia, primary hypogonadism, and delayed sexual development. In a patient with Leydig cell hypoplasia and hypogonadism, a T-to-A mutation in position 1874 of the LH receptor gene was found.[94] Testicular histology in this man revealed the absence of mature Leydig cells; the seminiferous tubules had thickened basal lamina and spermatogenic arrest at the elongated spermatid stage.[95] Female members of the kindred with LH receptor mutation revealed normal development of secondary sex characteristics, increased LH levels, and amenorrhea.

### Inactivating mutations of the FSH receptor gene

It would be expected that a loss-of-function mutation of the gene for the human FSH receptor (2p21) would be associated with hypergonadotropic ovarian dysgenesis. In 1995, a search for linkage in multiple affected Finnish families reported finding a C566T transition predicting an Ala189Val substitution. This mutation segregated perfectly with the disease phenotype of primary amenorrhea, arrest of follicular development, and infertility.[96] Expression of the gene in transfected cells showed almost no signal transduction. Compared with similar patients with ovarian dysgenesis who did not have the mutation, patients with the mutation were shorter and had more ovarian follicles.[97] In contrast to females, males with this mutation were fertile but had reduced sperm counts. Population studies have shown this mutation in about 1% of Finns, with geographical enrichment suggestive of a founder effect.

To date, five additional inactivating mutations have been described, including cases with double heterozygosity of mutations. The clinical features are slightly different, apparently due to differences in residual activity in the mutated proteins.

### Laboratory evaluation

A full blood count, including hemoglobin, urea and electrolytes, creatinine, fasting blood glucose, aspartate aminotransferase (AST), alanine aminotransferase (ALT), bilirubin, alkaline phosphatase, and urinalysis, should be performed as part of the general health evaluation.

The measurement of total serum testosterone level, preferably in an early-morning sample obtained between 8 and 11 a.m., remains the best biochemical test for the diagnosis of androgen deficiency. A total serum testosterone level of less than 200 ng/dL (7 nmol/L) in an early-morning serum sample in association with consistent symptoms is evidence of testosterone deficiency. An early-morning serum testosterone level greater than 350 ng/dL (12 nmol/L) makes the diagnosis of androgen deficiency unlikely. In men with serum testosterone levels between 200 and 350 ng/dL (7–12 nmol/L), the measurement of total testosterone level should be repeated, and the free testosterone level should be measured. In older men, and in patients with Klinefelter's syndrome and those in other clinical states that are associated with increased sex hormone–binding globulin (SHBG) levels, measurements of total testosterone level may underestimate the degree of testosterone deficiency. In these patients, an indirect calculation of free and bioavailable testosterone using the Vermeulen formula (this requires knowledge of the SHBG and albumin levels), or, if available, a direct measurement of the free testosterone level can be useful in unmasking testosterone deficiency.

Serum LH levels should be measured in men with low testosterone levels, because it can help in determining whether the site of lesion is in the testis or at the hypothalamic–pituitary site. Men with androgen deficiency can be classified as hypergonadotropic (high LH) or hypogonadotropic (low or inappropriately normal LH) based on their LH levels. An elevated LH level indicates a lesion at the testicular level. Common causes of primary testicular failure include Klinefelter's syndrome, HIV infection, uncorrected cryptorchidism, cancer chemotherapeutic agents, radiation, surgical orchiectomy, and prior infectious orchitis. A karyotype should be determined to exclude Klinefelter's syndrome in men with low testosterone and elevated LH levels.

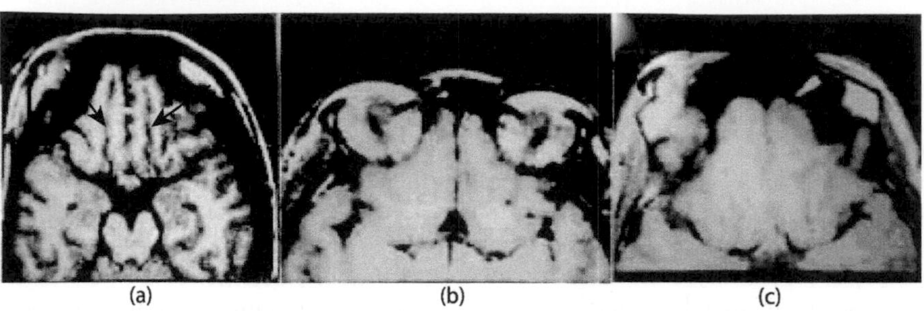


**Figure 17.2**
*MRI scans of a normal person and two patients with Kallmann's syndrome. (a) MRI section of a normal brain, with well-developed rhinencephalon and olfactory sulcus (arrows). (b and c) Sections of the rhinencephalon from patients with idiopathic hypogonadotropic hypogonadism and anosmia, showing poorly developed olfactory bulbs and absence of olfactory sulci. (From Klingmuller D et al.,* J Clin Endocrinol Metab, 65*, 581–4, 1987.)*

Men who have low testosterone levels but "inappropriately normal" or low LH levels have hypogonadotropic hypogonadism, their defect residing at the hypothalamic–pituitary site.[83] The causes of hypogonadotropic hypogonadism include space-occupying lesions of the hypothalamic–pituitary site, hyperprolactinemia, eating disorders, iron overload states such as hemochromatosis and hemosiderosis, excessive exercise, substance abuse, chronic illness, and a number of hypothalamic syndromes characterized by hypogonadotropic hypogonadism.[83] (See Chapter 16).

In men with hypogonadotropic hypogonadism, the physician should verify or exclude the presence of systemic illness, eating disorders, excessive exercise, and substance abuse. Serum prolactin level should be measured, and a magnetic resonance imaging (MRI) scan of the hypothalamic–pituitary region with a contrast agent should be obtained. Measurement of serum prolactin and MRI scan of the hypothalamic–pituitary region can help exclude the presence of a space-occupying lesion. Serum iron, transferrin saturation, and ferritin levels can be measured to exclude iron overload states such as hemochromatosis. Patients in whom all other detectable causes of hypogonadotropic hypogonadism have been excluded are classified as having IHH. Some men with IHH have hyposmia or anosmia, cleft palate, digital abnormalities, coloboma, and/or a single kidney, many of these associated features being pathognomonic of Kallmann's syndrome (Figure 17.2).[84] Several hypothalamic syndromes are associated with hypogonadotropic hypogonadism; these syndromes are recognized by a pattern of associated dysmorphic features (see chapter 16 on the inherited causes of IHH).

## *When should free testosterone levels be measured?*

Measurement of free testosterone levels can be useful in diagnosing androgen deficiency in men with alterations in SHBG levels.[85–88] Most of the circulating testosterone is bound to SHBG and albumin; only 0.5%–2.0% of circulating testosterone is unbound or "free." Total testosterone levels are affected by the prevalent SHBG concentrations. Alterations in SHBG levels due to normal aging,[85,86] obesity,[89,90] some types of medications, or chronic illness such as chronic liver disease, or on a congenital basis, can confound interpretation of total testosterone levels. Therefore, measurement of free testosterone levels, presumably reflecting the biologically active fraction, can be useful in the conditions discussed in the following subsections, particularly if the total testosterone levels are in the borderline zone.

### *Obesity*

Obese men have decreased SHBG levels. Most mildly to moderately obese men have lower serum total testosterone levels due to decreased SHBG concentrations;[89,90] their free testosterone concentrations are normal. Severely obese men may have hypogonadotropic hypogonadism due, in part, to increased estradiol levels (the result of increased aromatization of testosterone by adipose tissue) that suppress LH and FSH secretion.[90]

### *Older men*

Serum SHBG concentrations are increased in older men.[85,86] Therefore, total testosterone levels underestimate the degree of age-related decline in serum testosterone levels.

| Method | Potential merits and demerits | Utility |
|---|---|---|
| Tracer analog methods | These methods are affected by SHBG concentrations and therefore do not provide a true index of "free" testosterone | They are convenient to perform but should not be used because of concerns about validity |
| Equilibrium dialysis using tracer or direct measurement of dialyzed testosterone | Free testosterone levels measured by equilibrium dialysis have good clinical correlation. The equilibrium dialysis methods are technically demanding, affected by dialysis conditions, and available only from a few commercial laboratories | They are clinically useful if performed in a reliable laboratory |
| Bioavailable testosterone level (unbound plus albumin-bound testosterone fraction) | Measurement of bioavailable testosterone levels by ammonium sulfate precipitation has good clinical correlation | Clinically useful if performed in a reliable laboratory. The method is available only from a few commercial laboratories |
| Calculation of free testosterone levels by measurement of total testosterone and SHBG levels | Total testosterone and SHBG levels can be measured accurately and precisely by direct immunoassays. The validity of the algorithms used to calculate free testosterone from total testosterone and SHBG concentrations in men with chronic illness has not been established | Useful in healthy, young men, but validity not established in different illnesses that might affect SHBG concentrations and binding |

**Table 17.3**
*Methods for the measurement of serum-free testosterone levels.*

### *Chronic illness*

Serum SHBG concentrations are increased in HIV-infected men[27] and in some types of liver disease (e.g., cirrhosis associated with hepatitis C infection), but they may be decreased in men with nephrotic syndrome.

### *Hyperthyroidism*

SHBG concentrations are increased in hyperthyroidism, which is often associated with a raised total testosterone level.

## *The methods for free testosterone measurement (Table 17.3)*

Measurements of serum-free testosterone levels are fraught with difficulty and are not recommended as a general screening test. Serum-free testosterone levels should be measured only in specific clinical situations, as described in this chapter, and measurements should be obtained (1) from a reliable laboratory that has experience with the assay and (2) by using an appropriate assay that is not affected by the SHBG concentration.

The tracer analog methods are relatively inexpensive and convenient, but they are dependent on SHBG concentrations and, therefore, do not provide a true index of "free" testosterone.[88] They should not be used because of concerns about validity. Gas chromatography–mass spectrometry (GC-MS), although not available in routine laboratories, holds the greatest promise for accuracy and sensitivity, especially when measuring lower levels.

Free testosterone levels measured by equilibrium dialysis have good clinical correlation.[87,88] The equilibrium dialysis methods are technically demanding, affected by dialysis conditions, and available from only a few commercial laboratories.

Measurement of bioavailable testosterone levels by the ammonium sulfate precipitation method has good clinical correlation.[86]

Free testosterone concentrations can also be calculated from total testosterone and SHBG concentrations by using previously published algorithms. Total testosterone and SHBG levels can be measured accurately and precisely by direct immunoassays. The validity of the algorithms used to calculate free testosterone from total testosterone and SHBG concentrations in men with chronic illness has not been established; this method may be useful in healthy, young men, but its validity has not been established in different illnesses that might affect SHBG concentrations and binding.

## Treatment of androgen deficiency

Testosterone replacement therapy can be administered by using one of several available formulations with appropriate attention to its pharmacokinetics (Table 17.4). The benefits of testosterone replacement therapy have only been demonstrated in men who have androgen deficiency, as indicated by serum testosterone levels that are distinctly below the lower limit of the normal male range.

The dose of testosterone that is optimum for replacement is unknown, because we do not know the dose dependency of various androgen-dependent physiological processes. Although serum testosterone concentrations that are at the lower end of the normal male range can normalize sexual function in men, it is not clear whether low-normal testosterone levels can maintain bone mineral density and muscle mass. We also do not know whether serum testosterone concentrations in the high-normal range that might restore bone mineral density will adversely affect insulin sensitivity or plasma lipids. In light of these uncertainties, the current recommendation is to restore serum testosterone levels to the mid-normal range.

### Clinical pharmacology of the available androgen formulations and key points about testosterone replacement therapy (Table 17.4)

Testosterone replacement therapy should be guided in part by an understanding of the clinical pharmacology of the formulation used. Testosterone serves as a prohormone, and it is converted in the body to 17β-estradiol by the enzyme CyP450 aromatase and to 5α-dihydrotestosterone by the enzyme 5α-reductase. The effects of testosterone on bone resorption, plasma lipids, gonadotropin inhibition, and certain organizational effects on the brain require its conversion to estradiol. Similarly, 5α reduction of testosterone to 5α-dihydrotestosterone is obligatory for mediating its effects on the genital skin, the scrotum, the prostate, and the scalp. It is generally believed that testosterone may have direct effects on muscle and bone formation, since patients with 5α-reductase deficiency generally have good musculature. Therefore, while evaluating testosterone formulations, it is important to ascertain that the formulation being used can achieve physiological estradiol and dihydrotestosterone concentrations in addition to mid-normal testosterone concentrations.

### Orally administered, 17α-alkylated derivatives of testosterone (17α-methyltestosterone)

Testosterone is well absorbed after its oral administration, but it is quickly degraded during its passage through the liver. Therefore, it is not possible to achieve sustained blood levels of testosterone after oral administration of crystalline testosterone. 17α-Alkylated derivatives of testosterone are relatively resistant to hepatic degradation and can be given orally; however, because of the potential for hepatotoxicity, these formulations should not be used for testosterone replacement.[98,99] Hereditary angioedema due to C1 esterase deficiency is the only exception to this general recommendation; in this condition, oral 17α-alkylated androgens are useful because they stimulate hepatic synthesis of the C1 esterase inhibitor.

### Injectable testosterone esters

The esterification of testosterone at the 17β-hydroxy position makes the molecule hydrophobic and extends its duration of action.[100–102] De-esterification of testosterone esters occurs quickly in plasma, is not limiting, and cannot account for the long duration of action. It is the slow release of testosterone ester from its oily depot in the muscle that accounts for its extended duration. The longer the side chain and hydrophobicity of the ester, the greater the duration of action. Thus, testosterone enanthate and cypionate, with longer side chains, have longer durations of action compared to testosterone propionate.

Within 24 h after intramuscular administration of 200 mg testosterone enanthate or cypionate, serum testosterone levels rise into the high-normal or supraphysiological range and then gradually decline into the hypogonadal range over the next 2 weeks.[101,102] A bimonthly regimen of testosterone enanthate or cypionate results in "highs" and "lows" in serum testosterone levels that are attended by changes in the patient's mood, sexual desire, and activity and energy levels.

| Formulation | Regimen | Pharmacokinetic profile | DHT and estradiol | Advantages | Disadvantages |
|---|---|---|---|---|---|
| Testosterone enanthate or cypionate | 100 mg IM weekly or 200 mg IM every 2 weeks | After a single IM injection, serum testosterone levels rise into the supraphysiological range and then decline gradually into the hypogonadal range by the end of the dosing interval[101–103] | DHT and estradiol levels rise in proportion to the increase in testosterone levels. T/DHT and T/E2 ratios do not change | Corrects symptoms of androgen deficiency; relatively inexpensive, if self-administered; flexibility of dosing | Requires IM injection; peaks and valleys in serum testosterone levels |
| Scrotal testosterone patch[104,105] | One scrotal patch designed to nominally deliver 6 mg over 24 h, applied daily | Normalizes serum testosterone levels in many but not all androgen-deficient men | Serum estradiol levels are in the physiological male range, but DHT levels rise into the supraphysiological range. T/DHT ratio is significantly lower than in healthy men | Corrects symptoms of androgen deficiency | To promote optimum adherence of the patch, scrotal skin needs to be shaved; high DHT levels |
| Nongenital transdermal system[107,108] | One or two patches, designed to nominally deliver 5–10 mg testosterone over 24 h, applied daily on nonpressure areas | Restores serum testosterone, DHT, and estradiol levels into the physiological male range | T/DHT and T/estradiol levels are in the physiological male range | Ease of application, corrects symptoms of androgen deficiency, and mimics the normal diurnal rhythm of testosterone secretion. Lesser increase in hemoglobin than injectable esters | Serum testosterone levels in some androgen-deficient men may be in the low-normal range; these men may need application of two patches daily; skin irritation at the application site may be a problem for some patients |

**Table 17.4**
*Clinical pharmacology of the available androgen formulations and key points about testosterone replacement therapy.*

| *Formulation* | *Regimen* | *Pharmacokinetic profile* | *DHT and estradiol* | *Advantages* | *Disadvantages* |
|---|---|---|---|---|---|
| Testosterone gel | Testosterone gel containing 50–100 mg testosterone should be applied daily | Restores serum testosterone and estradiol levels into the physiological male range | Serum DHT levels are higher and T/DHT ratios are lower in hypogonadal men treated with the testosterone gel than in healthy eugonadal men | Corrects symptoms of androgen deficiency, provides flexibility of dosing, ease of application, good skin tolerability | Potential of transfer to a female partner or child by direct skin-to-skin contact; moderately high DHT levels |
| 17α-methyl testosterone[109] | Orally active, 17-α-alkylated compound that should not be used because of potential for liver toxicity | Orally active | | | Clinical responses variable; potential for liver toxicity; should not be used for treatment of androgen deficiency |

***Table 17.4*** **(Continued)**
*Clinical pharmacology of the available androgen formulations and key points about testosterone replacement therapy.*

The kinetics of testosterone enanthate and cypionate are identical. The serum levels of estradiol and dihydrotestosterone (metabolites that are derived by conversion from testosterone) are normal if testosterone replacement is physiological.

The recent introduction of intramuscular testosterone undecanoate (Nebido, Bayer, Leverkusen, Germany; 1 g) provides a convenient preparation with a long duration of action[103,104] The first two injections are given at an interval of 6 weeks, and thereafter at 3-month intervals. Nebido is made up in a 4 cc preparation that must be administered as a deep intramuscular injection. Occasional patients have reported coughing following injection, possibly the consequence of circulating oily droplets.

## Testosterone transdermal systems

Three transdermal testosterone patches are now commercially available: a scrotal testosterone patch (Testoderm, ALZA Corporation, Palo Alto, CA, USA) and two nongenital patches (Androderm, Watson-TheraTech, Salt Lake City, UT, USA; and Testoderm TTS, ALZA Corporation) (Table 17.4).

### *The scrotal transdermal system*

The scrotal transdermal system, when applied daily on the scrotal skin, can produce mid-normal serum testosterone levels in hypogonadal men 4–8 h after application of the patch, followed by a gradual decrease in serum testosterone levels over the next 24 h.[105] Serum estradiol levels are normal, but dihydrotestosterone levels are high in hypogonadal men treated with the scrotal testosterone patch, presumably due to the high rates of 5α reduction of testosterone to dihydrotestosterone during passage through the scrotal skin. Because testosterone effects on the prostate are mediated through its metabolite, dihydrotestosterone, there was initial concern that long-term exposure to high serum dihydrotestosterone levels might have deleterious effects on the prostate. However, long-term follow-up of men treated with the scrotal patch has not revealed an unusual increase in prostate problems.[106]

### *Nongenital patches*

One or two nongenital patches can be applied on the nonscrotal skin. Serum testosterone and estradiol levels are in the mid-normal range 4–12 h after application of the patch.[100,107] Unlike the scrotal patch, the nongenital patch produces physiological levels of serum dihydrotestosterone. Sexual function and a sense of well-being are restored in androgen-deficient men treated with the nongenital patch.

The transdermal systems are more expensive than testosterone esters. The expense of testosterone esters is increased if injections are given in a medical office; however, nearly all patients or their close family members can be taught to administer the injections. The use of nongenital patches may be associated with skin irritation in some individuals; the frequency of local skin reactions is greater with the Androderm patch than with the Testoderm patch.

### *Testosterone gel*

The US Food and Drug Administration (FDA) has approved a testosterone hydroalcoholic gel for the treatment of classical hypogonadism in men. The testosterone gel is available in 2.5 and 5 g unit doses that nominally deliver 25 and 50 mg of testosterone, respectively, to the application site. Initial pharmacokinetic studies[108] have demonstrated that 50, 75, and 100 mg doses applied daily to the skin can raise and maintain serum total and free testosterone concentrations into the mid- to high-normal range in healthy, hypogonadal men. Serum total and free testosterone concentrations are uniform throughout the 24 h application period.

The current recommendations are to start with a 75 mg dose and to adjust the dose based on the measurement of serum testosterone levels. If steady-state total testosterone concentrations exceed 800 ng/dL (>30 nmol/L) on this dose, the dose should be reduced to 50 mg daily. Conversely, if the serum testosterone concentrations are lower than 500 ng/dL (<18.7 nmol/L), then the dose should be increased to 100 mg daily.

The relative advantages of the testosterone gel are its ease of application, its invisibility after application, and the flexibility of dosing. The major concern about the use of the gel is the potential for transfer to one's sexual partner and to children, who may come in close contact with the patient. Initial studies have shown that significant transfer can occur to the female partner after vigorous and direct skin-to-skin contact. Less than 5% of treated individuals reported skin irritation at the application site.

Tostran (Prostakan) gel contains 2% testosterone (10 mg/mL) in a 60 g multidose dispenser and has been used successfully as a transcutaneously active preparation[109] delivery. The excipient contains butylhydroxytoluene and propylene glycol, and it overcomes the inconvenience of "one dose fits all." The site of application is the intact skin of the abdomen or inner thighs, preferably in the morning. Hands must be washed after application, and the application site should not be washed for 2 h.

### Testosterone undecanoate

This testosterone ester, when administered orally in oleic acid, is absorbed preferentially through the lymphatics into the systemic circulation and is spared first-pass degradation through the liver. Doses of 40–80 mg, given two or three times daily, are typically used. However, the clinical responses are variable in different individuals and on different days in the same individual. Serum dihydrotestosterone-to-testosterone ratios are higher in hypogonadal men treated with oral testosterone undecanoate, as compared to healthy eugonadal men.

### Testosterone implants

Implants of crystalline testosterone have been used for androgen replacement in men and women for over 60 years. The implants are inserted in the subcutaneous tissue (in the abdominal wall or buttock) by means of a trocar through a small skin incision after administration of a local anesthetic. Testosterone is released by surface erosion from the implant and absorbed into the systemic circulation. Four to six 200 mg implants can maintain serum testosterone concentrations in the mid- to high-normal range for up to 6 months. The need for skin incision for insertion and removal, spontaneous extrusions (2%–5%), and fibrosis at the site of implant insertion are potential drawbacks of this formulation.

## Novel androgen formulations

A number of novel androgen formulations with better pharmacokinetics or more selective activity profiles are under development. These novel delivery systems may provide greater convenience, a better physiological testosterone profile, or a longer duration of action. A biodegradable testosterone microsphere formulation has been shown to provide physiological testosterone levels for 10–11 weeks.

Efforts to develop nonsteroidal, selective androgen receptor modulators (SARMs) with defined properties represent a most exciting development. In a manner analogous to selective estrogen receptor modulators such as raloxifene, it may be possible to administer androgen agonists that exert the desired physiological effects on muscle, bone, and sexual function, but do not adversely affect the prostate and the cardiovascular system.

## *Contraindications for androgen administration in men*

Testosterone replacement is contraindicated or should be administered with caution in men with certain androgen-sensitive clinical disorders.

#### Prostate cancer

Prostate cancer is an androgen-dependent tumor, and androgen administration may promote tumor growth. Although testosterone administration is absolutely contraindicated in men with a history of active prostate cancer, in those who have had early disease eradicated by either radical prostatectomy or radiotherapy, testosterone replacement can be considered with careful monitoring of the prostate-specific antigen (PSA) level.

#### Benign prostatic hypertrophy with severe symptoms

Testosterone replacement can be administered safely to men with benign prostatic hypertrophy who have mild to moderate symptom scores. Androgen deficiency is associated with decreased prostate volume, and androgen replacement increases prostate volumes in those in age-matched controls.[110–112] In patients with preexisting, severe symptoms of benign prostatic hypertrophy, even small increases in prostate volume during testosterone administration may exacerbate obstructive symptoms. In these men, testosterone should either not be administered or be administered with caution, with careful and frequent monitoring of obstructive symptoms.

#### Erythrocytosis

Testosterone replacement, particularly when administered through the intramuscular route, is associated with an increase in red cell mass, presumably through its effects on erythropoietin and stem cell proliferation.[113–116]

Therefore, testosterone replacement should not be administered to men with a baseline hematocrit of 52% or greater without appropriate evaluation and treatment of erythrocytosis.

#### Sleep apnea

Testosterone can induce sleep apnea or exacerbate preexisting sleep apnea because of its neuromuscular effects on the upper airway,[117–122] and it should not be given to men with severe obstructive sleep apnea without appropriate evaluation and treatment of the sleep apnea.

#### Breast cancer

Because testosterone is converted to estrogen, it is contraindicated in patients with breast cancer.

## *Monitoring androgen replacement therapy*

Tables 17.5 and 17.6 list the clinical outcomes and laboratory tests that should be monitored in order to assess the adequacy and safety of testosterone replacement therapy.

| |
|---|
| Restoration and maintenance of sexual function |
| Induction and maintenance of secondary sex characteristics such as hair growth |
| Restoration of energy and sense of well-being |
| Restoration of serum testosterone level in the mid-normal range for healthy, eugonadal men |

**Table 17.5**
*Assessment of treatment efficacy.*

| |
|---|
| Clinical |
| Clinical evaluation should focus on ascertaining the presence of: |
| Breast tenderness or enlargement |
| Acne and oiliness of skin |
| Symptoms of sleep apnea |
| Symptoms of benign prostatic hypertrophy |
| Digital rectal examination for prostatic enlargement or nodules |
| Biochemical |
| Hemoglobin level |
| Serum PSA |

**Table 17.6**
*Monitoring of adverse effects.*

**Frequency of monitoring**
Evaluations of the clinical effectiveness and safety of testosterone replacement therapy should be performed 3 and 6 months after initiating testosterone therapy and annually thereafter.

## *Establishing the efficacy of testosterone replacement therapy (Table 17.5)*

### *Target testosterone levels*

We do not have a clinically useful biological marker of androgen action. The complexities of the diurnal, pulsatile, and circannual rhythms of testosterone make it difficult to mimic the endogenous pattern of testosterone secretion. Therefore, restoration of serum testosterone levels into the mid-normal range remains the goal of therapy.[107] Serum testosterone level should be measured 3 months after initiating therapy to assess the adequacy of therapy. In patients being treated with testosterone enanthate or cypionate, serum testosterone levels should be 400–700 ng/dL (15–26 nmol/L) 1 week after the injection. If nadir levels 14 days after the injection are low, the interval between injections may be shortened; a less preferred option is to increase the dose. In men on chronic transdermal therapy, serum testosterone levels 4–12 h after the patch application should be mid-normal. If serum testosterone levels are lower than 450 ng/dL (17 nmol/L) 4–8 h after patch application, the dose should be increased to two patches daily. In men being treated with testosterone gel, serum testosterone levels should be 450–800 ng/dL (17–30 nmol/L). If serum testosterone levels are outside this range, the dose should be appropriately adjusted.

### *Clinical evidence of efficacy*

Restoration of sexual function, secondary sex characteristics, energy level, and a sense of well-being are important objectives of testosterone replacement therapy. Therefore, it is important to ask the patient about sexual desire and activity, whether the patient has early-morning erections, and whether he is able to achieve and maintain erections that are adequate for sexual intercourse.

Some hypogonadal men continue to complain of sexual dysfunction even after testosterone replacement has been instituted; these patients can benefit from counseling. Hypogonadal men with prepubertal onset of androgen deficiency who are started on testosterone in their late 20s or their 30s may find it difficult to cope with their newfound sexuality and need counseling. If the patient has a sexual partner, it is crucial to include the partner in counseling because of the dramatic physical and sexual changes that occur with androgen treatment.

Facial hair growth in response to androgen replacement is variable and depends on the patient's racial background.

### *LH and FSH levels*

The usefulness of LH and FSH levels to assess the adequacy of testosterone replacement remains questionable. In men with hypergonadotropic hypogonadism, particularly those with Klinefelter's syndrome, it is uncommon for serum LH and FSH levels to be normalized by physiological replacement doses of testosterone that restore sexual function. Similarly, measurements of LH and FSH levels are not useful in men with hypogonadotropic hypogonadism, because in these men the feedback relationship between serum testosterone and LH secretion is perturbed because of the underlying hypothalamic–pituitary disorder.

### *Bone mineral density*

Institution of testosterone replacement therapy is associated with an increase in bone mineral density in androgen-deficient men. Men with IHH who have closed epiphyses experience an increase in cortical bone density, while those with open epiphyses demonstrate increases in both cortical and trabecular bone density after testosterone treatment. In adult men with androgen deficiency acquired after the completion of pubertal development, testosterone replacement induces an improvement primarily in the trabecular bone density. The bone density is, however, not normalized in most hypogonadal men by physiological testosterone replacement. The clinical utility of following bone mineral density in androgen-deficient men has not been demonstrated.

### *Body composition assessment*

Testosterone treatment is associated with an increase in lean body mass and muscle strength;[123–126] however, measurements of body composition are not clinically indicated at this time.

## *Monitoring potential adverse experiences (Table 17.6)*

Men receiving androgen replacement therapy should be monitored for potential adverse effects.

### *Hemoglobin levels*

Administration of testosterone to androgen-deficient men is typically associated with a 3%–5% increase in hemoglobin levels. Clinically significant polycythemia is uncommon in young hypogonadal men, but it can occur in men with sleep apnea, a significant smoking history, or COPD; in such patients, hemoglobin levels should be closely monitored after institution of testosterone replacement therapy. Testosterone administration in older men is associated with greater increments in hemoglobin than those observed in young, hypogonadal men. The magnitude of hemoglobin increase during testosterone therapy appears to be related to the magnitude of the peak serum testosterone levels. Testosterone replacement by means of a transdermal system has been reported to produce a lesser increase in hemoglobin levels than that associated with testosterone esters.

### *Digital examination of the prostate, and serum PSA levels (Table 17.7)*

Testosterone replacement therapy increases prostate volume and PSA levels to those seen in age-matched controls, but continued androgen treatment does not further increase prostate volume beyond that expected for age.[106,110-112,127,128] There is no evidence that testosterone replacement causes prostate cancer. However, androgen can exacerbate preexisting prostate cancer and should not be administered to men with a history of active prostate cancer. Many older men harbor microscopic foci of cancer in their prostates. In addition, older men with prostate cancer may have low testosterone levels.[129] We do not know whether long-term testosterone administration to older men will unmask microscopic foci of prostate cancer. This uncertainty is the main reason for periodic PSA measurements in men receiving testosterone replacement therapy.

Serum PSA levels are lower in testosterone-deficient men and are restored to normal following testosterone replacement;[106,110,127,128,130] however, serum PSA levels do not increase progressively in healthy hypogonadal men with replacement doses of testosterone. In two recent placebo-controlled trials of testosterone administration in older men, the change in serum PSA levels over a 3-year treatment period was not significantly different between placebo and testosterone-treated men.

Serum PSA levels tend to fluctuate when measured repeatedly in the same individual over time. Therefore, when serum PSA levels in androgen-deficient men on testosterone replacement therapy show a change from a previously measured value, the clinician has to decide whether the change warrants detailed evaluation of the patient for prostate cancer, or whether it is simply due to test-to-test variability in PSA measurement. The data from the Finasteride Study for Benign Prostatic Hypertrophy demonstrated that the 95% confidence interval for the change in PSA values measured 3–6 months apart is 1.4 ng/mL. Therefore, a change in PSA of >1.5 ng/mL between any two values measured 3–6 months apart in the same patient should be verified by a repeat PSA measurement. If the repeated measurement confirms a change of >1.5 ng/mL from the previous value, then that patient should be referred for urological evaluation. In addition, in patients in whom sequential PSA measurements are available for more than 2 years, the PSA velocity criterion can be used; a change of >0.75 ng/mL/year in PSA velocity is unusual in men with benign prostatic disease and warrants evaluation for prostate cancer. However, Carter has emphasized that the PSA velocity criterion should not be used for time periods <2 years.

### *Sleep apnea*

Testosterone can induce or exacerbate sleep apnea in some individuals, particularly those with obesity or COPD.[117–121] This appears to be due to the direct effects of testosterone on laryngeal muscles.

### *Evaluation of the local application site in men treated with transdermal patches and gel*

In patients being treated with a testosterone patch or testosterone gel, the application site should be inspected for local skin reactions, including erythema

| |
|---|
| 1. Enquire about symptoms of benign prostatic hypertrophy using an American Urologic Association (AUA) symptom questionnaire, perform a digital rectal examination, and obtain a baseline PSA measurement before initiating androgen replacement therapy |
| 2. Testosterone should not be administered to men with baseline PSA greater than 4 ng/mL, AUA symptom score >14, or a palpable abnormality on digital rectal examination without a urological evaluation |
| 3. The presence of benign prostatic hypertrophy by itself is not a contraindication for testosterone replacement therapy. However, testosterone should not be prescribed to men with AUA symptom score greater than 14 without a thorough urological evaluation |
| 4. After institution of testosterone replacement therapy, serum PSA measurement and digital rectal examination should be performed at 3 months, 9 months, and annually thereafter. In addition, at these points, an assessment of the symptoms of benign prostatic hypertrophy should be made by using the AUA symptom score |
| 5. There is considerable test-to-test variability in PSA measurements. A change in serum PSA level of greater than 1.5 ng/mL between two measurements 3–6 months apart should be verified by retesting. A persistent increase of 1.5 ng/mL or greater should warrant a urological evaluation to exclude prostate cancer. |
| 6. In men in whom sequential PSA levels are available over a period of greater than 2 years, PSA velocity can be calculated as the change from baseline in PSA levels divided by the elapsed time in years; PSA velocity is expressed as ng/mL/year. A PSA velocity of greater than 0.75 ng/mL/year should warrant a urological evaluation to exclude prostate cancer. However, PSA velocity criteria must not be applied to follow-up data of less than 2 years' duration. |

***Table 17.7***
*Guidelines for prostate follow-up in hypogonadal men receiving androgen replacement.*

and induration, that can occur in 5%–10% of patients receiving the nongenital patch. Blister formation is relatively rare. Local skin reactions are less common with the Testoderm patch than with the Androderm patch.

### *Cardiovascular risk assessment*

The long-term effects of testosterone supplementation on cardiovascular risk are unknown. Testosterone effects on plasma lipids depend on the dose (physiological or supraphysiological), the route of administration (oral or parenteral), and the formulation (whether aromatizable or not). Physiological testosterone replacement by an aromatizable androgen has a modest or no effect on plasma high-density lipoprotein (HDL). In middle-aged men with low testosterone levels, physiological testosterone replacement has been shown to improve insulin sensitivity and reduce visceral obesity. In epidemiological studies, serum testosterone concentrations are inversely related to waist-to-hip ratio and plasma HDL levels, which are surrogate markers for the risk of heart disease. These data suggest that physiological testosterone replacement may reduce cardiovascular risk in androgen-deficient men (as discussed further in this chapter). Indeed, a low testosterone level is not uncommon in patients with diabetes mellitus and/or metabolic syndrome, and numerous studies have reported an association between testosterone deficiency and visceral obesity, insulin resistance, and dyslipidemia.[131,132] In a 6-month study, transdermal testosterone replacement therapy was associated with beneficial effects on insulin resistance, total and LDL cholesterol, $Lp_{(a)}$, and sexual health in hypogonadal men (total testosterone <11 nmol/L or free testosterone of <255 pmol/L), lending support to the notion that testosterone may reduce cardiovascular risk in such patients.[109] While no specific recommendations can be made at this time, men receiving androgen replacement therapy should undergo cardiovascular risk assessment as part of their general health evaluation.

### *Breast enlargement*

Testosterone administration can induce breast enlargement due to testosterone conversion to estradiol, although this is an uncommon complication. Even with administration of supraphysiological doses of testosterone enanthate, less than 4% of men in a contraceptive trial developed detectable breast enlargement. Breast cancer is listed as a contraindication for testosterone replacement therapy, primarily because of concern that increased estrogen levels during testosterone treatment might exacerbate breast cancer growth. There are, however, few case reports of breast cancer occurring as a complication of testosterone treatment. Men with Klinefelter's syndrome have a higher risk of breast cancer than the general population.

**Testosterone therapy in late-onset hypogonadism**

It is now becoming increasingly recognized that older men with common medical conditions have a higher prevalence of borderline low serum testosterone levels; these conditions include obesity, metabolic syndrome, diabetes mellitus, osteoporosis, COPD, coronary heart disease, HIV, inflammatory conditions (e.g., arthritis), and cardiac, renal, and liver failure. These conditions have stronger associations with the finding of borderline low testosterone than aging *per se*. Late-onset hypogonadism (LOH) is a clinical and biochemical syndrome associated with aging-related comorbidities (especially obesity), and it is characterized by symptoms suggestive of testosterone deficiency and consistently low testosterone levels, after exclusion of classical causes for hypogonadism (e.g., Klinefelter syndrome, Kallmann syndrome, and pituitary tumors).

**Biochemical diagnosis**

National and international guidelines, recommendations, and position statements are available for the diagnosis of hypogonadism.[133] To establish the diagnosis, serum total testosterone levels should be measured before 11 a.m. because of the circadian rhythm. Readings below the reference range on at least two different occasions support a diagnosis of hypogonadism less than 8–12 nmol/L. Additional investigations include the measurement of gonadotropins and prolactin and the calculation of free testosterone when total testosterone is borderline. Methods for the calculation of free testosterone can be found at www.issam.ch.

**Treatment**

While testosterone treatment in patients with classical hypogonadism is effective and safe, some studies suggest that testosterone replacement in LOH may have some short-term benefits (improved body composition, greater bone density, increased lean body mass, reduced fat mass, and improved sexual function);[134] however, longer term studies of sufficient power to document clinical outcomes are lacking.[135] Although testosterone replacement therapy has been used effectively for many years in younger patients with classical hypogonadism without major adverse effects, this experience and the risk–benefit balance cannot be extrapolated to LOH.

Occult prostate cancer is common in elderly men. In the absence of long-term controlled studies, it is unclear whether testosterone therapy has adverse effects on the prostate. A history of prostatic symptoms should be taken, and measurement of PSA should be performed before commencing testosterone treatment in men older than 40 years. Currently, major international guidelines recommend continued surveillance with annual PSA measurement and, if the PSA level is abnormal, urological referral. Since testosterone replacement may cause secondary polycythemia, the hematocrit should be assessed before and annually after the beginning of therapy. The long-term effects of testosterone treatment on cardiovascular disease susceptibility are currently unknown,[23,136] and therefore testosterone replacement should be used cautiously in men with symptomatic cardiovascular disease.[137,138]

Modern testosterone preparations allow delivery of physiological doses to achieve better replacement therapy. The aim of testosterone treatment is to achieve serum testosterone levels within the mid-reference range.

# Erectile dysfunction in men

Erectile dysfunction is the inability of the male to attain and/or maintain an erection sufficient to allow sexual intercourse.[62,139,140] "Impotence" is a more general term that also includes libidinal, orgasmic, and ejaculatory dysfunction in addition to an inability to attain or maintain a penile erection.[62]

## Prevalence

Erectile dysfunction is a common problem, affecting 10–30 million men in the United States alone.[14,62,139–142] The prevalence of erectile dysfunction increases with age; it affects less than 3% of men younger than 45 years of age, but 75% of men over 80 years of age.[14,142]

Men suffering from other medical problems such as hypertension, diabetes, cardiovascular disease, and end-stage renal disease have a significantly higher prevalence of erectile dysfunction than healthy men.[14,62,142]

### The regulation of sexual function and the physiology of penile erection

Sexual function is a complex, multicomponent system that comprises central mechanisms for regulation of libido and arousability, and local mechanisms for the nitric oxide synthase activity in the cavernosal smooth muscle.[143] Therefore, it is possible that physiologically normal testosterone concentrations might be required for optimum penile rigidity. Orgasm and ejaculation are not androgen dependent and can occur without a full penile erection.

Normal penile erection requires coordinated involvement of the intact central and peripheral nervous systems, the corpora cavernosa and spongiosa, as well as a normal arterial blood supply and venous drainage (Figure 17.3).[144–147] The cavernosal arteries and their branches, the helicine arteries, provide blood flow to the penis.[147] Helicine arteries drain blood into the cavernosal sinuses.[144,145] Dilation of the helicine arteries increases the blood flow and pressure in the cavernosal sinuses.[144,145] Relaxation of the cavernosal smooth muscle that surrounds the cavernosal sinuses along with increased blood flow (from 10 cc/min when flaccid to 150 cc/min during tumescence) result in pooling of blood in the cavernosal spaces and penile engorgement. The expanding corpora cavernosa compress the venules against the rigid tunica albuginea, restricting the venous outflow from the cavernosal spaces. This facilitates entrapment of blood in the cavernosal sinuses (passive veno-occlusion) and achievement of a rigid erection.[144]

The relaxation of the cavernosal smooth muscle trabeculae is under the regulation of the autonomic nervous system.[144–149] Although cholinergic, adrenergic, and noradrenergic noncholinergic (NANC) mediators all play a role, the principal biochemical regulator of cavernosal smooth muscle relaxation is nitric oxide derived from the nerve terminals innervating the corpora cavernosa, endothelial lining of the penile arteries, and cavernosal sinuses.[144–149] Nitric oxide also induces arterial dilation. The actions of nitric oxide on the cavernosal smooth muscle and the arterial blood flow are mediated through the activation of guanyl cyclase and the production of cyclic guanosine monophosphate (cGMP).[144–150] The latter acts as an intracellular second messenger and causes smooth muscle relaxation by lowering intracellular calcium (Figure 17.4).[147]

A class of enzymes called cyclic nucleotide phosphodiesterases degrades cGMP into an inactive form, GMP.

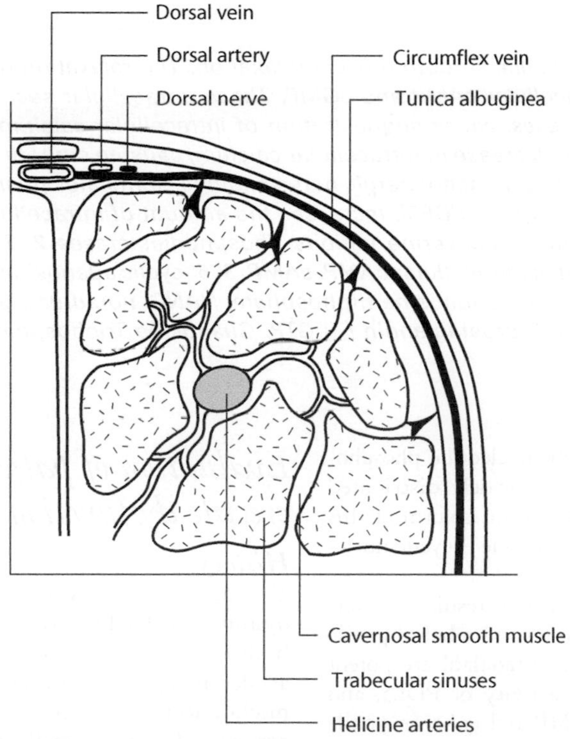


***Figure 17.3***
*Anatomy of penile erection. Corpora cavernosa are made up of trabecular spaces that are surrounded by cavernosal smooth muscle. Helicine arteries provide the arterial supply to the cavernosal spaces. The dorsal nerve provides sensory innervation to the penis. During erection, the relaxation of the trabecular smooth muscle and increased blood flow result in engorgement of the sinusoidal spaces in the corpora cavernosa. The expansion of the sinusoids compresses the venous return against the tunica albuginea, resulting in entrapment of blood. This imparts rigidity to the tumescent penis. (Adapted from Lue TF,* N Engl J Med, 342, *1802–13, 2000.)*

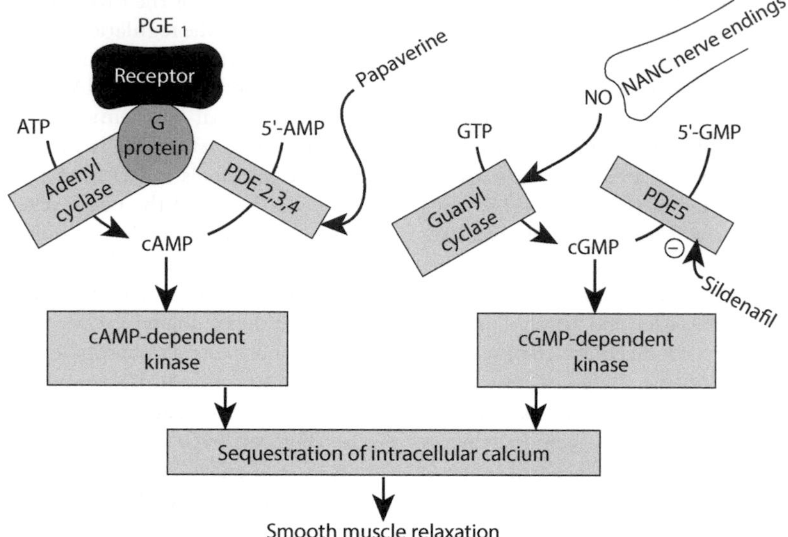


***Figure 17.4***
*Biochemical mechanisms of penile smooth muscle relaxation. The relaxation of the cavernosal smooth muscle is regulated by intracellular cAMP and cGMP. These intracellular second messengers, by activation of specific protein kinases, cause sequestration of intracellular calcium and closure of calcium channels. This results in a net decrease in intracellular calcium, causing smooth muscle relaxation. Nitric oxide, released by noradrenergic, noncholinergic nerve endings, stimulates guanyl cyclase. Sildenafil, by inhibiting phosphodiesterase type 5 (PDE5), increases the amount of intracellular cGMP. Prostaglandin E1 stimulates cAMP generation. Papaverine inhibits phosphodiesterases 2, 3, and 4 (PDE 1,2,3), and thereby increases the amount of intracellular cAMP. cAMP; 3′,5′-cyclic adenosine monophosphate; cGMP; 3′,5′-guanyl monophosphate; ATP, adenosine triphosphate; NANC, noradrenergic, noncholinergic nerve endings; NO, nitric oxide; PGE1, prostaglandin E1; GTP, Guanosine Triphosphate; 5′ AMP, 5′ adenosine monophosphate.*

There are many isoforms of cyclic nucleotide phosphodiesterases, and these isoforms are widely distributed throughout the body; the predominant isoform of this enzyme in the cavernosal smooth muscle is cyclic nucleotide phosphodiesterase 5 (PDE5).[140,144,147]

Hydrolysis of cGMP by this enzyme results in reversal of the smooth muscle relaxation and relief of penile erection. Sildenafil, vardenafil, and tadalafil are potent and selective inhibitors of the activity of PDE5, and they prevent breakdown of cGMP and enhance penile erection.[148]

Additional cGMP-independent pathways, some of which proceed through cyclic adenosine monophosphate (cAMP)-dependent mechanisms, also contribute to trabecular smooth muscle relaxation. For instance, prostaglandin E1, normally synthesized by corpus cavernosum smooth muscle, can increase intracellular cAMP concentration and potentiate smooth muscle relaxation.[144–151]

## *Evaluation of patients with erectile dysfunction (Table 17.8)*

### *History*

The diagnostic workup of the patient with erectile dysfunction should start with an evaluation of general health.[139,140] General medical history should be directed at identifying etiological factors as well as factors that might affect the selection and response to therapy. The presence of diabetes mellitus, coronary artery disease, peripheral vascular disease, and hypertension may suggest a vascular cause. A history of stroke, spinal cord or back injury, multiple sclerosis, or dementia may point to a neurological disorder. Also relevant are a history of pelvic trauma, prostate surgery, or priapism. Social history should include ascertainment of recreational drug abuse—particularly alcohol, cocaine, marijuana, and tobacco. Information about medications, particularly

*History*

A. Ascertain psychosexual history of:
   1. The strength of marital relationship and marital discord
   2. Depression
   3. Stress
   4. Performance anxiety

B. Ascertain etiological factors, such as:
   1. The presence of diabetes mellitus, hypertension, end-stage renal disease, peripheral vascular disease
   2. History of spinal cord injury, stroke, or Alzheimer's disease
   3. Prostate or pelvic surgery
   4. Pelvic injury
   5. Concomitant medications such as antihypertensive, antidepressant, antipsychotic; antiandrogens such as flutamide, casadex, cyproterone acetate, and cimetidine; inhibitors of androgen production such as ketoconazole and GnRH agonists
   6. The use of recreational drugs such as alcohol, cocaine, opiates, and tobacco

C. Ascertain factors that might affect choice of therapy and the patient's response to it such as:
   1. Coexisting coronary artery disease and its symptoms and severity
   2. The use of nitrates for angina
   3. Exercise tolerance
   4. The use of vasodilators for hypertension or congestive heart failure

*Physical examination*

1. Ascertain signs of androgen deficiency such as loss of secondary sex characteristics, eunuchoidal proportions, small testicular volume, or breast enlargement
2. Neurological findings of spinal cord lesion, previous stroke, or peripheral neuropathy; genital and perineal sensation
3. Palpation of femoral and pedal pulses, and evidence of lower extremity ischemia
4. Penile examination to exclude Peyronie's disease

*Laboratory evaluation*

1. Brachial penile blood pressure index
2. Intracavernosal injection of vasodilator
3. Duplex ultrasonography
4. Pelvic arteriography
5. Cavernosography

***Table 17.8***
*Diagnostic evaluation of erectile dysfunction.*

antihypertensives, antiandrogens, antidepressants, and antipsychotics, is important, because almost one-fourth of all cases of impotence can be attributed to medications. Psychiatric illnesses such as depression or psychosis, or drugs used to treat these disorders, might be associated with sexual dysfunction.

A detailed sexual history, including the nature of relationships, partner expectations, situational erectile failure, performance anxiety, and marital discord, should be elicited (Table 17.8).[139,140] It is important to distinguish between inability to achieve erection, changes in sexual desire, failure to achieve orgasm and ejaculation, and dissatisfaction with a sexual relationship. The physician should inquire about the onset, duration, and quality of erections and the presence of nocturnal and early-morning erections.

### Physical examination

A directed physical examination should assess secondary sex characteristics, the presence or absence of breast enlargement, and testicular volume. An evaluation of femoral and pedal pulses can provide clues to the presence of peripheral vascular disease (Table 17.8).

The neurological examination should focus on the presence of motor weakness, perineal sensation, rectal sphincter tone, and the bulbocavernosus reflex. The examination of the penile shaft should ascertain any unusual curvature or palpable chordee, and the patient should be asked about any significant deviation of the penile shaft during tumescence.

### Laboratory tests

The workup of the man with erectile dysfunction should start with a general health evaluation.[139,140] Measurements of hemoglobin, white blood count, AST, ALT, bilirubin, alkaline phosphatase, blood urea nitrogen (BUN), and creatinine can provide useful information about general health and the presence of liver and kidney disease.

### Evaluation of penile vasculature and blood flow

There are several tests that can evaluate the integrity of penile vasculature and blood flow.[139,140] Of these, the penile brachial blood pressure index is the simplest. For computation of this index, brachial and penile blood pressure measurements are taken on both sides with the patient in the supine position before and after leg exercise.[152–155] The ratio of the penile-to-brachial systolic blood pressure is calculated on both sides under these conditions. An abnormal response is defined as any penile-to-brachial systolic blood pressure ratio of $<0.65$ or a decrease in the index of $>0.15$ after exercise. The penile brachial blood pressure index is a relatively specific but not very sensitive marker of vascular insufficiency.[152–155] This index can provide a useful clue to the presence of vascular insufficiency, which should then be further investigated by duplex sonography or angiography. Recent publications have raised questions about the reproducibility and accuracy of this index.[154]

Intracavernosal injection of a vasoactive amine such as prostaglandin E1 can be helpful in men for whom this mode of therapy is being considered.[139,140] This procedure can show whether the patient will respond to this therapeutic modality and facilitate patient education about the procedure and its potential side effects. Failure to respond to intracavernosal injection can raise the suspicion of vascular insufficiency or a venous leak that might need further evaluation and treatment. The penile brachial blood pressure index and the response to intracavernosal injection may diverge in about 20% of men with vascular problems. A venous leak should be suspected in these individuals.

Most men with erectile dysfunction do not need duplex color sonography, cavernosography, or pelvic angiography.[139,140] These procedures should be performed only in patients where the results of these tests would alter the management or prognosis, and only by those with considerable experience with their use. For instance, angiography could be useful in a young man.

### Nocturnal penile tumescence

Although recording of nocturnal penile tumescence (NPT) can help differentiate organic from psychogenic impotence, this test is expensive, labor-intensive, and not required in most men with erectile dysfunction. A history of nighttime or early-morning erections, or a stamp test, has a high correlation with erections recorded by an NPT device.

### Diagnostic tests to exclude androgen deficiency and hypothalamic–pituitary lesions

There is considerable debate about the usefulness and cost-effectiveness of hormonal evaluation and the extent to which androgen deficiency should be investigated in men presenting with erectile dysfunction. Eight to ten percent of men with erectile dysfunction have low testosterone levels; the prevalence of androgen deficiency increases with advancing age.[53,65–67,71]

The prevalence of low testosterone levels is not significantly different between men who present with erectile dysfunction and an age-matched healthy population.[53] These data are consistent with the proposal that erectile dysfunction and androgen deficiency are two common but independently distributed disorders.[53]

It is important to exclude androgen deficiency in this patient population for several reasons.[68] First, androgen deficiency is a correctable cause of sexual dysfunction, and many, though not all, men with erectile dysfunction and low testosterone levels would respond to testosterone replacement. Second, hypogonadism might have additional deleterious effects on the individual's health; for instance, hypogonadism might contribute to osteoporosis; loss of muscle mass and function; increased risk of disability, falls, and fracture; insulin resistance; and cardiovascular disease. Therefore, regardless of the presence of sexual dysfunction, androgen deficiency should be corrected by appropriate hormone replacement therapy. Further, androgen deficiency might be a manifestation of a serious underlying disease, such as HIV infection or a hypothalamic–pituitary space-occupying lesion, and needs evaluation.

In large studies,[53,65,67] only a small fraction of men with erectile dysfunction and low testosterone levels have been found to have space-occupying lesions of the hypothalamic–pituitary region. In one large survey, all of the hypothalamic–pituitary lesions were found in men with serum testosterone levels less than 150 ng/dL (<5.6 nmol/L).[67] Therefore, the cost-effectiveness of the diagnostic workup to rule out an underlying lesion of the hypothalamic–pituitary region can be increased by limiting the workup to men with serum testosterone levels less than 150 ng/dL (<5.6 nmol/L).

## Treatment of erectile dysfunction

The selection of the therapeutic modality should be based on the underlying etiology, patient preference, the nature and strength of the patient's relationship with his sexual partner, and the absence or presence of underlying cardiovascular disease and other comorbid conditions.[139,140] A stepwise approach that first utilizes noninvasive therapies that are easier to use and have fewer adverse effects and then progresses to therapies that require injections or surgical interventions only after the first-line choices have been exhausted can minimize risk and increase patient acceptance (Table 17.9). The physician should discuss the risks and benefits of all the diagnostic procedures and therapies with the couple.

1. All patients and their sexual partners can benefit from and should receive psychosexual counseling
2. First-line therapies:
   (a) Sildenafil citrate
   (b) Vacuum constriction devices
3. Second-line therapies:
   (a) Intracavernosal injection of alprostadil
   (b) Intracavernosal injections of other vasoactive amines
4. Third-line therapies:
   (a) Penile prosthesis
   (b) Vascular surgery

***Table 17.9***
*A stepwise approach to treatment of erectile dysfunction.*

The treatment of associated medical disorders should be optimized. In men with diabetes mellitus, efforts to optimize glycemic control should be instituted, although improving glycemic control may not improve sexual function. In men with hypertension, control of blood pressure should be optimized, and, if possible, the therapeutic regimen should be modified to remove antihypertensive drugs that impair sexual function. This strategy is not always possible, because almost all antihypertensive agents have been associated with sexual dysfunction; the frequency of this adverse event is less with converting enzyme inhibitors than with other agents.

All patients with erectile dysfunction can benefit from and should receive psychosexual counseling.

## First-line therapies

### Psychosexual counseling

Counseling is always indicated in both psychogenic and organic impotence. It can help decrease performance anxiety and increase the patient's ability to cope with the problem.[139,140] Involving the partner in the counseling can help dispel misperceptions about the problem, decrease stress, enhance intimacy and the ability to talk about sex, and increase the chances of a successful outcome of therapy. Counseling sessions are also helpful in uncovering conflicts in relationships, psychiatric problems, alcohol and drug abuse, and significant misperceptions about sex. Although psychobehavioral therapy has been claimed to relieve depression and anxiety, there is a striking paucity of outcome data on the effectiveness of this therapeutic modality.

### Sildenafil

Sildenafil is a selective type 5 phosphodiesterase inhibitor that is a safe and effective first-line oral treatment for erectile dysfunction.[156–161]

#### Mechanism of action

Sildenafil blocks the hydrolysis of cGMP induced by nitric oxide.[156,157] Therefore, sildenafil action requires an intact nitric oxide response, as well as constitutive synthesis of cGMP by the cells. By selectively inhibiting cGMP catabolism in the cavernosal smooth muscle cells, sildenafil restores the natural erectile response to sexual stimulation, but it does not produce an erection in the absence of such stimulation.

The intactness of the nitric oxide production pathway and sexual stimulation are both necessary for sildenafil to successfully induce an erection.

### Efficacy

The efficacy of sildenafil was demonstrated in a randomized dose–response study[151] in which 532 men with organic, psychogenic, or mixed erectile dysfunction were randomized to receive placebo or 25, 50, or 100 mg sildenafil for 24 weeks. In this dose–response study,[151] patients on sildenafil performed better in terms of increased rigidity, frequency of vaginal penetration, and maintenance of erection. Increasing doses of sildenafil were associated with higher mean scores for the questions assessing frequency of penetration and maintenance of erections after sexual penetration. In a follow-up dose escalation study,[151] 329 men were randomly assigned to receive placebo or 50 mg sildenafil for 12 weeks. At each follow-up, the dose of sildenafil was increased or decreased by 50%, depending upon the therapeutic response or side effects. Sixty-four percent of attempts at intercourse were successful for the men receiving sildenafil, as compared to 22% for men receiving placebo. The mean numbers of successful attempts per month were 5.9 for men receiving sildenafil and 1.5 for those receiving placebo. The mean scores for orgasms, intercourse satisfaction, and overall satisfaction were also significantly higher in the sildenafil group than in the placebo group.[151]

Sildenafil has been shown to be effective in men with diabetes mellitus in a separate clinical trial.[68] In this randomized clinical trial, 268 men with diabetes mellitus and erectile dysfunction received either placebo or sildenafil for 12 weeks. Fifty-six percent of men receiving sildenafil reported improved erections, compared with 10% of those receiving placebo ($P < 0.001$). The percentage of men reporting at least one successful attempt at intercourse was 61% for the sildenafil group versus 22% for the placebo group. This study[68] demonstrated that sildenafil is an effective treatment for erectile dysfunction in patients with diabetes mellitus.

Sildenafil is also effective in men with erectile dysfunction due to a variety of other causes, including spinal cord injury and prostatectomy.[158,159] In general, baseline sexual function and the etiology of sexual dysfunction are good predictors of response to therapy;[158] however, there is no baseline characteristic that predicts absolute failure to respond to sildenafil therapy. Therefore, a therapeutic trial of sildenafil is warranted in all patients except those in whom it is contraindicated.[158]

### Adverse effects associated with sildenafil therapy shown in Table 17.10

In clinical trials, the adverse effects that have been reported with greater frequency in sildenafil-treated men than placebo-treated men include headaches, flushing, dyspepsia, respiratory tract disorders, and visual disturbances.[160] Sildenafil does not affect semen characteristics.[161–168] No cases of priapism were noted in any of the pivotal clinical trials.

| Adverse event | Sildenafil (%) | Placebo (%) |
|---|---|---|
| Headache | 16 | 4 |
| Flushing | 10 | 1 |
| Dyspepsia | 7 | 2 |
| Rate of discontinuation | 2.5 | 2.3 |

*Source:* Morales A, et al., *International Journal of Impotence Research* 10, 69–74, 1998.
*Note:* Most adverse effects were reported to be mild to moderate in intensity and transient. In other studies, visual disturbances resulting in blue–green color-tinged vision, increased light perception, blurred vision, and myalgias have also been reported in association with the use of sildenafil.

**Table 17.10**
*Common adverse events associated with the use of sildenafil in men with erectile dysfunction.*

### Hemodynamic effects of sildenafil citrate

In postmarketing surveillance, several instances of myocardial infarction and sudden death were reported[162–168] in men using sildenafil. Forty-four of the 130 deaths reported by the FDA from March to November 1998 occurred in temporal relation to the ingestion of sildenafil;[162–168] 16 of these deaths occurred in individuals who were taking nitrates. Because most men presenting with erectile dysfunction also have a high prevalence of cardiovascular risk factors, it is unclear whether these events were causally related to the ingestion of sildenafil, underlying heart disease, or both.[168]

In a rigorously controlled study,[169] oral administration of 100 mg sildenafil to men with severe coronary artery disease produced only small decreases in systemic blood pressure and no significant changes in cardiac output, heart rate, coronary blood flow, and coronary artery diameter. This led the American Heart Association to conclude that the preexistence of coronary artery disease by itself does not constitute a contraindication for the use of sildenafil.[168]

### Guidelines for the use of sildenafil in men with coronary artery disease are shown in Table 17.11[46,168]

Before prescribing sildenafil, it is crucial to assess cardiovascular risk factors. If the patient has hypertension

1. Sildenafil is absolutely contraindicated in men taking long-acting or short-acting nitrate drugs on a regular basis.
2. If the patient has stable coronary artery disease, is not taking long-acting nitrates, and uses short-acting nitrates only infrequently, the use of sildenafil should be guided by careful consideration of risks.
3. All men taking nitrates should be warned about the risks of the potential interaction between nitrates and sildenafil. The patients should also be warned that concurrent recreational use of inhaled nitrates or poppers could result in marked hypotension that could be serious or even fatal.
4. Sildenafil is contraindicated within 24 h of the ingestion of any form of nitrate.
5. In men with preexisting coronary artery disease, the risks of inducing cardiac ischemia during sexual activity should be assessed before prescribing sildenafil. This assessment may include a stress test.
6. Men who are taking a combination antihypertensive medication should be warned about the possibility of sildenafil-induced hypotension. This is of particular concern in men with congestive heart failure who have low blood volume or who are receiving complex regimens that include vasodilators or diuretics.

*Source:* Bhasin S, Swerdloff RS, *Endocrine Rev*, 7, 106–14, 1986.

***Table 17.11***
***American College of Cardiology and American Heart Association recommendations for the use of sildenafil by men with cardiac disease.***

or symptomatic coronary artery disease, the treatment of those clinical disorders should be optimized.[140,168] The physician must inquire about the use of nitrates, because sildenafil is absolutely contraindicated in individuals taking any form of nitrates or nitrites on a daily basis.

Sildenafil can be used in men who use nitrates infrequently. However, sildenafil should not be used within 24 h of the use of nitrates.[168]

In men with preexisting coronary artery disease, sexual activity can induce coronary ischemia;[167] these individuals should undergo assessment of their exercise tolerance. One practical way to assess exercise tolerance is to have the patient climb one or two flights of stairs. If the individual can safely climb one or two flights of stairs without angina or excessive shortness of breath, he can probably engage in sexual intercourse with a stable partner without similar symptoms. Exercise testing before prescribing sildenafil may be indicated in some men with significant heart disease to assess the risk of inducing cardiac ischemia during sexual activity.[168]

In men with congestive heart failure, on vasodilator drugs, or on complex regimens of antihypertensive drugs, it is advisable to monitor blood pressure after initial administration of sildenafil.[168]

There have been extensive reviews published on the safety of sildenafil therapy.[170–177]

### *Drug–drug interactions*

Sildenafil is metabolized mostly by the P450 2C9 and the P450 3A4 pathways.[168] Cimetidine and erythromycin, inhibitors of P450 3A4, increase the plasma concentrations of sildenafil. Protease inhibitors may also alter the activity of the P450 3A4 pathway and affect the clearance of sildenafil.[168]

Conversely, sildenafil is an inhibitor of the P450 2C9 metabolic pathway, and its administration could potentially affect the metabolism of drugs metabolized by this system, such as warfarin and tolbutamide.[168]

The most serious interactions of sildenafil are with the nitrates. The vasodilator effects of nitrates are augmented by sildenafil; this also applies to inhaled forms of nitrates such as amyl nitrate or nitrite, which are sold under the street name "poppers." Concomitant administration of the two drugs can cause a potentially fatal decrease in blood pressure.[168]

### *Therapeutic regimens*

In most men with erectile dysfunction, sildenafil should be started at an initial dose of 25 mg. If this dose does not produce any adverse effects, then the dose should be increased to 50 mg.[168] Further dose adjustment should be guided by the therapeutic response to therapy and occurrence of adverse effects. Increments in unit dose should be limited to 25 mg at one time. Typically, unit doses higher than 100 mg are not recommended. To minimize the risk of hypotension and adverse cardiovascular events in association with the use of sildenafil, the American Heart Association has prepared a list of recommendations (Table 17.11), which should followed rigorously.[168]

Sildenafil should be taken at least 1 h before sexual intercourse. It should not be taken more than once in any 24 h period.

## *Cost-effectiveness of sildenafil use for erectile dysfunction*

A number of studies have evaluated the economic cost of treating erectile dysfunction in men in managed-care organizations.[178-180] These analyses, using a prevalence-based cost-of-illness approach, have concluded that sildenafil and vacuum constriction devices are the most cost-effective of all the available therapeutic options in the managed-care setting and should be considered as first-line strategies.[178–180]

### Tadalafil (Cialis®)

Tadalafil (Cialis®) dosed at 5–20 mg two to three times a week orally has a prolonged duration of action, lasting up to 36 hours, enabling thrice weekly dosing, where appropriate. It should be used with caution in those who are likely to have prolonged erections (e.g., diseases such as sickle cell anemia, multiple myeloma or leukaemia, or a history of recurrent prolonged erections), men with an abnormal or deformed penis, heart disease, serious liver problems, or serious kidney problems.

It should not be used in patients with angina who are taking nitrate drugs, serious heart disease or a recent heart attack or stroke, low blood pressure or uncontrolled high blood pressure, those advised that sexual activity is not advisable because of health problems (e.g., heart problems or a recent stroke), or people who have previously experienced loss of vision because of nonarteritic anterior ischemic optic neuropathy (NAION). The dose is 5–20 mg.

Tadalafil is a substrate of and predominantly metabolized by CYP3A4 and drugs that inhibit CYP3A4 can increase tadalafil exposure. For example, ketoconazole (400 mg daily), a selective and potent inhibitor of CYP3A4, increases tadalafil 20-mg single-dose exposure (AUC) by 312% and Cmax by 22%, relative to the values for tadalafil 20 mg alone.

Ritonavir (200 mg twice daily), an inhibitor of CYP3A4, CYP2C9, CYP2C19, and CYP2D6, increases tadalafil 20-mg single-dose exposure (AUC) by 124% with no change in Cmax, relative to the values for tadalafil 20 mg alone. Based on these results, in patients taking concomitant potent CYP3A4 inhibitors, the dose of CIALIS should not exceed 10 mg, and the drug should not be administered at less than 72 hr intervals.

### Vardenafil (Levitra)

The dose is 5–20 mg, and it has an identical mode of action to sildenafil. Caution should be exerted in patients with bleeding disorders, or active peptic ulceration, and those in whom there is a susceptibility to prolongation of the QT interval

Certain drugs are contraindicated with vardenafil. These include α-blockers (e.g., doxazosin) and nitrates (e.g., isosorbide, nitroglycerin), and certain antiarrhythmics (e.g., amiodarone, procainamide, quinidine, sotalol) because the risk of irregular heartbeat may be increased

Azole antifungals (e.g., itraconazole), HIV protease inhibitors (e.g., indinavir, ritonavir), macrolide antibiotics (e.g., erythromycin), or telithromycin may increase the risk of vardenafil's side effects. In contrast, rifampin may decrease vardenafil's effectiveness.

### Vacuum devices for inducing erection

Commercially available vacuum devices consist of a plastic cylinder, a vacuum pump, and an elastic constriction band.[139,140] The plastic cylinder fits over the penis and is connected to a vacuum pump. The vacuum within the cylinder draws blood into the penis, producing an erection. An elastic band slipped around the base of the penis traps the blood in the penis, maintaining an erection as long as the rubber band is retained around the base. The constriction band should not be left in place for more than 30 min. These devices are safe, relatively inexpensive, and reasonably effective. These devices impair ejaculation, resulting in entrapment of semen. They are difficult and awkward for some patients to use. Some couples dislike the lack of spontaneity engendered by the use of these devices. Partner cooperation is usually important for the successful use of these devices.[181–188]

### Testosterone replacement in androgen-deficient men presenting with erectile dysfunction

Testosterone replacement in healthy, young, androgen-deficient men restores sexual function.[10,13,14,189–196] In healthy young men, relatively low-normal levels of serum testosterone can maintain sexual function.[10,193,196] In male rats,[194,195] a decrease in serum testosterone concentrations to castration levels is associated with marked impairment of all measures of mating behavior, and testosterone replacement to levels that are at the lower end of the adult male range normalizes all measures of mating behavior.

In general, supraphysiological doses of testosterone do not further improve sexual function. It is possible that increasing testosterone levels above the physiological range might increase arousability; however, this has not been conclusively demonstrated.

Androgen deficiency and erectile dysfunction are two common but independently distributed clinical disorders in middle-aged and older men that often coexist in the same patient. Eight to ten percent of men presenting with erectile dysfunction have low testosterone levels.[53,65–67,69] The prevalence of low testosterone levels is not significantly different between middle-aged and older men with impotence and those without impotence.[53] Testosterone administration is unlikely to improve sexual function in men with normal testosterone levels. Therefore, indiscriminate use of testosterone replacement in all older men with erectile dysfunction is not warranted. However, it is important to exclude testosterone deficiency in older men presenting with erectile dysfunction. Androgen deficiency may be a manifestation of an underlying disease such as a pituitary tumor. In addition, therapies directed just at erectile dysfunction in men will not correct androgen deficiency, which, if left uncorrected, will have deleterious effects on bone, muscle, energy level, and sense of well-being.

Many, but not all, impotent men with low testosterone levels experience improvements in their libido and overall sexual activity with androgen replacement therapy.[68,197] The response to testosterone supplementation even in this group of men is variable,[53,65–67,69] because of the coexistence of other disorders such as diabetes mellitus, hypertension, cardiovascular disease, and psychogenic factors.[53] A meta-analysis[197] of the usefulness of androgen replacement therapy concluded that testosterone administration is associated with greater improvements in sexual function than those associated with placebo in men with erectile dysfunction and low testosterone levels.[197]

Erectile dysfunction in middle-aged and older men is often a multifactorial disorder. Common causes of erectile dysfunction in men include diabetes mellitus, hypertension, medication, peripheral vascular disease, psychogenic factors, and end-stage renal disease. These factors often coexist in the same patient. Therefore, it is not surprising that testosterone treatment might not improve sexual function in all men with androgen deficiency.

Testosterone treatment does not improve sexual function in impotent men who have normal testosterone levels.[66] We do not know whether testosterone replacement improves sexual function in impotent men with borderline serum testosterone levels.

## *Second-line therapies*

### ***Intraurethral therapies***

#### *Intraurethral prostadil*

**Mechanism of action**

Alprostadil is a stable, synthetic form of prostaglandin E1 which causes an increase in cAMP levels and thereby promotes cavernosal smooth muscle relaxation.

**Efficacy**

Alprostadil, when applied into the urethra, has been shown to improve erectile function in approximately 43% of patients with organic impotence in placebo-controlled, double-blind clinical trials.[198–200] Use of a constriction device after application of transurethral alprostadil can increase the efficacy of this form of therapy.

**Treatment regimen**

Typically, the initial dose of 500 μg is applied in the doctor's office. The patient should be observed for clinical response and adverse effects such as decrease in blood pressure and local bleeding. The dose of alprostadil can be increased to 1000 μg per application or decreased to 250 μg, depending upon the clinical response and the adverse effects.

**Potential complications of transurethral alprostadil.** Common side effects of transurethral alprostadil therapy are penile pain and urethral burning.[198–200] Urethral bleeding and priapism are unusual side effects of transurethral alprostadil.

**Relative merits and demerits of transurethral therapy.** The major shortcomings of transurethral alprostadil are its relatively low and inconsistent response rates as well as penile pain. The advantages include local application and low incidence of systemic complications.

#### *Intracavernosal injection of vasoactive amines (Table 17.12)*

Several formulations of alprostadil are commercially available (e.g., CaverJect, Pfizer, New York, NY, USA; Prostin VR, Pfizer; and Edex, Auxilium, Chesterbrook, PA, USA). In addition, a combination of phentolamine, papaverine, and alprostadil is also available (Trimix).

#### *Intracavernosal alprostadil*

**Mechanism of action**

Alprostadil increases cAMP generation and thereby causes cavernosal smooth muscle relaxation.

**Efficacy**

Intracavernosal injections of alprostadil can result in successful erection in almost 75% of treated men. It is more effective than papaverine and phentolamine.

1. The patient should be instructed on how to inject the medication, and he should be educated about the risks of this form of therapy.
2. Physicians who wish to prescribe intracavernosal injections must have contingency plans and a designated urologist to handle emergencies related to complications of intracavernosal injections, such as priapism.
3. It is advisable to administer the first injection in the physician's office and observe the blood pressure and heart rate response. This provides an excellent opportunity for educating the patient, observing adverse effects, and determining whether the patient will respond to this form of therapy.
4. The dose of the vasoactive substance should be adjusted to achieve an erection that is sufficient for sexual intercourse but that does not last for more than 30 min.
5. The patient should be advised that priapism and fibrosis are potential complications of intracavernosal therapy.
6. After the injection, the patient should compress the injection site to minimize the risk of hematoma formation and subsequent fibrosis.
7. If the erection does not abate in 30 min, the patient should be instructed to take a tablet of pseudoephedrine or an intracavernosal injection of phenylephrine. If this is not effective, the patient should either call a designated urologist or come to the emergency room.
8. Intracavernosal therapy is not suitable for patients with psychiatric disorders, hypercoagulable states, or sickle cell disease, and for those who are receiving anticoagulant therapy.

***Table 17.12***
*Checklist before administering intracavernosal therapy.*

#### Regimens

The usual dose range is 5–20 μg. The first injection should be administered in the physician's office; this can help determine whether the patient will respond to this form of therapy. This can also be useful for educating the patient about the technique and potential adverse effects.

#### Potential side effects

Common side effects of intracavernosal alprostadil injections are painful erections, hyperalgesia, priapism, and fibrosis. The incidence of priapism and fibrosis is lower than that observed with papaverine.

#### Relative merits and demerits

High rates of efficacy and low incidence of priapism are the main advantages of alprostadil over other forms of intracavernosal therapies. However, the need for intracavernosal injection, painful erections, and the need for urological backup in the event of priapism are its relative drawbacks.

### *Papaverine*

#### Mechanism of action

Papaverine is an antispasmodic agent and exerts its action as a nonselective phosphodiesterase inhibitor. As such, it would be expected to increase both cAMP and cGMP levels within the trabecular smooth muscle cell, resulting in an increase in penile blood inflow, cavernous artery diameter, and cavernosal smooth muscle relaxation.

#### Efficacy

Intracavernous injection of vasoactive substances has been shown to be an effective treatment of organic erectile dysfunction in 50%–80% of treated patients.

#### Dose regimen

The usual dose regimen is 15–60 mg.

#### Potential complications

Up to 50% of men discontinue this kind of therapy due to the inconvenience of injections, needle phobia, and side effects such as plaque or nodule formation, hematoma, and infection. The incidence of priapism and corporal fibrosis is high (up to one-third of treated men).

#### Relative merits and demerits

Papaverine is not commercially available in the United States. A topical preparation of papaverine has been studied and is not as effective as intracavernosal injection.[14] High rates of priapism and fibrosis make it an unacceptable choice in an internist's practice without adequate urological backup.

### *α-Adrenergic receptor blockers*

The sympathetic α-adrenergic receptors are thought to mediate and maintain corpus cavernosum tone in a detumescent state. All three subtypes of α-adrenergic receptors are expressed in human corpus cavernosum. Phentolamine, an α1- and α2-adrenergic antagonist, has been used alone and in combination with other agents for the treatment of erectile dysfunction.

#### Efficacy

When given alone, phentolamine is not very effective in producing rigid erections. However, in combination with papaverine, it is highly effective in producing successful erections in over 75% of treated men.

#### Dose regimen

One-half to one milligram of phentolamine is usually given in combination with 30 mg papaverine.

#### Potential complications

Major side effects of phentolamine are hypotension and palpitations due to reflex tachycardia. When given in combination with papaverine, it can induce priapism and fibrosis.

## *Third-line therapies*

### ***Penile prosthesis***

Insertion of penile prostheses should be limited to men who have failed other forms of therapy. The available prosthetic devices are of three types: inflatable, semi-rigid, and malleable. The major complications of prosthetic devices include infections, erosions, and the risk of mechanical failure. Penile prostheses have a finite life span and need replacement in 5–10 years. They produce an unnatural erection. Because of the concern about silicone implants, their use has decreased significantly in recent years. Migration of silicone particles to regional lymph nodes has been reported, although we do not know whether this migration has any adverse health consequences.

### *Newer therapeutic approaches under development*

A number of novel selective phosphodiesterase inhibitors are under development. Milrinone is a selective type 3 phosphodiesterase inhibitor in human corpus cavernosum. Rolipram is a selective type 4 phosphodiesterase inhibitor.

Doxazocin, an α-adrenergic blocker, was evaluated for its potential in enhancing the effects of intracavernosal therapy; results showed limited efficacy. Chlorpromazine, deliquamine, moxysylate, prazosin, and yohimbine have not been shown to be efficacious in large-scale, placebo-controlled, randomized clinical trials. Trazodone has been shown to cause priapism and induce erection when injected intracavernosally. Oral trazodone has been used to treat psychogenic erectile dysfunction.

Apomorphine, a dopamine receptor agonist, is known to induce erection when administered orally. Side effects, including nausea and vomiting, may be unacceptable.

Endothelin is a potent vasoconstrictor and is synthesized by trabecular smooth muscle cells. Therefore, endothelin receptor antagonists may be useful in the treatment of erectile dysfunction. Most of the studies to date have been in animal models. In future, gene therapy holds promise for the management of impotence.

### *Gene therapy for erectile dysfunction*

This represents an evolving field that is currently in the preclinical phase of investigation. As proof of concept, however, somatic gene transfer has been possible in animal studies, with the tissue-specific overexpression of potassium channels, nitric oxide synthase, and vascular endothelial growth factor. This type of approach may be applicable to humans provided that safe vectors become available.[201]

# *Infertility and subfertility in men*

Infertility, defined as the inability of a couple to achieve pregnancy despite unprotected intercourse for a period of greater than 12 months, affects 10%–15% of couples.[202–207] In a third of infertile couples, the primary problem resides in the male partner; in a third, in the female partner; and in the remaining third, in both the male and the female partner.[203–207]

## *Germ cell development in the testis*

The process of spermatogenesis takes place in the seminiferous tubules of the testis and is divided into three major stages[207] (Figure 17.5): spermatogonial replication, meiosis, and spermiogenesis. During the first stage, the spermatogonial stem cells divide mitotically several times to give rise to successive generations of spermatogonia, of which there are at least three main types in the human tubules: the dark type A, the pale type A, and type B.[207] The type B spermatogonia proliferate to give rise to primary spermatocytes at the preleptotene stage of meiosis, in which DNA is actively synthesized.

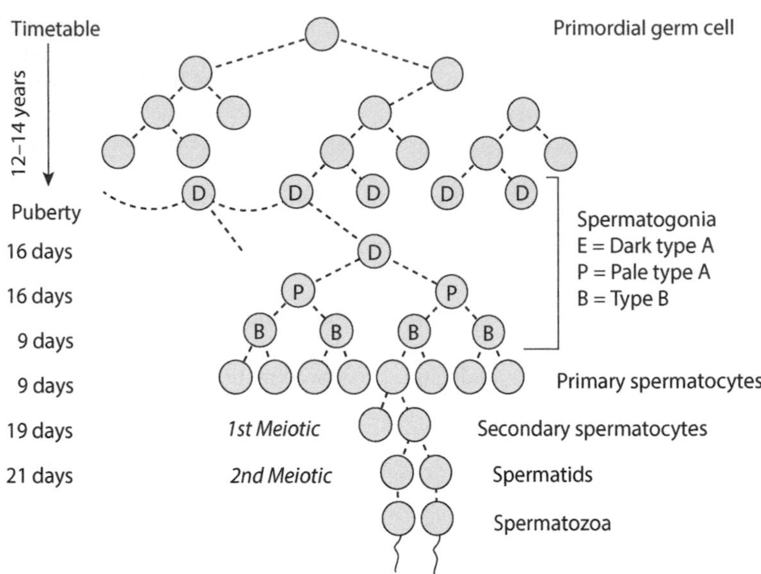


***Figure 17.5***
*Stages of spermatogenesis in the human testis. After the migration of germ cells into the gonadal ridges is complete during embryogenesis, there are approximately 300,000 germ cells per gonad. The primordial germ cells differentiate and undergo mitotic divisions, so that at the time of puberty there are approximately 6 million germ cells in each testis. The germ cell development is arrested at the stage of spermatogonia dark type A. With sexual maturation, each spermatogonium differentiates and gives rise to 16 primary spermatocytes. Each primary spermatocyte enters meiosis and gives rise to four haploid spermatids. The spermatids are initially round, and they undergo a series of differentiation steps that include the reorganization of the nucleus and cytoplasm and the development of a flagellum, resulting in the formation of spermatozoa. Each spermatogonium gives rise to 64 spermatozoa. (Adapted from Griffin JE et al., (eds.)* Williams Textbook of Endocrinology, *8th edn., Saunders, Philadelphia, 1992, pp. 810.)*

The second stage is the process of meiosis, which consists of two successive divisions of the spermatocyte accompanied by only one duplication of chromosomes (Figure 17.5). At the completion of meiosis, four spermatids are produced, each containing a single, or haploid, set of chromosomes. The final stage of spermatogenesis is called spermiogenesis, which involves a complex process of structural transformation and differentiation of the spermatid. During spermiogenesis, the chromatin of the spermatid condenses into a compact mass of dense granules, and the nucleus becomes invested by a membranous derivative of the Golgi apparatus, the acrosome, which contains enzymes that will digest a path for the sperm to penetrate the outer vestments of the egg. The cytoplasm elongates and surrounds the flagellum, which sprouts from a centriole. At the time of sperm formation, most of the cytoplasm is cast off in the form of a residual body. The spermatid completes its metamorphosis into a spermatozoon by forming a complex tail by the axonemal complex of two inner-singlet and nine outer-doublet microtubules. In men, the total duration of spermatogenesis has been evaluated at between 60–74 days.[207]

Normal spermatogenesis requires complex interactions between germ cells and various somatic cells, such as Sertoli and Leydig cells, and the synergistic actions of the pituitary gonadotropins LH and FSH. LH, after binding to its G protein–coupled receptor, stimulates the production of testosterone by the Leydig cells; high intratesticular testosterone concentrations are essential for the initiation and maintenance of spermatogenesis within the testis. FSH initiates function in immature Sertoli cells by stimulating the formation of the blood–testis barrier and the secretion of a wide range of proteins and growth factors, such as androgen-binding protein, inhibin, activin, stem cell factor, plasminogen activator, transferrin, sulfated glycoproteins, and lactate.[208] Once spermatogenesis is established in the adult testis, Sertoli cells become less responsive to FSH.

Failure of spermatogenesis can result from impaired secretion or action of LH and FSH or from intrinsic defects in spermatogenesis within the testis. While a multitude of acquired causes can impair spermatogenesis, there is reason to believe that a genetic basis exists in a majority of infertile men. It is worth emphasizing that the molecular defects that result in infertility in a majority of infertile men remain unknown. Although the number of human genes known to be implicated in the pathophysiology of infertility is small, a significantly larger database exists for the mouse and *Drosophila*. For instance, 2400 *Drosophila* loci have been implicated in male sterility! It is certain that additional autosomal and X- and Y-specific candidate genes that are associated with defects of germ cell replication, meioisis, or spermiogenesis will be discovered in man.

# Pathogenesis of infertility

Common causes of infertility are listed in Table 17.13. Several large surveys of infertile men have been published.[202–207,209] Although differences exist in the frequency of various etiological factors in surveys from different centers, based in part on patient referral patterns, the nature and extent of investigation, and geography, these surveys are in agreement that subfertility and infertility in men form a heterogeneous group of disorders.[209] A specific cause of infertility is not determinable in most men. Most infertile men have idiopathic oligozoospermia or male factor infertility.

Of infertile men, 15%–20% are azoospermic. An additional 10% have severe oligozoospermia (sperm density less than 1 million/mL). Correctable or treatable causes of infertility, such as gonadotropin deficiency and obstruction, are present in only a small number of men.

Although varicoceles are present in 10%–30% of men with infertility, their role, if any, in the pathophysiology of male infertility remains controversial.

## Diagnosis

### History

In the diagnostic workup of infertility, it is important to evaluate both the male and the female partner simultaneously (Figures 17.6 and 17.7).[210] The history should focus on duration of infertility, previous evidence of fertility in the man or the woman, contraceptive use, sexual function, and the frequency and timing of intercourse in relation to the menstrual cycle. The inquiry should also be directed at ascertaining the timing of pubertal development, shaving frequency, hair loss, and hair distribution. A history of scrotal trauma, genitourinary infection, sexually transmitted disease, and scrotal or inguinal surgery may also be pertinent. Details of other medical problems such as erectile dysfunction, diabetes mellitus, and autonomic neuropathy that might be associated with retrograde ejaculation should be obtained.

### Physical examination

Physical examination should focus on determining whether the patient has evidence of androgen deficiency. The measurements of body proportions (height-to-span

| *Diagnosis* | *Incidence (%)* |
|---|---|
| Idiopathic infertility | 60–80 |
| Primary testicular failure (chromosomal disorders including Klinefelter's syndrome, undescended testis, irradiation, orchitis, drugs) | 8–10 |
| Genital tract obstruction (congenital absence of vas, vasectomy, epididymal obstruction) | 5 |
| Coital disorders | <1 |
| Hypogonadotropic hypogonadism (pituitary adenomas, panhypopituitarism, idiopathic hypogonadotropic hypogonadism, hyperprolactinemia) | 3–4 |
| Varicocele[a] | 15–35 |
| Others (sperm autoimmunity, drugs, toxins, systemic illness) | 5 |

*Source:* Adapted from Baker HW et al., Relative incidence of etiologic factors in male infertility. In: Santen RJ, Swedloff RS, eds. *Reproductive Dysfunction: Diagnosis and Management of Hypogonadism,* Marcel Dekker, New York, 341–72, 1986. With permission.

[a] Although the prevalence of varicocele in infertile men is higher than in the general population, it is not known whether the presence of varicocele causes or contributes to infertility.

**Table 17.13**
*Major etiologic diagnoses in infertile men.*

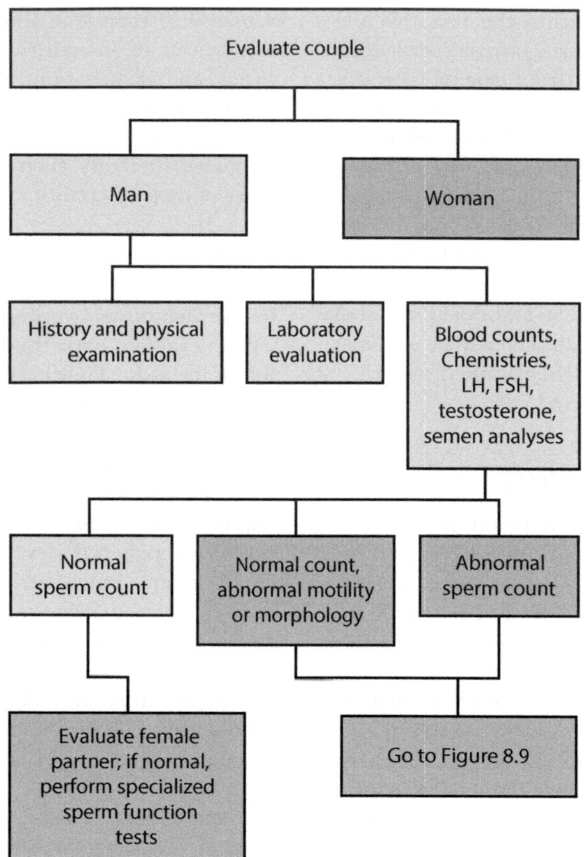


***Figure 17.6***
*Evaluation of an infertile couple. LH, luteinizing hormone; FSH, follicle-stimulating hormone.*

and upper segment-to-lower segment ratio); voice (high pitched or not); hair distribution, including escutcheon; muscle mass; and body habitus, and the absence or presence of gynecomastia, can point to hypogonadism. Measurement of testicular volume by the Prader orchidometer is an important part of the evaluation. The presence of cryptorchidism, varicocele, or nodularity of the vas deferens should be recorded. A digital rectal examination for assessment of prostate size should be performed.

### *Laboratory evaluation*

An algorithm for the evaluation is provided in Figure 17.8. Initial evaluation should focus on assessment of general health and include a complete blood count, blood chemistries, and urinalysis.[210]

## *Semen analysis*

Three or more semen samples should be obtained by masturbation after a 48 h abstinence period. Semen should be assessed for volume, sperm density and count, sperm motility, and sperm morphology.[211,212] According to the World Health Organization,[211] a normal semen specimen in 1987 should have a volume of more than 2 mL, sperm density of greater than 20 million/mL, and a total sperm count of 40 million per ejaculate. More than 50% of sperm should show forward motility, and more than 30% of cells should have normal morphology. This was revised in 2010 and the new ranges are shown in Table 17.14.

The significance of leukocytes in the semen is not clear. The presence of leukocytes in the semen does not necessarily indicate accessory gland infection.

## *Hormonal evaluation*

Measurement of testosterone, LH, and FSH can help in the diagnosis of hypogonadism and determine whether hypogonadism is hypogonadotropic or hypergonadotropic[210] (Figures 17.7 through 17.9).

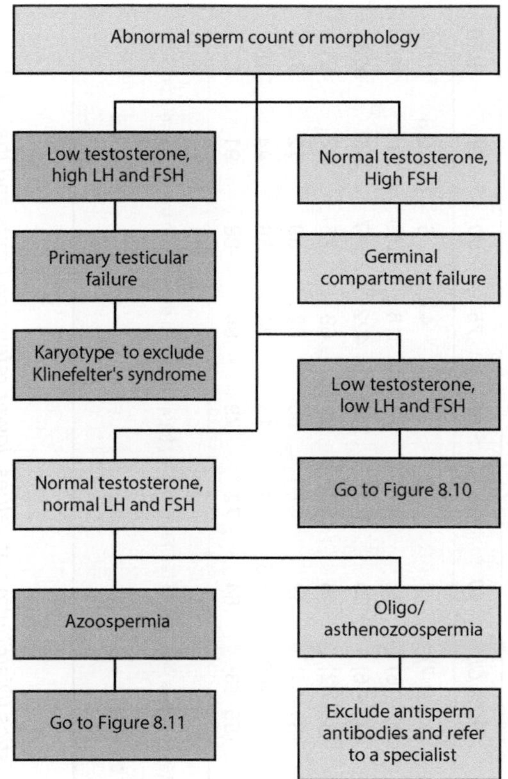


***Figure 17.7***
*Evaluation of an infertile man with abnormal sperm count and morphology. LH, luteinizing hormone; FSH, follicle-stimulating hormone.*

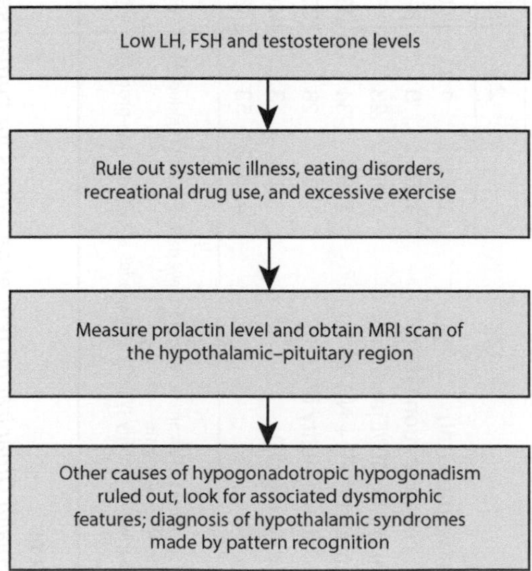


***Figure 17.8***
*An algorithm for further evaluation of men with hypogonadotropic hypogonadism.*

| | *N* | *Centiles* | | | | | | | | | | |
|---|---|---|---|---|---|---|---|---|---|---|---|---|
| | | *2.5* | *(95% CI)* | *5* | *(95% CI)* | *10* | *25* | *50* | *75* | *90* | *95* | *97.5* |
| Semen volume (ml) | 1941 | 1.2 | (1.0–1.3) | 1.5 | (1.4–1.7) | 2 | 2.7 | 3.7 | 4.8 | 6 | 6.8 | 7.6 |
| Sperm concentration ($10^6$/ml) | 1859 | 9 | (8–11) | 15 | (12–16) | 22 | 41 | 73 | 116 | 169 | 213 | 259 |
| Total number ($10^6$/Ejaculate) | 1859 | 23 | (18–29) | 39 | (33–46) | 69 | 142 | 255 | 422 | 647 | 802 | 928 |
| Total motility (PR + NP, %)* | 1781 | 34 | (33–37) | 40 | (38–42) | 45 | 53 | 61 | 69 | 75 | 78 | 81 |
| Progressive motility (PR, %)* | 1780 | 28 | (25–29) | 32 | (31–34) | 39 | 47 | 55 | 62 | 69 | 72 | 75 |
| Normal forms (%) | 1851 | 3 | (2.0–3.0) | 4 | (3.0–4.0) | 5.5 | 9 | 15 | 24.5 | 36 | 44 | 48 |
| Vitality (%) | 428 | 53 | (48–56) | 58 | (55–63) | 64 | 72 | 79 | 84 | 88 | 91 | 92 |

*Note:* The values are from unweighted raw data. For a two-sided distribution the 2.5th and 97.5th centiles provide the reference limits; for a one-sided distribution the fifth centile provides the lower reference limit.
*PR, progressive motility (WHO, 1999 grades a + b); NP, non-progressive motility (WHO, 1999 grade c).

***Table 17.14***
*World Health Organization reference values for human semen characteristics (Distribution of values, lower reference limits and their 95% CI for semen parameters from fertile men whose partners had a time-to-pregnancy of 12 months or less).*

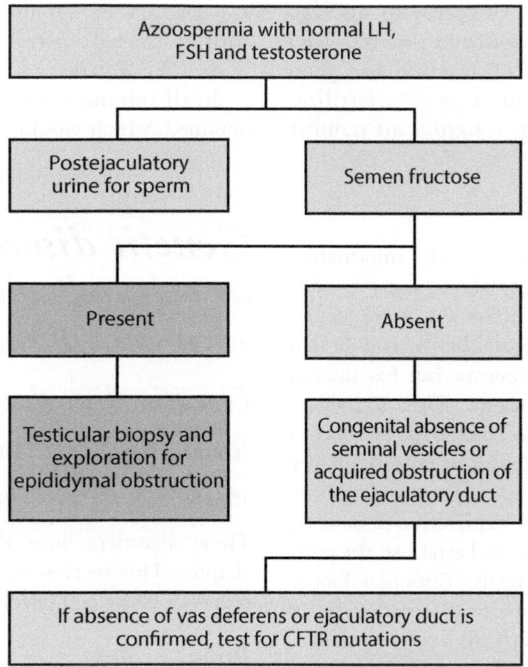


***Figure 17.9***
*Evaluation of azoospermic men with normal LH, FSH, and testosterone levels. CFTR: cystic fibrosis transmembrane conductance regulator.*

High LH and FSH levels in the presence of low testosterone concentrations suggest primary testicular failure. In these men, a karyotype should be performed to exclude the presence of Klinefelter's syndrome (47,XXY) or its variants. A normal karyotype, however, does not exclude the possibility of mosaicism (46,XY/47,XXY).

Elevated testosterone and elevated LH levels in a man who appears hypogonadal suggest androgen insensitivity. Analysis of skin fibroblasts for androgen binding or analysis of peripheral lymphocyte DNA can help to confirm mutations in androgen receptor or 5α-reductase genes. An isolated increase in serum FSH levels with normal LH and testosterone levels suggests failure of the germ cell compartment.

If the patient has hypogonadotropic hypogonadism, a history of eating disorders, excessive exercise, and systemic illness should be looked for (Figure 17.8). Serum prolactin levels should be measured, and an MRI scan of the hypothalamic–pituitary region should be obtained to exclude a space-occupying lesion. In older men with mild hypogonadotropic hypogonadism, the search for additional causes of hypogonadotropism is often unrewarding, and the cost-effectiveness of extensive pituitary evaluation has not been established. Older men with severe hypogonadotropic hypogonadism and with serum testosterone levels less than 150 ng/dL (5.2 nmol/L) should be evaluated for the presence of a pituitary pathology by obtaining prolactin measurements and an MRI scan.

Men with azoospermia and normal LH and testosterone levels may have an obstructive lesion, such as congenital absence of the vas deferens or epididymis, or an acquired obstruction (Figure 17.9). In such patients, postejaculatory urine should be checked to exclude retrograde ejaculation, and seminal fructose should be measured. Very low fructose concentrations suggest the absence of seminal vesicles or obstruction. In such patients, exploration and testicular biopsy should be performed to rule out obstruction or germ cell failure. If the absence of vas deferens or seminal vesicles is confirmed, then the individual should be tested for mutations in the cystic fibrosis conductance regulator (CFTR) gene.

In men who have normal hormone levels and low or normal sperm count, specialized sperm function tests are indicated. Various sperm function tests, including the cervical mucus penetration test, acrosome reaction, zona-free hamster egg penetration test, human zona pellucida binding test, and specialized sperm biochemistry, are used in specialized andrology laboratories. The clinical utility of the acrosome reaction is not clear. A positive hamster oocyte penetration test is indicative of the ability of sperm to undergo capacitation and acrosome reaction, and penetrate and fuse with the hamster egg. This reaction has good concordance with fertilization in an *in vitro* fertilization procedure. It has, however, a significant number of false-negative results.

### *Testicular biopsy*

Although testicular biopsy can provide information about the spermatogenic defect, there are very few instances where this procedure alters the management and prognosis. For instance, testicular biopsy is indicated in an infertile man who is azoospermic but has normal testosterone and LH concentrations. This individual should undergo further workup to exclude the presence of obstruction, including an examination of postejaculatory urine for sperm and seminal fructose. If seminal fructose is present, testicular biopsy and exploration should be performed to rule out obstruction and establish the presence of spermatogenesis in the testis. Testicular biopsy has also been used to retrieve sperm or spermatids for intracytoplasmic sperm injection (ICSI) in men with azoospermia in whom sperm cannot be obtained from the semen. Fertility has been achieved by intracytoplasmic injection of sperm obtained from testicular biopsy in men with azoospermia associated with Klinefelter's syndrome or other causes.

### *Computer-aided sperm analysis*

Many computer-aided sperm analysis systems are commercially available. These systems are convenient, but they offer no real advantage over manual methods for assessment of sperm morphology. These automated systems are susceptible to error in the estimation of sperm concentration.

### *Genetic testing*

Because genetic disorders account for a significant fraction of infertile men, genetic testing of the infertile man and of the offspring will become increasingly important, especially in those couples who are being considered for ICSI. As mentioned in the "Hormonal Evaluation" section, infertile men with congenital absence of the vas deferens or seminal vesicles should be screened for mutations in the CFTR gene. Infertile men with azoospermia or severe oligozoospermia in whom the cause of infertility cannot be ascertained should be screened for Y chromosome microdeletions. Offspring born through the use of ICSI have a higher frequency of sex chromosome aneuploidy than the general population; in addition, the prevalence of sex chromosome disorders is 6–10-fold higher among infertile men, especially those with azoospermia. This has led some to conclude that infertile men with nonobstructive azoospermia should undergo karyotype analysis. Men with postmeiotic germ cell arrest may have mutations in the *CREM* gene.

In all instances, a detailed family history should be obtained, which would then guide genetic testing.

# *Genetic disorders associated with infertility in man (Table 17.15)*

## *Genetic disorders associated with impaired gonadotropin secretion or action*

These disorders have already been discussed in this chapter. This section will focus only on the genetic disorders of germ cell development.

### *Primary defects of spermatogenesis*

#### *Sex chromosome disorders*

Approximately 5% of infertile men carry chromosome abnormalities; of these, a majority involve sex chromosomes (4% on average), and 1% involve the autosomes.[213–216] The prevalence of sex chromosomal and autosomal abnormalities in infertile men is 15 and 6 times higher, respectively, than in the general population.[217,218]

#### *Klinefelter's syndrome*

Klinefelter's syndrome is the most common chromosomal disorder associated with male infertility and is found in 1:500 to 1:1000 live-born males throughout all ethnic groups.[217,218] The most frequent karyotype in men with Klinefelter's syndrome is 47,XXY (93%), but 46,XY/47,XXY; 48,XXXY; 48,XXYY; and 49,XXXXY karyotypes have also been reported.[26,219,220] The XXY chromosomal constitution has been described in other mammals such as mouse, Chinese hamster, cat, dog, sheep, ox, and pig, and it is associated with sterility. The testes of 47,XXY animals are devoid of germ cells.[26,220]

Azoospermia is the rule in men with Klinefelter's syndrome who have the 47,XXY karyotype. Men with mosaicism may have germ cells in their testes, especially at a younger age.

Testicular histology in men with Klinefelter's syndrome shows hyalinization of seminiferous tubules and absence of spermatogenesis.[25,26] Patients with mosaicism may have normal-sized testes and spermatogenesis at puberty. However, progressive degeneration and hyalinization of seminiferous tubules take place after puberty.

| *Genetic or chromosomal disorder* | *Genotype* | *Hormonal profile* | *Histology* | *Semen* |
|---|---|---|---|---|
| Klinefelter's syndrome | 47,XXY, 46,XY/47,XXY | Low or low-normal testosterone, increased LH and FSH | Hyalinization of seminiferous tubules, absence of germ cells, normal or hyperplastic Leydig cells | Azoospermia |
| Y chromosome microdeletions | 46,XY, microdeletions of AZFa, AZFb, AZFc, AZFd regions | Usually normal or low-normal testosterone, normal LH, and normal or increased FSH | Variable. Some men may have Sertoli cell–only phenotype, others have germ cell arrest | Azoospermia or severe oligozoospermia |
| Bilateral congenital absence of vas deferens | Mutations of the *CFTR* gene | Usually normal testosterone, LH and FSH | Testicular histology tends to be normal, but patients have obstructive azoospermia | Azoospermia. May or may not have clinical features of cystic fibrosis |
| *CREM* mutations | Mutations of the *CREM* gene | Normal testosterone and LH, normal or elevated FSH | Germ cell arrest at the spermatid stage early in spermiogenesis | Azoospermia |
| Thalassemia | Mutations of one or more β-globin gene(s) | Typically have hypogonadotropic hypogonadism with low testosterone, and low LH and FSH; occasionally primary testicular failure may also occur | | Azoospermic, depending on degree of gonadotropin deficiency |
| Sickle cell disease | Mutations of the globin gene | May have primary testicular failure due to testicular infarcts resulting in low testosterone and high LH and FSH. Some patients may have iron overload and hypogonadotropic hypogonadism | Testicular infarcts | May have oligozoospermia, depending on the severity of the disease and the degree of LH and FSH deficiency |

***Table 17.15***
*Relatively common chromosomal and genetic disorders in infertile men in which genetic testing is possible.*

In some men, the tubular dysgenesis is patchy; degenerating tubules are interspersed with apparently normal tubules. The Leydig cells appear to be increased, although their function is impaired.

The 47,XXY karyotype in patients with Klinefelter's syndrome results from nondysjunction during the first meiotic division in one of the parents. Nondysjunction of maternal chromosomes is the cause of the 47,XXY karyotype in two-thirds of affected men. Advanced maternal age is a risk factor for nondysjunction. The mechanism by which an extra X chromosome renders patients infertile is not known. In male germ cells, inactivation of the single X chromosome in primary spermatocytes of heterogametic males is necessary for spermatogenesis to proceed through meiosis. The necessity for X inactivation in male germ cell differentiation in heterogametic species is not clearly understood; however, inactivation of the single X may be necessary for normal sex chromosome pairing or to prevent expression of some X-linked genes that are detrimental to spermatogenesis.

The hypogonadism associated with Klinefelter's syndrome can range from mild to severe, leading to a wide variation in clinical presentation. Penile length in these patients appears to be inversely correlated with length of the CAG repeats in the androgen receptor.[221] The phenotype in the adult is, in addition to severely impaired spermatogenesis and varying degrees of hypogonadism, manifested by a tall body habitus with sparse body and facial hair, gynecomastia, diminished libido, and small testes. In childhood, common presenting features can include delayed speech development, learning difficulties in school, unusually rapid growth in mid-childhood, and truncal obesity. The cause of language difficulties often encountered in individuals with Klinefelter's syndrome has been investigated by high-resolution MRI, which has demonstrated a relative reduction in the left temporal gray matter compared with control subjects.[222] Of interest is that individuals who had been treated with testosterone had larger temporal lobe volumes than those not receiving testosterone; indeed, it appears that testosterone improves verbal fluency scores of Klinefelter's syndrome patients.

The hypothalamic–pituitary–testicular axis in boys with Klinefelter's syndrome can appear normal until puberty, with no apparent differences in the levels of testosterone, LH, or FSH when compared to controls.[223] However, at the onset of puberty and subsequently, laboratory analysis reveals normal or low-normal testosterone and elevated gonadotropin levels, with FSH elevated to a greater extent than LH. Treatment consists of testosterone therapy to improve virilization, sexual function, bone density, and quality of life. Gynecomastia is treated by cosmetic surgery after androgen replacement therapy has begun. New approaches to the treatment of infertility in the patients have involved testicular sperm extraction (TESE) using microsurgical techniques to identify occasion foci of spermatogenesis and the use of subsequent ICSI.[224] However, disappointingly, analysis of spermatozoa obtained by testicular biopsy in individuals with Klinefelter's syndrome has revealed an increased prevalence of sperm with an additional X chromosome, and higher rates of aneuploidy and trisomy 21.[225,226] Preimplantation genetic diagnosis (PGD) is generally offered to couples with Klinefelter's syndrome who undergo successful TESE and ICSI. This technique allows for selecting chromosomally abnormal embryos in order to avoid transferring abnormal embryos. In a comparison of PGD in 113 embryos from 20 couples with Klinefelter's syndrome with 578 embryos from control couples with X-linked disease undergoing PGD for gender determination, a significantly higher percentage of sex chromosome (13.2% vs. 3.1%) and autosome (15.6% vs. 5.2%) abnormalities in embryos from Klinefelter's syndrome couples as compared with the X-linked couples was found.[227] With respect to the sex chromosome abnormalities, monosomy X, monosomy Y, 47,XXX, 47,XYY, and mosaicisms were identified. Interestingly, no embryo with 47,XXY from Klinefelter's syndrome couples was identified.

Studies have shown that in adults with Klinefelter's syndrome, overall age-matched mortality is roughly doubled, mainly from nonneoplastic diseases of the cardiovascular, respiratory, and digestive systems, and from diabetes, with an increase in the incidence of breast cancer (20-fold higher), extragonadal germ cell tumors (posterior mediastinum), and autoimmune diseases. Taurodontism (an enlargement of the pulp in molar teeth), predisposing one to premature dental caries, is seen in almost 50% of Klinefelter's syndrome patients. Early varicose veins are also a feature of Klinefelter's syndrome, as is an increased risk of deep vein thrombosis.

### *Noonan's syndrome: the male Turner's syndrome*

These patients have the 46,XY karyotype, male external genitalia, and the clinical stigmata of Turner's syndrome.[228] The condition is autosomal dominant or occasionally sporadic in nature, and it is characterized by short stature, hypertelorism, downward-slanting eyes, ptosis, strabismus, low-set ears with thickened helices, a high nasal bridge, micrognathia (a triangular-shaped face due to an abnormally small lower jaw), a high arched palate, a low hairline, and dental malocclusion. The condition is caused by mutations in genes in the Ras–MAPK signaling pathway.

Approximately 50% of men with Noonan's syndrome have mutations in the *PTPN11* (protein tyrosine phosphatase nonreceptor type 11) gene,[229] and the remainder have mutations in the *SOS1* (son of sevenless homolog 1), *RAF1*, or *KRAS* genes. The testis size is reduced, the Leydig cell function is impaired, gonadotropins are raised, and there is delayed puberty. Sterility and cryptorchidism (seen in 50%) are common.

### *XYY syndrome*

There is a higher frequency of the 47,XYY karyotype in men with tall stature and nodular cystic acne, among prisoners and mental hospital patients.[230] The mean intelligence quotient and educational level are lower in 47,XYY individuals than in healthy controls.

### *Mixed gonadal dysgenesis (45,X/46,XY)*

The patients with mixed gonadal dysgenesis usually have a 45,X/46,XY karyotype, a testis on one side, and a streak gonad on the other.[231] Some degree of ambiguity in the genitalia is usual. The phenotypic males with mixed gonadal dysgenesis often have abdominal testes with normal Leydig cells but without any germ cells.[231] The dysgenetic gonad is at high risk for neoplastic degeneration.

### *XX males*

These patients have a male phenotype and normal-looking testes, but they are azoospermic and have high LH and FSH levels.[232,233] The portion of the Y chromosome that contains the Sry may be translocated onto the X chromosome or an autosome; a few patients may be mosaics and carry some 46,XY cell lines. However, because they lack other Y-specific genes required for spermatogenesis, they are sterile.

### *The Y chromosome microdeletion syndrome*

Large deletions of the Y chromosome that can be seen under the microscope in late prophase and hence are detectable on routine karyotype are uncommon in infertile men. However, submicroscopic deletions of the long arm of the Y chromosome, which are not detectable on karyotype and hence are called "microdeletions," are present in 5%–10% of azoospermic men.[234–246] These microdeletions can be detected by PCR-based sequence-tagged site mapping or by Southern hybridization. The initial studies had focused on infertile men with severe defects of spermatogenesis (i.e., those with azoospermia). However, more recent studies have shown that Y deletions are also present in oligozoospermic men.[247,248] Most infertile men with Y deletions have severe defects of spermatogenesis (i.e., they have either azoospermia or severe oligozoospermia).[249–251] Although the total number of infertile men with Y deletions who have been studied in detail is small, most of these patients have had testicular volumes of less than 15 mL and elevated FSH levels. The testicular histologies in the small number of reported cases of Y deletions have revealed either Sertoli cells only or germ cell arrest phenotypes. The limited number of patients in whom testicular histology has been examined has not allowed a correlation between the location and size of the deletion and the histological phenotype. However, Vogt et al.[252] have reported that three loci can be identified in Yq, termed AZFa, AZFb, and AZFc, wherein deletions are associated with specific testicular histopathology.

Two Y-specific candidate gene families have been cloned by deletion mapping of infertile men with Yq deletions and proposed as candidates for the putative AZF locus, the *RBM* (RNA-binding motif containing) gene family[247,253] and the *DAZ* (deleted in azoospermia) gene family.[250,254–256] Both are multiple-copy gene families[256,257] that contain the RNA-binding motif. The *RBM* gene family has more than 30 copies spread throughout the Y chromosome, most of the copies being located in deletion intervals 6A and 6B. At least two members of the *RBM* gene family, *RBM-1* and *RBM-2*, are expressed in the testis.[257] The presence of the RNA-binding motif in the predicted protein sequence suggests that these genes play a role in RNA processing; however, the precise role of the RBM proteins in germ cell development remains unclear.

The *DAZ* gene family is also a multiple-copy gene family.[256] The mouse and *Drosophila* homologs of *DAZ* have been mapped to chromosomes 17 and 3, respectively.[254,258] An autosomal homolog of *DAZ* has also been identified in the human and mapped to chromosome 3.[234,259] The homologs of the autosomal *DAZ*-like gene, *DAZL1*, are present in all mammalian species; *DAZ* homologs are present only on the Y chromosomes of great apes and Old World monkeys. Mutations of the *DAZL1* gene in *Drosophila*, *boule*, are associated with meiotic arrest and azoospermia.[254]

Similarly, *DAZL1* mutations in knockout mice are associated with sterility, providing further evidence for the role of this gene product in germ cell development.[235]

In infertile men with *DAZ* deletions, both meiotic arrest and Sertoli cell–only phenotypes have been described; it is possible that germ cell degeneration may occur secondarily.

The precise physiological function and role of the *RBM* and *DAZ* gene families in human spermatogenesis remain unclear. The RNA molecules that are the targets of these RNA-binding proteins have not been identified.

Using DAZ as bait in a two-hybrid system, Tsui et al.[306] identified two novel proteins, *DAZ*-associated proteins (DAZAP) 1 and 2, that interact with *DAZ* and *DAZL1*. The *DAZAP* genes have been mapped to chromosomal regions 19p13.3 and 2q33–q34.

Although deletions involving the *DAZ* genes appear to be the most frequent, a large proportion of Y deletions are outside the *DAZ* region; some of these involve the *RBM* gene. Additional candidate gene families, including *BPY2, CDY1, PRY,* and *TTY2*, have been identified in the AZFc region of the Y chromosome.[236] The role of these additional Y-specific gene families in germ cell development and infertility is not understood. It is also not clear how deletions of one or two copies of the *RBM* or *DAZ* genes could explain infertility when there are multiple copies of these genes elsewhere on the Y chromosome. A significant proportion of infertile men with *DAZ* deletions are oligospermic and not azoospermic. Furthermore, only 5%–10% of infertile men have Y deletions. These data suggest that additional Y-specific and autosomal genes may be involved in other infertility phenotypes.[236]

### *The length of the polyglutamine tract in the androgen receptor protein and infertility*[237-240]

The length of the CAG trinucleotide repeat in exon 1 of the androgen receptor gene that encodes for the polyglutamine tract in the androgen receptor protein is polymorphic in humans.[237–241] *In vitro* studies have demonstrated that the transactivational activity of the androgen receptor protein is related inversely to the length of the polyglutamine tract. Individuals with very long tracts have spinobulbal muscular atrophy (Kennedy's disease), a degenerative disease of the spinal cord neurons. However, several reports indicate that men with idiopathic oligozoospermia have a higher likelihood of having longer polyglutamine tracts than fertile men.[237–239] For instance, in one study of 153 infertile men and 72 healthy controls, Yong et al.[239] reported that 20% of infertile men have reduced androgenicity because of a long CAG repeat length in exon 1 of the androgen receptor gene. These authors have proposed that long polyglutamine tracts are associated with increased risk of infertility and reduced risk of prostate cancer. Conversely, these authors assert that short polyglutamine tracts are associated with increased transactivational activity, increased risk of prostate cancer, and reduced risk of infertility. Dadze et al.,[240] on the other hand, found no relationship between the CAG repeat length and impaired spermatogenesis in a sample of infertile men of German origin. Therefore, the validity of this hypothesis remains to be verified.

### *Autosomal gene defects and male infertility*

#### *Cyclic adenosine 3′,5′-monophosphate-response element modulator gene expression and spermatogenic arrest*[241]

The cAMP-response element modulator gene codes for a transcription factor that is expressed in postmeiotic germ cells and is important for physiological regulation of the balance between differentiation and apoptosis during normal germ cell development.[241–245] Mice that are null for CREM protein are sterile and reveal spermatogenic arrest at the first step of spermiogenesis.[245] Late spermatids are absent, and there is an increase in the number of apoptotic germ cells in the seminiferous tubules of *CREM*-mutant mice.[245] Normal spermatogenesis in fertile men is characterized by a switch from CREM repressors to CREM activator isoforms in postmeiotic germ cells. *In situ* hybridization studies on testicular biopsies obtained from infertile men with germ cell arrest have demonstrated the absence of activator isoforms of CREM in postmeiotic germ cells and increased apoptosis.[241–244] These data suggest that germ cell arrest could result from failure of this normal transition from repressor to activator isoforms of CREM in the seminiferous tubule.

#### *Bilateral congenital absence of vas deferens and the CFTR mutations*

Mutations in the coding region of the *CFTR* gene may result in congenital absence of the vas deferens without causing the classic pulmonary disease.[246] Fifty to seventy percent of men with congenital absence of the vas deferens harbor mutations of the *CFTR* gene. About 50% are homozygous for a common cystic fibrosis gene abnormality such as F508, and some have compound heterozygosity.

#### *Gonadal dysfunction associated with sickle cell disease and thalassemia*

A significant proportion of men with sickle cell disease have low testosterone levels. The majority of men with sickle cell disease and low testosterone levels suffer from primary testicular dysfunction.[261] It is assumed that testicular dysfunction results from microinfarcts in the testis because of the vaso-occlusive disease. However, hypogonadotropic hypogonadism due to hypothalamic–pituitary dysfunction has also been reported in men with sickle cell disease.

The pituitary and gonadal dysfunction occurs in thalassemia due to iron deposition in these tissues.[262] Hypogonadotropic hypogonadism is the predominant form of androgen deficiency syndrome in men with thalessemia and can be treated effectively with gonadotropin

| |
|---|
| Clomiphene and antiestrogens |
| Varicocelectomy |
| LH and FSH |
| Testosterone rebound |
| Antibiotics |
| Vitamins and minerals |
| Artificial insemination by husband's sperm |
| Low-dose glucocorticoid therapy |

*Source:* Adapted from Burger HG, Baker HW, *Annu Rev Med*, 38, 29–40, 1987. With permission.

**Table 17.16**
***Treatment modalities whose beneficial effects have not been demonstrated in male factor infertility.***

replacement therapy. Pituitary and testicular overload and the resulting hypogonadism can be prevented by prophylactic iron-chelating therapy.

*Testicular dysfunction in myotonic dystrophy*

Myotonic dystrophy is an autosomal dominant disorder associated with CTG repeats in the dystrophin gene. Testicular atrophy occurs in 75% of these men, primarily due to degeneration of the seminiferous tubules. Although Leydig cells are preserved, serum testosterone levels are low in many patients due to primary testicular failure.[263]

*Subfertility associated with diabetes*

Men with diabetes mellitus may experience infertility if they have retrograde ejaculation due to autonomic neuropathy or if they have poor glycemic control. Impotence is common in men who have had diabetes for more than 10 years.

# Treatment

## The role of the internist in the management of the infertile couple

The internist can play an important role in the treatment of infertile men by initiating a rational diagnostic evaluation and referring those who require more specialized care.[264] The internist should focus on ascertaining a specific treatable cause of infertility, even though specific treatment modalities may be applicable to only a fraction of infertile men. In this regard, it is particularly important to identify and treat gonadotropin deficiency, because hormone replacement therapy in this disorder is highly effective. Similarly, it is also useful to quickly ascertain whether the patient has untreatable sterility in which case the couple should be appropriately counseled about adoption or artificial insemination with donor sperm. One of the most useful roles that an internist can play is to present to the couple a realistic prognosis, the pros and cons of different treatment options, and estimates of costs, and to guide the couple away from interventions that have not been shown to be effective (Table 17.16).

## Gonadotropin treatment of men with hypogonadotropic hypogonadism

### Preparations

hCG and human menopausal gonadotropin (hMG) preparations have been commercially available for over three decades.[265–269] hCG is purified from the urine of pregnant women, being secreted primarily by the human placenta during pregnancy. hMG is derived from the urine of postmenopausal women. While hCG primarily stimulates Leydig cell testosterone production by interacting with LH–hCG receptors, hMG contains LH and FSH activities in almost equal proportions (Table 17.15).

## Treatment modalities whose beneficial effects have not been demonstrated in male factor infertility

Highly purified preparations of hLH and hFSH, derived from human cadaver pituitary, had become available for research studies from the National Pituitary Agency of the National Institute of Diabetes and Digestive and Kidney Diseases. However, the occurrence of a "slow virus" degenerative disease (Creutzfeldt–Jakob disease) in a few patients treated with earlier preparations of human growth hormone (HGH)[260] led to the withdrawal and cessation of the use of all human pituitary hormones for therapeutic purposes. A highly purified hFSH preparation is commercially available, and, although extensively used in gynecological applications, it is now available for use in medicine with hypogonadotropic hypogonadism.[270–273] The mature β subunit of rhFSH has seven fewer amino acids than are reported in the literature, but it has similar oligosaccharide structures as purified urinary hFSH preparation (Follitropin Beta: Puregon).[271]

Recombinant hFSH is also indistinguishable from purified urinary hFSH in its biological activity *in vitro* and *in vivo*. rhFSH is available in ampoules containing 75 IU (approximately 7.5 μg FSH), which accounts for >99% of protein content. The pharmacokinetics of urinary hFSH and recombinant hFSH are similar.

## Biological effects of gonadotropin therapy

Pharmacological doses of hCG, when administered to normal men, lead to biphasic testosterone and estradiol responses.[274–277] When 1500–6000 units of hCG are given intramuscularly to normal adult men, an initial peak in serum testosterone levels can be observed 2 h later, with a sustained peak at 72–96 h. Serum testosterone levels may remain elevated for as long as 6 days after a single hCG injection. Serum estradiol levels also exhibit a similar biphasic response. It should be noted that the biphasic testosterone and estradiol responses are characteristic of only postpubertal, normally virilized men.[274–279] In prepubertal boys or hypogonadotropic men not previously primed with gonadotropins, only a monophasic increase in serum testosterone, peaking.

72–96 h after hCG injection, can be seen, and there is significant latency before testosterone levels begin to rise. Smals et al.[274] have suggested that an early testosterone response in normally virilized postpubertal men results from testosterone release from a readily releasable pool of preformed hormone and/or a rapid induction of mature enzymatic machinery. Wang et al.[277] demonstrated that hypogonadotropic men who were previously primed with hCG treatment also exhibit a biphasic testosterone response to LH infusion, consistent with the proposal that maturation of the biphasic adult pattern is a function of prior gonadotropin priming of the testis.

Multiple injections of pharmacological doses of hCG lead to diminished testosterone response to subsequent hCG injections, a phenomenon referred to as "desensitization."[274–276] Desensitization to hCG can be seen under several different clinical and experimental circumstances: first, multiple daily hCG injections do not result in higher serum testosterone levels than single daily injections; and, second, men with hCG-secreting neoplasia do not usually have elevated serum testosterone levels.[274]

It has long been known that in prepubertal males, hCG, when given alone, widens the seminiferous tubules and increases the number of primary spermatocytes.[280,281]

However, spermatogenesis does not progress to completion, and germ cell development remains arrested. The addition of hMG to patients on hCG results in an increase in testis size, progression of germ cell development, completion of spermiogenesis, and the appearance of sperm in the ejaculate.

## Therapeutic aspects

The two best predictors of success of gonadotropin therapy in hypogonadotropic men are testicular volume at presentation and the time of onset of hypogonadotropism (prepubertally or postpubertally). In general, the larger the testis size, the greater the likelihood of success; best responses are seen in men with initial testicular volume greater than 8 mL.[82,282] Similarly, patients who became hypogonadotropic after puberty (e.g., because of a pituitary tumor, surgery, or irradiation) experience higher overall success rates than those who have never undergone pubertal changes.[82,282]

The presence of a coincidental or associated primary testicular abnormality will, of course, attenuate the testicular response to gonadotropin therapy. Some patients with IHH may also have cryptorchidism; earlier studies[283,284] indicated that these patients did not respond well to hCG therapy, leading to an erroneous speculation that there may be dual defects in IHH, the first hypothalamic and the second testicular.

Although a variety of treatment regimens are being used, there is no consensus on what constitute the optimum dose and schedule of gonadotropin administration. Published data and empirical clinical experience indicate that a reasonable starting dose is 1000–1500 IU[82,282–284] given intramuscularly three times weekly. Serum testosterone levels should be measured 6–8 weeks later, 48–72 h after an hCG injection, in order to adjust and optimize the regimen. The goal should be to adjust the dose to achieve serum testosterone levels in the mid-normal range. Sperm counts should be monitored on a monthly basis. It may take several[82,282–284] months for spermatogenesis to be restored, and patients often get very impatient and prematurely disappointed. Therefore, it is very important to forewarn patients about the potential length and expense of the treatment, and to provide conservative estimates of success rates.

If, after 6 months of therapy with hCG alone, serum testosterone levels are in the mid-normal range but the sperm concentrations are low, it is time to add FSH. This can be done by using hMG, highly purified FSH, or recombinant FSH. The selection of FSH dose is empirical. A common practice is to start with the addition of 0.5 to 1 ampoule of hMG (1 ampoule = 75 IU LH plus 75 IU FSH) three times each week in conjunction with the hCG injections. If, after 3 months of combined treatment, sperm densities are still low, the dose of hMG should be increased to 1 or 2 ampoules. It may occasionally take 18–24 months or longer for spermatogenesis to be restored. Physiologically, it may make more sense to use FSH first to increase the pool of Sertoli cells, which support spermatogenesis, prior to adding hCG, and studies are in progress to determine whether the outcome is superior with this strategy rather than the other one discussed here. There are also ongoing studies investigating the use of modified long-acting FSH analogs (FSH-CTP, or corifollitropin), which have to be injected only every two weeks, in the induction of spermatogenesis.

Spermatogenesis-inducing therapy is expensive but is otherwise well tolerated. The development of antibodies to hCG is not a common event.[285–288] Braunstein et al.[285] found no evidence of antibodies in 41 people treated with hCG for weight reduction. Another study found antibodies in less than 1% of men treated with short courses of hCG.[286] There are only a handful of case reports of treatment failure due to the development of anti-hCG antibodies.[285–288]

In men with postpubertal onset of hypogonadotropism, spermatogenesis can usually be reinitiated by hCG alone, and the success rates are high.[82] In contrast, men in whom hypogonadotropic hypogonadism developed prior to the completion of pubertal maturation usually do not respond to hCG alone but require combined treatment with hCG and hMG for longer duration, and their overall success rates are lower. Prior androgen therapy appears not to affect subsequent responsiveness to gonadotropin therapy.[289]

The degree of gonadotropin deficiency, as reflected by the pretreatment testicular volume, is an important determinant of the response to gonadotropin therapy. In general, men with testicular volumes greater than 8 mL have higher response rates than those with testicular volumes less than 4 mL.[282]

An open-label clinical trial by the Spanish Collaborative Group on Male Hypogonadotropic Hypogonadism[270] evaluated the efficacy of self-administered highly purified hFSH (150 IU three times a week) and hCG (2500 IU twice a week) in men with IHH. Serum testosterone concentrations were normalized in all but one patient. Testicular volume increased threefold during treatment, and 80% of men who were initially azoospermic achieved a positive sperm count. The maximum sperm density during treatment was 25±8 million/mL. Three men developed gynecomastia.

## Pulsatile GnRH therapy

Pioneering studies by Knobil's group[290–292] had predicted that pulsatile administration of GnRH would be required to maintain normal LH and FSH output from the pituitary. Continuous infusion of GnRH in monkeys, made hypogonadotropic by radiofrequency lesions of the hypothalamic GnRH-secreting nuclei, downregulates LH and FSH secretion. Synthetic GnRH is commercially available for therapy of patients with hypogonadotropism due to GnRH deficiency.[293] However, the success of GnRH therapy assumes normal pituitary and gonadal function. The agonist analogs of GnRH are not useful for restoring gonadotropin secretion, because after an initial short-lived stimulatory phase, GnRH agonists downregulate pituitary LH and FSH output.[294–296]

A large number of clinical studies utilizing GnRH in a variety of treatment regimens have demonstrated successful induction of puberty by pulsatile administration of low doses of GnRH. Therapy is usually started with an initial dose of 25 ng/kg per pulse, administered subcutaneously every 2 h by a portable, and FSH levels need to be monitored. The dose of GnRH may need to be increased until serum testosterone levels in the mid-normal range are reached. There is considerable variability in the GnRH dose requirement among different subjects, and doses ranging from 25 to 200 ng/kg may be required to induce virilization.[278] Once pubertal changes have been initiated, the dose of GnRH can be reduced without any adverse effects on serum testosterone, LH, and FSH levels.

The gonadotropin secretion and gonadal function can be maintained for extended periods of time (months to years) in a majority of carefully selected patients with IHH by pulsatile GnRH therapy.[278,279,297] Development of anti-GnRH antibodies is an uncommon occurrence, but it can be a cause of treatment failure. Increases in sperm counts and testicular volume have been reported in over 70% of treated men, and improvements in sexual function and virilization can be induced in over 90% of subjects. Some of the patients with IHH have associated cryptorchidism, and these men might have an additional testicular defect. Local cutaneous infections do occur, but they are infrequent and minor. While induction of virilization by pulsatile GnRH administration in patients with IHH has provided important insights into the mechanisms of puberty and regulation of gonadotropin secretion by GnRH, this approach has no particular advantage over the traditional gonadotropin therapy.[283,284] Carrying a portable infusion device can be cumbersome, and follow-up of these patients often requires considerable physician supervision and laboratory monitoring.

Liu et al.[282] compared an hCG–hMG regimen with pulsatile GnRH therapy regarding its efficacy in inducing spermatogenesis. After 2 years of therapy, 40% of GnRH-treated men and 80% of the hCG–hMG treated men produced sperm. The sperm concentrations in all men were below $5 \times 10^6$/mL and were comparable in the two groups. In another retrospective review,[283,284] hCG–hMG and pulsatile GnRH therapy were found to be equally effective in inducing spermatogenesis. Spermatogenesis was induced in 54 of 57 courses of therapy, and pregnancies occurred in 26 of 36 courses. The two therapies did not significantly differ in terms of the time to first appearance of sperm or pregnancy rates. These and other data[283,284] demonstrate that both pulsatile GnRH therapy and traditional gonadotropin replacement therapy are equally effective in inducing spermatogenesis in men with IHH.

## Azoospermia

The presence of azoospermia, total teratozoospermia, and primary testicular failure with azoospermia indicates a poor prognosis.[298] In these instances, adoption and artificial insemination using donor sperm are reasonable options.[202,298]

With the advent of ICSI, the prognosis for these men has improved. There are several case reports of successful pregnancies in partners of men with Klinefelter's syndrome using intracytoplasmic injection of sperm retrieved from testicular biopsy into the oocyte.[299–301] Palermo et al.[300] have reported high success rates with the use of ICSI using spermatozoa surgically retrieved from azoospermic men. These investigators report clinical pregnancy rates of 49% for nonobstructive cases and 57% for testicular spermatozoa obtained from men with obstructive azoospermia.[300] Success rates vary considerably among centers, depending upon patient selection and experience with the procedure.

Couples who are undergoing ICSI using testicular spermatozoa should be counseled about the risks of sex chromosome aneuploidy and other genetic disorders being transmitted to the offspring through ICSI. Also, it is best to present a realistic prognosis and dampen expectations at the very outset.

### *Should varicoceles be treated surgically or left alone in infertile men?*

Varicoceles are present in 10%–30% of infertile men; however, they are also common in men of known fertility.[302] Therefore, the role of varicoceles in the pathophysiology of male infertility remains unclear.[302–307] Although many uncontrolled studies have reported improvements in sperm density and sperm motility after varicocele resection, these data are difficult to interpret because of the lack of appropriate control groups. Most varicocele studies have lacked scientific rigor and are uninterpretable. Only a few controlled clinical trials have been performed, and these trials have failed to show significantly greater improvements in fertility after surgical resection of varicoceles than after counseling alone.[304] Therefore, there are insufficient data to support a recommendation for surgical resection of varicoceles in most infertile men.

The expert opinion among urologists favors surgical correction of varicoceles in adolescent boys; the rationale is that there is catch-up growth of the testes after varicocelectomy which might not occur without the surgical correction. However, prospective data from controlled clinical trials are lacking.

### *Intracytoplasmic sperm injection for male factor infertility*

ICSI, first used successfully in 1992 for the treatment of infertility, has become a widely used treatment modality worldwide.[308] Tens of thousands of infertile couples have undergone this procedure since then, at hundreds of centers around the world.[264,308–310] A recent survey convened by the European Society of Human Reproduction and Embryology[308] has reported that the fertilization rates obtained with ejaculated, epididymal, and testicular spermatozoa for 1995 were 64%, 62%, and 52%, respectively. Eighty to ninety percent of couples had embryo transfer, and the viable pregnancy rates were 21% for ejaculated, 22% for epididymal, and 19% for testicular sperm. The incidence of multiple gestation was 30%–40%. The pregnancy rates were similar for obstructive and nonobstructive azoospermia.[308]

There has been considerable concern about the possibility of transmitting genetic disorders from the parents to the offspring born through the use of ICSI.

Reassuringly, the perinatal outcome of children born after ICSI was not significantly different from those born after *in vitro* fertilization or natural conception.[263,308–310] A small increase in frequency of congenital malformations has been explained on the basis of the higher prevalence of multiple births. When multiplicity is taken into account, the incidence of major or minor malformations is not increased.[264,308–310] There is, however, a small but significant increase in the frequency of chromosome aneuploidy, especially sex chromosome aneuploidy, among the offspring of ICSI. Data from the Swedish Medical Birth Registry[264,311] have also demonstrated an increase in relative risk of hypospadias. Long-term data on the mental and physical well-being of children born through the use of ICSI are not available.

Therefore, a large body of carefully collected data indicates that ICSI is a safe treatment modality that can be effective in many cases of male factor infertility.[311]

However, ICSI is an expensive and complicated procedure. Couples should undergo extensive counseling before they are referred for ICSI. They should also be advised to undergo genetic counseling and testing.

# References


1. Finkelstein JS, Klibanski A, Neer RM, et al. Osteoporosis in men with idiopathic hypogonadotropic hypogonadism. *Ann Intern Med* 1987; **106**(3): 354–61.
2. Katznelson L, Finkelstein JS, Schoenfeld DA, et al. Increase in bone density and lean body mass during testosterone administration in men with acquired hypogonadism. *J Clin Endocrinol Metab* 1996; **81**(12): 4358–65.
3. Stepan JJ, Lachman M, Zverina J, et al. Castrated men exhibit bone loss: Effect of calcitonin treatment on biochemical indices of bone remodeling. *J Clin Endocrinol Metab* 1989; 69(3): 523–7.
4. Boonen S, Vanderschueren D, Cheng XG, et al. Age-related (type II) femoral neck osteoporosis in men: Biochemical evidence for both hypovitaminosis D- and androgen deficiency-induced bone resorption. *J Bone Miner Res* 1997; 12(12): 2119–26.
5. Kenny AM, Gallagher JC, Prestwood KM, et al. Bone density, bone turnover, and hormone levels in men over age 75. *J Gerontol A Biol Sci Med Sci* 1998; 53(6): M419–25.
6. Stanley HL, Schmitt BP, Poses RM, et al. Does hypogonadism contribute to the occurrence of a minimal trauma hip fracture in elderly men? *J Am Geriatr Soc* 1991; 39(8): 766–71.
7. Bhasin S, Bremner WJ. Clinical review 85: Emerging issues in androgen replacement therapy. *J Clin Endocrinol Metab* 1997; **82**(1): 3–8.
8. Katznelson L, Rosenthal DI, Rosol MS, et al. Using quantitative CT to assess adipose distribution in adult men with acquired hypogonadism. *Am J Roentgenol* 1998; **170**(2): 423–7.
9. Mauras N, Hayes V, Welch S, et al. Testosterone deficiency in young men: Marked alterations in whole body protein kinetics, strength, and adiposity. *J Clin Endocrinol Metab* 1998; **83**(6): 1886–92.
10. Bagatell CJ, Heiman JR, Rivier JE, et al. Effects of endogenous testosterone and estradiol on sexual behavior in normal young men [published erratum appears in *J Clin Endocrinol Metab* 1994; **78**(6): 1520]. *J Clin Endocrinol Metab* 1994; **78**(3): 711–16.
11. Carani C, Granata AR, Bancroft J, et al. The effects of testosterone replacement on nocturnal penile tumescence and rigidity and erectile response to visual erotic stimuli in hypogonadal men. *Psychoneuroendocrinology* 1995; **20**(7): 743–53.
12. Cunningham GR, Hirshkowitz M, Korenman SG, et al. Testosterone replacement therapy and sleep-related erections in hypogonadal men. *J Clin Endocrinol Metab* 1990; **70**(3): 792–7.
13. Davidson JM, Camargo CA, Smith ER. Effects of androgen on sexual behavior in hypogonadal men. *J Clin Endocrinol Metab* 1979; **48**(6): 955–8.
14. Kwan M, Greenleaf WJ, Mann J, et al. The nature of androgen action on male sexuality: A combined laboratory–self-report study on hypogonadal men. *J Clin Endocrinol Metab* 1983; **57**(3): 557–62.
15. Salmimies P, Kockott G, Pirke KM, et al. Effects of testosterone replacement on sexual behavior in hypogonadal men. *Arch Sex Behav* 1982; 11(4): 345–53.
16. Barrett-Connor E, Khaw KT. Endogenous sex hormones and cardiovascular disease in men. A prospective population-based study. *Circulation* 1988; **78**(3): 539–45.
17. Marin P, Holmang S, Jonsson L, et al. The effects of testosterone treatment on body composition and metabolism in middle-aged obese men. *Int J Obes Relat Metab Disord* 1992; **16**(12): 991–7.
18. Marin P. Testosterone and regional fat distribution. *Obes Res* 1995; **3**(Suppl 4): 609S–12S.
19. Marin P, Oden B, Bjorntorp P. Assimilation and mobilization of triglycerides in subcutaneous abdominal and femoral adipose tissue in vivo in men: Effects of androgens. *J Clin Endocrinol Metab* 1995; **80**(1): 239–43.
20. Seidell JC, Bjorntorp P, Sjostrom L, et al. Visceral fat accumulation in men is positively associated with insulin, glucose, and C-peptide levels, but negatively with testosterone levels. *Metabolism* 1990; **39**(9): 897–901.
21. Gray A, Feldman HA, McKinlay JB, et al. Age, disease, and changing sex hormone levels in middle-aged

men: Results of the Massachusetts Male Aging Study. *J Clin Endocrinol Metab* 1991; 73(5): 1016–25.

22. Gray A, Berlin JA, McKinlay JB, et al. An examination of research design effects on the association of testosterone and male aging: Results of a meta-analysis. *J Clin Epidemiol* 1991; 44(7): 671–84.
23. Wu FCW, Tajar A, Beynon JM, et al. Identification of late-onset hypogonadism in middle-aged and elderly men. *New Eng J Med* 2010; **363**: 123–35.
24. Tajar A, Huhtienhami I, O'Neill TW, et al. Characteristics of androgen deficiency in late onset hypogonadism: Results from the European Male Aging Study. *J Clin Endocrinol Metab* 2012; **97**(5): 1508–16.
25. Bandmann HJ, Breit R, Perwein E. *Klinefelter's Syndrome*. Berlin: Springer-Verlag; 1984.
26. Paulsen CA, Gordon DL, Carpenter RW, et al. Klinefelter's syndrome and its variants: A hormonal and chromosomal study. *Recent Prog Horm Res* 1968; **24**: 321–63.
27. Arver S, Sinha-Hikim I, Beall G, et al. Serum dihydrotestosterone and testosterone concentrations in human immunodeficiency virus-infected men with and without weight loss. *J Androl* 1999; **20**(5): 611–18.
28. Coodley GO, Loveless MO, Nelson HD, et al. Endocrine function in the HIV wasting syndrome. *J Acquir Immune Defic Syndr* 1994; 7(1): 46–51.
29. Dobs AS, Dempsey MA, Ladenson PW, et al. Endocrine disorders in men infected with human immunodeficiency virus. *Am J Med* 1988; **84**(3 Pt 2): 611–16.
30. Dobs AS, Few WL III, Blackman MR, et al. Serum hormones in men with human immunodeficiency virus-associated wasting. *J Clin Endocrinol Metab* 1996; **81**(11): 4108–12.
31. Grinspoon S, Corcoran C, Lee K, et al. Loss of lean body and muscle mass correlates with androgen levels in hypogonadal men with acquired immunodeficiency syndrome and wasting. *J Clin Endocrinol Metab* 1996; **81**(11): 4051–8.
32. Laudat A, Blum L, Guechot J, et al. Changes in systemic gonadal and adrenal steroids in asymptomatic human immunodeficiency virus-infected men: Relationship with the CD4 cell counts. *Eur J Endocrinol* 1995; **133**(4): 418–24.
33. Berns JS, Rudnick MR, Cohen RM. A controlled trial of recombinant human erythropoietin and nandrolone decanoate in the treatment of anemia in patients on chronic hemodialysis. *Clin Nephrol* 1992; **37**(5): 264–7.
34. Chopp RT, Mendez R. Sexual function and hormonal abnormalities in uremic men on chronic dialysis and after renal transplantation. *Fertil Steril* 1978; **29**(6): 661–6.
35. Handelsman DJ, Dong Q. Hypothalamo–pituitary gonadal axis in chronic renal failure. *Endocrinol Metab Clin North Am* 1993; **22**(1): 145–61.
36. Casaburi R. Rationale for anabolic therapy to facilitate rehabilitation in chronic obstructive pulmonary disease. *Baillières Clin Endocrinol Metab* 1998; **12**(3): 407–18.
37. Bhasin S, Storer TW, Asbel-Sethi N, et al. Effects of testosterone replacement with a nongenital, transdermal system, Androderm, in human immunodeficiency virus-infected men with low testosterone levels. *J Clin Endocrinol Metab* 1998; **83**(9): 3155–62.
38. Bhasin S, Storer TW, Javanbakht M, et al. Testosterone replacement and resistance exercise in HIV-infected men with weight loss and low testosterone levels. *JAMA* 2000; **283**(6): 763–70.
39. Grinspoon S, Corcoran C, Askari H, et al. Effects of androgen administration in men with the AIDS wasting syndrome. A randomized, double-blind, placebo-controlled trial. *Ann Intern Med* 1998; **129**(1): 18–26.
40. MacAdams MR, White RH, Chipps BE. Reduction of serum testosterone levels during chronic glucocorticoid therapy. *Ann Intern Med* 1986; **104**(5): 648–51.
41. Reid IR, Ibbertson HK, France JT, et al. Plasma testosterone concentrations in asthmatic men treated with glucocorticoids. *Br Med J (Clin Res Ed)* 1985; **291**(6495): 574.
42. Trachtenberg J, Halpern N, Pont A. Ketoconazole: A novel and rapid treatment for advanced prostatic cancer. *J Urol* 1983; **130**(1): 152–3.
43. Pont A, Williams PL, Azhar S, et al. Ketoconazole blocks testosterone synthesis. *Arch Intern Med* 1982; **142**(12): 2137–40.
44. Johnson DE, Babaian RJ, Swanson DA, et al. Medical castration using megestrol acetate and minidose estrogen. *Urology* 1988; **31**(5): 371–4.
45. Venner P. Megestrol acetate in the treatment of metastatic carcinoma of the prostate. *Oncology* 1992; 49(Suppl 2): 22–7.
46. Bhasin S, Swerdloff RS. Mechanisms of gonadotropin-releasing hormone agonist action in the human male. *Endocrine Rev* 1986; 7(1): 106–14.
47. Kim WH, Swerdloff RS, Bhasin S. Regulation of alpha and rat luteinizing hormone-beta messenger ribonucleic acids during gonadotropin-releasing hormone agonist treatment in vivo in the male rat. *Endocrinology* 1988; **123**(4): 2111–16.
48. Okonmah AD, Bradshaw WG, Couceyro P, et al. The effect of neuroleptic drugs on serum testosterone level in the male rat. *Gen Pharmacol* 1986; 17(2): 235–8.
49. Rinieris P, Hatzimanolis J, Markianos M, et al. Effects of treatment with various doses of haloperidol on the pituitary–gonadal axis in male schizophrenic patients. *Neuropsychobiology* 1989; **22**(3): 146–9.
50. Halbreich U, Palter S. Accelerated osteoporosis in psychiatric patients: Possible pathophysiological processes. *Schizophr Bull* 1996; **22**(3): 447–54.

51. Carter HB, Pearson JD, Metter EJ, et al. Longitudinal evaluation of serum androgen levels in men with and without prostate cancer. *Prostate* 1995; 27(1): 25–31.
52. Ferrini RL, Barrett-Connor E. Sex hormones and age: A cross-sectional study of testosterone and estradiol and their bioavailable fractions in community-dwelling men. *Am J Epidemiol* 1998; 147(8): 750–4.
53. Korenman SG, Morley JE, Mooradian AD, et al. Secondary hypogonadism in older men: Its relation to impotence. *J Clin Endocrinol Metab* 1990; 71(4): 963–9.
54. Morley JE, Kaiser FE, Perry HM III, et al. Longitudinal changes in testosterone, luteinizing hormone, and follicle-stimulating hormone in healthy older men. *Metabolism* 1997; 46(4): 410–13.
55. Simon D, Preziosi P, Barrett-Connor E, et al. The influence of aging on plasma sex hormones in men: The Telecom Study. *Am J Epidemiol* 1992; 135(7): 783–91.
56. Tenover JS. Effects of testosterone supplementation in the aging male. *J Clin Endocrinol Metab* 1992; 75(4): 1092–8.
57. Tsitouras PD, Martin CE, Harman SM. Relationship of serum testosterone to sexual activity in healthy elderly men. *J Gerontol* 1982; 37(3): 288–93.
58. Morley JE, Perry HM III, Kaiser FE, et al. Effects of testosterone replacement therapy in old hypogonadal males: A preliminary study. *J Am Geriatr Soc* 1993; 41(2): 149–52.
59. Sih R, Morley JE, Kaiser FE, et al. Testosterone replacement in older hypogonadal men: A 12-month randomized controlled trial. *J Clin Endocrinol Metab* 1997; 82(6): 1661–7.
60. Snyder PJ, Peachey H, Hannoush P, et al. Effect of testosterone treatment on body composition and muscle strength in men over 65 years of age. *J Clin Endocrinol Metab* 1999; 84(8): 2647–53.
61. Snyder PJ, Peachey H, Hannoush P, et al. Effect of testosterone treatment on bone mineral density in men over 65 years of age. *J Clin Endocrinol Metab* 1999; 84(6): 1966–72.
62. Urban RJ, Bodenburg YH, Gilkison C, et al. Testosterone administration to elderly men increases skeletal muscle strength and protein synthesis. *Am J Physiol* 1995; 269(5 Pt 1): E820–6.
63. Tenover JL. Testosterone for all? The 80th Endocrine Society Meetings, New Orleans. S8–1, 1998.
64. Benet AE, Melman A. The epidemiology of erectile dysfunction. *Urol Clin North Am* 1995; 22(4): 699–709.
65. Buvat J, Lemaire A. Endocrine screening in 1,022 men with erectile dysfunction: Clinical significance and cost-effective strategy. *J Urol* 1997; 158(5): 1764–7.
66. Carani C, Zini D, Baldini A, et al. Effects of androgen treatment in impotent men with normal and low levels of free testosterone. *Arch Sex Behav* 1990; 19(3): 223–34.
67. Citron JT, Ettinger B, Rubinoff H, et al. Prevalence of hypothalamic–pituitary imaging abnormalities in impotent men with secondary hypogonadism. *J Urol* 1996; 155(2): 529–33.
68. Hajjar RR, Kaiser FE, Morley JE. Outcomes of long-term testosterone replacement in older hypogonadal males: A retrospective analysis. *J Clin Endocrinol Metab* 1997; 82(11): 3793–6.
69. Kaiser FE, Viosca SP, Morley JE, et al. Impotence and aging: Clinical and hormonal factors. *J Am Geriatr Soc* 1988; 36(6): 511–19.
70. Morales A, Johnston B, Heaton JP, et al. Testosterone supplementation for hypogonadal impotence: Assessment of biochemical measures and therapeutic outcomes. *J Urol* 1997; 157(3): 849–54.
71. Lugg JA, Rajfer J. Drug therapy for erectile dysfunction. *AUA Update* 1996; 15: 290.
72. Morley JE. Sex hormones and diabetes. *Diabetes Metab Rev* 1998; 6: 6–15.
73. Morley JE, Perry HM III. Androgen deficiency in aging men. *Med Clin North Am* 1999; 83(5): 1279–89.
74. van der Walt LA, Wilmsen EN, Jenkins T. Unusual sex hormone patterns among desert-dwelling hunter-gatherers. *J Clin Endocrinol Metab* 1978; 46(4): 658–63.
75. Sherman BM, Halmi KA, Zamudio R. LH and FSH response to gonadotropin-releasing hormone in anorexia nervosa: Effect of nutritional rehabilitation. *J Clin Endocrinol Metab* 1975; 41(1): 135–42.
76. Comerci GD. Medical complications of anorexia nervosa and bulimia nervosa. *Med Clin North Am* 1990; 74(5): 1293–310.
77. Mozaffarian GA, Higley M, Paulsen CA. Clinical studies in an adult male patient with 'isolated follicle stimulating hormone (FSH) deficiency'. *J Androl* 1983; 4(6): 393–8.
78. Ballabio A, Bardoni B, Carrozzo R, et al. Contiguous gene syndromes due to deletions in the distal short arm of the human X chromosome. *Proc Natl Acad Sci U S A* 1989; 86(24): 10001–5.
79. Hardelin JP, Levilliers J, Young J, et al. Xp22.3 deletions in isolated familial Kallmann's syndrome. *J Clin Endocrinol Metab* 1993; 76(4): 827–31.
80. Rebuffe-Scrive M, Marin P, Bjorntorp P. Effect of testosterone on abdominal adipose tissue in men. *Int J Obes* 1991; 15(11): 791–5.
81. Burris AS, Rodbard HW, Winters SJ, et al. Gonadotropin therapy in men with isolated hypogonadotropic hypogonadism: The response to human chorionic gonadotropin is predicted by initial testicular size. *J Clin Endocrinol Metab* 1988; 66(6): 1144–51.
82. Finkel DM, Phillips JL, Snyder PJ. Stimulation of spermatogenesis by gonadotropins in men with

hypogonadotropic hypogonadism. *N Engl J Med* 1985; 313(11): 651–5.

83. Whitcomb RW, Crowley WF Jr. Clinical review 4: Diagnosis and treatment of isolated gonadotropin-releasing hormone deficiency in men. *J Clin Endocrinol Metab* 1990; **70**(1): 3–7.
84. Klingmuller D, Dewes W, Krahe T, et al. Magnetic resonance imaging of the brain in patients with anosmia and hypothalamic hypogonadism (Kallmann's syndrome). *J Clin Endocrinol Metab* 1987; **65**(3): 581–4.
85. Longcope C, Goldfield SR, Brambilla DJ, et al. Androgens, estrogens, and sex hormone-binding globulin in middle-aged men. *J Clin Endocrinol Metab* 1990; 71(6): 1442–6.
86. Nankin HR, Calkins JH. Decreased bioavailable testosterone in aging normal and impotent men. *J Clin Endocrinol Metab* 1986; **63**(6): 1418–20.
87. Rosner W. Errors in the measurement of plasma free testosterone. *J Clin Endocrinol Metab* 1997; **82**(6): 2014–15.
88. Sinha-Hikim I, Arver S, Beall G, et al. The use of a sensitive equilibrium dialysis method for the measurement of free testosterone levels in healthy, cycling women and in human immunodeficiency virus-infected women [published erratum appears in *J Clin Endocrinol Metab* 1998; **83**(8): 2959]. *J Clin Endocrinol Metab* 1998; **83**(4): 1312–18.
89. Glass AR, Swerdloff RS, Bray GA, et al. Low serum testosterone and sex-hormone-binding-globulin in massively obese men. *J Clin Endocrinol Metab* 1977; **45**(6): 1211–19.
90. Zumoff B, Strain GW, Miller LK, et al. Plasma free and non-sex-hormone-binding-globulin-bound testosterone are decreased in obese men in proportion to their degree of obesity. *J Clin Endocrinol Metab* 1990; 71(4): 929–31.
91. Morley JE, Charlton E, Patrick P, et al. Validation of a screening questionnaire for androgen deficiency in aging males. *Metabolism* 2000; 49(9): 1239–42.
92. Themmen AP, Martens JW, Brunner HG. Gonadotropin receptor mutations. *J Endocrinol* 1997; **153**(2): 179–83.
93. Latronico AC, Anasti J, Arnhold IJ, et al. Brief report: Testicular and ovarian resistance to luteinizing hormone caused by inactivating mutations of the luteinizing hormone-receptor gene. *N Engl J Med* 1996; 334(8): 507–12.
94. Laue L, Wu SM, Kudo M, et al. A nonsense mutation of the human luteinizing hormone receptor gene in Leydig cell hypoplasia. *Hum Mol Genet* 1995; 4(8): 1429–33.
95. Laue LL, Wu SM, Kudo M, et al. Compound heterozygous mutations of the luteinizing hormone receptor gene in Leydig cell hypoplasia. *Mol Endocrinol* 1996; **10**(8): 987–97.
96. Aittomaki K, Lucena JL, Pakarinen P, et al. Mutation in the follicle-stimulating hormone receptor gene causes hereditary hypergonadotropic ovarian failure. *Cell* 1995; **82**(6): 959–68.
97. Aittomaki K, Herva R, Stenman UH, et al. Clinical features of primary ovarian failure caused by a point mutation in the follicle-stimulating hormone receptor gene. *J Clin Endocrinol Metab* 1996; **81**(10): 3722–6.
98. Bagheri SA, Boyer JL. Peliosis hepatis associated with androgenic-anabolic steroid therapy. A severe form of hepatic injury. *Ann Intern Med* 1974; **81**(5): 610–18.
99. Yoshida EM, Erb SR, Scudamore CH, et al. Severe cholestasis and jaundice secondary to an esterified testosterone, a non-C17 alkylated anabolic steroid. *J Clin Gastroenterol* 1994; **18**(3): 268–70.
100. Dobs AS, Meikle AW, Arver S, et al. Pharmacokinetics, efficacy, and safety of a permeation-enhanced testosterone transdermal system in comparison with bi-weekly injections of testosterone enanthate for the treatment of hypogonadal men. *J Clin Endocrinol Metab* 1999; **84**(10): 3469–78.
101. Snyder PJ, Lawrence DA. Treatment of male hypogonadism with testosterone enanthate. *J Clin Endocrinol Metab* 1980; **51**(6): 1335–9.
102. Sokol RZ, Palacios A, Campfield LA, et al. Comparison of the kinetics of injectable testosterone in eugonadal and hypogonadal men. *Fertil Steril* 1982; **37**(3): 425–30.
103. Edelstein D, Basaria S. Testosterone undecanoate in the treatment of male hypogonadism. *Expert Opin Pharmacother* 2010; 11: 2095–106.
104. Minnemann T, Schubet M, Hubler D, et al. A four year efficacy and safety study of the long-acting parenteral testosterone undecanoate. *Aging Male* 2007; 10: 155–8.
105. Cunningham GR, Cordero E, Thornby JI. Testosterone replacement with transdermal therapeutic systems. Physiological serum testosterone and elevated dihydrotestosterone levels. *JAMA* 1989; **261**(17): 2525–30.
106. Behre HM, Von Eckardstein S, Kliesch S, et al. Long-term substitution therapy of hypogonadal men with transscrotal testosterone over 7–10 years. *Clin Endocrinol (Oxf)* 1999; **50**(5): 629–35.
107. Meikle AW, Mazer NA, Moellmer JF, et al. Enhanced transdermal delivery of testosterone across nonscrotal skin produces physiological concentrations of testosterone and its metabolites in hypogonadal men. *J Clin Endocrinol Metab* 1992; 74(3): 623–8.
108. Wang C, Berman N, Longstreth JA, et al. Pharmacokinetics of transdermal testosterone gel in hypogonadal men: Application of gel at one site versus four sites: A General Clinical Research Center Study. *J Clin Endocrinol Metab* 2000; **85**(3): 964–9.
109. Jones TH, Arver S, Behre H, et al. Testosterone replacement in hypogonadal men with type 2 diabetes and/or metabolic syndrome (the TIMES2 study). *Diabetes Care* 2011; 34(4): 828–37.
110. Cooper CS, Perry PJ, Sparks AE, et al. Effect of exogenous testosterone on prostate volume, serum and

semen prostate specific antigen levels in healthy young men. *J Urol* 1998; 159(2): 441–3.
111. Meikle AW, Arver S, Dobs AS, et al. Prostate size in hypogonadal men treated with a nonscrotal permeation-enhanced testosterone transdermal system. *Urology* 1997; 49(2): 191–6.
112. Sasagawa I, Nakada T, Kazama T, et al. Volume change of the prostate and seminal vesicles in male hypogonadism after androgen replacement therapy. *Int Urol Nephrol* 1990; 22(3): 279–84.
113. Rencricca NJ, Solomon J, Fimian WJ Jr, et al. The effect of testosterone on erythropoiesis. *Scand J Haematol* 1969; 6(6): 431–6.
114. Naets JP, Wittek M. The mechanism of action of androgens on erythropoiesis. *Ann N Y Acad Sci* 1968; 149(1): 366–76.
115. Fried W, Marver D, Lange RD, et al. Studies on the erythropoietic stimulating factor in the plasma of mice after receiving testosterone. *J Lab Clin Med* 1966; 68(6): 947–51.
116. Dexter DD, Dovre EJ. Obstructive sleep apnea due to endogenous testosterone production in a woman. *Mayo Clin Proc* 1998; 73(3): 246–8.
117. Cistulli PA, Grunstein RR, Sullivan CE. Effect of testosterone administration on upper airway collapsibility during sleep. *Am J Respir Crit Care Med* 1994; 149(2 Pt 1): 530–2.
118. Emery MJ, Hlastala MP, Matsumoto AM. Depression of hypercapnic ventilatory drive by testosterone in the sleeping infant primate. *J Appl Physiol* 1994; 76(4): 1786–93.
119. Grunstein RR. Metabolic aspects of sleep apnea. *Sleep* 1996; 19(10 Suppl): S218–20.
120. Matsumoto AM, Sandblom RE, Schoene RB, et al. Testosterone replacement in hypogonadal men: Effects on obstructive sleep apnoea, respiratory drives, and sleep. *Clin Endocrinol (Oxf)* 1985; 22(6): 713–21.
121. Schneider BK, Pickett CK, Zwillich CW, et al. Influence of testosterone on breathing during sleep. *J Appl Physiol* 1986; 61(2): 618–23.
122. Tripathy D, Shah P, Lakshmy R, et al. Effect of testosterone replacement on whole body glucose utilisation and other cardiovascular risk factors in males with idiopathic hypogonadotrophic hypogonadism. *Horm Metab Res* 1998; 30(10): 642–5.
123. Bhasin S, Storer TW, Berman N, et al. Testosterone replacement increases fat-free mass and muscle size in hypogonadal men. *J Clin Endocrinol Metab* 1997; 82(2): 407–13.
124. Brodsky IG, Balagopal P, Nair KS. Effects of testosterone replacement on muscle mass and muscle protein synthesis in hypogonadal men—a clinical research center study. *J Clin Endocrinol Metab* 1996; 81(10): 3469–75.
125. Wang C, Eyre DR, Clark R, et al. Sublingual testosterone replacement improves muscle mass and strength, decreases bone resorption, and increases bone formation markers in hypogonadal men—a clinical research center study. *J Clin Endocrinol Metab* 1996; 81(10): 3654–62.
126. Bhasin S, Tenover JS. Age-associated sarcopenia issues in the use of testosterone as an anabolic agent in older men. *J Clin Endocrinol Metab* 1997; 82(6): 1659–60.
127. Hanash KA, Mostofi KF. Androgen effect on prostate specific antigen secretion. *J Surg Oncol* 1992; 49(3): 202–4.
128. Svetec DA, Canby ED, Thompson IM, et al. The effect of parenteral testosterone replacement on prostate specific antigen in hypogonadal men with erectile dysfunction. *J Urol* 1997; 158(5): 1775–7.
129. Morgentaler A, Bruning CO III, DeWolf WC. Occult prostate cancer in men with low serum testosterone levels. *JAMA* 1996; 276(23): 1904–6.
130. Winters SJ, Atkinson L. Serum LH concentrations in hypogonadal men during transdermal testosterone replacement through scrotal skin: Further evidence that ageing enhances testosterone negative feedback. The Testoderm Study Group. *Clin Endocrinol (Oxf)* 1997; 47(3): 317–22.
131. Ding EL, Song Y, Malik VS, et al. Sex differences of endogenous sex hormones and risk of type 2 diabetes: A systematic review and meta-analysis. *JAMA* 2006; 295: 1288–99.
132. Guay A, Jacobson J. The relationship between testosterone levels, the metabolic syndrome (by two criteria) and insulin resistance in a population of men with organic erectile dysfunction. *J Sex Med* 2007; 4: 1046–55.
133. Bhasin S, Cunningham GR, Hayes FJ, et al. Testosterone therapy in men with androgen deficiency syndromes: An Endocrine Society clinical practise guideline. *J Clin Endocrinol Metab* 2010; 95: 2536–59.
134. Bouloux PM, Legros JJ, Elbers JM, et al. Effects of oral testosterone undecanoate therapy on bone mineral density and body composition in 322 aging men with symptomatic testosterone deficiency: A 1-year, randomized, placebo-controlled, dose-ranging study. *Aging Male* 2013; 16(2): 38–47.
135. Wang C, Nieschlag E, Swerdloff R, et al. Investigation, treatment and monitoring of late-onset hypogonadism in males: ISA, ISSAM, EAU, EAA and ASA recommendations. *Eur J Endocrinol* 2008; 159: 507–14.
136. Fernandez-Balsells MM, Murad HM, Lane M, et al. Adverse effects of testosterone therapy in adult men: A systematic review and meta-analysis. *J Clin Endocrinol Metab* 2010; 95: 2560–75.
137. Basaria S, Coviello AD, Travison TG, et al. Adverse events associated with testosterone administration. *N Engl J Med* 2010; 363(2): 109–22.
138. Dhatariya K, Nagi D, Jones TH. ABCD position statement on the management of hypogonadal males with type 2 diabetes. *Practical Diabetes* 2010; 27: 408–12.

139. NIH Consensus Conference. Impotence. NIH Consensus Development Panel on Impotence. *JAMA* 1993; **270**(1): 83–90.
140. Lue TF. Erectile dysfunction. *N Engl J Med* 2000; **342**(24): 1802–13.
141. Furlow WL. Prevalence of impotence in the United States. *Med Aspects Hum Sex* 1985; **19**: 13–16.
142. Feldman HA, Goldstein I, Hatzichristou DG, et al. Impotence and its medical and psychosocial correlates: Results of the Massachusetts Male Aging Study. *J Urol* 1994; **151**(1): 54–61.
143. Lugg JA, Rajfer J, Gonzalez-Cadavid NF. Dihydrotestosterone is the active androgen in the maintenance of nitric oxide-mediated penile erection in the rat. *Endocrinology* 1995; **136**(4): 1495–501.
144. Andersson KE, Wagner G. Physiology of penile erection. *Physiol Rev* 1995; **75**(1): 191–236.
145. Christ GJ. The penis as a vascular organ. The importance of corporal smooth muscle tone in the control of erection. *Urol Clin North Am* 1995; **22**(4): 727–45.
146. Lue TF, Tanagho EA. Hemodynamics of erection. In: Tanagho EA, Lue TF, McClure RD, eds. *Contemporary Management of Impotence and Infertility*. Baltimore: Williams and Wilkins; 1988, pp. 28–38.
147. Naylor AM. Endogenous neurotransmitters mediating penile erection. *Br J Urol* 1998; **81**(3): 424–31.
148. Goldstein I, Lue TF, Padma-Nathan H, et al. Oral sildenafil in the treatment of erectile dysfunction. Sildenafil Study Group [published erratum appears in *N Engl J Med* 1998; **339**(1): 59]. *N Engl J Med* 1998; **338**(20): 1397–404.
149. Rajfer J, Aronson WJ, Bush PA, et al. Nitric oxide as a mediator of relaxation of the corpus cavernosum in response to nonadrenergic, noncholinergic neurotransmission. *N Engl J Med* 1992; **326**(2): 90–4.
150. McDonald LJ, Murad F. Nitric oxide and cyclic GMP signaling. *Proc Soc Exp Biol* Med 1996; **211**(1): 1–6.
151. Nehra A, Barrett DM, Moreland RB. Pharmacotherapeutic advances in the treatment of erectile dysfunction. *Mayo Clin Proc* 1999; **74**(7): 709–21.
152. Ruutu ML, Virtanen JM, Lindstrom BL, et al. The value of basic investigations in the diagnosis of impotence. *Scand J Urol Nephrol* 1987; **21**(4): 261–5.
153. Takasaki N, Kotani T, Miyazaki S, et al. [Measurement of penile brachial index (PBI) in patients with impotence]. *Hinyokika Kiyo* 1989; **35**(8): 1365–8.
154. Aitchison M, Aitchison J, Carter R. Is the penile brachial index a reproducible and useful measurement? *Br J Urol* 1990; **66**(2): 202–4.
155. Mueller SC, Wallenberg-Pachaly H, Voges GE, et al. Comparison of selective internal iliac pharmacoangiography, penile brachial index and duplex sonography with pulsed Doppler analysis for the evaluation of vasculogenic (arteriogenic) impotence. *J Urol* 1990; **143**(5): 928–32.
156. Rendell MS, Rajfer J, Wicker PA, et al. Sildenafil for treatment of erectile dysfunction in men with diabetes: A randomized controlled trial. Sildenafil Diabetes Study Group. *JAMA* 1999; **281**(5): 421–6.
157. Boolell M, Allen MJ, Ballard SA, et al. Sildenafil: An orally active type 5 cyclic GMP-specific phosphor diesterase inhibitor for the treatment of penile erectile dysfunction. *Int J Impot Res* 1996; **8**(2): 47–52.
158. Moreland RB, Goldstein I, Traish A. Sildenafil, a novel inhibitor of phosphodiesterase type 5 in human corpus cavernosum smooth muscle cells. *Life Sci* 1998; **62**(20): PL309–18.
159. Giuliano F, Hultling C, el Masry WS, et al. Randomized trial of sildenafil for the treatment of erectile dysfunction in spinal cord injury. Sildenafil Study Group. *Ann Neurol* 1999; **46**(1): 15–21.
160. Jarow JP, Burnett AL, Geringer AM. Clinical efficacy of sildenafil citrate based on etiology and response to prior treatment. *J Urol* 1999; **162**(3 Pt 1): 722–5.
161. Dinsmore WW, Hodges M, Hargreaves C, et al. Sildenafil citrate (Viagra) in erectile dysfunction: Near normalization in men with broad-spectrum erectile dysfunction compared with age-matched healthy control subjects [published erratum appears in *Urology* 1999; **53**(5): 1072]. *Urology* 1999; **53**(4): 800–5.
162. Morales A, Gingell C, Collins M, et al. Clinical safety of oral sildenafil citrate (VIAGRA) in the treatment of erectile dysfunction. *Int J Impot Res* 1998; **10**(2): 69–73.
163. Aversa A, Mazzilli F, Rossi T, et al. Effects of sildenafil (Viagra) administration on seminal parameters and post-ejaculatory refractory time in normal males. *Hum Reprod* 2000; **15**(1): 131–4.
164. Feenstra J, Drie-Pierik RJ, Lacle CF, et al. Acute myocardial infarction associated with sildenafil. *Lancet* 1998; **352**(9132): 957–8.
165. Zusman RM, Morales A, Glasser DB, et al. Overall cardiovascular profile of sildenafil citrate. *Am J Cardiol* 1999; **83**(5A): 35C–44C.
166. Arora RR, Timoney M, Melilli L. Acute myocardial infarction after the use of sildenafil. *N Engl J Med* 1999; **341**(9): 700.
167. Muller JE, Mittleman A, Maclure M, et al. Triggering myocardial infarction by sexual activity. Low absolute risk and prevention by regular physical exertion. Determinants of Myocardial Infarction Onset Study Investigators. *JAMA* 1996; **275**(18): 1405–9.
168. Cheitlin MD, Hutter AM Jr, Brindis RG, et al. Use of sildenafil (Viagra) in patients with cardiovascular disease. Technology and Practice Executive Committee [published erratum appears in *Circulation* 1999; **100**(23): 2389]. *Circulation* 1999; **99**(1): 168–77.
169. Herrmann HC, Chang G, Klugherz BD, et al. Hemodynamic effects of sildenafil in men with severe coronary artery disease. *N Engl J Med* 2000; **342**(22): 1622–6.

170. Padma-Nathan H, Steers WD, Wicker PA. Efficacy and safety of oral sildenafil in the treatment of erectile dysfunction: A double-blind, placebo-controlled study of 329 patients. Sildenafil Study Group. *Int J Clin Pract* 1998; **52**(6): 375–9.
171. Goldenberg MM. Safety and efficacy of sildenafil citrate in the treatment of male erectile dysfunction. *Clin Ther* 1998; **20**(6): 1033–48.
172. Conti CR, Pepine CJ, Sweeney M. Efficacy and safety of sildenafil citrate in the treatment of erectile dysfunction in patients with ischemic heart disease. *Am J Cardiol* 1999; **83**(5A): 29C–34C.
173. Osterloh IH, Collins M, Wicker P, et al. Sildenafil citrate (VIAGRA): Overall safety profile in 18 double-blind, placebo controlled, clinical trials. *Int J Clin Pract Suppl* 1999; **102**: 3–5.
174. Young J. Sildenafil citrate (VIAGRA) in the treatment of erectile dysfunction: A 12-week, flexible-dose study to assess efficacy and safety. *Int J Clin Pract Suppl* 1999; **102**: 6–7.
175. Goldstein I. A 36-week, open label, non-comparative study to assess the long-term safety of sildenafil citrate (VIAGRA) in patients with erectile dysfunction. *Int J Clin Pract Suppl* 1999; **102**: 8–9.
176. Kloner RA. Cardiovascular risk and sildenafil. *Am J Cardiol* 2000; **86**(2A): 57F–61F.
177. McMahon CG, Samali R, Johnson H. Efficacy, safety and patient acceptance of sildenafil citrate as treatment for erectile dysfunction. *J Urol* 2000; 164(4): 1192–6.
178. McGarvey MR. Tough choices: The cost-effectiveness of sildenafil. *Ann Intern Med* 2000; **132**(12): 994–5.
179. Smith KJ, Roberts MS. The cost-effectiveness of sildenafil. *Ann Intern Med* 2000; **132**(12): 933–7.
180. Tan HL. Economic cost of male erectile dysfunction using a decision analytic model: For a hypothetical managed-care plan of 100,000 members. *Pharmacoeconomics* 2000; 17(1): 77–107.
181. Witherington R. Vacuum devices for the impotent. *J Sex Marital Ther* 1991; 17(2): 69–80.
182. Lewis JH, Sidi AA, Reddy PK. A way to help your patients who use vacuum devices. *Contemp Urol* 1991; 3(12): 15–21.
183. Morley JE. Management of impotence. Diagnostic considerations and therapeutic options. *Postgrad Med* 1993; 93(3): 65–72.
184. Morales A. Nonsurgical management options in impotence. *Hosp Pract (Off Ed)* 1993; **28**(3A): 15–20, 23.
185. Lewis RW, Witherington R. External vacuum therapy for erectile dysfunction: Use and results. *World J Urol* 1997; 15(1): 78–82.
186. Ganem JP, Lucey DT, Janosko EO, et al. Unusual complications of the vacuum erection device. *Urology* 1998; 51(4): 627–31.
187. Finelli A, Hirshberg ED, Radomski SB. The treatment choice of elderly patients with erectile dysfunction. *Geriatr Nephrol Urol* 1998; **8**(1): 15–19.
188. Oakley N, Moore KT. Vacuum devices in erectile dysfunction: Indications and efficacy. *Br J Urol* 1998; **82**(5): 673–81.
189. Skakkebaek NE, Bancroft J, Davidson DW, et al. Androgen replacement with oral testosterone undecanoate in hypogonadal men: A double blind controlled study. *Clin Endocrinol (Oxf)* 1981; 14(1): 49–61.
190. McClure RD, Oses R, Ernest ML. Hypogonadal impotence treated by transdermal testosterone. *Urology* 1991; **37**(3): 224–8.
191. Nankin HR, Lin T, Osterman J. Chronic testosterone cypionate therapy in men with secondary impotence. *Fertil Steril* 1986; 46(2): 300–7.
192. Arver S, Dobs AS, Meikle AW, et al. Improvement of sexual function in testosterone deficient men treated for 1 year with a permeation enhanced testosterone transdermal system. *J Urol* 1996; **155**(5): 1604–8.
193. Buena F, Swerdloff RS, Steiner BS, et al. Sexual function does not change when serum testosterone levels are pharmacologically varied within the normal male range. *Fertil Steril* 1993; 59(5): 1118–23.
194. Bhasin S, Fielder T, Peacock N, et al. Dissociating antifertility effects of behavior in male rats. *Am J Physiol* 1988; **254**(1 Pt 1): E84–91.
195. Fielder TJ, Peacock NR, McGivern RF, et al. Testosterone dose-dependency of sexual and nonsexual behaviors in the gonadotropin-releasing hormone antagonist-treated male rat. *J Androl* 1989; **10**(3): 167–73.
196. Bhasin S. The dose-dependent effects of testosterone on sexual function and on muscle mass and function. *Mayo Clin Proc* 2000; **75**(Suppl): S70–5.
197. Jain P, Rademaker AW, McVary KT. Testosterone supplementation for erectile dysfunction: Results of a meta-analysis. *J Urol* 2000; **164**(2): 371–5.
198. Engelhardt PF, Plas E, Hubner WA, et al. Comparison of intraurethral liposomal and intracavernosal prostaglandin-E1 in the management of erectile dysfunction. *Br J Urol* 1998; **81**(3): 441–4.
199. Kim ED, McVary KT. Topical prostaglandin-E1 for the treatment of erectile dysfunction. *J Urol* 1995; **153**(6): 1828–30.
200. Peterson CA, Bennett AH, Hellstrom WJ, et al. Erectile response to transurethral alprostadil, prazosin and alprostadil–prazosin combinations. *J Urol* 1998; **159**(5): 1523–7.
201. Yoshimura N, Kato R, Michael B, et al. Gene therapy as future treatment of erectile dysfunction. *Expert Opin Biol Ther* 2010; **10**(9): 1305–14.
202. Bhasin S, de Kretser DM, Baker HW. Clinical review 64: Pathophysiology and natural history of male infertility. *J Clin Endocrinol Metab* 1994; **79**(6): 1525–9.

203. de Kretser DM, Burger HG, Fortune D, et al. Hormonal, histological and chromosomal studies in adult males with testicular disorders. *J Clin Endocrinol Metab* 1972; **35**(3): 392–401.
204. Lamb DJ, Niederberger CS. Animal models that mimic human male reproductive defects. *Urol Clin North Am* 1994; **21**(3): 377–87.
205. Jaffe T, Oates RD. Genetic abnormalities and reproductive failure. *Urol Clin North Am* 1994; **21**(3): 389–408.
206. Skakkebaek NE, Giwercman A, de Kretser D. Pathogenesis and management of male infertility. *Lancet* 1994; **343**(8911): 1473–9.
207. Heller CG, Clermont Y. Kinetics of the germinal epithelium in man. *Recent Prog Horm Res* 1964; **20**: 545–75.
208. Griswold MD. Protein secretions of Sertoli cells. *Int Rev Cytol* 1988; **110**: 133–56.
209. Baker HW, Burger HG, de Kretser DM, et al. Relative incidence of etiologic factors in male infertility. In: Santen RJ, Swedloff RS, eds. *Reproductive Dysfunction: Diagnosis and Management of Hypogonadism*. New York: Marcel Dekker; 1986, pp. 341–72.
210. Swerdloff RS, Boyers SP. Evaluation of the male partner of an infertile couple. An algorithmic approach. *JAMA* 1982; **247**(17): 2418–22.
211. World Health Organization. *Laboratory Manual for the Examination of Human Semen and Semen–Cervical Mucus Interaction*. Cambridge: Cambridge University Press; 1987.
212. Wang C, Chan SY, Ng M, et al. Diagnostic value of sperm function tests and routine semen analyses in fertile and infertile men. *J Androl* 1988; 9(6): 384–9.
213. Zuffardi O, Tiepolo L. Frequencies and types of chromosome abnormalities associated with human male infertility. In: Crosignani PG, Rubin BL, eds. *Genetic Control of Gametic Production and Function*. New York: Academic Press; 1982, pp. 261–73.
214. Kjessler B. *Karyotype, Meiosis and Spermatogenesis in a Sample of Men Attending an Infertility Clinic*. Basel: S. Karger; 1966.
215. Chandley AC. The chromosomal basis of human infertility. *Br Med Bull* 1979; **35**(2): 181–6.
216. Koulischer L, Schoysman R. Studies of the mitotic and meiotic chromosomes in infertile males. *J Genet Hum* 1975; **23**(Suppl): 58–70.
217. Jacobs PA, Melville M, Ratcliffe S, et al. A cytogenetic survey of 11,680 newborn infants. *Ann Hum Genet* 1974; **37**(4): 359–76.
218. Hamerton JL, Canning N, Ray M, et al. A cytogenetic survey of 14,069 newborn infants. I. Incidence of chromosome abnormalities. *Clin Genet* 1975; **8**(4): 223–43.
219. Bryns JP, Kleckowska A, van den Berghe H. *The X Chromosome and Sexual Development: Clinical Aspects*. New York: Alan R. Liss; 1983.
220. Huckins C, Bullock LP, Long JL. Morphological profiles of cryptorchid XXY mouse testes. *Anat Rec* 1981; 199(4): 507–18.
221. Zinn AR, Ramos P, Elder FF, et al. Androgen receptor CAGn repeat length influences phenotype of 47,XXY (Klinefelter) syndrome. *J Clin Endocrinol Metab* 2005; 90(9): 5041–6.
222. Patwardham AJ, Eliez S, Bender B, et al. Brain morphology in Klinefelter's syndrome: Extra X chromosome and testosterone supplementation. *Neurology* 2000; **54**: 2218–23.
223. Winter JS. Androgen therapy in Klinefelter syndrome during adolescence. *Birth Defects* 1991; **26**: 234–45.
224. Aksglaede L, Juul A. Testicular function and fertility in men with Klinefelter syndrome: A review. *Eur J Endocrinol* 2013; **168**(4): R67–76.
225. Bergere M, Wainer R, Nataf V, et al. Biopsied testes cells of four 47,XXY patients: Fluorescence in-situ hybridization and ICSI results. *Human Reprod* 2002; **17**: 32–7.
226. Hennebicq S, Pelletier R, Bergues U, Rousseaux S. Risk of trisomy 21 in offspring of patients with Klinefelter's syndrome. *Lancet* 2001; **30**: 2104–5.
227. Staessen C, Tournaye H, Van Assche E, et al. PGD in 47,XXY Klinefelter's syndrome patients. *Human Reprod* 2003; **9**: 319–30.
228. Sharland M, Burch M, McKenna WM, et al. A clinical study of Noonan syndrome. *Arch Dis Child* 1992; 67(2): 178–83.
229. Papadopoulou A, Issakidis M, Gole E, et al. Phenotypic spectrum of 80 Greek patients referred as Noonan syndrome and PTPN11 mutation analysis: The value of initial clinical assessment. *Eur J Pediatr* 2012; **171**(1): 51–8.
230. Santen RJ, DeKretser DM, Paulsen CA, et al. Gonadotropins and testosterone in the XYY syndrome. *Lancet* 1970; 2(7668): 371.
231. Davidoff F, Federman DD. Mixed gonadal dysgenesis. *Pediatrics* 1973; **52**(5): 725–42.
232. Page DC, Brown LG, de la Chapelle A. Exchange of terminal portions of X and Y-chromosomal short arms in human XX males. *Nature* 1987; **328**(6129): 437–40.
233. Page DC, de la CA, Weissenbach J. Chromosome Y-specific DNA in related human XX males. *Nature* 1985; **315**(6016): 224–6.
234. Chai NN, Phillips A, Fernandez A, et al. A putative human male infertility gene DAZLA: Genomic structure and methylation status. *Mol Hum Reprod* 1997; 3(8): 705–8.
235. Ruggiu M, Speed R, Taggart M, et al. The mouse Dazla gene encodes a cytoplasmic protein essential for gametogenesis. *Nature* 1997; **389**(6646): 73–7.
236. Saut N, Terriou P, Navarro A, et al. The human Y chromosome genes BPY2, CDY1 and DAZ are not

essential for sustained fertility. *Mol Hum Reprod* 2000; 6(9): 789–93.
237. Lim HN, Chen H, McBride S, et al. Longer polyglutamine tracts in the androgen receptor are associated with moderate to severe undermasculinized genitalia in XY males. *Hum Mol Genet* 2000; 9(5): 829–34.
238. Tut TG, Ghadessy FJ, Trifiro MA, et al. Long polyglutamine tracts in the androgen receptor are associated with reduced trans-activation, impaired sperm production, and male infertility. *J Clin Endocrinol Metab* 1997; **82**(11): 3777–82.
239. Yong EL, Ghadessy F, Wang Q, et al. Androgen receptor transactivation domain and control of spermatogenesis. *Rev Reprod* 1998; 3(3): 141–4.
240. Dadze S, Wieland C, Jakubiczka S, et al. The size of the CAG repeat in exon 1 of the androgen receptor gene shows no significant relationship to impaired spermatogenesis in an infertile Caucasoid sample of German origin. *Mol Hum Reprod* 2000; 6(3): 207–14.
241. Tamai KT, Monaco L, Nantel F, et al. Coupling signalling pathways to transcriptional control: Nuclear factors responsive to AMP. *Recent Prog Horm Res* 1997; **52**: 121–39.
242. Peri A, Krausz C, Cioppi F, et al. Cyclic adenosine 3′,5′-monophosphate-responsive element modulator gene expression in germ cells of normo- and oligo-azoospermic men. *J Clin Endocrinol Metab* 1998; **83**(10): 3722–6.
243. Lin WW, Lamb DJ, Lipshultz LI, et al. Absence of cyclic adenosine 3′:5′ monophosphate responsive element modulator expression at the spermatocyte arrest stage. *Fertil Steril* 1998; 69(3): 533–8.
244. Weinbauer GF, Behr R, Bergmann M, et al. Testicular cAMP responsive element modulator (CREM) protein is expressed in round spermatids but is absent or reduced in men with round spermatid maturation arrest. *Mol Hum Reprod* 1998; 4(1): 9–15.
245. Blendy JA, Kaestner KH, Weinbauer GF, et al. Severe impairment of spermatogenesis in mice lacking the CREM gene. *Nature* 1996; **380**(6570): 162–5.
246. Anguiano A, Oates RD, Amos JA, et al. Congenital bilateral absence of the vas deferens. A primarily genital form of cystic fibrosis. *JAMA* 1992; **267**(13): 1794–7.
247. Reijo R, Alagappan RK, Patrizio P, et al. Severe oligozoospermia resulting from deletions of azoo-spermia factor gene on Y chromosome. *Lancet* 1996; 347(9011): 1290–3.
248. Pryor JL, Kent-First M, Muallem A, et al. Microdeletions in the Y chromosome of infertile men. *N Engl J Med* 1997; 336(8): 534–9.
249. Nagafuchi S, Namiki M, Nakahori Y, et al. A minute deletion of the Y chromosome in men with azoospermia. *J Urol* 1993; **150**(4): 1155–7.
250. Najmabadi H, Huang V, Yen P, et al. Substantial prevalence of microdeletions of the Y-chromosome in infertile men with idiopathic azoospermia and oligozoospermia detected using a sequence-tagged site-based mapping strategy. *J Clin Endocrinol Metab* 1996; **81**(4): 1347–52.
251. Henegariu O, Hirschmann P, Kilian K, et al. Rapid screening of the Y chromosome in idiopathic sterile men, diagnostic for deletions in AZF, a genetic Y factor expressed during spermatogenesis. *Andrologia* 1994; 26(2): 97–106.
252. Vogt P, Chandley AC, Hargreave TB, et al. Microdeletions in interval 6 of the Y chromosome of males with idiopathic sterility point to disruption of AZF, a human spermatogenesis gene. *Hum Genet* 1992; **89**(5): 491–6.
253. Martinez MC, Bernabe MJ, Gomez E, et al. Screening for AZF deletion in a large series of severely impaired spermatogenesis patients. *J Androl* 2000; 21(5): 651–5.
254. Eberhart CG, Maines JZ, Wasserman SA. Meiotic cell cycle requirement for a fly homologue of human deleted in azoospermia. *Nature* 1996; **381**(6585): 783–5.
255. Reijo R, Seligman J, Dinulos MB, et al. Mouse autosomal homolog of DAZ, a candidate male sterility gene in humans, is expressed in male germ cells before and after puberty. *Genomics* 1996; **35**(2): 346–52.
256. Saxena R, Brown LG, Hawkins T, et al. The DAZ gene cluster on the human Y chromosome arose from an autosomal gene that was transposed, repeatedly amplified and pruned. *Nat Genet* 1996; 14(3): 292–9.
257. Najmabadi H, Chai N, Kapali A, et al. Genomic structure of a Y-specific ribonucleic acid binding motif-containing gene: A putative candidate for a subset of male infertility. *J Clin Endocrinol Metab* 1996; **81**(6): 2159–64.
258. Cooke HJ, Lee M, Kerr S, et al. A murine homologue of the human DAZ gene is autosomal and expressed only in male and female gonads. *Hum Mol Genet* 1996; 5(4): 513–16.
259. Yen PH, Chai NN, Salido EC. The human autosomal gene DAZLA: Testis specificity and a candidate for male infertility. *Hum Mol Genet* 1996; 5(12): 2013–17.
260. Fradkin JE, Schonberger LB, Mills JL, et al. Creutzfeldt–Jakob disease in pituitary growth hormone recipients in the United States. *JAMA* 1991; **265**(7): 880–4.
261. Abbasi AA, Prasad AS, Ortega J, et al. Gonadal function abnormalities in sickle cell anemia. Studies in adult male patients. *Ann Intern Med* 1976; **85**(5): 601–5.
262. Kletzky OA, Costin G, Marrs RP. Gonadotropin insufficiency in patients with thalassemia major. *J Clin Endocrinol Metab* 1979; **48**(6): 901–5.
263. Takeda R, Ueda M. Pituitary–gonadal function in male patients with myotonic dystrophy—serum testosterone levels and histological damage of the testis. *Acta Endocrinol (Copenh)* 1977; **84**(2): 382–9.

264. Wennerholm UB, Bergh C, Hamberger L, et al. Obstetric outcome of pregnancies following ICSI, classified according to sperm origin and quality. *Hum Reprod* 2000; **15**(5): 1189–94.
265. Heller CG, Elson WO. Classification of male hypogonadism and discussion of the pathologic physiology, diagnosis and treatment. *J Clin Endocrinol Metab* 1948; **8**: 345–66.
266. MacLeod J, Pazianos A, Ray BS. Restoration of human spermatogenesis by menopausal gonadotropins. *Lancet* 1964; **1**(7344): 1196–7.
267. Santen RJ, Paulsen CA. Hypogonadotropic eunuchoidism. II. Gonadal responsiveness to exogenous gonadotropins. *J Clin Endocrinol Metab* 1973; **36**(1): 55–63.
268. Gemzell C, Kiessler G. Treatment of infertility after partial hypophysectomy with human pituitary gonadotropins. *Lancet* 1964; **1**(7344): 44–7.
269. Johnson SG. A study of human testicular function by the use of human menopausal gonadotropin and human chorionic gonadotropin in male hypogonadotropic eunuchoidism and infantilism. *Acta Endocrinol (Copenh)* 1966; **53**: 315–41.
270. Burgues S, Calderon MD. Subcutaneous self-administration of highly purified follicle stimulating hormone and human chorionic gonadotropin for the treatment of male hypogonadotrophic hypogonadism. Spanish Collaborative Group on Male Hypogonadotropic Hypogonadism. *Hum Reprod* 1997; **12**(5): 980–6.
271. Recombinant Human FSH Product Development Group. Recombinant follicle stimulating hormone: Development of the first biotechnology product for the treatment of infertility. *Hum Reprod Update* 1998; **4**(6): 862–81.
272. Liu PY, Turner L, Rushford D, et al. Efficacy and safety of recombinant human follicle stimulating hormone (Gonal-F) with urinary human chorionic gonadotropin for induction of spermatogenesis and fertility in gonadotropin-deficient men. *Hum Reprod* 1999; **14**(6): 1540–5.
273. Zitzmann M, Nieschlag E. Hormone substitution in male hypogonadism. *Mol Cell Endocrinol* 2000; **161**(1–2): 73–88.
274. Smals AG, Pieters GF, Drayer JI, et al. Leydig cell responsiveness to single and repeated human chorionic gonadotropin administration. *J Clin Endocrinol Metab* 1979; **49**(1): 12–14.
275. Padron RS, Wischusen J, Hudson B, et al. Prolonged biphasic response of plasma testosterone to single intramuscular injections of human chorionic gonadotropin. *J Clin Endocrinol Metab* 1980; **50**(6): 1100–4.
276. Saez JM, Forest MG. Kinetics of human chorionic gonadotropin-induced steroidogenic response of the human testis. I. Plasma testosterone: Implications for human chorionic gonadotropin stimulation test. *J Clin Endocrinol Metab* 1979; **49**(2): 278–83.
277. Wang C, Paulsen CA, Hopper BR. Acute steroidogenic responsiveness to human luteinizing hormone in hypogonadotropic hypogonadism. *J Clin Endocrinol Metab* 1980; **51**(6): 1269–73.
278. Hoffman AR, Crowley WF Jr. Induction of puberty in men by long-term pulsatile administration of low-dose gonadotropin-releasing hormone. *N Engl J Med* 1982; **307**(20): 1237–41.
279. Whitcomb RW, Crowley WF Jr. Male hypogonadotropic hypogonadism. *Endocrinol Metab Clin North Am* 1993; **22**(1): 125–43.
280. Bergada C, Mancini RE. Effect of gonadotropins on the induction of spermatogenesis in human prepubertal testis. *J Clin Endocrinol Metab* 1973; **37**(6): 935–43.
281. Mancini RE, Seiguer AC, Lloret AP. Effect of gonadotropins on the recovery of spermatogenesis in hypophysectomized patients. *J Clin Endocrinol Metab* 1969; **29**(4): 467–78.
282. Liu L, Banks SM, Barnes KM, et al. Two-year comparison of testicular responses to pulsatile gonadotropin-releasing hormone and exogenous gonadotropins from the inception of therapy in men with isolated hypogonadotropic hypogonadism. *J Clin Endocrinol Metab* 1988; **67**(6): 1140–5.
283. Buchter D, Behre HM, Kliesch S, et al. Pulsatile GnRH or human chorionic gonadotropin/human menopausal gonadotropin as effective treatment for men with hypogonadotropic hypogonadism: A review of 42 cases. *Eur J Endocrinol* 1998; **139**(3): 298–303.
284. Kliesch S, Behre HM, Nieschlag E. High efficacy of gonadotropin or pulsatile gonadotropin-releasing hormone treatment in hypogonadotropic hypogonadal men. *Eur J Endocrinol* 1994; **131**(4): 347–54.
285. Braunstein GD, Bloch SK, Rasor JL, et al. Characterization of antihuman chorionic gonadotropin serum antibody appearing after ovulation induction. *J Clin Endocrinol Metab* 1983; **57**(6): 1164–72.
286. Nieschlag E, Bernitz S, Topert M. Antigenicity of human chorionic gonadotropin preparations in men. *Clin Endocrinol (Oxf)* 1982; **16**(5): 483–8.
287. Sokol RZ, McClure RD, Peterson M, et al. Gonadotropin therapy failure secondary to human chorionic gonadotropin-induced antibodies. *J Clin Endocrinol Metab* 1981; **52**(5): 929–32.
288. Claustrat B, David L, Faure A, et al. Development of anti-human chorionic gonadotropin antibodies in patients with hypogonadotropic hypogonadism. A study of four patients. *J Clin Endocrinol Metab* 1983; **57**(5): 1041–7.
289. Burger HG, de Kretser DM, Hudson B, et al. Effects of preceding androgen therapy on testicular response to human pituitary gonadotropin in hypo-gonadotropic hypogonadism: A study of three patients. *Fertil Steril* 1981; **35**(1): 64–8.

290. Belchetz PE, Plant TM, Nakai Y, et al. Hypophysial responses to continuous and intermittent delivery of hypothalamic gonadotropin-releasing hormone. *Science* 1978; **202**(4368): 631–3.
291. Knobil E. The neuroendocrine control of the menstrual cycle. *Recent Prog Horm Res* 1980; **36**: 53–88.
292. Wildt L, Hausler A, Marshall G, et al. Frequency and amplitude of gonadotropin-releasing hormone stimulation and gonadotropin secretion in the rhesus monkey. *Endocrinology* 1981; **109**(2): 376–85.
293. Spratt DI, Hoffman AR, Crowley WF Jr. Hypogonadotropic hypogonadism. In: Santen RJ, Swerdloff RS, eds. *Male Reproductive Dysfunction*. New York: Marcel Dekker; 1986, pp. 227–49.
294. Moore MP, Smith R, Donald RA, et al. The effects of different dose regimes of D-SER(TBU)6–LHRH-EA10 (HOE 766) in subjects with hypogonadotrophic hypogonadism. *Clin Endocrinol (Oxf)* 1981; **14**(1): 93–7.
295. Laron Z, Dickerman Z, Ben Zeev Z, et al. Long-term effect of D-Trp6-luteinizing hormone-releasing hormone on testicular size and luteinizing hormone, follicle-stimulating hormone, and testosterone levels in hypothalamic hypogonadotropic males. *Fertil Steril* 1981; **35**(3): 328–31.
296. Vickery BH. Comparison of the potential for therapeutic utilities with gonadotropin-releasing hormone agonists and antagonists. *Endocrine Rev* 1986; **7**(1): 115–24.
297. Spratt DI, Finkelstein JS, O'Dea LS, et al. Long-term administration of gonadotropin-releasing hormone in men with idiopathic hypogonadotropic hypogonadism. A model for studies of the hormone's physiologic effects. *Ann Intern Med* 1986; **105**(6): 848–55.
298. Burger HG, Baker HW. The treatment of infertility. *Annu Rev Med* 1987; **38**: 29–40.
299. Bourne H, Stern K, Clarke G, et al. Delivery of normal twins following the intracytoplasmic injection of spermatozoa from a patient with 47,XXY Klinefelter's syndrome. *Hum Reprod* 1997; **12**(11): 2447–50.
300. Palermo GD, Schlegel PN, Hariprashad JJ, et al. Fertilization and pregnancy outcome with intracyto plasmic sperm injection for azoospermic men. *Hum Reprod* 1999; 14(3): 741–8.
301. Palermo GD, Schlegel PN, Sills ES, et al. Births after intracytoplasmic injection of sperm obtained by testicular extraction from men with nonmosaic Klinefelter's syndrome. *N Engl J Med* 1998; **338**(9): 588–90.
302. Crosignani PG, Rubin BL. Optimal use of infertility diagnostic tests and treatments. The ESHRE Capri Workshop Group. *Hum Reprod* 2000; **15**(3): 723–32.
303. Ismail MT, Sedor J, Hirsch IH. Are sperm motion parameters influenced by varicocele ligation? *Fertil Steril* 1999; 71(5): 886–90.
304. Nieschlag E, Hertle L, Fischedick A, et al. Update on treatment of varicocele: Counselling as effective as occlusion of the vena spermatica. *Hum Reprod* 1998; **13**(8): 2147–50.
305. Culha M, Mutlu N, Acar O, et al. Comparison of testicular volumes before and after varicocelectomy. *Urol Int* 1998; **60**(4): 220–3.
306. Asci R, Sarikaya S, Buyukalpelli R, et al. The outcome of varicocelectomy in subfertile men with an absent or atrophic right testis. *Br J Urol* 1998; **81**(5): 750–2.
307. Segenreich E, Israilov S, Shmuele J, et al. Evaluation of the relationship between semen parameters, pregnancy rate of wives of infertile men with varicocele, and gonadotropin-releasing hormone test before and after varicocelectomy. *Urology* 1998; **52**(5): 853–7.
308. Tarlatzis BC, Bili H. Intracytoplasmic sperm injection. Survey of world results. *Ann N Y Acad Sci* 2000; **900**: 336–44.
309. Bonduelle M, Camus M, De Vos A, et al. Seven years of intracytoplasmic sperm injection and follow-up of 1987 subsequent children. *Hum Reprod* 1999; 14(Suppl 1): 243–64.
310. Wennerholm UB, Bergh C, Hamberger L, et al. Incidence of congenital malformations in children born after ICSI. *Hum Reprod* 2000; **15**(4): 944–8.
311. Devroey P, Vandervorst M, Nagy P, et al. Do we treat the male or his gamete? *Hum Reprod* 1998; 13(Suppl 1): 178–85.

# 18

# Amenorrhea and hirsutism

*Stephen Franks*

## *Introduction*

Amenorrhea and hirsutism are two of the commonest presenting symptoms to a reproductive endocrine clinic, reflecting the high prevalence of these symptoms in the female population. If they occur together, amenorrhea and hirsutism are very likely to represent manifestations of polycystic ovary syndrome (PCOS) that is by far the commonest endocrine disorder in women of reproductive age. In this chapter, amenorrhea and hirsutism are considered, but the significance of the coincidence of these symptoms is discussed in detail in the context of PCOS.

## *Amenorrhea*

Amenorrhea is conventionally defined as absence of periods for 6 months or more. Amenorrhea can be further categorized as primary amenorrhea in a woman who has never menstruated and secondary amenorrhea in a woman who has had at least one period. With the exception of a small proportion of cases in which there is a congenital or acquired genital tract abnormality, amenorrhea is indicative of anovulation and most commonly reflects a disorder of gonadotropin regulation or PCOS. As one might expect, the proportion of young women who have a congenital abnormality of ovarian development (such as Turner syndrome) or of the genital tract is greater in women with primary amenorrhea than in women with secondary amenorrhea (such congenital abnormalities accounting for about 60% of cases of primary amenorrhea); otherwise, there is considerable overlap in causes of primary and secondary amenorrhea.[1] In adolescent girls, there is little distinction between delayed menarche (defined as no periods by 16 years of age) and primary amenorrhea, but it is important to assess the stage of pubertal development in girls with delayed menarche. The causes of secondary amenorrhea are summarized in Table 18.2.

## *Causes of amenorrhea*

The common causes of amenorrhea are shown in Tables 18.1 and 18.2. Causes can be classified, functionally, into three major groups: primary ovarian failure (POF), now more commonly called primary ovarian insufficiency (POI); deficiency or disordered regulation of gonadotropins; and PCOS in which the mechanism of anovulation is uncertain. For a more comprehensive list of endocrine causes of amenorrhea, see the review by Unuane et al.[2]

The prevalence of the various causes of amenorrhea varies somewhat from clinic to clinic, but overall, the most common causes of secondary amenorrhea are functional disorders of gonadotropin regulation, PCOS, and POI. Primary pituitary deficiency of gonadotropins is rare, but it is important to note that although pituitary tumors (other than hyperprolactinemia) are uncommon causes of amenorrhea, it may be an early, or even presenting symptom in women who have acromegaly,[3] Cushing disease,[4] or nonfunctioning pituitary adenomas. In such cases, the length of the history and concurrence of other symptoms and signs are often the most important clues that there may be a less common underlying cause for the amenorrhea. For example, although PCOS is by far the commonest cause of amenorrhea with hirsutism, one would be more suspicious of a diagnosis of Cushing

A. Primary ovarian or genital tract disorders
   - Gonadal dysgenesis (most commonly Turner syndrome)
   - Genital (Müllerian) tract abnormalities
   - Disorders of sexual development (DSDs)

B. Hypothalamic/pituitary disorders
   - Deficiency of gonadotropin-releasing hormone

*Note:* Plus any of the causes of secondary amenorrhea

***Table 18.1***
*Causes of primary amenorrhea.*

A. Primary ovarian insufficiency
   - Genetic
   - Autoimmune
   - Irradiation or chemotherapy
   - Idiopathic

B. Secondary ovarian dysfunction
   i. Disorders of gonadotropin regulation
      Organic
      - Hyperprolactinemia
      - Kallmann's syndrome and its variants
      - Destructive lesions of hypothalamus
      Functional
      - Weight loss
      - Exercise
      - Idiopathic
   ii. Gonadotropin deficiency
      - Pituitary tumor
      - Pituitary surgery or irradiation
      - Granulomatous/ inflammatory infiltration

C. Polycystic ovary syndrome

D. Genital tract abnormalities

***Table 18.2***
*Causes of secondary amenorrhea.*

syndrome in a woman who presented in her mid-thirties with a short history of these symptoms without any previous such history.

In a series of 100 consecutive patients presenting to a single reproductive endocrine clinic (at St. Mary's Hospital, Imperial College Healthcare National Health Service [NHS] Trust) with amenorrhea,[1] the single most common cause was a hypothalamic disorder of gonadotropin regulation mainly due to weight loss or excessive exercise (35%). Twenty other patients had evidence of disordered gonadotropin regulation resulting from hyperprolactinemia (11 cases) or of unknown origin (9 cases). Thirty-two percent had PCOS and 11% had POF.

## *Primary ovarian failure*

POF, usually defined as the menopause occurring at or before the age of 40 years, or its alternative term POI, affects about 1% of women. It is characterized by raised (menopausal) serum levels of follicle-stimulating hormone (FSH). Most cases are idiopathic, and a clear-cut underlying cause for POF is evident in only in about one-third of women. Among those women with an identifiable cause of POF, women who are survivors of cancer treatment are probably the most common cases in which a specific diagnosis can be made. Improved treatment of cancer, both in children and adults, has led to an increase in the number of women presenting with ovarian failure due to radiotherapy or chemotherapy. Genetic causes of POF usually involve the X chromosome, but there are increasing reports of autosomal abnormalities.[5] Absence of a second X chromosome, XO, or Turner's syndrome leads to premature depletion of oocytes during the first decade of life and typically presents as POF. However, some patients have a mosaic karyotype (45XX, 45X) and present later with POF. Other karyotypic abnormalities associated with POF include small deletions of the short or long arm of the X chromosome or gene mutations on the X chromosome. Although most women with XXX have normal ovarian function, a few will develop POF. Abnormalities in the *FMR1* gene (on the long arm of the X chromosome) are one of the most genetic causes of POF.[5] The recognition of *FMR1* polymorphisms as a cause of POF followed the observation that POF occurred commonly in heterozygous carriers of fragile X syndrome.[6] A genetic mutation in the FSH receptor has also been identified as a rare cause of POF presenting with primary amenorrhea.

It is estimated that about 30% of women with POF have an autoimmune cause for POF. Detection of autoantibodies is uncommon in POF, but the strong association with other autoimmune endocrinopathies, such as thyroid disease, provides good, if indirect, evidence for an autoimmune component to POF.[7]

## *Disordered regulation of gonadotropins*

Organic causes of gonadotropin-releasing hormone (GnRH) deficiency are well characterized but relatively uncommon causes of anovulation, whereas functional causes are common.[8] Weight loss, excess exercise, and psychological stress can have a profound effect on the hypothalamic GnRH pulse generator and lead to a fall in FSH and luteinizing hormone (LH) secretion and abolition of ovulatory cycles. These women may present with various forms of cycle irregularity but most commonly with amenorrhea. The typical endocrine picture is low (sometimes normal) circulating levels of FSH and LH, with inappropriately low serum estradiol. On ultrasound, the endometrium is thin and the ovaries are typically small with very few antral follicles, but they may contain multiple follicles that resemble the appearance of a midpubertal ovary.[9] Cycle disturbance may persist, even when weight is regained or stressful lifestyle factors are removed. Some women who present with hypothalamic amenorrhea do not have a clear-cut history of vigorous exercise, anorexia, or bulimia, and they often have a normal body mass index (BMI) at the time of presentation. These women are often high achievers who put little time aside for relaxing and socializing. Before any medical therapy is considered, it is important to address the psychological issues that may be behind the hypothalamic disturbance.[8]

### *Hyperprolactinemia (see Chapter 1)*

Hyperprolactinemia is the commonest pituitary disorder causing amenorrhea. It is often due to an autonomous prolactin-secreting pituitary tumor. Despite this, it can also be regarded as a disorder of gonadotropin regulation because the mechanism of anovulation involves an adverse effect of raised prolactin on the normal hypothalamic control of gonadotropin secretion.[10] The characteristic endocrine profile is a persistently raised serum prolactin, with low gondotropins and low estrogen production.

### *Polycystic ovary syndrome*

PCOS is the commonest cause of anovulatory infertility.[11,12] It frequently presents with amenorrhea, or, more commonly, with oligomenorrhea. It is typically associated with excess androgen production so that hirsutism is also a common presenting feature, as is discussed in more detail below. In contrast to patients with other causes of amenorrhea, amenorrheic women with PCOS are not estrogen-deficient; their serum estradiol levels tend to be in the normal early-mid follicular phase range.

The etiology of PCOS remains unclear, but both genetic and environmental (particularly nutritional) factors are involved.[13] The evidence for a genetic basis is strong, but PCOS is a complex endocrine disorder and it is likely that more than one or probably several genes are involved.[14,15] Many logical candidate genes in the steroidogenic and metabolic pathways have been explored, but no locus has emerged from such studies as having a convincing etiological contribution to the syndrome. However, recent genome-wide association studies (GWASs) have suggested some promising candidate loci, including those on chromosome 2 close to the genes encoding gonadotropin receptors. The role of dietary factors is best illustrated by the higher prevalence of symptoms amongst overweight or obese women with PCOS, compared with those in lean women with the syndrome.[16,17] The classic definition of PCOS is the combination of anovulation with clinical and/or biochemical evidence of hyperandrogenism but studies based on ultrasonographic identification of polycystic ovaries suggested that this definition needs to be broadened. The spectrum of presentation of patients with PCOS includes women with hirsutism who have regular cycles as well as nonhirsute women with anovulation. These findings led to the revision of diagnostic criteria for PCOS.[18] The most common biochemical feature of each of these groups is raised serum concentrations of testosterone and other androgens. Hypersecretion of LH is common, particularly in anovulatory women, and is a specific but not very sensitive index of the syndrome; many patients with all other clinical and biochemical features of PCOS have normal LH levels. The diagnosis is made primarily on clinical and ultrasonographic criteria. The finding of a raised level of testosterone, LH, or both merely complements the clinical diagnosis.

Nevertheless, it is important to measure serum testosterone in hirsute women because a greatly increased serum testosterone level (i.e., more than twice the upper limit of the normal range) is an indication for further investigation. More serious causes of hirsutism, such as Cushing syndrome and adrenal or ovarian tumors are rare but may masquerade as PCOS (indeed, polycystic ovaries are commonly found on ultrasonography in these conditions), and a serum testosterone is a useful screening procedure. A short history of hirsutism or rapid worsening of hyperandrogenic symptoms should alert the investigator to the probability of one of these much less common but more serious causes.

### *A metabolic disorder in PCOS*

PCOS is now known to be associated with a characteristic metabolic disorder comprising hyperinsulinemia, insulin resistance, and dyslipidemia.[11,12,19,20] There is an interaction between the effect of PCOS and that of obesity so that the metabolic abnormalities in women with PCOS are amplified to a much greater degree by obesity than is the case for weight-matched control subjects.

The metabolic abnormalities also appear to be a particular feature of those with the classic syndrome (i.e., hyperandrogenism and anovulation), whereas equally hyperandrogenemic women with polycystic ovaries but regular menses tend to have normal insulin secretion and action.[21]

These findings have significant implications for long-term health. Between 15% and 30% of obese young women with PCOS have impaired glucose tolerance or frank, type 2 diabetes mellitus (T2DM), and it is estimated that women with PCOS have a two- to fourfold increase in risk for T2DM.[16,20] As far as investigation of metabolic abnormalities in women with PCOS is concerned, it is suggested that an oral glucose tolerance test should be performed routinely in obese women with PCOS (BMI >30 kg/m$^2$).[20] Nevertheless, all obese subjects with PCOS must be considered to be at risk of T2DM and should be offered dietary advice.

## Investigation of amenorrhea

Investigation of patients with amenorrhea or oligomenorrhea generally requires only a small number of tests[1] (Table 18.3). A single blood sample is taken for the measurement of FSH, LH, and prolactin, and a detailed pelvic ultrasound scan is helpful in assessing ovarian and endometrial morphology. In patients presenting with amenorrhea, it is also necessary to assess estrogen production, either by direct measurement of serum estradiol or by performing a progestogen withdrawal test. If patients are also complaining of symptoms of hyperandrogenism (acne, hirsutism, alopecia), serum testosterone should be measured. It is debatable whether thyroid function tests (i.e., a baseline serum measurement of thyroid-stimulating hormone [TSH]) should be performed routinely in women with amenorrhea or anovulatory menses. Abnormal thyroid function tests may be no more common in women with menstrual disorders than in an age-matched, female population with regular, ovulatory menses. But because thyroid disease is common among the female population, and TSH measurement is certainly indicated in patients with POF and hyperprolactinemic amenorrhea, both of which are associated with primary hypothyroidism, it is the practice in my clinic to measure thyroid function routinely.

- Serum FSH (LH)
- Serum prolactin
- Assessment of estrogen production (serum estradiol, progestogen withdrawal test)
- Testosterone
- Serum TSH
- Pelvic ultrasonography

***Table 18.3***
*Investigation of amenorrhea.*

## Management of patients with amenorrhea

Management of patients with amenorrhea or oligomenorrhea includes the following three categories: treatment of infertility, treatment of hormone (estrogen and/or progesterone) deficiency, and treatment of the consequences of hormone excess (e.g., hirsutism due to hyperandrogenism and galactorrhea due to hyperprolactinemia) (Figure 18.1).

### Induction of ovulation

The choice of treatment for induction of ovulation depends on making the appropriate diagnosis. For women with POF, there is no point in trying to stimulate ovulation; here, the emphasis should be on hormone replacement therapy (HRT). Infertility in women with POF can only effectively be treated by egg donation in the context of an assisted reproductive technology (ART) program.

For women with functional hypothalamic disorders of gonadotropin regulation, it is important to treat any underlying cause. For women with weight loss–related or exercise-related amenorrhea, it is not simply a matter of advising that they eat more healthily or exercise less vigorously; psychological support is very important in management.[8] Even in those with idiopathic "functional hypothalamic amenorrhea," psychotherapy may be indicated and can be effective.[22] In some cases, women with hypothalamic amenorrhea who have regained weight, reduced exercise, and benefited from psychological therapies do not resume menses. It is then appropriate to induce ovulation using pulsatile GnRH therapy, the more physiological approach, or exogenous gonadotropins, equally effective but carrying the greater risk of multiple follicle development.

In women with PCOS, induction of ovulation can be accomplished in 75%–80% of cases by the use of antiestrogens, typically clomiphene citrate, the treatment of first choice for anovulatory women with PCOS.[23–25] The conventional starting dose is 50 mg/day for 5 days (from day 2 onward) after a spontaneous period of

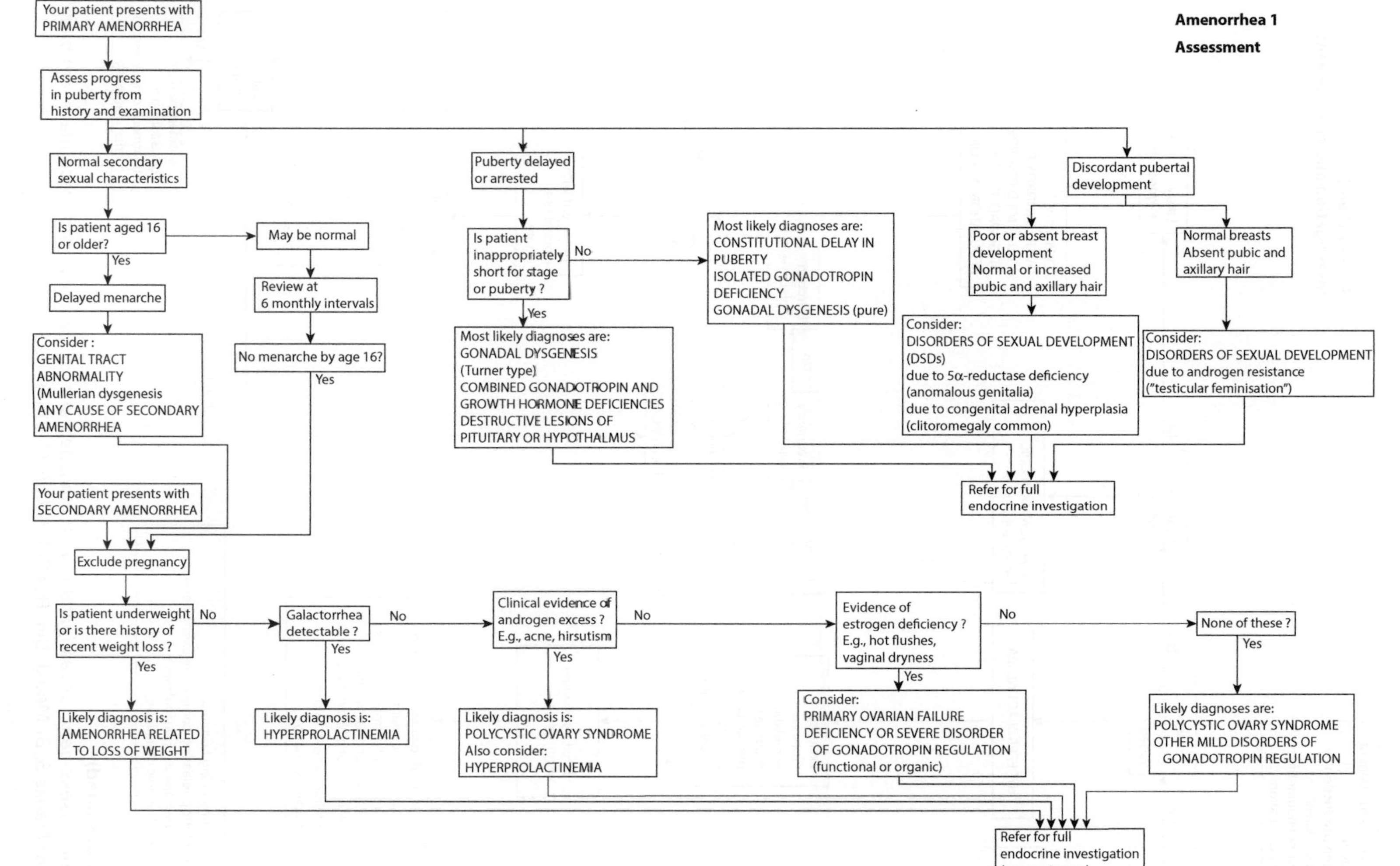


***Figure 18.1***
*Algorithm for assessment, investigation and management of primary and secondary amenorrhea. (Updated from Franks S,* Br Med J (Clin Res Ed) *294(6575); 815–9, 1987.)*

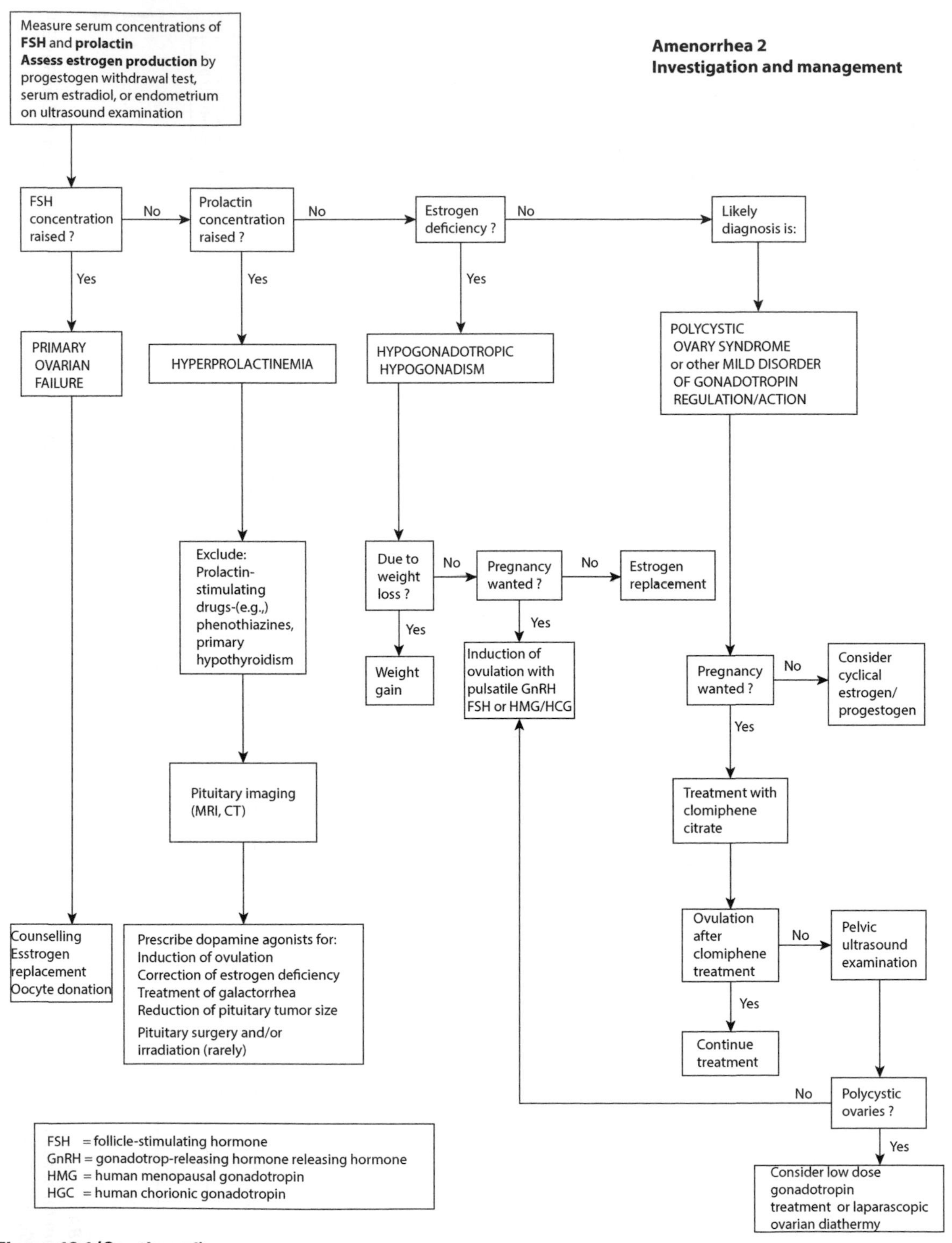


***Figure 18.1* (Continued)**

*Algorithm for assessment, investigation and management of primary and secondary amenorrhea (Updated from Franks S,* Br Med J (Clin Res Ed) *294(6575); 815–9, 1987.*)

progestogen-induced withdrawal bleed. It is prudent to monitor the first cycle of treatment by ultrasound tracking and endocrine tests to determine whether ovulation has occurred and whether there has been either a poor response (no dominant follicle emerging) or an excessive response (too many follicles). The dose can then be adjusted accordingly, but there is no clear evidence that increasing the dose above 100 mg/day can improve the ovulation and pregnancy rate. Management of clomiphene-resistant subjects is more difficult. Laparoscopic ovarian diathermy can be effective,[26] but in many centers the treatment of choice in clomiphene nonresponders is low-dose FSH,[25] with careful ultrasonographic monitoring of the ovarian response.[27]

### *Hormone replacement therapy (see Chapter 5)*

In women with POF or with hypothalamic amenorrhea who do not wish to conceive, the associated estrogen deficiency requires treatment both to control symptoms (hot flushes, vaginal dryness) and to prevent long-term consequences of estrogen deficiency, notably osteopenia and osteoporosis. In the absence of definitive comparative studies, there is no clear consensus about whether estrogen replacement in young women should be by conventional HRT or by combined oral contraceptive (COC)[5] and often personal preferences of doctor and patient tend to dictate the choice. Although there remains concern about the potential adverse effects of long-term estrogen replacement to women receiving HRT after the natural menopause, there is no evidence that estrogen treatment in young women increases the risk of breast disease or cardiovascular disease over and above that seen in women having spontaneous cycles or those on oral contraceptive.

### *Regulation of menses*

Regulation of menses may be an issue in amenorrheic women with PCOS in whom there is a risk of unopposed estrogen production (i.e., without the protective effect of progesterone) leading to endometrial hyperplasia and increased long-term risk of uterine cancer. At the very least, endometrial thickness should be monitored regularly; in the absence of data, the interval is somewhat arbitrary but perhaps every 3–6 months. In addition, in most cases, it is advisable to give cyclical progestogens or prescribe COC.

## *Hirsutism (see Chapters 1, 10)*

The definition of hirsutism in women is excessive terminal hair in a male pattern distribution.[28,29] The effect of excess body hair in an individual woman depends not only on its extent and severity but also on cultural influences.[30] The effects of androgen excess on the hair follicle is affected by ethnic origin, with hirsutism being a more prevalent symptom of hyperandrogenism in women from the Indian subcontinent and from Mediterranean countries than it is in those of northern European or east Asian origin. Virilization is an extreme manifestation of androgen excess that may include not only hirsutism but also frontotemporal balding, clitoromegaly, and deepening of the voice. It is more likely to be indicative of a more serious cause of androgen excess, such as androgen-secreting tumor, than is "simple" hirsutism.

In taking a careful history regarding duration and severity of hair growth, it is important to assess its impact on daily life,[30] including asking how much time the woman spends in removing body hair, and by which method. Severe hirsutism has a serious adverse effect on social interactions in that affected women are very likely to be depressed.[31–33] In terms of assessment of hirsutism in the clinic, it is useful to use the Ferriman–Gallwey chart (Table 18.4) that provides a simple scoring system for assessment of distribution and severity of excess body hair.[28,30]

Circulating testosterone is largely protein-bound either to sex hormone–binding globulin (SHBG) (about 80%) or albumin (about 19%). Only about 1% of testosterone is therefore "free" in the circulation, and it is the free fraction of testosterone that is considered to be the bioavailable form.[34] It is still not clear whether protein-bound (especially albumin-bound) testosterone is also biologically available, but it is well-recognized that changes in the serum concentrations of SHBG affect testosterone bioactivity.

## *Causes of hirsutism*

The common causes of hirsutism are summarized in Table 18.5. PCOS accounts for most cases,[11,12,35,36] including not only women with the classic combination of oligomenorrhea and hirsutism but also women who have regular cycles and hirsutism.[11] Nearly 90% of women with hirsutism and regular cycles, who may previously have been regarded as having idiopathic hirsutism,[11,35] have polycystic ovaries. Hyperthecosis is a somewhat nebulous entity, mainly based on histological appearance, which, especially in premenopausal women, probably represents an extreme of the polycystic ovary. In hyperthecosis, there are "islands" of theca cells within the stroma, as well as in follicles, and these islands are presumed to contribute to excess androgen production. In postmenopausal women, these foci of stromal

| Site | Grade | Definition |
|---|---|---|
| 1. Upper lip | 1 | A few hairs at outer margin |
| | 2 | A small moustache at outer margin |
| | 3 | A moustache extending halfway from outer margin |
| | 4 | A moustache extending to midline |
| 2. Chin | 1 | A few scattered hairs |
| | 2 | Scattered hairs with small concentrations |
| | 3 & 4 | Complete cover, light and heavy |
| 3. Chest | 1 | Circumareolar hairs |
| | 2 | With midline in addition |
| | 3 | Fusion of these areas, with three-quarters cover |
| | 4 | Complete cover |
| 4. Upper back | 1 | A few scattered hairs |
| | 2 | Rather more, still scattered |
| | 3 & 4 | Complete cover, light and heavy |
| 5. Lower back | 1 | A sacral tuft of hair |
| | 2 | With some lateral extension |
| | 3 | Three-quarters cover |
| | 4 | Complete cover |
| 6. Upper abdomen | 1 | A few midline hairs |
| | 2 | Rather more, still midline |
| | 3 & 4 | Half and full cover |
| 7. Lower abdomen | 1 | A few midline hairs |
| | 2 | A midline streak of hair |
| | 3 | A midline band of hair |
| | 4 | An inverted V-shaped growth |
| 8. Arm | 1 | Sparse growth affecting not more than a quarter of the limb surface |
| | 2 | More than this; cover still incomplete |
| | 3 & 4 | Complete cover, light and heavy |
| 9. Forearm | 1–4 | Complete cover of dorsal surface; 2 grades and 2 of heavy growth |
| 10. Thigh | 1–4 | As for arm |
| 11. Leg | 1–4 | As for arm |

***Table 18.4***
*Semiquantitative assessment of hirsutism using the Ferriman–Gallwey score.*

androgen production may be further activated by high circulating levels of LH. Androgen-secreting tumors of the ovary are rare, but it is clearly important to make an early diagnosis based on history and, usually, greatly elevated serum levels of testosterone.

Women with PCOS who are overweight are more likely to be hirsute than those who are lean,[37,38] and weight gain is often associated with an increase in the extent and severity of hirsutism. Conversely, hirsutism may improve in women who lose weight.[17,39] Hyperinsulinemia in PCOS may contribute to the severity of hirsutism by a direct effect of insulin on androgen production by the ovary and by suppressing production of SHBG and thereby increasing bioavailability of testosterone.

The most common adrenal cause of hirsutism is nonclassical (late-onset) congenital adrenal hyperplasia (CAH) due to deficiency of the 21-hydroxylase enzyme.[29,40] The less common, classical (early-onset, salt-losing) form of CAH is usually diagnosed in

Ovarian
- PCOS (>80%)
- Ovarian tumors (sex cord stromal tumors; Sertoli–Leydig cell tumors; adrenal-like tumors of the ovary) (<1%)

Adrenal
- Congenital adrenal hyperplasia (classical 1%; nonclassical [late-onset] 3%)
- Cushing syndrome (<1%)
- Adrenal tumors (adenoma, carcinoma) (<1%)

Idiopathic
- With raised androgens (5%)
- Without raised androgens (7%)

***Table 18.5***
*Causes of hirsutism.*

infancy (or even *in utero*), and early treatment can prevent development of symptoms and signs of androgen excess. Late-onset CAH may be difficult to distinguish clinically from PCOS because the presentation on nonclassical 21-hydroxylase deficiency can be identical to that of PCOS.[40] Thus, it may present as hirsutism (with or without menstrual disturbances) accompanied by elevated levels of LH and testosterone and polycystic ovaries on ultrasound. It is debatable whether measurement of 17-hydroxyprogesterone (17-OHP) in a random sample or after a short Synacthen test (SST) should be part of the routine testing of patients with hirsutism (see below). Other important adrenal causes include Cushing syndrome and adrenal tumors, but these causes are rare, and important clues to diagnosis such as short duration, severe symptoms, and highly elevated serum testosterone levels may be gleaned from history and initial investigations. In 10%–15% of women with hirsutism, there is no obvious underlying cause; in such cases, a diagnosis of idiopathic hirsutism is appropriate.

## Investigation of hirsutism

It is arguable that no investigations are needed in women who have mild, long-standing hirsutism and who have regular menstrual cycles (Table 18.6).[29] They are likely to have polycystic ovaries or idiopathic hirsutism. The main reason for measuring serum testosterone in a woman with hirsutism is to exclude more serious causes of androgen excess. Women with chronic hirsutism and regular cycles are likely to have normal or modestly elevated serum levels of testosterone. Currently available commercial testosterone immunoassays are unreliable for measuring levels in the normal female range,[41] so many laboratories have turned to tandem mass spectrometry (TMS) assays. Generally, the finding of a testosterone level within the normal range, by any method, is unlikely to be indicative of serious pathology. It is higher levels that should prompt further investigation, particularly those that are >2 SDs outside the normal range. Measurement of SHBG and calculation of the free testosterone (T) index (total T/SHBG × 100) are not routinely indicated in the investigation of hirsutism.

In moderate hirsutism, particularly if associated with oligomenorrhea or amenorrhea, PCOS is by far the commonest cause, and this clinical diagnosis should be supported by ultrasonography and endocrine tests: serum testosterone, LH, and FSH in the first instance. The differential diagnosis includes nonclassical CAH, but it is debatable whether it is necessary routinely to perform the specific diagnostic tests for 21-hydroxylase deficiency. The chance of a positive diagnosis depends on the expected background prevalence of CAH in the local population, and even if the diagnosis is made, management of hirsutism is not likely to be any different from that in women with PCOS. The definitive test for CAH is measurement of 17-OHP before and during a standard SST that may be supplemented by genetic screening.

It is important to perform further tests in women who present with severe hirsutism, women with a short duration of hirsutism, and women whose serum testosterone is more than twice the upper limit of the normal range. If the serum testosterone level is in the male range (i.e., >10 nmol/L), a tumor of the ovary or adrenal should be suspected. In rare instances, very high testosterone levels may occur in women with PCOS and severe insulin resistance; in such cases, the presence of acanthosis nigricans is a helpful diagnostic sign.

Measurement of DHEAS is helpful if an adrenal source of androgen excess is suspected. A 24 h urine free cortisol measurement is a useful screening test for Cushing syndrome.[29] Imaging of the ovaries and adrenals by ultrasound or magnetic resonance imaging (MRI) is necessary in cases where a tumor is suspected. Selective venous catheterization is rarely required and, if needed, should only be performed in endocrine centers with extensive experience of this technique. The use of other tests depends on clinical and biochemical pointers, for example, fasting insulin levels in women with PCOS, acanthosis nigricans, and very high testosterone levels.

| | |
|---|---|
| Mild, chronic hirsutism, regular cycles | No tests? (testosterone, pelvic ultrasonography) |
| Moderate hirsutism with or without cycle disturbance | Testosterone, LH, FSH, ultrasonography |
| Severe hirsutism, short history, testosterone >5 nmol/L[a] | DHEAS, 17-OHP, dexamethasone suppression, 24 h urine free cortisol, ovarian and/or adrenal imaging, fasting glucose/insulin |

[a] Extensive investigation should be reserved for more severe cases or cases with a short history of hirsutism or with markedly elevated serum testosterone (more than twice upper limit of normal range for the lab). DHEAS, dehydroepiandrosterone sulfate; 17OHP (usually measured before and during an SST).

***Table 18.6***
*Investigation of hirsutism.*

## Management of hirsutism

It is important in the management of hirsutism to use the combined approach of physical methods of hair removal and, where indicated, medication, usually hormonal therapy[29,42] (Table 18.7). The various methods of hair removal should be discussed with the patient. It may be appropriate to refer patients to a dermatologist, if he or she has a special interest in the management of hirsutism. Electrolysis or laser hair removal is often very effective; unfortunately, such treatment is rarely available within the NHS.

In a mild hirsutism, hair removal by shaving or depilatory creams may suffice. An alternative for treatment of facial hirsutism is the ornithine decarboxylase inhibitor eflornithine (Vaniqa®).[43] It may take up to 3 months of use to demonstrate significant reduction in hair growth, and it should be discontinued after 4 months of treatment if there is no noticeable improvement. Eflornithine is probably most effective in combination with laser hair removal.[44]

Endocrine management of hirsutism usually means use of combined oral contraceptives to suppress ovarian androgen production and therefore lowering of serum testosterone levels. This approach may suffice in women with mild-to-moderate hirsutism, but in more severe hirsutism, additional benefit can be achieved by the use of an androgen receptor inhibitor, such as cyproterone acetate or spironolactone.[29,45,46] Co-cyprindiol (initially marketed as Dianette®) is a combined hormonal preparation containing cyproterone acetate (2 mg) and is licensed for the treatment of severe acne as well as moderately severe hirsutism. However, the data suggesting that co-cyprindiol is associated with a greater risk of venous thromboembolism than third-generation "pills" remain controversial,[47] and, in practice, it is a useful, usually well tolerated, and effective treatment for hirsutism.

Hair removal
- Creams, shaving, electrolysis, laser

Topical inhibition of hair growth
- Eflornithine

Suppression of androgen secretion and/or action
- Oral contraceptives
- Antiandrogens: cyproterone acetate (including co-cyprindiol); spironolactone; flutamide
- 5α-reductase inhibitors: finasteride

***Table 18.7***
*Management of hirsutism.*

The antiandrogen flutamide may also be effective but is not recommended for treatment of hirsutism because of potential hepatotoxicity. Finasteride is an inhibitor of 5α-reductase, which converts testosterone to the more potent androgen dihydrotestosterone, but its efficacy in treating hirsutism is difficult to evaluate because of a lack of appropriately powered randomized controlled trials.[48] Metformin has been claimed to reduce hair growth, but systematic analysis of the results of studies points to only a small and clinically insignificant effect.[49,50]

Suppression of ovarian function by long-acting analogs of GnRH agonists is largely ineffective and unnecessary, as is oophorectomy. The exceptions are those rare cases where hirsutism results from hyperthecosis or androgen-secreting ovarian tumors. Because, in hyperthecosis, testosterone secretion remains LH-dependent, suppression of LH with long-acting agonist analogs of GnRH lowers testosterone. Indeed, this treatment is useful both in diagnosis and management, although alternatives for treatment are antiandrogens and oophorectomy.

Management of symptoms of hirsutism due to nonclassical CAH is probably best accomplished by using the combination of physical hair removal and antiandrogens, as for PCOS. There is little evidence to suggest that the use of glucocorticoids is more effective in these circumstances. The one situation in which glucocorticoid suppression may be helpful is if women with nonclassical CAH are hoping to conceive. In such circumstances, the endometrium in spontaneous and induced menstrual cycles may remain thin because of higher than normal progesterone concentrations in the follicular phase.

In summary, hirsutism is a very common and distressing problem. Its most common cause is PCOS, but a carefully obtained history will provide indicators of rare but more serious causes, such as androgen-secreting tumors. Investigations should be targeted to the clinical presentation. Optimum management requires a combination of physical hair removal, hormonal treatments, and, where necessary, psychological support.

## References


1. Franks. Primary and secondary amenorrhea. *BMJ.* 1987;294:815–18.
2. Unuane D, Tournaye H, Velkeniers B, Poppe K. Endocrine disorders & female infertility. *Best Pract Res Clin Endocrinol Metab* 2011;25(6):861–73.
3. Johnson MR, McGregor AM. Endocrine disease and pregnancy. *Baillieres Clin Endocrinol Metab* 1990;4(2):313–32.
4. Lado-Abeal J, Rodriguez-Arnao J, Newell-Price JD, Perry LA, Grossman AB, Besser GM, et al. Menstrual abnormalities in women with Cushing's disease are correlated with hypercortisolemia rather than raised circulating androgen levels. *J Clin Endocrinol Metab* 1998;83(9):3083–8.
5. Goswami D, Conway GS. Premature ovarian failure. *Hum Reprod Update* 2005;11(4):391–410.
6. Conway GS, Payne NN, Webb J, Murray A, Jacobs PA. Fragile X premutation screening in women with premature ovarian failure. *Hum Reprod* 1998;13(5):1184–7.
7. Conway GS, Kaltsas G, Patel A, Davies MC, Jacobs HS. Characterization of idiopathic premature ovarian failure. *Fertil Steril* 1996;65(2):337–41.
8. Berga S, Naftolin F. Neuroendocrine control of ovulation. *Gynecol Endocrinol* 2012;28(Suppl 1):9–13.
9. Adams J, Franks S, Polson DW, Mason HD, Abdulwahid N, Tucker M, et al. Multifollicular ovaries: Clinical and endocrine features and response to pulsatile gonadotropin releasing hormone. *Lancet* 1985;2(8469–70):1375–9.
10. Polson DW, Sagle M, Mason HD, Adams J, Jacobs HS, Franks S. Ovulation and normal luteal function during LHRH treatment of women with hyperprolactinaemic amenorrhea. *Clin Endocrinol (Oxf).* 1986;24(5):531–7.
11. Franks S. Polycystic ovary syndrome. *N Engl J Med* 1995;333(13):853–61.
12. Ehrmann DA. Polycystic ovary syndrome. *N Engl J Med* 2005;352(12):1223–36.
13. Franks S. Genetic and environmental origins of obesity relevant to reproduction. *Reprod Biomed Online* 2006;12(5):526–31.
14. Franks S, McCarthy M. Genetics of ovarian disorders: Polycystic ovary syndrome. *Rev Endocr Metab Disord.* 2004;5(1):69–76.
15. Urbanek M. The genetics of the polycystic ovary syndrome. *Nat Clin Pract Endocrinol Metab.* 2007;3(2):103–11.
16. Moran LJ, Misso M, Wild RA, Norman RJ. Impaired glucose tolerance, type 2 diabetes and metabolic syndrome in polycystic ovary syndrome: A systematic review and meta-analysis. *Hum Reprod Update* 2010;16:347–63.
17. Kiddy DS, Hamilton-Fairley D, Bush A, Short F, Anyaoku V, Reed MJ, et al. Improvement in endocrine and ovarian function during dietary treatment of obese women with polycystic ovary syndrome. *Clin Endocrinol (Oxf)* 1992;36(1):105–11.
18. Rotterdam ESHRE/ASRM-Sponsored PCOS Consensus Workshop Group. Revised 2003 consensus on diagnostic criteria and long-term health risks related to polycystic ovary syndrome (PCOS). *Hum Reprod* 2004;19(1):41–17.
19. Dunaif A. Insulin resistance and the polycystic ovary syndrome: Mechanism and implications for pathogenesis. *Endocr Rev* 1997;18(6):774–800.
20. Fauser BC, Tarlatzis BC, Rebar RW, Legro RS, Balen AH, Lobo R, et al. Consensus on women's health aspects of polycystic ovary syndrome (PCOS): The Amsterdam ESHRE/ASRM-sponsored 3rd PCOS Consensus Workshop Group. *Fertil Steril* 2012;97(1):28–38.
21. Barber TM, Wass JA, McCarthy MI, Franks S. Metabolic characteristics of women with polycystic ovaries and oligo-amenorrhea but normal androgen levels: Implications for the management of polycystic ovary syndrome. *Clinical Endocrinology* 2007;66(4):513–17.
22. Berga SL, Marcus MD, Loucks TL, Hlastala S, Ringham R, Krohn MA. Recovery of ovarian activity in women with functional hypothalamic amenorrhea

who were treated with cognitive behavior therapy. *Fertil Steril*. 2003; **80**(4): 976-81

23. Balen AH. Induction of ovulation in the management of polycystic ovary syndrome. *Mol Cell Endocrinol* 2013;373(1–2):77–82.
24. Kousta E, White DM, Franks S. Modern use of clomiphene citrate in induction of ovulation. *Hum Reprod Update* 1997;3(4):359–65.
25. Thessaloniki ESHRE/ASRM-Sponsored PCOS Consensus Workshop Group. Consensus on infertility treatment related to polycystic ovary syndrome. *Hum Reprod* 2008; 23(3):462–77.
26. Farquhar C, Brown J, Marjoribanks J. Laparoscopic drilling by diathermy or laser for ovulation induction in anovulatory polycystic ovary syndrome. *Cochrane Database Syst Rev*. 2012;6:CD001122. doi: 10.1002/14651858.CD001122.pub4. Review.
27. White DM, Polson DW, Kiddy D, Sagle P, Watson H, Gilling-Smith C, et al. Induction of ovulation with low-dose gonadotropins in polycystic ovary syndrome: An analysis of 109 pregnancies in 225 women. *J Clin Endocrinol Metab* 1996;81(11):3821–4.
28. Ferriman D, Gallwey JD. Clinical assessment of body hair growth in women. *J Clin Endocrinol Metab* 1961;21:1440–7.
29. Koulouri O, Conway GS. Management of hirsutism. *BMJ* 2009;338:b847.
30. Yildiz BO, Bolour S, Woods K, Moore A, Azziz R. Visually scoring hirsutism. *Hum Reprod Update* 2010;16(1):51–64.
31. Barth JH, Catalan J, Cherry CA, Day A. Psychological morbidity in women referred for treatment of hirsutism. *J Psychosom Res* 1993;37(6):615–19.
32. Archer JS, Chang RJ. Hirsutism and acne in polycystic ovary syndrome. *Best Pract Res Clin Obstet Gynaecol* 2004;18(5):737–54.
33. Jones GL, Hall JM, Balen AH, Ledger WL. Health-related quality of life measurement in women with polycystic ovary syndrome: A systematic review. *Hum Reprod Update* 2008;14(1):15–25.
34. Pardridge WM. Serum bioavailability of sex steroid hormones. *Clin Endocrinol Metab* 1986;15(2):259–78.
35. Adams J, Polson DW, Franks S. Prevalence of polycystic ovaries in women with anovulation and idiopathic hirsutism. *Br Med J (Clin Res Ed)* 1986;293(6543):355–19.
36. Azziz R, Sanchez LA, Knochenhauer ES, Moran C, Lazenby J, Stephens KC, et al. Androgen excess in women: Experience with over 1000 consecutive patients. *J Clin Endocrinol Metab* 2004;89(2):453–62.
37. Kiddy DS, Sharp PS, White DM, Scanlon MF, Mason HD, Bray CS, et al. Differences in clinical and endocrine features between obese and non-obese subjects with polycystic ovary syndrome: An analysis of 263 consecutive cases. *Clin Endocrinol (Oxf)* 1990;32(2):213–20.
38. Barber TM, McCarthy MI, Wass JA, Franks S. Obesity and polycystic ovary syndrome. *Clin Endocrinol (Oxf)* 2006;65(2):137–45.
39. Pasquali R, Antenucci D, Casimirri F, Venturoli S, Paradisi R, Fabbri R, et al. Clinical and hormonal characteristics of obese amenorrheic hyperandrogenic women before and after weight loss. *J Clin Endocrinol Metab* 1989;68(1):173–9.
40. Bidet M, Bellanne-Chantelot C, Galand-Portier MB, Tardy V, Billaud L, Laborde K, et al. Clinical and molecular characterization of a cohort of 161 unrelated women with nonclassical congenital adrenal hyperplasia due to 21-hydroxylase deficiency and 330 family members. *J Clin Endocrinol Metab* 2009;94(5):1570–8.
41. Rosner W, Vesper H. Toward excellence in testosterone testing: A consensus statement. *J Clin Endocrinol Metab* 2010;95(10):4542–8.
42. Koulouri O, Conway GS. A systematic review of commonly used medical treatments for hirsutism in women. *Clin Endocrinol (Oxf)* 2008;68(5):800–5.
43. Wolf JE, Jr., Shander D, Huber F, Jackson J, Lin CS, Mathes BM, et al. Randomized, double-blind clinical evaluation of the efficacy and safety of topical eflornithine HCl 13.9% cream in the treatment of women with facial hair. *Int J Dermatol* 2007;46(1):94–8.
44. Lapidoth M, Dierickx C, Lanigan S, Paasch U, Campo-Voegeli A, Dahan S, et al. Best practice options for hair removal in patients with unwanted facial hair using combination therapy with laser: Guidelines drawn up by an expert working group. *Dermatology* 2010;221(1):34–42.
45. Barth JH, Cherry CA, Wojnarowska F, Dawber RP. Spironolactone is an effective and well tolerated systemic antiandrogen therapy for Hirsute women. *J Clin Endocrinol Metab* 1989;68(5):966–70.
46. Barth JH, Cherry CA, Wojnarowska F, Dawber RP. Cyproterone acetate for severe hirsutism: Results of a double-blind dose-ranging study. *Clin Endocrinol (Oxf)* 1991;35(1):5–10.
47. Franks S, Layton A, Glasier A. Cyproterone acetate/ethinyl estradiol for acne and hirsutism: Time to revise prescribing policy. *Hum Reprod* 2008;23(2):231–2.
48. Swiglo BA, Cosma M, Flynn DN, Kurtz DM, Labella ML, Mullan RJ, et al. Clinical review: Antiandrogens for the treatment of hirsutism: A systematic review and metaanalyses of randomized controlled trials. *J Clin Endocrinol Metab* 2008;93(4):1153–60.
49. Costello MF, Shrestha B, Eden J, Johnson NP, Sjoblom P. Metformin versus oral contraceptive pill in polycystic ovary syndrome: A Cochrane review. *Hum Reprod* 2007;22(5):1200–9.
50. Franks S. When should an insulin sensitizing agent be used in the treatment of polycystic ovary syndrome? *Clin Endocrinol (Oxf)* 2011;74(2):148–51.

# 19

# Endocrine problems in pregnancy

*Anjali Amin, Stephen Robinson*

## *Introduction*

Endocrine complications in pregnancy are common and potentially life-threatening. Their prevention and treatment require an understanding of the physiology of pregnancy and its relation to the pathophysiology of the condition. Pregnancy is associated with extensive maternal physiological changes to accommodate the needs of the mother and fetus. The maternal endocrine adaptations in pregnancy have both causal and reactive elements. Many of the endocrine diseases occurring in women of childbearing age can lead to subfertility; therefore, preexisting endocrine conditions may need special interventions to facilitate ovulation. If these conditions remain untreated, they can lead to serious morbidity and mortality for both mother and fetus; therefore, early recognition is imperative.

Endocrine complications in pregnancy represent a useful paradigm to address all medical complications of pregnancy. After addressing the pathophysiology of the condition in pregnancy, it is useful to consider each of the maternal issues, fetal issues, obstetric issues, and finally the effect of having the condition in pregnancy in the long term for the condition itself. Gestational age may need to be considered, in diagnosis and management, particularly for surgical procedures that may be necessary during pregnancy (Box 19.1).

The diagnosis of endocrine conditions presenting during pregnancy can pose challenges because biochemical testing may be limited in pregnancy. Adult nonpregnant reference ranges may not be accurate in pregnancy. In addition, certain radiological investigations may be contraindicated in pregnancy, adding to the difficulties surrounding the diagnosis.

## *Thyroid disease*

Pregnancy results in major alterations in maternal thyroid hormone physiology. Human chorionic gonadotrophin (hCG), produced by the syncytiotrophoblasts of the developing placenta, has a high degree of homology with thyroid-stimulating hormone (TSH) and can stimulate the TSH receptor.[1] During the first trimester, the high concentration of hCG stimulates the thyroid in terms of growth and function, resulting in a suppressed TSH in several normal pregnancies.[2,3] Some mothers may go on to develop a high tri-iodothyronine (T3) and free T3. Later in pregnancy as estrogen rises, so does the thyroid-binding globulin,[4] due to reduced catabolism.[5] Consequently, total thyroxin (T4) concentrations are increased in the mother, although free T4 usually remains normal or slightly low.[6] The fetus places high iodine demands on the mother; therefore, the mother may become relatively iodine deficient as a consequence of fetal demands and urinary loss. Rising TSH and maternal goiter consequent to relative iodine deficiency is not uncommon in iodine-deficient areas.[6] Relative iodine deficiency is found in many countries, including the United Kingdom.[7] Increased thyroid hormone production is only possible with adequate iodine availability.[8] Furthermore, the increase in maternal glomerular filtration rate results in higher iodine requirements because iodine is passively excreted; the ideal intake defined by the World Health Organization (WHO) is 250 μg daily.[9] In addition, expansion of plasma volume results in a lower serum albumin concentration.[10] As a consequence of these physiological changes, normal reference ranges from a nonpregnant population are not valid in pregnancy. Hence, cautious interpretation of thyroid function

**Box 19.1** *Endocrine complications in pregnancy*

When considering endocrine diseases of pregnancy, it is useful to consider the interaction of maternal–placental–fetal physiology on the pathophysiology of the disease on

- Pregnancy outcomes
- Maternal outcomes
- Fetal outcomes
- The natural history of the disease itself

tests in pregnancy needs to be made[11] (Figure 19.1). The role of thyroid in pregency is as follows:

1. In normal pregnancy, hCG, produced by the corpus luteum, stimulates the maternal thyroid in terms of growth and function. hCG has great homology with TSH. This hCG effect can cause enough thyroid hormone production to reduce or even suppress TSH production by the pituitary. The mother is relatively hyperthyroid in normal pregnancy, even when there is no thyroid pathology.
2. Thyroid hormones are carried by several proteins, but the majority is carried by thyroid-binding globulin. Thyroid-binding globulin production is increased by estrogen, leading to an increased need for thyroid hormones. The normal hypothalamic pituitary thyroid axis can adapt and produce more thyroid hormone. The mother with less capacity of the thyroid to adapt may become relatively hypothyroid and would need to increase thyroid hormone replacement to compensate.
3. The fetoplacental unit takes up iodine. This uptake can cause an iodine-insufficient mother to become an iodine-deficient mother. In turn, this can cause growth in the thyroid. Thyroxine does cross the placenta, but the flow is limited by placental type 3 monodeiodinases. The placenta does not have the same flexibility for T3 transfer.
4. Maternal production of TSH receptor antibody is able to cross the placenta, and in excess, this can cause fetal goiter and fetal thyrotoxicosis. This can occur in utero, presenting with fetal tachycardia, and then continue into the first 2 weeks of life. However, the thyrotoxicosis is not then maintained.

Thyroid disease is one of the most common endocrine abnormalities found in pregnancy. Maternal thyroid disease can have adverse effects on the pregnancy and the fetus.[12] The most frequently encountered disorders include thyrotoxicosis, hypothyroidism, and thyroid nodules.

## Thyrotoxicosis (see Chapter 13)

Thyrotoxicosis is a constellation of symptoms, signs, and risks resulting from excessive amounts of thyroid hormones. Thyrotoxicosis occurs in approximately

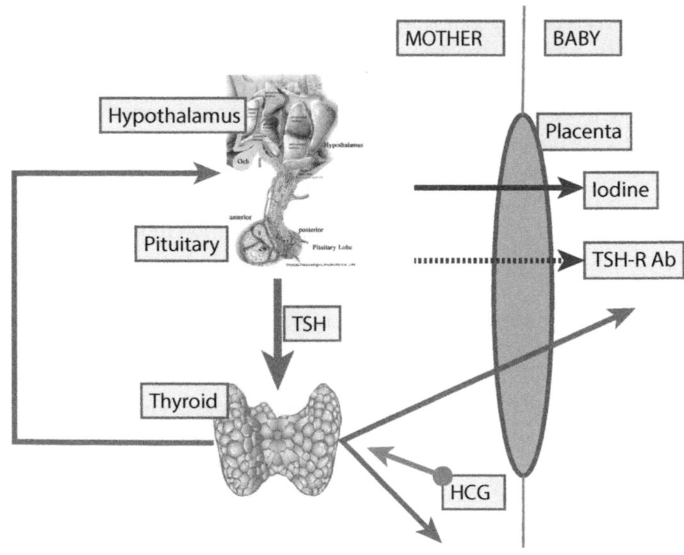


***Figure 19.1***
*The thyroid in pregnancy.*

0.2% of all pregnancies.[13] Autoimmune thyroid disease (AITD) or Graves' disease accounts for the majority of these cases in areas with sufficient iodine intake,[14] especially in women of reproductive age. Other causes of hyperthyroidism include multinodular goiter and autonomously functioning nodules; hyperthyroidism may be seen early in a destructive thyroiditis such as postviral, Hashimoto's, or postpartum thyroiditis. In cases of a low or suppressed serum TSH, the distinction between normal physiological changes of pregnancy and hyperemesis gravidarum and hyperthyroidism must be made.[12]

Preexisting AITD frequently improves during pregnancy, which is likely to be related to alterations in immune mechanisms. Conversely, cases of AITD occur more frequently during the postpartum period than at other times in women of childbearing age,[15] In the period after birth, exacerbation of immune reactivity normally occurs between 3 and 12 months,[16] leading to recurrence of disease. Clinical improvement tends to be in the second and third trimester, which is thought to be related to the reduction in levels of circulating thyroid-stimulating immunoglobulins.[17]

Preexisting ophthalmopathy often improves in pregnancy, due to a relative immune suppression, with a potential for deterioration in the postpartum period.

### *Pregnancy issues*

Untreated thyrotoxicosis may adversely affect the pregnancy, with increased rates of miscarriage, low birth weight, prematurity, eclampsia, and congenital birth defects.[18–20] The incidence of small, for gestational age, infants is higher in mothers who remain hyperthyroid compared with those who were euthyroid through their pregnancy.[20] The mother may proceed to thyroid storm, especially at a time of intercurrent stress such as miscarriage or general anesthetic. The placenta presents a relative barrier to high maternal circulating thyroid hormone concentrations. However, the immunoglobulin G (IgG) antibody responsible for AITD (TSH receptor-stimulating antibody, TRAB) may cross the placenta. At the end of the pregnancy, this may then cause a fetal goiter with consequent face presentation and fetal thyrotoxicosis; the latter typically persists for the duration of time it takes for the maternally derived TRAB to be cleared, usually between 3 and 12 weeks. TRAB represents the crucial difference when compared with gestational thyrotoxicosis. Stimulating maternal TRABs can cross the placenta and cause both fetal hyperthyroidism and fetal goiter in 1%–5% of neonates born to mothers with AITD.[19,21] The placenta represents a barrier to maternally derived thyroid hormones.

### *Diagnosis*

The hypermetabolic state of pregnancy can make the diagnosis of thyrotoxicosis difficult. Heat intolerance, warm skin, tachycardia, emotional lability, weight loss, diarrhea, and significant tachycardia and systolic flow murmurs may occur but may be seen in normal pregnancy, too.[13,17] Features of AITD include thyroid-associated ophthalmopathy, smooth goiter with bruit, and family history of autoimmune thyroid disease.

Gestational thyrotoxicosis may be found alone or with hyperemesis gravidarum and can occur at any stage in pregnancy but typically does not persist beyond 20 weeks of gestation.[22] Hyperemesis gravidarum occurs in 0.3%–1% of pregnancies and is characterized by nausea and vomiting, resulting in >5% weight loss, ketonuria, dehydration, and electrolyte and liver abnormalities in severe cases.[23,24] Any woman presenting with hyperemesis gravidarum should have her thyroid function checked, although few women will need treatment for the thyroid function. Distinguishing gestational thyrotoxicosis from AITD may be difficult but is supported by lack of evidence of autoimmunity, goiter, and negative TRAB.[12] TSH can be transiently suppressed related to the high concentrations of hCG[25,26] and the T3 and T4 concentrations variably elevated.

The diagnosis of thyrotoxicosis is made based on clinical findings and thyroid function tests. TSH is suppressed with elevated free T4 and T3 concentrations. Nuclear imaging with technetium uptake scan cannot be performed in pregnancy. Thyroid peroxidase and TRABs are measured in an effort to separate AITD and gestational thyrotoxicosis. Furthermore, TRABs may cross the placenta and stimulate the fetal thyroid.[21] The likelihood of developing fetal hyperthyroidism requiring treatment is related to the level of maternal stimulating TRAB levels.[27] Levels greater than five times control values make both intrauterine and neonatal thyrotoxicosis likely. Hence, these antibodies should be measured either before pregnancy or by the end of the second trimester in women with current AITD, those with a previous history and treatment with radioiodine therapy or thyroidectomy, and those with a previous neonate with AITD.[12] In normal labor, the fetus must flex the neck to present the lowest skull diameter to the pelvis; a fetal goiter prevents this flexion. A fetal thyroid ultrasound can be carried out to investigate fetal goiter when TRABs are positive. Women with hyperthyroidism could consider a definitive approach before conception (Box 19.2).

### *Treatment*

β-Blockers are important for symptom control and for rate control in the presence of significant maternal tachycardia. If the free T3 is >10 pmol/L, many physicians

**Box 19.2** *The management of hyperthyroidism in pregnancy*

- Propylthiouracil (PTU) could be considered in the first trimester; carbimazole subsequently.
- The lowest dose of thionamide should be used, aiming to keep free T3 and Free T4 at the upper end of normal.
- Positive maternal TSH receptor antibody measured in the second trimester indicates fetal thyroid ultrasound at 34 weeks of gestation.

would consider antithyroid medication but would only be able to confirm the diagnosis of autoimmune thyrotoxicosis retrospectively. First-line treatment is medical, with one of the thionamide derivatives, carbimazole or PTU. Current Endocrine Society Practice guidelines suggest PTU as first-line treatment, especially during first-trimester organogenesis because methimazole has rarely been linked with congenital abnormalities.[12,28,29] This is notoriously difficult to ensure because many women may not have their thyroid function checked until their booking visit, which classically in the United Kingdom does not occur until 12 weeks of gestation. There are no data suggesting the change to PTU in early pregnancy is associated with reduced malformation; furthermore, PTU is associated with hepatitis that does not necessarily resolve on therapy discontinuation. It has been suggested that methimazole crosses the placenta at a greater rate than PTU,[30] although this has not been confirmed.[31] PTU is favored for new diagnoses because it does not cross into breast milk; however, if a mother presents taking carbimazole, many physicians do not change medication in pregnancy.[32] Methimazole may rarely have fetal side effects, including aplasia cutis, although PTU is known to have more maternal effects such as hepatitis.[33] Antithyroid drugs need dose titration, based on TSH and T4 values. Doses of antithyroid drugs should maintain the maternal free T4 in the upper nonpregnant reference range. Block-and-replace regimens should not be used in pregnancy because carbimazole can cross the placenta but the replacing thyroxin does not; therefore, there is potential for fetal hypothyroidism. Doses of <20 mg of carbimazole or 150 mg of PTU are considered unlikely to affect the fetus.

Surgical treatment should be considered in women who are unable to tolerate medical treatment because of allergy or severe adverse reaction, women who do not respond to medical treatment or require persistently high doses of medication, and women noncompliant to therapy. Surgery is ideally performed in the second trimester when organogenesis is complete; however, the dangers of severe untreated maternal thyrotoxicosis are considerable and surgery can be performed in the third trimester. Adequate β-blockade is essential before such surgery. Surgery is however associated with an increased risk of spontaneous abortion or premature delivery.[34]

Radioactive iodine treatment has no role in pregnancy because it crosses the placenta and hence may ablate the fetal thyroid and has a risk of teratogenicity in terms of radiation dose.

A mother who had AITD in the past and was treated with surgery or radioactive iodine may still have TSH receptor antibodies despite being hypothyroid and taking thyroxin.[21] One could be alerted to this scenario with the presence of active thyroid-associated ophthalmopathy. The fetus of such a pregnancy may become thyrotoxic and develop a goiter *in utero*. Fetal tachycardia exceeding 160 beats per minute after 22 weeks of gestation can be used as evidence of intrauterine thyrotoxicosis. Treatment of the mother with antithyroid medication should be adjusted to maintain a fetal heart rate of 140 beats per minute or so. Untreated, the weight of such infants is often low; the birth may be preterm, with microcephaly and cerebroventricular enlargement. Neonates have hyperphagia, diarrhea, and they may be irritable, with frontal bossing and a triangular facies. Neonatal hyperthyroidism occurs in approximately 5% of neonates of mothers with AITD.[21] TSH and T4 ought to be measured in the cord blood of babies born to mothers with a history of AITD. If the mother has been on treatment with antithyroid drugs at the end of her pregnancy, clinical signs of neonatal thyrotoxicosis may be unapparent at birth, presenting only a few days after delivery, due to protection of the fetus by the maternal antithyroid drugs. Neonatal hyperthyroidism should be treated promptly with antithyroid medication and β blockade. Either propylthiouracil 5–10 mg/kg/day or carbimazole 0.5–1 mg/kg/day should be administered every 8 h to inhibit thyroid hormone synthesis. In severely ill infants, propranolol 2 mg/kg/day may be helpful in slowing the heart and reducing hyperactivity. The disease is self-limiting.

## Familial gestational hyperthyroidism

Familial gestational hyperthyroidism is an extremely rare cause of thyrotoxicosis in pregnancy and is caused by an autosomal dominant mutation in the thyrotropin receptor that is hypersensitive to the effects of hCG.[35] There is a family history of thyrotoxicosis in pregnancy.

The thyrotoxicosis begins to improve as hCG concentrations fall, and it resolves postpartum. The symptoms and signs are similar to those seen with autoimmune thyrotoxicosis, without the autoimmune phenomena such as exophthalmos, anti-TSH receptor antibody positivity, and lymphocytic infiltration of the thyroid gland. Treatment is the same as for AITD.

## Hypothyroidism (Box 19.3) (see Chapter 13)

Hypothyroidism, or underactive thyroid, is found when the thyroid gland fails to produce or secrete sufficient thyroid hormones, T4 and T3. The definition of sufficient depends on pregnancy; the fetus appears to require near perfect maternal function compared with the nonpregnant state. Primary hypothyroidism is common in women of childbearing age, with a prevalence of 2%–3% of women during pregnancy.[12]

### Pregnancy issues

Normal maternal thyroid function is essential to both mother and the developing fetus. Untreated maternal hypothyroidism is associated with an increased risk of obstetric complications and adverse neonatal outcomes.[12] Abnormal maternal thyroid function is particularly important during the first 12–14 weeks of gestation, when fetal brain development relies heavily on placental transfer of maternal thyroid hormone.[36] The severely hypothyroid mother is at increased risk of pre eclampsia.[37] When the mother is hypothyroid, the fetus is at increased risk of congenital anomalies, low birth weight, and stillbirth. Severe MH is associated with cognitive delay in early childhood.[38] Even mild MH is associated with lower developmental IQ score in children at the age of 6 years.[39] Mothers with treated hypothyroidism demonstrate no such risk. Adverse maternal and fetal outcomes secondary to thyroid dysfunction during pregnancy may justify screening for thyroid function early in pregnancy and treating with levothyroxine if the mother is found to be hypothyroid. By contrast, a well-powered study of nearly 22,000 women at 12 weeks of gestation demonstrated no benefit for fetal brain development for screening and management and treatment for maternal hypothyroidism in pregnancy, compared with no screening.[40] There is a higher prevalence of subclinical hypothyroidism in women who deliver before 32 weeks and an association between thyroid autoimmunity and adverse obstetric outcome independent of thyroid function.[41] Higher maternal TSH levels even within the reference range have been linked to a higher risk of miscarriage, fetal and neonatal distress, and preterm delivery.[42,43] To date, there is no solid evidence to advocate universal screening of maternal TSH.

It is reported that the mother with positive thyroid peroxidase antibodies is at increased risk of miscarriage even when euthyroid; this intriguing area is under investigation, and no treatment with thyroxin in euthyroid mothers is recommended at present.[44]

> **Box 19.3** *The management of hyperthyroidism in pregnancy*
>
> - Maternal hypothyroidism (MH) is an important cause of maternal and fetal morbidity.
> - When recognized before pregnancy, MH should be managed with a first-trimester increment in thyroxin replacement, with an aim to keep the TSH <2.5 mIU/L.
> - There is no evidence base for screening for MH in an unselected population.
> - Women with positive thyroid peroxidase antibodies may have an increased miscarriage rate; the use of thyroxin treatment in these women may reduce the high miscarriage rate. There are insufficient data to suggest this as policy.

### Diagnosis

The diagnosis can be made with symptoms and signs of maternal hypothyroidism; most MH is diagnosed with the TSH, in conjunction with free T3 and free T4 hormones. The range for T4 during pregnancy differs from the nonpregnant range, in part due to the doubling of thyroid-binding globulin concentration in pregnancy. During the first trimester, serum hCG levels rise and peak toward the end of the first trimester.[45] The stimulating effect of hCG on the TSH receptor leads to a drop in TSH levels in the first trimester of pregnancy,[6] with a concomitant rise in fetal (f)T4 and fT3.

### Treatment

Subclinical hypothyroidism (when the TSH is elevated with a normal free T4) detected before pregnancy should be treated as for primary hypothyroidism.[46] Treatment is with levothyroxine and is the treatment of choice in pregnancy or outwith pregnancy, generally starting at 100 μg daily, but higher doses may be used to render the mother euthyroid quickly. The dose of thyroxin should be altered to keep the TSH at the lower end of the normal range. Guidelines for diagnosis from the Endocrine Society recommend that the TSH should be kept <2.5 mU/L in the first trimester and <3 mU/L in the second and third trimesters.[12] The etiology of hypothyroidism is important in determining the timing and magnitude of thyroid hormone replacement in pregnancy.[47] In women with preexisting hypothyroidism, levothyroxine dosage will normally need to be increased, with data showing that most pregnant women will require a 30% increase in levothyroxine dose in the first trimester once conception is confirmed to decrease the risk of maternal hypothyroidism and its effects on the fetus, and about a 50% increase by 16–20 weeks, with 75%–85% of women requiring higher doses of levothyroxine during their pregnancy.[48,49] This, however, does not account for the underlying etiologies of hypothyroidism that are of relevance because an empirical increase in levothyroxine dose could lead to under or overreplacement with potential detrimental effects on mother and baby.[47] In the postpartum period, doses will generally return to prepregnancy doses.

## Goiter (Box 19.4)

In areas of iodine deficiency, thyroid size has been shown to enlarge during pregnancy, compared with those areas with sufficient iodine.[50] This relationship is thought to be related to autoregulatory mechanisms of iodine on thyroid growth. hCG has intrinsic thyroid-stimulating activity, particularly in the first trimester, with subsequent effects on thyroid enlargement.[51]

Thyroid nodules may present during pregnancy, although many probably represent the presentation of preexisting nodules. There may be enlargement of nodules during pregnancy and presentation of new nodules,[52] and this may be the result of the negative iodine balance that occurs during pregnancy.[53]

Thyroid cancers diagnosed during pregnancy have been associated with a poor prognosis compared with tumors that developed in nongravid periods, with some reports of a higher rate of recurrent or persistent disease in patients with thyroid cancer related to pregnancy[54]; other studies suggest that pregnancy does not cause thyroid cancer recurrence in survivors of papillary thyroid cancer with no structural or biochemical evidence of disease persistence at time of conception.[55] Evidence, however, suggests that there is no difference in overall survival, death caused by thyroid cancer, or recurrence in patients with pregnancy-related differentiated thyroid cancer.[56]

**Box 19.4** *Key points for goiter management in pregnancy*

- Most cases of goiter are physiological in pregnancy.
- A solitary thyroid nodule, in a euthyroid woman, should be investigated with ultrasound and fine-needle aspiration cytology. Surgery for malignant nodules can be normally and safely delayed until after pregnancy.

### Diagnosis

An ultrasound of the thyroid should be carried out in the first instance for a new palpable thyroid mass. If this is a solitary mass, a fine-needle aspiration with cytological examination should be performed.

### Treatment

The multidisciplinary team is of utmost importance in the management of thyroid cancer in pregnancy. Thyroid cancer found in pregnancy follows a similar pattern to nonpregnancy states; the prognosis is good for the majority presenting under the age of 40 years.[57] The Endocrine Society Guidelines recommend that when malignant thyroid nodules are diagnosed in the first or early second trimester, the pregnancy should continue with surgery being offered in the second trimester when there are improved chances of fetal viability.[12] Radioactive iodine scans or treatment are not possible nor generally needed in pregnancy. Pregnant women, who have been treated for low-risk differentiated thyroid cancer and regarded as free of disease, require little more than routine TSH monitoring and periodic clinical examination.[58] Thyroglobulin levels can vary significantly during pregnancy depending on trimester; however, the overall levels remain within the normal nonpregnant reference range.[59,60] Women who have high-risk differentiated thyroid cancer or who have had recurrence prepregnancy require more intensive follow-up with measurement of unstimulated thyroglobulin[58] and neck ultrasonography and repeated analyses of thyroid function.[61]

# Adrenal disease

The maternal adrenal glands do not change morphologically during pregnancy. However, pregnancy has a profound effect on adrenal steroidogenesis. Maternal glucocorticoid production is up regulated to provide increased concentrations of estrogens and cortisol necessary for the mother and also for fetal development. Maternal corticotropin-releasing hormone (CRH) concentrations rise during the second and third trimester, mostly resulting from placental production. Adrenocorticotropic hormone (ACTH) concentrations rise during the first trimester, with a further increase during labor. Serum cortisol

**Box 19.5** *Key points for adrenal disease management in pregnancy*

- The normal ranges for many adrenal tests, including dynamic tests, are poorly described.
- Cushing's syndrome is rare in pregnancy, but early recognition and treatment are essential to avoid morbidity and mortality in pregnancy.
- Pheochromocytoma, if untreated, has major maternal mortality. Medical and surgical management can be considered in pregnancy.
- Congenital adrenal hyperplasia is an important cause of infertility; treatment requires appropriate management in pregnancy, especially to avoid virilization of the affected female fetus.
- Glucocorticoid insufficiency will require careful management to address the stress of pregnancy events.

values increase during pregnancy, largely the result of the response to increased cortisol-binding globulin concentrations, induced by rising estradiol levels. In addition the renin–angiotensin–aldosterone pathway is stimulated, accommodating the 50% increase in maternal circulating volume without resulting in hypertension. The placenta plays a vital role in these complex changes.

Adrenal disease in pregnancy (Box 19.5) is rare and encompasses several different conditions that result from hormonal excess and deficiency. The diagnosis is often difficult in pregnancy, because dynamic tests may be meaningless due to normal physiological changes in pregnancy.

## *Cushing's syndrome (see Chapter 1)*

Cushing's syndrome results from excess exposure to glucocorticoid. Most cases relate to exogenous cortisol; Cushing's syndrome is relatively rare when the production of cortisol is endogenous. Cushing's syndrome may be a primary adrenal disorder associated with low ACTH (40%–50% of pregnancy cases) or from ACTH drive either from the pituitary (Cushing's disease, 30% of pregnancy cases)[62,63] or an ectopic ACTH source. Pregnancy occurring in women with Cushing's syndrome is rare, with only about 150 cases in the literature;[64] this is felt to be due to anovulation caused by the high serum cortisol levels.

### *Pregnancy issues*

Untreated Cushing's syndrome has poor maternal and fetal outcomes. It increases the rates of spontaneous abortion, perinatal death, premature birth, and intrauterine growth retardation.[62,65] The fetoplacental unit can reduce fetal exposure from excess maternal steroids through the protective action of placental type 2 11β-hydroxysteroid dehydrogenase. This can be overwhelmed by excess maternal steroids that, crossing to the fetus, may be associated with intrauterine growth restriction.

### *Diagnosis*

Symptoms and signs of Cushing's syndrome can sometimes be subtle, because they are often features that may also be common in pregnancy, such as abdominal striae, emotional lability, edema, and impaired glucose tolerance. The striae tend to be more pigmented and wider, and they may occur outside of the abdominal wall. Other features include proximal myopathy, hypertension, hirsutism, acne, and bruising.

Diagnosis can be difficult in pregnancy, because normal reference ranges vary considerably. There are wide trimester-specific changes in urine free cortisol in pregnancy. An overnight dexamethasone suppression test is not reliable in pregnancy, and false-positive values may occur in pregnancy. The low-dose dexamethasone suppression test is the definitive diagnostic test for the syndrome. In the differential diagnosis of Cushing's syndrome, one should consider that adrenal adenoma is responsible for 40%–50% in pregnancy compared with 15% outwith pregnancy. ACTH suppression, usually diagnostic of an adrenal cause outwith pregnancy, may be unsuppressed in half of pregnant mothers with a primary adrenal cause. The high-dose dexamethasone suppression test has increased utility in pregnancy. Magnetic resonance imaging (MRI) of the adrenal or pituitary will be performed depending on results.[66] Inferior petrosal sinus sampling is safe and useful in pregnancy when indicated.

### *Treatment*

Untreated Cushing's syndrome is associated with significant fetal and maternal morbidity. Surgery may achieve remission, even with surgery late in the third trimester, but the fetal prognosis remains guarded. In cases of pituitary-driven Cushing's disease, transsphenoidal surgery is the treatment of choice. Surgery should be considered for adrenal lesions (see section "Pheochromocytoma"). There are few safety data on the use of medical treatments in Cushing's syndrome. Metyrapone,[67,68] a glucocorticoid synthesis inhibitor, has been used successfully in pregnancy, with no reports of congenital malformations. Ketoconazole, an antifungal steroidogenesis inhibitor, has also been used in pregnancy without causing congenital malformations; however, there are reports of intrauterine growth retardation and antiandrogenic effects.[69,70]

## Pheochromocytoma (see Chapter 21)

Pheochromocytoma is associated with excess production of catecholamines, usually from an adrenal neuroendocrine tumor; however, 15% may be found in sympathetic ganglia, so-called paragangliomas. These tumors are very rare in pregnancy, with a reported incidence of <0.002% pregnancies,[71] but they can be life-threatening for mother and fetus. Pheochromocytoma can be associated with multiple endocrine neoplasia type 2.

### Pregnancy issues

Pheochromocytoma in pregnancy was previously associated with maternal and fetal mortality rates of up to 50%.[72] A more recent review has suggested a vast improvement, with the maternal mortality rate dropping to 4% and the fetal mortality rate dropping to 11%.[73]

### Diagnosis

Most patients with a new diagnosis of pheochromocytoma present in a similar manner to severe preeclampsia. They may exhibit unstable hypertension, proteinuria, headaches, sweating, and tachycardia. It may present with a hypertensive crisis, occurring during induction of anesthesia, labor, or surgery. Failure to consider pheochromocytoma may result in death.

Diagnosis is made with 24 h urine collection for catecholamines and metanephrines. Plasma catecholamines can also be measured. If these results are positive, then imaging should be undertaken in the form of MRI scanning preferably, although CT scanning may occasionally be justified. Isotope scans such as $^{131}$I-labeled metaiodobenzylguanidine (MIBG) are contraindicated during pregnancy.

### Treatment

Treatment is in the form of long-term α-adrenergic blockade, preferably with phenoxybenzamine that provides long acting, stable, noncompetitive blockade.[74] Its starting dose is generally 10 mg twice daily, with dose titration until the hypertension is controlled. Phenoxybenzamine crosses the placenta, with some reports of perinatal depression and transient hypotension[75]; however, other studies have shown it to be safe for the fetus.[76] In addition, approximately 1% of the dose of phenoxybenzamine may enter the mother's milk.[77] β-Blockade can be given for persistent maternal tachycardia or arrhythmias, but only after full α-blockade. Hypertensive emergencies can be treated with intravenous phentolamine or sodium nitroprusside. The definitive treatment for pheochromocytoma is surgical removal, ideally before 24 weeks of gestation after α-blockade administration, although there is a higher risk of miscarriage in the first trimester. After 24 weeks of gestation, the size of the uterus makes abdominal exploration and resection of the tumor more difficult. Retroperitoneoscopic removal would theoretically seem ideal but has not been utilized in pregnancy, possibly because the uterus is also retroperitoneal. Ideally, delivery of the baby needs to be after fetal maturity has been achieved. Vaginal delivery has been associated with higher rates of maternal mortality than for caesarean sections,[78] which may be the result of catecholamine release secondary to pain and uterine contractions.[75] Many women can be safely treated with α-adrenergic blockade and the condition managed surgically after pregnancy, but the key is early diagnosis.[79]

## Congenital adrenal hyperplasia (see Chapter 18)

Congenital adrenal hyperplasia (CAH) encompasses a group of inherited conditions (autosomal recessive) caused by a defect in one of the five enzymes involved at different stages of the conversion of cholesterol into cortisol within the adrenal cortex. Of the different types of CAH, only women with 21-hydroxylase (21-OHD) deficiency, 11-hydroxylase (11-OHD) deficiency, and 3-β-hydroxy steroid dehydrogenase (3-β-HSD) deficiency are able to become pregnant, because the other deficiencies result in infertility. Women who are fertile may have oligo-ovulation, leading to reduced fertility rates, depending on the severity of the CAH. Pregnancy rates in women with simple virilizing CAH are about 50%.[80] Ovulation induction may be necessary in this group. Risk of transmission to the fetus depends upon the carrier status of the father, and ideally the risk should be assessed before pregnancy. Once the mother is pregnant, prenatal diagnosis of the three enzyme deficiencies is recommended, because prenatal treatment of the neonate with corticosteroid suppression is now possible, to prevent virilization of the affected female fetus. Dexamethasone seems to be associated with a reduction in fetal virilization without significant maternal or fetal adverse effects,[81] although some prefer to use hydrocortisone or prednisolone due to reports of low birth weight with dexamethasone.[82] The Endocrine Society currently recommends using a glucocorticoid that is metabolized by the placenta, such as hydrocortisone, to avoid glucocorticoid and adrenal suppression of the fetus (Grade 1b evidence). The society also recommends measurement of androstenedione, testosterone, and 17β-hydroxyprogesterone in the mother every 2–3 weeks, and glucocorticoid dosage adjusted to maintain concentrations within the reference range for the stage of pregnancy. Even if androgen production cannot be suppressed to normal, placental aromatase protects the fetal genitalia and the brain from masculinization. Glucocorticoid supplementation is required during labor as for other causes of glucocorticoid deficiency.

## Adrenal insufficiency (see Chapters 5, 13)

Primary adrenal insufficiency (Addison's disease) is a rare disease of reduced adrenal steroid (both gluco- and mineralocorticoid) production.[83] The number of births in women diagnosed with adrenal insufficiency is falling with time. The most common cause of primary adrenal insufficiency in pregnancy is autoimmune in origin. Other causes such as tuberculosis, metastases, hemorrhage, or infarction are rare. Secondary adrenal insufficiency from pituitary causes are much more common.

### Pregnancy issues

The fetoplacental unit is relatively safe in maternal hypocortisolemia; the danger to the mother is from acute steroid deficiency. However, there is some evidence to suggest that mothers with autoimmune adrenal insufficiency have an increased risk of caesarean section and preterm delivery.[84]

### Diagnosis

Clinical manifestations of adrenal insufficiency mimic many of those found normally early in pregnancy. Symptoms include weakness, dizziness, syncope, hyperpigmentation, nausea, and vomiting. It is important to recognize symptoms early, because adrenal crisis can arise at times of stress such as labor or an intercurrent infection.

### Treatment

Corticosteroid use is safe both in pregnancy and in breast feeding, with higher doses required if the patient is vomiting and during labor. All patients with adrenal insufficiency ought to have an emergency supply of intramuscular hydrocortisone, with advice on how to administer it. This may be imperative in the first trimester, when hyperemesis classically occurs, potentially leading to missed oral doses of corticosteroid. Some have suggested a need for increased hydrocortisone in the final trimester because there is an increase in cortisol-binding globulin, but this is disputed.[85] Fludrocortisone dose may need to be increased in pregnancy; plasma renin activity is not informative in pregnancy.[85] During labor, adequate saline hydration is needed, and hydrocortisone 25 mg should be administered intramuscularly 6 hourly. If labor is prolonged, the dose of hydrocortisone should be augmented to 100 mg 6 hourly, or as a continuous intravenous infusion (2–3 mg/h). After delivery, the dose can be reduced to maintenance within 3 days.

## Pituitary disease (Box 19.6) (see Chapter 1)

Pituitary hyperplasia stimulated by estrogen can cause the anterior pituitary to increase in size in normal pregnancy.[86] Involution of the enlarged pituitary takes longer in the breastfeeding mother. There is an associated increase in prolactin concentrations to 2–3000 mU/L during normal pregnancy; values can remain elevated in the breastfeeding mother, especially at the time of suckling. Concentrations of luteinizing hormone and follicle-stimulating hormone are suppressed by maternal estrogen through pregnancy.[87] Throughout pregnancy, the placenta secretes both human placental lactogen and

**Box 19.6** *Pituitary disease in pregnancy*

- Functioning and nonfunctioning pituitary tumors may, rarely, need surgical management in pregnancy to protect the optic chiasm.
- Intrapartum pituitary blood loss with pituitary necrosis (Sheehan's syndrome) is less common with modern obstetric care. Anterior pituitary dysfunction with failure of lactation with amenorrhea should alert carers to this possibility.
- Lymphocytic hypophysitis is most common in late pregnancy and early postpartum. Anterior and posterior pituitary dysfunction are seen. MRI is often characteristic.
- Hypopituitarism will cause subfertility; therefore, adequate treatment before pregnancy will be necessary. Adequate glucocorticoid for stress must be planned. Oxytocinase in late pregnancy may cause the need for increased desmopressin dosing in cranial diabetes insipidus.

a specific placental growth hormone (GH), although total GH concentrations remain unchanged in pregnancy. Concentrations of antidiuretic hormone (ADH) are unchanged in pregnancy[88]; however, placental vasopressinase metabolizes ADH, therefore turnover is higher.[89]

## Mass

All pituitary tumors have the propensity to enlarge during pregnancy, due to estrogen effect on lactotroph numbers.[90] Tumors may be functioning or nonfunctioning. The most common functioning tumors in pregnancy are prolactinomas. Nonfunctioning tumors commonly tend to arise from gonadotrophs; however, it is the lactotroph hyperplasia occurring during pregnancy that may cause mass effect, namely compression of the optic chiasm. If any of the pituitary tumors reach a size where they are causing visual field loss, surgery ought to be considered. The decision will be influenced by gestational age and risk of a general anesthetic. Radiotherapy is contraindicated in pregnancy.

## Prolactinoma (Box 19.7)

Hyperprolactinemia can be consequent on normal pregnancy, breastfeeding, stalk disconnection with loss of dopaminergic suppression of lactotroph prolactin secretion, dopamine antagonist therapy, in addition to lactotroph pituitary adenomas. Prolactinomas are the most common functional pituitary tumors found in pregnancy.[91,92] Significant hyperprolactinemia commonly causes subfertility and treatment restores ovulation in 90% of cases (Figure 19.2a and b).

**Box 19.7** *Prolactinomas in pregnancy*

- A lactotroph adenoma with hyperprolactinemia has an adverse effect on fertility that can be addressed with bromocriptine or cabergoline.
- Inevitably, dopamine agonists will be used in early pregnancy; both seem safe, although the evidence for bromocriptine is greater.
- Macroadenomas are more likely than treated macroadenomas or microadenomas to enlarge in late pregnancy.
- MRI and visual field assessment should be used to direct dopamine agonist therapy in pregnancy.

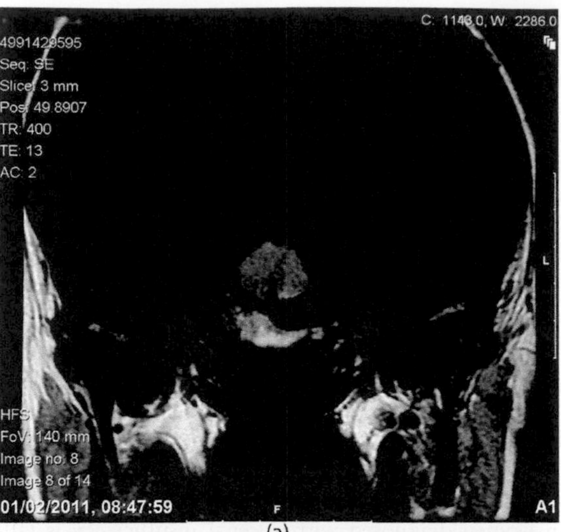


(a)

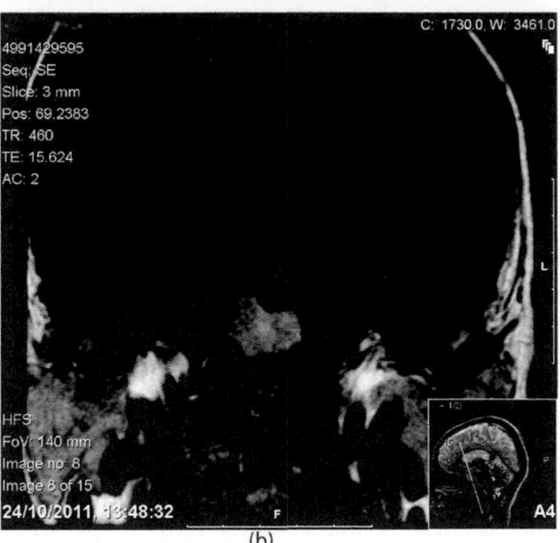


(b)

***Figure 19.2***
*(a and b) MRI illustrates a pituitary with prolactinoma in pregnancy. The lactotroph hyperplasia on the background of the pituitary adenoma has caused the pituitary to enlarge and compress the optic chiasm. After pregnancy, the pituitary becomes smaller and no longer compresses the optic chiasm.*

### Diagnosis

Prolactinomas may present with galactorrhea, anovulation, and amenorrhea with subfertility. Mass effects such as headaches and visual field defects are less common with prolactinoma compared to other pituitary tumors, as the endocrine changes often present before mass effects.

Diagnosis in pregnancy is unusual as significant hyperprolactinemia will have contributed to anovulation. However, presentation of such an adenoma with pituitary apoplexy sometimes occurs.

### Treatment

Lactotroph hyperplasia during normal pregnancy can cause an already enlarged pituitary macroadenoma to grow and compress the optic chiasm. The risk of tumor growth is considerably reduced if diagnosed and treated before conception and if necessary through pregnancy. In general, dopamine receptor agonists are discontinued once pregnancy is confirmed. Bromocriptine and almost certainly cabergoline are safe in terms of spontaneous abortion, fetal malformation, premature delivery, multiple birth, and the long term for the infant.[93–95] Bromocriptine has been used through pregnancy when there is a large tumor with possibility of chiasmal compression without adverse effect, but with less experience.

Enlargement of prolactinomas is seen in about 2.7% of microadenomas, 22.9% of untreated macroadenomas, and 4.8% of pretreated macroadenomas.[96] In the presence of a large and growing pituitary mass, most physicians would start or continue bromocriptine in pregnancy; in most instances, this treatment is successful. The measurement of prolactin concentrations is noncontributory. The mass size should be monitored at 28 weeks with an MRI scan, although gadolinium enhancement is avoided, especially before 24 weeks, gestation. Visual fields should be serially assessed in such women, although prolactin concentration has no value. In general, the effects of large pituitary masses improve after delivery, with shrinkage of the tumor. There are some particular concerns about cabergoline and valvular heart disease, although the dangers of a large pituitary are more certain; ideally, women should have been investigated particularly with an echocardiogram before pregnancy.

## Sheehan's syndrome

This is a rare disease caused by postpartum ischemic necrosis of the pituitary gland after postpartum hemorrhage, resulting in varying degrees of anterior pituitary dysfunction.

### Diagnosis

The limited pituitary circulation in the portal veins from the hypothalamus may be exposed by the physiological enlargement of the pituitary in normal pregnancy. If particularly large, especially with a prolactinoma or the lactotroph hyperplasia in normal pregnancy, the pituitary is sensitive to changes in maternal blood pressure. A large maternal blood loss, for example, after postpartum hemorrhage, can lead to pituitary necrosis. Laboratory tests reveal anterior pituitary hormone deficiencies. This is usually made based upon history and examination. Electrolyte abnormalities, particularly hyponatremia, may be present, because cortisol is required for free water excretion.[97]

### Treatment

Treatment is conservative with replacement of anterior pituitary hormones. The excellent obstetric care, particularly afforded to women in developed countries over the past 50 years, has been associated with considerable reduction in the incidence of this life-altering disease.

## Acromegaly

Increased GH production by somatotroph cells in the pituitary, or acromegaly, is rare in pregnancy. The hyperprolactinemia associated in 30% with acromegaly and pituitary dysfunction has some effect on the menstrual cycle.[98,99] In women diagnosed before pregnancy, treatment with dopamine receptor agonists to correct the high concentrations of prolactin may be necessary to induce ovulation.[100]

### Diagnosis

The condition may present with mass effect and visual field loss. Glucose intolerance, hypertension, and cardiac disease (both cardiomyopathy and coronary artery disease) are features that worsen during pregnancy. All of these features need monitoring during pregnancy, with visual field testing once every trimester.

Diagnosis can be difficult in pregnancy because conventional assays are unable to distinguish between maternal and placental GH. Insulin-like growth factor (IGF)-I values are less helpful in the diagnosis of acromegaly in pregnancy, because concentrations increase in the latter half of normal pregnancies anyway.[101] Maternal GH does not cross the placenta; hence, acromegaly has little effect on the fetus. Macrosomia is sometimes seen in acromegalic pregnancies; however, this is thought to be related to the glucose intolerance seen in the mother.

### Treatment

Most newly diagnosed patients will not require treatment in pregnancy. Dopamine receptor agonists can be used before pregnancy as mentioned previously; however, there is little reason to continue treatment through pregnancy. Somatostatin analogs cross the placenta and hence are not recommended, although they have been used with no cases of fetal malformations reported.[102] Somatostatin receptors are present in many tissues, including the brain; hence, there is a technical risk to the developing fetus. Enlarging tumors causing visual field loss may be an indication for surgery, although the risk to the fetus from the anesthetic will need to be considered and will depend on gestational age. Acromegalic women should be able to breastfeed.

## Hypopituitarism (see Chapter 1)

Hypopituitarism prepregnancy can result from several different causes such as pituitary tumors, vascular causes, trauma, infiltrative causes, and after radiotherapy. Commonly, the gonadotrophs are affected, resulting in fertility problems, although hormonal manipulation and *in vitro* fertilization have revolutionized the lives of women of childbearing age. Steroid and thyroid hormone ought to be given as necessary. Most women will require an increase in their dose of thyroid hormone during pregnancy. Glucocorticoid must be adjusted to cope with stressful events in pregnancy.

During pregnancy, hypopituitarism may present as a result of enlargement of an existing pituitary tumor, lymphocytic hypophysitis, or pituitary infarction. Symptoms and signs can be confused with those occurring normally in pregnancy, for example, lethargy, nausea, and vomiting. Dynamic pituitary function tests have little role due to the normal physiological changes that occur during pregnancy, making results uninterpretable in many cases. Lack of treatment is associated with poor pregnancy outcomes. In cases of acute hypopituitarism, glucocorticoid must always be started first. Thyroxine replacement therapy can be commenced later, after the patient's condition has stabilized. GH replacement therapy has no place in pregnancy.

Diabetes insipidus is less common, particularly as a new diagnosis in pregnancy. Treatment is with desmopressin, shown to be safe in pregnancy. Monitoring of treatment should be based on symptoms, serum and urine osmolalities, and plasma sodium. In patients diagnosed with diabetes insipidus before pregnancy, doses of desmopressin will need to be increased toward the latter end of the pregnancy, due to increased clearance of desmopressin by vasopressinase (oxytocinase), an enzyme produced by the placenta that rapidly inactivates desmopressin and oxytocin.

Autoimmune or lymphocytic hypophysitis presents peripartum with issues such as headache and visual disturbance. There can be both anterior pituitary dysfunction with life-threatening hypocortisolemia and posterior pituitary dysfunction with diabetes insipidus.[103] Lymphocytic hypophysitis is most common in pregnancy (in 30%–50% of cases), with most cases occurring in the second and third trimester or within the first 6 months after delivery.[104] Patients can present severely ill with both local effects, such as headache, and systemic effects, particularly from glucocorticoid deficiency.

## Calcium disorders (Box 19.8) (see Chapter 11)

Pregnancy is associated with profound changes in calcium and parathyroid hormone physiology. Intact parathyroid hormone (PTH) levels decline in the first half of pregnancy, reaching a nadir in the second trimester and then rising thereafter. There is a drop in total serum calcium, with no change in the maternal ionized calcium concentration, pregnancy-related hypercalciuria, and increased maternal calcium absorption from the gut, particularly in the second and third trimesters. Calcium is actively transported across the placenta, facilitated by PTH-related peptide, with the fetal skeleton using this for bone mineralization. Maternal levels of parathyroid hormone–related protein (PTHrp) rise during pregnancy, most probably of fetal origin, although PTHrp is also found in amniotic fluid, amnion, chorion, placenta, and uterus. The placenta produces 1,25-dihydroxyvitamin D [1,25$(OH)_2$D] (it is a high expressor of 1-β-hydroxylase) that enters the maternal circulation and regulates calcium absorption from the gut. Hypovitaminosis D, with or without

**Box 19.8** *Calcium disorders in pregnancy*

- Sustained maternal hypercalcemia is usually due to primary hyperparathyroidism. The hypercalcemia may seriously affect fetal parathyroid gland development, and surgery should be considered in pregnancy.
- Hypoparathyroidism with hypocalcemia is usually postsurgical. Treatment with active vitamin D metabolites should be monitored closely through pregnancy.
- Vitamin D deficiency is common, especially in sun exposure–reduced groups in northern latitudes. Supplementation of the whole population and treatment of vitamin D–deficient groups is probably important but lacks evidence-based hard outcomes, as opposed to surrogate outcomes.

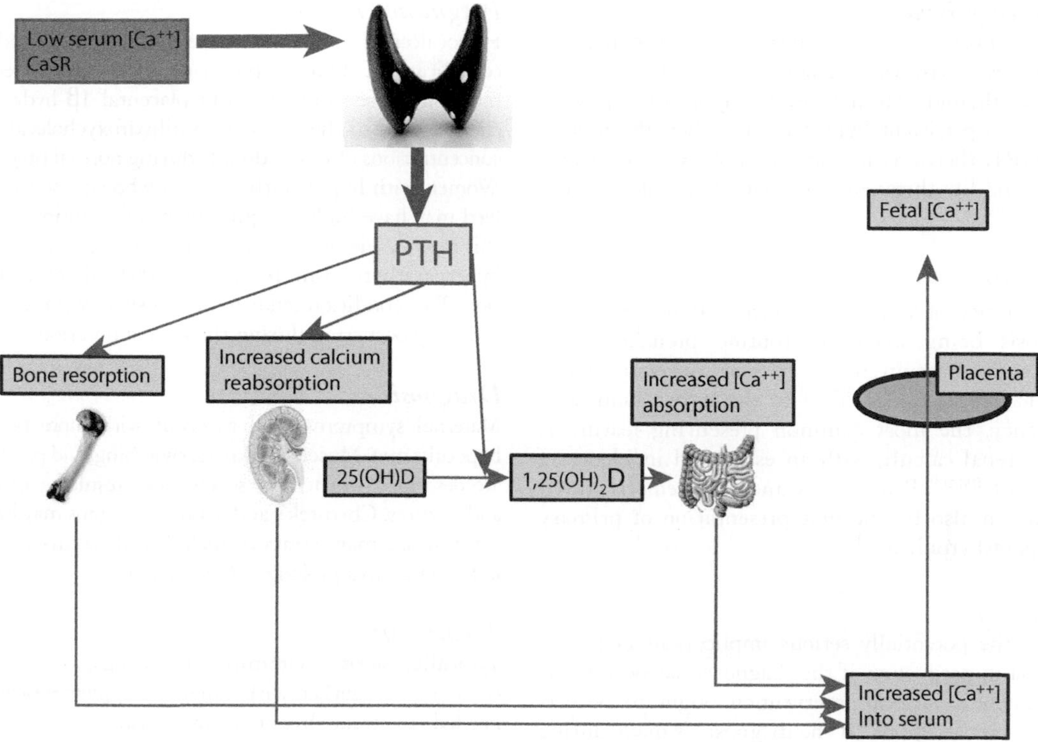


***Figure 19.3***
*Maternofetal calcium metabolism. In general, a low serum calcium is sensed by parathyroid calcium-sensing receptors, causing the production of PTH. PTH may then (1) increase bone resorption, increasing calcium concentration; (2) increase calcium reabsorption from filtrate back into plasma, thereby increasing plasma calcium concentration; and (3) increase conversion of 25-hydroxy vitamin D to the active 1,25(OH)$_2$D. This causes increased calcium absorption in the gut, again leading to increased calcium concentration in the plasma. In normal pregnancy a main physiological effect is increased gut sensitivity to vitamin D, allowing increased maternal absorption of vitamin D. This is at a time when there is maternal bone remodeling, increased calcium loss in the urine, and fetoplacental uptake of calcium. When a mother with vitamin D deficiency consumes calcium with vitamin D, her existing secondary appropriate hyperparathyroidism can lead to temporary hypercalcemia. This may be seen by measuring calcium after the consumption of calcium and vitamin D in a vitamin D–deficient mother during pregnancy. Calcium is taken up by the fetus. If the mother and fetus are vitamin D deficient, the fetus then can become reliant on maternal transplacental calcium to maintain plasma calcium. After delivery, when this calcium supply is removed from the fetus, the neonate may become hypocalcemic and even suffer hypocalcemic seizures.*

secondary hyperparathyroidism, is common in pregnancy. Despite being a relatively rare cause of hypocalcemia in pregnancy, vitamin D concentrations are important in many nonclassical actions. (Figure 19.3).

## Hypercalcemia

Primary hyperparathyroidism (PHPT) is the most common cause of hypercalcemia during pregnancy[105]; malignancy is a rare cause of hypercalcemia in pregnancy. PHPT is rare, with fewer than 200 cases reported in the literature,[106] although it is probably underreported. The diagnosis of mild PHPT may be missed, due to the movement of maternal calcium to the fetal skeleton. Reported frequencies of 60% maternal and 80% fetal complications in pregnancy may overestimate the real risk but demonstrate the risks of this condition.[106]

### Pregnancy issues

Fetal complications include intrauterine growth retardation, low birth weight, and preterm delivery. The fetal parathyroid may not develop appropriately when exposed to persistent hypercalcemia when the mother has PHPT; therefore, neonates may show signs of prolonged and life-threatening neonatal hypocalcemia and tetany.[107,108]

### Diagnosis

The majority of women are asymptomatic, with the diagnosis being made on routine prenatal blood tests or postpartum if the neonate develops symptomatic hypocalcemia. Due to the hypercalciuria of pregnancy, the most common presenting feature is that of renal calculi, with an estimated incidence of 24%–26%.[108,109] Pancreatitis and hyperemesis gravidarum can also be the first presentation of primary hyperparathyroidism.

### Treatment

Due to the potentially serious implications of hypercalcemia in pregnancy, if the diagnosis has been made prepregnancy, surgical intervention ought to be carried out preconception. If the diagnosis is made during pregnancy, the management will depend on the level of hypercalcemia, the presence of complications, and gestation; a calcium concentration of 2.85 mmol/L has been used as a guide to the need for surgical intervention in pregnancy.[110] It is widely accepted that mild asymptomatic PHPT can be managed conservatively, with neonatal monitoring for hypocalcemia. Good hydration is important with conservative management. In patients that cannot be managed conservatively, ultrasound scanning can be used to localize the parathyroid adenoma if it is present. Sestamibi scanning using the radioactive isotope Tc-99m is not recommended in pregnancy. If surgery is contemplated, then minimally invasive parathyroidectomy is ideal when the adenoma is localized; although ideally performed in the second trimester, in the presence of severe hypercalcemia, modern anesthetic practice can safely enable third trimester surgery.

## Hypoparathyroidism

The most common causes of hypoparathyroidism in pregnancy are postthyroidectomy or autoimmune causes; other causes include hypomagnesemia. PTH exerts its effect on both the kidney and bone, whereas reduced concentrations or defective action of PTH results in hypocalcemia and hyperphosphatemia.

### Pregnancy issues

Hypocalcemia can result in several maternal and fetal complications. During pregnancy, vitamin D requirements increase gradually, and placental 1β-hydroxylase converts this to the active 1,25 dihydroxycholecalciferol, concentrations of which double during normal pregnancy. Women with hypoparathyroidism who choose to breastfeed may have higher requirements of vitamin D during this period. The fetus can develop subsequent secondary hyperparathyroidism, resulting in skeletal demineralization. This condition tends to be transient, with resolution normally occurring during the neonatal period.

### Diagnosis

Maternal symptoms tend to occur with more profound hypocalcemia. Muscle weakness, twitching, and paresthesia are described, with more severe cases resulting in tetany and seizures. Chvostek's and Trousseau's signs may be present. Cardiac manifestations include arrhythmias, particularly related to a prolonged QT interval.

### Treatment

Typically, active vitamin D analogs, calcitriol or α-calcidol, together with calcium supplementation are needed to treat hypoparathyroidism. These analogs should be monitored at least monthly in pregnancy and immediately postpartum to react to the physiological changes.[111] In cases of severe hypocalcemia, intravenous calcium may have to be administered, particularly during labor, because if untreated there is an increased risk of tetany. This is thought to be related to hyperventilation during labor, resulting in an acute fall in ionized calcium.

Vitamin D and calcium may be ineffective in treating hypocalcemia associated with hypomagnesemia. Treatment with magnesium supplements, considered safe in pregnancy, is more likely to correct the low calcium values.

## Hypovitaminosis D

Vitamin D is consumed in the diet and largely produced after the action of ultraviolet B (UVB) on skin; the active metabolite $1,25(OH)_2D$ can be considered a hormone, because it is released into the blood in response to a specific stimulus, having classical actions on calcium and bone metabolism through a specific receptor. Vitamin D also has an increasing repertoire of nonclassical actions, from insulin action and insulin secretion to immune modulation and lung development. Maternal hypovitaminosis D is common especially in dark-skinned or covered skin women in northern latitudes.

### *Pregnancy issues*

Low maternal concentrations of vitamin D are associated with reduced fetal bone mass (neonatal rickets) and in neonatal hypocalcemia. Vitamin D concentrations are particularly low in premature babies, because the third trimester is a critical time for transplacental vitamin D transfer. Preeclampsia and caesarean section are more common. The longer term issues with childhood asthma and infection are being defined.

### *Diagnosis*

It is not known whether screening is beneficial or indeed whether vitamin D should be supplemented in all women or only in symptomatic women diagnosed with vitamin D and parathormone estimation.

### *Treatment*

All pregnant women could be supplemented with calcium and vitamin D 800 IU/day. Treatment of vitamin D–deficient women with up to 20,000 IU/week appears safe and appropriate in women with vitamin D deficiency.

## *Summary*

Endocrine disorders in pregnancy are common, with potential consequences for both mother and fetus if left untreated. These conditions vary from the common to the very rare, and some may impact on fertility, thereby reducing their prevalence in pregnancy.

Preexisting conditions may require additional support to achieve successful conception. There should also be a plan for their management in pregnancy. These conditions may require specialist input during pregnancy, particularly because there may be implications for the baby.

New diagnoses can be difficult to make in pregnancy, because symptoms may be varied and may occasionally be assigned to pregnancy physiology. Once a diagnosis has been made, further investigation may be limited in pregnancy and may have to be deferred until the postpartum period unless treatment is needed for maternal and fetal health.

## *References*


1. Glinoer D, de Nayer P, Bourdoux P, Lemone M, Robyn C, van Steirteghem A, et al. Regulation of maternal thyroid during pregnancy. *J Clin Endocrinol Metab*. 1990;71(2):276–87.
2. Kosugi S, Mori T. TSH receptor and LH receptor, 1995. *Endocr J*. 1995;42(5):587–606.
3. Glinoer D, De Nayer P, Robyn C, Lejeune B, Kinthaert J, Meuris S. Serum levels of intact human chorionic gonadotropin (HCG) and its free alpha and beta subunits, in relation to maternal thyroid stimulation during normal pregnancy. *J Endocrinol Invest*. 1993;16(11):881–8.
4. Ain KB, Mori Y, Refetoff S. Reduced clearance rate of thyroxine-binding globulin (TBG) with increased sialylation: A mechanism for estrogen-induced elevation of serum TBG concentration. *J Clin Endocrinol Metab*. 1987;65(4):689–96.
5. Glinoer D. Pregnancy and iodine. *Thyroid*. 2001;11(5):471–81.
6. Glinoer D. The regulation of thyroid function in pregnancy: Pathways of endocrine adaptation from physiology to pathology. *Endocr Rev*. 1997;18(3):404–33.
7. Vanderpump MP, Lazarus JH, Smyth PP, Laurberg P, Holder RL, Boelaert K, et al. Iodine status of UK schoolgirls: A cross-sectional survey. *Lancet*. 2011;377(9782):2007–12.
8. Yarrington C, Pearce EN. Iodine and pregnancy. *J Thyroid Res*. 2011;2011:934104.
9. Dafnis E, Sabatini S. The effect of pregnancy on renal function: Physiology and pathophysiology. *Am J Med Sci*. 1992;303(3):184–205.

*10. Feldt-Rasmussen U, Bliddal Mortensen AS, Rasmussen AK, Boas M, Hilsted L, Main K. Challenges in interpretation of thyroid function tests in pregnant women with autoimmune thyroid disease. *J Thyroid Res*. 2011;2011:598712.

11. Lee RH, Spencer CA, Mestman JH, Miller EA, Petrovic I, Braverman LE, et al. Free T4 immunoassays are flawed during pregnancy. *Am J Obstet Gynecol*. 2009;200(3):260 e1–6.

*12. Abalovich M, Amino N, Barbour LA, Cobin RH, De Groot LJ, Glinoer D, et al. Management of thyroid dysfunction during pregnancy and postpartum: An Endocrine Society Clinical Practice Guideline. *J Clin Endocrinol Metab*. 2007;92(8 Suppl):S1–47.

13. Burrow GN. Thyroid function and hyperfunction during gestation. *Endocr Rev*. 1993;14(2):194–202.
14. Laurberg P, Pedersen KM, Vestergaard H, Sigurdsson G. High incidence of multinodular toxic goitre in the elderly population in a low iodine intake area vs. high incidence of Graves' disease in the young in a high iodine intake area: Comparative surveys of thyrotoxicosis epidemiology in East-Jutland Denmark and Iceland. *J Intern Med*. 1991;229(5):415–20.
15. Azizi F. Effect of methimazole treatment of maternal thyrotoxicosis on thyroid function in breast-feeding infants. *J Pediatr*. 1996;128(6):855–8.


* Key or Classic references.

16. Amino N, Tanizawa O, Mori H, Iwatani Y, Yamada T, Kurachi K, et al. Aggravation of thyrotoxicosis in early pregnancy and after delivery in Graves' disease. *J Clin Endocrinol Metab.* 1982;55(1):108–12.
17. Mestman JH. Hyperthyroidism in pregnancy. *Clin Obstet Gynecol.* 1997;40(1):45–64.
18. Papendieck P, Chiesa A, Prieto L, Gruneiro-Papendieck L. Thyroid disorders of neonates born to mothers with Graves' disease. *J Pediatr Endocrinol Metab.* 2009;22(6):547–53.
19. Weetman AP. Graves' disease. *N Engl J Med.* 2000;343(17):1236–48.
20. Mitsuda N, Tamaki H, Amino N, Hosono T, Miyai K, Tanizawa O. Risk factors for developmental disorders in infants born to women with Graves disease. *Obstet Gynecol.* 1992;80(3 Pt 1):359–64.
21. Laurberg P, Nygaard B, Glinoer D, Grussendorf M, Orgiazzi J. Guidelines for TSH-receptor antibody measurements in pregnancy: Results of an evidence-based symposium organized by the European Thyroid Association. *Eur J Endocrinol.* 1998;139(6):584–6.
22. Rodien P, Jordan N, Lefevre A, Royer J, Vasseur C, Savagner F, et al. Abnormal stimulation of the thyrotrophin receptor during gestation. *Hum Reprod Update.* 2004;10(2):95–105.
23. Goodwin TM. Hyperemesis gravidarum. *Clin Obstet Gynecol.* 1998;41(3):597–605.
24. Niebyl JR. Clinical practice. Nausea and vomiting in pregnancy. *N Engl J Med.* 2010;363(16):1544–50.
25. Goodwin TM, Montoro M, Mestman JH. Transient hyperthyroidism and hyperemesis gravidarum: Clinical aspects. *Am J Obstet Gynecol.* 1992;167(3):648–52.
26. Haddow JE, McClain MR, Lambert-Messerlian G, Palomaki GE, Canick JA, Cleary-Goldman J, et al. Variability in thyroid-stimulating hormone suppression by human chorionic [corrected] gonadotropin during early pregnancy. *J Clin Endocrinol Metab.* 2008;93(9):3341–7.
27. Jurczynska J, Zieleniewski W. [Clinical implications of occurrence of antithyroid antibodies in pregnant women and in the postpartum period]. *Przegl Lek.* 2004;61(8):864–7.
28. Clementi M, Di Gianantonio E, Pelo E, Mammi I, Basile RT, Tenconi R. Methimazole embryopathy: Delineation of the phenotype. *Am J Med Genet.* 1999;83(1):436.
29. Johnsson E, Larsson G, Ljunggren M. Severe malformations in infant born to hyperthyroid woman on methimazole. *Lancet.* 1997;350(9090):1520.
30. Marchant B, Brownlie BE, Hart DM, Horton PW, Alexander WD. The placental transfer of propylthiouracil, methimazole and carbimazole. *J Clin Endocrinol Metab.* 1977;45(6):1187–93.
31. Mortimer RH, Cannell GR, Addison RS, Johnson LP, Roberts MS, Bernus I. Methimazole and propylthiouracil equally cross the perfused human term placental lobule. *J Clin Endocrinol Metab.* 1997;82(9):3099–102.
32. Wing DA, Millar LK, Koonings PP, Montoro MN, Mestman JH. A comparison of propylthiouracil versus methimazole in the treatment of hyperthyroidism in pregnancy. *Am J Obstet Gynecol.* 1994;170(1 Pt 1):90–5.
33. Pearce SH. Spontaneous reporting of adverse reactions to carbimazole and propylthiouracil in the UK. *Clin Endocrinol (Oxf).* 2004;61(5):589–94.
34. Pekonen F, Lamberg BA, Ikonen E. Thyrotoxicosis and pregnancy. An analysis of 43 pregnancies in 42 thyrotoxic mothers. *Ann Chir Gynaecol.* 1978;67(1):1–7.
35. Rodien P, Bremont C, Sanson ML, Parma J, Van Sande J, Costagliola S, et al. Familial gestational hyperthyroidism caused by a mutant thyrotropin receptor hypersensitive to human chorionic gonadotropin. *N Engl J Med.* 1998;339(25):1823–6.
36. Casey BM, Dashe JS, Wells CE, McIntire DD, Byrd W, Leveno KJ, et al. Subclinical hypothyroidism and pregnancy outcomes. *Obstet Gynecol.* 2005;105(2):239–45.
37. Leung AS, Millar LK, Koonings PP, Montoro M, Mestman JH. Perinatal outcome in hypothyroid pregnancies. *Obstet Gynecol.* 1993;81(3):349–53.
38. Henrichs J, Bongers-Schokking JJ, Schenk JJ, Ghassabian A, Schmidt HG, Visser TJ, et al. Maternal thyroid function during early pregnancy and cognitive functioning in early childhood: The generation R study. *J Clin Endocrinol Metab.* 2010;95(9):4227–34.
*39. Haddow JE, Palomaki GE, Allan WC, Williams JR, Knight GJ, Gagnon J, et al. Maternal thyroid deficiency during pregnancy and subsequent neuropsychological development of the child. *N Engl J Med.* 1999;341(8):549–55.
40. Lazarus JH, Bestwick JP, Channon S, Paradice R, Maina A, Rees R, et al. Antenatal thyroid screening and childhood cognitive function. *N Engl J Med.* 2012;366(6):493–501.
41. Lao TT. Thyroid disorders in pregnancy. *Curr Opin Obstet Gynecol.* 2005;17(2):123–7.
42. Benhadi N, Wiersinga WM, Reitsma JB, Vrijkotte TG, Bonsel GJ. Higher maternal TSH levels in pregnancy are associated with increased risk for miscarriage, fetal or neonatal death. *Eur J Endocrinol.* 2009;160(6):985–91.
43. Stagnaro-Green A, Chen X, Bogden JD, Davies TF, Scholl TO. The thyroid and pregnancy: A novel risk factor for very preterm delivery. *Thyroid.* 2005;15(4):351–7.
44. Prummel MF, Wiersinga WM. Thyroid autoimmunity and miscarriage. *Eur J Endocrinol.* 2004;150(6):751–5.
45. Barnhart KT, Sammel MD, Rinaudo PF, Zhou L, Hummel AC, Guo W. Symptomatic patients with an early viable intrauterine pregnancy: HCG curves redefined. *Obstet Gynecol.* 2004;104(1):50–5.
46. Klein RZ, Haddow JE, Faix JD, Brown RS, Hermos RJ, Pulkkinen A, et al. Prevalence of thyroid

deficiency in pregnant women. *Clin Endocrinol (Oxf)*. 1991;35(1):41–6.
47. Loh JA, Wartofsky L, Jonklaas J, Burman KD. The magnitude of increased levothyroxine requirements in hypothyroid pregnant women depends upon the etiology of the hypothyroidism. *Thyroid*. 2009;19(3):269–75.
48. Mandel SJ, Larsen PR, Seely EW, Brent GA. Increased need for thyroxine during pregnancy in women with primary hypothyroidism. *N Engl J Med*. 1990;323(2):91–6.
49. Alexander EK, Marqusee E, Lawrence J, Jarolim P, Fischer GA, Larsen PR. Timing and magnitude of increases in levothyroxine requirements during pregnancy in women with hypothyroidism. *N Engl J Med*. 2004;351(3):241–9.
*50. Berghout A, Wiersinga W. Thyroid size and thyroid function during pregnancy: An analysis. *Eur J Endocrinol*. 1998;138(5):536–42.
51. Glinoer D. What happens to the normal thyroid during pregnancy? *Thyroid*. 1999;9(7):631–5.
52. Kung AW, Chau MT, Lao TT, Tam SC, Low LC. The effect of pregnancy on thyroid nodule formation. *J Clin Endocrinol Metab*. 2002;87(3):1010–14.
53. Rosen IB, Korman M, Walfish PG. Thyroid nodular disease in pregnancy: Current diagnosis and management. *Clin Obstet Gynecol*. 1997;40(1):81–9.
54. Vannucchi G, Perrino M, Rossi S, Colombo C, Vicentini L, Dazzi D, et al. Clinical and molecular features of differentiated thyroid cancer diagnosed during pregnancy. *Eur J Endocrinol*. 2010;162(1):145–51.
55. Hirsch D, Levy S, Tsvetov G, Weinstein R, Lifshitz A, Singer J, et al. Impact of pregnancy on outcome and prognosis of survivors of papillary thyroid cancer. *Thyroid*. 2010;20(10):1179–85.
56. Alves GV, Santin AP, Furlanetto TW. Prognosis of thyroid cancer related to pregnancy: A systematic review. *J Thyroid Res*. 2011;2011:691719.
57. Moosa M, Mazzaferri EL. Outcome of differentiated thyroid cancer diagnosed in pregnant women. *J Clin Endocrinol Metab*. 1997;82(9):2862–6.
58. Imran SA, Rajaraman M. Management of differentiated thyroid cancer in pregnancy. *J Thyroid Res*. 2011;2011:549609.
59. Soldin OP, Tractenberg RE, Hollowell JG, Jonklaas J, Janicic N, Soldin SJ. Trimester-specific changes in maternal thyroid hormone, thyrotropin, and thyroglobulin concentrations during gestation: Trends and associations across trimesters in iodine sufficiency. *Thyroid*. 2004;14(12):1084–90.
60. Hara Y, Tanikawa T, Sakatsume Y, Sato K, Ikeda H, Ishii J, et al. Decreased serum thyroglobulin levels in the late stage of pregnancy. *Acta Endocrinol (Copenh)*. 1986;113(3):418–23.
*61. Mazzaferri EL. Approach to the pregnant patient with thyroid cancer. *J Clin Endocrinol Metab*. 2011;96(2):265–72.
62. Buescher MA, McClamrock HD, Adashi EY. Cushing syndrome in pregnancy. *Obstet Gynecol*. 1992;79(1):130–7.
63. Pickard J, Jochen AL, Sadur CN, Hofeldt FD. Cushing's syndrome in pregnancy. *Obstet Gynecol Surv*. 1990;45(2):87–93.
64. Vilar L, Freitas Mda C, Lima LH, Lyra R, Kater CE. Cushing's syndrome in pregnancy: An overview. *Arq Bras Endocrinol Metabol*. 2007;51(8):1293–302.
65. Aron DC, Schnall AM, Sheeler LR. Cushing's syndrome and pregnancy. *Am J Obstet Gynecol*. 1990;162(1):244–52.
66. Oldfield EH, Doppman JL, Nieman LK, Chrousos GP, Miller DL, Katz DA, et al. Petrosal sinus sampling with and without corticotropin-releasing hormone for the differential diagnosis of Cushing's syndrome. *N Engl J Med*. 199126;325(13):897–905.
67. Connell JM, Cordiner J, Davies DL, Fraser R, Frier BM, McPherson SG. Pregnancy complicated by Cushing's syndrome: Potential hazard of metyrapone therapy. Case report. *Br J Obstet Gynaecol*. 1985;92(11):1192–5.
68. Hana V, Dokoupilova M, Marek J, Plavka R. Recurrent ACTH-independent Cushing's syndrome in multiple pregnancies and its treatment with metyrapone. *Clin Endocrinol (Oxf)*. 2001;54(2):277–81.
69. Amado JA, Pesquera C, Gonzalez EM, Otero M, Freijanes J, Alvarez A. Successful treatment with ketoconazole of Cushing's syndrome in pregnancy. *Postgrad Med J*. 1990;66(773):221–3.
70. Berwaerts J, Verhelst J, Mahler C, Abs R. Cushing's syndrome in pregnancy treated by ketoconazole: Case report and review of the literature. *Gynecol Endocrinol*. 1999;13(3):175–82.
71. Chestnut DH. *Obstetric Anesthesia: Principles and Practice*. 2nd ed. St. Louis: Mosby; 1999.
72. Schenker JG, Chowers I. Pheochromocytoma and pregnancy. Review of 89 cases. *Obstet Gynecol Surv*. 1971;26(11):739–47.
73. Ahlawat SK, Jain S, Kumari S, Varma S, Sharma BK. Pheochromocytoma associated with pregnancy: Case report and review of the literature. *Obstet Gynecol Surv*. 1999;54(11):728–37.
74. Harper MA, Murnaghan GA, Kennedy L, Hadden DR, Atkinson AB. Phaeochromocytoma in pregnancy. Five cases and a review of the literature. *Br J Obstet Gynaecol*. 1989;96(5):594–606.
75. Santeiro ML, Stromquist C, Wyble L. Phenoxybenzamine placental transfer during the third trimester. *Ann Pharmacother*. 1996;30(11):1249–51.
76. Lyons CW, Colmorgen GH. Medical management of pheochromocytoma in pregnancy. *Obstet Gynecol*. 1988;72(3 Pt 2):450–1.

77. Aplin SC, Yee KF, Cole MJ. Neonatal effects of long-term maternal phenoxybenzamine therapy. *Anesthesiology*. 2004;100(6):1608–10.
78. Schenker JG, Granat M. Phaeochromocytoma and pregnancy — an updated appraisal. *Aust N Z J Obstet Gynaecol*. 1982;22(1):1–10.
79. Burgess GE 3rd. Alpha blockade and surgical intervention of pheochromocytoma in pregnancy. *Obstet Gynecol*. 1979;53(2):266–70.
80. Stikkelbroeck NM, Beerendonk CC, Willemsen WN, Schreuders-Bais CA, Feitz WF, Rieu PN, et al. The long term outcome of feminizing genital surgery for congenital adrenal hyperplasia: Anatomical, functional and cosmetic outcomes, psychosexual development, and satisfaction in adult female patients. *J Pediatr Adolesc Gynecol*. 2003;16(5):289–96.
81. Merce Fernandez-Balsells M, Muthusamy K, Smushkin G, Lampropulos JF, Elamin MB, Abu Elnour NO, et al. Prenatal dexamethasone use for the prevention of virilization in pregnancies at risk for classical congenital adrenal hyperplasia because of 21-hydroxylase (CYP21A2) deficiency: A systematic review and meta-analyses. *Clin Endocrinol (Oxf)*. 2010;73(4):436–44.
*82. Seckl JR. Glucocorticoid programming of the fetus; adult phenotypes and molecular mechanisms. *Mol Cell Endocrinol*. 2001;185(1–2):61–71.
83. Lebbe M, Arlt W. What is the best diagnostic and therapeutic management strategy for an Addison patient during pregnancy. *Clinical Endocrinology*. 2013;78:497–502.
84. Bjornsdottir S, Cnattingius S, Brandt L, Nordenstrom A, Ekbom A, Kampe O, et al. Addison's disease in women is a risk factor for an adverse pregnancy outcome. *J Clin Endocrinol Metab*. 2010;95(12):5249–57.
85. Quinkler M, Hahner S. What is the best long-term management strategy for patients with primary adrenal insufficiency? *Clin Endocrinol (Oxf)*. 2012;76(1):21–5.
86. Gonzalez JG, Elizondo G, Saldivar D, Nanez H, Todd LE, Villarreal JZ. Pituitary gland growth during normal pregnancy: An in vivo study using magnetic resonance imaging. *Am J Med*. 1988;85(2):217–20.
87. Jeppsson S, Rannevik G, Liedholm P, Thorell JI. Basal and LRH-stimulated secretion of FSH during early pregnancy. *Am J Obstet Gynecol*. 1977;127(1):32–6.
88. Fisher DA. Maternal-fetal neurohypophyseal system. *Clin Perinatol*. 1983;10(3):695–707.
89. Barron WM. Water metabolism and vasopressin secretion during pregnancy. *Baillieres Clin Obstet Gynaecol*. 1987;1(4):853–71.
90. Scheithauer BW, Sano T, Kovacs KT, Young WF, Jr., Ryan N, Randall RV. The pituitary gland in pregnancy: A clinicopathologic and immunohistochemical study of 69 cases. *Mayo Clin Proc*. 1990;65(4):461–74.
91. Casanueva FF, Molitch ME, Schlechte JA, Abs R, Bonert V, Bronstein MD, et al. Guidelines of the Pituitary Society for the diagnosis and management of prolactinomas. *Clin Endocrinol (Oxf)*. 2006;65(2):265–73.
92. Kars M, Dekkers OM, Pereira AM, Romijn JA. Update in prolactinomas. *Neth J Med*. 2010;68(3):104–12.
93. Krupp P, Monka C. Bromocriptine in pregnancy: Safety aspects. *Klin Wochenschr*. 1987;65(17):823–7.
94. Raymond JP, Goldstein E, Konopka P, Leleu MF, Merceron RE, Loria Y. Follow-up of children born of bromocriptine-treated mothers. *Horm Res*. 1985;22(3):239–46.
95. Stalldecker G, Mallea-Gil MS, Guitelman M, Alfieri A, Ballarino MC, Boero L, et al. Effects of cabergoline on pregnancy and embryo-fetal development: Retrospective study on 103 pregnancies and a review of the literature. *Pituitary*. 2010;13(4):345–50.
96. Holmgren U, Bergstrand G, Hagenfeldt K, Werner S. Women with prolactinoma — effect of pregnancy and lactation on serum prolactin and on tumour growth. *Acta Endocrinol (Copenh)*. 1986;111(4):452–9.
97. Huang YY, Ting MK, Hsu BR, Tsai JS. Demonstration of reserved anterior pituitary function among patients with amenorrhea after postpartum hemorrhage. *Gynecol Endocrinol*. 2000;14(2):99–104.
98. Katznelson L, Kleinberg D, Vance ML, Stavrou S, Pulaski KJ, Schoenfeld DA, et al. Hypogonadism in patients with acromegaly: Data from the multi-centre acromegaly registry pilot study. *Clin Endocrinol (Oxf)*. 2001;54(2):183–8.
99. Grynberg M, Salenave S, Young J, Chanson P. Female gonadal function before and after treatment of acromegaly. *J Clin Endocrinol Metab*. 2010;95(10):4518–25.
100. Herman-Bonert V, Seliverstov M, Melmed S. Pregnancy in acromegaly: Successful therapeutic outcome. *J Clin Endocrinol Metab*. 1998;83(3):727–31.
*101. Bronstein MD, Paraiba DB, Jallad RS. Management of pituitary tumors in pregnancy. *Nat Rev Endocrinol*. 2011;7(5):301–10.
102. Colao A, Merola B, Ferone D, Lombardi G. Acromegaly. *J Clin Endocrinol Metab*. 1997;82(9):2777–81.
103. Caturegli P, Newschaffer C, Olivi A, Pomper MG, Burger PC, Rose NR. Autoimmune hypophysitis. *Endocr Rev*. 2005;26(5):599–614.
104. Thodou E, Asa SL, Kontogeorgos G, Kovacs K, Horvath E, Ezzat S. Clinical case seminar: Lymphocytic hypophysitis: Clinicopathological findings. *J Clin Endocrinol Metab*. 1995;80(8):2302–11.
105. Kristoffersson A, Dahlgren S, Lithner F, Jarhult J. Primary hyperparathyroidism in pregnancy. *Surgery*. 1985;97(3):326–30.

106. Schnatz PF, Curry SL. Primary hyperparathyroidism in pregnancy: Evidence-based management. *Obstet Gynecol Surv*. 2002;57(6):365–76.
107. Jaafar R, Yun Boo N, Rasat R, Latiff HA. Neonatal seizures due to maternal primary hyperparathyroidism. *J Paediatr Child Health*. 2004;40(5–6):329.
108. Moniz CF, Nicolaides KH, Tzannatos C, Rodeck CH. Calcium homeostasis in second trimester fetuses. *J Clin Pathol*. 1986;39(8):838–41.
109. Carella MJ, Gossain VV. Hyperparathyroidism and pregnancy: Case report and review. *J Gen Intern Med*. 1992;7(4):448–53.
110. Norman J, Politz D, Politz L. Hyperparathyroidism during pregnancy and the effect of rising calcium on pregnancy loss: A call for earlier intervention. *Clin Endocrinol (Oxf)*. 2009;71(1):104–9.
111. Caplan RH, Beguin EA. Hypercalcemia in a calcitriol-treated hypoparathyroid woman during lactation. *Obstet Gynecol*. 1990;76(3 Pt 2):485–9.

# 20

# Fluid and electrolyte disorders

*Ploutarchos Tzoulis, Pierre-Marc G. Bouloux*

## Physiology of water balance

Human cellular function depends on constant tonicity of the extracellular fluid. Water homeostasis is very accurately controlled to maintain plasma osmolality within a remarkably narrow range of 282–298 mOsm/kg.[1] Osmolality is defined as the concentration of all the solutes in a given weight of water. Total plasma osmolality is estimated as follows: Posm (mOsm/kg $H_2O$) = 2 × [serum Na (mmol/L) + glucose (mmol/L) + blood urea nitrogen (BUN) (mmol/L)]. Effective osmolality or tonicity of the plasma applies only to the effective solutes. Effective solutes are impermeable to cell membranes; are restricted to the extracellular fluid (ECF) compartment; and create osmotic pressure gradients across cell membranes, leading to osmotic movement of water from the intracellular fluid (ICF) to the ECF.[2]

Sodium (Na) is the predominant effective solute and the most important osmotically active cation. Plasma Na concentrations are physiologically maintained within a narrow range of 135–145 mmol/L, despite great variations in Na and water intake. The main determinants of serum sodium (sNa) are Na intake, Na output, water intake, and water output that is dependent on the ability to excrete excess water in dilute urine.[3] Because disorders of Na balance are rare, hyponatremia is usually due to a defect in water homeostasis. Water homeostasis is maintained through arginine vasopressin (AVP) and thirst.

### AVP–Aquaporins

AVP is a nine-amino acid peptide hormone that is synthesized in the magnocellular and parvocellular neurosecretory neurons of the paraventricular nuclei (PVNs) and supraoptic nuclei (SONs) of the hypothalamus. AVP is stored within neurosecretory granules in the posterior pituitary gland and is released into the circulation in response to specific stimuli. AVP binds to the V2-receptor (V2R) in the basolateral membrane of the principal cells of collecting ducts of the kidney and initiates cAMP-mediated activation of AQP2 water channels.[4] As a result, AVP leads to renal water reabsorption through increase of collecting duct water permeability. AVP stimulates three G protein–coupled receptors: V1a receptors (V1aRs) that are mainly vascular, V1b receptors (V1bRs) in the anterior pituitary, and V2 receptors (V2Rs) in the kidney. AVP binding to V1aRs leads to smooth vessel contraction, whereas stimulation of V1bRs by AVP releases adrenocorticotrophic hormone (ACTH).[5]

The discovery of aquaporin (AQP) water channels by Agre et al.[6] elucidated the mechanism by which water crosses biological membranes. Thirteen mammalian AQPs have been identified to date; they are specialized membrane transport proteins that mediate transport of water across cell membranes.[7] AQPs have six membrane-spanning domains and they are organized as shown in Figure 20.1.[8]

AQP2 is the predominant AVP-regulated water channel in the kidney and plays a key role in the control of collecting duct water permeability. There are short-term and long-term regulatory systems of water permeability and AQP2 by AVP. Short-term regulation occurs within few minutes and takes place through trafficking of AQP2 from intracellular storage vesicles to the apical plasma membrane, allowing reabsorption of water from lumen to the cell.[8] The long-term regulation

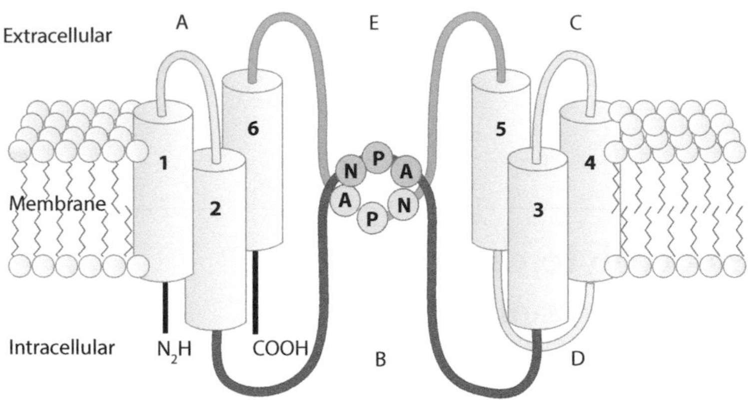


***Figure 20.1***
*AQP is a transmembrane protein with two intramembrane loops (B and E) and three extramembrane loops (A, C, and D). An asparagine-proline-alanine (NPA) motif is contained in each of the highly conserved B and E loops. These loops fold into the lipid bilayer in an "hourglass" manner that forms a pore. (Adapted from Chen YC et al.,* Biology of the Cell/Under the Auspices of the European Cell Biology Organization, *97, 357–71, 2005.)*

occurs within hours to days through increase of the number of the water channels in the cell. AVP binds to V2Rs on the basolateral plasma membrane of the collecting duct. The agonist-occupied V2R activates adenylate cyclase; the resultant increase in cAMP leads to activation of PKA (Protein Kinase A). Increasing levels of PKA phosphorylates transcription factors such as CREB-P ([cAMP-Response Element]-binding protein); these factors bind to CRE in the promoter of the AQP2 gene to increase gene transcription.[9]

## *Regulation of AVP release*

AVP secretion is primarily regulated by plasma osmolality. Osmoreceptors are located within the circumventricular organs, specifically in the subfornical organ (SFO) and the organum vasculosum laminae terminalis (OVLT).[1] Neural signals are transmitted from the osmoreceptors to the sites of AVP synthesis (supraoptic and paraventricular nuclei).

There are three basic principles behind osmoregulation of AVP secretion. The first principle is that there is an osmotic threshold (mean 284.3 mOsm/kg in a healthy man) at which AVP release into the plasma starts. The second principle is that there is a linear and very close relationship between plasma osmolality and plasma AVP. The slope of this line is a measure of the sensitivity of the AVP-osmoreceptor and AVP-releasing unit.[10] The third principle is that the threshold and the slope of the regression line vary considerably between individuals due to genetic factors, but they are highly reproducible within an individual.[11]

This osmoregulatory system is very sensitive. Changes of ≤1% in plasma osmolality are sufficient to cause significant increases in plasma AVP levels, and increases in plasma osmolality of only 5–10 mOsm/kg $H_2O$ (2%–4%) above the osmotic threshold lead to maximal antidiuresis. Urine osmolality is directly proportional to plasma AVP concentrations, but urine volume is inversely related to AVP levels (Figure 20.2).[2]

Age has a significant effect on osmoregulation of AVP release. Osmoreceptor sensitivity (the slope of AVP regression line) is much greater in the old subjects compared with young subjects, but free water clearances are the same. This may be a compensatory mechanism for the reduced renal ability to conserve water in aging man.[12]

There is also nonosmotic control of AVP release. Baroreceptors are located in the left atrium, aortic arch, and carotid sinus. Severe plasma volume reductions of >20%–25% are a potent stimulus of AVP release and override osmotic regulatory system.[10] Modest reductions in effective arterial volume shift the relationship between osmolality and AVP release to the left (Figure 20.3).[2]

## *Thirst*

Thirst can be stimulated by four different signals: increased plasma osmolality detected by osmoreceptors in the anterior hypothalamus, decreased blood volume detected by cardiac baroreceptors, decreased arterial blood pressure with concomitant increased plasma levels of angiotensin II that binds to

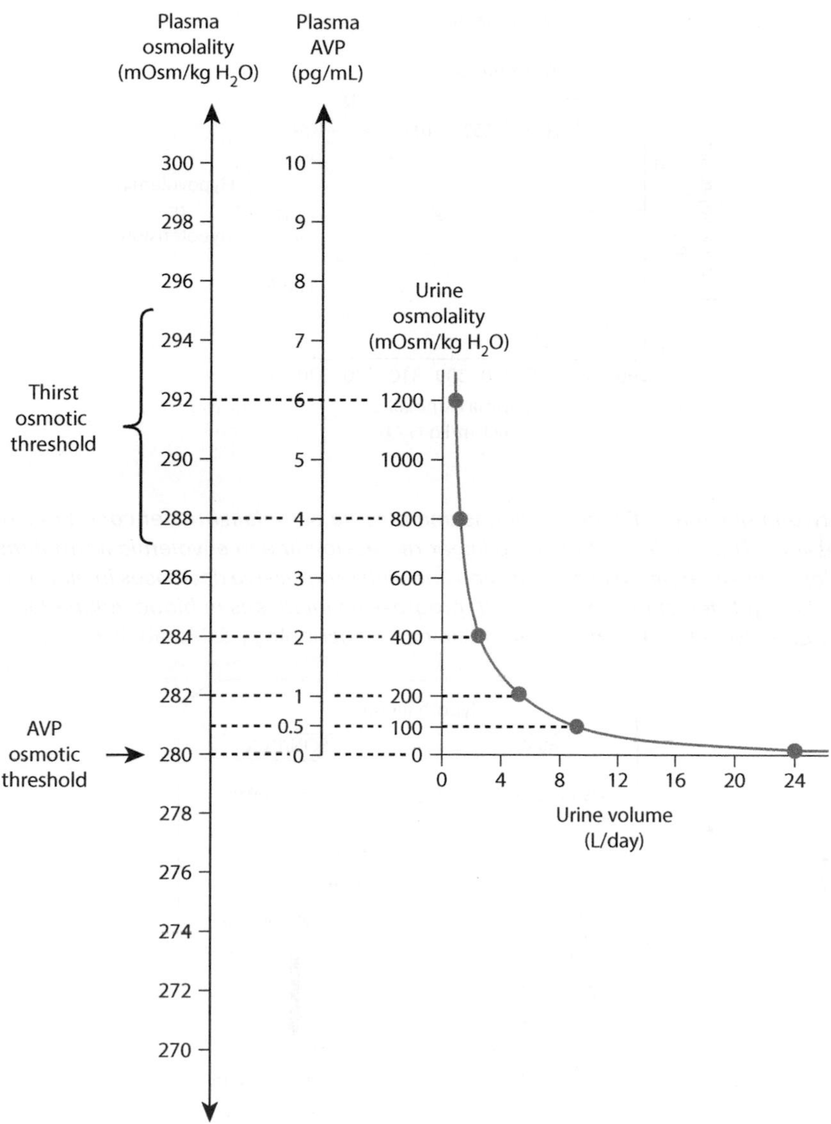


***Figure 20.2***
*Representation of physiological relationships between plasma osmolality, plasma AVP levels, urine osmolality, and urine volume. (Adapted from Verbalis JG et al.,* Best Practice & Research Clinical Endocrinology & Metabolism, *17, 471–503, 2003.)*

receptors in the subfornical organ, and increased gastric Na load detected by Na receptors in the abdominal viscera.[13]

Osmoregulation of thirst is the main determinant of thirst and shares the same principles with the osmoregulation of AVP release. Thirst sensation is mild when plasma osmolality is within the normal range to replace insensible losses and maintain water homeostasis. When plasma osmolality is above the osmotic threshold for the individual, there is very intense thirst response to increase fluid intake.

The act of drinking inhibits rapidly AVP release and thirst before any changes in plasma osmolality. This inhibition occurs through oropharyngeal receptors that activate neural inputs to the hypothalamus.[1] This is a defense mechanism to prevent overhydration.

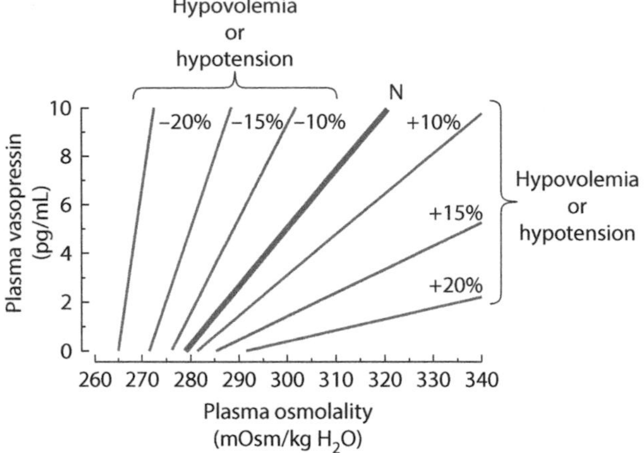


***Figure 20.3***
*Relationship between plasma AVP concentrations and plasma osmolality under conditions of varying blood volume and pressure. The line N illustrates the linear regression line in euvolemic normotensive adults. The lines to the left depict the changes in this regression line with progressive decreases in blood volume/pressure, and the lines to the right depict the changes with progressive increases in blood volume/pressure. (Adapted from Verbalis JG et al.,* Best Practice & Research Clinical Endocrinology & Metabolism, *17, 471–503, 2003.)*

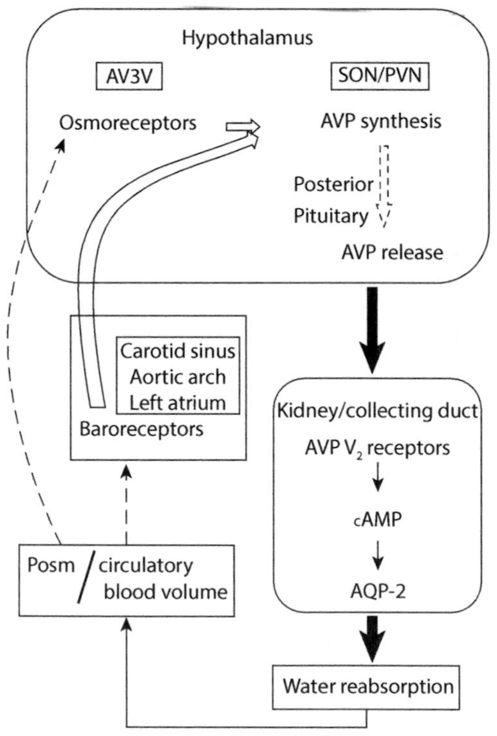


***Figure 20.4***
*Overview of AVP-mediated water homeostasis. AV3V, SON/PVN, cAMP, AQP-2; AV3V, anteroventral third ventricle region of hypothalamus; SON, supraoptic nuclei; PVN, paraventricular nuclei; AVP, arginine vasopressin; cAMP, cyclic AMP; AQP-2, aquaporin-2. (Adapted from Ishikawa SE, Schrier RW,* Clinical Endocrinology, *58, 1–17, 2003.)*

Overall, body water homeostasis is achieved mainly through constant AVP-mediated changes in urine concentration and volume in response to plasma osmolality (Figure 20.4).[4] Thirst plays the role of the backup defense mechanism.

# Hyponatremia (see Severe hyponatremia, Chapter 24)

Hyponatremia is defined as an sNa concentration of <135 mmol/L (normal range, 135–145 mmol/L) and is the most frequent electrolyte disorder seen in clinical practice. Hyponatremia almost always represents an excess of water in relation to Na in the extracellular fluid.[14] The two commonest mechanisms are by depletion of total body Na in excess of water losses (hypovolemic hyponatremia) or excess of body water (euvolemic or hypervolemic hyponatremia).

## Epidemiology

Hyponatremia is a common occurrence in hospitalized patients. The incidence of hyponatremia during acute hospital admission has been reported at 30%–42%.[15] sNa <130 mmol/L has been observed at 2.6%–6.2% of inpatients.[15,16]

Also, hyponatremia is common among older individuals in the community. Measurement of Na levels in 5179 subjects aged ≥55 years from the population-based Rotterdam study showed that the prevalence of hyponatremia was 7.7% and in the subgroup of aged ≥75 years was 11.6%.[17]

Increasing age is a strong independent risk factor for developing hyponatremia (Figure 20.5).[18] Several factors contribute to the increased risk of hyponatremia in the elderly: decreased total body water, age-related impaired diluting capacity of the kidney, age-related decrease in glomerular filtration rate and thereby increased passive reabsorption of fluid, impaired kidney ability to conserve Na, increased AVP levels at baseline and also in response to osmotic stimuli, and iatrogenic factors (e.g., polypharmacy, losing control of fluid intake).[19]

Hyponatremia, even mild (sNa 130–135 mmol/L), is associated with significantly increased in-hospital and long-term mortality as well as increased length of hospital stay.[20,21] Hyponatremia is a poor prognostic marker in patients with acute ST elevation myocardial infarct,[22] with heart failure,[23,24] with cirrhosis,[25] and with cancer.[26] It is not known whether a causal relationship between hyponatremia and mortality exists or whether hyponatremia is just a marker of severity of illness that is not causally related to mortality.[27,28] Another possibility is that hyponatremia may contribute to organ dysfunction and therefore indirectly contribute to excess mortality, but there is limited data about the effect of hyponatremia on other organs, such as the heart.[29]

## Clinical presentation

Symptoms and signs of hyponatremia vary and depend on the severity of hyponatremia, the rate of decline in sNa concentration, and the patient's age and sex. Usually, patients with mild hyponatremia (sNa 130–135 mmol/L) are asymptomatic or have subtle symptoms. Nonneurological symptoms, such as nausea, vomiting,

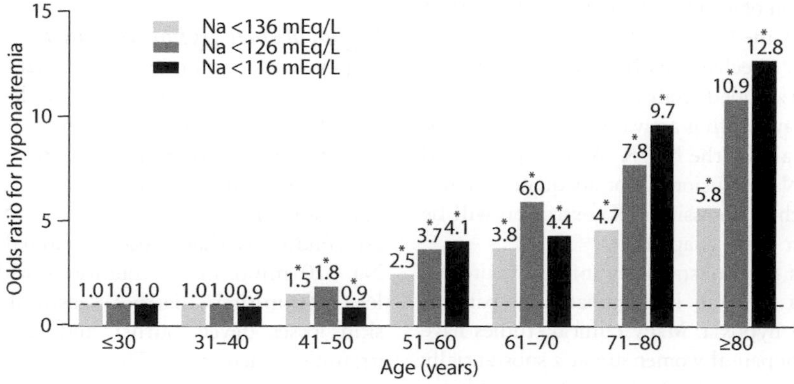


**Figure 20.5**
*Association between age and the odds of developing hospital-acquired hyponatremia. Odds ratios >1.0 signify increased risk compared with subjects <30 years. (Adapted from Hawkins RC,* Clinica Chimica Acta; International Journal of Clinical Chemistry*, 337, 169–72, 2003.)*

malaise, thirst, and weakness, are more common in moderate hyponatremia (sNa 125–130 mmol/L). In cases of severe hyponatremia (sNa <125 mmol/L), central nervous system symptoms dominate, with development of headache, muscle cramps, lethargy, restlessness, agitation, disorientation, and apathy. In cases of severe or rapidly evolving hyponatremia, seizures, coma, brainstem herniation, respiratory arrest, and death can occur.[30]

Patients with chronic hyponatremia were described as "asymptomatic" until a few years ago. Recent evidence has suggested that chronic hyponatremia is not a benign condition. Even mild hyponatremia is associated with impairment in cognitive function, gait disturbances, and high incidence of falls.[31] Several studies have shown that chronic hyponatremia is related to increased risk of bone fractures.[32–34] Animal and *in vitro* data suggest that hyponatremia may *per se* reduce bone mineral density and cause osteoporosis through increase in bone resorption.[35]

### Hyponatremic encephalopathy

The severity of symptoms depends to a large extent on the rapidity of fall of plasma Na levels. In acute hyponatremia, water starts immediately to move into cells to achieve osmotic equilibrium. In brain, this initial swelling starts the process of extrusion of intracellular solutes. If solute extrusion is successfully achieved, osmotic equilibrium will be maintained between brain and plasma, and the patient will remain asymptomatic or mildly symptomatic. However, if adequate solute extrusion is not accomplished, water will continue to move into the brain, and this osmotic movement can lead to brain edema, raised intracranial pressure, and eventual tentorial herniation.[36]

The movement of water into brain cells appears to be mediated by a specific type of water-selective channel, the aquaporin AQP4, that has been identified in the brain. The action of antidiuretic hormone (ADH) on AQP in the brain is mediated via V1Rs.[36]

There are many mechanisms by which osmotically active solutes are extruded from brain during hyponatremia. The pathway which is activated first is the extrusion of Na from brain by the $Na^+/K^+$/ATPase pump and Na channels.[37] If Na extrusion is not adequate to lower brain osmolality, then potassium (K) extrusion will be stimulated to assist brain adaptation.

The two factors that substantially influence outcome in terms of brain damage in hyponatremic patients are female sex and hypoxia. Many clinical studies have shown that premenopausal women are at a substantially greater risk of dying or developing permanent brain damage from symptomatic hyponatremia than are either postmenopausal women or men of any age. Eighty percent of all patients with symptomatic hyponatremia who die or experience brain damage are women and the odds ratio for women versus men is 28:1.[38] The net effect of female sex hormones is to prevent brain adaptation while stimulating water influx into the brain. First, both estrogens and progesterone inhibit the $Na^+/K^+$/ATPase pump that plays an important role in extrusion of Na from cells. Second, female sex hormones also increase circulating levels of ADH and are responsible for the water retention. ADH has also two direct effects on the brain: it increases water movement into the brain and it significantly increases vascular smooth muscle contractility, decreases cerebral blood flow, and leads to brain tissue hypoxia. Thus, the ability of premenopausal females to appropriately adapt to hyponatremia may depend in large part on the time of the menstrual cycle at which hyponatremia develops.[39] It is worth mentioning that elderly men tend to be resistant to the effects of hyponatremic encephalopathy. Men have larger skulls than women, and by the age of 60 years, their brain has shrunk substantially more than in women; thus, they have a lot more space in their skulls to adapt to brain edema.

Hypoxia is a major factor contributing to brain damage in patients with hyponatremia. Hypoxia leads to a failure of increase in Na/-K/-ATPase transport activity. Hypoxia is also a major stimulus for increased secretion of ADH that directly increases water movement into the brain and as well as decreases brain production of ATP.[39]

## Causes of hyponatremia

After clinical and biochemical evaluation of extracellular volume status, hyponatremia is classified as hypovolemic, euvolemic, and hypervolemic. Each of these three types of hyponatremia can be due to a wide variety of causes (Table 20.1).[40]

### Hypovolemic hyponatremia

Hypovolemic hyponatremia is characterized by extracellular volume depletion with Na loss exceeding water loss. The reduced effective arterial blood volume is a potent stimulant of AVP secretion.

Hypovolemic hyponatremia is caused by extrarenal losses of Na or renal losses of Na. The commonest conditions that cause extrarenal Na losses (urine Na <20 mmol/L) are conditions with gastrointestinal losses (vomiting, diarrhea, gastrointestinal bleeding), skin losses (fever, burns), and losses in third space (trauma, pancreatitis). The commonest conditions that cause renal Na losses (urine Na >40 mmol/L) are thiazide diuretics, mineralocorticoid deficiency, cerebral salt wasting, and salt-wasting nephropathy.[3]

Four to eleven percent of patients on thiazide diuretics develop hyponatremia, and they are in some cases

| | Urinary Na <20 mmol/L | Urinary Na >40 mmol/L |
|---|---|---|
| Hypovolemic | Gastrointestinal (GI) losses | Diuretics |
| | Mucosal losses | Addison's disease |
| | Pancreatitis | Cerebral salt wasting |
| | Na depletion postdiuretics | Salt-wasting nephropathy |
| Euvolemic | Hypothyroidism | Syndrome of inappropriate antidiuretic hormone secretion (SIADH) |
| | SIADH with ongoing fluid restriction | ACTH deficiency |
| | Primary polydipsia | |
| | Inappropriate fluid replacement | |
| Hypervolemic | Cirrhosis | Cardiac failure or cirrhosis on diuretic therapy |
| | Cardiac failure | |
| | Nephrotic syndrome | |

*Source:* Adapted from Hannon MJ, Thompson CJ, *European Journal of Endocrinology/European Federation of Endocrine Societies*, 162, S5–12, 2010.

***Table 20.1***
*Causes of hyponatremia.*

hypovolemic and in other cases euvolemic. The three main factors implicated in thiazide-induced hyponatremia are increased water intake, reduced free water clearance, and renal $Na^+$ and $K^+$ loss. Thiazide diuretics impair diluting ability in several ways. Diuretics may reduce glomerular filtration rate and enhance reabsorption of Na and water in the proximal nephron, diminishing fluid delivery to the distal diluting sites. In some cases thiazide-induced volume depletion stimulates nonosmotic AVP release. In addition, thiazides may directly enhance water permeability and water reabsorption in the collecting duct.[41] Thiazide diuretics act by inhibiting reabsorption of Na and Cl from the distal convoluted tubule by blocking the thiazide-sensitive Na/Cl cotransporter; thus, they are electrolyte deficient in terms of Na and K.[41] Water retention caused by impaired water excretion combined with cation depletion may result in severe hyponatremia.

In primary adrenal insufficiency, hyponatremia is attributed to mineralocorticoid and glucocorticoid deficiency. Mineralocorticoid deficiency leads to renal salt wasting, extracellular fluid volume depletion, and reduction of cardiac output. Nonosmotic stimulation of AVP release through baroreceptors leads to hyponatremia.[42]

## *Euvolemic hyponatremia*

Euvolemic hyponatremia is usually due to SIADH, but other less common causes are inappropriate fluid replacement with hypotonic fluids, excessive water intake in primary polydipsia, glucocorticoid deficiency, and severe hypothyroidism.

Secondary adrenocortical insufficiency should always be considered in patients with hyponatremia in the context of traumatic brain injury (TBI) or subarachnoid hemorrhage (SAH). In the acute phase after SAH, 7%–14% develop ACTH deficiency, and acute adrenal insufficiency may account for up to 10% of cases of acute hyponatremia post-SAH.[43] Early morning cortisol (F) of <300 nmol/L in the context of the acutely ill patient with SAH is highly suggestive of acute adrenal insufficiency; early morning F levels of 300–500 nmol/L in combination with other features, such as hypoglycemia, hypotension, or slow clinical progression, raises the clinical suspicion of acute F deficiency and a trial of glucocorticoid therapy should be considered.[44] In the setting of acute TBI, 10%–16% develop acute ACTH deficiency, but this is rarely the cause of hyponatremia in this context.[44,45] A study of acutely ill patients with severe hyponatremia due to hypopituitarism with secondary adrenal insufficiency found that there were no subjects with ACTH deficiency who had basal plasma F >439 nmol/L.[46]

Hyponatremia in secondary adrenal insufficiency is attributed mainly to inappropriate secretion of AVP. F is a physiological tonic inhibitor of AVP secretion[46]; animal and human postmortem studies have shown that AVP expression in hypothalamic neurons is strongly suppressed by glucocorticoids.[47] A second factor is that patients with secondary adrenal insufficiency have reductions in cardiac output and mean arterial pressure that cause nonosmotic AVP release.[42,48] Also, release of AVP increases significantly the expression of AQP2 mRNA and protein in the kidney, but the AQP2 mRNA expression is more manifest in the kidney than that expected from the plasma AVP levels. The mechanisms underlying this exaggerated effect of AQP2 in the kidney are not well understood.[49] In addition, in glucocorticoid deficiency, there is upregulation of Na transporters in the proximal tubule that limit fluid delivery to the distal diluting segment of the kidney.[50]

The differences between hyponatremia due to primary and hyponatremia due to secondary adrenal insufficiency are shown in Table 20.2.[51]

In clinical practice, hyponatremia due to hypothyroidism occurs in the context of severe hypothyroidism and myxoedema. An important factor in the impaired ability to dilute urine is the nonosmotic release of AVP; hypothyroid subjects have inappropriately high circulating levels of AVP and they do not suppress their AVP levels following an oral water load.[42,52] Decreased heart rate and myocardial contractility contribute to reduced cardiac output that leads to nonosmotic release of AVP via carotid sinus baroreceptors.[53] Also, reduction in plasma renal flow and in glomerular filtration rate leads to diminished delivery of water to the distal diluting segment of the kidney; the greater the impairment in renal function, the more likely is the development of hyponatremia.[53] There is another mechanism of diminished fluid delivery to the distal part of the nephron; hypothyroidism causes marked upregulation of renal cortex AQP1 and thus increases proximal tubular reabsorption of water.[52] Overall, the predominant mechanism is the nonosmotic release of AVP and subsequent increase in expression of renal AQP2, but there are also reduced distal fluid delivery and several tubular defects.

## *SIADH*

SIADH is defined as the syndrome when AVP is not appropriately suppressed when sNa levels fall below the osmotic threshold for physiological AVP secretion.[40] SIADH is characterized by slight extracellular volume expansion that is not clinically detectable.

To diagnose a patient with SIADH, the patient should meet all the diagnostic criteria summarized in Table 20.3.[54,55]

SIADH is classified to four different types as shown in Figure 20.6.[56]

i. Type A is the commonest. It is characterized by erratic, excessive secretion of AVP and loss of linear relationship between plasma osmolality and AVP secretion. The wide fluctuations in AVP levels do not usually lead to large changes in urine osmolality because urine osmolality tends to be fixed at the highest possible level. It occurs in about 30%–40% of patients with SIADH and especially in patients with malignancy. This form is typically associated with small cell lung cancer and leads to more severe hyponatremia.
ii. Type B occurs in about 30% of patients and is characterized by a slow, constant "leak" of AVP at levels below normal osmotic threshold but a linear relationship between plasma osmolality and AVP secretion above osmotic threshold. The levels of urine osmolality tend to be fixed at a lower level

| | *Primary adrenal insufficiency* | *Secondary adrenal insufficiency* |
|---|---|---|
| Volume status | Hypovolemia | Euvolemia |
| Serum K | High or normal | Normal |
| Serum renin activity | High | Normal |
| Serum ACTH | High | Low |
| Serum urea | High or normal | Low or normal |
| Serum urate | High or normal | Low or normal |
| Fractional excretion (FE) urea | Low or normal | High or normal |
| FE urate | Low or normal | High or normal |

*Source:* Modified from Liamis G et al., *Annals of Medicine*, 43, 179–87, 2011.

***Table 20.2***
*Differential diagnosis of hyponatremia due to primary and secondary adrenal insufficiency.*

| |
|---|
| Essential diagnostic criteria for SIADH |
| • sNa <135 mmol/L |
| • Serum osmolality <275 mOsm/kg |
| • Urine osmolality >100 mOsm/kg |
| • Urine Na >40 mmol/L (provided the patient is not on salt restriction) |
| • Euvolemic |
| • Normal adrenal and thyroid function |
| • No use of diuretics within past week |
| Additional diagnostic criteria for SIADH |
| • Serum urate <0.24 mmol/L |
| • FENa >1% and FEurea >55% |
| • Failure to improve sNa by >5 mmol/L and increase of FENa by >0.5% after test infusion of 2 L of isotonic saline over 24 h |

*Source:* Adapted from Thompson C et al., *Best Practice & Research Clinical Endocrinology & Metabolism*, 26, S7–15, 2012; Ellison DH, Berl T, *The New England Journal of Medicine*, 356, 2064–72, 2007.

***Table 20.3***
*Essential and additional criteria for the diagnosis of hyponatremia due to SIADH.*

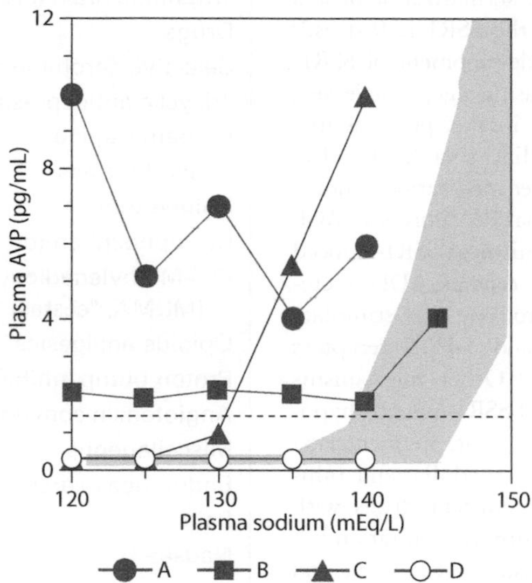


***Figure 20.6***
*Osmoregulation of AVP in patients with SIADH is depicted for types A, B, C, and D. (Adapted from Robertson GL,* The American Journal of Medicine, *119, S36–42, 2006.)*

than in type A. This pattern suggests damage to the posterior pituitary or to the inhibitory neurons of osmoregulation in the hypothalamus.

iii. Type C is well known as "reset osmostat" and occurs in about 30% of patients. The close linear relationship between plasma osmolality and AVP secretion is maintained, and the patient is able to fully suppress AVP production. Unlike types A and B, the urine osmolality varies markedly with changes in hydration and plasma Na levels. The abnormality lies at the osmotic threshold for AVP secretion that is lower than normal. This is due to downward resetting of the osmoregulatory system. These patients are protected against the progression to severe hyponatremia.

iv. Type D is a rare clinical phenomenon characterized by undetectable AVP levels. In some cases, it is the gain-of-function mutations of the AVP V2R that lead to constant activation of V2R.[40] Other potential causes are postreceptor defects in trafficking of the AQP2 water channels or secretion of an antidiuretic compound other than AVP.

The most common causes of SIADH are as follows: (1) malignancies, (2) pulmonary disorders, (3) disorders of central nervous system, (4) drugs, and (5) miscellaneous. The causes of SIADH that are frequently encountered in clinical practice are listed in Table 20.4.

Drug-induced hyponatremia is among the commonest and preventable causes of hyponatremia. SSRIs and serotonin and noradrenaline reuptake inhibitors (SNRIs) cause hyponatremia relatively frequent. Most patients develop hyponatremia within 30 days after the start of the SSRI, with a median time to onset of 13–21 days[57,58], and mean time to normalization of sNa concentration upon cessation of the SSRI is 9 days.[58] Recognized risk factors for the development of SSRI-induced hyponatremia are increasing age, female sex, low body weight, excessive fluid intake, previous history of hyponatremia, low baseline sNa levels <138 mmol/L, and treatment with other medications known to cause hyponatremia (e.g., thiazide diuretics, ACE inhibitors)[57–61]. The main mechanism of SSRI-induced hyponatremia is by increase of central ADH secretion; SSRIs increase levels of serotonin and stimulate 5-hydroxytryptophan (5-HT)1c and 5-HT2 receptors that activate ADH secretion.[62,63] Other mechanisms involved in the pathophysiology of SSRI-induced hyponatremia are a resetting of the osmostat, augmentation of the effect of ADH in the renal medulla, and inhibition of the metabolism of concomitant drugs with subsequent increase in their serum concentration.[57,64] Serum electrolytes should be measured at baseline and after 3–4 weeks in high-risk groups, such as the elderly (>65 years), and in subjects with low body weight and low baseline sNa.[65,66]

| |
|---|
| Malignancies |
| Small-cell-lung cancer |
| Mesothelioma |
| GI tract cancer (stomach, duodenum, pancreas) |
| Genitourinary tract cancer (ureter, bladder, prostate) |
| Lymphoma |
| Nasopharyngeal carcinoma |
| Pulmonary causes |
| Pneumonia |
| Tuberculosis |
| Lung abscess |
| Respiratory failure |
| Central nervous system disorders |
| Meningitis/encephalitis |
| SAH |
| Subdural hematoma |
| Cerebrovascular accident |
| Tumor |
| Abscess |
| Traumatic brain injury |
| Drugs |
| Selective serotonin reuptake inhibitors (SSRIs) |
| Tricyclic antidepressants |
| Carbamazepine |
| Phenothiazines |
| Haloperidol |
| Cyclophosphamide |
| (3,4-Methylenedioxy-*N*-methylamphetamine) (MDMA, "ecstasy") |
| Opioids analgesics |
| Proton pump inhibitors (PPIs) |
| Angiotensin convertase (ACE) inhibitors |
| Miscellaneous |
| Endurance exercise (postmarathon) |
| Pain |
| Nausea |

***Table 20.4***
*Causes of SIADH that are frequently encountered in clinical practice.*

Ecstasy (MDMA) has found widespread use in young adults. It has been associated with hyponatremia and can lead to coma and in some cases to death. A variety of factors are involved in the pathogenesis of ecstasy-associated hyponatremia and include advice to drink copious amounts of low-solute-content fluids to prevent dehydration, ecstasy-induced thirst, ecstasy-induced increased release of AVP that is mediated via ecstasy-induced release of serotonin,[67] increased sweat Na losses and ecstasy-related delay in gastrointestinal motility, which may lead to passive absorption of large amounts of water in the intestinal lumen.[68,69]

### Hypervolemic hyponatremia

Hypervolemic hyponatremia is characterized by expansion of extracellular volume with water retention exceeding Na retention.

The three commonest causes of hypervolemic hyponatremia are congestive cardiac failure, cirrhosis, and nephrotic syndrome. The main mechanism is nonosmotic release of AVP. Arterial baroreceptors sense arterial underfilling (either due to reduced cardiac output or due to arterial vasodilation) and activate the neurohumoral axis as a compensatory response to maintain arterial perfusion. The neurohumoral response has three components: baroreceptor-mediated AVP release to retain water, activation of the renin–angiotensin–aldosterone system to retain Na, and stimulation of the sympathetic nervous system to increase systemic and arterial vascular resistance.[42] The classical picture is that of renal Na retention with urine Na <20 mmol/L.

In hypervolemic hyponatremia due to renal failure, kidneys are not able to conserve Na with urine Na >40 mmol/L.

| | |
|---|---|
| Hypervolemia | Peripheral edema |
| | Ascites |
| | Raised jugular venous pressure |
| | Pulmonary edema |
| Euvolemia | Absence of clinical signs of volume |
| | Expansion/depletion |
| Hypovolemia | Dry mucous membranes |
| | Reduced skin turgor |
| | Invisible jugular venous pressure |
| | Reduction in systolic blood pressure by >20 mmHg after standing for 1 min |
| | Increase in heart rate by >20 beats/min or >10% after standing for 1 min |

**Table 20.5**
*Classification of volume status according to clinical signs.*

## Evaluation of patients with hyponatremia

The evaluation of the patient with hyponatremia should include medical history, detailed drug history, physical examination, and appropriate laboratory investigations.

### Clinical assessment

The first step in a patient with hyponatremia is the assessment of volume status. This is the key to the differential diagnosis and appropriate management of hyponatremia. Status should be assessed by clinical parameters, such as jugular venous pressure, skin turgor, mucous membranes, postural changes in blood pressure, and heart rate. Common clinical signs that facilitate the accurate classification of volume status are as shown in Table 20.5.

In clinical practice, it can be very difficult to differentiate between euvolemia and mild volume depletion. Even in the context of a clinical study, the clinical evaluation for diagnosing hypovolemia has been found to have sensitivity as low as 41% and specificity of 80%.[70] The clinical prediction of extracellular fluid volume status is unsatisfactory, and physicians should take into account the limitations of physical examination of hyponatremic patients.

### Laboratory evaluation

The second step is laboratory evaluation. Laboratory tests that should be performed in patients with hyponatremia are listed in the following sections.

#### *Serum osmolality*

First, it is necessary to determine whether the patient has hypotonic or nonhypotonic hyponatremia. Hypo-osmolar state is defined as serum osmolality <280 mOsm/kg.

In most cases, hyponatremia reflects a state of hypotonicity. But normotonic or even hypertonic hyponatremia occurs in the context of pseudohyponatremia or translocational hyponatremia.

Pseudohyponatremia is classically seen in the context of marked hyperlipidemia or hypertriglyceridemia or paraproteinemia. In these cases, serum osmolality remains normal at >280 mOsm/kg.

Translocational hyponatremia occurs in the presence of osmotically active substances (high glucose levels or patients during a mannitol infusion). An increase in serum osmolality leads to movement of water from the cells to the extracellular fluid and subsequently a decrease in serum Na levels by dilution. Acute hyperglycemia decreases the sNa concentration due to an immediate extracellular shift of water because glucose is restricted to the extracellular space. Thus, patients with severe hyperglycemia have hypertonic hyponatremia. It has been proposed that sNa should be corrected for hyperglycemia by adding 1.6 mmol/L for every 5.6 mmol/L increase of glucose levels above the normal range.[71] Experimental studies have shown that the degree of hyponatremia varies among individuals with acute hyperglycemia and becomes more pronounced with marked hyperglycemia. A correction factor of adding 2.4 mmol/L in the Na concentration for every 5.6 mmol/L increase in glucose concentration is more accurate than the 1.6 correction factor that was derived from theoretical predictions. Because of the curvilinear association between glucose levels and Na levels, the 2.4 correction factor performs very well especially in the clinically important ranges of serum glucose >24.4 mmol/L.[72]

### *Urine osmolality*

In the patient with hypotonic hyponatremia, the ability of the kidneys to dilute urine needs to be assessed. Urine osmolality (U-Osm) <100 mOsm/kg suggests normal water excretion as appropriate response to hypotonic hyponatremia. ADH production is fully and appropriately suppressed, resulting in a maximally dilute urine. This occurs in primary polydipsia and sometimes in reset osmostat syndrome.

A urine osmolality >100 mOsm/kg suggests an inappropriate response to hypotonic hyponatremia. The patient has an impaired ability to excrete water and is unable to maximally dilute urine. This occurs in conditions with impairment of water excretion (SIADH, hypervolemic and hypovolemic hyponatremia).

Urine-specific gravity (U-SG) is often used in clinical practice as a bedside tool to estimate urine osmolality. Three methods for measuring U-SG are currently available: refractometry, hydrometry, and cation exchange on a reagent strip. The U-SG indicates the number and weight of solute particles in urine, whereas the U-Osm is determined only by the number of particles in the solution.

At urine pH of 7.0 and with a U-SG of 1.010, we can predict a U-Osm of approximately 320 mOsm/kg $H_2O$ using either method. For an increase in SG of 0.01, the predicted osmolality increases by about 181 or 203 mOsm/kg $H_2O$ based on whether the U-SG is measured by reagent strip or by refractometry, respectively.[73] The relationship between U-SG and U-Osm is illustrated in Figure 20.7.[74]

Variations in pH, glucose, protein, hemoglobin, bilirubin, ketones, and urobilinogen affect the linear correlation between U-SG and U-Osm significantly, hence it is difficult to predict the osmolality with any degree of certainty in the presence of these factors. The relationship between U-SG and U-Osm is affected by pH when U-SG is measured using reagent strip but not to the same extent when it is measured using refractometry.[73]

U-SG can be used reliably at the bedside as a good estimate of urine osmolality in clean urine samples and can facilitate the close monitoring of patients with hyponatremia and their response to treatment. In pathological urine samples, U-SG gives unreliable estimate of urine osmolality.

### *Urine Na*

With hypotonic hyponatremia and an impaired ability to dilute urine, the effective arterial blood volume as well as the renal Na losses need to be assessed.

In terms of differentiating between hypovolemic and euvolemic state, a Na <20 mmol/L in a spot urine sample usually suggests volume depletion (provided there is no

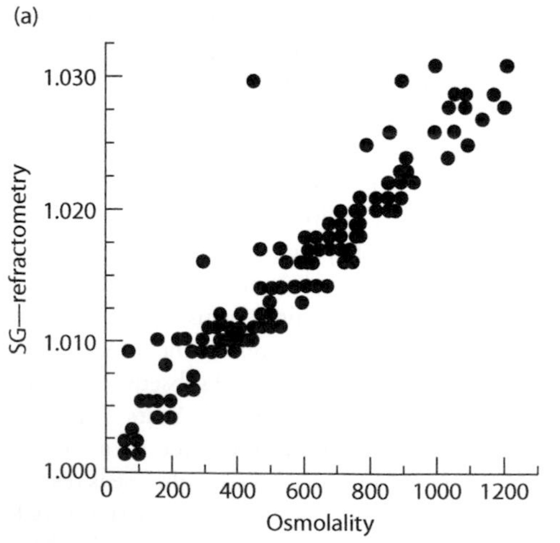


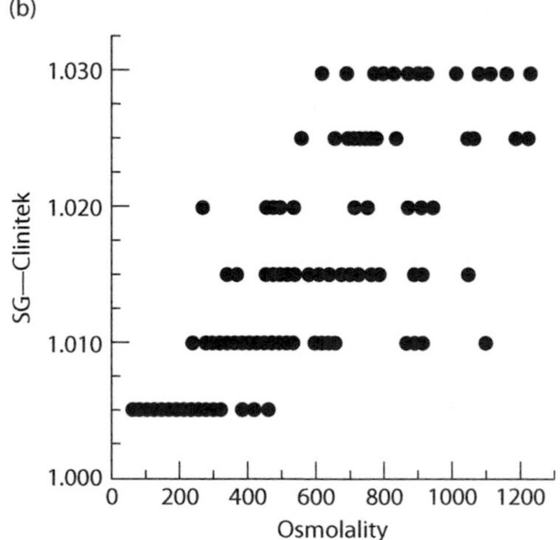


***Figure 20.7***
*Relationship between U-Osm (urine osmolality) measured in mOsm/kg and U-SG (urine specific gravity) measured with a refractometer (a) as well as U-SGmeasured with an automatic readout of the Bayer dipstick (b). (Adapted from de Buys Roessingh AS et al.,* Archives of Disease in Childhood, *85, 155–7, 2001.)*

renal salt wasting), but elderly patients can have urine Na values as high as 50–60 mmol/L because of reduced renal conservation of Na in response to a reduced effective blood volume. A urine Na >40 mmol/L suggests a euvolemic state, but euvolemic patients with very low solute intake or salt depletion can have much lower urine Na values.[75] An equivocal urine Na of 20–40 mmol/L is not useful in terms of determining volume status.

In the hyponatremic patient, urine Na measurement can identify the origin of Na losses (extrarenal losses if Na is <20 mmol/L and renal losses if urine is Na >40 mmol/L).[54]

### *Serum urea, creatinine, and uric acid*

Serum urea and the urea:creatinine ratio are of some value in discriminating between hypovolemia and euvolemia, especially when creatinine is normal. Urea levels tend to rise in volume depletion and be low in euvolemic state. Serum urea and urea:creatinine ratio tend to rise with age, and there is a significant overlap in values between SIADH and hypovolemic hyponatremia, which limits their utility. It has been shown that older subjects have a more important decrease in urea clearance (by 56%) than in urea production (by 27%), leading to an increase in plasma urea of 29%. Patients <40 years old with SIADH present with higher mean FEurea (58% ± 14%) compared with patients >70 years old with SIADH (mean FEurea 44% ± 15%).[76]

Serum uric acid levels are of great value in differentiating between euvolemia and volume depletion. A serum uric acid <0.24 mmol/L has a positive predictive value of 73%–100% for SIADH, whereas uric acid >0.32 mmol/L is strongly suggestive of volume depletion. Reduced serum urate levels results from water retention, volume expansion, and associated decrease in proximal Na reabsorption that indirectly reduces urate reabsorption, which is located mainly in the proximal tubule.[77,78]

### *Serum F and thyroid function tests*

The possibility of adrenal insufficiency (primary or secondary) should be excluded. If a morning or random F is not unequivocally normal, dynamic assessment of glucocorticoid reserve is strongly recommended, usually in the form of a short corticotrophin (Synacthen 250 mg IM) test.[79] TSH and free T4 are recommended to check thyroid function.

### *Fractional excretion of sodium (FENa), urea (FEurea), potassium (FEk), and urate (FEurate)*

Fractional excretion of FENa, FEurea, FEk, and FEurate are calculated as shown below

FENa = (Una × Pcrea) × 100/(Pna × Ucrea)
FEurea = (Uurea × Pcrea) × 100/(Purea × Ucrea)
FEk = (UK × Pcrea) × 100/(PK × Ucrea)
FEurate = (Uurate × Pcrea) × 100/(Purate × Ucrea)

In view of the multiple parameters that affect urine Na, the combination of several clearance ratios can be an adjunctive tool. FENa is a more reliable parameter for natriuresis than is urine Na and an FENa >1% suggests SIADH or diuretic use. It has been shown that the combination of low FENa <0.5% and low FEurea <55% is the best biochemical way to identify hypovolemic individuals who respond to isotonic saline infusion.[70,80]

In patients on diuretics, the differential diagnosis of hyponatremia can pose major challenges. Diuretics inhibit tubular Na reabsorption and increase urinary Na excretion; as a result, urine Na and FENa are usually high. Urine Na and FENa have limited diagnostic utility in differentiating a diuretic effect from SIADH.[70] An FEurate value of >12% has a positive predictive value of 100% in diagnosing SIADH in patients on diuretics, whereas FEurate <8% excludes SIADH.[81] The reason that FEurate has high diagnostic accuracy in patients on diuretics is that diuretic therapy does not affect the transport mechanisms of urate, localized exclusively in the proximal tubule.

FEK could be of value in detecting diuretic use in patients whose home treatment is unknown or who deny diuretic use. Patients on diuretics have FEK values >17%.[70]

### *Serum copeptin*

Recent studies have shown that the measurement of plasma copeptin has diagnostic utility in the differential diagnosis of hyponatremia. Copeptin is derived from the same precursor peptide as AVP and is released in equimolar amounts together with AVP. Plasma AVP measurement is not part of the diagnostic evaluation of hyponatremia because of preanalytical and analytical problems as well as lack of reliable assays. Copeptin has been shown to be a reliable surrogate marker of AVP secretion.[82]

There are two potential roles of plasma copeptin in the differential diagnosis of hyponatremia. First, suppressed levels of copeptin can reliably distinguish patients with primary polydipsia in contrast to other causes of hyponatremia where copeptin is elevated. Second, the copeptin to urine Na ratio has been shown to be superior to the established criteria in discriminating volume depleted from normovolemic hyponatremic patients. Copeptin/urine Na × 100 <30 pmol/mmol has 85% sensitivity and 87% specificity in identifying normovolemic patients with hyponatremia.[82]

*Diagnostic trial of isotonic saline*

In a large number of cases, there is uncertainty about the volume status of the patient. In these cases, a trial of isotonic fluids infusion (2 L of 0.9% saline over 24 h) is strongly recommended because it can be a very useful diagnostic and therapeutic tool.

It has been shown that a test infusion with isotonic saline in patients with SIADH rarely causes significant sNa reduction, despite the fact that urinary osmolality usually exceeds administered fluid osmolality. It is rarely hazardous, so long as urine osmolality is <538 mOsm/kg $H_2O$ and urine Na + K is below Na concentration of the infused isotonic saline (154 mmol/L). The safety of a trial of isotonic saline in SIADH is attributed to the incapacity of the kidney to use only electrolytes to elaborate a given urinary osmolality.[83]

Increase in sNa by at least 5 mmol/L usually suggests hypovolemic state, whereas increase of sNa by <5 mmol/L indicates euvolemia. Studies have shown that this cutoff can be misleading in up to 30% of cases, however, either because some patients with SIADH and serum osmolality <300 mOsm/kg respond very well to isotonic saline or because some hypovolemic patients with severe salt depletion do not respond well.[78] In terms of using FENa criteria, an increase of FENa by <0.5% suggests hypovolemia, whereas an increase of FENa by >0.5% suggests euvolemia. It is proposed that the isotonic saline infusion test only allows a reliable classification of hyponatremia, as far as both these sNa and FENa criteria are taken into account.

### Radiological investigations

Patients with SIADH should be investigated further to identify the underlying cause. Common radiological investigations include chest X-ray (to identify pulmonary causes), computed tomography (CT) or magnetic resonance imaging (MRI) of the brain to identify central nervous system (CNS) causes, and CT imaging of lungs and abdomen to identify possible malignancy. Positron emission tomography (PET)/CT may represent the most sensitive means of detecting a neoplasm.

## Management

Appropriate management requires prompt and appropriate diagnosis of the type and cause of hyponatremia, identification of the cause, and treatment of the underlying disease being of paramount importance.

The desired rate of correction of hyponatremia needs to be taken into account when considering management options for hyponatremia. In acute hyponatremia (onset <48 h), patients may present with alarming neurological findings because of cerebral edema. In these cases, rapid correction of sNa is necessary.[84] In chronic hyponatremia (onset >48 h), rapid correction of sNa may cause osmotic demyelination syndrome (OMS). This is a syndrome when patients develop myelinolysis most often in the pons with associated quadriparesis, pseudobulbar palsy, and locked-in syndrome (central pontine myelinolysis) but they also sometimes develop myelinonysis in other areas such as the thalamus, internal capsule, deep cerebral cortex, and cerebellum (extrapontine myelinolysis).[85] OMS can be avoided by limiting correction of chronic hyponatremia to <10–12 mmol/L in 24 h and <18 mmol/L in 48 h. Patients with malnutrition, alcoholism, or advanced liver disease may be especially susceptible to OMS, and in these patients the correction of sNa should be <8 mmol/L in 24 h.[86]

### Diagnosis of hypovolemic hyponatremia

Accurate diagnosis of hypovolemic hyponatremia, particularly when subtle, is essential and pivotal to correct management. As stated, it can be extremely difficult to differentiate it from euvolemia. Treatment is by correction of volume deficit with isotonic (0.9%) saline; the relative water excess will correct itself.

In addition, all diuretics should be withheld. In cases of confirmed or suspected mineralocorticoid deficiency, corticosteroids should be administered urgently.

### Management of euvolemic hyponatremia

In euvolemic hyponatremia, the currently available therapeutic options are hypertonic saline, fluid restriction, demeclocycline, and AVP-receptor antagonists. The most important determinant guiding therapy is whether the patient has severe neurological symptoms or not.

In patients with hyponatremia-related severe neurological presentations such as seizures or reduced consciousness level, rapid correction is needed. The only way to accomplish this promptly is with a hypertonic (3%) saline infusion, although overcorrection must be avoided if additional neurological sequelae are to be avoided. The patient should be monitored closely by a clinician with expertise in fluid disorders in a high dependency/intensive care unit (ICU) setting (with sNa monitoring every 2 h). The recommended starting dose is a low rate infusion of 0.5–2.0 mL/kg/h with titration according to sNa levels every 2 h.[87] It is necessary and appropriate to correct acutely to safe levels rather than to normal levels.[86]

In cases without severe neurological manifestations, fluid restriction has been the mainstay of treatment for hyponatremia due to SIADH. The principal disadvantage is that a significant proportion of patients find it very difficult to comply with fluid restriction due to thirst. Fluid restriction of 500–1200 mL/day is recommended according to the severity of hyponatremia, urine output, and urine electrolytes. The second drawback of this approach is that it usually takes several days to lead to significant increase in sNa levels.

An alternative treatment option is demeclocycline. Demeclocycline inhibits the action of vasopressin on the distal collecting tubule of the kidney and causes nephrogenic diabetes insipidus in most patients. The disadvantages of demeclocycline are (1) it is not effective in some patients and the response of each individual is unpredictable, (2) the onset of action is variable and usually longer than 3 days, and (3) it can cause profound polyuria and associated kidney injury.[86]

AVP-receptor antagonists were recently introduced in clinical practice. Tolvaptan, the only drug of this class currently licensed in Europe, is an oral, selective, nonpeptide antagonist that blocks AVP binding to V2Rs and activation of receptors at the renal collecting tubules. The result is water excretion without changing the total electrolyte excretion ("aquaresis"). Tolvaptan has been shown to be effective in raising and maintaining sNa in patients with hypervolemic and euvolemic hyponatremia.[88] The cost of vaptans has limited its clinical use in many centers. The possibility of overrapid correction of hyponatremia has also been of concern, but no cases of osmotic demyelination have been reported hitherto. The drug should be started in a hospital setting due to the need for dose titration and close monitoring of sNa and volume status. The starting dose is 15 mg once daily, increasing to a maximum of 60 mg daily as tolerated to achieve the desired Na concentration. Patients who do not perceive thirst should not be treated with this agent, and patients on treatment should have access to water. Monitoring of Na should take place within 4–6 h of administration, and overcorrection diagnosed if the Na rises by more than 6 mmol/L in the first 6 h or 8 mmol/L in the first 6–12 h. Infusion of a hypotonic solution may be necessary in such patients, and the dosage reduced or the drug stopped. The drug is metabolized by the CYP3A4 pathway, and clinicians should be aware of coadministration of drugs that are metabolized by this pathway. Overall, it remains to be seen whether AVP-receptor antagonists will become the mainstay of treatment of SIADH instead of fluid restriction.

Ongoing research is needed to assess the effect of treatment of hyponatremia on mortality, length of hospital stay, and patient's quality of life. Studies on the efficacy and safety of vaptans versus fluid restriction would be helpful in terms of defining the role of vaptans in the treatment of hyponatremia due to SIADH.[89]

### Urine osmolality and urine: Plasma electrolyte ratios

Urine osmolality as well as urine plasma/electrolyte ratio (U/P ratio) can inform treatment decisions. In cases of high urine osmolality >600 mOsm/kg $H_2O$, water restriction should be severe, and these patients are most likely to benefit from use of vaptans. Patients with relatively low and fixed urine osmolality at 300–400 mOsm/kg $H_2O$ can be managed effectively by less severe water restriction.[78]

Another recommended approach is to use the simplified U/P ratio as defined by the sum of urine Na and urine K concentration from a spot collection divided by the plasma Na (U/P ratio = UNa + UK/PNa).

If this ratio is <0.5, 1000 mL fluid restriction is recommended. If the ratio is 0.5–1.0, 500 mL fluid restriction is recommended. If the ratio is >1.0, then no electrolyte-free water is excreted, and theoretically patient should minimize fluid intake to 0 mL. This approach could guide the recommended volume of fluid restriction and predict the response of the patient.[90] This formula could also predict patients likely to be refractory to fluid restriction who would most benefit from vasopressin receptor antagonists (U/P ratio >1.0).[84]

### Management of hypervolemic hyponatremia

In hypervolemic hyponatremia, the mainstays of treatment are Na restriction and diuretics. Loop diuretics (furosemide, bumetanide) are primarily used with the addition of K-sparing diuretics (spironolactone) as treatment for secondary hyperaldosteronism, especially in patients with cirrhosis.

## Hypernatremia

Hypernatremia is defined as an sNa concentration exceeding 145 mmol/L and is a common electrolyte disorder. Hypernatremia is always associated with hyperosmolality and represents a state of relative excess of Na to water in the extracellular fluid.

## Epidemiology

The incidence of hypernatremia in hospitalized patients is 1%–2%.[91,92] Hypernatremia usually occurs in infants, the elderly, patients with altered mental status, and intubated patients because they have impaired thirst or limited access to water.[93]

Hypernatremia that precedes hospitalization is mainly a geriatric disease and often occurs in patients living in nursing homes. Hospital-acquired hypernatremia is not a geriatric disease because these patients have a mean age of 59 years.[92] Hospital-acquired hypernatremia has been regarded as an indicator of quality of care and results usually from inadequate provision of electrolyte-free water combined with an inability to increase oral water intake in response to hypertonicity. These patients have impaired mental status and impaired thirst perception or are unable to regulate their water intake because they are intubated. In addition, they have increased free-water losses due to their impaired renal concentrating capacity as well as increased enteral or insensible losses.[92]

Hypernatremia is a common electrolyte disorder in critically ill patients in ICUs. Two percent of patients are hypernatremic on admission to the ICU and 7% develop hypernatremia during the ICU stay.[94]

Patients with sNa levels >150 mmol/L have a high inpatient mortality rate of 37%–48%.[92,94–96] Traditionally, hypernatremia has been proposed as a marker of the severity of the underlying disease. The increased mortality has been attributed to the severity of the underlying disease, but several retrospective studies have shown an independent effect of hypernatremia on mortality. Causal relationship has not been proved, but the adverse effects of hypernatremia on various physiological functions may contribute to excess mortality.[97] Overall, it is difficult to separate the effect of hypernatremia from the effect of the underlying disease, but the strong association of hypernatremia with excess mortality is likely to be a combination of the effects of the underlying disease and the harmful consequences of hypernatremia *per se*.[98]

## Clinical presentation

The severity of symptoms of hypernatremia depends on the value of sNa and the rapidity of onset of hypernatremia. Patients with hypernatremia present with neurological symptoms and signs that include lethargy, irritability, restlessness, muscle weakness, seizures, and coma. Hypernatremia and therefore hyperosmolality lead to a shift of free water from the intracellular to the extracellular space. This shift leads to brain cell shrinkage that can result in vascular rupture and permanent neurological deficit in severe cases.[99]

Hypernatremia has also effects on other physiological functions. Hyperosmolality disturbs insulin-mediated glucose use and potentially contributes to the development of hyperglycemia. Also, hypernatremia has a negative effect on left ventricular contractility.[97]

## Causes

Hypernatremia is always associated with hyperosmolar state. Thirst is the major defense mechanism against

| |
|---|
| Pure water loss |
| Unreplaced insensible losses due to adipsia or limited access to water |
| Diabetes insipidus (cranial or nephrogenic) |
| Hypotonic fluid losses |
| Cutaneous losses (burns, excessive sweating) |
| GI losses (viral gastroenteritis, osmotic diarrhea, vomiting) |
| Renal losses (loop diuretics, osmotic diuresis, postobstructive diuresis, polyuric phase of acute tubular necrosis) |
| Na gain |
| Fluid infusion (Na bicarbonate, feeding, replacement of insensible losses with isotonic saline) |
| Na-rich enemas, emetics, intrauterine injection, dialysis |
| Ingestion of salt, sea water, baking soda, salt tablets |
| Primary hyperaldosteronism |
| Cushing's syndrome |
| Transient shift of water |
| After rigorous exercise or prolonged seizures |

**Table 20.6**
*Causes of hypernatremia.*

development of hypernatremia. A rise in serum osmolality leads to severe thirst and secretion of ADH and therefore increases water intake and reduces water loss.

Hypernatremia represents a water deficit in relation to the Na stores. The pathophysiology of hypernatremia includes water loss—pure water loss or hypotonic fluids loss—or Na gain or both or in rare cases transient shift of water to intracellular compartment. The causes of hypernatremia are classified in Table 20.6.

### *Pure water loss*

Inadequate intake of water is the commonest cause of hypernatremia. This applies to infants, the elderly, and patients with reduced consciousness level who cannot replace their insensible losses through skin and respiration.

Another cause of pure water deficit is adipsia, or impaired thirst. Patients with hypothalamic disease (e.g., tumors, radiotherapy, sarcoidosis) can have a defect in their hypothalamic osmoreceptors and associated hypodipsia or adipsia.

Diabetes insipidus causes impaired ability to concentrate urine, and as a result, polyuria with dilute urine. Central diabetes insipidus is characterized by reduced ADH secretion and nephrogenic diabetes insipidus by resistance of collecting tubules of the kidneys to the action of ADH. Patient with diabetes insipidus do not develop hypernatremia as long as they are able to maintain fluid intake adequate to compensate for the water loss.[99]

### *Hypotonic fluid losses*

Cutaneous causes of hypotonic fluid losses are burns and excessive sweating. Commonest causes of GI losses are forms of diarrhea when diarrheal fluid is hypotonic compared with serum. This applies mainly to viral and bacterial gastroenteritis and osmotic diarrhea related to lactulose use.

Renal losses of hypotonic fluids are mainly osmotic diuresis (due to hyperglycemia, uremia, or mannitol administration) and loop diuretics. Also, patients with renal insufficiency can have impaired concentrating ability of the kidney.

### *Na gain*

Na gain is rarely the only cause of hypernatremia. The commonest causes are iatrogenic due to administration of hypertonic fluids (Na bicarbonate or feeding preparations) or due to replacement of insensible losses with isotonic fluids or due to intrauterine installation of hypertonic saline for the termination of pregnancy or due to use of high Na dialysate in dialysis or due to administration of Na-rich antimicrobials (fosfomycin, voriconazole).[97] In infants, accidental or nonaccidental salt poisoning (1 teaspoon of salt) can cause very severe hypernatremia with serum Na >180 mmol/L.

Patients with primary hyperaldosteronism commonly have chronic, mild hypernatremia with sNa concentrations <150 mmol/L. Their hypernatremia is corrected by either medical or surgical treatment of the hyperaldosteronism. In comparison with normal subjects, secretion of ADH is not induced in these patients until higher than normal levels of plasma osmolality were reached (290.8 ± 1.3 vs. 284.2 ± 0.9 mOsm/kg). Thus, in patients with primary hyperaldosteronism, in comparison with normal subjects, the threshold at which ADH is secreted is shifted to the right, but the slope of the line comparing ADH levels and plasma osmolality is similar as shown in Figure 20.8.[100,101] This phenomenon has been described as adjustment of the osmostat to the right of normal and has rarely been noted in conditions other than primary hyperaldosteronism. The mechanisms behind this phenomenon have not been clearly explained; the sustained volume expansion in patients with primary hyperaldosteronism may diminish receptor sensitivity or mineralocorticoids, and hypokalemia may affect the osmostat.[101]

A rare endocrine cause of mild hypernatremia is Cushing's syndrome, especially due to ectopic ACTH release. In this context, high F secretion exceeds the metabolic capacity of 11β-hydroxysteroid-dehydrogenase (11-βHSD2) or very high circulating levels of ACTH inhibit 11-βHSD2. As a result, inhibition of conversion of F to inactive cortisone (E) allows access of excess F to the renal tubular mineralocorticoid receptor (MR). This induced excess mineralocorticoid state can cause hypernatremia through a similar mechanism with primary hyperaldosteronism.[102]

### *Combination of water loss and Na gain*

This combination has been reported in a large proportion of hypernatremic patients in the ICU setting. Common abnormalities in these critically ill patients are hypokalemia, hypercalcemia, and renal damage that affect the concentrating ability of the kidney as well as hyperglycemia and uremia that cause osmotic diuresis. Apart from negative water balance, these patients often have positive Na balance due to fluid resuscitation with 0.9% saline and use of Na bicarbonate.[97]

### *Transient shift of water*

Rigorous exercise or seizures can cause transient hypernatremia for 10–15 min. Degradation of glycogen to smaller active molecules such as lactate increases intracellular osmolality, causing shift of water from the extracellular to the intracellular compartment.

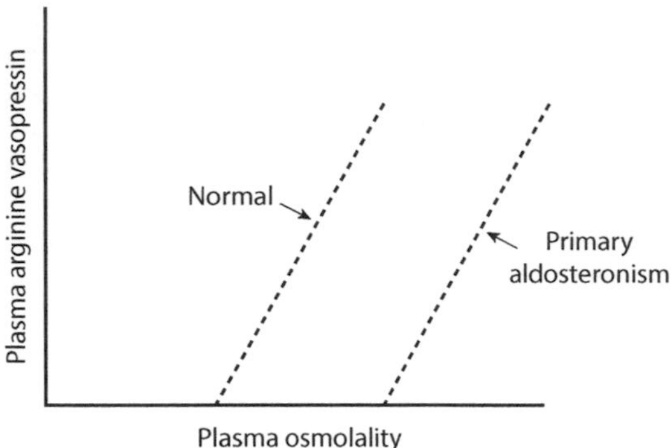


***Figure 20.8***
*Diagram showing shift of osmostat to the right of normal in patients with primary hyperaldosteronism. (Adapted from Gregoire JR,* Mayo Clinic Proceedings, *69, 1108–10, 1994.)*

# *Evaluation of patient*

Evaluation of the patient with hypernatremia includes taking a medical history, clinical examination, and appropriate investigations.

The aim is first to classify the patient according to the total body Na (TBNa) into low TBNa or normal TBNa or high TBNa and then to identify the exact causes.[103] The cause is often evident from the history. Clinical assessment of volume status is of paramount importance to determine whether the patient is hypovolemic. Measurement of fluid input and output is essential to guide the treatment of hypernatremia. Recommended laboratory tests in all patients are serum Na, K, urea, creatinine, osmolality, glucose, and calcium (Ca).

In cases, where the etiology of hypernatremia is unclear, measurement of urine osmolality and Na can be of great value. In patients with low TBNa (e.g., due to renal or GI hypotonic fluid losses), there will be clinical signs of hypovolemia, urine Na will be low (<20 mmol/L) if the patient is not on diuretics, and urine osmolality will be appropriately high (>800 mOsm/kg $H_2O$). In patients with normal TBNa (e.g., due to pure water loss in diabetes insipidus or in unreplaced insensible losses), there will be no clinical signs of volume contraction and urine Na will vary according to the Na intake. Urine osmolality will not be appropriately elevated in the context of diabetes insipidus (<300 mOsm/kg $H_2O$ in complete diabetes insipidus and 300–600 mOsm/kg $H_2O$ in partial diabetes insipidus) or will be appropriately elevated in the cases of unreplaced insensible losses. In patients with increased TBNa (e.g., after hypertonic solutions or salt tablets), urine Na will be high (typically >100 mmol/L) with elevated urine osmolality.[103]

There are some additional diagnostic tools to distinguish euvolemic from hypovolemic patients and guide treatment. In patients not receiving diuretics, FENa <0.5% strongly suggests extracellular volume depletion. In patients receiving diuretics that make the interpretation of urine biochemical parameters unreliable, the ratio of serum urea to serum creatinine has been proposed as a tool to discriminate hypovolemic from euvolemic hypernatremia. A value of urea (measured in mg/dL; 1 μmol/L = 2.8 mg/dL)/creatinine (measured in mg/dL; 1 μmol/L = 0.01 mg/dL) ratio >57 has been shown to differentiate hypovolemic subjects from euvolemic with a sensitivity of 96.5% and specificity of 100%.[95] This ratio has limitations in situations such as acute hemorrhage, sever liver damage, and catabolic states.

# *Management*

Adequate treatment of hypernatremia requires managing the underlying cause and correcting sNa levels. In terms of addressing the cause, measures such as control of hyperglycemia, withholding diuretics or lactulose, correcting hypercalcemia or hypokalemia, and discontinuation of hypertonic fluids should first be undertaken.[93]

Two important factors need to be considered in the management of hypernatremia: the volume status and the rapidity of onset of hypernatremia. Accurate assessment of the volume status is crucial. In cases of symptomatic hypovolemia, resuscitation with isotonic fluids is the first step of action to restore the effective vascular volume and the adequate perfusion of vital organs. In a second stage and after the patient is cardiovascularly stable, 5% dextrose is recommended to correct the water deficit. Euvolemic patients should be treated by administration of free water in the form of a 5% dextrose solution. In the rare context of hypervolemic patients due to Na gain, they should be treated with loop diuretics to induce natriuresis, and subsequent fluid losses should be replaced with fluids hypotonic to their urine.[97]

With respect to the rapidity of onset, hypernatremia should be differentiated into acute (onset within last 48 h) and chronic (onset >48 h). In cases where hypernatremia has developed within hours (e.g., iatrogenic due to hypertonic infusion) and no compensatory mechanisms have begun, Na levels should be corrected at a rate of 1 mmol/L/h. In cases of chronic hypernatremia, the maximal rate of correction of sNa levels should be 0.5 mmol/L/h.[99] Studies of different rates of correction of hypernatremia in children have shown that the maximum safe rate of correction of sNa is 10–12 mmol/L/24 h to prevent the risk of cerebral edema and seizures.[104–110]

# Physiology of K balance

K is the most abundant cation in the body. Under normal circumstances, 98% of the total body K is located in the ICF and only 2% in the ECF of an adult. The ratio between intracellular and extracellular K is the major determinant of the resting membrane potential and is regulated primarily by the $Na^+,K^+$-ATPase pump located on the plasma membrane of most cells.[111] Intracellular K takes part in multiple vital functions, including regulation of cell volume, acid–base balance, protein synthesis, enzymatic function, and cell growth.[112]

Serum K levels are tightly regulated within the narrow range of 3.5–5.0 mmol/L. The daily intake of K is on average 60–100 mmol. Under normal circumstances, K excretion equals daily intake. 90%–95% of K is excreted by the kidneys and only 5%–10% is excreted through the GI tract (Figure 20.9).[112]

## Acute regulation

The acute regulation of K homeostasis takes place through cellular shifts of K. Dietary K is absorbed by the bowel, enters the ECF, and is rapidly distributed to the ICF. This rapid movement of K from the ECF to the ICF is necessary because it prevents rapid postprandial increases in serum K. The two main hormones that maintain the high ratio of intracellular to extracellular K are insulin and catecholamines. Both insulin and catecholamines increase cellular K uptake by stimulating cell membrane $Na^+,K^+$-ATPase.[113] Postprandial insulin release stimulates $Na^+,K^+$-ATPase activity, mainly through translocation of $Na^+,K^+$-ATPase from intracellular stores to the cell surface and as a result promotes intracellular shift of K, most importantly in the skeletal muscle. Also, insulin stimulates $Na^+,K^+$-ATPase activity indirectly through stimulation of $Na^+/H^+$ exchanger activity. For insulin, there is a feedback system in which hyperkalemia stimulates insulin secretion and hypokalemia inhibits insulin secretion.[113] Catecholamines activate β2-adrenergic receptors to increase K cellular uptake and activate α1-adrenergic receptors to decrease K cellular uptake by directly affecting $Na^+$, $K^+$-ATPase activity in muscle and liver.[112,114]

In addition, thyroid hormones and aldosterone contribute to the transcellular distribution of K. Aldosterone increases $Na^+$, $K^+$-ATPase activity and

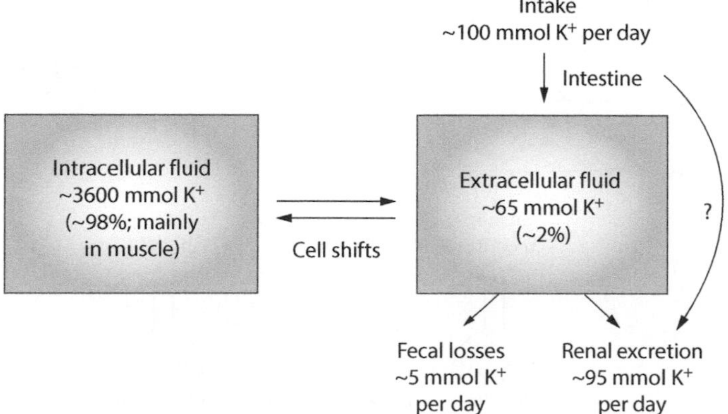


***Figure 20.9***
*Distribution of $K^+$ in the body. The pool of $K^+$ in the ECF is determined by input from the GI system and output in urine and stools, as well as the distribution between the ECF and the ICF compartments. (Adapted from Unwin RJ et al.,* Nature Reviews Nephrology, *7, 75–84, 2011.)*

promotes K influx to the cells as a result of enhanced Na entry through $Na^+/H^+$ transporters. Thyroid hormones stimulate synthesis of $Na^+$, $K^+$-ATPase, thus thyrotoxicosis can lead to hypokalemia.[113] Sudden increases in osmolality can promote K efflux from the cells to the ECF, resulting in a rise in serum K levels. Finally, the acid–base status of the plasma has a significant impact on transcellular shifts of K through multiple ion transport pathways, such as $Na^+$-$H^+$, $Na^+$, $K^+$-ATPase, and $Cl^-$-$HCO_3$.[115] The mechanisms of K shift between ICF and ECF are illustrated in Figure 20.10.[112]

## *Chronic regulation*

The kidneys are the regulators of the long-term K homeostasis. Under normal circumstances, most filtered K is reabsorbed by the proximal convoluted tubule and the loop of Henle, and only about 10% of filtered K arrives at the distal convoluted tubule. Control over the amount of K excreted in the urine resides mainly in the connecting tubule and cortical collecting duct. Connecting tubule cells and principal cells of the cortical collecting duct secrete K, while A-type intercalated cells of the collecting duct can reabsorb K.[116] Under normal circumstances, the amount of K secreted by the connecting tubule and principal cells of the collecting duct determines the amount of K excreted in the urine.[112] Renal K secretion depends mainly on aldosterone action and the urine flow rate.

The mechanism of K secretion by principal cells, as illustrated in Figure 20.11,[117] is that Na is reabsorbed through amiloride-sensitive epithelial Na channels (ENaCs) in the apical membrane of the principal cells; Na entry depolarizes the apical membrane, and this negative charge in the lumen promotes K secretion through various channels, mainly low-conductance renal outer medullary K (ROMK) channels. Aldosterone has a very important role; it stimulates K secretion by increasing activity of ENaCs.[118]

$K^+$ is taken up into cells across the basolateral membrane via $Na^+$, $K^+$-ATPases. $Na^+$ reabsorption via ENaCs depolarizes the apical membrane potential and provides the driving force for $K^+$ secretion through apical ROMK channels. Thus, increased $Na^+$ delivery would stimulate $K^+$ secretion. Aldosterone increases Na reabsorption via ENaCs to stimulate $K^+$ secretion.

In addition to the K excretion rate regulated by aldosterone action, the second important factor is urine flow rate. Urine flow rate to the collecting duct depends

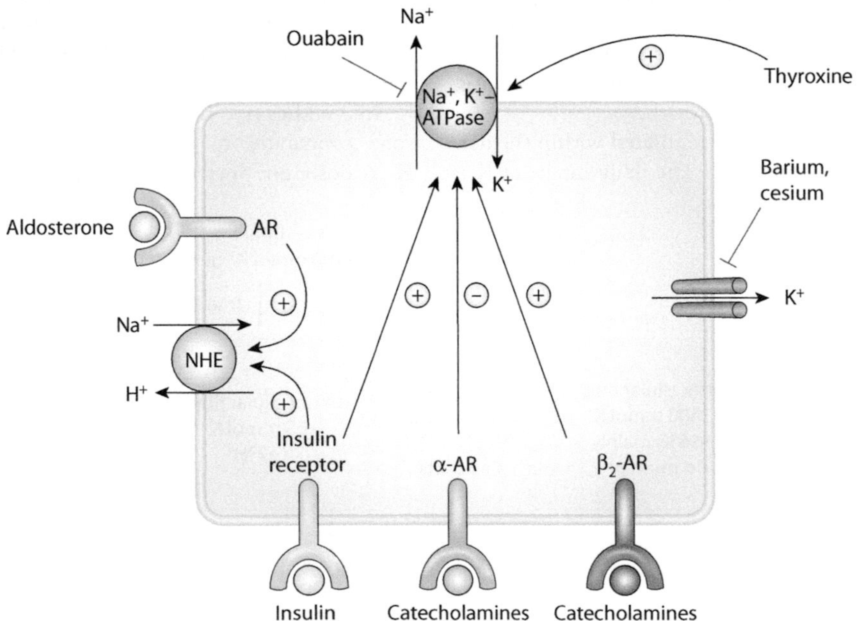


***Figure 20.10***
*Cellular shifts in K. α-AR, α-adrenergic receptor; β2-AR, β2-adrenergic receptor; AR, aldosterone receptor; $H^+$, hydrogen; $K^+$, potassium; $Na^+$, sodium; NHE, $Na^+/H^+$ exchanger. (Adapted from Unwin RJ et al.,* Nature Reviews Nephrology, *7, 75–84, 2011.)*

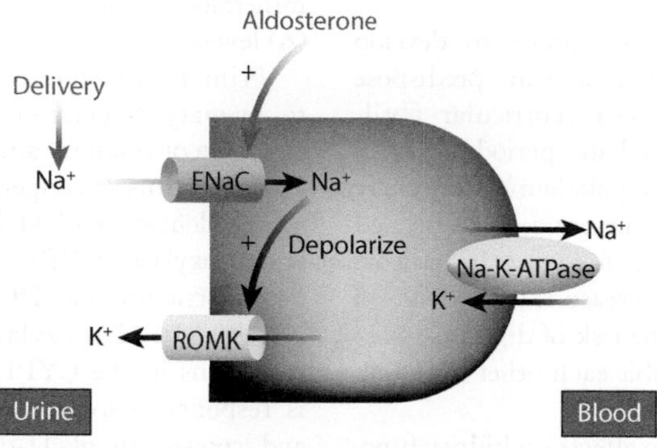


***Figure 20.11***
*K secretion in the distal nephron. $K^+$, potassium; $Na^+$, sodium; ENaC, epithelial sodium channel; ROMK, renal outer medullary potassium; Na,K-ATPase; sodium-potassium adenosine triphosphatase. (Adapted from Huang CL, Kuo E,* Journal of the American Society of Nephrology, *18, 2649–52, 2007.)*

mainly on the excretion of osmoles, such as urea, Na, and Cl. Increased urine flow rate stimulates further reabsorption of Na and causes further depolarization of the apical membrane; thus, it increases K secretion.[112] Flow-induced increases in K secretion are mediated by large-conductance big K (BK or Maxi-K) channels.

# Hypokalemia

Hypokalemia is a common electrolyte disturbance in hospitalized patients. Hypokalemia is defined as plasma K concentration <3.5 mmol/L.

## Epidemiology

The estimated incidence of hypokalemia in hospitalized patients is 12%–21%, whereas the percentage of inpatients with serum K <3.0 mmol/L is 3.4%–5.2%.[119–121] Female sex and increasing age are associated with increased incidence of hypokalemia.[121] Hypokalemia is very common in patients on peritoneal dialysis, patients with infectious diseases, and patients on diuretics. Patients with hypokalemia have frequently other electrolyte abnormalities, such as hypomagnesemia, hyponatremia, and hypophosphatemia.[120]

## Clinical presentation

Hypokalemia is classified according to the serum K levels as mild (3.0–3.5 mmol/L), moderate (2.5–3.0 mmol/L), and severe (<2.5 mmol/L). The severity of symptoms depends on the severity of hypokalemia and the rapidity of the onset of hypokalemia. Mild hypokalemia is usually asymptomatic, and the severity of symptoms increases as plasma K levels decline. Clinical manifestations of hypokalemia are mainly related to the effects of low plasma K on muscles and cardiac myocytes function.

Mild-to-moderate hypokalemia can cause myalgia and muscle weakness. Patients with severe hypokalemia can develop muscle necrosis, paralysis, and rhabdomyolysis. Plasma K levels <2.0 mmol/L can be related with ascending paralysis, respiratory muscle weakness leading to respiratory failure, and involvement of gastrointestinal muscles resulting in ileus.

Hypokalemia and paralysis is defined as an acute loss of muscle power associated with plasma K concentration <3.0 mmol/L. This clinical presentation can be due to hypokalemic periodic paralysis (HPP) or non-HPP. HPP is due to an acute shift of K into the cells and is divided into familial periodic paralysis (FPP), thyrotoxic periodic paralysis (TPP), and sporadic periodic paralysis (SPP). HPP is a form of periodic paralysis characterized by the absence of K wasting or an acid–base disorder and the presence of recurrent attacks with positive family history or clinical thyrotoxicosis. Non-HPP is characterized by a large deficit of K with high K excretion and usually an acid–base abnormality.[122,123]

In cardiac myocytes, hypokalemia reduces K conductance and results in prolonged repolarization phase of the cardiac action potential, reflected as prolonged QT interval in the electrocardiogram (ECG). Classical changes observed in the ECG of patients with hypokalemia are early T wave flattening or inversion followed by ST segment depression and a prominent U wave, which occurs at the end of the T wave and can be difficult to distinguish from it.[116]

Patients with hypokalemia are prone to develop various arrhythmias. Hypokalemia can predispose to ventricular tachycardia or even ventricular fibrillation, especially in the immediate period after an acute myocardial infarction. Hypokalemia, especially when accompanied by hypomagnesemia, is associated with an increased risk of *torsades de pointes*. In patients on digoxin, hypokalemia can increase the incidence of arrhythmias and also increase the risk of digitalis toxicity because K and digoxin inhibit each other's binding at the $Na^+$, $K^+$-ATPase pump.[116]

Finally, hypokalemia has also effects on kidney function and glucose metabolism. Hypokalemia can cause downregulation of the water channel AQP2 in the collecting duct, thereby resulting in impairment of the concentrating ability of the kidneys and nephrogenic diabetes insipidus.[111] Also, hypokalemia has a negative impact on glucose handling through impairment of insulin secretion and tissue sensitivity to insulin.

## Causes

Hypokalemia can be classified via five main causes: (1) shift of K from the ECF to the ICF, (2) increased renal losses, (3) increased extrarenal losses, (4) minimal K intake, and (5) Hypomagnesemia.

### Transcellular shifts in K

Medication is the commonest cause of transcellular shifts of K. β2-Sympathomimetic drugs, such as bronchodilators and pseudoephedrine anticongestants, cause reduction of plasma K for up to 4 h.[113] Theophylline and caffeine decrease serum K levels by stimulating the release of catecholamines and by increasing $Na^+$,$K^+$-ATPase activity through inhibiting cellular phosphodiesterase.[113] Insulin-related hypokalemia due to K shift to the cells is a clinical problem in cases of insulin overdose and in the context of the treatment of diabetic ketoacidosis.

HPP, either as FPP or TPP, is caused by a shift of K into the cells. Also, rapid decrease of serum K by 1.0 mmol/L occurs in delirium tremens due to release of large amounts of epinephrine, β2-adrenergic stimulation and associated transcellular shift of K.[113]

### Increased renal losses

The two main mechanisms are through increased mineralocorticoid activity or through increased distal delivery of Na or nonreabsorbed anions. Increased mineralocorticoid activity could be due to primary hyperaldosteronism (hyporeninemic), secondary hyperaldosteronism (hyperreninemic), or uncommon conditions with excess mineralocorticoid activity and suppressed aldosterone (A) levels.

Primary mineralocorticoid excess occurs mainly due to primary hyperaldosteronism (due to A-producing adenoma or bilateral adrenal hyperplasia).

Rare forms of congenital adrenal hyperplasia (CAH) due to deficiency of 11 β-hydroxylase (CYP11β1) or 17 α-hydroxylase (CYP17α) result in increased levels of deoxycorticosterone (DOC) and excess mineralocorticoid activity. 11β-Hydroxylase deficiency results from several mutations in the CYP11B1 gene, and 11β-hydroxylase is responsible for conversion of 11-deoxycortisol to F and conversion of 11-deoxycorticosterone to corticosterone. Without this enzyme activity, A and F levels are low (Figure 20.12).[124] Low F stimulates ACTH secretion that leads to accumulation of precursors, including DOC, 11-deoxycortisol (11-DOC), and 17α-hydroxyprogesterone (17-OHP). DOC is a mineralocorticoid that at supraphysiologic levels promotes salt retention, volume expansion, and arterial hypertension. 17α-Hydroxylase deficiency is a rare autosomal recessive disorder (frequency of <1% of the total cases of CAH) that affects both adrenal and gonadal steroid production. These patients have increased ACTH levels and increased mineralocorticoids (DOC, corticosterone) with low levels of A and hypokalemic alkalosis.[124]

Patients with Cushing's syndrome secondary to ectopic ACTH secretion frequently develop a state of mineralocorticoid excess defined by hypertension and hypokalemic alkalosis. These patients exhibit both high levels of F and E, indicating that 11β-HSD2 function is intact but saturated by the high substrate levels of circulating F, resulting in F spillover to act on the MR[125] (Figure 20.13).

Apparent mineralocorticoid excess (AME) is a rare disorder and is inherited in an autosomal recessive manner. Partial or complete inactivation of the enzyme 11β-HSD2 results in illicit activation of the MR by F in A target tissues, rendering F a potent mineralocorticoid. Presentation is usually during neonatal life or childhood with low birth weight, failure to thrive, short stature, severe hypertension, and hypokalemic metabolic alkalosis. Biochemically, blood test abnormalities comprise hypokalemia, suppressed renin, and undetectable aldosterone levels. Some patients have a milder variant (type II AME) and present in late adolescence or early adulthood with a milder clinical phenotype of hypertension and hypokalemia.[125]

Excessive ingestion of licorice can cause a similar clinical syndrome with AME. Licorice flavoring is used in sweets in Europe and in chewing tobacco in the United States and sufficient quantities may lead to significant

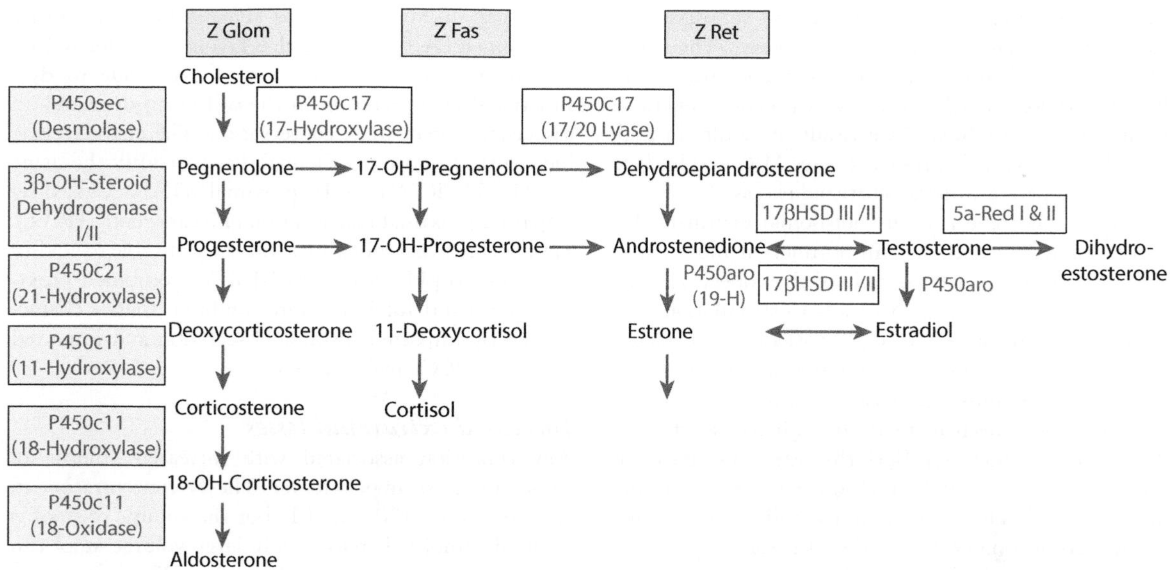


***Figure 20.12***

*Adrenal steroid synthesis. Z Glom, zona glomerulosa; Z Fas, zona fasciculata; Z Ret, zona reticularis; 19-H, 19-hydroxylase; HSD, hydroxysteroid dehydrogenase; P450aro, aromatase; 5α-Red, 5α-reductase. (Adapted from Melcescu E et al.,* Hormone and Metabolic Research, *44, 867–78, 2012.)*

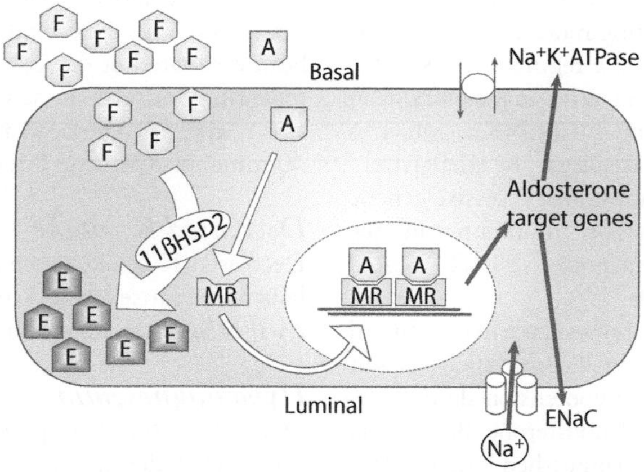


***Figure 20.13***

*Mineralocorticoid action in the target cell of the cortical collecting duct. The mineralocorticoid receptor (MR) binds F and A with equal affinity, but plasma F concentrations exceed those of A by 100–1000-fold. Selective binding and activation of the MR by A is ensured by the action of the enzyme 11β-HSD2. This enzyme converts hormonally active F to hormonally inactive E and protects the MR from F. Upon binding of A to the MR, the MR-A complex stimulates upregulation of the ENaC channels and the basolateral $Na^+$,$K^+$-ATPase. (Adapted from Hammer F, Stewart PM,* Best Practice & Research Clinical Endocrinology & Metabolism, *20, 337–53, 2006.)*

hypertension, hypokalemia, edema, and suppression of the renin–angiotensin–aldosterone system. The active component of licorice, glycyrrhetinic acid, has a very low affinity for the MR but is a very potent competitive inhibitor of 11β-HSD2. As a result, it results in high renal levels of F, which then activates MRs and leads to a state of apparent mineralocorticoid excess.[126]

Liddle syndrome is a rare autosomal dominant disorder characterized by a gain-of-function mutation of the ENaC of the principal cells of the collecting duct. Excessive reabsorption of Na leads to stimulation of K secretion and hypokalemia. These patients are characterized by volume overload and hypertension in the setting of suppressed renin–angiotensin–aldosterone axis.[116]

The second mechanism is through increased distal delivery of Na and water. Both thiazide and loop diuretics block Cl-associated Na reabsorption and, as a result, increase distal delivery of Na to the collecting duct and distal reabsorption of Na, further destabilizing the apical membrane and stimulating K secretion.[113]

Bartter syndrome is a group of rare genetic disorders (types I, II, III, IV, V) with physiologic features consistent with a primary renal tubular defect in the thick ascending limb of the loop of Henle where NaCl is primarily reabsorbed by the Na-K-2Cl cotransporter (NKCC2). Bartter syndrome is caused by dysfunction of various ion transport channels, including inactivating mutations in the gene for the NKCC2 in the thick ascending limb (type I Bartter); inactivating mutations in the gene for ROMK channels, which are a regulator of NKCC2 activity (type II Bartter); and inactivating mutations in the gene for the renal Cl channel (CLCNKB), which is another regulator of NKCC2 activity (type III Bartter).

Gitelman syndrome is an autosomal recessive genetic disorder due to loss-of-function mutations in the thiazide-sensitive Na,Cl cotransporter (NCCT) located in the distal convoluted tubule.[127]

Bartter and Gitelman syndromes have many clinical features in common, such as hypokalemic alkalosis, salt wasting, and normotension or hypotension despite elevated levels of plasma renin and aldosterone. Bartter and Gitelman syndromes can be distinguished based on laboratory parameters, including serum magnesium (Mg) and urinary Ca. All patients with Gitelman syndrome have hypomagnesemia, compared with 20%–30% of cases of Bartter syndrome. Gitelman syndrome is characterized by hypocalciuria in contrast to normocalciuria or hypercalciuria in Bartter syndrome. Interestingly, Bartter resembles the effects of loop diuretics and Gitelman the effects of thiazide diuretics.[128]

Three types of renal tubular acidosis (RTA type 1, type 2, and type 3) produce hypokalemia in combination with hyperchloremic metabolic acidosis of normal anion gap because of various abnormalities in tubular function. RTA type I (distal RTA) is characterized by an impairment in acidification of urine due to dysfunctional acid secretion in the collecting duct and an associated defect in K conservation. The characteristic biochemical finding is the inability to acidify the urine to pH <5.5. RTA type II (proximal RTA) is caused by impaired proximal reabsorption of bicarbonate ($HCO_3$). Patients have bicarbonaturia, but they are able to acidify the urine to pH <5.3. Type III RTA (combined proximal and distal RTA) is a rare condition that is characterized by impaired distal acid secretion and impaired proximal $HCO_3$ reabsorption.[116]

### Increased extrarenal losses

Any condition associated with increased volume of stool can cause hypokalemia. The K concentration in the stool is 50–100 mmol/L, but the volume of stool is normally small; therefore, only large volume stool can lead to significant extrarenal K losses. The commonest conditions are secretory diarrhea, laxative abuse, and high-output stoma.

In very rare occasions, significant K losses arise from sweat. This occurs in conditions with increased K concentration in the sweat such as cystic fibrosis or in conditions with excessive amounts of sweat such as strenuous exertion in an extremely hot weather. The mean sweat loss of an American football player during a 2 h practice session in 28°C and 65% relative humidity has been estimated at 4.8 L, and the mean sweat loss for a male runner under the same conditions is about 1.5 L/h; as a result, an American football player can lose up to 40 mmol of K during 2 h of intensive training.[129]

### Decreased K intake

Decreased K intake alone can very rarely lead to hypokalemia because kidneys are capable of minimizing any renal K losses to maintain K homeostasis.

### Hypomagnesemia

More than 50% of patients with clinically significant hypokalemia have concomitant Mg deficiency. Concomitant Mg deficiency aggravates hypokalemia and renders it refractory to treatment by K. Hypomagnesemia impairs the activity of $Na^+$-$K^+$-ATPase and causes depletion of the intracellular K stores.[113]

Mg deficiency contributes to hypokalemia mainly by enhancing renal K secretion as a result of reduction of Mg-dependent inhibition of ROMK channels. In the cortical collecting duct cells, K is secreted into luminal fluid via apical (ROMK and BK) channels. At the physiologic intracellular Mg concentration, ROMK conducts more K ions inward than outward (inward rectifying).

This is because intracellular Mg binds ROMK and blocks K efflux and secretion and in this way limits K efflux. This unique inward-rectifying property of ROMK renders intracellular Mg levels a critical determinant of ROMK-mediated K secretion in the distal nephron. Changes in intracellular Mg concentration over the physiologic-pathophysiologic range would significantly affect K secretion.[117]

The causes of hypokalemia are summarized in Table 20.7.

| Causes of hypokalemia |
|---|
| **Transcellular shift** |
| Drugs |
| β2-Adrenergic agonists: bronchodilators (salbutamol, terbutaline), decongestants (pseudoephedrine) |
| Insulin |
| Theophylline |
| Caffeine |
| Verapamil intoxication |
| Nondrug causes |
| HPP |
| Metabolic alkalosis |
| Autonomic causes (catecholamines release) |
| **Increased renal losses** |
| Primary mineralocorticoid excess |
| Primary hyperaldosteronism |
| Cushing's syndrome |
| 11β-Hydroxylase deficiency |
| 17α-Hydroxylase deficiency |
| Hyperreninemic hyperaldosteronism |
| Malignant hypertension |
| Renovascular hypertension |
| Renin-secreting tumors |
| Apparent mineralocorticoid excess |
| 11β-HSD2 deficiency |
| Excessive ingestion of licorice |
| Liddle syndrome |
| Increased distal delivery of Na |
| Diuretics (thiazide, loop diuretics) |
| Bartter syndrome |
| Gitelman syndrome |
| Increased distal delivery of anions |
| RTA type 1 |
| RTA type 2 |
| RTA type 3 |
| **Increased extrarenal losses** |
| GI losses |
| Secretory diarrhea (cholera, salmonella) |
| Laxative abuse |
| VIPoma |
| Ileostomy |
| Sweat losses |
| Strenuous exercise in hot climate |
| Cystic fibrosis |
| **Decreased K intake** |
| **Hypomagnesemia** |

***Table 20.7***
*Causes of hypokalemia.*

## *Evaluation of patient*

The duration of hypokalemia and the clinical context should always be considered. Often, the etiology of hypokalemia is apparent such as in patients with transient acute hypokalemia caused by K shift in the context of diabetic ketoacidosis treated with large amounts of insulin. All patients with hypokalemia should have serum Mg levels measured because hypomagnesemia very often coexists with hypokalemia.

In patients with no apparent etiology of hypokalemia, assessment of the renal response to hypokalemia is recommended to identify the source of K losses. There are four methods to assess urinary K excretion: (1) K concentration in a 24 h urine collection, (2) K concentration in a spot urine sample, (3) urine K-creatinine ratio, and (4) transtubular K gradient (TTKG).

The first method is based on the measurement of K excretion rate in a 24 h urine sample. Values <15–20 mmol/day suggest an extrarenal cause of K depletion. The disadvantages of this traditional approach are that obtaining a 24 h collection is time-consuming, collections are often incomplete, and also 24 h collection delays K therapy that should be given promptly in the setting of a medical emergency.[118,122]

The second method is the measurement of K concentration in a spot urine sample, and it is has the advantage of convenience. Urine K concentration <20 mmol/L usually suggests extrarenal losses and urine K >20 mmol/L renal losses, but there is a great overlap between renal and extrarenal causes of K loss. It can be often misleading because it does not take into account the urine volume, and many patients with hypokalemia have polyuria. Polyuria due to thirst or concentrating defect in cases of chronic hypokalemia leads to a low value for the urine K concentration even if significant renal K wasting is present.[122]

The third method is the urine K (Uk)/creatinine (Ucrea) ratio. Uk/Ucrea >1.5, when both variables are measured in mmol/L, distinguishes hypokalemia due to renal K wasting from nonrenal K loss. Provided creatinine is excreted at a near constant rate, this ratio corrects for variations in urine volume. The other caveat is that this ratio should be interpreted with caution in cases of very low or very high muscle mass because creatinine is derived from muscle mass.[130]

The fourth method is the estimation of TTKG. This is a semiquantitative assessment of K in the cortical collecting duct because it corrects K in the urine for the amount of reabsorbed water in the medullary collecting duct. TTKG is calculated by dividing the urine:plasma K concentration ratio by the urine:plasma osmolality ratio according to the following formula: urine K/plasma K × plasma Osm/urine Osm. Values <2 suggest nonrenal causes. TTKG is invalid if urine Osm is lower than plasma Osm.[118]

If hypokalemia is due to renal K losses, the next step is the assessment of acid–base status by measurement of serum pH, serum HCO3, blood pressure, plasma renin activity and aldosterone is recommended. In cases of metabolic acidosis, measurement of urine chloride is indicated.

In the group of patients with chronic hypokalemia, normotension, alkalosis, and hyperreninemic hyperaldosteronism of uncertain origin, a thiazide test can be extremely useful to differentiate Gitelman syndrome from Bartter syndrome. After an overnight fast, the patient is kept recumbent for 4 h and is invited to drink tap water (10 mL/kg of body weight) to facilitate spontaneous voiding. After two 30-min basal clearances, 50 mg of hydrochlorothiazide (HCT) is administered orally, and six additional 30 min clearances are performed. Blood samples are collected at 60 and 240 min, and urine is collected every 30 min by spontaneous voiding and analyzed for Na, Cl, K, and creatinine. The maximal diuretic-induced increase over basal in the subsequent 3 h of fractional excretion of chloride (FECl) is calculated as the maximal FECl at any point during 3 h post-HCT administration minus the mean of the two basal FECl. Patients with Gitelman syndrome have blunted diuretic effect as indicated by much lower Na and Cl postdiuretic urine excretion. A maximal diuretic-induced increase of FECl of <2.3% has a diagnostic sensitivity of 93% and specificity of 100% for the diagnosis of Gitelman syndrome.[131] In addition, genetic testing is available for all known genes responsible for Gitelman syndrome and Bartter syndrome.

## Management

The main considerations in the treatment of hypokalemia are the presence and severity of symptoms and the levels of serum K. There is a wide variation in the physiologic effects of K deficit; ECG and muscle strength monitoring are essential. The appropriate preparation of K, route of administration, and rate of administration depend on the clinical context.

The principle underlying the rate of K replacement is that it should be carried out gradually. Rapid administration of K is potentially dangerous unless there is a life-threatening situation. Bolus injection of K should never be given because it can precipitate cardiac arrest. The estimation of the size of the K deficit is difficult because ECF concentration does not always reflect accurately K body stores, and empiric replacement with frequent monitoring of serum K levels is recommended. Cautious replacement should take place to avoid the risk of developing hyperkalemia posthypokalemia, a response that occurs in as many as 16% of hypokalemic inpatients.[120]

Mg levels in the serum should be routinely measured because 40% of hypokalemic patients have concomitant hypomagnesemia.[132] In cases of hypomagnesemia, Mg should be replaced to avoid the problem of refractory K repletion because Mg replacement reduces renal K losses.

In mild asymptomatic hypokalemia (serum K 3.0–3.5 mmol/L), oral K replacement is preferred. Oral K chloride at dosages 60–80 mmol/day is initiated and sometimes needs up-titration to 100–150 mmol/day if there are continuing K losses. Liquid or effervescent forms of KCl are often not well tolerated due to strong, unpleasant taste. Slow-release tablets of KCl are better tolerated, but in rare cases they can lead to ulcerative lesions and hemorrhage in the GI tract; they need to be swallowed with plenty of fluid during meals.[133,134]

In patients with serum K <3.0 mmol/L who are asymptomatic, intravenous or oral KCl replacement should be administered. Mg replacement is recommended (with oral magnesium glycerophosphate or gluconate) if serum Mg levels are low.

In patients with serum K <3.0 mmol/L and life-threatening arrhythmia (ventricular tachycardia or digoxin toxicity with unstable cardiac rhythm or acute myocardial infarct and significant ventricular ectopy), intravenous KCl at a rate of 20 mmol/h should be administered.[135] If cardiac arrest is imminent, even more rapid administration of 5–10 mmol KCl over 5–15 min may be used. In these cases of rapid intravenous KCl replacement, cardiac monitoring in an ICU is advisable.[133] In cases of cardiac arrest and hypokalemia, intravenous KCl at a rate of 20 mmol over 2–3 min can be administered.[135] In the context of hypokalemia and life-threatening arrhythmias, intravenous magnesium sulfate (10 mmol over 30 min) should always be administered, even before hypomagnesemia is confirmed biochemically.[135]

The most commonly used K salt is KCl because it is very effective, especially when there is concomitant Cl loss. Alternatively $KHCO_3$ can be used if hypokalemia coexists with metabolic acidosis, and $KPO_4$ can be considered in cases of diabetic ketoacidosis with combined K and $PO_4$ depletion.[133]

Finally, hypokalemia is often iatrogenic and should be prevented whenever possible. Patients with diuretic-induced hypokalemia should be re-evaluated in terms of need for diuretic therapy and addition of K-sparing diuretic (amiloride or spironolactone) should be considered. Other patients at high risk of developing hypokalemia are patients on renal replacement therapy who can develop hypokalemia toward the end or immediately after a session of hemodialysis.[133]

# Hyperkalemia

Hyperkalemia is defined as plasma K concentration >5.0 mmol/L. Hyperkalemia is classified as mild (K 5.1–5.9 mmol/L), moderate (K 6.0–6.4 mmol/L), and severe (K >6.5 mmol/L).

## Epidemiology

The incidence of hyperkalemia in hospitalized patients is 7.0%–10.0% for plasma K >5.0 mmol/L, 2.8%–3.3% for K >5.5 mmol/L, and 1.4%–1.5% for K >6.0 mmol/L.[121,136,137] Increasing age is strongly associated with increased incidence of hyperkalemia.[121] Some studies have shown slightly higher incidence of hyperkalemia in males compared with females.[121,136] Hyperkalemia is often multifactorial and is commonly associated with kidney disease, K-sparing diuretics, and K supplements.

## Clinical presentation

Hyperkalemia is often asymptomatic. The clinical manifestations of hyperkalemia are due to the effects on elevated K levels on skeletal muscle cells and cardiac myocytes function. In general, the severity of clinical manifestations and ECG changes reflects the absolute levels of serum K and the rapidity of onset of hyperkalemia.

In terms of muscle weakness, severe hyperkalemia may present with ascending muscle weakness progressing to flaccid paralysis, paraesthesia, and depressed tendon reflexes. Usually, respiratory muscles and cranial nerve function are intact.

In terms of cardiac conduction abnormalities, hyperkalemia causes increased K conductance in cardiac myocytes and rapid repolarization that is reflected typically as a tall, peaked (tented) T wave or in some cases as large amplitude T wave (T wave greater than or equal to that of the R wave in more than one lead). This is the first change seen at levels of K >5.5–6.5 mmol/L. At K levels >6.5–7.5 mmol/L, the PR interval becomes prolonged, and there is reduction in the amplitude of P wave that can finally disappear. The QRS complex widens when K levels are >7.0–8.0 mmol/L.[138] These changes can progress to loss of sinoatrial conduction with onset of a wide complex "sine wave" (S and T waves merging) ventricular rhythm.[139] Patients with severe hyperkalemia can die due to ventricular fibrillation, asystole, or wide pulseless idioventricular rhythm. The serial ECG changes that occur in hyperkalemia are illustrated in Figure 20.14.[138]

## Causes

Hyperkalemia occurs due to transcellular shift of K, increase in K intake, or decrease in renal excretion of K. Hyperkalemia is often multifactorial, but almost always there is a defect in kidney function. About three quarters of hospitalized patients with hyperkalemia have an element of kidney failure, and medications contribute in 30%–60% of cases.[140]

Spurious hyperkalemia or pseudohyperkalemia in the serum is defined as a marked elevation of serum K levels in the absence of elevated K levels in the plasma and in the absence of clinical evidence of electrolyte imbalance. Pseudohyperkalemia is considered in cases when serum K levels exceed plasma K levels by >0.4 mmol/L.[141] Difficulty in collecting blood sample with prolonged tourniquet application, repeated fist clenching during venipuncture, shaking of blood samples, long storage of samples, and exposure of samples to low temperatures can cause spurious hyperkalemia. Hematological disorders such as thrombocytosis, pronounced leukocytosis, and red cell disorders (e.g., stomatocytosis or spherocytosis) are related with leakage of K from platelets *in vitro* during clotting or white blood cell breakdown *in vitro* or red cell lysis, respectively, and can result in serum pseudohyperkalemia.[142]

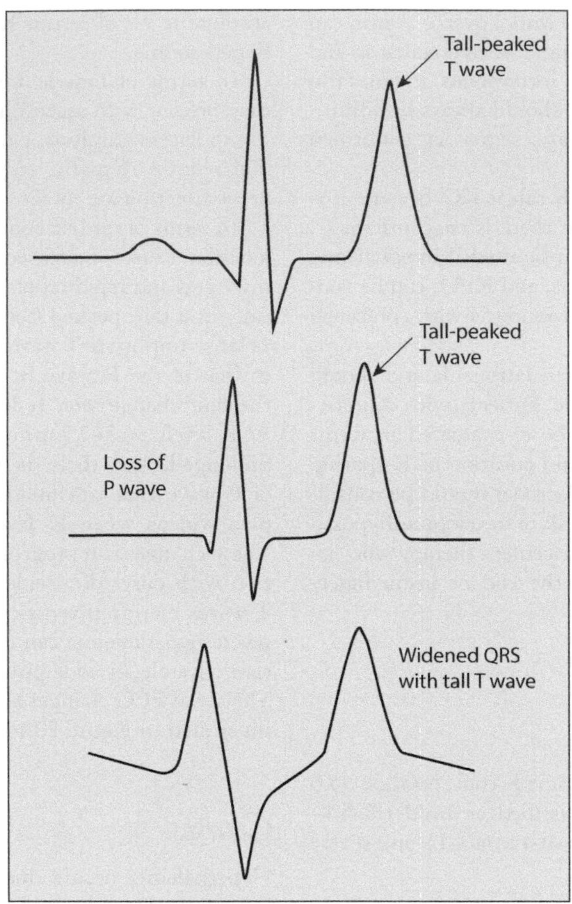


***Figure 20.14***
*Serial ECG changes in hyperkalemia. QRS. (Adapted from Slovis C, Jenkins R,* British Medical Journal*, 324, 1320–3, 2002.)*

The three groups of causes of true hyperkalemia are as follows:

1. Transcellular shift of K. The commonest causes are due to metabolic acidosis or in the context of hyperosmolality, especially hyperglycemic hyperosmolar state.
2. Increase in K intake. Increased K intake due to oral/intravenous K supplements or K content of nasogastric feeding/total parenteral nutrition contributes to 15%–30% of cases of hyperkalemia.[136,140]
3. Decrease in K renal excretion. This is the most important etiology of hyperkalemia. Effective K excretion requires A action and sufficient distal delivery of Na and water within the nephron. This is classified to causes due to decreased mineralocorticoid activity or reduced tubular ability to secrete K or oliguric renal failure.

Primary hypoaldosteronism occurs in Addison's disease and in classic salt-wasting form of congenital adrenal hyperplasia (due to severe 21-hydroxylase deficiency). Many drugs, such as direct renin inhibitors (e.g., aliskiren [Rasilez]), ACE inhibitors, and angiotensin II receptor blockers (ARBs) interact with the renin–angiotensin–aldosterone axis and cause hyperreninemic hypoaldosteronism.

Heparin-induced hyperkalemia is frequently underappreciated despite it occuring in approximately 7%–8% of heparin-treated patients. Heparin (both unfractionated and low molecular weight) is a potent, reversible inhibitor of A production.[143] This effect is specific only for the zona glomerulosa; all other corticosteroids are not affected. Heparin interferes with adrenal A production through several different mechanisms. The most important mechanism is mediated by reduction in both number and affinity of angiotensin II receptors in the zona glomerulosa.[144] Heparin-induced A suppression presents within 2–3 days and is marked by days 4–6. After discontinuation of heparin, serum A levels return to baseline over approximately the same period.

Patients with diabetes and chronic renal impairment due to diabetic nephropathy can exhibit reduction in the synthesis of active renin and hyporeninemic hypoaldosteronism. There are various factors that contribute to hyporeninemia in these patients: volume expansion in these patients can suppress the renin–angiotensin–aldosterone axis, decreased levels of prostaglandins reduce renin release, conversion of the precursor prorenin to active renin is impaired and diabetic autonomic neuropathy is often associated with a low renin state.[145]

Nonsteroidal anti-inflammatory drugs (NSAIDs) cause hyporeninemia through impairment of prostaglandin synthesis in the juxtaglomerular apparatus.[116]

Pseudohypoaldosteronism type 1 (PHA1) is a rare condition characterized by renal resistance to the actions of A; patients exhibit salt wasting, hyperkalemia, and metabolic acidosis, despite elevated serum A levels. It is caused by loss-of-function mutations in ENaC (autosomal recessive PHA1) or MC-R (autosomal dominant PHA1).

Pseudohypoaldosteronism type 2 (PHA2: Gordon's syndrome) is a rare autosomal dominant disorder characterized by hypertension, hyperkalemia, and metabolic acidosis with normal renal function, caused by mutations in *WNKT1* and *-4*. The WNK1 and WNK4 proteins regulate channels in the cell membrane that control the transport of Na or K into and out of cells, primarily in the kidneys.

The WNK4 protein normally blocks Na and K channels, thereby decreasing Na reabsorption and K secretion. The WNK1 protein normally stops WNK4's inhibition of Na channels, thereby increasing Na reabsorption. The WNK1 protein also inhibits K channels, thereby decreasing K secretion.

Mutations in the *WNK1* gene increase the activity of the gene and lead to excess WNK1 protein expression. The excess protein abnormally increases Na reabsorption and blocks K secretion. These effects lead to increased circulating Na and K levels, causing hypertension and hyperkalemia.

Mutations in the *WNK4* gene lead to an abnormal protein that no longer inhibits Na channels but inhibits K channels more strongly. Like *WNK1* gene mutations, mutations in the *WNK4* gene lead to increased Na reabsorption and decreased K secretion, resulting in hypertension and hyperkalemia.

In these patients, thiazide diuretics rapidly ameliorate all clinical findings. In contrast to PHA1, serum A levels are low or normal, but there is a degree of A resistance.[146]

| |
|---|
| **Transcellular K shift** |
| Metabolic acidosis |
| Hyperosmolality |
| Insulin deficiency |
| β Blockers |
| **Increase in K intake** |
| Intravenous/oral K replacement |
| Nasogastric feeding/parenteral nutrition |
| **Decrease in K renal excretion** |
| Hyperreninemic hypoaldosteronism |
| Addison's disease |
| Classical CAH (CYP21A) |
| ACE inhibitors, ARBs, direct renin inhibitors |
| Heparin |
| Hyporeninemic hypoaldosteronism |
| Diabetic nephropathy |
| Chronic interstitial nephritis |
| NSAIDs |
| Cyclosporine |
| Human immunodeficiency infection |
| Aldosterone resistance |
| Pseudohypoaldosteronism |
| Spironolactone, eplerenone |
| Impaired tubular K secretion |
| Amiloride |
| Trimethoprim |
| Oliguric renal failure |

***Table 20.8***
*Classification of hyperkalemia.*

Amiloride and trimethoprim act in a similar manner by inhibiting competitively ENaCs in the distal nephron. As a consequence, the transepithelial voltage is reduced and renal K secretion is inhibited.[147]

The causes of hyperkalemia are summarized in Table 20.8.

## *Evaluation of patient*

The initial diagnostic approach includes clinical history, detailed drug history, and physical examination. The physiological impact of hyperkalemia on ECG changes and muscle weakness must be documented. Urgent therapy may be mandated based on ECG changes, levels of K, and rapidity of onset of hyperkalemia. Absence of ECG changes does not exclude the need for immediate intervention because progression to lethal arrhythmias can be unpredictable and lethal.[148] Hyperkalemia should always be treated first before its cause is investigated. Often, the etiology is apparent, for example, in patients who are on nephrotoxic drugs or have oliguric renal failure.

In cases of normal renal function and absence of predisposing factors (such as K supplementation or K raising drugs), spurious hyperkalemia should be suspected and excluded. Simultaneous measurement of serum K, plasma K (sample anticoagulated with lithium heparin), and full blood count should be performed.[142] Serum K greater than plasma K by >0.4 mmol/L indicates pseudohyperkalemia.

In cases the cause of hyperkalemia is not evident, a stepwise approach is recommended. The first step is to assess the renal response to hyperkalemia. TTKG <6–8 (and usually <5) indicates inappropriate renal response and suggests renal cause of hyperkalemia; TTKG >6–8 (and usually >10) suggests a nonrenal cause.[149,150] In cases when urine osmolality is lower than plasma osmolality, TTKG is not reliable. The next step in cases of reduced renal K excretion is measurement of A and renin activity.

# Treatment

## Acute treatment of hyperkalemia

The three main approaches for acute therapy of hyperkalemia are (1) opposing the toxic effects of K on the cardiac membrane, (2) shifting of K into cells, and (3) removing K from the body.

### *Opposing the toxic effects of K on the cardiac membrane*

The most effective way to antagonize the toxic effects of hyperkalemia on the myocardium and stabilize the cardiac membrane is intravenous infusion of Ca salts. Ca salts are used in all patients with ECG changes associated with hyperkalemia and sometimes in patients with K levels >6.0 mmol/L, even in the absence of ECG changes. Patients should have continuous ECG monitoring because ECG changes can develop and progress rapidly. Calcium chloride contains more Ca (6.8 mmol in 10 mL) than calcium gluconate (2.2 mmol in 10 mL) and has greater bioavailability. Calcium gluconate is usually preferred because of reduced risk to cause tissue injury if extravasation occurs, apart from cases of imminent cardiac arrest when calcium chloride is usually used.[135,148] Ca salts do not lower K levels in the plasma. Ten milliliters of 10% calcium gluconate is infused intravenously over 2–5 min. The onset of effect is at 1–3 min and the duration is 30–60 min. If no improvement in ECG changes is observed within 10 min, intravenous infusion of calcium gluconate can be repeated. In patients on digoxin treatment, intravenous calcium gluconate should be infused with caution over 30 min because Ca could potentiate digoxin toxicity.[135]

### *Shifting of K into cells*

Insulin stimulates the $Na^+,K^+$-ATPase pump, resulting in intracellular uptake of K. Ten units of regular soluble insulin intravenously with 50 mL of 50% dextrose (25 g of glucose) has been the standard treatment for acute hyperkalemia, but some studies have reported high incidence of delayed hypoglycemia (30–60 min postinsulin), especially in patients with severe kidney disease.[151] The alternative regimen is 10 units of insulin with 40 g of glucose, which can reduce the possibility of hypoglycemia.[152] Insulin infusion results in 0.7–1.0 mmol/L reduction in K levels. The time of onset is 15–20 min, with a peak effect at 30–60 min, and the duration of action is 4–6 h.[135] The effect of insulin on K levels is independent of its effect on glucose levels. Uremia reduces its glucose-lowering action, but it does not affect its hypokalemic action.[152] Administration of intravenous glucose without insulin is not recommended because supraphysiological levels of insulin are needed for its hypokalemic action, which many patients will not achieve by endogenous production of insulin.

Nebulized β2-adrenergic agonists stimulate the enzyme adenyl cyclase and increase the conversion of ATP to 3′5′-cyclic AMP that stimulates the $Na^+,K^+$-ATPase pump, resulting in intracellular shift of K.[153] Ten milligrams of nebulized salbutamol leads to 0.5–0.8 mmol/L reduction in K levels. The onset of action is 15–30 min, with peak effect at 90 min and a duration of action of 4–6 h. Salbutamol should be used very cautiously, especially in these doses that are much higher than the doses used for bronchodilation in patients with tachyarrhythmias or ischemic heart disease, because it can increase myocardial oxygen consumption, exacerbate tachycardia, and cause tremor.[154] Twenty percent to 40% of patients do not have adequate response to salbutamol for unclear reasons, and it is not possible to predict who will fail to respond.[151]

Sodium bicarbonate does not lower K levels in the plasma. It has a role in the acute management of hyperkalemia only in the context of severe metabolic acidosis with pH <7.2.[154]

A combined regimen of intravenous insulin with glucose plus nebulized salbutamol is recommended because it causes more pronounced reduction in K levels and also reduces the frequency of insulin-induced hypoglycemic episodes.[148,151,153]

*Removing K from the body*

Calcium resonium, an exchange resin, is a cross-linked polymer with negatively charged units that exchanges Ca for K across the intestinal wall. It is slow-acting and it is not useful in the acute treatment of hyperkalemia.[135] Intravenous fluids should be considered in cases of volume depletion because they can improve renal perfusion and increase urinary K excretion.

Dialysis is the most effective means for removal of K. Hemodialysis is more effective than peritoneal dialysis and can reduce K levels by 1.0–1.2 mmol/L in the first 60 min if K-free dialysate is used.[148] Rebound hyperkalemia is a frequent phenomenon several hours posthemodialysis.

All patients who receive treatment for acute hyperkalemia should have close monitoring of plasma K levels, and appropriate measures should be taken to prevent the recurrence of hyperkalemia.

### *Chronic treatment of hyperkalemia*

The three main approaches to the chronic treatment of hyperkalemia are (1) removing drugs inducing hyperkalemia, (2) restriction in K intake, and (3) improving K removal from the body.

*Removing drugs inducing hyperkalemia*

The commonest preventable causes of hyperkalemia are medications, and most patients with hyperkalemia and estimated glomerular filtration rate (eGFR) >15 mL/min have drug-induced hyperkalemia. Extensive review of drug history is required to identify any medications interfering with the action of aldosterone or β-adrenergic agonists or insulin. Medications involved in the renin–angiotensin–aldosterone axis should be reviewed, such as direct renin antagonists, ACE inhibitors, angiotensin II receptor antagonists, and MC-RMR antagonists.

Also, nonselective β-blockers can contribute to hyperkalemia in patients on renal replacement therapy.

*Restriction in K intake*

Patients on dialysis should have restricted dietary K intake at 40–50 mmol or 1.5–2.0 g/day.[155]

*Improving K removal from body*

Patients on dialysis can develop increased plasma K levels during prolonged fasting due to low endogenous insulin levels. Patients on hemodialysis who fast in preparation for a diagnostic test or an operation should be treated with intravenous infusion of glucose and insulin to prevent hyperkalemia.[156]

Addition of thiazide or loop diuretics should be considered in selected patients to increase renal excretion of K.

Addition of laxatives should be considered to avoid constipation because uremic patients eliminate up to 25% of K intake via the GI tract.

## *References*


1. McKenna K, Thompson C. Osmoregulation in clinical disorders of thirst appreciation. *Clinical Endocrinology* 1998; 49(2): 139–52.
2. Verbalis JG. Disorders of body water homeostasis. *Best Practice & Research Clinical Endocrinology & Metabolism* 2003; 17(4): 471–503.
3. Reynolds RM, Seckl JR. Hyponatraemia for the clinical endocrinologist. *Clinical Endocrinology* 2005; **63**(4): 366–74.
4. Ishikawa SE, Schrier RW. Pathophysiological roles of arginine vasopressin and aquaporin-2 in impaired water excretion. *Clinical Endocrinology* 2003; **58**(1): 1–17.
5. Russell JA. Bench-to-bedside review: Vasopressin in the management of septic shock. *Critical Care* 2011; 15(4): 226.
6. Agre P, Preston GM, Smith BL, et al. Aquaporin CHIP: The archetypal molecular water channel. *The American Journal of Physiology* 1993; **265**(4 Pt 2): F463–76.
7. Verkman AS. Aquaporins in clinical medicine. *Annual Review of Medicine* 2012; **63**: 303–16.
8. Chen YC, Cadnapaphornchai MA, Schrier RW. Clinical update on renal aquaporins. *Biology of the Cell/Under the Auspices of the European Cell Biology Organization* 2005; 97(6): 357–71.
9. Nielsen S, Kwon TH, Christensen BM, et al. Physiology and pathophysiology of renal aquaporins. *Journal of the American Society of Nephrology: JASN* 1999; 10(3): 647–63.
10. Baylis PH, Thompson CJ. Osmoregulation of vasopressin secretion and thirst in health and disease. *Clinical Endocrinology* 1988; 29(5): 549–76.
11. Thompson CJ, Selby P, Baylis PH. Reproducibility of osmotic and nonosmotic tests of vasopressin secretion in men. *The American Journal of Physiology* 1991; **260**(3 Pt 2): R533–9.
12. Helderman JH, Vestal RE, Rowe JW, et al. The response of arginine vasopressin to intravenous ethanol and hypertonic saline in man: The impact of aging. *Journal of Gerontology* 1978; **33**(1): 39–47.
13. Stricker EM, Sved AF. Thirst. *Nutrition* 2000; **16**(10): 821–6.
14. Adrogue HJ, Madias NE. Hyponatremia. *The New England Journal of Medicine* 2000; **342**(21): 1581–9.
15. Upadhyay A, Jaber BL, Madias NE. Incidence and prevalence of hyponatremia. *The American Journal of Medicine* 2006; 119(7 Suppl 1): S30–5.

16. Hoorn EJ, Lindemans J, Zietse R. Development of severe hyponatraemia in hospitalized patients: Treatment-related risk factors and inadequate management. *Nephrology, Dialysis, Transplantation: Official Publication of the European Dialysis and Transplant Association – European Renal Association* 2006; **21**(1): 70–6.
17. Liamis G, Rodenburg EM, Hofman A, et al. Electrolyte disorders in community subjects: Prevalence and risk factors. *The American Journal of Medicine* 2013; **126**(3): 256–63.
18. Hawkins RC. Age and gender as risk factors for hyponatremia and hypernatremia. *Clinica Chimica Acta; International Journal of Clinical Chemistry* 2003; **337**(1–2): 169–72.
19. Miller M. Hyponatremia and arginine vasopressin dysregulation: Mechanisms, clinical consequences, and management. *Journal of the American Geriatrics Society* 2006; **54**(2): 345–53.
20. Gill G, Huda B, Boyd A, et al. Characteristics and mortality of severe hyponatraemia—a hospital-based study. *Clinical Endocrinology* 2006; **65**(2): 246–9.
21. Clayton JA, Le Jeune IR, Hall IP. Severe hyponatraemia in medical in-patients: Aetiology, assessment and outcome. *QJM: Monthly Journal of the Association of Physicians* 2006; **99**(8): 505–11.
22. Goldberg A, Hammerman H, Petcherski S, et al. Hyponatremia and long-term mortality in survivors of acute ST-elevation myocardial infarction. *Archives of Internal Medicine* 2006; **166**(7): 781–6.
23. Rusinaru D, Tribouilloy C, Berry C, et al. Relationship of serum sodium concentration to mortality in a wide spectrum of heart failure patients with preserved and with reduced ejection fraction: An individual patient data meta-analysis(dagger): Meta-Analysis Global Group in Chronic heart failure (MAGGIC). *European Journal of Heart Failure* 2012; **14**(10): 1139–46.
24. Gheorghiade M, Abraham WT, Albert NM, et al. Relationship between admission serum sodium concentration and clinical outcomes in patients hospitalized for heart failure: An analysis from the OPTIMIZE-HF registry. *European Heart Journal* 2007; **28**(8): 980–8.
25. Jenq CC, Tsai MH, Tian YC, et al. Serum sodium predicts prognosis in critically ill cirrhotic patients. *Journal of Clinical Gastroenterology* 2010; **44**(3): 220–6.
26. Doshi SM, Shah P, Lei X, Lahoti A, Salahudeen AK. Hyponatremia in hospitalized cancer patients and its impact on clinical outcomes. *American Journal of Kidney Diseases: The Official Journal of the National Kidney Foundation* 2012; **59**(2): 222–8.
27. Chawla A, Sterns RH, Nigwekar SU, et al. Mortality and serum sodium: Do patients die from or with hyponatremia? *Clinical Journal of the American Society of Nephrology: CJASN* 2011; **6**(5): 960–5.
28. Waikar SS, Mount DB, Curhan GC. Mortality after hospitalization with mild, moderate, and severe hyponatremia. *The American Journal of Medicine* 2009; **122**(9): 857–65.
29. Hoorn EJ, Zietse R. Hyponatremia and mortality: How innocent is the bystander? *Clinical Journal of the American Society of Nephrology: CJASN* 2011; **6**(5): 951–3.
30. Douglas I. Hyponatremia: Why it matters, how it presents, how we can manage it. *Cleveland Clinic Journal of Medicine* 2006; **73**(Suppl 3): S4–12.
31. Renneboog B, Musch W, Vandemergel X, et al. Mild chronic hyponatremia is associated with falls, unsteadiness, and attention deficits. *The American Journal of Medicine* 2006; **119**(1): 71. e1–8.
32. Hoorn EJ, Rivadeneira F, van Meurs JB, et al. Mild hyponatremia as a risk factor for fractures: The Rotterdam Study. *Journal of Bone and Mineral Research: The Official Journal of the American Society for Bone and Mineral Research* 2011; **26**(8): 1822–8.
33. Kinsella S, Moran S, Sullivan MO, et al. Hyponatremia independent of osteoporosis is associated with fracture occurrence. *Clinical Journal of the American Society Nephrology* 2010; **5**(2): 275–80.
34. Gankam Kengne F, Andres C, Sattar L, et al. Mild hyponatremia and risk of fracture in the ambulatory elderly. *QJM: Monthly Journal of the Association of Physicians* 2008; **101**(7): 583–8.
35. Verbalis JG, Barsony J, Sugimura Y, et al. Hyponatremia-induced osteoporosis. *Journal of Bone and Mineral Research: The Official Journal of the American Society for Bone and Mineral Research* 2010; 25(3): 554–63.
36. Fraser CL, Arieff AI. Epidemiology, pathophysiology, and management of hyponatremic encephalopathy. *The American Journal of Medicine* 1997; **102**(1): 67–77.
37. Fraser CL, Sarnacki P. Na+-K+-ATPase pump function in rat brain synaptosomes is different in males and females. *The American Journal of Physiology* 1989; **257**(2 Pt 1): E284–9.
38. Ayus JC, Wheeler JM, Arieff AI. Postoperative hyponatremic encephalopathy in menstruant women. *Annals of Internal Medicine* 1992; 117(11): 891–7.
39. Arieff AI. Influence of hypoxia and sex on hyponatremic encephalopathy. *The American Journal of Medicine* 2006; 119(7 Suppl 1): S59–64.
40. Hannon MJ, Thompson CJ. The syndrome of inappropriate antidiuretic hormone: Prevalence, causes and consequences. *European Journal of Endocrinology/European Federation of Endocrine Societies* 2010; **162**(Suppl 1): S5–12.
41. Hix JK, Silver S, Sterns RH. Diuretic-associated hyponatremia. *Seminars in Nephrology* 2011; **31**(6): 553–66.
42. Schrier RW. Vasopressin and aquaporin 2 in clinical disorders of water homeostasis. *Seminars in Nephrology* 2008; **28**(3): 289–96.

43. Hannon MJ, Finucane FM, Sherlock M, et al. Clinical review: Disorders of water homeostasis in neurosurgical patients. *The Journal of Clinical Endocrinology and Metabolism* 2012; 97(5): 1423–33.
44. Hannon MJ, Sherlock M, Thompson CJ. Pituitary dysfunction following traumatic brain injury or subarachnoid haemorrhage – in "Endocrine Management in the Intensive Care Unit". *Best Practice & Research Clinical Endocrinology & Metabolism* 2011; 25(5): 783–98.
45. Agha A, Rogers B, Mylotte D, et al. Neuroendocrine dysfunction in the acute phase of traumatic brain injury. *Clinical Endocrinology* 2004; 60(5): 584–91.
46. Diederich S, Franzen NF, Bahr V, et al. Severe hyponatremia due to hypopituitarism with adrenal insufficiency: Report on 28 cases. *European Journal of Endocrinology/European Federation of Endocrine Societies* 2003; 148(6): 609–17.
47. Erkut ZA, Pool C, Swaab DF. Glucocorticoids suppress corticotropin-releasing hormone and vasopressin expression in human hypothalamic neurons. *The Journal of Clinical Endocrinology and Metabolism* 1998; 83(6): 2066–73.
48. Chen YC, Cadnapaphornchai MA, Summer SN, et al. Molecular mechanisms of impaired urinary concentrating ability in glucocorticoid-deficient rats. *Journal of the American Society of Nephrology: JASN* 2005; 16(10): 2864–71.
49. Saito T, Ishikawa SE, Ando F, et al. Vasopressin-dependent upregulation of aquaporin-2 gene expression in glucocorticoid-deficient rats. *American Journal of Physiology Renal Physiology* 2000; 279(3): F502–8.
50. Wang W, Li C, Summer SN, et al. Molecular analysis of impaired urinary diluting capacity in glucocorticoid deficiency. *American Journal of Physiology Renal Physiology* 2006; 290(5): F1135–42.
51. Liamis G, Milionis HJ, Elisaf M. Endocrine disorders: Causes of hyponatremia not to neglect. *Annals of Medicine* 2011; 43(3): 179–87.
52. Chen YC, Cadnapaphornchai MA, Yang J, et al. Nonosmotic release of vasopressin and renal aquaporins in impaired urinary dilution in hypothyroidism. *American Journal of Physiology Renal Physiology* 2005; 289(4): F672–8.
53. Hanna FW, Scanlon MF. Hyponatraemia, hypothyroidism, and role of arginine-vasopressin. *Lancet* 1997; 350(9080): 755–6.
54. Thompson C, Berl T, Tejedor A, et al. Differential diagnosis of hyponatraemia. *Best Practice & Research Clinical Endocrinology & Metabolism* 2012; 26(Suppl 1): S7–15.
55. Ellison DH, Berl T. Clinical practice. The syndrome of inappropriate antidiuresis. *The New England Journal of Medicine* 2007; 356(20): 2064–72.
56. Robertson GL. Regulation of arginine vasopressin in the syndrome of inappropriate antidiuresis. *The American Journal of Medicine* 2006; 119(7 Suppl 1): S36–42.
57. Liu BA, Mittmann N, Knowles SR, et al. Hyponatremia and the syndrome of inappropriate secretion of antidiuretic hormone associated with the use of selective serotonin reuptake inhibitors: A review of spontaneous reports. *Canadian Medical Association Journal* 1996; 155(5): 519–27.
58. Kirchner V, Silver LE, Kelly CA. Selective serotonin reuptake inhibitors and hyponatraemia: Review and proposed mechanisms in the elderly. *Journal of Psychopharmacology* 1998; 12(4): 396–400.
59. Fabian TJ, Amico JA, Kroboth PD, et al. Paroxetine-induced hyponatremia in older adults: A 12-week prospective study. *Archives of Internal Medicine* 2004; 164(3): 327–32.
60. Movig KL, Leufkens HG, Lenderink AW, et al. Association between antidepressant drug use and hyponatraemia: A case-control study. *British Journal of Clinical Pharmacology* 2002; 53(4): 363–9.
61. Jacob S, Spinler SA. Hyponatremia associated with selective serotonin-reuptake inhibitors in older adults. *The Annals of Pharmacotherapy* 2006; 40(9): 1618–22.
62. Spigset O, Hedenmalm K. Hyponatraemia and the syndrome of inappropriate antidiuretic hormone secretion (SIADH) induced by psychotropic drugs. *Drug Safety* 1995; 12(3): 209–25.
63. Roxanas MG. Mirtazapine-induced hyponatraemia. *The Medical Journal of Australia* 2003; 179(8): 453–4.
64. Romero S, Pintor L, Serra M, et al. Syndrome of inappropriate secretion of antidiuretic hormone due to citalopram and venlafaxine. *General Hospital Psychiatry* 2007; 29(1): 81–4.
65. Wilkinson TJ, Begg EJ, Winter AC, et al. Incidence and risk factors for hyponatraemia following treatment with fluoxetine or paroxetine in elderly people. *British Journal of Clinical Pharmacology* 1999; 47(2): 211–17.
66. Dodd S, Malhi GS, Tiller J, et al. A consensus statement for safety monitoring guidelines of treatments for major depressive disorder. *The Australian and New Zealand Journal of Psychiatry* 2011; 45(9): 712–25.
67. Simmler LD, Hysek CM, Liechti ME. Sex differences in the effects of MDMA (ecstasy) on plasma copeptin in healthy subjects. *The Journal of Clinical Endocrinology and Metabolism* 2011; 96(9): 2844–50.
68. Campbell GA, Rosner MH. The agony of ecstasy: MDMA (3,4-methylenedioxymethamphetamine) and the kidney. *Clinical Journal of the American Society of Nephrology: CJASN* 2008; 3(6): 1852–60.
69. Cherney DZ, Davids MR, Halperin ML. Acute hyponatraemia and 'ecstasy': Insights from a quantitative and integrative analysis. *QJM: Monthly Journal of the Association of Physicians* 2002; 95(7): 475–83.
70. Musch W, Thimpont J, Vandervelde D, et al. Combined fractional excretion of sodium and urea better predicts

response to saline in hyponatremia than do usual clinical and biochemical parameters. *The American Journal of Medicine* 1995; 99(4): 348–55.
71. Katz MA. Hyperglycemia-induced hyponatremia—calculation of expected serum sodium depression. *The New England Journal of Medicine* 1973; **289**(16): 843–4.
72. Hillier TA, Abbott RD, Barrett EJ. Hyponatremia: Evaluating the correction factor for hyperglycemia. *The American Journal of Medicine* 1999; **106**(4): 399–403.
73. Imran S, Eva G, Christopher S, et al. Is specific gravity a good estimate of urine osmolality? *Journal of Clinical Laboratory Analysis* 2010; 24(6): 426–30.
74. de Buys Roessingh AS, Drukker A, Guignard JP. Dipstick measurements of urine specific gravity are unreliable. *Archives of Disease in Childhood* 2001; **85**(2): 155–7.
75. Milionis HJ, Liamis GL, Elisaf MS. The hyponatremic patient: A systematic approach to laboratory diagnosis. *Canadian Medical Association Journal* 2002; **166**(8): 1056–62.
76. Musch W, Verfaillie L, Decaux G. Age-related increase in plasma urea level and decrease in fractional urea excretion: Clinical application in the syndrome of inappropriate secretion of antidiuretic hormone. *Clinical Journal of the American Society of Nephrology: CJASN* 2006; **1**(5): 909–14.
77. Musch W, Decaux G. Utility and limitations of biochemical parameters in the evaluation of hyponatremia in the elderly. *International Urology and Nephrology* 2001; **32**(3): 475–93.
78. Decaux G, Musch W. Clinical laboratory evaluation of the syndrome of inappropriate secretion of antidiuretic hormone. *Clinical Journal of the American Society of Nephrology: CJASN* 2008; **3**(4): 1175–84.
79. Smith JC, Siddique H, Corrall RJ. Misinterpretation of serum cortisol in a patient with hyponatraemia. *British Medical Journal* 2004; **328**(7433): 215–16.
80. Musch W, Hedeshi A, Decaux G. Low sodium excretion in SIADH patients with low diuresis. *Nephron Physiology* 2004; **96**(1): P11–18.
81. Fenske W, Stork S, Koschker AC, et al. Value of fractional uric acid excretion in differential diagnosis of hyponatremic patients on diuretics. *The Journal of Clinical Endocrinology and Metabolism* 2008; **93**(8): 2991–7.
82. Fenske W, Stork S, Blechschmidt A, et al. Copeptin in the differential diagnosis of hyponatremia. *The Journal of Clinical Endocrinology and Metabolism* 2009; **94**(1): 123–9.
83. Musch W, Decaux G. Treating the syndrome of inappropriate ADH secretion with isotonic saline. *QJM: Monthly Journal of the Association of Physicians* 1998; **91**(11): 749–53.
84. Peri A, Combe C. Considerations regarding the management of hyponatraemia secondary to SIADH. *Best Practice & Research Clinical Endocrinology & Metabolism* 2012; **26**(Suppl 1): S16–26.
85. Murase T, Sugimura Y, Takefuji S, et al. Mechanisms and therapy of osmotic demyelination. *The American Journal of Medicine* 2006; **119**(7 Suppl 1): S69–73.
86. Verbalis JG, Goldsmith SR, Greenberg A, et al. Hyponatremia treatment guidelines 2007: Expert panel recommendations. *The American Journal of Medicine* 2007; **120**(11 Suppl 1): S1–21.
87. Sherlock M, Thompson CJ. The syndrome of inappropriate antidiuretic hormone: Current and future management options. *European Journal of Endocrinology/ European Federation of Endocrine Societies* 2010; **162**(Suppl 1): S13–18.
88. Schrier RW, Gross P, Gheorghiade M, et al. Tolvaptan, a selective oral vasopressin V2-receptor antagonist, for hyponatremia. *The New England Journal of Medicine* 2006; **355**(20): 2099–112.
89. Hoorn EJ, Bouloux PM, Burst V. Perspectives on the management of hyponatraemia secondary to SIADH across Europe. *Best Practice & Research Clinical Endocrinology & Metabolism* 2012; **26**(Suppl 1): S27–32.
90. Furst H, Hallows KR, Post J, et al. The urine/plasma electrolyte ratio: A predictive guide to water restriction. *The American Journal of the Medical Sciences* 2000; **319**(4): 240–4.
91. Snyder NA, Feigal DW, Arieff AI. Hypernatremia in elderly patients. A heterogeneous, morbid, and iatrogenic entity. *Annals of Internal Medicine* 1987; **107**(3): 309–19.
92. Palevsky PM, Bhagrath R, Greenberg A. Hypernatremia in hospitalized patients. *Annals of Internal Medicine* 1996; **124**(2): 197–203.
93. Adrogue HJ, Madias NE. Hypernatremia. *The New England Journal of Medicine* 2000; **342**(20): 1493–9.
94. Lindner G, Funk GC, Schwarz C, et al. Hypernatremia in the critically ill is an independent risk factor for mortality. *American Journal of Kidney Diseases: The Official Journal of the National Kidney Foundation* 2007; **50**(6): 952–7.
95. Liamis G, Tsimihodimos V, Doumas M, et al. Clinical and laboratory characteristics of hypernatraemia in an internal medicine clinic. *Nephrology, Dialysis, Transplantation: Official Publication of the European Dialysis and Transplant Association – European Renal Association* 2008; **23**(1): 136–43.
96. Alshayeb HM, Showkat A, Babar F, et al. Severe hypernatremia correction rate and mortality in hospitalized patients. *The American Journal of the Medical Sciences* 2011; **341**(5): 356–60.
97. Lindner G, Funk GC. Hypernatremia in critically ill patients. *Journal of Critical Care* 2012.
98. Funk GC, Lindner G, Druml W, et al. Incidence and prognosis of dysnatremias present on ICU admission. *Intensive Care Medicine* 2010; **36**(2): 304–11.

99. Agrawal V, Agarwal M, Joshi SR, et al. Hyponatremia and hypernatremia: Disorders of water balance. *The Journal of the Association of Physicians of India* 2008; 56: 956–64.
100. Robertson GL. Physiology of ADH secretion. *Kidney International Supplement* 1987; 21: S20–6.
101. Gregoire JR. Adjustment of the osmostat in primary aldosteronism. *Mayo Clinic Proceedings* 1994; 69(11): 1108–10.
102. Torpy DJ, Mullen N, Ilias I, et al. Association of hypertension and hypokalemia with Cushing's syndrome caused by ectopic ACTH secretion: A series of 58 cases. *Annals of the New York Academy of Sciences* 2002; 970: 134–44.
103. Kumar S, Berl T. Sodium. *Lancet* 1998; 352(9123): 220–8.
104. Kahn A, Brachet E, Blum D. Controlled fall in natremia and risk of seizures in hypertonic dehydration. *Intensive Care Medicine* 1979; 5(1): 27–31.
105. Hoorn EJ, Betjes MG, Weigel J, et al. Hypernatraemia in critically ill patients: Too little water and too much salt. *Nephrology, Dialysis, Transplantation: Official Publication of the European Dialysis and Transplant Association – European Renal Association* 2008; 23(5): 1562–8.
106. Adrogue HJ, Madias NE. Aiding fluid prescription for the dysnatremias. *Intensive Care Medicine* 1997; 23(3): 309–16.
107. Liamis G, Kalogirou M, Saugos V, et al. Therapeutic approach in patients with dysnatraemias. *Nephrology, Dialysis, Transplantation: Official Publication of the European Dialysis and Transplant Association – European Renal Association* 2006; 21(6): 1564–9.
108. Barsoum NR, Levine BS. Current prescriptions for the correction of hyponatraemia and hypernatraemia: Are they too simple? *Nephrology, Dialysis, Transplantation: Official Publication of the European Dialysis and Transplant Association – European Renal Association* 2002; 17(7): 1176–80.
109. Nguyen MK, Kurtz I. A new quantitative approach to the treatment of the dysnatremias. *Clinical and Experimental Nephrology* 2003; 7(2): 125–37.
110. Lindner G, Schwarz C, Kneidinger N, et al. Can we really predict the change in serum sodium levels? An analysis of currently proposed formulae in hypernatraemic patients. *Nephrology, Dialysis, Transplantation: Official Publication of the European Dialysis and Transplant Association – European Renal Association* 2008; 23(11): 3501–8.
111. Rastegar A, Soleimani M. Hypokalaemia and hyperkalaemia. *Postgraduate Medical Journal* 2001; 77(914): 759–64.
112. Unwin RJ, Luft FC, Shirley DG. Pathophysiology and management of hypokalemia: A clinical perspective. *Nature Reviews Nephrology* 2011; 7(2): 75–84.
113. Gennari FJ. Hypokalemia. *The New England Journal of Medicine* 1998; 339(7): 451–8.
114. Brown MJ, Brown DC, Murphy MB. Hypokalemia from beta2-receptor stimulation by circulating epinephrine. *The New England Journal of Medicine* 1983; 309(23): 1414–19.
115. Aronson PS, Giebisch G. Effects of pH on potassium: New explanations for old observations. *Journal of the American Society of Nephrology: JASN* 2011; 22(11): 1981–9.
116. Hoskote SS, Joshi SR, Ghosh AK. Disorders of potassium homeostasis: Pathophysiology and management. *The Journal of the Association of Physicians of India* 2008; 56: 685–93.
117. Huang CL, Kuo E. Mechanism of hypokalemia in magnesium deficiency. *Journal of the American Society of Nephrology* 2007; 18(10): 2649–52.
118. Halperin ML, Kamel KS. Potassium. *Lancet* 1998; 352(9122): 135–40.
119. Paice BJ, Paterson KR, Onyanga-Omara F, et al. Record linkage study of hypokalaemia in hospitalized patients. *Postgraduate Medical Journal* 1986; 62(725): 187–91.
120. Crop MJ, Hoorn EJ, Lindemans J, Zietse R. Hypokalaemia and subsequent hyperkalaemia in hospitalized patients. *Nephrology, Dialysis, Transplantation: Official Publication of the European Dialysis and Transplant Association – European Renal Association* 2007; 22(12): 3471–7.
121. Hawkins RC. Gender and age as risk factors for hypokalemia and hyperkalemia in a multiethnic Asian population. *Clinica Chimica Acta; International Journal of Clinical Chemistry* 2003; 331(1–2): 171–2.
122. Lin SH, Lin YF, Chen DT, et al. Laboratory tests to determine the cause of hypokalemia and paralysis. *Archives of Internal Medicine* 2004; 164(14): 1561–6.
123. Lin SH, Lin YF, Halperin ML. Hypokalaemia and paralysis. *QJM: Monthly Journal of the Association of Physicians* 2001; 94(3): 133–9.
124. Melcescu E, Phillips J, Moll G, et al. 11Beta-hydroxylase deficiency and other syndromes of mineralocorticoid excess as a rare cause of endocrine hypertension. *Hormone and Metabolic Research* 2012; 44(12): 867–78.
125. Hammer F, Stewart PM. Cortisol metabolism in hypertension. *Best Practice & Research Clinical Endocrinology & Metabolism* 2006; 20(3): 337–53.
126. Farese RV, Jr., Biglieri EG, Shackleton CH, et al. Licorice-induced hypermineralocorticoidism. *The New England Journal of Medicine* 1991; 325(17): 1223–7.
127. Shaer AJ. Inherited primary renal tubular hypokalemic alkalosis: A review of Gitelman and Bartter syndromes. *The American Journal of the Medical Sciences* 2001; 322(6): 316–32.
128. Unwin RJ, Capasso G. Bartter's and Gitelman's syndromes: Their relationship to the actions of loop and thiazide diuretics. *Current Opinion in Pharmacology* 2006; 6(2): 208–13.

129. Godek SF, Bartolozzi AR, Godek JJ. Sweat rate and fluid turnover in American football players compared with runners in a hot and humid environment. *British Journal of Sports Medicine* 2005; **39**(4): 205–11; discussion: 11.
130. Groeneveld JH, Sijpkens YW, Lin SH, et al. An approach to the patient with severe hypokalaemia: The potassium quiz. *QJM: Monthly Journal of the Association of Physicians* 2005; **98**(4): 305–16.
131. Colussi G, Bettinelli A, Tedeschi S, et al. A thiazide test for the diagnosis of renal tubular hypokalemic disorders. *Clinical Journal of the American Society of Nephrology: CJASN* 2007; **2**(3): 454–60.
132. Whang R, Whang DD, Ryan MP. Refractory potassium repletion. A consequence of magnesium deficiency. *Archives of Internal Medicine* 1992; **152**(1): 40–5.
133. Kim GH, Han JS. Therapeutic approach to hypokalemia. *Nephron* 2002; **92**(Suppl 1): 28–32.
134. Cohn JN, Kowey PR, Whelton PK, et al. New guidelines for potassium replacement in clinical practice: A contemporary review by the National Council on Potassium in Clinical Practice. *Archives of Internal Medicine* 2000; **160**(16): 2429–36.
135. Alfonzo AV, Isles C, Geddes C, et al. Potassium disorders—clinical spectrum and emergency management. *Resuscitation* 2006; **70**(1): 10–25.
136. Paice B, Gray JM, McBride D, et al. Hyperkalaemia in patients in hospital. *British Medical Journal (Clinical Research Edition)* 1983; **286**(6372): 1189–92.
137. Stevens MS, Dunlay RW. Hyperkalemia in hospitalized patients. *International Urology and Nephrology* 2000; **32**(2): 177–80.
138. Slovis C, Jenkins R. ABC of clinical electrocardiography: Conditions not primarily affecting the heart. *British Medical Journal* 2002; **324**(7349): 1320–3.
139. Montague BT, Ouellette JR, Buller GK. Retrospective review of the frequency of ECG changes in hyperkalemia. *Clinical Journal of the American Society of Nephrology: CJASN* 2008; **3**(2): 324–30.
140. Acker CG, Johnson JP, Palevsky PM, et al. Hyperkalemia in hospitalized patients: Causes, adequacy of treatment, and results of an attempt to improve physician compliance with published therapy guidelines. *Archives of Internal Medicine* 1998; **158**(8): 917–24.
141. Sevastos N, Theodossiades G, Archimandritis AJ. Pseudohyperkalemia in serum: A new insight into an old phenomenon. *Clinical Medicine & Research* 2008; **6**(1): 30–2.
142. Smellie WS. Spurious hyperkalaemia. *British Medical Journal* 2007; **334**(7595): 693–5.
143. Oster JR, Singer I, Fishman LM. Heparin-induced aldosterone suppression and hyperkalemia. *The American Journal of Medicine* 1995; **98**(6): 575–86.
144. Thomas CM, Thomas J, Smeeton F, et al. Heparin-induced hyperkalemia. *Diabetes Research and Clinical Practice* 2008; **80**(2): e7–8.
145. Grande Villoria J, Macias Nunez JF, Miralles JM, et al. Hyporeninemic hypoaldosteronism in diabetic patients with chronic renal failure. *American Journal of Nephrology* 1988; **8**(2): 127–37.
146. Geller DS. Mineralocorticoid resistance. *Clinical Endocrinology* 2005; **62**(5): 513–20.
147. Perazella MA. Trimethoprim-induced hyperkalaemia: Clinical data, mechanism, prevention and management. *Drug safety: An International Journal of Medical Toxicology and Drug Experience* 2000; **22**(3): 227–36.
148. Kim HJ, Han SW. Therapeutic approach to hyperkalemia. *Nephron* 2002; **92**(Suppl 1): 33–40.
149. Ethier JH, Kamel KS, Magner PO, et al. The transtubular potassium concentration in patients with hypokalemia and hyperkalemia. *American Journal of Kidney Diseases: The Official Journal of the National Kidney Foundation* 1990; **15**(4): 309–15.
150. Hollander-Rodriguez JC, Calvert JF, Jr. Hyperkalemia. *American Family Physician* 2006; **73**(2): 283–90.
151. Allon M, Copkney C. Albuterol and insulin for treatment of hyperkalemia in hemodialysis patients. *Kidney International* 1990; **38**(5): 869–72.
152. Ahee P, Crowe AV. The management of hyperkalaemia in the emergency department. *Journal of Accident & Emergency Medicine* 2000; **17**(3): 188–91.
153. Lens XM, Montoliu J, Cases A, et al. Treatment of hyperkalaemia in renal failure: Salbutamol v. insulin. *Nephrology, Dialysis, Transplantation: Official Publication of the European Dialysis and Transplant Association – European Renal Association* 1989; 4(3): 228–32.
154. Kamel KS, Wei C. Controversial issues in the treatment of hyperkalaemia. *Nephrology, Dialysis, Transplantation: Official Publication of the European Dialysis and Transplant Association – European Renal Association* 2003; **18**(11): 2215–18.
155. Allon M. Hyperkalemia in end-stage renal disease: Mechanisms and management. *Journal of the American Society of Nephrology: JASN* 1995; 6(4): 1134–42.
156. Allon M. Treatment and prevention of hyperkalemia in end-stage renal disease. *Kidney International* 1993; 43(6): 1197–209.

# 21

# Endocrine hypertension

*Frances McManus, John M. Connell, Marie Freel*

## *Introduction*

Hypertension is well recognized as an important risk factor for the development of cardiovascular disease. This relationship has been further highlighted by a recent meta-analysis demonstrating that hypertension accounts for more than 7 million excess deaths per year worldwide.[1] The majority (>90%) of cases of hypertension have no clear underlying cause and are due to a combination of genetic and environmental factors, termed "essential" or "primary" hypertension. A significant number of endocrine conditions, including acromegaly, primary hyperparathyroidism, and hyperthyroidism, are associated with hypertension, but the underlying mechanisms in these circumstances are unclear.

In contrast, there are several examples of endocrine disease in which hypertension features prominently as a direct result of hormonal abnormalities. In particular, excess production of aldosterone (primary aldosteronism [PA]) is now accepted to be the commonest cause of secondary hypertension, highlighting the importance of endocrine disease in this disorder. This chapter focuses on PA and other diseases of the endocrine system that are directly associated with high blood pressure.

## *Mineralocorticoid hypertension (see Chapter 10)*

The case study involved a 33-year-old man who was referred to a hypertension clinic with a 2-year history of poorly controlled hypertension despite good compliance with three antihypertensive agents (bisoprolol, 10 mg daily; amlodipine, 10 mg daily; and ramipril, 10 mg daily). He was otherwise well with no significant past medical history and no family history of hypertension.

At the clinic, he was lean, with a body mass index (BMI) of 24 kg/m$^2$. Blood pressure was 148/110 mm/Hg supine. Serum potassium was low at 2.9 mmol/L (normal range, 3.5–5 mmol/L).

Given his young age and lack of risk factors, he was screened for secondary causes of hypertension. The presence of hypokalemia increased clinical suspicion of PA, and an aldosterone-to-renin ratio (ARR) was measured. Plasma aldosterone was 650 pmol/L (100–400 pmol/L) and plasma renin (as plasma renin concentration [PRC]) was 1.2 mIU/L (0–40 mIU/L), giving an ARR of 542 (>35 suspicious).

His medications were discontinued, and he was commenced on doxazosin 16 mg daily and verapamil SR 240 mg daily as well as potassium supplementation to allow further evaluation of his aldosterone status. A repeat ARR remained elevated, and a saline suppression test demonstrated a baseline aldosterone of 1100 pmol/L that failed to suppress significantly after 2 L of intravenous aldosterone (810 pmol/L). Subsequent adrenal computed tomography (CT) demonstrated a 1.5-cm left-sided adrenal adenoma (Figure 21.1). He underwent a laparoscopic adrenalectomy. One year after surgery, his blood pressure was 126/74 mm/Hg on no medications and plasma potassium was 5 mmol/L.

## *Background*

Although several corticosteroids produced by the adrenal gland have mineralocorticoid function (Figure 21.2), aldosterone is the most potent and predominant human mineralocorticoid. Aldosterone binds to the mineralocorticoid receptor (MR), a nuclear hormone receptor, and causes it to translocate to the nucleus, interact with the respective response elements, and induce a change in transcriptional activity that leads to an increase in activity of the epithelial sodium channel in the distal convoluted tubule (DCT) (Figure 21.3).[2] Excess mineralocorticoid results in retention of sodium chloride and water, with obligate loss of potassium and hydrogen ions to maintain electrical neutrality. The resultant clinical picture is of hypertension, metabolic alkalosis, and hypokalemia.

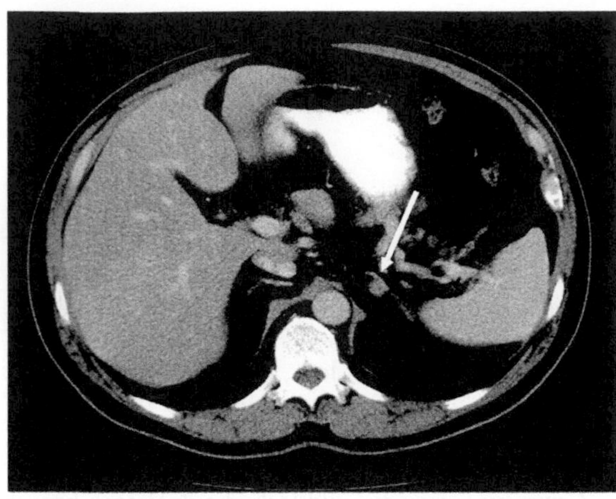

***Figure 21.1***
*CT of abdomen demonstrating a small left-sided adrenal adenoma (arrow).*

The most common cause of mineralocorticoid hypertension is autonomous production of aldosterone (PA) that can arise from many pathological mechanisms. The incidence of PA in general, and the proportion of each subtype, varies according to the population studied. In a European population, PA accounts for 5%–15% of cases of hypertension.[3,4] More rarely, mineralocorticoid hypertension can be caused by inappropriate activation of the MR by alternative ligands, or by abnormal activation of aldosterone-induced proteins downstream to the receptor.

## *Consequences of excess aldosterone: cardiovascular system*

The consequences of excess aldosterone production on epithelial tissue are well recognized (e.g., electrolyte abnormalities, and hypertension). However, it is less well recognized that excess aldosterone is associated with increased cardiovascular morbidity. Animal models of aldosterone excess have been shown to develop cardiac, renal, and cerebrovascular damage in the context of a high-salt diet.[5] This effect has been confirmed in patients with PA who have been shown to develop

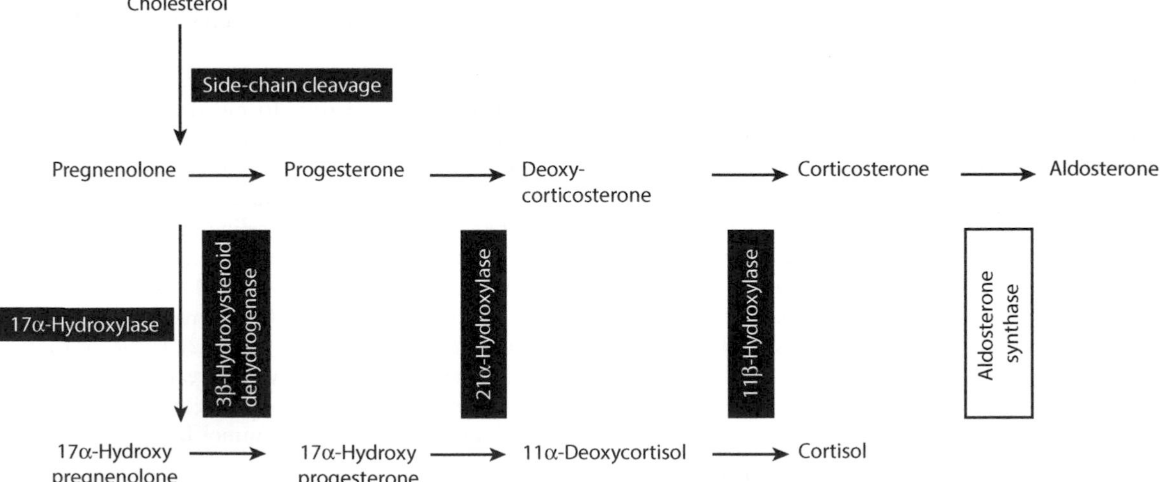


***Figure 21.2***
*Adrenal glucocorticoid and mineralocorticoid pathways. Aldosterone synthase is expressed only in adrenal glomerulosa cells. Although both 11β-hydroxylase and aldosterone synthase can undertake the 11-hydroxylation of deoxycorticosterone and 11-deoxycortisol, only aldosterone synthase can undertake the 18-hydroxylation and 18-methyloxidation that are the final rate-limiting steps in the synthesis of aldosterone.*

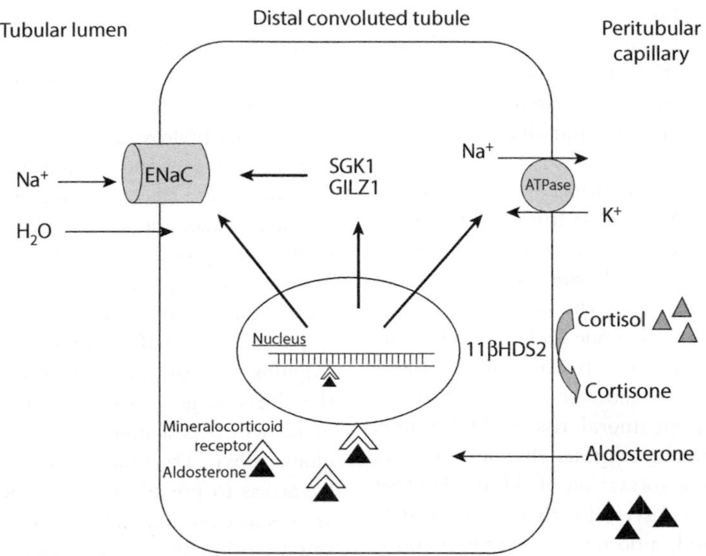


***Figure 21.3***
*Classical genomic action of aldosterone. Aldosterone binds to the MR (MR is protected from the alternative ligand cortisol by the enzyme 11βHSD2), and the hormone–receptor complex is translocated to the nucleus where it binds to DNA, resulting in increased transcription of aldosterone-induced proteins. These proteins include the relevant ion channels themselves (ENaC, $Na^+$–$K^+$-ATPase) and various proteins that modulate and prolong the action of ENaC. For example, serum and glucocorticoid-induced kinase-1 (SGK1) and glucocorticoid-induced leucine zipper protein-1 (GILZ1) act to inhibit the ENaC regulatory complex that, in a basal state, promotes the degradation of ENaC. (From Soundararajan R et al.,* J Biol Chem, *285, 30363–9, 2010.)*

more cardiovascular complications that essential hypertensive patients matched for clinical parameters, including blood pressure.[6] Further evidence exists for the detrimental effect of aldosterone, even where aldosterone is elevated but remains in the normal range. For instance, data from the Framingham cohort demonstrated increasing levels of plasma aldosterone and increased ratio of aldosterone to renin, although below the criteria for the diagnosis of PA, are associated with increased risk of future hypertension.[7] Finally, blockade of the MR is associated with reduced mortality in the context of heart failure[8] and after myocardial infarction.[9]

A variety of mechanisms have been proposed to explain the cardiovascular consequences of excess aldosterone, including stimulation of collagen, promotion of vascular remodeling, and activation of macrophages and other proinflammatory humeral factors. A proposed link between the metabolic syndrome and excess aldosterone has also been suggested to contribute to excess cardiovascular damage. The hypokalemia sometimes observed in the context of aldosterone excess is a possible linking mechanism, potentially leading to a blunted insulin response, but the evidence for this relationship is inconsistent.[10,11]

Regardless of the mechanism, both animal and human studies are consistent in the fact that there appears to be a synergy between elevated aldosterone and a high-salt diet. In fact, many experimental models only demonstrated the harmful effects of aldosterone excess in the presence of excess salt intake. Therefore, although aldosterone is an important factor in the development of hypertension and other adverse cardiovascular phenotypes, the influence of environmental factors is also crucial.

# *Causes of PA*

## *Sporadic PA*

The relative prevalence of causes of PA varies by geographical location, but the majority are sporadic, regardless of the population studies. In a Caucasian population, the most common cause of sporadic PA is bilateral adrenal hyperplasia, accounting for approximately 60%, whereas an aldosterone-producing adenoma accounts for 35% of patients with PA. In contrast, in a Japanese cohort, aldosterone-producing adenoma (APA) accounts for the majority of PA cases[12] (about 80%).

The etiology of these conditions remains largely unknown, and whether APAs arise from nodular adrenal glands or whether the two conditions are independent is a matter of much debate. However, it has been shown that tissue around the resected adenoma differs from normal adrenal tissue and has undergone remodeling with reduced vascularization and zona glomerulosa hyperplasia.[13] In contrast, a comparison of the transcriptome of peritumoral tissue, APA tissue, and normal adrenal tissue suggests that it is not an intermediate step in the formation of APAs. Another interesting phenomenon observed is that, in contrast to what would be expected, aldosterone synthase expression elsewhere in the adrenal gland is not suppressed and indeed is persistently expressed in aldosterone-producing cell clusters, sometimes quite distant to the adenoma.[13,14]

A significant advance in the understanding of the pathogenesis of APAs was made in the identification of the genetic defect in familial hyperaldosteronism type III (FHA 3; see below).[15] The discovery that somatic mutations in a gene encoding a potassium channel (KCNJ5) is present in around one-third of sporadic APAs[16,17] provides fertile ground for further investigation. This discovery builds on work that has revealed the role of TWIK-related acid-sensitive $K^+$ (TASK) channels in the regulation of aldosterone secretion. TASK channels are two-pore, four-transmembrane domain potassium channels. A TASK subunit knockout mouse exhibited features of autonomous aldosterone production.[18]

Elimination of functional TASK channels caused the membrane potential of the glomerulosa cells to be significantly more depolarized, and it is proposed that this leads to continuous calcium channel activity and increased sensitivity to angiotensin II and abnormal adrenal cortex zonation, that is, ectopic expression of aldosterone synthase in the high-capacity fasciculata layer.[19] Despite these advances, there remain many unanswered questions around the sequence of pathological events that lead to PA, where aldosterone production is independent of the renin–angiotensin system.

### Familial syndromes

Familial syndromes are a rare cause of PA. However, their etiology gives insight into the control and regulation of aldosterone in both health and disease.

#### FHA 1 (glucocorticoid-remediable aldosteronism [GRA])

GRA is an autosomal dominant, monogenic disorder caused by a hybrid gene comprising the regulatory element of 11β-hydroxylase, which catalyzes the final steps of cortisol synthesis, and it is normally expressed in the zona fasciculata, and the coding region of aldosterone synthase, which catalyzes the final steps of aldosterone production in the zona glomerulosa. This gives rise to a phenotype of early onset hypertension and mineralocorticoid excess.[20] Aldosterone is produced in response to adrenocorticotropic hormone (ACTH) rather than its usual principal trophins potassium and angiotensin II; but importantly, the chimeric gene is expressed ectopically in the fasciculata, which is a much higher output system than the glomerulosa. This allows the gene product inappropriate access to greater quantities of 11-deoxycorticosterone as a substrate for substantial aldosterone production. Importantly, therefore, it is not only that the gene is under regulation by ACTH that produces a state of mineralocorticoid excess but also the aberrant locus of enzyme expression and structure of the gland that causes dysregulated corticosteroid production, thus highlighting the necessity of strict anatomical and functional zonation.

#### FHA 2

FHA 2 is also an autosomal dominant disorder leading to clustering of PA within families. Although the gene defect causing FHA 2 has not been discovered, linkage analysis of affected families has suggested an association between markers within cytogenetic band 7p22 and this phenotype.[21] It is currently diagnosed if patients have at least two relatives with hyperaldosteronism and screening for FHA 1 (GRA) is negative.

#### FHA 3 (KCNJ5)

FHA 3 has recently been characterized in a single affected family where three members had severe, early onset hypertension and massive bilateral adrenal hyperplasia. The discovery that germline mutations in the KCNJ5 gene lead to autosomal dominant hyperaldosteronism has provided a clear genetic cause of this condition in a small cohort of patients. More importantly, as discussed above, it has provided novel mechanistic insight into the normal control of aldosterone and possible pathogenic mechanism in patients with nonfamilial APAs.

## PA: Approach to diagnosis

Because PA is a relatively common secondary cause of hypertension, with excess cardiovascular mortality compared with hypertensive controls and specific management issues, there is a clear case for investigation of hypertensive patients at high risk. However, the diagnosis of PA can cause confusion because there are few specific clinical symptoms and the biochemical tests can be obscured by confounding factors. The Endocrine Society's recently published guidelines[22] suggest screening for PA using simultaneous measurements of renin and aldosterone (to give the ARR) in patients with moderate to severe or resistant hypertension, or otherwise felt to be at high risk, as shown in Figure 21.4. If this initial test if positive, confirmatory testing followed by the subtype diagnosis should proceed.

### *Screening test*

As can be seen from the illustrative case, the initial screening test of ARR can be performed without the need for stopping antihypertensive medication in patients with severe hypertension (with the exceptions of spironolactone, eplerenone, and amiloride) because the likely effects of these agents on renin and aldosterone measurements (Table 21.1) can be allowed for. It should be measured on an unrestricted sodium intake, which should not require adjustment from normal for the majority of patients.

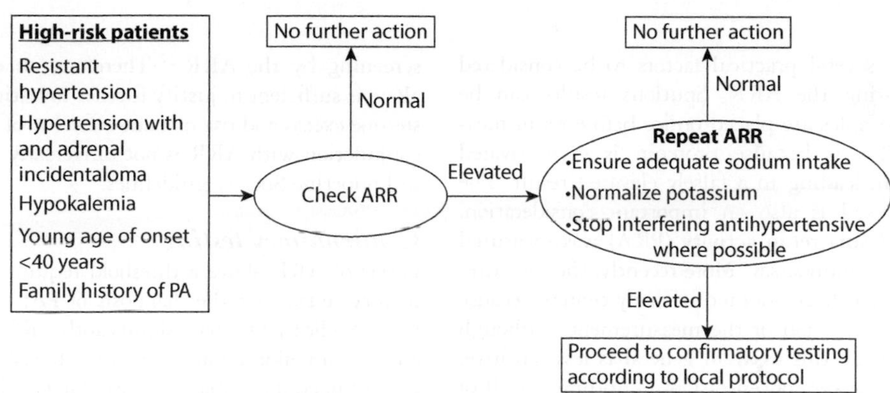


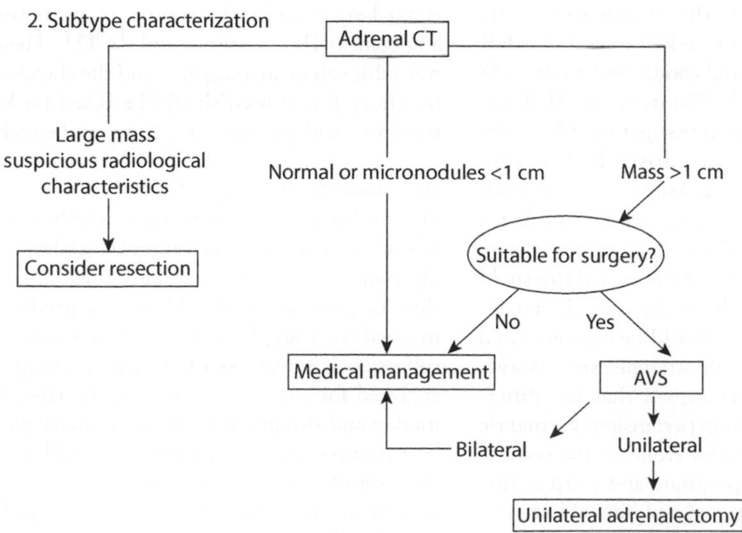


***Figure 21.4***
*Suggested algorithm for the investigation and management of PA. ARR, aldosterone-to-renin ratio; AVS, adrenal vein sampling.*

| Drug | Effect on plasma renin | Effect on ARR |
|---|---|---|
| β blockers | Reduce | Increase |
| Diuretic | Increase | Reduce |
| ACE inhibitors | Increase | Reduce |
| ARB | Increase | Reduce |
| Calcium channel blockers | Increase/none | Reduce/none |
| Mineralocorticoid receptor antagonists | Increase | Increase |
| Direct renin inhibitors | PRA: reduced<br>PRC: increased | Increased<br>Reduced |

***Table 21.1***
*Response of ARR to commonly used antihypertensives.*

There are several practical factors to be considered when measuring the ARR. Spurious results can be obtained if samples are placed on ice before renin measurement. This is because prorenin is cryoactivated to form renin, leading to a falsely elevated result. The renin assay used is also an important consideration. Previously, plasma renin activity (PRA) was measured using a radioimmunoassay. More recently, the measurement of PRC has been adopted in many centers because this allows automation of the measurement. Although more economical, this assay in general is less sensitive, particularly at lower concentrations.[23] Adding cut-off of minimum plasma aldosterone concentration before further confirmatory testing has been proposed to minimize false-positive results; however, this is not universally accepted. The cut-off values for aldosterone and ARR are dependent on local assays and conditions: a ratio >35 (renin as PRC in μU/mL) and >750 (renin as PRA ng/mL/h) should stimulate further investigation. One criticism of the ARR is that it is often driven by low-renin levels rather than high plasma aldosterone, a criticism that has led to debate as to how (or indeed if) some forms of PA differ from "low-renin" essential hypertension. Therefore, it has been proposed that a minimal threshold of plasma aldosterone (>15 ng/dL or 416 pmol/L) in conjunction with an elevated ARR should be demonstrated before further investigation for aldosterone excess is warranted.[24] However, it could be argued that the difference between PA and low-renin hypertension is semantic and that a "normal" plasma aldosterone in the context of a suppressed renin is in appropriate and justifies further investigation. Moreover, use of a plasma aldosterone cut-off may lower the sensitivity of the ARR to detect PA given that, in at least one study, plasma aldosterone levels of <15 ng/dL (416 pmol/L) were found in more than a third of patients confirmed to have PA after initial screening by the ARR.[25] Therefore, an elevated ARR alone is sufficient to justify further investigation of aldosterone excess and use of a cut-off value of aldosterone in conjunction with ARR is not universally recommended in Endocrine Society guidelines.

## *Confirmatory testing*

Levels of ARR above a threshold require further confirmatory testing for the diagnosis of PA; to perform this test, medications that significantly affect the renin–angiotensin–aldosterone system (RAAS) should be discontinued if possible as occurred in our illustrative case. The purpose of the confirmatory test is to establish autonomous secretion of aldosterone, meaning that aldosterone is no longer under the control of its normal trophins, angiotensin II, potassium, and ACTH. There are several ways this can be investigated, and the choice of which confirmatory test is used should be based on local practice, resources, and patients' compliance and suitability.

### *Oral sodium loading test*

Oral sodium intake is increased (with sodium chloride tablet if necessary) to >200 mmol (6 g)/day, for 3 days. The high-salt diet can increase kaliuresis and hypokalemia; therefore, potassium should be measured daily and normalized with supplementation, if necessary. A 24-h urine collection is undertaken from the morning of day 3 and analyzed for sodium (to ensure compliance with sodium intake) and urinary aldosterone. Urinary aldosterone can be measured by radioimmunoassay (aldosterone 18-oxo-glucuronide), but this measurement is less accurate than measuring aldosterone metabolites by liquid or gas chromatography and tandem mass spectroscopy, a method that is becoming more widely available. Autonomous secretion of aldosterone is confirmed if urinary aldosterone excretion exceeds 33 nmol/day (12 μg/24 h).

This test is of limited value in patients with renal disease, because aldosterone 18-oxo-glucuronide is a renal metabolite, and its excretion may not rise in patients with renal disease. However, the main limitation of this test is the inherent inaccuracies of 24-h urine collections in most patients.

### *Intravenous saline infusion test*

In this test, 2 L of 0.9% sodium chloride solution is infused intravenously over 4 h into the recumbent patient, with monitoring of blood pressure and heart rate throughout. Again, potassium must be corrected before the start of this procedure. After 4 h, blood is drawn for measurement of plasma aldosterone. Levels <139 pmol/L (5 ng/dL) make PA less likely, values between 139 and 277 pmol/L (5 and 10 ng/dL) are indeterminate, and levels >277 pmol/L (10 ng/dL) make a diagnosis of PA highly likely. The main disadvantage of this test is the volume of intravenous fluid infused, which may be dangerous in patients with cardiac failure. This is the confirmatory test of choice in our center and clearly demonstrated persistent aldosterone production in the case at the beginning of the chapter.

### *Fludrocortisone suppression test*

Fludrocortisone acetate (0.1 mg every 6 h) is administered for 4 days, and in addition, the oral sodium intake is maintained at an intake of >200 mmol/day using sodium chloride supplementation. As in all cases, potassium is monitored regularly and supplemented as required. Plasma renin should be suppressed, and failure to suppress the upright (10 a.m.) aldosterone at day 4 to <166 pmol/L (6 ng/dL) on day 4 confirms the diagnosis of PA. To exclude a confounding effect of ACTH stimulation on aldosterone secretion, it is suggested that plasma cortisol measured at 10 a.m. should be lower than the 7 a.m. level. Although the fludrocortisone suppression test is considered by some to be the most sensitive of the confirmatory tests, it has several disadvantages. There is a significant risk of hypokalemia and consequent dysrhythmia; as such, its use should be restricted to centers with expertise and facilities to cope with complications. In light of this, most centers undertake this test as an inpatient, which has cost and resource implications.

### *Captopril challenge*

The captopril challenge consists of measurement of plasma renin and aldosterone before and 2 h after a single dose of captopril (25 mg). This would normally be expected to suppress aldosterone by >30%, but in PA, aldosterone will remain high. However, this test has been reported to be less sensitive than salt suppression methods; thus, it is rarely used.

## *Subtype characterization of PA: Further tests*

Having confirmed autonomous secretion of aldosterone, the next clinical challenge is to diagnose the subtype of PA. Further imaging is important to exclude an aldosterone-secreting carcinoma as well as to inform management, which is clearly different depending on the underlying cause of aldosterone excess. Lateralizing the site of excess aldosterone production is the next step and, ideally, this step requires adrenal vein sampling.

### ***Imaging***

The imaging modality of choice is CT. This technique has advantages over magnetic resonance imaging (MRI) in the assessment of spatial resolution and it is less expensive. In contrast, MRI has the advantage that it does not involve radiation exposure that, in some patients, may be more appropriate.

An APA is usually a small (<2-cm), lipid-rich tumor with a typical appearance on CT, corresponding to <10 Hounsfield units (measurement of density) with a rapid wash-out phase (>50% at 5 min) after the administration of contrast agent. Bilateral adrenal hyperplasia can appear as either micro (<1-cm) or macro (>1-cm) adenomas or a combination of the two. Patients with idiopathic hyperaldosteronism can appear normal or demonstrate nodular change on adrenal CT. Unfortunately, CT cannot be solely used to distinguish between unilateral disease, amenable to adrenalectomy, and bilateral or idiopathic disease, which should be managed medically. For example, nonfunctioning adrenal adenomas are relatively common in older patients and radiologically indistinguishable from APAs. Small APAs may not be seen on CT and the incorrect diagnosis of idiopathic hyperaldosteronism reached; and conversely, areas that look like microadenomas may in fact represent area of hyperplasia. As a result of these limitations, a more accurate method of lateralization of aldosterone secretion is required to avoid inappropriate surgery in patients with bilateral disease or withholding curative surgery to patients who may benefit. The exception to this sequence of investigations is in patients under the age of 40 years, in whom an adrenal adenoma of >1 cm is identified as occurred in the case at the beginning of the chapter. In these patients, it would be reasonable to proceed to adrenalectomy without further investigation.

### ***Lateralizing aldosterone secretion***

The standard investigation to confirm aldosterone excess is adrenal vein sampling (AVS). AVS is a technically demanding procedure that is difficult to access out with tertiary referral centers. Even in this setting, protocols differ between centers, technical expertise is not always consistent, and results are variable. An extensive data-gathering exercise is underway to assess many aspects of the use of AVS (Adrenal Vein Sampling International study, AVIS), and the first report from this group has indicated that although this is a safe technique, complications (e.g., adrenal vein rupture) occurred least frequently in operators who performed the most tests.[26]

One of the main differences in protocol between centers involves the use of ACTH stimulation. The rationale for this is to reduce the influence of stress-induced stimulation of aldosterone production (from endogenous ACTH), which may obscure the results. In addition, the adrenal veins, particularly the right, are difficult to cannulate; cannulation can be confirmed by measuring cortisol gradients between the adrenal vein and the inferior vena cava, and some centers perform this measurement during the procedure to improve successful cannulation rates. Proponents of ACTH stimulation suggest that this approach maximizes the central–peripheral cortisol gradient and provides further reassurance that the vein was successfully cannulated. Adrenal vein sampling can be sequential or simultaneous, with increasing levels of technical expertise required for simultaneous measurements.

The AVIS data report that half the centers used ACTH stimulation, either as a bolus or continuous infusion. However, interpretation of results differed significantly between centers, even within the stimulated and unstimulated protocols.[26] The Endocrine Society guidelines suggest that the aldosterone concentration from the left and right adrenal vein should be divided by their respective cortisol concentrations to correct for any dilutional effects of contamination from either suboptimal sampling or collateral circulation.[22] In the context of ACTH stimulation, a cortisol-corrected aldosterone ratio from high to low should be >4:1 to indicate unilateral hypersecretion. This is based on data that suggest this cut-off has a sensitivity of 95% and specificity of 100%.[27] Where ACTH stimulation is not used, the guideline suggests either a ratio of 2:1 or a gradient between peripheral aldosterone concentration and the suspect adrenal of 2.5 times, as long as the contra lateral adrenal demonstrates suppressed aldosterone production as indicated by an aldosterone concentration no higher than the peripheral circulation.

Given these difficulties, the prospect of another tool to differentiate unilateral, surgically curable disease from bilateral disease is appealing. The use of $^{11}$C-metomidate as a radiotracer in positron emission tomography (PET)-CT could be useful in this situation. Recent data have demonstrated sensitivity and specificity of 76% (CI 59–93) and 87% (CI 69–104) using this noninvasive technique that requires less technical expertise.[28] The use of $^{11}$C-metomidate PET is be limited to centers with access to a cyclotron, but this promising diagnostic test may be used more frequently in the future.

## Treatment for PA

### Surgery

In patients with unilateral disease who are otherwise medically fit, surgical resection of the affected adrenal gland is the treatment of choice. This offers the possibility of curing hyperaldosteronism, although it is important to be aware that not all patients achieve complete remission of hypertension. Cure rates are variable (30%–70%), and given the diagnostic difficulties discussed above, this is not surprising.[24] Factors that are associated with cure are younger age, fewer antihypertensives preoperatively, shorter duration of hypertension, and absence of a family history of high blood pressure.[29] Despite these problems, with careful patient selection, the majority of patients have either no or a substantially reduced requirement for antihypertensive therapy postoperatively.

Adrenalectomy is usually carried out laparoscopically, and this surgery offers the advantage of shorter inpatient stay and reduced morbidity. Preoperatively, electrolytes should be normalized and blood pressure treated, preferably with an MR antagonist. This treatment has the effect of both addressing the specific actions of aldosterone excess and possibly allowing the renin–angiotensin system to recover, reducing the chance of hypoaldosteronism postoperatively.

### Medical therapies

In patients with bilateral disease, or patients with APA and unsuitable for a surgical procedure, medical therapy with aldosterone antagonists is the cornerstone of therapy. Spironolactone is an effective MR antagonist, although is not specific and also acts as an antagonist for the androgen and progesterone receptors. These properties account for the side effects that can limit its use, particularly at high doses (gynecomastia, sexual dysfunction in males, and menstrual irregularity in women). Eplerenone is more specific for the MR but is less potent, requiring higher doses. Both should be started at low dose (25 mg once daily for spironolactone, twice daily eplerenone) and titrated slowly with monitoring of plasma potassium. Once aldosterone action is appropriately suppressed, plasma renin should rise, and this rise can be a useful way to monitor the titration regime. If adequate control of hypertension is not achieved with mineralocorticoid antagonists alone, amiloride is an appropriate and relatively effective antihypertensive. By blocking the epithelial sodium in the DCT, it is a rational second-line agent. Calcium channel blockers and diuretics are also reasonable to use in combination with MR antagonists; however, unless plasma renin (and angiotensin II) is released from the inhibitory effects of excessive action of aldosterone, angiotensin-converting enzyme (ACE) inhibitors, and ARB antagonists are unlikely to impact blood pressure control.

## Other forms of mineralocorticoid hypertension

Although PA is the major cause of mineralocorticoid hypertension, there are many other conditions that cause hypertension with excessive retention of salt and water.

### Liddle's syndrome

Liddle's syndrome is a rare, autosomal dominant condition and associated with moderate-to-severe hypertension presenting in childhood, arising from over activation of the epithelial sodium channel (ENaC). In common with PA, patients are hypokalemic with a metabolic alkalosis and have a low plasma renin, but in this case plasma aldosterone concentrations are low.[30] The genetic abnormality lies on chromosome 16, and "gain-of-function mutations" identified to date lie in the cytoplasmic C-terminal tails of the β- and γ-subunits of ENaC.[31] These mutations result in loss of an adaptor motif that interacts with neural precursor cell-expressed, developmentally down regulated 4-2 (Nedd4-2). Nedd4-2 ligates a ubiquitin "tag" to the ENaC that targets it for internalization and subsequent destruction. This induces constitutive activity of the ENaC in the cortical collecting duct, as if activated by aldosterone. Importantly, in this condition, spironolactone is *not* effective because activation of ENaC is not due to excessive aldosterone levels and is independent of the MR. However, the ENaC is amiloride sensitive, and this is the treatment of choice in these patients.

### Pseudohypoaldosteronism type 2 (Gordon's syndrome)

Pseudohypoaldosteronism type 2, or Gordon's syndrome, is characterized by hypertension, hyperkalemia, metabolic acidosis, normal renal function, and low or low-normal plasma renin activity and normal or elevated aldosterone concentrations.[32] In addition, patients with this condition, which is inherited in an autosomal dominant manner, are exquisitely sensitive to thiazide diuretics, suggesting a gain-of-function mutation in the thiazide-sensitive NaCl transporter in the distal convoluted tubule (DCT). However, the mutation lies not within the gene encoding the transporter itself, but rather on chromosomes 12 and 17 that each encodes a With No Lysine Kinase (WNK).[33] The discovery of the molecular and genetic mechanisms behind this condition has provided valuable insight into the physiological regulation of blood pressure via sodium and potassium transport in the distal nephron. WNK1 and -4 localize to the DCT and cortical collecting duct and are involved in the regulation of the NaCl transporter acting via a kinase cascade, leading to loss of inhibition of the NaCl transporter and increased expression at the apical surface (Figure 21.3). This may be of relevance in the regulation of blood pressure at a population level because there have been many studies implicating variation in genes encoding WNKs as well as other regulators of the NaCl transport to blood pressure variation.[34–37] In addition, these targets may also present novel opportunities for pharmacological therapy of hypertension.

### Activation of MR by alternative ligands

Although aldosterone is the predominant mineralocorticoid in humans in health, other steroid compounds can activate the MR if produced in excessive quantities. For example, in patients with congenital adrenal hyperplasia caused by 11β-hydroxylase or 17α-hydroxylase deficiencies, mineralocorticoid hypertension is observed in the context of low plasma aldosterone levels. In this situation, the MR is activated by deoxycorticosterone that is produced in excessive quantities. Cortisol can also occupy the MR, but in health this is prevented from being a ligand by the action of 11β-hydroxysteroid dehydrogenase. This enzyme protects the MR from inappropriate activation by metabolizing cortisol to inactive cortisone[38] (Figure 21.5). In the absence of this enzyme, activation of MR by cortisol, which circulates in significantly greater concentrations than aldosterone, leads to salt and water retention and elevated blood pressure. The syndrome of apparent mineralocorticoid excess (SAME) was first identified in 1979.[39] The underlying etiology was confirmed to be mutation in the gene coding for 11β-hydroxysteroid dehydrogenase type 2 (11βHSD2).[40] Reduced activity of 11βHSD2 can also be an acquired phenomenon in the presence of substances (glycyrrhetinic acid, contained in licorice) that inhibit 11βHSD2.

Finally, abnormalities of the MR can lead to mineralocorticoid hypertension. An autosomal dominant missense mutation in the MR gene, S810L, leads to increased ligand promiscuity of the receptor such that it is able to be occupied by a range of steroids, including those that have not undergone 21-hydroxylation, for example, progesterone.[41] Because progesterone is the major hormone of pregnancy, hypertension, which is usually evident prepregnancy, is dramatically exacerbated by the rise in activation of MR.

# *Glucocorticoid hypertension (see Chapter 1)*

Cardiovascular disease, and, in particular, hypertension, is a major cause of morbidity and death in patients with cortisol excess. Hypertension is found in up to 70% of subjects with Cushing's syndrome, and this can be particularly severe in patients with ectopic ACTH.[42] In one small study estimating cardiovascular risk in 49 patients with active Cushing's syndrome, it was found that 85% of subjects were hypertensive, 42% had diabetes, and 41% were obese.[43] In addition, exogenously administered glucocorticoid can also lead to high blood pressure that can develop rapidly within 24–48 h of exposure to oral hydrocortisone or dexamethasone.[44] The pathogenesis of hypertension in these circumstances is not fully understood and is due to many factors.

## *Hemodynamic features*

There have been several studies in humans and animals to clarify the hemodynamic consequences of synthetic (dexamethasone) and naturally occurring steroids (cortisol and corticosterone). These studies suggest that such steroids exert disparate effects on the circulation, although they still do not fully explain the hemodynamic and hypertensive consequences of corticosteroids. For instance, both human and rat studies have shown that administration of dexamethasone results in hypertension with an elevated total peripheral resistance (TPR) but no effect on cardiac output, heart rate, or stroke volume.[45,46] However, pretreatment of such subjects with the vasodilator minoxidil fails to prevent dexamethasone-induced hypertension, despite a significant reduction in TPR.[46] In contrast, hydrocortisone (cortisol) administration in humans leads to hypertension in association with an increased cardiac output and renal vascular resistance with no effect on TPR or heart rate.[44,45] Again, however, reduction in cardiac output using the β-adrenergic blocker atenolol failed to ameliorate cortisol-induced hypertension.[45]

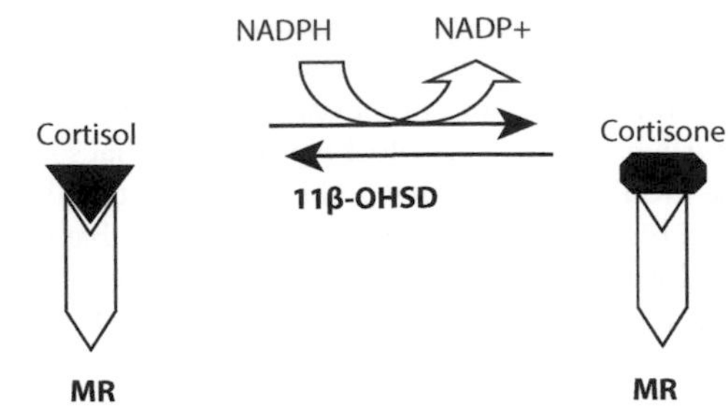


***Figure 21.5***
*The 11β-hydroxysteroid dehydrogenase system. 11βHSD can interchangeably convert cortisol to its inactive metabolite cortisone. The type 2 isoform of the enzyme is found mainly in the kidney and catalyzes the oxidation step (cortisol–cortisone) that protects the MR from occupation by cortisol because cortisone fails to activate the MR.*

## *Increased plasma volume/ MR binding*

It is widely accepted that retention of sodium and water is the major mechanism by which cortisol excess leads to hypertension. In normal circumstances, the MR is protected from continual activation by glucocorticoid, which binds the MR with equal affinity to aldosterone but is far more abundant in the circulation, by the enzyme 11βHSD2. This enzyme converts cortisol to its inactive metabolite cortisone, and cortisone does not transactivate the MR (Figure 21.5). It has been suggested that high serum cortisol concentrations, characteristic of Cushing's syndrome, "overwhelm" the 11βHSD2 system, allowing cortisol to activate the MR, thereby causing hypertension due to the retention of urinary sodium and subsequent expansion of plasma volume.

However, a definite causal relationship between cortisol-induced water/sodium retention and hypertension has not yet been demonstrated. For example, inhibition of the MR using spironolactone failed to prevent cortisol-induced sodium retention or hypertension in normal volunteers or ACTH-induced hypertension in rats.[47,48] Moreover, assessment of a range of synthetic steroids (including prednisolone, dexamethasone, and triamcinolone) demonstrated induction of hypertension without significant plasma volume expansion and retention of urinary sodium.[49] Therefore, the exact contribution of cortisol-mediated MR activation to the development of glucocorticoid-mediated hypertension remains unclear.

## Other mechanisms

More recent evidence has suggested a role for oxidative stress and the nitric oxide (NO) system in glucocorticoid-induced hypertension. For example, ACTH- and dexamethasone-induced hypertension in rats is associated with reduced levels of plasma nitrate and nitrite (NO metabolites). At the molecular level, *in vitro* studies of cultured human endothelial cells and rat aorta, kidney, and liver have demonstrated that exposure to dexamethasone results in down regulation of endothelial NO synthase mRNA and protein.[50,51]

## Glucocorticoid resistance

Glucocorticoid resistance is a rare, genetic disorder characterized by hypercortisolemia without the characteristic phenotype of cortisol excess. The syndrome is inherited in an autosomal recessive or dominant manner, and the most common genetic defects identified exist within the glucocorticoid receptor gene.[52] This causes reduced peripheral activity of cortisol, and the ensuing compensatory increase in ACTH drive results in stimulated production of cortisol as well as adrenal androgens and ACTH-dependent mineralocorticoids deoxycorticosterone and corticosterone by the adrenal cortex.

The clinical presentation is similar to that of congenital adrenal hyperplasia due to 11β-hydroxylase deficiency. Female subjects present with features of virilization and males with precocious puberty and infertility, whereas both sexes present with classic mineralocorticoid hypertension with hypokalemic alkalosis. Hypertension in these cases is mediated primarily by elevated DOC and corticosterone that, in turn, lead to suppression of renin and aldosterone production. However, clinical features can vary in severity, and some subjects are relatively asymptomatic.[52]

Table 21.2 outlines the classical biochemical features that can help make the diagnosis of familial glucocorticoid resistance. There are many biochemical features that overlap with true cortisol excess, and discrimination relies on a lack of classical features of cortisol excess (lack of striae, centripetal obesity, thin or bruised skin); assessment of bone mineral density that is often increased in glucocorticoid resistance; and demonstration of a preserved diurnal rhythm and response to thyrotropin-releasing hormone (TRH) stimulation, both of which are absent in Cushing's syndrome.[53]

Familial glucocorticoid resistance can be treated by dexamethasone to suppress ACTH production; the treatment of hypertension may also require addition of MR antagonists.

## Adrenal carcinoma

Adrenocortical carcinoma (ACC) is a rare but extremely aggressive endocrine malignancy. The incidence is approximately 1–2 cases per million per year in Europe and North America, with a prevalence of 4–12 cases per million.[54] At least 65% of ACCs are secretory, and most commonly produce excess cortisol (40%) or cortisol with adrenal androgens (25%). Therefore, hypertension in association with ACC is usually glucocorticoid-dependent, although there are rare cases of pure aldosterone or DOC-producing ACC.

# Catecholamine excess (see Chapters 7, 9, 10, 24)

A 36-year-old woman was referred to the endocrine outpatient clinic with a 3-year history of increasing anxiety, sweats, intermittent headache, and hypertension. She was on no regular medications and had no relevant past

| | *Cushing's syndrome* | *Glucocorticoid resistance* |
|---|---|---|
| Classical Cushingoid features | Usually present | Absent |
| Bone mineral density | Decreased | Normal or increased |
| Diurnal rhythm of cortisol production | Absent | Maintained |
| TRH test | No TSH response | Normal TSH response |
| Insulin tolerance testing | No ACTH/cortisol/growth hormone (GH) response | Normal |

***Table 21.2***
*Key clinical and biochemical features distinguishing Cushing's syndrome from glucocorticoid resistance.*

medical or family history. Positive findings on examination included a resting pulse of 110 beats per minute, supine blood pressure of 162/110 mm/Hg, and standing blood pressure of 139/85 mm/Hg.

The patient underwent biochemical evaluation for catecholamine excess, and the results are summarized in Table 21.3. Subsequent adrenal CT showed a heterogeneous, large left-sided adrenal mass (Figure 21.6) in keeping with pheochromocytoma, and $^{123}$I-metaiodobenzylguanidine (MIBG) scintigraphy demonstrated that this mass was MIBG avid with no evidence of extra-adrenal disease.

The patient subsequently underwent a laparoscopic left adrenalectomy. Preoperatively, she required treatment with phenoxybenzamine 120 mg daily in divided doses with the addition of labetalol 200 mg twice daily a few days before surgery. Preoperative blood pressure was 128/74 mm/Hg (supine) and 89/62 mm/Hg (erect).

After surgery, symptoms resolved and biochemistry normalized (Table 21.3). The pathology of the excised adrenal gland was found to be in keeping with pheochromocytoma, with a relatively low mitotic count (<3 per high-power field [HPF]), but evidence of vascular invasion within adrenal and extra-adrenal soft tissue. Thus, she underwent adjuvant therapy in the form of 10,000 MBq of $^{131}$I-MIBG. She still undergoes regular surveillance, but there is no evidence of recurrence 4 years after surgery.

## Background

Rarely, episodic or persistent hypertension can develop as a consequence of tumors of the chromaffin cells of the adrenal medulla or sympathetic ganglia that are referred to as "pheochromocytoma" and "paraganglioma," respectively. Such tumors produce and metabolize catecholamines but are sometimes nonsecretory. As a result, it is believed that many pheochromocytomas are diagnosed at postmortem; in one series of 54 autopsy-proven cases of pheochromocytoma from the Mayo Clinic, there were no clinical features in at least 50%.[55]

The overall prevalence of pheochromocytoma is unknown, although it is estimated to exist in 0.05%–0.2% of hypertensive subjects with an annual incidence of 0.8 per 100,000 person-years. Pheochromocytoma typically occurs in the fourth or fifth decade and is equally common in men and women.

## Pathogenesis and pathology

The majority of pheochromocytomas (about 90%) arise in the adrenal medulla. Extra-adrenal pheochromocytomas (paragangliomas) can arise anywhere from the

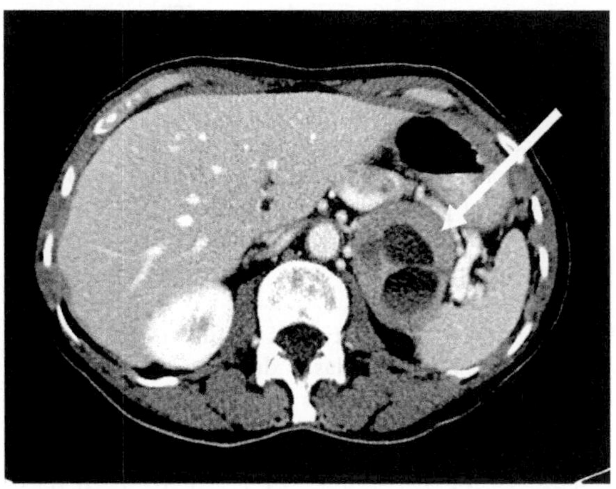

**Figure 21.6**
*Adrenal CT of patient with pheochromocytoma demonstrating a large, heterogeneous left-sided adrenal mass (arrow).*

| | | Diagnosis | Postoperative | Normal range |
|---|---|---|---|---|
| 24-h urine | Norepinephrine | 24,596 | 251 | <900 nmol/24 h |
| | Epinephrine | <50 | <50 | <230 nmol/24 h |
| | Dopamine | 12,616 | 1418 | <330 nmol/24 h |
| | Free normetanephrine | 10,818 | 159 | <650 nmol/24 h |
| | Free metanephrine | 61 | 65 | <350 nmol/24 h |
| Plasma | Normetanephrine | 19,219 | 515 | 120–1180 pmol/L |
| | Metanephrine | 187 | 190 | 80–150 pmol/L |

**Table 21.3**
*Pre- and postoperative biochemistry of a patient with pheochromocytoma*

base of the skull to pelvis, although the majority occur around the abdominal aorta or kidneys.

Typically, pheochromocytomas are cystic and/or hemorrhagic in appearance, with areas of necrosis, calcification, or both (Figure 21.7). Most tumors are at least 2–3 cm by time of diagnosis, although the size is variable; there have been tumors of up to 20 cm reported and smaller tumors can be diagnosed, especially in the context of screening of those with a genetic predisposition to pheochromocytoma (see below).[56]

The pathology of pheochromocytomas is unusual in that there are no absolute histological criteria for differentiating benign from malignant pheochromocytomas, and these tumors can never be specifically classified as benign. The 2004 World Health Organization (WHO) criteria define malignancy by the presence of metastases, not local invasion.[57] Even extensive invasion, although potentially lethal, is a poor predictor of metastases, and a lack of apparent invasion does not preclude the development of metastases.

It remains a challenge to recognize the malignant potential of tumors where metastases have not been identified at the time of diagnosis. Several scoring systems derived from invasion, histological growth patterns, cytological features, mitotic activity, and other characteristics have been proposed.[58] One important study showed that >70% of such tumors could be classified correctly on the basis of four factors: (1) extra-adrenal location, (2) coarse nodularity, (3) confluent necrosis, and (4) absence of hyaline globules.[59] These features, as well as the presence of a higher mitotic count (>3 per 20 HPF, 400×), five atypical mitotic figures, absence of sustentacular cells as identified by S100 staining, and an MIB-1 labeling index of >2.5% are all used by the U.K. Royal College of Pathologists to identify malignant potential of pheochromocytomas.[60] A new system for stratifying pheochromocytoma (Pheochromocytoma of the Adrenal gland Scoring Scale or PASS) uses weighted analysis of a range of features to separate benign from malignant lesions[61] (Table 21.4). However, there are conflicting reports as to its reliability, and it is not routinely used in histopathology reports of pheochromocytoma in the United Kingdom.

Finally, immunohistochemistry may be of use in situations where the histological features are ambiguous to clarify the presence of an adrenocortical or adrenomedullary tumor. For example, chromogranin is negative in cortical tumors and almost always positive in pheochromocytomas.[60]

## Genetics

Traditionally, pheochromocytomas were said to follow the "rule of tens": 10% are extra-adrenal, 10% bilateral, 10% malignant, and 10% genetic. Although much of this rule still applies, it is now recognized that >10% (and probably nearer to 25%) of tumors have an underlying genetic basis.[62]

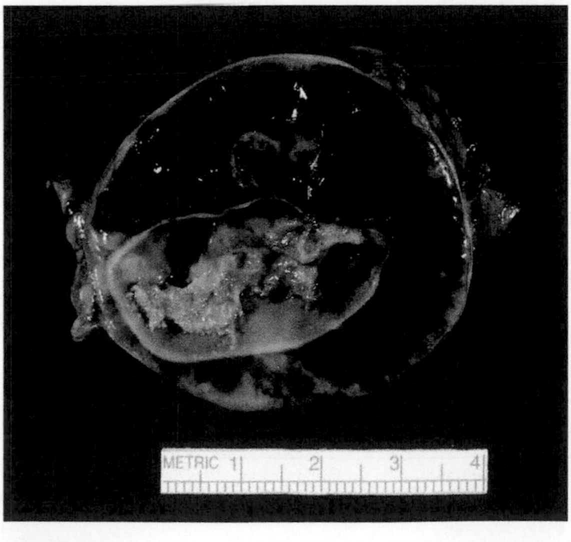

**Figure 21.7**
*Typical appearance of pheochromocytoma after adrenalectomy. Note the hemorrhagic and cystic components.*

| Feature | Score |
|---|---|
| Large nests of cells or diffuse growth >10% tumor volume | 2 |
| Necrosis (confluent or central in large cell nests) | 2 |
| High cellularity | 2 |
| Cellular monotony | 2 |
| Presence of spindle-shaped tumor cells | 2 |
| Mitotic figures (>3 per HPF) | 2 |
| Extension of tumor into adjacent fat | 2 |
| Vascular invasion | 1 |
| Capsular invasion | 1 |
| Profound nuclear pleomorphism | 1 |
| Nuclear hyperchromasia | 1 |
| Total possible score | 20 |

**Table 21.4**
*Pheochromocytoma of the Adrenal gland Scoring Scale (PASS score).*

The genetic syndromes associated with pheochromocytomas are summarized in Table 21.5. Pheochromocytomas occurs in up to 50% of subjects with multiple endocrine neoplasia (MEN), 10%–20% of those with von Hippel–Lindau (VHL), and rarely in neurofibromatosis type 1 (0.1%–5%).[63]

The clinical phenotype of pheochromocytoma associated with VHL and MEN2 differ, largely due to the difference in biochemical phenotype. MEN2 patients tend to be more symptomatic, with a higher incidence of hypertension, mainly because the tumors of such patients express phenylethanolamine *N*-methyltransferase (PNMT), the enzyme that converts norepinephrine to epinephrine, and tyrosine hydroxylase, a rate-limiting enzyme of catecholamine biosynthesis (Figure 21.8). As a result, pheochromocytomas of MEN2 patients tend to secrete epinephrine, whereas VHL patients produce higher levels of norepinephrine.[64]

More recently, familial pheochromocytoma and paraganglioma syndromes have been identified due to mutations in the succinate dehydrogenase (SDH) (succinate:ubiquinone oxidoreductase) subunit genes [SDHB, SDHC, SDHD, SDHAF2 (SDH5), SDHA] that compose portions of mitochondrial complex II. Mitochondrial complex II is a tumor suppressor gene involved in the electron transport chain and the tricarboxylic acid (TCA) cycle.

The genetics of pheochromocytoma and paraganglioma is a rapidly changing and evolving field.

| *Syndrome* | *Gene and mode of inheritance* | *Clinical features* | *Risk of pheochromocytoma (%)* | *Risk of malignancy (%)* |
|---|---|---|---|---|
| MEN2A/2B | RET oncogene/ AD | Medullar thyroid cancer, primary hyperparathyroidism pheochromocytoma (mucosal neuromas in 2B) | 50 | Usually benign |
| VHL | VHL tumor suppressor gene/AD | Retinal angioma, cerebellar and spinal hemangioblastoma, clear cell renal cell carcinoma, renal and pancreatic cysts, pheochromocytoma | 10–15 | 5 |
| NF1 | NF1 gene/AD | Café au lait patches, axillary freckling, cutaneous neurofibromas, Lisch nodules, optic glioma, pheochromocytoma | 2 | |
| SDH | B subunit/AD | Extra-adrenal and adrenal pheochromocytoma, GIST, head and neck PGL | 45% have disease by 40 years; 80% lifetime risk | 30–70 |
| | C subunit/AD | Head and neck PGL, GIST | Rare | Uncertain |
| | D subunit/ maternal imprinting | Head and neck PGL, benign extra-adrenal and adrenal pheochromocytoma, GIST | Rare | Uncertain |
| | 5 (SDHAF2)/AD | Head and neck PGL | | |

*NF, neurofibromatosis; SDH, succinate dehydrogenase; GIST, gastrointestinal stromal tumors; AD, autosomal dominant.*

***Table 21.5***
*Summary of major genetic syndromes associated with pheochromocytoma and paraganglioma (PGL).*

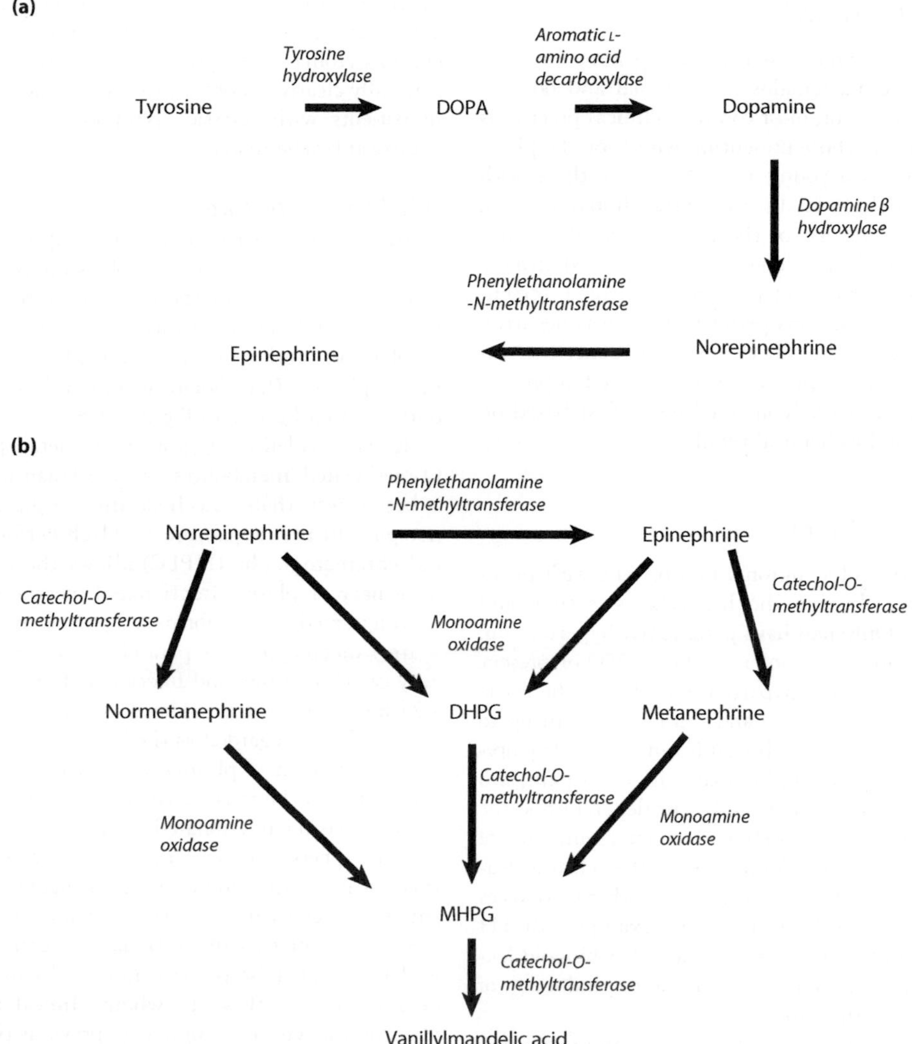


***Figure 21.8***
*(a) Catecholamine biosynthesis. (b) Catecholamine metabolism. DOPA- 3,4 dihydroxyphenylalanine; DHPG-3,4-dihydroxyphenylethyleneglycol; MHPG- 3-methoxy-4-hydroxyphenylethyleneglycol.*

For example, in 2010, loss-of-function mutations in the FP/TMEM127 gene were identified in 2% of patients with familial and sporadic pheochromocytoma, but not paraganglioma. TMEM127 is a negative regulator of mammalian target of rapamycin (mTOR) effector proteins.[65] In addition, mutations within the SDH5 (SDHA2) gene have recently been identified as causing familial paraganglioma syndromes in one kindred first identified in the 1980s.[66] SDH5 is important for the flavination and function of SDHA. However, this genetic syndrome remains extremely rare, and only one further kindred has been identified so far.

In 2011, loss-of-function mutations in the MAX gene were identified in three patients with familial pheochromocytoma.[67] MAX is a component of the MYC-MAX-MXD1 transcription factors that regulate cell proliferation, differentiation, and apoptosis. In an extension of this study, MAX mutations were found in 5 (8.5%) of 59 patients with suspected familial pheochromocytoma (based on age of onset <30 years, bilateral pheochromocytoma, or positive family history).

## Whom to screen?

The question of who to screen for a genetic cause of pheochromocytoma remains controversial and no consensus exists. Current, most common clinical practice is to offer testing to those presenting with sporadic pheochromocytoma at a young age (<50 years), those with bilateral or malignant disease, extra-adrenal tumors, positive family history, or those with clinical features leading to suspicion of one of the associated genetic syndromes. In our case of pheochromocytoma, screening for genetic causes was performed and was negative. Some centers screen for all the available genetic mutations, whereas others perform a more staged approach, screening for most likely affected genes first based on the clinical and biochemical profile.[68]

## Clinical features

The classic triad of symptoms in a patient with pheochromocytoma are episodic headache, sweating, and tachycardia.[69] Only half have paroxysmal hypertension, and the rest can be normotensive (5%–15%) or present with apparent essential hypertension.[70] Headache is the commonest clinical feature and can be found in up to 90% of patients.[70] Other clinical features include palpitations, tremor, pallor, abdominal pain, chest pain, and anxiety. Broadly, symptoms and signs depend upon the location of the tumor as well as the relative amounts of catecholamine secreted. More rarely, other clinical features can be found due to cosecretion of other substances in addition to catecholamines. For example, ACTH cosecretion can lead to development of Cushingoid features and hypoglycemia can occur due to production of insulin-like growth factor-2.

Increasingly, asymptomatic pheochromocytomas are being identified in patients who undergo abdominal imaging for unrelated reasons but are found to have an adrenal mass (so-called "incidentaloma"). Some reports are estimating that up to 50% of pheochromocytomas may be asymptomatic, although a series from the Mayo Clinic reported that 15 of 150 (10%) pheochromocytoma patients were discovered incidentally by abdominal CT.[71]

## Diagnosis

Pheochromocytoma is rarely confirmed in patients in whom such a diagnosis is suspected. For instance, one case series describes confirmed pheochromocytoma in only 1 of 300 patients who had undergone diagnostic evaluation.[72] There are a wide variety of potential differential diagnoses but pheochromocytoma can usually be easily excluded; a useful rule is that if a pheochromocytoma is symptomatic, then the biochemistry is usually clearly abnormal, so this diagnosis is excluded in patients with "classic" symptoms with normal or equivocal biochemistry.

### Biochemical testing

There has been much debate over the optimal biochemical test to diagnose or exclude pheochromocytoma and, as yet, no consensus exists. However, most institutions rely on a combination of measurements of urinary catecholamines and urinary and/or plasma fractionated metanephrines. Catecholamine biosynthesis and metabolites are highlighted in Figure 21.8.

Recent evidence suggests that metanephrines, the O-methylated metabolites of catecholamines, may be a better test than catecholamines (e.g., epinephrine, norepinephrine, dopamine).[73] High-performance liquid chromatography (HPLC) allows the measurement of urinary or plasma fractionated metanephrines, that is, (conjugated + free) normetanephrine and (conjugated + free) metanephrine separately. Measurement of urinary catecholamines and fractionated metanephrines in a 24-h urine sample provides 98% sensitivity and specificity and so is regarded as the best first-line test.[74]

Measurement of plasma fractionated metanephrines is accepted as the most sensitive test (96%–100%), and normal plasma fractionated metanephrines effectively excludes pheochromocytoma. However, specificity of this test is unsatisfactory and is estimated to be 77% in patients older than 60 years.[75] Reliance solely on measurement of plasma unfractionated metanephrines can lead to a high false-positive rate, and this test should be restricted to those in whom clinical suspicion of pheochromocytoma is high (e.g., previous pheochromocytoma, underlying genetic predisposition, or a typical adrenal mass on abdominal imaging).

Suppression testing using clonidine (α2-adrenergic receptor antagonist) or pentolinium (ganglion blocker) can occasionally be used to confirm or exclude a diagnosis of pheochromocytoma, especially in cases where there is suspicion of a falsely positive increase in plasma catecholamines/fractionated metanephrines. In patients with true pheochromocytoma, plasma catecholamines/fractionated metanephrines fail to suppress after administration of clonidine or pentolinium.[76] In practice, however, these tests are rarely required or performed.

In addition to catecholamines, chromaffin cells contain other peptides, such as chromogranins and neuropeptide Y, and ATP and calcium. Chromogranin A is increased in 80% of patients with pheochromocytoma, although this is not specific and can be increased in many other conditions and neuroendocrine tumors.[77] Its main role, therefore, is not in confirming diagnosis but as a useful marker of possible tumor recurrence.

### Imaging

Ideally, imaging to locate a catecholamine-secreting tumor should be performed after a biochemical diagnosis has been established and not before. CT and MRI are most commonly used, and both techniques have high sensitivity (98%–100%) but lower specificity (70%) in detecting pheochromocytoma. Because 95% of pheochromocytomas are located within the abdomen and pelvis, imaging can usually be restricted to this area initially and extended to the thorax, head, and neck if initial imaging is negative.[78]

On CT, pheochromocytomas typically have a heterogeneous appearance, with Hounsfield units of >20 and can often contain cystic components or areas of calcification (Figure 21.6). On T2-weighted MRI, tumors are again often heterogeneous and are bright on appearance.

Functional imaging, using radiolabeled catecholamine analogs, can be a useful adjunct in the diagnosis or staging of pheochromocytoma. MIBG is a structural analog of norepinephrine; 85% of adrenal pheochromocytomas are positive on $^{123}$I-MIBG imaging, although this value is lower for malignant, familial, and extra-adrenal tumors.[79] MIBG scanning is useful to confirm whether an adrenal lesion is likely to be a pheochromocytoma; to identify metastatic disease; and, occasionally, to locate an extra-adrenal pheochromocytoma where plain imaging has been negative. Finally, it is useful to establish MIBG positivity in a patient who may subsequently require high dose $^{131}$I-MIBG therapy for malignant pheochromocytoma or, as in our case, adjuvant $^{131}$I-MIBG therapy if thought to be at higher risk of recurrence.

$^{111}$In-octreotide scanning can also be useful, although only about 25% of adrenal pheochromocytoma demonstrate significant uptake. Its main use is in imaging of head and neck paragangliomas of which 75% demonstrate positive uptake.[79] PET scanning using various $^{18}$F-labeled tracers (especially $^{18}$F-fluorodeoxyglucose) is useful mainly in identifying metastatic disease.

## Management

Unless there is a significant contraindication, pheochromocytoma should be managed surgically in the first instance. However, patients must be initially managed medically to control symptoms and blood pressure but, most importantly, to minimize the risk of intraoperative hemodynamic instability.

α-Antagonists, such as phenoxybenzamine, are the mainstay of treatment as illustrated in the case. Phenoxybenzamine is a nonselective, irreversible α-adrenoceptor antagonist that blocks the vasoconstrictor effects of catecholamines. The main role of α blockade is to allow expansion of intravascular volume that is reduced in pheochromocytoma due to vasoconstrictor hypertension and compensatory pressure natriuresis. The dose of phenoxybenzamine is slowly increased according to blood pressure for several weeks before surgery; the target blood pressure is usually about 120/80 mm/Hg seated with a systolic blood pressure >90 mm/Hg on standing. Immediately before surgery, patients may require admission for intravenous saline to further expand plasma volume.[80] Once sufficiently α-blocked, patients with pheochromocytoma may require the addition of a selective β1-antagonist to offset excessive tachycardia. Patients with tumors that secrete mainly norepinephrine are less likely to require β blockers, whereas patients with tumors that produce significant levels of epinephrine may often require higher doses.

Laparoscopic adrenalectomy is the surgical procedure of choice to resect pheochromocytoma (if tumor diameter is <8 cm). This now carries a low perioperative morbidity and mortality rate if performed by a surgeon with sufficient experience. Cortical-sparing adrenalectomy has been performed in selected cases, mainly in patients with MEN 2 and VHL disease.[81] However, this is not standard clinical practice, because of concerns about the risk of local recurrence. In most cases, blood pressure is usually normal (without α and β blockade) by the time of hospital discharge but hypertension can occasionally persist for up to 4–8 weeks after surgery. However, persistent hypertension can occur in rare cases. The mechanism for this remains speculative but may be as a consequence of persisting hemodynamic changes; resetting of baroceptors; structural vascular or renal changes; or, most commonly, due to coexisting essential hypertension.[80]

### Malignant pheochromocytoma

As mentioned, the presence of metastatic disease is the only absolute evidence of malignant pheochromocytoma. However, the presence of underlying SDHB mutations along with certain histopathological features described previously may also suggest high malignant potential. The prognosis of malignant pheochromocytoma is variable; although the mean 5-year survival is 50%, about half of these patients have an aggressive disease, with death occurring within 1–3 years; the other half has a more indolent form of disease, with a life expectancy of up to 20 years.

There is no cure for metastatic pheochromocytoma, and the focus of treatment is on slowing disease progression. Therapeutic $^{131}$I-MIBG, when associated with $^{123}$I-MIBG uptake on a diagnostic scan, can be useful; however, only about 30%–70% of patients respond, and effects are usually temporary, necessitating repeated dosing or alternative therapies. In addition, some centers, including our own, advocate the use of a single dose of adjuvant $^{131}$I-MIBG in subjects felt to be at higher risk of local recurrence (demonstration of capsular or vascular invasion on pathology). Combination chemotherapy (usually with cyclophosphamide, vincristine, and dacarbazine) can also be considered in progressive disease, but only about 50% of patients respond to treatment, and there is controversy as to whether this regimen extends survival.[82] There is a clear need for innovative therapies for the treatment of metastatic pheochromocytoma, but the rarity of such tumors mean randomized clinical trials of novel treatments are difficult to perform. However, recent small-scale studies report an encouraging response to the tyrosine kinase inhibitor sunitinib, and further studies are in progress.[83]

## Follow-up

Postoperative catecholamines should be checked within a few weeks of surgery once acute effects of surgery have passed. It is recognized that follow-up of patients should be life long with an annual assessment of blood pressure, symptoms, and catecholamine levels because patients with pheochromocytoma are at increased risk of a second tumor, recurrence at the original site, or the development of distant metastases that may appear many years after the initial presentation.

## Conclusions

Hypertension due to endocrine causes is now the commonest cause of secondary hypertension, largely due to increased recognition of and screening for PA. It is important for clinicians to be alert to clinical or biochemical features that may increase the likelihood of an underlying endocrine cause for hypertension to allow targeted selection of appropriate patients to undergo screening for secondary causes of hypertension.

## References

1. Lawes CM, Vander HS, Rodgers A, et al. Global burden of blood-pressure-related disease, 2001. *Lancet* 2008;371:1513–18.
2. Soundararajan R, Pearce D, Hughey RP, et al. Role of epithelial sodium channels and their regulators in hypertension. *J Biol Chem* 2010;285:30363–9.
3. Rossi GP, Bernini G, Caliumi C, et al. A prospective study of the prevalence of primary aldosteronism in 1,125 hypertensive patients. *J Am Coll Cardiol* 2006;48:2293–300.
4. Lim PO, Dow E, Brennan G, et al. High prevalence of primary aldosteronism in the Tayside hypertension clinic population. *J Hum Hypertens* 2000;14:311–15.
5. Rocha R, Stier CT, Jr., Kifor I, et al. Aldosterone: A mediator of myocardial necrosis and renal arteriopathy. *Endocrinology* 2000;141:3871–8.
6. Milliez P, Girerd X, Plouin PF, et al. Evidence for an increased rate of cardiovascular events in patients with primary aldosteronism. *J Am Coll Cardiol* 2005;45:1243–8.
7. Newton-Cheh C, Guo CY, Gona P, et al. Clinical and genetic correlates of aldosterone-to-renin ratio and relations to blood pressure in a community sample. *Hypertension* 2007;49:846–56.
8. Pitt B, Zannad F, Remme WJ, et al. The effect of spironolactone on morbidity and mortality in patients with severe heart failure. Randomized Aldactone Evaluation Study Investigators. *New Engl J Med* 1999;341:709–17.
9. Pitt B. Aldosterone blockade in patients with acute myocardial infarction. *Circulation* 2003;107:2525–7.
10. Matrozova J, Steichen O, Amar L, et al. Fasting plasma glucose and serum lipids in patients with primary aldosteronism: A controlled cross-sectional study. *Hypertension* 2009;53:605–10.
11. Fallo F, Della MP, Sonino N, et al. Adiponectin and insulin sensitivity in primary aldosteronism. *Am J Hyperten* 2007;20:855–61.
12. Nishikawa T, Omura M, Ito H, et al. Prevalence of primary aldosteronism among Japanese hypertensive patients. *J Hypertens - Suppl* 2002;20:S172.
13. Boulkroun S, Samson-Couterie B, Dzib JF, et al. Adrenal cortex remodeling and functional zona glomerulosa hyperplasia in primary aldosteronism. *Hypertension* 2010;56:885–92.
14. Nishimoto K, Nakagawa K, Li D, et al. Adrenocortical zonation in humans under normal and pathological conditions. *J Clin Endocrinol Metab* 2010;95: 2296–305.
15. Choi M, Scholl UI, Yue P, et al. K+ channel mutations in adrenal aldosterone-producing adenomas and hereditary hypertension. *Science* 2011;331:768–72.

16. Boulkroun S, Beuschlein F, Rossi GP, et al. Prevalence, clinical, and molecular correlates of KCNJ5 mutations in primary aldosteronism. *Hypertension* 2012;59:592–8.
17. Azizan EAB, Murthy M, Stowasser M, et al. Somatic mutations affecting the selectivity filter of KCNJ5 are frequent in 2 large unselected collections of adrenal aldosteronomas. *Hypertension* 2012;59:587–91.
18. Davies LA, Hu C, Guagliardo NA, et al. TASK channel deletion in mice causes primary hyperaldosteronism. *Proc Natl Acad Sci U S A* 2008;105:2203–8.
19. Heitzmann D, Derand R, Jungbauer S, et al. Invalidation of TASK1 potassium channels disrupts adrenal gland zonation and mineralocorticoid homeostasis. *EMBO J* 2008;27:179–87.
20. Lifton RP, Dluhy RG, Powers M, et al. A chimaeric 11 beta-hydroxylase/aldosterone synthase gene causes glucocorticoid-remediable aldosteronism and human hypertension. *Nature* 1992;355:262–5.
21. Lafferty AR, Torpy DJ, Stowasser M, et al. A novel genetic locus for low renin hypertension: Familial hyperaldosteronism type II maps to chromosome 7 (7p22). *J Med Genet* 2000;37:831–5.
22. Funder JW, Carey RM, Fardella C, et al. Case detection, diagnosis, and treatment of patients with primary aldosteronism: An endocrine society clinical practice guideline. *J Clin Endocrinol Metab* 2008;93:3266–81.
23. Dorrian CA, Toole BJ, Alvarez-Madrazo S, et al. A screening procedure for primary aldosteronism based on the Diasorin Liaison automated chemiluminescent immunoassay for direct renin. *Ann Clin Biochem* 2010;47:3–9.
24. Young WF. Primary aldosteronism: Renaissance of a syndrome. *Clin Endocrinol* 2007;66:607–18.
25. Stowasser M, Gordon RD. Primary aldosteronism—careful investigation is essential and rewarding. *Mol Cell Endocrinol* 2004;217:33–9.
26. Rossi GP, Barisa M, Allolio B, et al. The Adrenal Vein Sampling International Study (AVIS) for identifying the major subtypes of primary aldosteronism. *J Clin Endocrinol Metab* 2012;97(5):1606–14.
27. Young WF, Stanson AW, Thompson GB, et al. Role for adrenal venous sampling in primary aldosteronism. *Surgery* 2004;136:1227–35.
28. Burton TJ, Mackenzie IS, Balan K, et al. Evaluation of the sensitivity and specificity of 11C-metomidate positron emission tomography (PET)-CT for lateralizing aldosterone secretion by Conn's adenomas. *J Clin Endocrinol Metab* 2012;97:100–9.
29. Sawka AM, Young WF, Thompson GB, et al. Primary aldosteronism: Factors associated with normalization of blood pressure after surgery. *Ann Intern Med* 2001;135:258–61.
30. Liddle GW. A familial renal disorder simulating primary aldosteronism but with negligible aldosterone secretion. *T Assoc Am Physician* 1963;76:199–213.
31. Shimkets RA, Warnock DG, Bositis CM, et al. Liddle's syndrome: Heritable human hypertension caused by mutations in the beta subunit of the epithelial sodium channel. *Cell* 1994;79:407–14.
32. Gordon RD. The syndrome of hypertension and hyperkalemia with normal glomerular filtration rate: Gordon's syndrome. *Aust N Z J Med* 1986;16:183–4.
33. Wilson FH, Disse-Nicodeme S, Choate KA, et al. Human hypertension caused by mutations in WNK kinases. *Science* 2001;293:1107–12.
34. Tobin MD, Raleigh SM, Newhouse S, et al. Association of WNK1 gene polymorphisms and haplotypes with ambulatory blood pressure in the general population. *Circulation* 2005;112:3423–9.
35. Newhouse SJ, Wallace C, Dobson R, et al. Haplotypes of the WNK1 gene associate with blood pressure variation in a severely hypertensive population from the British Genetics of Hypertension study. *Hum Mol Genet* 2005;14:1805–14.
36. Newhouse S, Farrall M, Wallace C, et al. Polymorphisms in the WNK1 gene are associated with blood pressure variation and urinary potassium excretion. *PLoS One* 2009;4:e5003.
37. Wang Y, O'Connell JR, McArdle PF, et al. Whole-genome association study identifies STK39 as a hypertension susceptibility gene. *Proc Natl Acad Sci U S A* 2009;106:226–31.
38. Edwards CR, Stewart PM, Burt D, et al. Localisation of 11 beta-hydroxysteroid dehydrogenase—tissue specific protector of the mineralocorticoid receptor. *Lancet* 1988;2:986–9.
39. Ulick S, Levine LS, Gunczler P, et al. A syndrome of apparent mineralocorticoid excess associated with defects in the peripheral metabolism of cortisol. *J Clin Endocrinol Metab* 1979;49:757–64.
40. Stewart PM, Corrie JE, Shackleton CH, et al. Syndrome of apparent mineralocorticoid excess. A defect in the cortisol-cortisone shuttle. *J Clin Invest* 1988;82:340–9.
41. Geller DS, Farhi A, Pinkerton N, et al. Activating mineralocorticoid receptor mutation in hypertension exacerbated by pregnancy. *Science* 2000;289:119–23.
42. Newell-Price J. Cushing's syndrome. In: Wass J, Stewart PM, eds. *Oxford Textbook of Endocrinology and Diabetes*. Oxford University Press, Oxford, UK 2011.
43. Mancini T, Kola B, Mantero F, et al. High cardiovascular risk in patients with Cushing's syndrome according to 1999 WHO/ISH guidelines. *Clin Endocrinol* 2004;61:768–77.

44. Connell JM, Whitworth JA, Davies DL, et al. Effects of ACTH and cortisol administration on blood pressure, electrolyte metabolism, atrial natriuretic peptide and renal function in normal man. *J Hypertens* 1987;5:425–33.
45. Pirpiris M, Sudhir K, Yeung S, et al. Pressor responsiveness in corticosteroid-induced hypertension in humans. *Hypertension* 1992;19(6 Pt 1):567–74.
46. Ong SL, Zhang Y, Sutton M, et al. Hemodynamics of dexamethasone-induced hypertension in the rat. *Hypertens Res—Clin E* 2009;32:889–94.
47. Williamson PM, Kelly JJ, Whitworth JA. Dose-response relationships and mineralocorticoid activity in cortisol-induced hypertension in humans. *J Hypertens* 1996;14:S37–41.
48. Li M, Wen C, Fraser T, et al. Adrenocorticotrophin-induced hypertension: Effects of mineralocorticoid and glucocorticoid receptor antagonism. *J Hypertens* 1999;17:419–26.
49. Connell JM, Whitworth JA, Davies DL, et al. Haemodynamic, hormonal and renal effects of adrenocorticotrophic hormone in sodium-restricted man. *J Hypertens* 1988;6:17–23.
50. Wen C, Li M, Fraser T, et al. L-Arginine partially reverses established adrenocorticotrophin-induced hypertension and nitric oxide deficiency in the rat. *Blood Pressure* 2000;9:298–304.
51. Wallerath T, Witte K, Schafer SC, et al. Down-regulation of the expression of endothelial NO synthase is likely to contribute to glucocorticoid-mediated hypertension. *Proc Natl Acad Sci U S A* 1999;96:13357–62.
52. Lamberts SW, Koper JW, Biemond P, et al. Cortisol receptor resistance: The variability of its clinical presentation and response to treatment. *J Clin Endocrinol Metab* 1992;74:313–21.
53. Lamberts SW, van Rossum E. Glucocorticoid resistance. In: Wass J, Stewart PM, eds. *Oxford Textbook of Endocrinology and Diabetes.* Oxford University Press, Oxford, UK 2011.
54. Allolio B, Fassnacht M. Clinical review: Adrenocortical carcinoma: Clinical update. *J Clin Endocrinol Metab* 2006;91:2027–37.
55. Sutton MG, Sheps SG, Lie JT. Prevalence of clinically unsuspected pheochromocytoma. Review of a 50-year autopsy series. *Mayo Clin Proc* 1981;56:354–60.
56. Tischler AS, Kimura N, McNicol AM. Pathology of pheochromocytoma and extra-adrenal paraganglioma. *Ann N Y Acad Sci* 2006;1073:557–70.
57. DeLellis R, Lloyd R, Heitz P, et al. *Tumours of Endocrine Organs.* Lyon: IARC Press; 2004.
58. Pacak K, Eisenhofer G, Ahlman H, et al. Pheochromocytoma: Recommendations for clinical practice from the First International Symposium. October 2005. *Nat Clin Pract Endocrinol Metab* 2007;3:92–102.
59. Linnoila RI, Keiser HR, Steinberg SM, et al. Histopathology of benign versus malignant sympathoadrenal paragangliomas: Clinicopathologic study of 120 cases including unusual histologic features. *Hum Pathol* 1990;21:1168–80.
60. Moonim M, Johnson S, McNicol AM. *Cancer Dataset for the Histological Reporting of Adrenal Cortical Carcinoma and Phaeochromocytoma/Paraganglioma. 2nd ed.* Royal College of Pathologists Carlton House Terrace, London; 2012.
61. Thompson LD. Pheochromocytoma of the Adrenal gland Scaled Score (PASS) to separate benign from malignant neoplasms: A clinicopathologic and immunophenotypic study of 100 cases. *Am J Surg Pathol* 2002;26:551–66.
62. Neumann HP, Bausch B, McWhinney SR, et al. Germline mutations in nonsyndromic pheochromocytoma. *N Engl J Med* 2002;346:1459–66.
63. Dluhy RG. Pheochromocytoma — death of an axiom. *N Engl J Med* 2002;346:1486–8.
64. Eisenhofer G, Walther MM, Huynh TT, et al. Pheochromocytomas in von Hippel-Lindau syndrome and multiple endocrine neoplasia type 2 display distinct biochemical and clinical phenotypes. *J Clin Endocrinol Metab* 2001;86:1999–2008.
65. Yao L, Schiavi F, Cascon A, et al. Spectrum and prevalence of FP/TMEM127 gene mutations in pheochromocytomas and paragangliomas. *JAMA* 2010;304:2611–19.
66. Bayley JP, Kunst HP, Cascon A, et al. SDHAF2 mutations in familial and sporadic paraganglioma and phaeochromocytoma. *Lancet Oncol* 2010;11:366–72.
67. Comino-Mendez I, Gracia-Aznarez FJ, Schiavi F, et al. Exome sequencing identifies MAX mutations as a cause of hereditary pheochromocytoma. *Nat Genet* 2011;43:663–7.
68. Erlic Z, Neumann HP. When should genetic testing be obtained in a patient with phaeochromocytoma or paraganglioma? *Clin Endocrinol* 2009;70:354–7.
69. Bravo EL. Pheochromocytoma: New concepts and future trends. *Kidney Int* 1991;40:544–56.
70. Manger WM, Gifford RW. Pheochromocytoma. *J Clin Hypertens* 2002;4:62–72.
71. Kudva YC, Young WF, Jr., Thompson GB, et al. Adrenal incidentaloma: An important component of the clinical presentation spectrum of benign sporadic adrenal pheochromocytoma. *Endocrinologist* 1999;9:77–80.
72. Fogarty J, Engel C, Russo J, et al. Hypertension and phaeochromocytoma testing: The association with anxiety disorders. *Arch Fam Med* 1994;3:55–60.
73. Lenders JW, Pacak K, Walther MM, et al. Biochemical diagnosis of pheochromocytoma: Which test is best? *JAMA* 2002;287:1427–34.
74. Boyle JG, Davidson DF, Perry CG, et al. Comparison of diagnostic accuracy of urinary free metanephrines, vanillyl mandelic acid, and catecholamines and plasma

catecholamines for diagnosis of pheochromocytoma. *J Clin Endocrinol Metab* 2007;92:4602–8.

75. Sawka AM, Jaeschke R, Singh RJ, et al. A comparison of biochemical tests for pheochromocytoma: Measurement of fractionated plasma metanephrines compared with the combination of 24-hour urinary metanephrines and catecholamines. *J Clin Endocrinol Metab* 2003;88:553–8.
76. Brown MJ, Allison DJ, Jenner DA, et al. Increased sensitivity and accuracy of phaeochromocytoma diagnosis achieved by use of plasma-adrenaline estimations and a pentolinium-suppression test. *Lancet* 1981;1:174–7.
77. Cotesta D, Caliumi C, Alo P, et al. High plasma levels of human chromogranin A and adrenomedullin in patients with pheochromocytoma. *Tumori* 2005;91:53–8.
78. Bravo EL. Evolving concepts in the pathophysiology, diagnosis, and treatment of pheochromocytoma. *Endocr Rev* 1994;15:356–68.
79. van der Harst E, de Herder WW, Bruining HA, et al. [(123)I]metaiodobenzylguanidine and [(111)In] octreotide uptake in benign and malignant pheochromocytomas. *J Clin Endocrinol Metab* 2001;86:685–93.
80. Young WF, Jr. Adrenal causes of hypertension: Pheochromocytoma and primary aldosteronism. *Rev Endocr Metab Dis* 2007;8:309–20.
81. Diner EK, Franks ME, Behari A, et al. Partial adrenalectomy: The National Cancer Institute experience. *Urology* 2005;66:19–23.
82. Nomura K, Kimura H, Shimizu S, et al. Survival of patients with metastatic malignant pheochromocytoma and efficacy of combined cyclophosphamide, vincristine, and dacarbazine chemotherapy. *J Clin Endocrinol Metab* 2009;94:2850–6.
83. Joshua AM, Ezzat S, Asa SL, et al. Rationale and evidence for sunitinib in the treatment of malignant paraganglioma/pheochromocytoma. *J Clin Endocrinol Metab* 2009;94:5–9.

# 22

# Obesity

*Ahmed Yousseif, Efthimia Karra, Sofia Rahman, Rachel L. Batterham*

## Introduction

In the past 30 years, the prevalence of obesity has increased to epidemic proportions, making obesity a major public health concern. In 2008, a systematic meta-analysis from 199 countries estimated that 1.46 billion adults were overweight, with 502 million individuals being obese worldwide. In the United Kingdom, 56% of women and 65% of men are overweight, and 24% of all adults are obese. Even more concerning is that the prevalence of obesity in children aged between 2 and 15 years has risen by 12% since 1995, with 170 million children globally classified as overweight or obese.[1–3,5–10]

Obesity and overweight are a direct cause of and major risk factor for several diseases, such as type 2 diabetes mellitus (T2DM), dyslipidemia, hypertension, cardiovascular disease, obstructive sleep apnea, musculoskeletal disorders, and certain forms of cancer.[1–3,5–10] Treatment of obesity is challenging, and the increasing obesity prevalence reflects failure of existent preventative and treatment strategies and the need for more effective therapies for obesity management.

## Definition and classification of obesity

Obesity is defined as abnormal or excessive fat accumulation that may impair health.[1] Based on this definition, women and men are classified as obese when their total body fat percentage reaches or exceeds 30% and 25%, respectively.

However, because direct quantification of body fat requires specialized equipment (e.g., dual-energy X-ray absorptiometry [DEXA]), body mass index (BMI) is commonly used as a surrogate to assess the degree of overweight and obesity. BMI is a measure of a person's weight relative to their height and is calculated by dividing the body weight in kilograms by the square of their height in meters (kg/m$^2$).

According to the World Health Organization (WHO) 2006 obesity classification, overweight is defined as BMI >25 kg/m$^2$ and obesity as a BMI of >30 kg/m$^2$. The BMI formula calculation is also follows: BMI = body weight (kg)/height$^2$ (m$^2$).

## Obesity classification

Obesity can be classified by BMI intervals and related aggregate risk of mortality, on the basis of the anatomical phenotypes, or by etiologic criteria.[1,2]

### BMI intervals

The recommended obesity classifications for BMI adopted by the National Institute of Health (NIH) and WHO are as follows:

- Underweight: BMI <18.5 kg/m$^2$
- Normal weight: BMI ≥18.5–24.9 kg/m$^2$
- Overweight: BMI ≥25.0–29.9 kg/m$^2$
- Obesity: BMI ≥30 kg/m$^2$

Obesity is then categorized as

- Obesity Class I: BMI of 30.0–34.9 kg/m$^2$
- Obesity Class II: BMI of 35.0–39.9 kg/m$^2$
- Obesity Class III: BMI ≥40 kg/m$^2$ (severe, extreme, or morbid obesity)

The diagnostic BMI cut-offs for overweight and obesity are based on data showing that BMI and mortality are interlinked via a J-shaped association. Thus, the relationship between BMI and risk allows identification of several levels of risk (risk stratification) that can be used to guide selection of therapy.[2,11–13] Although BMI is highly practical and the most widely used bodyweight assessment tool, it is limited by the lack of distinction between fat mass and lean mass. In addition, BMI lacks sensitivity to the gender and ethnic-related differences in relative body fatness. The arbitrary diagnostic BMI cut-offs are derived from data collected on whites, but have been widely adopted, as ethnic-based cut-offs are currently unavailable.[15] However, there is racial variation in the definition of overweight and obesity. In South Asian populations, the level of risk in terms of percentage of body fat is reached at a much lower BMI, whereas the opposite occurs in blacks compared with whites. In particular, the mean BMI associated with the development of an adverse metabolic profile is estimated at 21 kg/m$^2$ in South Asians. Thus, the WHO and NIH guidelines are currently applied to whites, Hispanics, and blacks. For Asians, overweight is defined as a BMI between 23 and 24.9 kg/m$^2$ and obesity as a BMI >25 kg/m$^2$. Finally, when interpreting BMI values, clinicians should be aware that BMI may overestimate the degree of obesity in individuals who are very muscular (e.g., professional athletes or bodybuilders).

## *Anatomical phenotypes*

The most common anatomical classification of obesity is based is on a prevalence of visceral or subcutaneous fat deposition. It is well established that visceral adiposity (also called central adiposity, android, or male-type obesity) is a major risk factor for the metabolic complications of obesity, whereas subcutaneous fat seems to be more benign. Therefore, in addition to measuring BMI, waist circumference should be measured to assess abdominal/central obesity. Patients with visceral obesity are at increased risk for heart disease, T2DM, hypertension, and dyslipidemia.

Waist circumference should be measured with a flexible tape placed on a horizontal plane at the level of the iliac crest as seen from the anterior view.[14] In adults with a BMI of 25–34.9 kg/m$^2$, a waist circumference >102 cm (40 in.) for men and 88 cm (35 in.) for women is associated with a greater risk. In patients with a BMI ≥35 kg/m$^2$, measurement of waist circumference is less helpful because it adds little to the predictive power of the disease risk classification of BMI; almost all individuals with this BMI also have an abnormal waist circumference. Like with BMI, there is ethnic variability in waist circumference values that predict increased risk. For example, South Asians have more total fat and visceral fat and therefore may be at higher risk of developing T2DM for a given BMI than whites. As such, in Asian females a waist circumference >80 cm and in Asian males a value >90 cm are considered abnormal.

The ratio of waist circumference to hip circumference (WHR) is an additional indirect way of assessing the degree of central versus peripheral obesity. WHO states that abdominal obesity is defined as a WHR >0.90 for males and >0.85 for females.

## *Etiology*

Based on its etiology, obesity can be classified as primary, when no obvious reason can be identified, or secondary, when there is an identifiable underlying etiology. Secondary obesity may occur in the context of endocrine pathologies, such as polycystic ovarian syndrome, Cushing's syndrome, hypothyroidism, hypothalamic defects, and growth hormone deficiency. Moreover, secondary obesity can be iatrogenic, either secondary to pharmacologic treatments, such as some antipsychotic, antidepressants, and some antiepileptic agents or steroid treatment; or due to hypothalamic injury, surgery, or both (Table 22.1).

Much of the BMI variance within a population can be explained by genetic factors (Tables 22.1 and 22.2); with twin and adoption studies revealing 40%–80% heritability for the obese phenotype. Genetic forms of obesity can be subdivided into those occurring within syndromes featuring obesity and those resulting from monogenic causes of obesity.[21] The latter are rare and affect a minority of people; however, studies of affected individuals and the implicated genes provide insight in the mechanisms regulating energy homeostasis. Finally, in the last decade genome-wide association studies (GWASs) have identified obesity risk-alleles that tend to occur at higher frequencies compared with monogenic forms of obesity but that have a smaller effect on BMI. Variation within the fat mass and obesity-associated (*FTO*) gene and the melanocortin-4 receptor (*MC4R*) gene are such examples.[22,23]

However, the fundamental reasons underpinning the current obesity pandemic are increased energy intake (overeating) in combination with reduced physical activity. Feeding behavior is governed by homeostatic drives that trigger food intake in the presence of energy deficits and hedonistic feeding stimuli,

| |
|---|
| Neuroendocrine obesity |
| Hypothalamic obesity |
| Cushing's syndrome |
| Polycystic ovarian syndrome |
| Hypogonadism |
| Growth hormone deficiency |
| Hypothyroidism |
| Pseudohypoparathyroidism |
| Iatrogenic |
| Drugs that cause weight gain |
| Hypothalamic surgery |
| Genetic forms of obesity |
| Genetic syndromes that feature obesity |
| Prader–Willi |
| Bardet–Biedl |
| Biemond syndrome II |
| Alstrom syndrome |
| Albright hereditary osteodystrophy |
| Fragile X syndrome |
| Germinal cell aplasia Sertoli cell-only syndrome |
| Simpson dysmorphia |
| Monogenic causes of obesity |
| Leptin deficiency |
| Leptin receptor deficiency |
| Pro-opiomelanocortin deficiency |
| Melanocortin-4 receptor deficiency |
| Prohormone covertase-1 deficiency |
| Neurotrophin receptor TrkB |
| Polymorphisms linked to obesity |
| Fat mass and obesity-associated (*FTO*) gene |
| Melanocortin-4 receptor (*MC4R*) gene |
| Social, behavioral, and dietary factors |
| Ethnicity |
| Socioeconomic stratus |
| Psychological factors |
| Sedentary lifestyle |
| Calorie-dense western diet |
| Restrained eaters |

***Table 22.1***
*Etiology of overweight and obesity.*

which result to food intake independently of caloric depletion. In our current "obesogenic" environment with its abundance of affordable energy-dense, palatable foods, reward-driven feeding overrides depletion signals and overpowers the physiological mechanisms regulating energy homeostasis. This, coupled with limited physical activity and more sedentary lifestyles, is the fundamental reason underlying the global obesity pandemic.

## *Obesity-associated morbidity and mortality*

Overweight and obesity are associated with several comorbid conditions. In particular, obesity increases the risk of impaired glucose tolerance, T2DM, dyslipidemia, cardiovascular disease, hypertension, and obstructive sleep apnea by approximately two to three fold. In addition, patients with obesity are at increased relative risk of cholelithiasis, nonalcoholic steatohepatitis (NASH), hyperuricemia, gout, osteoarthritis, irregular menses, and male and female subfertility and infertility. Obesity is associated with increased cancer risk, such as postmenopausal breast cancer, endometrial cancer, colonic cancer, and increased overall anesthetic operative risk. Furthermore, obesity impacts on the individual's psychosocial function and depression is common in severe obesity, particularly in younger patients and in women.

Finally, in addition to increased morbidity, many epidemiological studies have established that obesity is associated with increased mortality. The association between BMI and cause-specific mortality was illustrated in the Prospective Studies Collaboration analysis. In the upper BMI range (25–50 kg/m$^2$), each 5 kg/m$^2$ increase in BMI was associated with a significant increase in mortality from each of the following disorders:

- Ischemic heart disease (hazard ratio [HR] 1.39) and stroke (HR 1.39)
- T2DM (HR 2.16)
- Nonneoplastic chronic kidney disease (HR 1.59)
- Respiratory diseases (HR 1.20)
- Neoplastic disease (HR 1.10), with a significant association between BMI and mortality for several forms of cancer, such as colonic, kidney, liver, breast, endometrial, and prostatic cancer

| | Clinical features additional to obesity | Gene/locus |
|---|---|---|
| **Monogenic causes of obesity** | | |
| Leptin deficiency | Hypogonadism, impaired T-cell immune function, frequent infections, advanced skeletal maturation | *LEP* gene; 7q31 |
| Leptin receptor deficiency | Hypogonadism | *LEPR* gene; 1p31 |
| Melanocortin-4 receptor deficiency | Accelerated growth, increased lean body mass, bone density, and linear growth | *MC4R* gene; 18q22 |
| Pro-opiomelanocortin deficiency | Hypopigmentation, isolated ACTH deficiency | *POMC* gene; 2p23.3 |
| Prohormone convertase-1 deficiency | Hypogonadism, postprandial hypoglycemia, elevated plasma proinsulin levels | *PCSK1* gene; 5q15-q21 |
| Neurotrophic tyrosine kinase, receptor type 2 deficiency | Hyperactivity, developmental delay, impaired pain sensation, impaired memory | *NTRK2* gene; 9q22.1 |
| **Genetic syndromes featuring obesity** | | |
| Prader–Willi | Diminished fetal activity, hypotonia, short stature, mental retardation, small hands and feet, hypogonadism | Lack of paternal segment 15q11.2-q12 |
| Albright's hereditary osteodystrophy (pseudohypoparathyroidism) | Short stature, short fourth and fifth metacarpals, round face, mild mental retardation | Germline mutation in gene encoding the G protein α subunit; *GNAS1* gene |
| Alstrom syndrome | Retinal dystrophy, neurosensory deafness, diabetes | 2p13 |
| Bardet–Biedl syndrome | Hypogonadism, retinal dystrophy, mental retardation, structural renal abnormalities, or functional renal impairment | Genetically heterogeneous, 14 different genes implicated (referred to as *BBS* genes) |
| Fragile X syndrome | Prominent jaw, large ears, high-pitched speech, macroorchidism, mental retardation | Xq27.3 |
| **Variation in genes associated with obesity** | | |
| Fat mass and obesity associated (*FTO*) | 16q12.2 | |
| Transmembrane protein 18 (*TMEM18*) | 2p25.3 | |
| SH2B adaptor protein 1 (*SH2B1*) | 16p11.2 | |
| Brain-derived neurotrophic factor (*BDNF*) | 11p13 | |

***Table 22.2***
*Genetic forms of obesity.*

Overall, it is estimated that obesity reduces life expectancy by about 9 years and accounts for 30,000 deaths in the United Kingdom per annum.

# *Pathophysiology of obesity*

## *Energy homeostasis regulation*

Energy homeostasis refers to the complex, coordinated processes required to maintain constant internal conditions of energy balance status in the face of external variation in the environment. Regulation of energy homeostasis encompasses regulation of both energy intake and energy expenditure. Body fat accumulation occurs when energy intake exceeds energy expenditure. Under stable conditions, energy intake and expenditure are exquisitely matched. A cumulative small deviation in either energy intake or energy expenditure, such as 20-kcal daily intake excess or 1% reduction in expended energy would result in approximately 1-kg weight gain in a year or >50 kg over the span of adult life. However, in a given environment, bodyweight is kept remarkably stable during most of the human adult life, despite large fluctuations in daily caloric intake. This apparent stability of bodyweight in the majority of adults is proof of the existence of a powerful system controlling bodyweight.[17]

### *The gut–brain axis in the regulation of energy homeostasis*

Neuronal circuits in the central nervous system (CNS) play a critical role in orchestrating the control energy homeostasis.[16] In particular, neural regulators sense acute fuel influx and body energy/fat stores and consequently generate appropriate signals to the neural circuits that control feeding and energy expenditure. These signals in their turn trigger adaptive alterations of energy intake and energy expenditure. This process involves constant bidirectional exchange of information between the brain and the gut or the so-called gut–brain axis. In addition, environmental cues and genes influence all aspects of energy balance.

Long-term humoral signals (such as leptin and insulin) and short-term hormonal signals (such as the gut hormones ghrelin, peptide YY [PYY], and glucagon-like peptide 1 [GLP-1]) originating from the periphery act on the CNS to influence feeding behavior. The main central regions involved are the hypothalamus, in particular, the arcuate hypothalamic nucleus, and the dorsal vagal complex in the brain stem (Figure 22.1). The arcuate hypothalamic nucleus integrates signals from the periphery and from the brainstem. The arcuate nucleus contains two distinct subsets of neuronal populations that control food intake. One acts as a stimulus to feeding, and these neurons contain neuropeptide Y (NPY) and agouti-related peptide (AgRP). Both NPY and AgRP stimulate food intake when injected into the CNS. The second subset of neurons acts as an inhibitor of food intake. These neurons contain α-melanocyte–stimulating hormone (α-MSH) and cocaine- and amphetamine-regulated transcript (CART). Direct administration of either α-MSH or CART into the CNS inhibits food intake. When one of these neuronal subsets is activated, the other is inactive. Due to an altered blood–brain barrier, these neurons are responsive to acute circulating hunger and satiety signals such as ghrelin and PYY, respectively, but they are also responsive to signals of long-term body energy stores, such as leptin and insulin. From the arcuate nucleus, neurons project to the paraventricular nucleus. The paraventricular nucleus receives input from the brainstem and the lateral hypothalamus; in addition, it projects to the pituitary gland and is interconnected with cortical (cognitive) and limbic (reward-processing) brain regions.

Peripheral neural signals originating from the gastrointestinal (GI) tract, the viscera, and adipose tissue also relay information to the CNS regarding the absence or acute flux of nutrients and energy deposits. Neural signals are composed of vagal afferents that are activated by chemo- and baroreceptors of the gut and the viscera and transmit information to the brainstem, where visceral inputs are integrated.

Beyond the homeostatic control of feeding, food intake is also controlled by circadian rhythms, food-related learning experiences, and food memories, with the latter being controlled by cortical areas. More importantly, in our current obesogenic environment characterized by a plethora of easily accessible calorie-dense, palatable foods and an abundance of powerful food cues, the control of food intake is complicated by the notion of hedonistic feeding. In contrast to homeostatic eating that occurs in the presence of caloric deficits, hedonic feeding is independent of energy balance status and is purely driven by the pleasantness and rewarding aspects of food. Sophisticated research studies using modern imaging techniques, such as functional magnetic resonance imaging (fMRI), have demonstrated that cortical and mesolimbic reward-processing brain regions are implicated in the control of feeding behavior.[19,20] Figure 22.1 is a diagrammatic illustration of the gut–brain axis in its role of regulating energy balance status.

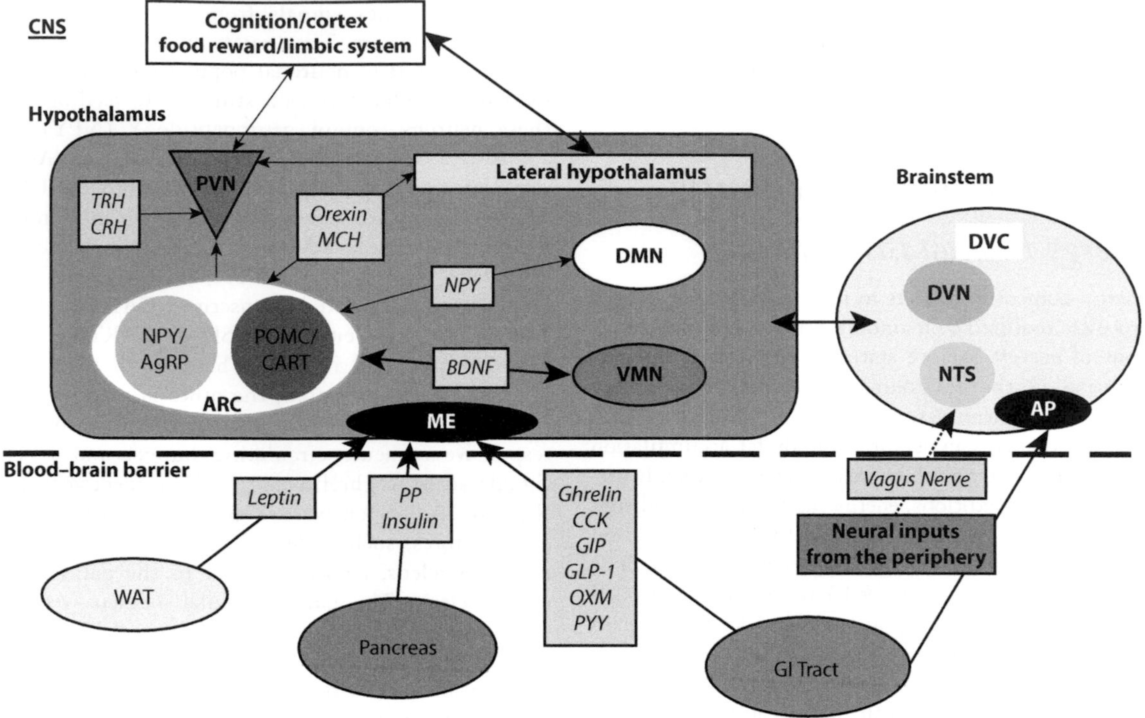


***Figure 22.1***

*Schematic representation of the gut–brain axis. Reciprocally connected neuronal circuits in the CNS play a critical role in orchestrating the control of energy homeostasis. Peripheral signals originating from the gut and adipose tissue relay information to the CNS about nutrient influx/deficit and energy-store status. These signals mediate the gut–brain crosstalk either directly via neural pathways or via the bloodstream due to the presence of an incomplete blood–brain barrier at the median eminence (ME) and area postrema (AP). ARC, arcuate nucleus; BDNF, brain-derived neurotrophic factor; CCK, cholecystokinin; CRH, corticotrophin-releasing hormone; DVC, dorsal vagal complex; DMN, dorsomedial nucleus; DVN, the dorsal motor nucleus of vagus; GI, gastrointestinal tract; GIP, glucose-dependent insulinotropic peptide; GLP-1, glucagon-like peptide-1; MCH, melanin-concentrating hormone; NPY/AgRP, Neuropeptide Y/Agouti-related peptide; NTS, nucleus of the tractus solitarius; OXM, oxyntomodulin; POMC/CART, pro-opiomelanocortin/cocaine- and amphetamine-regulated transcript; PP, pancreatic polypeptide; PVN, paraventricular nucleus; PYY, peptide YY; TRH, thyrotropin-releasing hormone; VMN, ventromedial hypothalamic nucleus; WAT, white adipose tissue.*

# *Leptin and the gut hormones ghrelin, PYY, and GLP-1 (Table 22.3)*

## *Leptin*

Leptin is secreted from the adipose tissue in proportion to the fat mass. Circulating leptin crosses the blood–brain barrier and reaches the hypothalamic NPY neurons, where it binds to the leptin receptor. Its actions induce satiety and negatively regulate fat mass. Loss of function mutations of the leptin gene or the leptin receptor gene cause severe obesity in rodents and humans.

## *Ghrelin*

Ghrelin, often referred to as the "hunger hormone," is a 28-amino acid peptide with unique orexigenic properties. It is derived from preproghrelin and is mainly produced from the *X/A*-like cells of the stomach and to a lesser degree from the small intestine.[18] Ghrelin undergoes unique posttranslational acylation in which the serine-3 residue is covalently linked to octanoic

| Gut hormone | Principal site of release | Factors affecting release | Role of hormone in bodyweight regulation |
|---|---|---|---|
| Ghrelin | X/A-like cells in gastric mucosa | ↑Fasting<br>↓Macronutrient intake<br>↑Diet-induced weight loss<br>↓Bariatric surgery<br>↑Sleep deprivation | Unique orexigenic hormone<br>↑Food intake<br>Role as meal initiator |
| PYY | L-cells in distal gut | ↓Fasting<br>↑Macronutrient intake<br>↑Bariatric surgery<br>↑Exercise | ↑Satiety<br>↑Energy expenditure |
| Pancreatic polypeptide (PP) | F-cells in pancreatic islets | ↓Fasting<br>↑Macronutrient intake<br>↑Exercise<br>↓Somatostatin | ↑Satiety<br>↑Energy expenditure |
| GLP-1 | L-cells in distal gut | ↑Macronutrient-intake<br>↓Caloric restriction<br>↑Bariatric surgery | ↑Satiety<br>↑Glucose-mediated insulin release (incretin effect) |
| OXM | L-cells in distal gut | ↑Macronutrient-intake | ↑Satiety<br>↑Energy expenditure |
| Cholecystokinin (CCK) | L-cells in duodenum and jejunum | ↑Fat-and protein-enriched chyme<br>↓Bile acids | ↑Satiety |
| Amylin | β-cells in pancreatic islets; cosecreted with insulin | ↑Food intake | ↑Satiety |

***Table 22.3***
*GI hormones regulating food intake.*

acid forming acyl-ghrelin. This posttranslational acylation is essential for ghrelin activation, allowing the peptide to cross the blood–brain barrier and bind to its receptor.

Circulating ghrelin concentrations increase with fasting and decrease after nutrient ingestion. Acute peripheral or central ghrelin administration to rats stimulates food intake, and similarly, in humans, peripherally infused ghrelin increases appetite and food intake. In rodents, chronic ghrelin administration causes hyperphagia and increased adiposity. Ghrelin also has prodiabetic properties. Specifically, it acts by stimulating insulin counterregulatory hormones, suppressing the insulin-sensitizing hormone adiponectin, blocking hepatic insulin signalling, and inhibiting insulin secretion, all of which acutely elevate blood glucose levels.

## PYY

PYY is a 36-amino acid peptide synthesized by the L-cells of the distal GI tract.[18] Two main forms of PYY have been described: PYY1-36 and PYY3-36. PYY3-36 is the predominant circulating form, arising from cleavage of the N-terminal Tyr–Pro residues from the full-length peptide PYY1-36 by the enzyme dipeptidyl-peptidase IV (DPPIV). Peripherally administered PYY3-36 inhibits food intake in rodents and normal weight and obese humans. Continuous or intermittent chronic PYY3-36 administration reduces adiposity and body weight gain in rodents. Obese subjects display an attenuated meal-stimulated PYY response and require a greater caloric load to achieve a similar postprandial PYY concentration in comparison with normal weight subjects. In addition to regulating appetite and body weight, PYY exerts glucoregulatory properties. Specifically in rodents, PYY3-36 enhances insulin-induced glucose disposal independently of food intake and bodyweight.

## GLP-1

GLP-1 is one of the peptides arising from posttranslational processing of preproglucagon. GLP-1 is also synthesized by the L-cells, predominantly located at the distal GI tract. In humans, oral but not intravenous administration of glucose stimulates GLP-1 release. The main physiological role of GLP-1 is that of an incretin hormone, stimulating insulin release in response to nutrient ingestion. GLP-1 enhances all steps of insulin biosynthesis and in addition exerts glucoregulatory properties by decelerating gastric emptying; inducing glucose-dependent inhibition of glucagon secretion; and stimulating pancreatic β-cell proliferation, thereby promoting differentiation of the islet progenitors and islet neogenesis in rodents. Several lines of evidence support a role for GLP-1 in appetite control and body weight regulation. Peripheral and central GLP-1 administration in rodents reduces food intake, whereas GLP-1 receptor antagonism increases food intake. Anorectic properties of GLP-1 have been reported in normal weight, overweight, and obese humans. Obese humans have been shown to exhibit attenuated postprandial GLP-1 release.

## Clinical evaluation of overweight and obese patients

Clinical evaluation for overweight and obesity should include measurement of bodyweight, BMI, waist circumference, and evaluation of overall medical risk. History-taking should include age at onset of weight gain, previous weight-loss attempts, change in dietary patterns, history of exercise, current and past medications, and history of smoking cessation. In addition to calculating BMI and measuring waist circumference, blood pressure should be measured, and a cardiovascular, respiratory, musculoskeletal, and abdominal examination undertaken. Biochemical assessment should include lipid profile and a fasting glucose measurement. Subsequent investigations or intervention, if necessary, is then based upon overall risk assessment.

## Genetic testing in the obesity clinic: Whom should we screen?

There is currently no consensus or established guidelines in relation to genetic screening for patients with obesity. Screening is mainly reserved for cases of severe, early onset obesity, obesity associated with hypothalamic symptomatology (hyperphagia, neuroendocrine dysfunction), features of syndromic forms of obesity, and various combinations of such cases.[24]

In cases of rapid-onset obesity, appropriate endocrine assessment to rule out underlying endocrine pathology (e.g., pituitary dysfunction, hypothyroidism, Cushing's, growth hormone deficiency, hypothalamic pathology) needs to take place before considering genetic screening. Thereafter, genetic screening work-up will depend on the clinical presentation, medical history, and family history. Presence of obesity in other family members suggests a dominant mutation or copy number variant (CNV) (i.e., deletion or duplication), whereas negative family history suggests either *de novo* mutation or autosomal recessive form. If history of intellectual impairment or a learning disability is present, then comparative genomic hybridization (CGH) could be undertaken. With CGH, CNVs can be identified in a wide-range manner, without the need to have *a priori* hypothesis. Candidate gene approach can be adopted if well-recognized associated features are present. MC4R deficiency accounts for 1%–6% of severe early onset obesity and should be undertaken first in cases of isolated severe obesity.

## Treatment for obesity

Lifestyle measures such as dieting, exercise, and behavioral modification are the cornerstone of weight-loss management. Caloric restriction is key, but in addition dietary modification/dietary macronutrient composition adjustment is important, because the latter could affect the release of endogenous regulators of appetite, thereby affecting feeding behavior. For example, Batterham et al.[4] demonstrated that in both normal weight and obese humans, high protein intake induced the greatest release of the anorectic hormone PYY and enhanced satiety, whereas in mice long-term augmentation of dietary protein resulted in increased plasma PYY levels, decreased food intake, and reduced adiposity.

However, dietary and lifestyle modifications usually result in at best modest weight loss and poor weight-loss maintenance. Behavioral interventions aimed at reducing calorie intake and increasing calories expended in daily physical activities can result in 9%–10% total body weight loss during the first 6 months of treatment. However, one third to two thirds of lost weight is regained within a year after the end of treatment and almost all weight is regained within 5 years posttreatment.

The goal of treatment is not only to reduce weight but also, more importantly, to improve the comorbid conditions associated with obesity. Patients should be made aware that obesity is a chronic disease requiring long-term treatment. Patients should also be informed that the efficacy of the current medication options is limited to 5%–10% bodyweight loss.[25,26,30] Thus, medication should not be viewed as a panacea for obesity treatment and should only be used as an adjunct to healthy lifestyle adaptations, including an increase in daily activity and a calorie-deficit diet.

## Obesity drugs

Drugs that have traditionally been used as weight-loss therapies include rimonabant, sibutramine, and orlistat. The U.S. Department of Health and Human Services, Food and Drug Administration (FDA), has recently approved Qsymia® for obesity treatment.[26]

Rimonabant (also known as SR141716) is an inverse agonist for the cannabinoid receptor rCB1. Rimonabant was marketed by Sanofi-Aventis in 2006 after receiving European Commission approval. It was used as weight-loss treatment in conjunction with diet and exercise in patients with BMI >30 kg/m$^2$ or BMI >27 kg/m$^2$ in the presence of comorbidities such as T2DM and dyslipidemia. However, in October 2008, the European Medicines Agency recommended the withdrawal of rimonabant due to serious psychiatric side effects, including suicidal ideation and suicide attempts.

Sibutramine is a reuptake inhibitor of serotonin, norepinephrine, and dopamine, thereby increasing their levels in synaptic clefts and promoting satiety. It was approved by the FDA in October 1997 for the treatment of obesity. However, in 2010 the FDA raised concerns that sibutramine increased the risk of myocardial infarctions and cerebrovascular accidents;[27] subsequently, sibutramine was withdrawn.

Orlistat inhibits pancreatic lipase and therefore alters fat absorption. As a result, about 30% of ingested fat is not digested and is excreted in feces. Orlistat is available in 120-mg capsules, and the recommended dose is 120 mg three times daily. However, a lower dose (60 mg), over-the-counter version is approved and available in the United Kingdom. In addition to inducing weight loss, orlistat is associated with improvement in serum lipid profile in a weight-independent manner. Systemic side effects are rare; however, absorption of fat-soluble vitamins may be decreased. Deficiency of fat-soluble vitamins (A, D, E, and K) and beta-carotene has been reported after orlistat treatment, with vitamin D being the most frequently affected. The most common side effects of orlistat are gastrointestinal, occurring in 15%–30% of patients and include intestinal cramps, flatus, and fecal incontinence. They tend to occur at the start of treatment and can be limited by reducing dietary fat intake (<30%). Severe liver injury has been reported in 13 cases with orlistat treatment. Formation of calcium oxalate stones with oxalate-induced acute kidney injury has also been reported; therefore, orlistat should be avoided in patients with a history of calcium oxalate stones.

Qsymia is a combination drug of low dose of the sympathomimetic drug phentermine and the antiepileptic drug topiramate. It is administered orally once daily. Qsymia was developed by Vivus, a California pharmaceutical company, and is indicated as an adjunct to a reduced calorie diet and increased physical activity for chronic weight management in adults with a BMI of ≥30 kg/m$^2$ or BMI of ≥27 kg/m$^2$ in the presence of at least one weight-related comorbidity, such as hypertension, T2DM, or dyslipidemia. In phase 2 and 3 clinical trials to date (EQUIP, CONQUER, SEQUEL studies), patients taking Qsymia in combination with a diet and lifestyle modification program have demonstrated statistically significant dose-dependent weight loss ranging between 5% and 10%, with associated improvements in glycemia and in cardiovascular risk factors. The most commonly reported side effects were tingling, dry mouth, constipation, and altered taste.

## Other drugs

### Diabetes drugs associated with weight loss

#### *Metformin*

In the Diabetes Prevention Program, a metformin-treated group experienced a mean weight loss of 2.5% compared with placebo over an average follow-up of 2.8 years, an effect that was maintained in a 10-year follow-up study. Thus, in overweight and obese patients with T2DM, metformin treatment is recommended for its dual benefits on glycemia and weight.

#### *Amylin*

Amylin is a peptide hormone cosecreted with insulin by the pancreatic beta islets in response to nutrient intake. Pramlintide is a synthetic analog of human amylin.

It has been shown to slow gastric emptying, reduce postprandial glucose levels, and improve hemoglobin A1C in patients with type 1 and T2DM. In addition, it has been reported to induce a modest weight loss compared with insulin and placebo (–0.8 kg and –2.27 kg, respectively).

### *GLP-1 analogs*

Exenatide is a long-acting synthetic peptide that is a GLP-1 receptor agonist, and liraglutide is a long-acting GLP-1 analog administered subcutaneously twice and once daily, respectively. They are currently available for adjunctive therapy for patients with T2DM who are inadequately controlled on oral agents. Dose-dependent weight loss has been reported in trials of exenatide in T2DM not well controlled on oral agents (~4.8 kg over 18 months in the absence of any dietetic or exercise interventions). In diabetes trials, liraglutide was associated with a significant reduction in weight up to 2.5 kg compared with placebo or glimepiride, whereas weight loss has also been reported in patients without diabetes who received liraglutide. In a 20-week randomized trial comparing liraglutide (administered subcutaneously in one of four daily doses, 1.2–3 mg), placebo, and open-label orlistat (120 mg orally three times daily) in 564 patients (mean BMI, 35 kg/m$^2$), weight loss increased with increasing doses of liraglutide, with mean weight loss ranging from 4.8 to 7.2 kg. Patients randomly assigned to any dose of liraglutide lost significantly more weight than those assigned to placebo (mean weight loss, 2.8 kg); whereas patients receiving the two highest doses of liraglutide (2.4 and 3.0 mg) lost significantly more weight than those assigned to orlistat (6.3, 7.2, and 4.1 kg, respectively). The two highest doses of liraglutide are higher than those currently prescribed for treatment of T2DM, and a greater proportion of patients taking these doses reported nausea (37%–47%) and vomiting (12%–14%).

### *Sympathomimetic drugs*

Sympathomimetic drugs reduce food intake by causing early satiety, acting by either stimulating the release of norepinephrine or inhibiting its reuptake into nerve terminals, such as phentermine, diethylpropion, benzphetamine, and phendimetrazine. Furthermore, they can act as norepinephrine and serotonin reuptake blockers (similar to sibutramine, discussed above) or as direct adrenergic receptors agonists (such as phenylpropanolamine, withdrawn from the market).

Phentermine and diethylpropion are associated with a relatively small risk of abuse. Phenylpropanolamine was removed from the market because of a small, but significant risk of hemorrhagic stroke in women. Ephedrine and ephedra alkaloids (Ma Huang) have been removed from the market. Low-dose phentermine is a component of the newly approved antiobesity agent Qsymia.

### *Antidepressants and antiepileptic drugs*

Bupropion, an antidepressant, is used during cessation of smoking to prevent weight gain. Fluoxetine, a selective serotonin reuptake inhibitor (SSRI), also used for the treatment of depression, has been reported to induce weight loss.

Topiramate, approved for use as an antiepileptic and for migraine treatment, has been shown in clinical studies to reduce weight with an average weight loss of 6.5% compared with 2% in the placebo arm. Topiramate is a component of the obesity drug Qsymia. Zonisamide, an antiepileptic agent with serotonergic and dopaminergic properties has been associated in clinical trials with weight loss but is not currently prescribed for the treatment of obesity.

However, in contrast to the drugs mentioned above, some antidepressants and some antiepileptic agents can cause weight gain, and this should be taken into consideration when prescribing antidepressant or antiepileptic medications in overweight or obese patients.

### *Belviq®*

Belviq is the marketing name for lorcaserin, which has also received FDA approval in 2012. Lorcaserin is a serotonin receptor agonist, highly selective for the 2C subtype of serotonin receptors. It decreases appetite, thereby decreasing body weight. Its efficacy seems to be comparable to that of orlistat in terms of weight loss, with the added benefit of reduction in cardiovascular disease surrogate markers, including blood pressure, heart rate, C-reactive protein (CRP), total cholesterol and low-density lipoprotein (LDL), fasting glucose, and insulin. The most common side effects attributed to this drug include headaches, nasopharyngitis, nausea, and dizziness. Lorcaserin is contraindicated in pregnancy and in patients with creatinine clearance <30 mL/min. Moreover, lorcaserin should not be coadministered with other serotoninergic agents due to increased risk of serotonin syndrome.

### *Dietary supplements*

Over-the-counter dietary supplements are widely used for weight loss, but there is limited evidence for their efficacy and safety. Such examples include ephedra, green tea, chromium, chitosan, and guar gum. Chitosan and guar gum are ineffective for weight loss, and their use should be discouraged. Similarly, Hoodia gordonii, a supplement derived from a South Africa desert plant, marketed and sold as an appetite suppressant, is also of unknown efficacy and safety. Clinicians should caution patients about use of dietary weight-loss formulations. Two compounded dietary supplements imported from Brazil, Emagrece Sim (also known as the Brazilian diet pill) and Herbathin, have been shown to contain prescription drugs, such as benzodiazepines, amphetamines, and fluoxetine. The FDA has issued a warning against their use, and clinicians should strongly discourage patients from using them.

### Human chorionic gonadotropin (hCG)

Injectable, oral, and sublingual preparations of hCG have been advertised as weight-loss aids. Among the values claimed for this treatment are loss of 1–2 pounds daily, absence of hunger, and maintenance of muscle tone. An integral component of the hCG diet is adherence to a very-low-calorie diet (500 kcal/day), and several randomized trials have shown that the hCG diet is not more effective than placebo in the treatment of obesity. Thus, hCG should not be used for the treatment of obesity.

### Experimental drugs

#### *Peptides*

There are several peptides that result in weight loss, either by a reduction in food intake or by increasing energy expenditure. None are currently approved by the FDA.

#### *Leptin*

Leptin is a peptide produced primarily in adipose tissue. Mice lacking leptin are obese (*ob/ob*). In humans with leptin deficiency, administration of physiological doses of leptin decreases food intake and causes weight loss. Obesity is associated with leptin resistance and hyperleptinemia. In a study of 47 obese women and men given placebo or varying doses of recombinant human leptin for 24 weeks, there was a weakly dose-dependent decrease in body weight, ranging from –1.3 kg in the placebo group to –1.4 kg in the 0.03-mg/kg group and –7.1 kg in the 0.30-mg/kg group.[28] Thus, these findings suggest that leptin resistance can be overcome with high doses of leptin, but whether the effect can be sustained remains unknown.

#### *PYY*

PYY is a peptide secreted from the L-cells of distal in response to nutrient intake and is suggested to play a role in mediating the weight-loss effects of bariatric surgery. In rodents and humans, acute PYY administration decreased appetite and food intake. However, in a 12-week trial of 133 obese patients randomly assigned to intranasal PYY (200 or 600 μg three times daily before meals) or placebo, in conjunction with diet and exercise, weight loss was similar in the placebo and 200-μg PYY groups; whereas weight loss could not be assessed in the 600-μg PYY group because of high dropout rate in this arm of the study (60%) due to nausea and vomiting. Studies are ongoing aimed at targeting the PYY system.

#### *Oxyntomodulin (OXM)*

OXM is a peptide also produced in L-cells of the GI tract. Like PYY, it also exerts anorectic properties and can induce weight loss.

### Anti-ghrelin targeting treatments

Two main characteristics of ghrelin render the peptide an attractive therapeutic target for obesity. First, ghrelin is the only known circulating orexigenic hormone, and second, it is a peptide that undergoes unique post-translational acylation with an octanoic acid being added. This acylation is necessary for ghrelin to cross the blood–brain barrier and for receptor binding. The enzyme mediating the acylation of ghrelin, ghrelin O-acyl-transferase (GOAT), has been recently characterized. Ghrelin antagonists have been evaluated in research studies, whereas more recently research efforts have focused on GOAT inhibition as an alternative way of targeting the ghrelin-GOAT system.

### Melanocortin-4 receptor agonists

The hypothalamic melanocortin system plays a key role in the control of body weight. Intranasal administration of the melanocortin sequence MSH/adrenocorticotropic hormone to normal weight subjects for 6 weeks decreased body fat by 1.7 kg. However, in a study of overweight men, where the same compound administered for 12 weeks there was no significant weight loss or adiposity decrease.[29]

### Serotonin agonists

Serotonin reduces food intake in animals and humans; thus, agonists to appropriate serotonin receptors are potentially valuable drugs. Lorcaserin is a selective agonist of the serotonin-2C receptor. Nonselective serotonergic agonists, such as fenfluramine and dexfenfluramine, also were shown to enhance weight loss in clinical trials. However, they increased the risk of serotonin-associated cardiac valvular disease, thought to occur through activation of serotonin receptor 2B. In addition to weight loss, lorcaserin had beneficial effects on surrogate markers of cardiovascular and diabetes risk, including systolic and diastolic blood pressure, heart rate, total and LDL cholesterol, CRP, fasting glucose, and circulating insulin levels.[31]

### Sympathomimetics

Tesofensine is a presynaptic inhibitor of norepinephrine, dopamine, and serotonin originally developed for the treatment of Parkinson's disease. Although its efficacy was limited for this application, study subjects were noted to experience significant weight loss. The efficacy and safety of tesofensine require further investigation.

## Bariatric surgery

In recent decades, the use of bariatric surgery to treat obesity has evolved significantly; currently, bariatric surgery is the single treatment modality inducing significant and sustainable weight loss.[32,33,34,38,39] The National Institute for Clinical Excellence (NICE) guidelines advocate consideration for bariatric surgery where nonsurgical therapies have failed in individuals with a BMI >40 kg/m$^2$ or with BMI >35 kg/m$^2$ and presence of other significant obesity-associated comorbidities that could be ameliorated by bariatric surgery.[36]

Bariatric procedures are divided into three categories based on their originally presumed mechanisms of action; malabsorptive, restrictive, and hybrid (or combination procedures).[32]

Malabsorptive procedures or pure bypass procedures include the jejunoileal bypass (JIB), duodenal–jejunal bypass (DJB), and biliopancreatic diversion (BPD) (Figure 22.2c, iv–vi). These operative techniques are associated with significant malabsorption and nutritional deficits; hence, their use has become limited.

Restrictive procedures, such as gastric banding (GB), vertical banded gastroplasty (VBG), and sleeve gastrectomy (SG) reduce gastric volume (Figure 22.2b, ii and iii). GB entails inserting a synthetic band with an inner inflatable balloon around the stomach below the gastroesophageal junction. The inner balloon diameter and hence the degree of gastric restriction is adjustable injecting saline into a subcutaneous port. In SG, a "sleeve" of stomach is resected leaving a small gastric tube with an intact pylorus. SG was originally described as a first-stage procedure followed by either biliopancreatic diversion-duodenal switch (BPD-DS) or Roux-en-Y gastric bypass (RYGB) in patients with a BMI >60 kg/m$^2$ or in high-risk patients. More recently, SG has been undertaken as a stand-alone bariatric procedure with early results suggesting that that SG results in comparable weight loss and resolution of comorbidities to RYGB.

Hybrid operations include RYGB and BPD-DS (Figure 22.2d, vii and viii). RYGB, the most commonly performed bariatric operation, is considered the most efficacious operative technique and is the "gold standard" treatment for severe obesity. RYGB involves dividing the stomach with a surgical stapler along the lesser curvature, creating a small gastric pouch. The small bowel is divided and is rearranged into a Y-configuration, and nutrients pass from the small upper stomach pouch, via a "Roux-limb." Bowel continuity is restored by an entero–entero anastomosis, between the excluded biliary limb and the alimentary limb, performed approximately 100 cm from the gastrojejunostomy (GJ). Hence, ingested nutrients bypass most of the stomach, duodenum, and the proximal jejunum. Biliary and pancreatic secretions enter the common channel and mix with the nutrients at the site of the entero–entero anastomosis. This procedure results in sustained weight loss and reduction in the obesity-related comorbidities, including improved glycemic control or even resolution of T2DM.

The most commonly performed bariatric procedures for the treatment of obesity currently include gastric banding, RYGBP, and SG. Figure 22.2 illustrates the normal anatomy of the gastrointestinal tract (Figure 22.2a) and the most common restrictive, malabsorptive, and hybrid bariatric procedures (Figure 22.2b through d). Figure 22.3 illustrates in more detail the GI tract manipulation in RYGB and SG.

### The bariatric patient pathway

NICE guidance recommends that bariatric surgery should be undertaken only by a multidisciplinary team (MDT) that can provide comprehensive preoperative assessment; information on the different procedures; regular postoperative assessment; management of comorbidities; psychological support before and after surgery; access to plastic surgery (i.e., apronectomy); and access to suitable equipment, and staff trained to use such equipment.[36]

The core professions or disciplines within the MDT should at least include specialist bariatric surgeon(s), bariatric nurse specialist(s), and specialist bariatric dietitian(s). In addition, there should be standing and immediate access to specialist physicians with interest in and commitment to metabolic medicine; psychologist(s)/psychiatrist(s) with specialist interest in bariatric surgery; and senior anesthetist(s) with experience of anaesthesia for bariatric surgery. Finally, a bariatric service should have access to referral to other specialists, including hepatologists, endocrinologists/diabetologists, respiratory physicians, hematologists, cardiothoracic physicians, plastic surgeons, and specialists in eating disorders. All patients require access to a full MDT, but many will not need to be seen by more than a few members. Figure 22.4 is a diagrammatic illustration of the current bariatric pathway in our bariatric center. Bariatric referral pathways and the

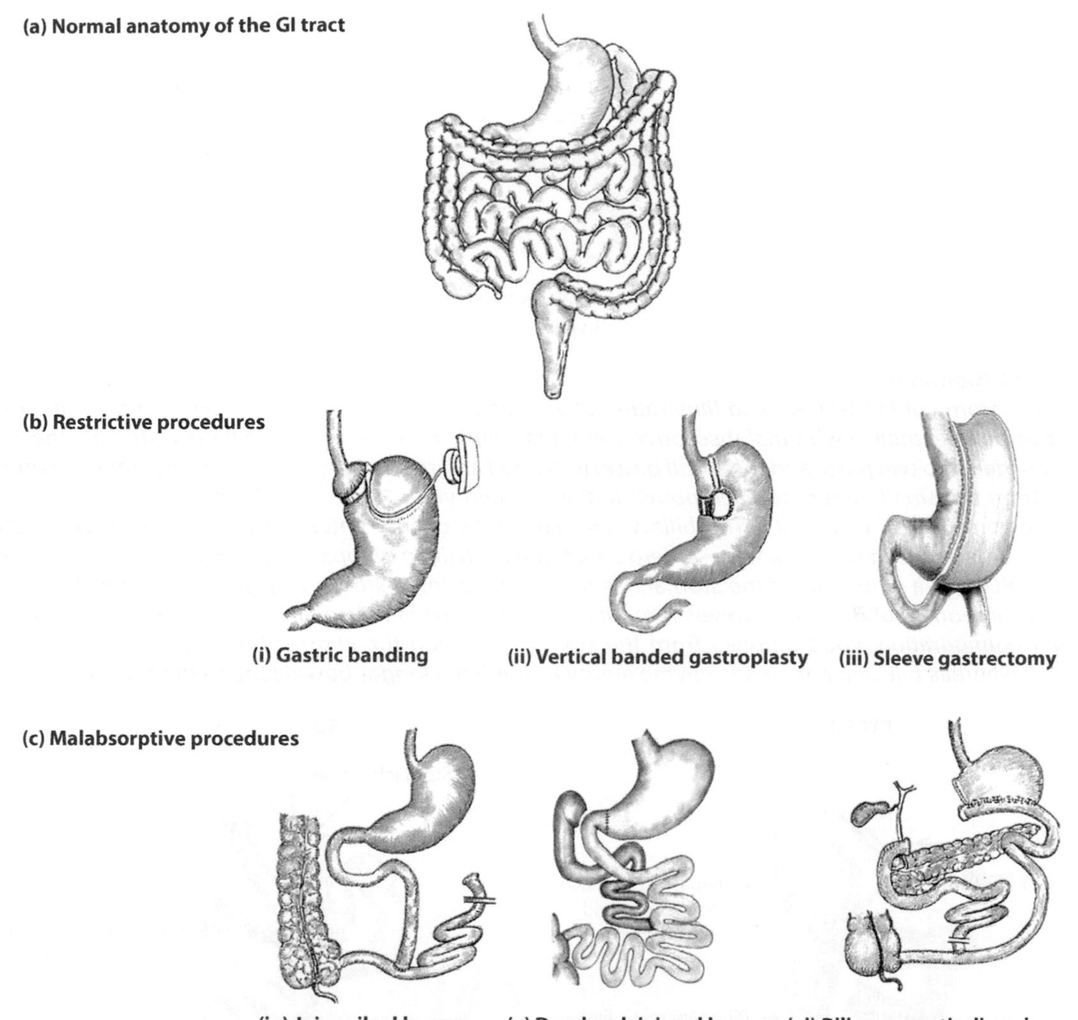


***Figure 22.2***
*Normal anatomy of the GI tract and illustration of various bariatric procedures. (a) Normal anatomy of the GI tract. In the normal GI tract, nutrients pass from the stomach into the duodenum and subsequently to the jejunum, ileum, and colon. (b) Restrictive procedures. (i) In gastric banding (GB), an inflatable silicon device is laparoscopically inserted below the gastroesophageal junction. The degree of gastric restriction can be adjusted by injecting saline into a subcutaneous port. (ii) In vertical banded gastroplasty (VBG), a small gastric pouch is constructed with the use of a band and staples. A small opening at the bottom of the pouch allows passage of nutrients to the small intestine. (iii) In sleeve gastrectomy (SG), a large portion of the stomach is resected leaving a "sleeve" of stomach behind. SG does not entail any bowel manipulation. (c) Malabsorptive procedures or bypass procedures. (iv) In jejunoileal bypass (JIB), the jejunum and ileum are bypassed. (v) In duodenal–jejunal bypass (DJB), the duodenum and jejunum are bypassed. (vi) In biliopancreatic diversion (BPD), part of the stomach is resected and the remaining stomach is then connected to the distal gut, thereby bypassing the duodenum and jejunum.*

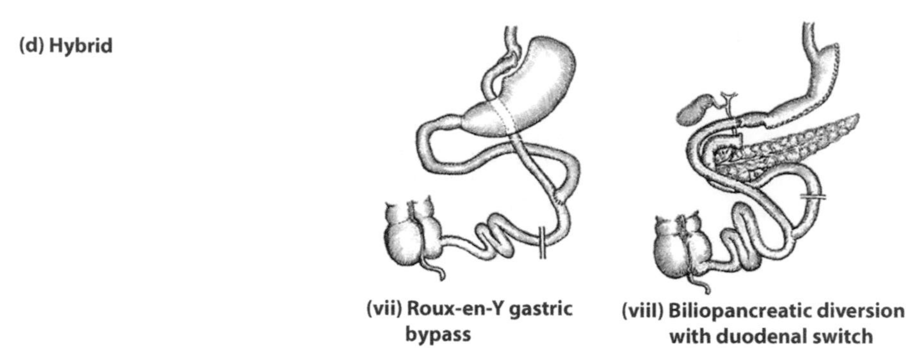


***Figure 22.2*** **(Continued)**
*Normal anatomy of the GI tract and illustration of various bariatric procedures. (d) Hybrid bariatric operations combine restrictive with malabsorptive elements. (vii) In Roux-en-Y gastric bypass (RYGB), the stomach is divided into two parts and the small bowel is divided and rearranged into a Y-configuration. Nutrients empty from the small upper stomach pouch to the jejunum via a "Roux-limb." An entero–entero anastomosis restores bowel continuity. The biliary and pancreatic chyme enter the common channel and mix with nutrients at the site of the entero–entero anastomosis. (viii) In biliopancreatic diversion with duodenal switch (BPD-DS), a large part of the stomach is removed leaving a sleeve of stomach behind. The malabsorptive component of BPD-DS involves rerouting a lengthy part of the small intestine, which is rearranged into a Y-configuration. Food empties from the stomach through the shorter bowel loop to the common channel; whereas bile and pancreatic chyme empty through the longer bowel loop to the common channel.*

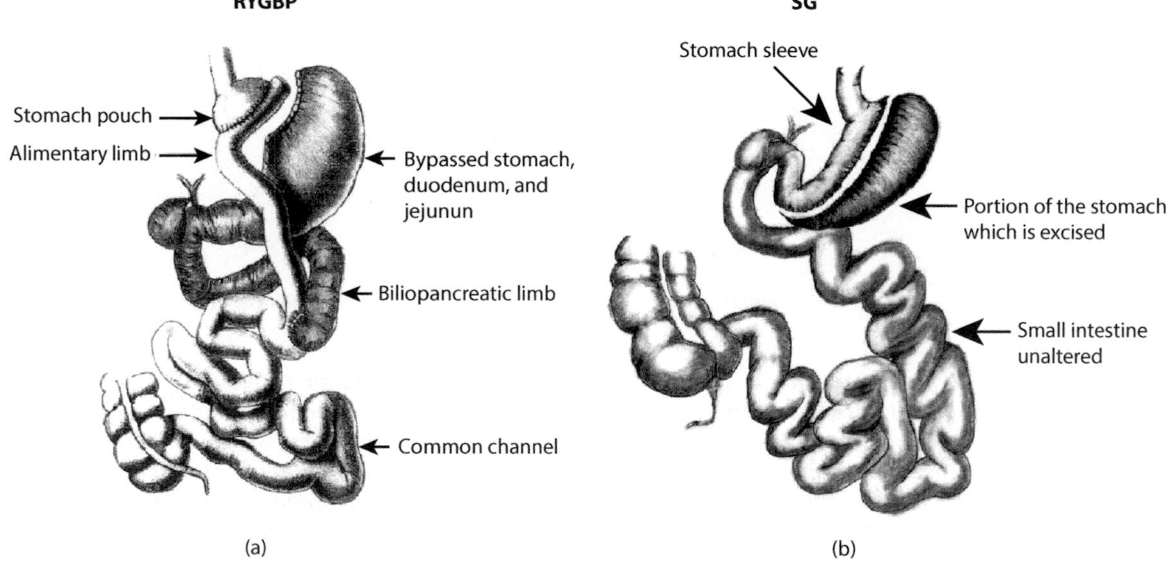


***Figure 22.3***
*GI tract anatomy post-Roux-en-Y gastric bypass (RYGB) and sleeve gastrectomy (SG). (a) In RYGBP, the stomach is divided and a small gastric pouch ~20 mL is constructed. The small bowel is also divided and rearranged into a Y-configuration. The ingested nutrients empty from the small upper stomach pouch to the mid-jejunum, thereby bypassing most of the stomach, the duodenum, and the proximal jejunum. Bowel continuity is restored by an entero-entero anastomosis. At the site of the entero-entero anastomosis, the biliary limb carrying the biliary and pancreatic chyme meets the alimentary limb that carries the nutrients, and the common channel is formed. (b) During SG, a large part of the stomach is resected, leaving only a sleeve of stomach behind. SG does not entail any intestinal manipulation.*

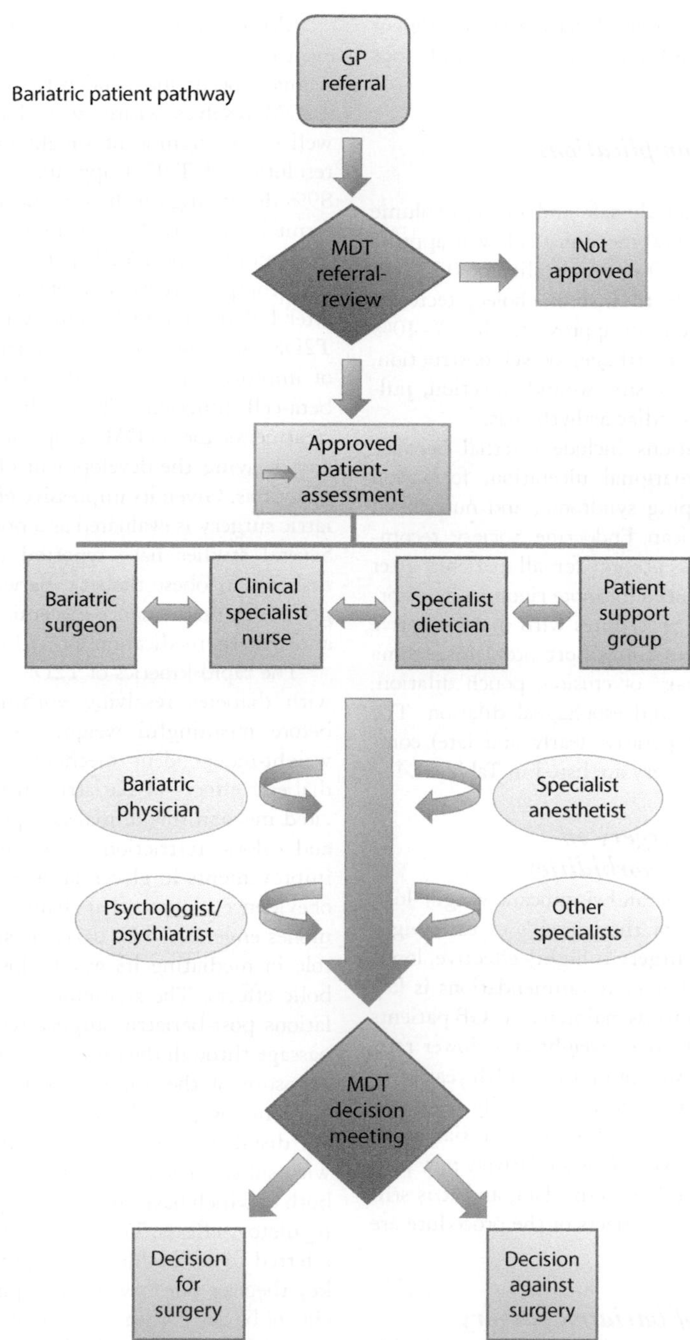


***Figure 22.4***
*Diagrammatic illustration of the bariatric patient pathway in our center. Bariatric referral pathways and the bariatric patient pathway may differ between different centers; however, they all share common foundations and key principles, including multidisciplinary approach [e.g., specialist bariatric surgeon(s), specialist bariatric dietician(s), specialist bariatric nurse(s), bariatric anesthetist(s), immediate access to bariatric physician(s), and access to referral to other specialists]. GP = general practitioner; MDT = multidisciplinary team.*

bariatric patient pathway may differ between different centers; however, they all share common foundations and key principles.[37]

### *Safety profile and complications of bariatric surgery*

Bariatric surgery is generally safe and in high-volume bariatric centers, in-hospital mortality is low at approximately of 0.14%, with 90-day mortality of 0.35%, a value that is comparable to that of cholecystectomy. Acute complications occur in approximately 5%–10% of cases and include hemorrhage, bowel obstruction, leak from the anastomotic site, wound infection, pulmonary embolism, and cardiac arrhythmias.

Long-term complications include internal hernias, anastomotic stenosis, marginal ulceration, formation fistulae, diarrhea, dumping syndrome, and nutritional deficiencies. The American Endocrine Society recommends vitamin supplementation for all patients after bariatric surgery with a need for more rigorous monitoring in those undergone procedures with malabsorptive element. GB patients can suffer port problems, stoma obstruction, band slippage or erosion, pouch dilation, gastroesophageal reflux, and esophageal dilation. The intraoperative and postoperative (early and late) complications of bariatric surgery are listed in Table 22.4.

### *Effects of bariatric surgery on weight and obesity comorbidities*

RYGB induces sustainable and significant weight loss, estimated at 60%–70% of the patient's excess weight over 2 years. Although surgery is highly effective, long-term compliance with dietary recommendations is key for weight loss and weight-loss maintenance. GB patients lose about 50% of their excess weight at a slower rate, often continuing to lose weight up to the fifth year post-surgery. Regular band adjustment is usually necessary to induce further weight loss. SG produces initial excess weight loss of 55%. However, SG is a relatively new procedure, with no available long-term data, and it is still under question whether the effects of the procedure are durable.

### *Metabolic benefits of bariatric surgery*

In addition to inducing significant and sustainable weight loss, bariatric surgery is associated with marked improvements in hyperlipidemia (70%), hypertension (62%), and obstructive sleep apnea (84%).[32,34] In addition, bariatric surgery results in substantial decrease of all-cause mortality (29% at 10-year follow-up), with decreased specific-cause mortality by 56% for coronary artery disease, 92% for diabetes, and 60% for cancer.[35]

RYGB surgery results in rapid amelioration and even complete resolution of T2DM. Remarkably, this seems to occur independently from weight loss, because T2DM resolves within several days of the procedure, well before significant weight loss occurs. The rate of resolution of T2DM appears to be between 64% and 89% depending on the type of bariatric procedure performed. Nevertheless, there is a trend toward better outcomes for the RYGB patients than the GB patients with complete remission reported in 70.1% at >2 years after RYGB and 58.3% after GB. The improvement in T2DM after weight loss is related to the dual effects of improvements in insulin sensitivity and pancreatic beta-cell function. The traditional focus of medical treatments for T2DM is optimizing glycemic control and delaying the development of diabetes-related complications. Given its impressive effects on glycemia, bariatric surgery is evaluated as a potential cure for T2DM. Several studies have reported complete resolution of diabetes in obese diabetic patients after bariatric surgery, with maintenance glycemia without the use of any antidiabetic medication for >10 years postsurgery.

The rapid kinetics of T2DM resolution after RYGB, with diabetes resolving within days to weeks even before meaningful weight loss occurs, implies that weight-independent mechanisms mediate these antidiabetic effects of bariatric surgery. The traditionally cited mechanisms of malabsorption, gastric restriction, and caloric restriction cannot explain these dramatic improvements in glycemia, whereas a cumulative body of evidence suggests that changes in circulating gut hormones engendered by bariatric surgery *per se* play a key role in mediating its weight loss and beneficial metabolic effects. The anatomical gastrointestinal manipulations post-bariatric surgery result in altered nutrient passage through the gut, thus translating to differential exposure of the gut enteroendocrine cells to luminal nutrients. Rapid delivery of partially digested chyme in the distal gut results in overstimulation of the L-cells with subsequent increased release of GLP-1 and PYY, both of which have anorectic properties and exert glucoregulatory effects. This hindgut overstimulation is often referred to as the hindgut hypothesis and is one of the key theories put forward to explain the metabolic benefits of bariatric surgery. Moreover, postoperative reductions in circulating ghrelin have been reported after bariatric surgery. Ghrelin increases appetite and is also implicated in the regulation of glycemia. Thus, given its physiological effects, ghrelin has been implicated as a mediator of the weight and metabolic outcomes of bariatric surgery as part of the ghrelin hypothesis. A final theory postulated to mediate the effects of bariatric surgery is referred to as the foregut exclusion

**Intraoperative complications**
**-Bleeding**
**-Splenic injury**: *More common with SG, usually controlled with hemostatic agents.*
**-Portal vein injury/thrombosis**
**-Bowel ischemia**: *Resulting from compromise of the mesentery root during transection or from internal hernias.*
**Early postoperative complications**
**-Bleeding:** *Typically at the anastomosis and/or staple lines; more often intraluminal.*
**-Wound infections:** *More common with open versus laparoscopic surgery (10%–15% vs. 3%–4%).*
**-Anastomotic leak:** *Usually occurs 1–4 weeks postsurgery; associated with high mortality rate. Patients often present with subtle symptoms/signs, such as low-grade fever, respiratory compromise, or unexplained tachycardia. Low index of suspicion is key for timely diagnosis. Can be radiographically confirmed by barium swallow or contrast computed tomography.*
**-Pulmonary embolism/deep venous thrombosis**
**-Pulmonary complications:** *Respiratory failure, atelectasis. The risk can be reduced with continuous positive airway pressure (CPAP) treatment of patients with obstructive sleep apnea (OSA) preoperatively.*
**-Cardiovascular complications:** *Myocardial infarction, arrhythmias, and heart failure.*
**Late postoperative complications**
**-Gastric remnant distension post-RYGB:** *Rare, but potentially fatal. Features include hiccups, left upper quadrant tympany, abdominal and/or shoulder pain, abdominal distension, tachycardia, shortness of breath. Radiographic assessment may reveal a large gastric air bubble. Treatment consists of emergency decompression with a gastrostomy tube or percutaneous gastrostomy with immediate operative exploration required if percutaneous drainage is not feasible, or if perforation is suspected.*
**-Stomal stenosis post-RYGB:** *Usually occurs several weeks after surgery. Symptoms include nausea, vomiting, dysphagia, gastroesophageal reflux, and inability to tolerate oral intake. The diagnosis is usually established by endoscopy or with upper GI series. Endoscopic balloon dilatation is usually successful, but surgical revision may be required.*
**-Marginal ulcers**
**-Cholelithiasis**
**-Nephrolithiasis**
**-Incisional hernias; internal hernias**
**-Blind loop syndrome post-RYGB**
**-Short bowel syndrome:** *Can result from small bowel resections for internal hernias or bowel obstruction from adhesions.*
**-Dumping syndrome**
**-Metabolic and nutritional derangements:** *Vitamin supplementation is routinely prescribed post-RYGB.*
**-Postoperative recurrent hyperinsulinemic hypoglycemia post-RYGB:** *Pancreatic nesidioblastosis has been proposed as the underlying mechanism.*
**-Change in bowel habits:** *Loose stool and diarrhea post-RYGB and constipation post-GB.*
**-Band erosion, band slippage or prolapse post-GB**
**-Port or tubing malfunction post-GB**
**-Narrowing or stenosis post-SG**

***Table 22.4***
*Complications of bariatric surgery.*

hypothesis. According to this hypothesis, the foregut produces an unknown anti-incretin molecule; therefore, bypass of the foregut after bariatric procedures, such as RYGBP, results in reduced production of this molecule, thereby negating its effects.

## Summary

In this chapter, we have provided an overview of the obesity prevalence, etiology, classification, pathophysiology, and current medical and surgical obesity treatment options. Main points are summarized as follows:

- The prevalence of obesity is increasing with epidemic proportions, especially over the past two decades, and currently the obesity crisis continues unabated. It is estimated that 1.46 billion people worldwide are overweight and 502 million are obese.
- Obesity and its associated comorbidities are a major public health problem, placing growing demands and a great financial burden on healthcare systems.
- In our current obesogenic environment, the main cause for the obesity pandemic is overconsumption of energy-dense, westernized foods coupled with more sedentary lifestyle.
- Lifestyle modification, behavioral interventions, and available pharmacotherapies for obesity management induce at best only modest weight loss, with poor weight-loss maintenance.
- Currently in the United Kingdom, only one drug, orlistat, is licensed for the treatment of overweight and obesity.
- Bariatric surgery is currently the only treatment modality inducing significant and sustained weight loss, leading to reduced morbidity and mortality.
- Bariatric surgery is associated with marked improvements in glycemia and even complete resolution of T2DM.
- There is currently a pressing need for effective preventative and treatment strategies to combat the obesity crisis.

## References


1. World Health Organization. Obesity and overweight. Geneva: World Health Organization, 2010.
2. National Institutes of Health (NIH), National Heart, Lung and Blood Institues (NHLBI). *The Practical Guide: Identification, Evaluation, and Treatment of Overweight and Obesity in Adults*. Bethesda: NIH, 2000. NIH Publication 004084.
3. Wang YC, McPherson K, Marsh T, et al. Health and economic burden of the projected obesity trends in the USA and the UK. *Lancet* 2011;378(9793):815–25.
4. Batterham RL, Heffron H, Kapoor S, et al. Critical role for peptide YY in protein-mediated satiation and body-weight regulation. *Cell Metab* 2006;4(3): 223–33.
5. Bray GA, Bellanger T. Epidemiology, trends, and morbidities of obesity and the metabolic syndrome. *Endocrine* 2006;29(1):109–17.
6. Finucane MM, Stevens GA, Cowan MJ, et al. National, regional, and global trends in body-mass index since 1980: Systematic analysis of health examination surveys and epidemiological studies with 960 country-years and 9.1 million participants. *Lancet* 2011;377(9765):557–67.
7. Swinburn BA, Sacks G, Hall KD, et al. The global obesity pandemic: Shaped by global drivers and local environments. *Lancet* 2011;378:804–14.
8. Calle EE, Thun MJ, Petrelli JM, et al. Body-mass index and mortality in a prospective cohort of U.S. adults. *N Engl J Med* 1999;341:1097–105.
9. Whitlock G, Lewington S, Sherliker P, et al. Body-mass index and cause-specific mortality in 900 000 adults: Collaborative analyses of 57 prospective studies. *Lancet* 2009;373:1083–96.
10. Adams KF, Schatzkin A, Harris TB, et al. Overweight, obesity, and mortality in a large prospective cohort of persons 50 to 71 years old. *N Engl J Med* 2006;355(8): 763–78.
11. Cornier MA, Despres JP, Davis N, et al. Assessing adiposity: A scientific statement from the American Heart Association. *Circulation* 2011;124(18):1996–2019.
12. Deurenberg P, Yap M, van Staveren WA. Body mass index and percent body fat: A meta analysis among different ethnic groups. *Int J Obes Relat Metab Disord* 1998;22(12):1164–71.
13. Gallagher D, Heymsfield SB, Heo M, et al. Healthy percentage body fat ranges: An approach for developing guidelines based on body mass index. *Am J Clin Nutr* 2000;72(3):694–701.
14. Janssen I, Katzmarzyk PT, Ross R. Waist circumference and not body mass index explains obesity-related health risk. *Am J Clin Nutr* 2004;79(3):379–84.
15. Razak F, Anand SS, Shannon H, et al. Defining obesity cut points in a multiethnic population. *Circulation* 2007;115(16):2111–18.
16. Schwartz MW, Woods SC, Porte D, Jr., et al. Central nervous system control of food intake. *Nature* 2000;404:661–71.
17. Berthoud HR, Morrison C. The brain, appetite, and obesity. *Annu Rev Psychol* 2008;59:55–92.

18. Karra E, Batterham RL. The role of gut hormones in the regulation of body weight and energy homeostasis. *Mol Cell Endocrinol* 2010;316:120–8.
19. Batterham RL, ffytche DH, Rosenthal JM, et al. PYY modulation of cortical and hypothalamic brain areas predicts feeding behaviour in humans. *Nature* 2007;450(7166):106–9.
20. Malik S, McGlone F, Bedrossian D, et al. Ghrelin modulates brain activity in areas that control appetitive behavior. *Cell Metab* 2008;7(5):400–9.
21. Farooqi S, O'Rahilly S. Genetics of obesity in humans. *Endocr Rev* 2006;27(7):710–18.
22. Frayling TM, Timpson NJ, Weedon MN, et al. A common variant in the FTO gene is associated with body mass index and predisposes to childhood and adult obesity. *Science (New York, NY)* 2007;316(5826):889–94.
23. Speliotes EK, Willer CJ, Berndt SI, et al. Association analyses of 249,796 individuals reveal 18 new loci associated with body mass index. *Nat Genet* 2010;42(11):937–48.
24. Phan-Hug F, Beckmann JS, Jacquemont S. Genetic testing in patients with obesity. *Best Pract Res Clin Endocrinol Metab* 2012; 26(2):133–43.
25. Leblanc ES, O'Connor E, Whitlock EP, et al. Effectiveness of primary care-relevant treatments for obesity in adults: A systematic evidence review for the U.S. Preventive Services Task Force. *Ann Intern Med* 2011;155:434–47.
26. Derosa G, Maffioli P. Anti-obesity drugs: A review about their effects and their safety. *Expert Opin Drug Saf* 2012;11:459–71.
27. James WP, Caterson ID, Coutinho W, et al. Effect of sibutramine on cardiovascular outcomes in over- weight and obese subjects. *N Engl J Med* 2010;363:905–17.
28. Heymsfield SB, Greenberg AS, Fujioka K, et al. Recombinant leptin for weight loss in obese and lean adults: A randomized, controlled, dose-escalation trial. *JAMA* 1999;282:1568–75.
29. Hallschmid M, Smolnik R, McGregor G, et al. Overweight humans are resistant to the weight-reducing effects of melanocortin 4-10. *J Clin Endocrinol Metab* 2006;91:522–5.
30. Rucker D, Padwal R, Li SK, et al. Long term pharmacotherapy for obesity and overweight: Updated meta-analysis. *BMJ* 2007;335:1194–9.
31. Chan EW, He Y, Chui CS, et al. Efficacy and safety of lorcaserin in obese adults: A meta-analysis of 1-year randomized controlled trials (RCTs) and narrative review on short-term RCTs. *Obes Rev* 2013;14(5):383–92.
32. Scott WR, Batterham RL. Roux-en-Y gastric bypass and laparoscopic sleeve gastrectomy: Understanding weight loss and improvements in type 2 diabetes after bariatric surgery. *Am J Physiol Regul Integr Comp Physiol* 2011;301:R15–27.
33. Sjostrom L, Narbro K, Sjostrom CD, et al. Effects of bariatric surgery on mortality in Swedish obese subjects. *N Engl J Med* 2007;357(8):741–52.
34. Sjostrom L, Lindroos AK, Peltonen M, et al. Lifestyle, diabetes, and cardiovascular risk factors 10 years after bariatric surgery. *N Engl J Med* 2004;351(26):2683–93.
35. Adams TD, Gress RE, Smith SC, et al. Long-term mortality after gastric bypass surgery. *N Engl J Med* 2007;357(8):753–61.
36. Specifying a bariatric surgical service for the treatment of people with severe obesity, 2012, www.nice.org.
37. BOMSS Standards for Clinical Services and Commissioning Guidelines, 2012, www.bomms.uk.
38. Van Gaal LF, De Block CE. Bariatric surgery to treat type 2 diabetes: What is the recent evidence? *Curr Opin Endocrinol Diabetes Obes* 2012; 19(5):352–8.
39. Terranova L, Busetto L, Vestri A, et al. Bariatric surgery: Cost-effectiveness and budget impact. *Obes Surg* 2012; 22(4):646–53.

# 23

# Endocrinology of aging

*Prasanth N. Surampudi, Christina Wang, Yanhe Lue, Ronald Swerdloff*

## Introduction

The endocrine system undergoes various complex changes as individuals advance in age. Age-related changes can be observed in thyroid function, gonadal function, pituitary dynamics, adrenal gland physiology, calcium metabolism, and glucose homeostasis. Many endocrine functions are intertwined, and any modulation or reduced function in one system can adversely affect other endocrine glands. The nature and extent of endocrine changes observed in individuals with aging are highly variable. The changes to the endocrine system depend on several factors, including gender, genetics, presence of other disease processes, accumulated effects of lifestyle, and environment.

The decreased endocrine function with aging is primarily due to changes in hormone secretion and reduced response of tissues to hormones. Aging causes a decrease in levels of some hormones and an increase in the levels of other hormones. Some hormone levels remain unchanged with aging. Hormones that decrease with aging include thyroid-stimulating hormone (TSH), testosterone, estrogen (E), growth hormone (GH), insulin-like growth factor (IGF)-I, dehydroepiandrosterone (DHEA), and melatonin. Hormones that decrease only to a small extent or remain unchanged with aging include cortisol, epinephrine, insulin, triiodothyronine (T3), and thyroxine (T4). Hormones that may increase with aging include follicle-stimulating hormone (FSH), luteinizing hormone (LH), norepinephrine, and parathyroid hormone. The major changes in circulating hormones that occur with aging are outlined in Table 23.1. The response of various tissues to these hormones also is altered (often decreases) with aging.

As individuals age, adults may live one-third of their life with some relative hormone deficiency. The reduced responsiveness of tissues to hormones and decline in hormone levels with aging make older men and women at risk of developing endocrine deficiencies and disorders. Thus, with aging, there is an increased prevalence of thyroid disorders (subclinical and clinical hypothyroidism and hyperthyroidism), hypogonadism, osteoporosis, and type 2 diabetes mellitus. These hormonal changes directly or indirectly also contribute to changes in body constitution and fat distribution (visceral obesity), muscle weakness, loss of cognitive function, reduction in sense of vitality, infertility, and sexual dysfunction.

Traditional treatment approaches aim to supplement deficient hormones to enhance the quality of life and promote longevity of the aging males. In certain cases, hormone replacement therapy (HRT) was found to be useful in improving health and well-being. Vitamin D replacement in older persons with low vitamin D levels prevents hip fracture, decreases falls, improves muscle strength, and increases the mean age at death. In certain cases, controversies exist about the effectiveness and safety of hormonal replacement therapy. The physician should obtain objective evidence of hormone deficiency, exclude secondary causes of endocrine dysfunction, and make an assessment of risks versus benefits of the replacement therapy before recommending HRT to older adults.

This chapter broadly covers endocrinological changes in aging men and women in thyroid, gonad, pituitary, and adrenal function. This chapter also summarizes the consequences of the hormonal changes, treatment options, and safety concerns of replacement therapy.

| Endocrine system | Hormone | Hormone changes with age |
|---|---|---|
| Hypothalamus | Corticotropin-releasing hormone (CRH) | Decreases with age |
| | Gonadotropin-releasing hormone (GnRH) | Decreases with age |
| | Growth hormone–releasing hormone (GHRH) | Decreases with age |
| Pituitary | Thyroid-stimulating hormone (TSH) | No change to slight decrease; decreased response to TRH stimulation |
| | Adrenocorticotropic hormone (ACTH) | Increases in amplitude; partly due to changes in CRH |
| | Growth hormone (GH) | Reduced GH pulse amplitude |
| | Luteinizing hormone (LH) | LH amplitude can decrease with age |
| | Follicle-stimulating hormone (FSH) | Increases in women; can increase or stay in normal range for men |
| Thyroid | Thyroxine (T4) | No significant change in level; decreased section but with decreased conversion to T3 |
| | Triiodothyronine (T3) | Slight decrease with age (decreased production and decreased conversion) |
| Gonadal | Estrogens | Estradiol decreases with age |
| | Androgens | Testosterone often decreases with age |
| Adrenal | Cortisol | Slightly elevated or no significant change |
| | Aldosterone | No significant change |
| | DHEA, DHEAS | Decreases with age; increase in the concentration of glucocorticoids compared with sex steroids |
| Liver | Insulin-like growth factor 1 (IGF-1) | Decreases with age; parallels decline in GH |
| | Leptin | No significant change to decreases with age |
| | Neuropeptide Y | No significant change to decreases with age |
| | Ghrelin | No significant change |

***Table 23.1***
*Hormonal changes with aging.*

# *Thyroid function and aging*

Thyroid physiology changes with age in otherwise healthy adults. TSH and T3 levels decline with increasing age with the TSH levels in older adults reported to be approximately 40% less than the levels in younger adults. Although thyroid disorders occur over the entire age range, they occur with increased prevalence in the elderly compared with young adults.[1,2] Older women showed higher prevalence of thyroid disorders compared with older men. The thyroid disorders observed in older adults include hyperthyroidism, hypothyroidism, and subclinical hyperthyroidism and hypothyroidism, and thyroid nodules. Early diagnosis and treatment of thyroid disorders is important because these disorders could increase risk of morbidity and mortality in aging subjects. It is important to distinguish direct age-related thyroid dysfunctions from disorders caused by malnutrition, illnesses, or drug side effects. Diagnosis of thyroid disorders in older adults is complex because the symptoms of thyroid disorders are often nonclassical and subtle, and they can resemble symptoms of certain diseases of the cardiovascular, gastrointestinal, and nervous systems.

## *Physiological changes of thyroid with aging*

Aging causes several anatomical and physiological changes in the thyroid. Gross and microscopic changes of the thyroid gland are observed with aging and include reduced size of follicles and increased fibrosis of the gland. Mass of the thyroid gland also decreases with increasing age. The hormonal changes observed with aging include a decrease in the levels of serum TSH and T3, and an increase in the levels of reverse (r)T3. In many instances, these decreased hormone levels are not associated with changes in the serum-free (F)T4, FT3, and T4 levels.[3]

The changes in the secretion of thyroid hormone levels are mainly due to aging-related alterations of the hypothalamic–pituitary system. There is reduced ability of thyrotropin-releasing hormone (TRH) to stimulate pituitary secretion with increasing age.[3–5] Reduced TSH levels result in a reduction of the secretion of T3 and T4 hormones. Peripheral T4 degradation is also reduced with aging, leading to no changes in serum T4 concentrations. As a result, serum T4 concentrations remain normal in healthy elderly subjects, and serum T3 shows an age-dependent decline.[3–5] Thyroid hormone action also appears to decline with aging as suggested by a lower oxygen consumption rate and a lower basal metabolic rate.

## *Hyperthyroidism and subclinical hyperthyroidism (see Chapters 13, 14)*

### *Hyperthyroidism*

Hyperthyroidism is defined as having symptoms of hyperthyroidism with low-serum levels of TSH, high T4, high FT4, and high T3. The prevalence of hyperthyroidism is estimated to be 0.5%–3% in the aging population.[4,6–9] Toxic multinodular goiter is a common cause of hyperthyroidism in older adults living in areas of low iodine intake;[10] Graves' disease is an important cause of hyperthyroidism in older adults living in regions of higher iodine intake.[8] In aged patients, hyperthyroidism may also be precipitated by excess iodine intake from drugs or radiographic contrast agents[4]; subacute thyroiditis can also be noted at an increased rate. Amiodarone-induced thyrotoxicosis type 1 occurs more often in individuals with Graves' disease. A unifocal toxic adenoma is a less common cause of hyperthyroidism in the elderly.

Older adults with hyperthyroidism display fewer signs and symptoms of hyperthyroidism compared with younger patients. Symptoms or signs of heat intolerance, orbitopathy, nervousness, or sinus tachycardia are seen less frequently. The decreased prevalence of elderly individuals with classical symptoms of hyperthyroidism could be due to concurrent medical conditions or medications such as β-blockers that can mask classical symptoms (e.g., sinus tachycardia). The classical symptoms of hyperthyroidism are often reduced in aging patients with Graves' disease, except for weight loss and atrial fibrillation.[11] Although apathetic hyperthyroidism is more common, the classical symptoms of hyperthyroidism may be seen older patients with more severe hyperthyroidism, and in smokers.[12]

There are important manifestations of hyperthyroidism that are seen more frequently in the elderly. Atrial fibrillation is an important age-related sign of hyperthyroidism.[13] In addition, older adults with hyperthyroidism experience an increased rate of gastrointestinal symptoms, such as diarrhea, loss of appetite, nausea, persistent vomiting; and neurological symptoms such as mania, depression, and cognitive impairment, including dementia.[14] Elevated T4 levels in the elderly are also associated with loss of bone density, increased fracture risk (e.g., hip and vertebral fractures), decreased physical function, and adverse impact on frailty.[15–17]

The diagnosis of hyperthyroidism in older adults may go unrecognized due to the less classical clinical signs and symptoms as well as variations in the classical presentation of laboratory tests. The TSH levels are generally lower in older adults with hyperthyroidism. The FT4 level is often elevated in most but not all elderly hyperthyroid patients. Thus, measurement of serum T3 levels is important in identifying some elderly men with hyperthyroidism because T3 thyrotoxicosis (i.e., elevated serum T3 with normal T4) is more common in the elderly. However, one should keep in mind that T3 elevations may be masked by the concomitant lowering of serum T3 by nonthyroidal illness and drugs (e.g., propranolol and iodinate contrast material). In these circumstances, thyrotoxicosis may blossom when the illness is corrected or the drugs are withdrawn that may lower T3 levels.

The use of radioactive iodine is preferred over antithyroid medications for the treatment of hyperthyroidism in older adults.[18] In addition, medications that offer rate control, such as β-blockers, should be added if the older adults have atrial fibrillation.[18]

### *Subclinical hyperthyroidism*

Subclinical hyperthyroidism is defined as a low serum TSH with an FT4 and FT3 in the upper end of the reference range.[19,20] Prevalence of subclinical hyperthyroidism is about 3%–8% in the older population.[7,21–24] The prevalence of subclinical hyperthyroidism depends on TSH cut-off values used to define the normal range, geographic area, iodine intake, and gender. It was found to be higher in older adults compared with young adults.[25] Several studies have also reported that the prevalence of subclinical hyperthyroidism is higher in women than in men[26] and lower in blacks than in whites.[9]

Overt and subclinical hyperthyroidism may be iatrogenic. The most common cause of subclinical hyperthyroidism is excessive replacement of thyroid hormone that is recognized as asymptomatic lower serum TSH levels <0.1 ng/dL.[27] Subclinical hyperthyroidism can also result from Graves' disease and toxic multinodular goiter. Subclinical hyperthyroidism may remain stable in patients over the age of 60 years because <0.5%–2% progress to overt hyperthyroidism.[28,29] One should also take into consideration other conditions that can influence the thyroid function tests, including dietary habits, fasting, nonthyroidal illness, and drugs (e.g., glucocorticoids, dopamine agonists).

Although free of classical symptoms, subclinical hyperthyroidism may increase long-term morbidity due to effects on the cardiovascular system, cognition, and risk of fractures.[25,30,31] Subclinical hyperthyroidism can aggravate preexisting heart disease and lead to cardiovascular morbidity (e.g., atrial fibrillation, impaired left ventricular diastolic filling, worsening of angina pectoris) but not necessarily lead to the development of left ventricular hypertrophy (LVH).[28,30,32–35] In the Prospective Study of Pravastatin in the Elderly at Risk (PROSPER) trial, subclinical hyperthyroidism was reported to increase the risk of cardiovascular complications when TSH was <0.1 ng/dL. Several longitudinal studies and cross-sectional studies have noted that individuals with subclinical hyperthyroidism are more predisposed to have cognitive dysfunction, but some studies have found conflicting results.[21,25,36] There was no clear association between subclinical hyperthyroidism and depression or between subclinical hyperthyroidism and impaired physical function.[21,25] Untreated subclinical hyperthyroidism can also result in increased bone turnover, decreased bone mineral density (BMD) (e.g., lower in femur and hip), and increased incidence of hip fractures (men > women).[31,37,38]

The need to treat subclinical hyperthyroidism in the elderly is controversial and depends on observing impaired cardiovascular, bone, or central nervous system clinical findings. Calcium, estrogen, bisphosphonates, or some combination of these agents may also be given to elderly women with decreased BMD and osteoporosis.[18,20] The decision to treat subclinical hyperthyroidism should not be based on the perception that there is an increased overall mortality risk.[39] Although some studies suggest that subclinical hyperthyroidism increases relative mortality risk, a larger number of studies do not seem to suggest increased cardiovascular and overall mortality risk.[21,22,30,39–42] If one elects to treat subclinical hyperthyroidism in the elderly, the treatment options are similar to those in younger patients (e.g., antithyroid drugs or radioactive iodine).

## *Hypothyroidism and subclinical hypothyroidism*

### *Hypothyroidism*

Hypothyroidism is a disorder resulting from the lower thyroid hormone level. The prevalence of hypothyroidism is found to vary significantly with age, gender, and race. A higher prevalence of hypothyroidism has been observed in older adults compared with young adults, and it can range from 6% to 14% in adults over 65 years of age.[7,43] The prevalence of overt hypothyroidism is higher in women than men.[7,9,44] In the Colorado thyroid disease prevalence study, the prevalence of hypothyroidism (based on elevated TSH levels) in adults over 75 years was reported to be 21% in women and 16% in men.[45]

Autoimmune (Hashimoto's) thyroiditis is one of the most common causes of hypothyroidism among the elderly.[4,46] Other important causes include postsurgical hypothyroidism and postradioiodine-induced hypothyroidism. The risk of developing hypothyroidism increases with age, postsurgery, and postradiation in elderly individuals. Of the individuals who undergo subtotal thyroidectomy, approximately 19% may be expected to develop hypothyroidism within the first 2 years.

The presentation of hypothyroidism in the elderly is often atypical and lacks the classic symptoms seen in younger patients.[47] In addition, it has a more insidious onset, and it often occurs concurrently with other disease pathologies that have similar signs and symptoms. The signs and symptoms such as fatigue, cold intolerance, constipation, and congestive heart failure can be attributed to other diseases, medication side effects, or to the process of aging itself. Complaints of low mood and low energy can often occur and can be confused with symptoms attributed to the diagnosis of depression, thereby increasing the concomitant use of antidepressive medications.[48] Individuals with myxedema coma are more often the elderly with concurrent illness. They may present with a stupor, seizures, respiratory depression, hypothermia, bradycardia, and metabolic abnormalities; the mortality rate in the older population can be very high.

Hypothyroidism can have adverse effects on the cardiovascular system, cardiometabolic parameters, and cognitive function and memory. Long-standing untreated hypothyroidism is associated with increased risk of atherosclerosis, increased arterial stiffness, and endothelial dysfunction, and coronary heart disease, and all-cause mortality.[49,50] Peripheral artery disease appears to be more adversely affected in hypothyroid males than females.[51] Hypothyroidism may induce insulin resistance that may lead to glucose and lipid abnormalities.[52] The clinical suspicion for hypothyroidism should also be increased in cases of persisting congestive heart failure and hyperlipidemia (e.g., elevated triglycerides).[4] Studies have shown that hypothyroidism can lead to a decline in several cognitive factors, including concentration, memory, visuospatial function, language, and executive function. The consensus on treatment of hypothyroidism to address cognitive decline is still evolving. Although some initial studies suggested that the treatment of hypothyroidism can result in beneficial effects on cognitive function, studies such as the Birmingham Elderly Thyroid Study did not report a beneficial impact from the treatment of hypothyroidism.[53,54]

Treatment of hypothyroidism independent of age is thyroid HRT. Levothyroxine (LT4) is the preferred drug of choice for the treatment of hypothyroidism.[18] The average replacement dose of LT4 is approximately 1.6 μg/kg.[18] It is preferable to give 20%–30% lower dose to older adults compared with that used in younger adults.

## *Subclinical hypothyroidism*

Subclinical hypothyroidism is by definition a laboratory diagnosis and is defined as an elevated TSH combined with a normal FT4 plus the absence of features of clinical hypothyroidism.[20] The prevalence of hypothyroidism was found to vary significantly with age, gender, and race. The prevalence of subclinical hypothyroidism is about 4%–8.5%, depending on the type of population.[9] Higher prevalence of subclinical hypothyroidism was observed in older adults compared with younger adults and was higher in women aged >60 years (~20%) compared with elderly men (8%).[55] The prevalence is lower in blacks than in whites.[9] The probability of progress from subclinical hypothyroidism to clinical hypothyroidism appears to be increased in individuals with higher levels of TSH, particularly true in females.[56–58]

The magnitude of TSH elevation at baseline is an indicator of the likely progression of subclinical hypothyroidism.[56] Potential consequences of subclinical hypothyroidism include cognitive impairment, changes in musculoskeletal function, changes in blood pressure, and cardiac metabolic abnormalities.[59] In several prospective trials, subclinical hypothyroidism was not significantly associated with impairment of cognitive function, or depression.[21,60,61] Subclinical hypothyroidism appears to increase the risk of hip fractures but does not increase risk of near-term mortality in individuals with hip fractures.[37,41] Other studies have also found no evidence for using LT4 replacement in subclinical hypothyroidism.[54] Aging individuals have a higher prevalence of sarcopenia, but in one cross-sectional study subclinical hypothyroidism could not be associated with effects on muscle mass, or strength in men and in women.[62] Mobility does not appear to be adversely affected by subclinical hypothyroidism.[63]

A cross-sectional study in Japan noted increased metabolic and cardiovascular disease (CVD) risk factors in individuals with subclinical hypothyroidism.[59] Although some studies have noted that the presence of subclinical hypothyroidism did not increase risk of blood pressure, other studies noted an increased prevalence of hypertension in women with subclinical hypothyroidism.[64–66] A small study has noted increases in intercellular adhesion molecule-1 concentrations in individuals with subclinical hypothyroidism.[67]

The overall effect on cardiovascular outcomes is variable and appears to be dependent on the degree of subclinical hypothyroidism. In some studies, no significant differences in cardiovascular outcomes and associated mortality were observed between the subclinical hypothyroidism and the euthyroid groups.[22,30] One may, however, need to differential between mild and moderate subclinical hypothyroidism in assessing the effects on cardiovascular risk factors and related mortality. In one study, they defined moderate subclinical hypothyroidism with TSH 6.1–10 mIU/mL and mild subclinical hypothyroidism with TSH: 3.1–6.0 mIU/mL and studied the impact on cardiovascular risk factors. In this study, they noted that individuals with moderate subclinical hypothyroidism have increased coronary heart disease prevalence and all-cause mortality.[49] A meta-analysis study observed an increased risk of coronary heart disease events and coronary heart disease mortality in individuals with TSH concentration of ≥10 mIU/L.[68] In a prospective study over 20 years, individuals with subclinical hypothyroidism (TSH 6.1–15 mIU/L) had increased incidence of ischemic heart disease events.[69] An increased incidence of heart failure was also observed in individuals with severe subclinical hypothyroidism (high TSH [>10] with normal T4).[70,71] A meta-analysis study of several randomized control studies did not report significant benefits with LT4 replacement therapy for individuals with cardiovascular morbidity.[72]

Treatment of subclinical hypothyroidism with thyroid replacement therapy (thyroxin) is controversial.[72] Some studies observed improvements in cardiovascular risk factors, such as insulin sensitivity, glucose metabolism, and soluble intercellular adhesion molecule-1 after treatment.[67] The American Association of Clinical Endocrinologists recommends treatment for patients only with TSH levels above 10 IU/mL or in patients with TSH levels between 5 and 10 IU/mL along with goiter or positive antithyroid peroxidase antibodies.[18]

### Thyroid nodules and cancer (see Chapter 15)

Multinodular goiters, or enlarged thyroid glands with multiple nodules, are much more common in older adults than in younger adults. Prevalence of thyroid nodules is higher in women compared with men. These nodules are generally benign and usually do not cause symptoms. Rarely, they become malignant; both papillary and follicular thyroid cancers are seen in the elderly. Surgery is the recommended treatment options for thyroid cancers. Because increased surveillance leads to more fine needle biopsies that lead to more surgeries, more information is necessary to balance benefit to risk of surgery in elderly patients with known small neoplasms or follicular lesions of ill-defined status.

## Gonadal function and aging

Aging affects the hypothalamic–pituitary–gonadal (HPG) axis at all levels, with significant changes in both male and female reproductive systems.

### Male gonadal function and aging (see Chapter 17)

Gonadal function in men often decreases with increasing age. Gonadal dysfunction in aging males often presents with decreased testosterone secretion and a decline of semen parameters.[73,74] There can be a decline in total testosterone (TT), free testosterone (FT), and bioavailable testosterone levels in aging males.[73,74] The waning of testosterone levels below the young adult reference range becomes more prevalent starting from age of 60 years.[73–77] A decline in gonadal function in aging men leads to disorders, such as hypogonadism, erectile dysfunction, and decreased fertility.

Testosterone and semen production are primarily dependent on the HPG axis. Gonadal dysfunction results in hormonal dysregulation and changes in cellular function within Leydig cells and Sertoli cells. The hypothalamus synthesizes and secretes gonadotropin-releasing hormone (GnRH) that acts on pituitary gland to produce LH and FSH. LH stimulates Leydig cells to produce testosterone. The decline in testosterone levels can be due to several factors: (1) decreased Leydig cell function, (2) decreased pituitary–hypothalamic axis function with loss of circadian variation, (3) increased levels of sex hormone–binding protein (SHBP) with age, (4) changes in testosterone receptors sensitivity, and (5) effects of altered cardiometabolic and inflammatory markers.[78–80]

The decreased testosterone levels may not only lead to hypogonadism but also adversely affect libido, and may lead to erectile dysfunction and decreased fertility. Although decreases in libido can contribute to erectile dysfunction, low levels of serum testosterone can also affect the strength of erections. The interplay between Sertoli cells, germ cells, and intratesticular testosterone is needed for spermatogenesis. A decrease in intratesticular testosterone along with changes in Sertoli cell function can lead to increased risk of infertility. Although the risk of infertility increases with age, it is less commonly reported in the older age group.

#### Hypogonadism in aging males

Hypogonadism in older men is a syndrome characterized by low serum testosterone levels and clinical symptoms that are often seen in younger hypogonadal men. Hypogonadism can be classified as primary, secondary, and mixed hypogonadism. Primary hypogonadism results from disorders of the testes. Secondary hypogonadism results from disorders of the hypothalamus and the pituitary. Mixed hypogonadism results from dual defects in the testes and in the pituitary–hypothalamic axis. Often, the type of hypogonadism in older men is either secondary or mixed hypogonadism.

Several longitudinal and cross-sectional studies (e.g., Baltimore Longitudinal Study of Aging [BLSA], Boston Area Community Health Survey [BACHS], European Male Aging Study [EMAS], and Massachusetts Male Aging Study [MMAS]) have determined the prevalence of hypogonadism in men.[73,74,81,82] The prevalence of hypogonadism in aging men appears to vary among studies, with low testosterone noted in 19% of men >60 years (BLSA) and 5.1% for men aged 70–79 years in one study (EMAS), but other studies have reported 18.4% among 70-year-old men (MMAS and BACHS). Some other studies have suggested that much of the increase in prevalence of hypogonadism with age is attributed to comorbid conditions.[83–85]

Symptoms and signs suggestive of hypogonadism include decreased libido, loss of vitality, increased visceral obesity, decreased muscle mass and strength, and decreased bone density.[86–88] Many hypogonadal aging men experience symptoms of low libido, changes in erectile function, and possibly changes in morning erection frequency, reduced sperm production (oligospermia), and sexual satisfaction.[89] In several studies, falling testosterone levels have been associated with declining strength and muscle mass.[90–93] There is a strong association between low bone density, bone loss, osteoporosis, and low testosterone levels in aging males.[13,14,94,95] There has also been an association of increased risk of fractures in men with hypogonadal states.[96–98]

Hypogonadism can contribute to dyslipidemia, hypertension, obesity, and diabetes, all of which increase the risk of cardiovascular disease.[99,100] A meta-analysis of observational studies noted that males with metabolic syndrome had lower TT and FT levels.[100] Low testosterone is associated with dyslipidemia, hypertension, obesity, and diabetes, all of which increase the risk of CVD.[101,102] Lower testosterone levels were associated with adverse changes to carotid intima medial thickness and ankle/brachial index as a measure of peripheral arterial disease and calcific aortic atheroma.[103–105]

Other nonspecific symptoms are decreased energy, motivation, and initiative; poor concentration and memory; mood changes and depression; and diminished physical or work capacity.[81,86–88] Aging hypogonadal men are at increased risk for depression.[106] Lower levels of testosterone appear to have an effect on spatial abilities, verbal abilities, and cognitive function.[107–111] This is of particular importance to the aging male who may experience changes in cognitive ability from other comorbidities such as vascular disease and other neurological pathologies.

The presence of measurable decline in serum testosterone (two low-serum a.m. testosterone levels before 10 a.m.) below the reference range for healthy, young adult men along with symptoms is indicative of hypogonadism. If the early morning serum TT) level is <250 ng/dL (8.5 nmol/L) (the normal reference range for TT in adult men is approximately 300–1000 ng/dL [0.2–34 nmol/L]), then patient is likely to be hypogonadal. A repeat TT measurement is required to confirm the diagnosis. Further evaluation is required if the TT is in the gray zone of 250–350 ng/dL (8.5–11.9 nmol/L) with FT levels and repeat TT level. If the results indicate a low TT levels, low FT levels, or both, then the patient is hypogonadal. These labs then should be followed with testing of the serum gonadotropins (LH, FSH) levels to help ascertain the anatomical level of hypogonadism. The diagnosis of hypogonadism in aging men should never be undertaken during an acute illness because it can result in temporarily low testosterone levels.[112,113]

The diagnosis of hypogonadism in aging men requires the clinician to consider etiologies such as hypothalamic and/or pituitary masses or infiltrative lesions, hyperprolactinemia, depression, chronic alcoholism, diabetes mellitus, and infiltrative diseases, such as hemochromatosis, and medications (e.g., opioids, anabolic steroids, glucocorticosteroids, antidepressants, cimetidine, spironolactone, antifungal drugs). Some functional disorders, such as exercise, malnutrition, and drugs, result in reversible hypogonadotropic hypogonadism (HH). Individuals who experience malnutrition (e.g., starvation, anorexia), activate mediators of inflammatory and stress responses, resulting in reduced hypothalamic secretion of GnRH.

There must be a definitive diagnosis of hypogonadism before the treatment is initiated. Borderline testosterone levels alone are not necessarily an indication to begin testosterone replacement therapy. There must be a combination of signs, symptoms, and issues with patient's quality of life.[113–115] There are several types of testosterone preparations that are currently available in the United States, including testosterone injections, scrotal and nonscrotal transdermal patches, oral testosterone, buccal testosterone, and testosterone gel preparations. Currently, testosterone injections and testosterone gel preparations are more commonly used in the United States.

The goal of testosterone therapy is to raise serum testosterone level into the mid-normal range [400–700 ng/dl, 13.6–23.8 nmol/L] with resolution or reduction in the symptoms of hypogonadism. Adjustments to the administration of testosterone dosage should be made when T >700 ng/dL (23.8 nmol/L) or T <350 ng/dL (11.9 nmol/L).[113,116–119] However, the ultimate goals of therapy are to reduce disease and disability, maintain or improve quality of life, and hopefully add vitality to the years.[120] The results of several studies indicate that testosterone therapy may provide several benefits, including improvements in muscle mass and strength, BMD, adiposity, lipid abnormalities, glucose control, cardiovascular disorders, sexual function, mood, and cognitive function.

The effects of testosterone replacement therapy on musculoskeletal system and on cognitive function have been studied. There are varying studies with respect to impact on muscle strength. Several studies found testosterone replacement therapy to be beneficial in improving muscle strength in hypogonadal older men.[121–125] Other studies did not observe significant improvements in muscle strength with testosterone therapy.[126–128] However, the improvements in muscle strength did not result in significant changes in functional ability. Testosterone replacement therapy was found to increase bone density in hypogonadal men.[121,129–131] The bone density increases, however, it may not reach normal adult bone mass.[132] Although BMD improves, the effect of testosterone replacement therapy on fracture risk is still unclear. None of the studies have been large enough to show a fracture risk reduction with testosterone replacement therapy. The effects of testosterone replacement therapy on measures of cognitive function and memory have shown mixed results.[133,134] Some studies have noted improvements in spatial memory.[110,111,135–137] The beneficial effects on cognition, memory, and visuospatial abilities were not seen in other randomized studies.[138–141] Randomized control trials of a longer duration are needed particularly in older hypogonadal men who are on testosterone replacement therapy to fully ascertain the benefits on cognitive performance.

Low testosterone is associated with dyslipidemia, hypertension, obesity, and diabetes, all of which increase the risk of CVD.[101,102] Testosterone therapy can have a beneficial effect on cardiometabolic risk factors. Several studies have noted that testosterone replacement therapy results in a reduction of body fat mass and waist circumference in hypogonadal men with and without obesity.[125,142–146] Several studies indicate a decrease in central adiposity in men with metabolic syndrome and/or type 2 diabetes with testosterone replacement therapy.[147–149] Testosterone therapy results in a small reduction in total cholesterol, some decrease in low-density lipoprotein (LDL) cholesterol, and a dose-dependent trend toward lower high-density lipoprotein (HDL).[143,147,150,151] In general, the effects on lipids are observed with higher dose testosterone treatment. The mechanisms that connect hypogonadism, insulin resistance, and type 2 diabetes are complicated and include inflammatory markers, oxidative stress, and many other possible underlying causes.[152] Several studies are reporting benefits for glucose control in men with concomitant hypogonadism and type 2 diabetes.[142,147,148,152–156]

Many of these studies suggest that there may be even neutral to beneficial effect of testosterone replacement therapy on the cardiovascular risk factors and adverse cardiovascular complications (e.g., angina).[157–161] Another randomized control study showed testosterone treatment in elderly patients with chronic heart failure improved various cardiac, respiratory, and muscular outcomes.[100,162] Other studies of testosterone replacement therapy have not demonstrated an increased incidence of CVD or events such as myocardial infarction, stroke, or angina.[163] There are meta-analyses trials of testosterone therapy and cardiovascular disease, but these trials generally have not been designed or adequately powered to detect effects on clinically significant cardiovascular events.[164] The true benefits of normalizing testosterone levels in hypogonadal men who have underlying cardiac disease are not fully understood and require further investigation.

The Endocrine Society guidelines do not recommend testosterone replacement therapy for those who have a history of severe lower urinary tract obstruction, untreated sleep apnea, prostate cancer or breast cancer, elevated hematocrit (e.g., >52%) and an American Urological Association International Prostate Symptom Score (IPSS) >19.[113]

## Female gonadal function and aging

Gonadal function in females declines with advancing age. It presents with decreased ovulation frequency and ovarian hormonal production. Estrogen and follicular production are dependent on the hypothalamus, pituitary, and ovaries (e.g., ovarian reserve). The decline in estrogen levels and ovarian function can occur gradually and become more prevalent starting in the early 40s to early 50s.

The Stages of Reproductive Aging Workshop (STRAW) classified various stages of the transition to menopausal and postmenopausal states.[165,166] Initially, one may notice changes in flow or length. This pattern becomes more frequent and periods can become more erratic early in perimenopausal phase. The menopausal transition (minimum 2–4 years) eventually progresses to prolonged amenorrhea (defined as >60 days).[165,166] The cessation of menses eventually occurs. Menopause is defined retrospectively after 12 months after cessation of menses.[167] Nearly all women reach menopause by the mid- to late-50s. The time period after menopause can be divided into early postmenopause (up to 5–8 years after menopause) and late menopause (rest of life).[165,166]

The transition from a reproductive stage to a postmenopausal period is marked by changes in hormone levels. The initial decline in ovarian hormone function results in decreased serum estradiol, and FSH and LH values that may increase or remain unchanged. The decline in antral follicles leads to decreased function of granulosa cells. This results in low levels of inhibin and subsequently leads to increases of FSH (cycle days 2–5). The patterns of variation of estradiol, FSH, and LH during the early menopausal transition were similar in different ethnicities.[168] In the Study of Women's Health Across the Nation (SWAN), the hormone levels differed when the results were stratified based on race and ethnicity.[168] This study also reported that the concentrations of estradiol appeared to be affected by body mass index (BMI) and stage of menopausal transition. The estradiol levels were lower among women with elevated BMI who were premenopausal and perimenopausal (early stage). This was unlike women in the late stages of the perimenopausal spectrum and postmenopausal women, where elevated BMI was associated with elevated levels of estrogen.

In the late stage of the menopausal transition, FSH can be >25 IU/L.[165,166] Subsequently, follicular release and activity ceases and estrogen falls further as LH and FSH both remain elevated. In the postmenopause state, FSH stabilizes and the ovaries may continue to produce hormones such as low levels of testosterone. Postmenopausal, most estradiol is the result of conversion of adrenal steroids to estradiol in adipose tissue.

### *Menopause in aging females*

As women undergo transition from perimenopause to menopause, they often report a variety of symptoms, including vaginal symptoms (e.g., dryness, dyspareunia), changes in cognitive and sleep function, decreased sense of vitality (e.g., variable complaints of fatigue), vasomotor symptoms (e.g., hot flushes and night sweats), and increased joint-related complaints (e.g., pains, stiffness).[169–171] The prevalence of vasomotor symptoms is high, but it varies with the definition of flushing and the population studied.[172–174] The flashes resolve in a majority of women within 4–5 years of onset.[175,176] The transition to menopause was noted to increase the likelihood of irritability, mood swings, and depressed mood compared with women who were in premenopause.[177,178]

There is still controversy as to the changes in sexual function associated with menopause and postmenopausal states. Vaginal symptoms such as dryness and dyspareunia can be seen in a significant number of women during the postmenopausal period.[169] Some were not able to associate the transition period of menopause with decreased sexual function (decreased libido and vaginal dryness) and decreased sleep.[170] Some have stated that the major decline in sexual function (e.g., libido) was noted in the postmenopausal state, with correlations with decline in estrogen and not with declines in testosterone.[179]

The changes in serum concentrations of estradiol in menopausal transition to postmenopause can result in many changes, including an increased risk of cardiovascular events and decreased BMD. During the postmenopausal period, the cardiovascular risk increases in women and can become near equivalent to males of similar age and risk factor profile.[180,181] There are changes in serum concentrations of atherogenic lipids with increases in LDL and total cholesterol increase and decreases in HDL. Some studies in postmenopausal women have noted that high gravidity was associated with reduced CVD and non-CHD CVD mortality.[182]

BMD decreases as the level of estrogen declines in the perimenopausal to postmenopausal transition. The age-related bone loss often begins in the fourth decade of life. The SWAN study reported that there were ethnic differences in the decline in bone density in premenopausal versus perimenopausal bone loss, but this decline was also affected by body weight.[183] Unlike in postmenopausal women, the BMD and rate of bone loss of premenopausal and early perimenopausal women is better correlated inversely with serum FSH than estradiol.[183] Bone loss becomes more pronounced as the menses become less frequent with rapid loss during the years shortly after the last menses.[183]

The Endocrine Society guidelines on postmenopausal therapy reports many benefits of estrogen therapy on relieving symptoms associated with menopause.[184] Standard doses of estrogen with or without a progestin can reduce the frequency and severity of hot flashes.[184] Nonhormonal alternatives (e.g., antidepressants, gabapentin) also appear to have some beneficial effects on hot flashes.[185,186] If needed, vaginal estrogen can be used for long-term therapy to relieve some of the symptoms.[187] The application of low doses of vaginal estradiol can relieve symptoms associated with vaginal atrophy. The use of transdermal estrogen has been associated with increased libido and sexually satisfying events per month.[184] Estrogen with or without a progestin can decrease early postmenopausal bone loss.[184] Estrogen therapy improves bone mass in late postmenopause (near equivalent to the bisphosphonates).[184] Selective estrogen receptor modulators such as raloxifene have also been found to improve BMD and reduce vertebral but not hip fractures.[184]

The type of HRT and route of administration can present different risks to postmenopausal women. The results from Women's Health Initiative (WHI) studies and other studies have noted that there is an increased risk of breast cancer with a combination estrogen–progestin therapy.[188,189] The risk of breast cancer was not noted when one used estrogen alone in postmenopausal men.[190,191] The risk of breast cancer was less with progesterone versus medroxyprogesterone.[192,193] The optimum dose and duration of progestin has not yet been established. In postmenopausal women, it is better to start with low dose of estrogen and consider tapering of HRT to help minimize breast cancer risks.[187] The risk of venous thromboembolism appeared to be increased in oral estrogen but not in transdermal formulations.[194–196] This finding was also noted in the E3N cohort.[197] The groups treated with HRT showed a decreased incidence of diabetes.[198,199] The type of HRT may influence the incidence of diabetes.[200] A meta-analysis study reported that HRT in nondiabetic postmenopausal women had reduced HRT, abdominal obesity, insulin resistance, new-onset diabetes, lipids, and blood pressure.[201]

Observations support the hypothesis that estrogen replacement may have a beneficial effect on the cardiovascular system with a reduction in CHD events when one starts therapy shortly after menopause but not many years after onset of menopause.[184] Initially, the WHI conducted a study in postmenopausal women regardless of years after menopause. The trial noted that women with estrogen–progestin replacement had an increased risk of coronary heart disease and stroke.[188] The trial noted that women with estrogen replacement alone had an increased risk of stroke.[202] Follow-up analysis of the WHI noted that increased risk of coronary heart disease and mortality increases when subjects are initiated with treatment after 10 years postmenopause.[191,203] Meta-analyses of randomized control trials noted that the increased CHD and mortality in older women was not seen in women who were started on therapy when they were between the ages of 50 and 59 years.[204,205] Estrogen replacement and selective estrogen receptor modulators do not reduce stroke incidence in older women with pre-existing vascular disease.[184] However, the type of HRT cannot yet be recommended for prevention of CVD.

# *GH deficiency and aging (see Chapter 5)*

GH is secreted by pituitary somatotrophs in a pulsatile manner. Growth hormone–releasing hormone (GHRH) stimulates the transcription of GH. Some of the other stimulatory factors on GH release include ghrelin, amino acids, hypoglycemia, slow waves during sleep, malnutrition, and stress. The maximal secretion of GH occurs during the night during slow-wave sleep, particularly when somatostatin release is diminished. GH acts both by direct action and indirectly through IGF-I. IGF-I is synthesized in both in the liver and in the periphery, and it circulates bound to several binding proteins, including insulin-like growth factor–binding protein (IGFBP)-3. The levels of IGF-I influence GH release by directly having inhibitory effects on the pituitary and hypothalamus. It also works indirectly by stimulating somatostatin, which has an inhibitory effect on GH release. The reduction of ghrelin (e.g., during digestion) and increase in circulating nonesterified free fatty acids also have inhibitory effects on GH secretion.

GH influences several aspects of body function, including production of IGF-1, metabolism (e.g., lipids, proteins, glucose, and insulin), and growth of bone, cartilage, and muscle. GH and IGF-I levels decrease by >50% in older adults of ≥60 years. Adults with GH deficiency (GHD) can experience fatigue, decreased general well-being, decreased mood, increased adiposity, increased insulin resistance, reduction of protein synthesis, relative decrease in muscle mass and strength, decreased bone density, increased risk of fracture, decreased insulin sensitivity, increased prevalence of impaired glucose tolerance, changes in lipid profile (e.g., increased LDL cholesterol and decreased HDL cholesterol), and in some severe cases can present with hypoglycemia.[206,207] GHD can also have adverse effects on cardiac health by influencing factors such as levels of atherogenesis and increased levels of plasminogen activator inhibitor type I.

GH secretion changes significantly over a lifetime.[208] GH levels are relatively low before puberty and increase to maximum levels (with secretion most prominent during the night sleeping phase) during puberty and adolescence.[209] GH secretion in adults falls by 14% with every advancing decade.[210] The serum IGF-I concentrations were found to decline with age in both genders after the age of 18 years.[211] In the Baltimore Longitudinal Study of Aging (BLSA) and the InCHIANTI, IGF-I declined approximately at the rate of 1.7 ng/mL/year in a linear manner with age in participants >50 years.[212] IGF-I was higher in men than women.[211,213]

The progressive decline in GH secretion has been termed the "somatopause." An extrapolation was made within a French study, and it projected that the annual incidence is 12 per million.[214] A Danish study reported that the expected incidence of adult onset GHD is 1.90 in males and 1.42 in females.[215] The symptoms of clinically significant somatopause (the decline in GH levels with symptoms of GHD) overlap with symptoms of other age-related disorders such as metabolic syndrome and late onset hypogonadism.[206,207] These comorbid conditions can place older people at risk for developing cardiovascular and osteoporotic conditions and reduce quality of life. One must observe for milder symptoms of adult onset GHD.[216]

## *Etiology of age-related decline in GH secretion and action*

The physiology of age-related decline in GH secretion is not completely established. Age does not affect GH pulse frequency, GH half-life, or basal GH release.[217–219] However, aging effects the amount of GH secreted in each pulse. Possible causes for the decline in GH levels with aging include reduced GHRH secretion, decline in pituitary responsiveness to GHRH due to multiple factors, and increased somatostatin secretion.[220–224] Several other factors have been reported to contribute to decline in GH/IGF-1 levels, including lack of exercise, sleep disorders, excessive food intake, increased levels of stress, increased adiposity, and influence of sex steroid such as low testosterone (in men).[208,225–228]

## Clinical consequences of age-related decline in GH and effects of GH replacement

GHD can result in decreased cognitive function (e.g., memory, concentration) and decreased sense of vitality. A meta-analysis of 13 studies does appear to show an association between decreased cognitive function and GHD.[229] The decline in cognitive function improved after treatment with GH.[229,230] The KIMS database revealed that GHD resulted in greater impairment of quality of life for women than men. Other studies have not found clear evidence of benefit on improved cognitive parameters, memory, or mood in normal elderly subjects.[231] The symptoms of GHD were found to be more subtle and impairment of quality of life relatively milder in subjects >60 years.[232]

GHD can also lead to alterations of body composition, and some parameters may improve with GH replacement. The effect of 10-year GH replacement on reduction in total body fat was transient in individuals with GHD.[233] There were improvements in lean body mass with GH replacement therapy.[234–236] Although low bone mass is infrequently seen in GHD in elderly, low IGF-I is associated with decreased bone density.[237–239] GH replacement improves lumbar spine and femoral neck BMD and seems to result in greater increases in the total body BMD in women than in men.[240,241] However, there appears to be greater reduction in incidence of fractures in men compared with women with GHD when on GH replacement.[242] The decline in muscle strength in GHD has been documented in the past by using several methods, including quadriceps and hand strength. GH replacement appears to help maintain muscle performance from age-related decline, it does not appear to actually increase muscle strength in muscle groups.[235,243–245]

Studies have reported that there is a higher incidence of cardiovascular risk factors, metabolic syndrome, and mortality in aging subjects with GHD.[246–249] There appears to be an increase in mortality rate among female subjects with GHD compared with male subjects.[250] The mortality rate of treated GHD subjects was reportedly similar to the mortality rate of normal subjects.[250,251] There were benefits to markers of metabolism, such as improved lipid profile and decreased hemoglobin AIc (HbAIc) with GH replacement.[233,252] The prevalence of metabolic syndrome does not decline with GH replacement in at least one study.[253] GH and IGF-I appear to influence cardiovascular factors such as endothelial progenitor cells.[254] The impact of GH replacement on cardiovascular outcomes is still a matter of debate, and larger studies are needed to elucidate the effects.

## GH deficiency treatment options for aging adults and safety concerns

The decision to treat GH deficiency is influenced by the lack of specificity of signs and symptoms, the variability in severity of symptoms, and the method of treatment. The diagnosis of GHD can be made based on symptoms and diagnostic tests. It is currently recommend that the insulin tolerance test (ITT; positive when GH ≤5.1 μg/L) and the GHRH-arginine test (positive when GH ≤4.1 μg/L) may be used to establish the diagnosis of GHD.[255] The GH Research Society, however, has noted that the induction of hypoglycemia is often contraindicated in the elderly; hence, it is preferable to use GHRH combined with arginine test. When GHRH is not be available or ITT is contraindicated, the glucagon stimulation test can be used.[255] In addition, one should be aware that the levels of IGF-I levels are often not as clearly delineated in aging individuals as in younger individuals. A normal IGF-1 does not exclude the diagnosis of GHD, whereas a low IGF-I level in the absence of underlying condition may suggest the diagnosis of GHD.[255]

Several treatment approaches have been examined to improve the GH deficiency in older adults. Treatment approaches examined include fasting, exercise, and use of certain amino acids and synthetic hormones. Exercise and caloric restriction will increase GH levels in part by reducing adipose tissue. However, the improvements observed in GH levels with exercise are lower in older adults than young adults. Amino acids such as arginine and lysine have been used by older adults to improve GH levels. No systematic studies were carried out to determine efficacy safety of the use of these amino acids.

GH is available as a prescription drug (e.g., human [h]GH), and administration of synthetic GH was found to improve GH and IGF-I levels, decrease adipose tissue, and marginally improve BMD in older adults.[256,257] The side effects from GH administration are similar in aging individuals to those observed with young GHD adults. They include fluid retention, joint and muscle pain, carpal tunnel syndrome (pressure on the nerve in the wrist causing hand pain and numbness), and type 2 diabetes mellitus.[255,256] Other less frequently reported side effects include headache, tinnitus, and benign intracranial hypertension.[255] hGH is approved for the treatment of GHD. hGH should be started at low doses and titrated based on clinical symptoms, IGF-I levels, and side effects to treatment.[255]

GHRH is not currently available in the United States. GHRH has been shown to restore spontaneous GH secretion and IGF-I levels in the elderly.[221] Administration of GHRH showed positive effects on body composition; however, an increase in physical performance scores was not observed.[222,224,258,259] GH-secretagogues (GHSs) are can be administered by subcutaneous, intranasal, or oral routes.[260] They stimulate GH secretion by acting both at the pituitary and the hypothalamic level on GHRH-secreting neurons.[260,261] Long-term studies with orally active GHS MK-677 showed improvements in IGF-I levels in elderly subjects.[262] Other observations of this study include (1) increase in lean body mass and (2) no changes in muscle strength.[262] Several side effects were reported with GHS therapy and include water retention, hypertension, headache, and metabolic dysfunction. Some of the side effects are dose-dependent.

# Adrenal function and aging

Aging causes changes in the adrenal gland morphology and altered regulation of the hypothalamic–pituitary–adrenal (HPA) axis; the latter leads to age-related changes in serum adrenal hormones such as cortisol, DHEA, and aldosterone. The different layers of the adrenal cortex (zona glomerulosa, zona fasciculata, and zona reticularis) undergo subtle change with age, including a reduction in the thickness of the zona reticularis and a relative increase in the outer cortical zones.[263]

There is an increased incidence and prevalence of adrenal gland nodules with age based on the autopsy and computed tomography (CT) imaging studies.[264] The adrenal hormonal changes with age include subtle increases in serum cortisol levels,[265] and significantly lower DHEA levels[266] with increasing age. The increased cortisol levels can adversely affect cognitive function, aggravate or produce sleep disorders, and increase the risk of osteoporosis in older adults.[265,267,268] Changes in aldosterone secretion are not common but can lead to mild to severe hyponatremia. Although its impact on mortality is less clear, alterations in plasma sodium levels can increase the risk of gait abnormalities, falls, fractures, and cognitive impairment.[269–271] The physiological roles of DHEA sulfate (S) are still being elucidated and currently postulated to include effects on the immune system, neurological system, bone, and cardiometabolic functions.[272,273]

## Etiology and related decline in adrenal hormones with age

Adrenal disorders observed in older adults are mainly due to changes in the secretion levels of cortisol and DHEA. Serum levels of DHEA and DHEAS fall dramatically with aging; in contrast, cortisol levels do not fall and may increase as men get older.

The HPA axis regulates the secretion of cortisol. The hypothalamus synthesizes and secretes corticotropin-releasing hormone (CRH) that subsequently regulates the pituitary gland to produce adrenocorticotropic hormone (ACTH). The sensitivity of the adrenal gland to ACTH pulses seems to be influenced by age and BMI.[274–276] Adrenal sensitivity to ACTH was decreased with increasing age.[277] The diminished hypothalamic pituitary sensitivity to feedback inhibition by cortisol can lead to increased levels of cortisol in both genders.[278,279]

The mechanisms responsible for the decline in DHEA levels are still unknown. Histomorphological analysis of adrenal specimens suggests that aging results in alterations within the adrenal cortex, resulting in a reduction in the size of the zona reticularis, and this may be responsible for the diminished production of DHEA.[263]

There are some alterations to the secretion patterns of renin–aldosterone axis, but these are different from the ACTH and cortisol axis. Although the plasma renin activity decreases with age, the plasma aldosterone levels appear not to change or may have modest changes below the clinical threshold.[280,281] Aldosterone serum concentrations often remain normal despite a small reduction in aldosterone secretion and this may be in part due to decreased clearance of aldosterone.[280,282]

## Cortisol changes and aging

Cortisol production has an ACTH-dependent circadian rhythm with peak levels in the early morning and a nadir at night. The mean 24-h serum cortisol concentrations can be elevated by up to 20% in both aging men and women; this is not accompanied by changes in corticosteroid-binding globulin.[279,283] The nocturnal nadir of serum cortisol concentrations in the elderly occurs at an earlier time than in younger subjects.

Cortisol, in aging individuals, may be affected by factors such as weight (slightly lower in obese), sleep abnormalities (slight elevation), and acute metabolic stress (increased).[284–288] The cortisol awakening response was slightly higher in aging subjects who experienced significant stress, such as in Alzheimer's patients, and social stressors (e.g., in the Whitehall II Study).[289,290] There may be an association between late life events and elevated secretion of morning cortisol and high diurnal variability of cortisol.[291,292]

Cortisol acts through specific intracellular receptors and affects numerous physiologic systems including cognitive function, immune function, glucose counter regulation, vascular tone, and bone metabolism. High levels of cortisol are known to contribute to increased risk of developing cognitive impairment, sleep disorders, and reduced BMD in older adults.[265,267,268]

Elevated cortisol levels appear to be associated with declining cognitive performance in aging individuals. The Vietnam Era Twin Study of aging showed an association with decline in executive measures, processing speed, and visual–spatial memory.[293] Many studies such as the Baltimore Memory Study have shown an association between impaired declarative memory function in nondemented older persons and elevated cortisol levels.[294–297] Data from the Longitudinal Aging Study Amsterdam revealed that elevated daytime cortisol levels can be associated with lower memory function and speed of information processing.[291] Some studies have suggested that an attenuated cortisol awakening response can also cause decreased cognitive performance but not declarative memory.[296,297]

Initial studies suggested that cortisol levels in aging individuals were inversely related to BMD, rate of bone loss, and risk of clinical fractures.[267,298] In aging individuals, cortisol appears to have gender-specific effects on BMD (measured by DEXA) with increased BMD loss in the lumbar spine of men and increased loss of BMD in the femur/hip of women.[299] In addition to changes in adrenal production of cortisol, studies have suggested that the cortisone conversion to cortisol and cortisol production within osteoblasts also appears to increase with age.[300] The use of exogenous steroids (e.g., steroid injections for arthritis, inhaled steroids for COPD or asthma) increases the levels of cortisol and contributes to decreased BMD.

Increased nocturnal cortisol levels are believed to contribute to sleep disorders in the elderly.[265] A small elevation in nocturnal cortisol levels was noted in aging individuals, particularly those with sleep abnormalities.[285–287] Finally, there is an association between the 24 h cortisol production rate and increased body fat in older men. Thus, the increase in HPA axis activity may play a role in the alterations in body composition with greater central fat distribution in aging subjects.[301]

## DHEA changes and aging

DHEA is the major steroid produced by the adrenal zona reticularis. In the serum, there are three forms of DHEA: (1) unconjugated DHEA, (2) sulfated DHEA (DHEAS), and (3) lipoidal DHEA. DHEA and DHEAS are the most abundant steroid hormones present in the body. DHEAS and DHEA levels appear to decrease from the third decade. By age 70, the levels are about 20% to 30% lower than those of young adults. The levels can be 80%–90% lower than those of younger individuals by the time one is greater than 80 years of age.[76,266,302] In aging populations, some studies have reported changes in diurnal variation (e.g., lower morning concentrations of DHEAS, higher nocturnal rate, burst frequency, and amplitude of DHEA) and appear to be cleared quickly from the circulation.[303] The levels of DHEA(S) appear to be higher in men compared to women.[303,304]

The physiological function of DHEA is not completely understood. It may have cardio protective, antidiabetic, anti-obesity properties and play a role in declining global function in aging subjects.[305–309] DHEA is thought to influence cardiovascular function. The decline in DHEA(S) has been associated with CVD and all cause of mortality.[310–312] The age-related decline in circulating DHEA(S) has led to a number of randomized trials to assess the effect of oral DHEA therapy in healthy elderly subjects and in those with comorbid conditions. DHEAS replacement therapy in aging adults did not show significant changes in cardiovascular risk factors, such as blood pressure, blood glucose, or improve insulin action.[313–317] While some studies have reported variable lowering of HDL and triglycerides in both genders, the reduction of HDL was not seen in men in another long-term longitudinal study with DHEA replacement.[318,319]

DHEA(s) levels have been associated with frailty, decreased physical function, and bone density. In the Hertfordshire Aging Study, lower levels of dehydroepiandrosterone sulfate (DHEAS) and higher cortisol: DHEAS ratios were all significantly associated with increased odds of frailty at 10-year follow-up.[320] A cross-sectional study in both genders not only found an association between DHEAS and frailty but also identified that this association between low DHEAS and frailty was attenuated with obesity (BMI >30 kg/m$^2$).[321] The replacement of DHEA does not significantly improve physical function, body composition, frailty, and an overall sense of well-being.[128,322–324] Replacement of DHEA in older subjects to produce DHEA levels similar to that of younger age groups has brought mixed results. DHEAS replacement resulted in some improvement in bone turnover and bone density in women but not in men.[325,326] The overall effect of DHEA replacement on BMD in elderly subjects is relatively small when compared with bisphosphonate therapy.[327]

In other studies, no distinct benefits of DHEA replacement in healthy older individuals were observed. In addition, studies also did not demonstrate improvement in well-being or cognition with DHEAS replacement.[322,323,325,328]

## *Aldosterone changes and aging (see Chapter 20)*

Hyponatremia is an electrolyte disturbance with sodium below 135. Hyponatremia can cause significant consequences for the aging individual including decreased cognitive function and increased risk of falls. The ability to retain sodium through reabsorption in the kidney plays an important role in maintaining normal sodium levels. Hypotonic hyponatremia can be categorized as hypovolemic, euvolemic, or hypervolemic.

This ability to retain sodium, and indirectly water, is directly influenced by aldosterone and renin. The site of action of aldosterone is on epithelial sodium channels (ENaC) in the principal cells of the collecting tubules.

The decrease in serum renin, renin activity, and aldosterone in aging individuals can result in hypoaldosteronism. The decline in secretion or action of renin and aldosterone is of particular importance when individuals have a type 4 renal tubular acidosis (RTA) or mild renal failure. Some older patients may have low-normal aldosterone values. The serum aldosterone concentrations and urinary aldosterone excretion should be checked in older hyponatremia patients to evaluate if primary aldosteronism is a cause of the hyponatremia. In addition to evaluating for hypoaldosteronism, the medications of elderly individuals should be reviewed. Medications such as thiazides and serotonin reuptake inhibitors are more likely to cause hyponatremia in the elderly than in other age groups.

## ***Summary and conclusions***

The goal of healthy aging is to limit the changes that increase frailty, cardiovascular risk, cognitive decline, and other comorbidities. While endocrine systems have substantial reserves in younger individuals, a combination of aging processes and life experienences (e.g., stress, diseases) can gradually reduce these reserves and lead to changes/alterations in various endorine systems (Table 23.2). The changes observed include a decline in the secretion of a number of hormones, an increase in the secretion of some other hormones, reduced tissue response to hormones, altered rates of hormone metabolism, and other pathological changes within the endocrine glands. Understanding the clinical effects of changes in endocrine function and activity may help in identifying therapies that limit disability and morbidity in aging individuals.

Hormones that decrease with aging include serum testosterone (total, free, and bioavailable); DHEA, DHEAS, GH, IGF-1; and vitamin D. Hormones that decrease only to a small extent or remain unchanged with aging include thyroid hormones T3 and T4, TSH, cortisol, and epinephrine. Hormones that may increase with aging include LH, fFSH, insulin, and ACTH. The individual effects of these hormonal changes vary significantly depending on several factors such as race, life style (e.g., food habits, exercise), gender, and genetics. These factors can exacerbate or minimize the impact of the aging process on endocrine function. As the body fails to adapt to further changes in cell loss and/or declines in hormonal function, the risk increases for developing several endocrine-related health problems such as thyroid abnormalities, hypogonadism (e.g., menopause in women, androgen deficiency in men), growth hormone deficiency, osteoporosis, and type 2 diabetes mellitus. Other effects include changes in body constitution, fat distribution (visceral obesity), muscle weakness, decline in cognitive functioning, and decline in sense of vitality.

The metabolism and many enzymatic processes are influenced by thyroid hormone and growth hormone levels. The alterations in thyroid hormone levels with aging can lead to an increased prevalence of age-related thyroid dysfunction. The thyroid-stimulating hormone in conjunction with the full panel of thyroid function tests should be used to make the diagnosis. However, the decreased peripheral degradation of T4 and slight decrease in plasma T3 concentrations have been associated with but not been causally related with functional changes in the aging process. The decreased levels of GH are in part due to changes in GHRH and IGF-binding proteins with aging. The clinical effects of GH in the process of aging can often seem to be nonspecific and overlap with other endocrine system effects. GH and IGF-1 have also been reported to play a role in the regulation and action of sex steroids. The GH

| Endocrine system | Clinical disorders | Associated labs | Clinical consequences |
|---|---|---|---|
| Thyroid | Hyperthyroidism | Decreased TSH increased T4 | Atrial fibrillation, diarrhea, constipation, loss of appetite, nausea and persistent vomiting or neurological symptoms, such as mania, depression, cognitive impairment, or incident dementia |
| | Subclinical hyperthyroidism | Decreased TSH, normal T4 | Pre-existing heart disease and can lead to atrial fibrillation, impaired left ventricular diastolic filling and worsening of angina pectoris, increased risk cognitive dysfunction, decreased BMD, and increased incidence of hip fractures |
| | Hypothyroidism | Increased TSH, decreased T4 | Decline in several cognitive factors such as concentration, memory, visuospatial function, language, and executive function; may induce insulin resistance, persistent hyperlipidemia, congestive heart failure, and macrocytic anemia |
| | Subclinical hypothyroidism | Increased TSH, normal T4 | Hypertension, cardiometabolic changes, cognitive impairment, insulin resistance, diabetes mellitus, dyslipidemia, and hyperuricemia |
| | Thyroid nodules | Otherwise normal thyroid function tests | If toxic: pattern is hyperthyroid; no symptoms if there is no mass effect; often benign; can have increased risk of cancer due to environmental exposure (e.g., radiation) |
| Gonadal | Hypogonadism (male) | Primary: elevated LH, FSH; low T Secondary: normal/low LH and FSH; low T | Include loss of vitality, visceral obesity, decreased libido, erectile dysfunction, decreased muscle mass and strength, decreased bone density, and mood changes, changes in cognitive function, increased cardiovascular risk |
| | Hypogonadism (female) | Primary: elevated LH, FSH; low E Secondary: normal/low LH and FSH; low E | Menopause, loss of vitality, decreased libido, decreased bone density, mood changes, changes in cognitive function, increased cardiovascular risk |
| Growth Hormone | Growth hormone deficiency | Low GH; Low IGF-1 | Decrease in muscle and bone mass, increased visceral fat, diminishing exercise and cardiac capacity, atherogenic alterations in lipid profile, thinning of skin, and many psychological and cognitive problems |
| Adrenal | Iatrogenic Cushing's syndrome | Low ACTH, elevated Cortisol | Cognitive impairment, sleep disorders, and reduced BMD |
| | DHEA disorders (still to be elucidated) | DHEA/DHEAS decline | Increased CVD risk, low BMD, depressed mood, insulin resistance, and decreased cognition |
| Bone | Osteopenia/ Osteoporosis | Low bone density T; Z; FRAX | Decreased height; increased risk of fractures |

***Table 23.2***
*Endocrine disorders and aging.*

deficiency should be diagnosed using a stimulatory test. GH replacement therapy is approved for adult onset GH deficiency in individuals with documentable low GH/IGF-1 levels and clinical symptoms.

Aging individuals also undergo several changes in the levels of adrenal and gonadal hormones. The levels of cortisol appear to be slightly elevated, and this appears to be dependent on life stressors (e.g., social stress, cognitive stress). While there is no significant decline in cortisol levels with age, DHEA(S) does decrease with age. The benefits for DHEA replacement therapy for elderly subjects are not yet established conclusively. With aging, the decreases in testosterone and estrogen have more definable and far-reaching clinical consequences. These changes can result in reduced sexual function (e.g., reduced libido, reduced sexual potency), adverse changes to body composition (e.g., decreased bone density, and muscle mass), increased risk of frailty, decreased cognitive function, and increased cardiovascular risk factors. The decreased bone density can be treated with SERMS, gonadal hormones (e.g., estrogens, testosterone), bisphosphonates, and, in certain instances GH replacement. The replacement therapy options with testosterone and estrogen for individuals with significant symptoms and low levels of hormones could be considered after careful evaluation of comorbidities. The treatments with testosterone and estrogen may also be beneficial to the cardiovascular system in certain age groups.[329]. Several studies are underway to investigate the benefits of the testosterone and estrogen replacement therapies for elderly men and women, respectively. A large multicentered NIH-sponsored double-blinded, placebo-controlled testosterone trial is currently underway in men over the age of 65 years, the purpose being to verify the benefits of testosterone replacement therapy on factors such as frailty, BMD, vitality, and coronary artery plaques.

The mechanisms that mediate age-related disruption of endocrine functions are still being elucidated. Many of the features of aging (e.g., visceral adiposity, decreased cognitive function, decreased BMD, sarcopenia, decreased sexual function, decreased sense of vitality, and increased cardiovascular risk factors) can be attributed to changes in thyroid function, growth hormone function, gonadal function, and adrenal function. Changes in any one particular organ system may not be a sole cause of multiple comorbidities associated with aging. The mechanisms that lead to age-related consequences are difficult to elucidate because of the overlapping interplay among the endocrine organs. Active intervention should be limited to individuals with clinical symptoms.

# References


1. Mariotti S, Chiovato L, Franceschi C, et al. Thyroid autoimmunity and aging. *Exp Gerontol* 1998;33:535–41.
2. Papaleontiou M, Haymart MR. Approach to and treatment of thyroid disorders in the elderly. *Med Clin North Am* 2012;96:297–310.
3. van Coevorden A, Laurent E, Decoster C, et al. Decreased basal and stimulated thyrotropin secretion in healthy elderly men. *J Clin Endocrinol Metab* 1989;69:177–85.
4. Mariotti S, Franceschi C, Cossarizza A, et al. The aging thyroid. *Endocr Rev* 1995;16:686–715.
5. Mazzoccoli G, Pazienza V, Piepoli A, et al. Hypothalamus-hypophysis-thyroid axis function in healthy aging. *J Biol Regul Homeost Agents* 2010;24:433–9.
6. Bannister P, Barnes I. Use of sensitive thyrotrophin measurements in an elderly population. *Gerontology* 1989;35:225–9.
7. Bensenor IM, Goulart AC, Lotufo PA, et al. Prevalence of thyroid disorders among older people: Results from the Sao Paulo Ageing & Health Study. *Cad Saude Publica* 2011;27:155–61.
8. Diez JJ. Hyperthyroidism in patients older than 55 years: An analysis of the etiology and management. *Gerontology* 2003;49:316–23.
9. Hollowell JG, Staehling NW, Flanders WD, et al. Serum TSH, T(4), and thyroid antibodies in the United States population (1988 to 1994): National Health and Nutrition Examination Survey (NHANES III). *J Clin Endocrinol Metab* 2002;87:489–99.
10. Carle A, Pedersen IB, Knudsen N, et al. Epidemiology of subtypes of hyperthyroidism in Denmark: A population-based study. *Eur J Endocrinol* 2011;164:801–9.
11. Nordyke RA, Gilbert FI, Jr., Harada AS. Graves' disease. Influence of age on clinical findings. *Arch Intern Med* 1988;148:626–31.
12. Boelaert K, Torlinska B, Holder RL, et al. Older subjects with hyperthyroidism present with a paucity of symptoms and signs: A large cross-sectional study. *J Clin Endocrinol Metab* 2010;95:2715–26.
13. Biondi B, Kahaly GJ. Cardiovascular involvement in patients with different causes of hyperthyroidism. *Nat Rev Endocrinol* 2010;6:431–43.
14. Kim JM, Stewart R, Kim SY, et al. Thyroid stimulating hormone, cognitive impairment and depression in an older korean population. *Psychiatry Investig* 2010;7:264–9.
15. van den Beld AW, Visser TJ, Feelders RA, et al. Thyroid hormone concentrations, disease, physical function, and mortality in elderly men. *J Clin Endocrinol Metab* 2005;90:6403–9.
16. Bauer DC, Ettinger B, Nevitt MC, et al. Risk for fracture in women with low serum levels of thyroid-stimulating hormone. *Ann Intern Med* 2001;134:561–8.

17. Yeap BB, Alfonso H, Chubb SA, et al. Higher free thyroxine levels are associated with frailty in older men. The Health In Men Study. *Clin Endocrinol (Oxf)* 2012;76:741–8.
18. Baskin HJ, Cobin RH, Duick DS, et al. American Association of Clinical Endocrinologists medical guidelines for clinical practice for the evaluation and treatment of hyperthyroidism and hypothyroidism. *Endocr Pract* 2002;8:457–69.
19. Shrier DK, Burman KD. Subclinical hyperthyroidism: Controversies in management. *Am Fam Physician* 2002;65:431–8.
20. Surks MI, Ortiz E, Daniels GH, et al. Subclinical thyroid disease: Scientific review and guidelines for diagnosis and management. *JAMA* 2004;291:228–38.
21. de Jongh RT, Lips P, van Schoor NM, et al. Endogenous subclinical thyroid disorders, physical and cognitive function, depression, and mortality in older individuals. *Eur J Endocrinol* 2011;165:545–54.
22. Sgarbi JA, Matsumura LK, Kasamatsu TS, et al. Subclinical thyroid dysfunctions are independent risk factors for mortality in a 7.5-year follow-up: The Japanese-Brazilian thyroid study. *Eur J Endocrinol* 2010;162:569–77.
23. Wilson S, Parle JV, Roberts LM, et al. Prevalence of subclinical thyroid dysfunction and its relation to socioeconomic deprivation in the elderly: A community-based cross-sectional survey. *J Clin Endocrinol Metab* 2006;91:4809–16.
24. Samuels MH. Subclinical thyroid disease in the elderly. *Thyroid* 1998;8:803–13.
25. Ceresini G, Lauretani F, Maggio M, et al. Thyroid function abnormalities and cognitive impairment in elderly people: Results of the Invecchiare in Chianti study. *J Am Geriatr Soc* 2009;57:89–93.
26. Parle JV, Franklyn JA, Cross KW, et al. Prevalence and follow-up of abnormal thyrotrophin (TSH) concentrations in the elderly in the United Kingdom. *Clin Endocrinol (Oxf)* 1991;34:77–83.
27. Peeters RP, Wouters PJ, van Toor H, et al. Serum 3,3',5'-triiodothyronine (rT3) and 3,5,3'-triiodothyronine/rT3 are prognostic markers in critically ill patients and are associated with postmortem tissue deiodinase activities. *J Clin Endocrinol Metab* 2005;90:4559–65.
28. Vadiveloo T, Donnan PT, Cochrane L, et al. The Thyroid Epidemiology, Audit, and Research Study (TEARS): Morbidity in patients with endogenous subclinical hyperthyroidism. *J Clin Endocrinol Metab* 2011;96:1344–51.
29. Sawin CT, Geller A, Kaplan MM, et al. Low serum thyrotropin (thyroid-stimulating hormone) in older persons without hyperthyroidism. *Arch Intern Med* 1991;151:165–8.
30. Cappola AR, Fried LP, Arnold AM, et al. Thyroid status, cardiovascular risk, and mortality in older adults. *JAMA* 2006;295:1033–41.
31. Turner MR, Camacho X, Fischer HD, et al. Levothyroxine dose and risk of fractures in older adults: Nested case-control study. *Brit Med J* 2011;342:d2238.
32. Kahaly GJ, Nieswandt J, Mohr-Kahaly S. Cardiac risks of hyperthyroidism in the elderly. *Thyroid* 1998;8:1165–9.
33. Auer J, Scheibner P, Mische T, et al. Subclinical hyperthyroidism as a risk factor for atrial fibrillation. *Am Heart J* 2001;142:838–42.
34. Sawin CT, Geller A, Wolf PA, et al. Low serum thyrotropin concentrations as a risk factor for atrial fibrillation in older persons. *N Engl J Med* 1994;331:1249–52.
35. Dorr M, Ittermann T, Aumann N, et al. Subclinical hyperthyroidism is not associated with progression of cardiac mass and development of left ventricular hypertrophy in middle-aged and older subjects: Results from a 5-year follow-up. *Clin Endocrinol (Oxf)* 2010;73:821–6.
36. Bensenor IM, Lotufo PA, Menezes PR, et al. Subclinical hyperthyroidism and dementia: The Sao Paulo Ageing & Health Study (SPAH). *BMC Public Health* 2010;10:298.
37. Lee JS, Buzkova P, Fink HA, et al. Subclinical thyroid dysfunction and incident hip fracture in older adults. *Arch Intern Med* 2010;170:1876–83.
38. Rosario PW. Bone and heart abnormalities of subclinical hyperthyroidism in women below the age of 65 years. *Arq Bras Endocrinol Metabol* 2008;52:1448–51.
39. Volzke H, Schwahn C, Wallaschofski H, et al. Review: The association of thyroid dysfunction with all-cause and circulatory mortality: Is there a causal relationship? *J Clin Endocrinol Metab* 2007;92:2421–9.
40. Haentjens P, Van Meerhaeghe A, Poppe K, et al. Subclinical thyroid dysfunction and mortality: An estimate of relative and absolute excess all-cause mortality based on time-to-event data from cohort studies. *Eur J Endocrinol* 2008;159:329–41.
41. Kalra S, Williams A, Whitaker R, et al. Subclinical thyroid dysfunction does not affect one-year mortality in elderly patients after hip fracture: A prospective longitudinal study. *Injury* 2010;41:385–7.
42. Waring AC, Harrison S, Samuels MH, et al. Thyroid function and mortality in older men: A prospective study. *J Clin Endocrinol Metab* 2012;97:862–70.
43. Flatau E, Trougouboff P, Kaufman N, et al. Prevalence of hypothyroidism and diabetes mellitus in elderly kibbutz members. *Eur J Epidemiol* 2000;16:43–6.
44. Empson M, Flood V, Ma G, et al. Prevalence of thyroid disease in an older Australian population. *Intern Med J* 2007;37:448–55.
45. Canaris GJ, Manowitz NR, Mayor G, et al. The Colorado thyroid disease prevalence study. *Arch Intern Med* 2000;160:526–34.
46. Dayan CM, Daniels GH. Chronic autoimmune thyroiditis. *N Engl J Med* 1996;335:99–107.

47. Almandoz JP, Gharib H. Hypothyroidism: Etiology, diagnosis, and management. *Med Clin North Am* 2012;96:203–21.
48. Kramer CK, von Muhlen D, Kritz-Silverstein D, et al. Treated hypothyroidism, cognitive function, and depressed mood in old age: The Rancho Bernardo Study. *Eur J Endocrinol* 2009;161:917–21.
49. McQuade C, Skugor M, Brennan DM, et al. Hypothyroidism and moderate subclinical hypothyroidism are associated with increased all-cause mortality independent of coronary heart disease risk factors: A PreCIS database study. *Thyroid* 2011;21:837–43.
50. Mariotti S, Cambuli VM. Cardiovascular risk in elderly hypothyroid patients. *Thyroid* 2007;17:1067–73.
51. Mazzeffi MA, Lin HM, Flynn BC, et al. Hypothyroidism and the risk of lower extremity arterial disease. *Vasc Health Risk Manag* 2010;6:957–62.
52. Dimitriadis G, Mitrou P, Lambadiari V, et al. Insulin action in adipose tissue and muscle in hypothyroidism. *J Clin Endocrinol Metab* 2006;91:4930–7.
53. Bono G, Fancellu R, Blandini F, et al. Cognitive and affective status in mild hypothyroidism and interactions with L-thyroxine treatment. *Acta Neurol Scand* 2004;110:59–66.
54. Parle J, Roberts L, Wilson S, et al. A randomized controlled trial of the effect of thyroxine replacement on cognitive function in community-living elderly subjects with subclinical hypothyroidism: The Birmingham Elderly Thyroid study. *J Clin Endocrinol Metab* 2010;95:3623–32.
55. Sawin CT, Chopra D, Azizi F, et al. The aging thyroid. Increased prevalence of elevated serum thyrotropin levels in the elderly. *JAMA* 1979;242:247–50.
56. Diez JJ, Iglesias P. Spontaneous subclinical hypothyroidism in patients older than 55 years: An analysis of natural course and risk factors for the development of overt thyroid failure. *J Clin Endocrinol Metab* 2004;89:4890–7.
57. Gopinath B, Wang JJ, Kifley A, et al. Five-year incidence and progression of thyroid dysfunction in an older population. *Intern Med J* 2010;40:642–9.
58. Imaizumi M, Sera N, Ueki I, et al. Risk for progression to overt hypothyroidism in an elderly Japanese population with subclinical hypothyroidism. *Thyroid* 2011;21:1177–82.
59. Ashizawa K, Imaizumi M, Usa T, et al. Metabolic cardiovascular disease risk factors and their clustering in subclinical hypothyroidism. *Clin Endocrinol (Oxf)* 2010;72:689–95.
60. Park YJ, Lee EJ, Lee YJ, et al. Subclinical hypothyroidism (SCH) is not associated with metabolic derangement, cognitive impairment, depression or poor quality of life (QoL) in elderly subjects. *Arch Gerontol Geriatr* 2010;50:e68–73.
61. Resta F, Triggiani V, Barile G, et al. Subclinical hypothyroidism and cognitive dysfunction in the elderly. *Endocr Metab Immune Disord Drug Targets* 2012;12:260–7.
62. Moon MK, Lee YJ, Choi SH, et al. Subclinical hypothyroidism has little influences on muscle mass or strength in elderly people. *J Korean Med Sci* 2010;25:1176–81.
63. Simonsick EM, Newman AB, Ferrucci L, et al. Subclinical hypothyroidism and functional mobility in older adults. *Arch Intern Med* 2009;169:2011–17.
64. Duan Y, Peng W, Wang X, et al. Community-based study of the association of subclinical thyroid dysfunction with blood pressure. *Endocrine* 2009;35:136–42.
65. Walsh JP, Bremner AP, Bulsara MK, et al. Subclinical thyroid dysfunction and blood pressure: A community-based study. *Clin Endocrinol (Oxf)* 2006;65:486–91.
66. Liu D, Jiang F, Shan Z, et al. A cross-sectional survey of relationship between serum TSH level and blood pressure. *J Hum Hypertens* 2010;24:134–8.
67. Kowalska I, Borawski J, Nikolajuk A, et al. Insulin sensitivity, plasma adiponectin and sICAM-1 concentrations in patients with subclinical hypothyroidism: Response to levothyroxine therapy. *Endocrine* 2011;40:95–101.
68. Rodondi N, den Elzen WP, Bauer DC, et al. Subclinical hypothyroidism and the risk of coronary heart disease and mortality. *JAMA* 2010;304:1365–74.
69. Razvi S, Weaver JU, Vanderpump MP, et al. The incidence of ischemic heart disease and mortality in people with subclinical hypothyroidism: Reanalysis of the Whickham Survey cohort. *J Clin Endocrinol Metab* 2010;95:1734–40.
70. Nanchen D, Gussekloo J, Westendorp RG, et al. Subclinical thyroid dysfunction and the risk of heart failure in older persons at high cardiovascular risk. *J Clin Endocrinol Metab* 2012;97:852–61.
71. Rodondi N, Bauer DC, Cappola AR, et al. Subclinical thyroid dysfunction, cardiac function, and the risk of heart failure. The Cardiovascular Health study. *J Am Coll Cardiol* 2008;52:1152–9.
72. Villar HC, Saconato H, Valente O, et al. Thyroid hormone replacement for subclinical hypothyroidism. *Cochrane Database Syst Rev* 2007;(3): CD003419. DOI: 10.1002/14651858.CD003419.pub2.
73. Harman SM, Metter EJ, Tobin JD, et al. Longitudinal effects of aging on serum total and free testosterone levels in healthy men. Baltimore Longitudinal Study of Aging. *J Clin Endocrinol Metab* 2001;86:724–31.
74. Araujo AB, Esche GR, Kupelian V, et al. Prevalence of symptomatic androgen deficiency in men. *J Clin Endocrinol Metab* 2007;92:4241–7.
75. Wu FC, Tajar A, Pye SR, et al. Hypothalamic-pituitary-testicular axis disruptions in older men are differentially linked to age and modifiable risk factors: The European Male Aging Study. *J Clin Endocrinol Metab* 2008;93:2737–45.

76. Gray A, Feldman HA, McKinlay JB, et al. Age, disease, and changing sex hormone levels in middle-aged men: Results of the Massachusetts Male Aging Study. *J Clin Endocrinol Metab* 1991;73:1016–25.
77. Feinberg AW, Feigel A, Shevkoplyas SS, et al. Muscular thin films for building actuators and powering devices. *Science* 2007;317:1366–70.
78. Wylie K, Froggatt N. Late onset hypogonadism, sexuality and fertility. *Hum Fertil (Camb)* 2010;13:126–33.
79. Rosner W. Sex steroids and the free hormone hypothesis. *Cell* 2006;124:455–6.
80. Traish AM, Saad F, Guay A. The dark side of testosterone deficiency: II. Type 2 diabetes and insulin resistance. *J Androl* 2009;30:23–32.
81. Wu FC, Tajar A, Beynon JM, et al. Identification of late-onset hypogonadism in middle-aged and elderly men. *N Engl J Med* 2010;363:123–35.
82. Araujo AB, O'Donnell AB, Brambilla DJ, et al. Prevalence and incidence of androgen deficiency in middle-aged and older men: Estimates from the Massachusetts Male Aging Study. *J Clin Endocrinol Metab* 2004;89:5920–6.
83. Kelleher S, Conway AJ, Handelsman DJ. Blood testosterone threshold for androgen deficiency symptoms. *J Clin Endocrinol Metab* 2004;89:3813–17.
84. Kapoor D, Aldred H, Clark S, et al. Clinical and biochemical assessment of hypogonadism in men with type 2 diabetes: Correlations with bioavailable testosterone and visceral adiposity. *Diabetes Care* 2007;30:911–17.
85. Zitzmann M, Faber S, Nieschlag E. Association of specific symptoms and metabolic risks with serum testosterone in older men. *J Clin Endocrinol Metab* 2006;91:4335–43.
86. Gooren LJ. Late-onset hypogonadism. *Front Horm Res* 2009;37:62–73.
87. Morales A, Tenover JL. Androgen deficiency in the aging male: When, who, and how to investigate and treat. *Urol Clin North Am* 2002;29:975–82, x.
88. Matsumoto AM. Andropause: Clinical implications of the decline in serum testosterone levels with aging in men. *J Gerontol A Biol Sci Med Sci* 2002;57:M76–99.
89. Meston CM. Aging and sexuality. *West J Med* 1997;167:285–90.
90. Srinivas-Shankar U, Wu FC. Frailty and muscle function: Role for testosterone? *Front Horm Res* 2009;37:133–49.
91. Breuer B, Trungold S, Martucci C, et al. Relationships of sex hormone levels to dependence in activities of daily living in the frail elderly. *Maturitas* 2001;39:147–59.
92. Baumgartner RN, Waters DL, Gallagher D, et al. Predictors of skeletal muscle mass in elderly men and women. *Mech Ageing Dev* 1999;107:123–36.
93. Morley JE, Kaiser FE, Perry HM 3rd, et al. Longitudinal changes in testosterone, luteinizing hormone, and follicle-stimulating hormone in healthy older men. *Metabolism* 1997;46:410–13.
94. Fink HA, Ewing SK, Ensrud KE, et al. Association of testosterone and estradiol deficiency with osteoporosis and rapid bone loss in older men. *J Clin Endocrinol Metab* 2006;91:3908–15.
95. Liu H, Paige NM, Goldzweig CL, et al. Screening for osteoporosis in men: A systematic review for an American College of Physicians guideline. *Ann Intern Med* 2008;148:685–701.
96. Meier C, Nguyen TV, Handelsman DJ, et al. Endogenous sex hormones and incident fracture risk in older men: The Dubbo Osteoporosis Epidemiology Study. *Arch Intern Med* 2008;168:47–54.
97. Smith MR. Treatment-related osteoporosis in men with prostate cancer. *Clin Cancer Res* 2006;12:6315s–19s.
98. Amin S, Zhang Y, Felson DT, et al. Estradiol, testosterone, and the risk for hip fractures in elderly men from the Framingham Study. *Am J Med* 2006;119:426–33.
99. Snyder PJ, Peachey H, Hannoush P, et al. Effect of testosterone treatment on bone mineral density in men over 65 years of age. *J Clin Endocrinol Metab* 1999;84:1966–72.
100. Brand JS, van der Tweel I, Grobbee DE, et al. Testosterone, sex hormone-binding globulin and the metabolic syndrome: A systematic review and meta-analysis of observational studies. *Int J Epidemiol* 2011;40:189–207.
101. Shabsigh R, Katz M, Yan G, et al. Cardiovascular issues in hypogonadism and testosterone therapy. *Am J Cardiol* 2005;96:67M–72M.
102. Nettleship JE, Jones RD, Channer KS, et al. Testosterone and coronary artery disease. *Front Horm Res* 2009;37:91–107.
103. Muller M, van den Beld AW, Bots ML, et al. Endogenous sex hormones and progression of carotid atherosclerosis in elderly men. *Circulation* 2004;109:2074–9.
104. Tivesten A, Mellstrom D, Jutberger H, et al. Low serum testosterone and high serum estradiol associate with lower extremity peripheral arterial disease in elderly men. The MrOS Study in Sweden. *J Am Coll Cardiol* 2007;50:1070–6.
105. Hak AE, Witteman JC, de Jong FH, et al. Low levels of endogenous androgens increase the risk of atherosclerosis in elderly men: The Rotterdam study. *J Clin Endocrinol Metab* 2002;87:3632–9.
106. Shores MM, Moceri VM, Sloan KL, et al. Low testosterone levels predict incident depressive illness in older men: Effects of age and medical morbidity. *J Clin Psychiatry* 2005;66:7–14.
107. Moffat SD, Zonderman AB, Metter EJ, et al. Longitudinal assessment of serum free testosterone concentration predicts memory performance and cognitive status in elderly men. *J Clin Endocrinol Metab* 2002;87:5001–7.
108. Thilers PP, Macdonald SW, Herlitz A. The association between endogenous free testosterone and

cognitive performance: A population-based study in 35 to 90 year-old men and women. *Psychoneuroendocrinology* 2006;31:565–76.
109. Muller M, Aleman A, Grobbee DE, et al. Endogenous sex hormone levels and cognitive function in aging men: Is there an optimal level? *Neurology* 2005;64:866–71.
110. Janowsky JS, Chavez B, Orwoll E. Sex steroids modify working memory. *J Cogn Neurosci* 2000;12:407–14.
111. Janowsky JS, Oviatt SK, Orwoll ES. Testosterone influences spatial cognition in older men. *Behav Neurosci* 1994;108:325–32.
112. Winters SJ, Kelley DE, Goodpaster B. The analog free testosterone assay: Are the results in men clinically useful? *Clin Chem* 1998;44:2178–82.
113. Bhasin S, Cunningham GR, Hayes FJ, et al. Testosterone therapy in men with androgen deficiency syndromes: An Endocrine Society clinical practice guideline. *J Clin Endocrinol Metab* 2010;95:2536–59.
114. Wang C, Nieschlag E, Swerdloff R, et al. Investigation, treatment, and monitoring of late-onset hypogonadism in males: ISA, ISSAM, EAU, EAA, and ASA recommendations. *J Androl* 2009;30:1–9.
115. Wang C, Nieschlag E, Swerdloff RS, et al. ISA, ISSAM, EAU, EAA and ASA recommendations: Investigation, treatment and monitoring of late-onset hypogonadism in males. *Aging Male* 2009;12:5–12.
116. Snyder PJ. Clinical use of androgens. *Annu Rev Med* 1984;35:207–17.
117. Snyder PJ, Lawrence DA. Treatment of male hypogonadism with testosterone enanthate. *J Clin Endocrinol Metab* 1980;51:1335–9.
118. Nieschlag E, Behre HM, Bouchard P, et al. Testosterone replacement therapy: Current trends and future directions. *Hum Reprod Update* 2004;10:409–19.
119. *Testosterone: Action, Deficiency, Substitution*. 3rd ed. Cambridge: Cambridge University Press; 2004.
120. Lunenfeld B, Nieschlag E. Testosterone therapy in the aging male. *Aging Male* 2007;10:139–53.
121. Svartberg J, Agledahl I, Figenschau Y, et al. Testosterone treatment in elderly men with subnormal testosterone levels improves body composition and BMD in the hip. *Int J Impot Res* 2008;20:378–87.
122. Page ST, Amory JK, Bowman FD, et al. Exogenous testosterone (T) alone or with finasteride increases physical performance, grip strength, and lean body mass in older men with low serum T. *J Clin Endocrinol Metab* 2005;90:1502–10.
123. Sih R, Morley JE, Kaiser FE, et al. Testosterone replacement in older hypogonadal men: A 12-month randomized controlled trial. *J Clin Endocrinol Metab* 1997;82:1661–7.
124. Perry HM 3rd, Miller DK, Patrick P, et al. Testosterone and leptin in older African-American men: Relationship to age, strength, function, and season. *Metabolism* 2000;49:1085–91.
125. Srinivas-Shankar U, Roberts SA, Connolly MJ, et al. Effects of testosterone on muscle strength, physical function, body composition, and quality of life in intermediate-frail and frail elderly men: A randomized, double-blind, placebo-controlled study. *J Clin Endocrinol Metab* 2010;95:639–50.
126. Clague JE, Wu FC, Horan MA. Difficulties in measuring the effect of testosterone replacement therapy on muscle function in older men. *Int J Androl* 1999;22:261–5.
127. Isidori AM, Giannetta E, Greco EA, et al. Effects of testosterone on body composition, bone metabolism and serum lipid profile in middle-aged men: A meta-analysis. *Clin Endocrinol (Oxf)* 2005;63:280–93.
128. Nair KS, Rizza RA, O'Brien P, et al. DHEA in elderly women and DHEA or testosterone in elderly men. *N Engl J Med* 2006;355:1647–59.
129. Behre HM, Kliesch S, Leifke E, et al. Long-term effect of testosterone therapy on bone mineral density in hypogonadal men. *J Clin Endocrinol Metab* 1997;82:2386–90.
130. Merza Z, Blumsohn A, Mah PM, et al. Double-blind placebo-controlled study of testosterone patch therapy on bone turnover in men with borderline hypogonadism. *Int J Androl* 2006;29:381–91.
131. Amory JK, Watts NB, Easley KA, et al. Exogenous testosterone or testosterone with finasteride increases bone mineral density in older men with low serum testosterone. *J Clin Endocrinol Metab* 2004;89:503–10.
132. Saggese G, Bertelloni S, Baroncelli GI. Sex steroids and the acquisition of bone mass. *Horm Res* 1997;48(Suppl 5):65–71.
133. Hogervorst E, Bandelow S, Combrinck M, et al. Low free testosterone is an independent risk factor for Alzheimer's disease. *Exp Gerontol* 2004;39:1633–9.
134. Beauchet O. Testosterone and cognitive function: Current clinical evidence of a relationship. *Eur J Endocrinol* 2006;155:773–81.
135. Tan RS, Pu SJ. A pilot study on the effects of testosterone in hypogonadal aging male patients with Alzheimer's disease. *Aging Male* 2003;6:13–17.
136. Cherrier MM, Craft S, Matsumoto AH. Cognitive changes associated with supplementation of testosterone or dihydrotestosterone in mildly hypogonadal men: A preliminary report. *J Androl* 2003;24:568–76.
137. Cherrier MM, Matsumoto AM, Amory JK, et al. Testosterone improves spatial memory in men with Alzheimer disease and mild cognitive impairment. *Neurology* 2005;64:2063–8.
138. Kenny AM, Bellantonio S, Gruman CA, et al. Effects of transdermal testosterone on cognitive function and health perception in older men with low bioavailable testosterone levels. *J Gerontol A Biol Sci Med Sci* 2002;57:M321–5.
139. Kenny AM, Fabregas G, Song C, et al. Effects of testosterone on behavior, depression, and cognitive function

in older men with mild cognitive loss. *J Gerontol A Biol Sci Med Sci* 2004;59:75–8.

140. Emmelot-Vonk MH, Verhaar HJ, Nakhai Pour HR, et al. Effect of testosterone supplementation on functional mobility, cognition, and other parameters in older men: A randomized controlled trial. *JAMA* 2008;299:39–52.
141. Yonker JE, Eriksson E, Nilsson LG, et al. Negative association of testosterone on spatial visualization in 35 to 80 year old men. *Cortex* 2006;42:376–86.
142. Marin P, Holmang S, Gustafsson C, et al. Androgen treatment of abdominally obese men. *Obes Res* 1993;1:245–51.
143. Jones TH, Saad F. The effects of testosterone on risk factors for, and the mediators of, the atherosclerotic process. *Atherosclerosis* 2009;207:318–27.
144. Allan CA, McLachlan RI. Androgens and obesity. *Curr Opin Endocrinol Diabetes Obes* 2010;17:224–32.
145. Calof OM, Singh AB, Lee ML, et al. Adverse events associated with testosterone replacement in middle-aged and older men: A meta-analysis of randomized, placebo-controlled trials. *J Gerontol A Biol Sci Med Sci* 2005;60:1451–7.
146. Munzer T, Harman SM, Hees P, et al. Effects of GH and/or sex steroid administration on abdominal subcutaneous and visceral fat in healthy aged women and men. *J Clin Endocrinol Metab* 2001;86:3604–10.
147. Kapoor D, Goodwin E, Channer KS, et al. Testosterone replacement therapy improves insulin resistance, glycaemic control, visceral adiposity and hypercholesterolaemia in hypogonadal men with type 2 diabetes. *Eur J Endocrinol* 2006;154:899–906.
148. Heufelder AE, Saad F, Bunck MC, et al. Fifty-two-week treatment with diet and exercise plus transdermal testosterone reverses the metabolic syndrome and improves glycemic control in men with newly diagnosed type 2 diabetes and subnormal plasma testosterone. *J Androl* 2009;30:726–33.
149. Kalinchenko SY, Tishova YA, Mskhalaya GJ, et al. Effects of testosterone supplementation on markers of the metabolic syndrome and inflammation in hypogonadal men with the metabolic syndrome: The double-blinded placebo-controlled Moscow study. *Clin Endocrinol (Oxf)* 2010;73:602–12.
150. Jones TH, Arver S, Behre HM, et al. Testosterone replacement in hypogonadal men with type 2 diabetes and/or metabolic syndrome (the TIMES2 study). *Diabetes Care* 2011;34:828–37.
151. Whitsel EA, Boyko EJ, Matsumoto AM, et al. Intramuscular testosterone esters and plasma lipids in hypogonadal men: A meta-analysis. *Am J Med* 2001;111:261–9.
152. Wang C, Jackson G, Jones TH, et al. Low testosterone associated with obesity and the metabolic syndrome contributes to sexual dysfunction and cardiovascular disease risk in men with type 2 diabetes. *Diabetes Care* 2011;34:1669–75.
153. Corona G, Monami M, Rastrelli G, et al. Type 2 diabetes mellitus and testosterone: A meta-analysis study. *Int J Androl* 2011;34:528–40.
154. Colangelo LA, Ouyang P, Liu K, et al. Association of endogenous sex hormones with diabetes and impaired fasting glucose in men: Multi-ethnic study of atherosclerosis. *Diabetes Care* 2009;32:1049–51.
155. Agledahl I, Hansen JB, Svartberg J. Impact of testosterone treatment on postprandial triglyceride metabolism in elderly men with subnormal testosterone levels. *Scand J Clin Lab Invest* 2008;68:641–8.
156. Aversa A, Bruzziches R, Francomano D, et al. Effects of testosterone undecanoate on cardiovascular risk factors and atherosclerosis in middle-aged men with late-onset hypogonadism and metabolic syndrome: Results from a 24-month, randomized, double-blind, placebo-controlled study. *J Sex Med* 2010;7:3495–503.
157. Chahla EJ, Hayek ME, Morley JE. Testosterone replacement therapy and cardiovascular risk factors modification. *Aging Male* 2011;14:83–90.
158. Mathur A, Malkin C, Saeed B, et al. Long-term benefits of testosterone replacement therapy on angina threshold and atheroma in men. *Eur J Endocrinol* 2009;161:443–9.
159. Malkin CJ, Pugh PJ, Morris PD, et al. Testosterone replacement in hypogonadal men with angina improves ischaemic threshold and quality of life. *Heart* 2004;90:871–6.
160. Nam UH, Wang M, Crisostomo PR, et al. The effect of chronic exogenous androgen on myocardial function following acute ischemia-reperfusion in hosts with different baseline levels of sex steroids. *J Surg Res* 2007;142:113–18.
161. Haddad RM, Kennedy CC, Caples SM, et al. Testosterone and cardiovascular risk in men: A systematic review and meta-analysis of randomized placebo-controlled trials. *Mayo Clin Proc* 2007;82:29–39.
162. Caminiti G, Volterrani M, Iellamo F, et al. Effect of long-acting testosterone treatment on functional exercise capacity, skeletal muscle performance, insulin resistance, and baroreflex sensitivity in elderly patients with chronic heart failure a double-blind, placebo-controlled, randomized study. *J Am Coll Cardiol* 2009;54:919–27.
163. Hajjar RR, Kaiser FE, Morley JE. Outcomes of long-term testosterone replacement in older hypogonadal males: A retrospective analysis. *J Clin Endocrinol Metab* 1997;82:3793–6.
164. Allan CA, McLachlan RI. Age-related changes in testosterone and the role of replacement therapy in older men. *Clin Endocrinol (Oxf)* 2004;60:653–70.
165. Soules MR, Sherman S, Parrott E, et al. Executive summary: Stages of Reproductive Aging Workshop

(STRAW) Park City, Utah, July, 2001. *Menopause* 2001;8:402–7.
166. Harlow SD, Gass M, Hall JE, et al. Executive summary of the Stages of Reproductive Aging Workshop + 10: Addressing the unfinished agenda of staging reproductive aging. *J Clin Endocrinol Metab* 2012;97:1159–68.
167. Soules MR. Development of a staging system for the menopause transition: A work in progress. *Menopause* 2005;12:117–20.
168. Randolph JF, Jr., Sowers M, Bondarenko IV, et al. Change in estradiol and follicle-stimulating hormone across the early menopausal transition: Effects of ethnicity and age. *J Clin Endocrinol Metab* 2004; 89:1555–61.
169. Dennerstein L, Dudley EC, Hopper JL, et al. A prospective population-based study of menopausal symptoms. *Obstet Gynecol* 2000;96:351–8.
170. Freeman EW, Sammel MD, Lin H, et al. Symptoms associated with menopausal transition and reproductive hormones in midlife women. *Obstet Gynecol* 2007;110:230–40.
171. Nelson HD, Haney E, Humphrey L, et al. Management of menopause-related symptoms. *Evid Rep Technol Assess (Summ)* 2005;1–6.
172. Hunter MS, Gentry-Maharaj A, Ryan A, et al. Prevalence, frequency and problem rating of hot flushes persist in older postmenopausal women: Impact of age, body mass index, hysterectomy, hormone therapy use, lifestyle and mood in a cross-sectional cohort study of 10,418 British women aged 54–65. *BJOG* 2012;119:40–50.
173. Green R, Santoro N. Menopausal symptoms and ethnicity: The Study of Women's Health Across the Nation. *Womens Health (Lond Engl)* 2009;5:127–33.
174. Thurston RC, Joffe H. Vasomotor symptoms and menopause: Findings from the Study of Women's Health across the Nation. *Obstet Gynecol Clin North Am* 2011;38:489–501.
175. Huang AJ, Grady D, Jacoby VL, et al. Persistent hot flushes in older postmenopausal women. *Arch Intern Med* 2008;168:840–6.
176. Kronenberg F. Hot flashes: Epidemiology and physiology. *Ann N Y Acad Sci* 1990;592:52–86; discussion 123–33.
177. Freeman EW. Associations of depression with the transition to menopause. *Menopause* 2010;17:823–7.
178. Freeman EW, Sammel MD, Lin H, et al. Symptoms in the menopausal transition: Hormone and behavioral correlates. *Obstet Gynecol* 2008;111:127–36.
179. Burger H. The menopausal transition—endocrinology. *J Sex Med* 2008;5:2266–73.
180. Kim HC, Greenland P, Rossouw JE, et al. Multimarker prediction of coronary heart disease risk: The Women's Health Initiative. *J Am Coll Cardiol* 2010;55:2080–91.
181. Deo R, Vittinghoff E, Lin F, et al. Risk factor and prediction modeling for sudden cardiac death in women with coronary artery disease. *Arch Intern Med* 2011;171:1703–9.
182. Jacobs MB, Kritz-Silverstein D, Wingard DL, et al. The association of reproductive history with all-cause and cardiovascular mortality in older women: The Rancho Bernardo Study. *Fertil Steril* 2012;97:118–24.
183. Neer RM. Bone loss across the menopausal transition. *Ann N Y Acad Sci* 2010;1192:66–71.
184. Santen RJ, Allred DC, Ardoin SP, et al. Postmenopausal hormone therapy: An Endocrine Society scientific statement. *J Clin Endocrinol Metab* 2010;95:s1–s66.
185. Loprinzi CL, Qin R, Balcueva EP, et al. Phase III, randomized, double-blind, placebo-controlled evaluation of pregabalin for alleviating hot flashes, N07C1. *J Clin Oncol* 2010;28:641–7.
186. Freeman EW, Guthrie KA, Caan B, et al. Efficacy of escitalopram for hot flashes in healthy menopausal women: A randomized controlled trial. *JAMA* 2011;305:267–74.
187. Martin KA, Manson JE. Approach to the patient with menopausal symptoms. *J Clin Endocrinol Metab* 2008;93:4567–75.
188. Rossouw JE, Anderson GL, Prentice RL, et al. Risks and benefits of estrogen plus progestin in healthy postmenopausal women: Principal results From the Women's Health Initiative randomized controlled trial. *JAMA* 2002;288:321–33.
189. Beral V, Reeves G, Bull D, et al. Breast cancer risk in relation to the interval between menopause and starting hormone therapy. *J Natl Cancer Inst* 2011;103:296–305.
190. Stefanick ML, Anderson GL, Margolis KL, et al. Effects of conjugated equine estrogens on breast cancer and mammography screening in postmenopausal women with hysterectomy. *JAMA* 2006;295:1647–57.
191. LaCroix AZ, Chlebowski RT, Manson JE, et al. Health outcomes after stopping conjugated equine estrogens among postmenopausal women with prior hysterectomy: A randomized controlled trial. *JAMA* 2011;305:1305–14.
192. Fournier A, Berrino F, Clavel-Chapelon F. Unequal risks for breast cancer associated with different hormone replacement therapies: Results from the E3N cohort study. *Breast Cancer Res Treat* 2008;107:103–11.
193. Fournier A, Fabre A, Mesrine S, et al. Use of different postmenopausal hormone therapies and risk of histology- and hormone receptor-defined invasive breast cancer. *J Clin Oncol* 2008;26:1260–8.
194. Canonico M, Oger E, Plu-Bureau G, et al. Hormone therapy and venous thromboembolism among postmenopausal women: Impact of the route of estrogen administration and progestogens: The ESTHER study. *Circulation* 2007;115:840–5.

195. Canonico M, Plu-Bureau G, Lowe GD, et al. Hormone replacement therapy and risk of venous thromboembolism in postmenopausal women: Systematic review and meta-analysis. *BMJ* 2008;336:1227–31.
196. Renoux C, Dell'aniello S, Garbe E, et al. Transdermal and oral hormone replacement therapy and the risk of stroke: A nested case-control study. *Brit Med J* 2010;340:c2519.
197. Canonico M, Fournier A, Carcaillon L, et al. Postmenopausal hormone therapy and risk of idiopathic venous thromboembolism: Results from the E3N cohort study. *Arterioscler Thromb Vasc Biol* 2010;30: 340–5.
198. Margolis KL, Bonds DE, Rodabough RJ, et al. Effect of oestrogen plus progestin on the incidence of diabetes in postmenopausal women: Results from the Women's Health Initiative Hormone Trial. *Diabetologia* 2004;47:1175–87.
199. Kanaya AM, Herrington D, Vittinghoff E, et al. Glycemic effects of postmenopausal hormone therapy: The Heart and Estrogen/progestin Replacement Study. A randomized, double-blind, placebo-controlled trial. *Ann Intern Med* 2003;138:1–9.
200. Bonds DE, Lasser N, Qi L, et al. The effect of conjugated equine oestrogen on diabetes incidence: The Women's Health Initiative randomised trial. *Diabetologia* 2006;49:459–68.
201. Salpeter SR, Walsh JM, Ormiston TM, et al. Meta-analysis: Effect of hormone-replacement therapy on components of the metabolic syndrome in postmenopausal women. *Diabetes Obes Metab* 2006;8:538–54.
202. Anderson GL, Limacher M, Assaf AR, et al. Effects of conjugated equine estrogen in postmenopausal women with hysterectomy: The Women's Health Initiative randomized controlled trial. *JAMA* 2004;291:1701–12.
203. Rossouw JE, Prentice RL, Manson JE, et al. Postmenopausal hormone therapy and risk of cardiovascular disease by age and years since menopause. *JAMA* 2007;297:1465–77.
204. Salpeter SR, Cheng J, Thabane L, et al. Bayesian meta-analysis of hormone therapy and mortality in younger postmenopausal women. *Am J Med* 2009;122:1016–22 e1.
205. Salpeter SR, Walsh JM, Greyber E, et al. Brief report: Coronary heart disease events associated with hormone therapy in younger and older women. A meta-analysis. *J Gen Intern Med* 2006;21:363–6.
206. Corpas E, Harman SM, Blackman MR. Human growth hormone and human aging. *Endocr Rev* 1993;14:20–39.
207. Prodam F, Pagano L, Corneli G, et al. Update on epidemiology, etiology, and diagnosis of adult growth hormone deficiency. *J Endocrinol Invest* 2008;31:6–11.
208. Veldhuis JD, Iranmanesh A, Bowers CY. Joint mechanisms of impaired growth-hormone pulse renewal in aging men. *J Clin Endocrinol Metab* 2005;90:4177–83.
209. Brook CG, Hindmarsh PC. The somatotropic axis in puberty. *Endocrinol Metab Clin North Am* 1992;21:767–82.
210. Iranmanesh A, Lizarralde G, Veldhuis JD. Age and relative adiposity are specific negative determinants of the frequency and amplitude of growth hormone (GH) secretory bursts and the half-life of endogenous GH in healthy men. *J Clin Endocrinol Metab* 1991;73:1081–8.
211. Bayram F, Gedik VT, Demir O, et al. Epidemiologic survey: Reference ranges of serum insulin-like growth factor 1 levels in Caucasian adult population with immunoradiometric assay. *Endocrine* 2011;40:304–9.
212. Maggio M, Ble A, Ceda GP, et al. Decline in insulin-like growth factor-I levels across adult life span in two large population studies. *J Gerontol A Biol Sci Med Sci* 2006;61:182–3.
213. Goodman-Gruen D, Barrett-Connor E. Epidemiology of insulin-like growth factor-I in elderly men and women. The Rancho Bernardo Study. *Am J Epidemiol* 1997;145:970–6.
214. Sassolas G, Chazot FB, Jaquet P, et al. GH deficiency in adults: An epidemiological approach. *Eur J Endocrinol* 1999;141:595–600.
215. Stochholm K, Gravholt CH, Laursen T, et al. Incidence of GH deficiency – a nationwide study. *Eur J Endocrinol* 2006;155:61–71.
216. Webb SM, Strasburger CJ, Mo D, et al. Changing patterns of the adult growth hormone deficiency diagnosis documented in a decade-long global surveillance database. *J Clin Endocrinol Metab* 2009;94:392–9.
217. Gentili A, Mulligan T, Godschalk M, et al. Unequal impact of short-term testosterone repletion on the somatotropic axis of young and older men. *J Clin Endocrinol Metab* 2002;87:825–34.
218. Iranmanesh A, South S, Liem AY, et al. Unequal impact of age, percentage body fat, and serum testosterone concentrations on the somatotrophic, IGF-I, and IGF-binding protein responses to a three-day intravenous growth hormone-releasing hormone pulsatile infusion in men. *Eur J Endocrinol* 1998;139:59–71.
219. Shah N, Aloi J, Evans WS, et al. Time mode of growth hormone (GH) entry into the bloodstream and steady-state plasma GH concentrations, rather than sex, estradiol, or menstrual cycle stage, primarily determine the GH elimination rate in healthy young women and men. *J Clin Endocrinol Metab* 1999;84:2862–9.
220. Russell-Aulet M, Jaffe CA, Demott-Friberg R, et al. In vivo semiquantification of hypothalamic growth hormone-releasing hormone (GHRH) output in humans: Evidence for relative GHRH deficiency in aging. *J Clin Endocrinol Metab* 1999;84:3490–7.
221. Corpas E, Harman SM, Pineyro MA, et al. Growth hormone (GH)-releasing hormone-(1-29) twice daily reverses the decreased GH and insulin-like growth

factor-I levels in old men. *J Clin Endocrinol Metab* 1992;75:530–5.

222. Khorram O, Laughlin GA, Yen SS. Endocrine and metabolic effects of long-term administration of [Nle27] growth hormone-releasing hormone-(1-29)-NH2 in age-advanced men and women. *J Clin Endocrinol Metab* 1997;82:1472–9.
223. Sherlock M, Toogood AA. Aging and the growth hormone/insulin like growth factor-I axis. *Pituitary* 2007;10:189–203.
224. Veldhuis JD, Patrie JT, Brill KT, et al. Contributions of gender and systemic estradiol and testosterone concentrations to maximal secretagogue drive of burst-like growth hormone secretion in healthy middle-aged and older adults. *J Clin Endocrinol Metab* 2004;89:6291–6.
225. Vahl N, Jorgensen JO, Jurik AG, et al. Abdominal adiposity and physical fitness are major determinants of the age associated decline in stimulated GH secretion in healthy adults. *J Clin Endocrinol Metab* 1996;81:2209–15.
226. Veldhuis JD, Erickson D, Iranmanesh A, et al. Sex-steroid control of the aging somatotropic axis. *Endocrinol Metab Clin North Am* 2005;34:877–93, viii.
227. Veldhuis JD, Liem AY, South S, et al. Differential impact of age, sex steroid hormones, and obesity on basal versus pulsatile growth hormone secretion in men as assessed in an ultrasensitive chemiluminescence assay. *J Clin Endocrinol Metab* 1995;80:3209–22.
228. Munzer T, Rosen CJ, Harman SM, et al. Effects of GH and/or sex steroids on circulating IGF-I and IGFBPs in healthy, aged women and men. *Am J Physiol Endocrinol Metab* 2006;290:E1006–13.
229. Falleti MG, Maruff P, Burman P, et al. The effects of growth hormone (GH) deficiency and GH replacement on cognitive performance in adults: A meta-analysis of the current literature. *Psychoneuroendocrinology* 2006;31:681–91.
230. Sathiavageeswaran M, Burman P, Lawrence D, et al. Effects of GH on cognitive function in elderly patients with adult-onset GH deficiency: A placebo-controlled 12-month study. *Eur J Endocrinol* 2007;156:439–47.
231. Liu H, Bravata DM, Olkin I, et al. Systematic review: The safety and efficacy of growth hormone in the healthy elderly. *Ann Intern Med* 2007;146:104–15.
232. Koltowska-Haggstrom M, Mattsson AF, Shalet SM. Assessment of quality of life in adult patients with GH deficiency: KIMS contribution to clinical practice and pharmacoeconomic evaluations. *Eur J Endocrinol* 2009;161(Suppl 1):S51–64.
233. Gotherstrom G, Bengtsson BA, Bosaeus I, et al. A 10-year, prospective study of the metabolic effects of growth hormone replacement in adults. *J Clin Endocrinol Metab* 2007;92:1442–5.
234. Harman SM, Blackman MR. The effects of growth hormone and sex steroid on lean body mass, fat mass, muscle strength, cardiovascular endurance and adverse events in healthy elderly women and men. *Horm Res* 2003;60:121–4.
235. Giannoulis MG, Sonksen PH, Umpleby M, et al. The effects of growth hormone and/or testosterone in healthy elderly men: A randomized controlled trial. *J Clin Endocrinol Metab* 2006;91:477–84.
236. Park JK, Hong JW, Kim CO, et al. Sustained-release recombinant human growth hormone improves body composition and quality of life in adults with somatopause. *J Am Geriatr Soc* 2011;59:944–7.
237. Murray RD, Columb B, Adams JE, et al. Low bone mass is an infrequent feature of the adult growth hormone deficiency syndrome in middle-age adults and the elderly. *J Clin Endocrinol Metab* 2004;89:1124–30.
238. Boonen S, Pye SR, O'Neill TW, et al. Influence of bone remodelling rate on quantitative ultrasound parameters at the calcaneus and DXA BMDa of the hip and spine in middle-aged and elderly European men: The European Male Ageing Study (EMAS). *Eur J Endocrinol* 2011;165:977–86.
239. Tritos NA, Greenspan SL, King D, et al. Unreplaced sex steroid deficiency, corticotropin deficiency, and lower IGF-I are associated with lower bone mineral density in adults with growth hormone deficiency: A KIMS database analysis. *J Clin Endocrinol Metab* 2011;96:1516–23.
240. Gotherstrom G, Bengtsson BA, Bosaeus I, et al. Ten-year GH replacement increases bone mineral density in hypopituitary patients with adult onset GH deficiency. *Eur J Endocrinol* 2007;156:55–64.
241. Elbornsson M, Gotherstrom G, Franco C, et al. Effects of 3-year GH replacement therapy on bone mineral density in younger and elderly adults with adult-onset GH deficiency. *Eur J Endocrinol* 2012;166:181–9.
242. Holmer H, Svensson J, Rylander L, et al. Fracture incidence in GH-deficient patients on complete hormone replacement including GH. *J Bone Miner Res* 2007;22:1842–50.
243. Gotherstrom G, Elbornsson M, Stibrant-Sunnerhagen K, et al. Muscle strength in elderly adults with GH deficiency after 10 years of GH replacement. *Eur J Endocrinol* 2010;163:207–15.
244. Widdowson WM, Gibney J. The effect of growth hormone (GH) replacement on muscle strength in patients with GH-deficiency: A meta-analysis. *Clin Endocrinol (Oxf)* 2010;72:787–92.
245. Giannoulis MG, Jackson N, Shojaee-Moradie F, et al. The effects of growth hormone and/or testosterone on whole body protein kinetics and skeletal muscle gene expression in healthy elderly men: A randomized controlled trial. *J Clin Endocrinol Metab* 2008;93:3066–74.
246. Sanmarti A, Lucas A, Hawkins F, et al. Observational study in adult hypopituitary patients with untreated

growth hormone deficiency (ODA study). Socioeconomic impact and health status. Collaborative ODA (Observational GH Deficiency in Adults) Group. *Eur J Endocrinol* 1999;141:481–9.
247. Verhelst J, Mattsson AF, Luger A, et al. Prevalence and characteristics of the metabolic syndrome in 2479 hypopituitary patients with adult-onset GH deficiency before GH replacement: A KIMS analysis. *Eur J Endocrinol* 2011;165:881–9.
248. Cannavo S, Marini F, Curto L, et al. High prevalence of coronary calcifications and increased risk for coronary heart disease in adults with growth hormone deficiency. *J Endocrinol Invest* 2011;34:32–7.
249. Itoh E, Hizuka N, Fukuda I, et al. Metabolic disorders in adult growth hormone deficiency: A study of 110 patients at a single institute in Japan. *Endocr J* 2006;53:539–45.
250. Stochholm K, Christiansen J, Laursen T, et al. Mortality and reduced growth hormone secretion. *Horm Res* 2007;68(Suppl 5):173–6.
251. van Bunderen CC, van Nieuwpoort IC, Arwert LI, et al. Does growth hormone replacement therapy reduce mortality in adults with growth hormone deficiency? Data from the Dutch National Registry of Growth Hormone Treatment in adults. *J Clin Endocrinol Metab* 2011;96:3151–9.
252. Schneider HJ, Klotsche J, Wittchen HU, et al. Effects of growth hormone replacement within the KIMS survey on estimated cardiovascular risk and predictors of risk reduction in patients with growth hormone deficiency. *Clin Endocrinol (Oxf)* 2011;75:825–30.
253. Attanasio AF, Mo D, Erfurth EM, et al. Prevalence of metabolic syndrome in adult hypopituitary growth hormone (GH)-deficient patients before and after GH replacement. *J Clin Endocrinol Metab* 2010;95:74–81.
254. Devin JK, Young PP. The effects of growth hormone and insulin-like growth factor-1 on the aging cardiovascular system and its progenitor cells. *Curr Opin Investig Drugs* 2008;9:983–92.
255. Molitch ME, Clemmons DR, Malozowski S, et al. Evaluation and treatment of adult growth hormone deficiency: An Endocrine Society clinical practice guideline. *J Clin Endocrinol Metab* 2011;96:1587–609.
256. Rudman D, Feller AG, Nagraj HS, et al. Effects of human growth hormone in men over 60 years old. *N Engl J Med* 1990;323:1–6.
257. Giordano R, Bonelli L, Marinazzo E, et al. Growth hormone treatment in human ageing: Benefits and risks. *Hormones (Athens)* 2008;7:133–9.
258. Vittone J, Blackman MR, Busby-Whitehead J, et al. Effects of single nightly injections of growth hormone-releasing hormone (GHRH 1-29) in healthy elderly men. *Metabolism* 1997;46:89–96.
259. Borst SE. Interventions for sarcopenia and muscle weakness in older people. *Age Ageing* 2004;33:548–55.
260. Ghigo E, Arvat E, Muccioli G, et al. Growth hormone-releasing peptides. *Eur J Endocrinol* 1997;136:445–60.
261. Ghigo E, Arvat E, Broglio F, et al. Endocrine and non-endocrine activities of growth hormone secretagogues in humans. *Horm Res* 1999;51(Suppl 3):9–15.
262. Murphy MG, Weiss S, McClung M, et al. Effect of alendronate and MK-677 (a growth hormone secretagogue), individually and in combination, on markers of bone turnover and bone mineral density in postmenopausal osteoporotic women. *J Clin Endocrinol Metab* 2001;86:1116–25.
263. Parker CR, Jr., Mixon RL, Brissie RM, et al. Aging alters zonation in the adrenal cortex of men. *J Clin Endocrinol Metab* 1997;82:3898–901.
264. Bovio S, Cataldi A, Reimondo G, et al. Prevalence of adrenal incidentaloma in a contemporary computerized tomography series. *J Endocrinol Invest* 2006;29:298–302.
265. Van Cauter E, Leproult R, Kupfer DJ. Effects of gender and age on the levels and circadian rhythmicity of plasma cortisol. *J Clin Endocrinol Metab* 1996;81:2468–73.
266. Vermeulen A. Dehydroepiandrosterone sulfate and aging. *Ann N Y Acad Sci* 1995;774:121–7.
267. Dennison E, Hindmarsh P, Fall C, et al. Profiles of endogenous circulating cortisol and bone mineral density in healthy elderly men. *J Clin Endocrinol Metab* 1999;84:3058–63.
268. Seeman TE, McEwen BS, Singer BH, et al. Increase in urinary cortisol excretion and memory declines: MacArthur studies of successful aging. *J Clin Endocrinol Metab* 1997;82:2458–65.
269. Chawla A, Sterns RH, Nigwekar SU, et al. Mortality and serum sodium: Do patients die from or with hyponatremia? *Clin J Am Soc Nephrol* 2011;6:960–5.
270. Tolouian R, Alhamad T, Farazmand M, et al. The correlation of hip fracture and hyponatremia in the elderly. *J Nephrol* 2012;25:789–93.
271. Renneboog B, Musch W, Vandemergel X, et al. Mild chronic hyponatremia is associated with falls, unsteadiness, and attention deficits. *Am J Med* 2006;119:71 e1–8.
272. Svec F, Porter JR. The actions of exogenous dehydroepiandrosterone in experimental animals and humans. *Proc Soc Exp Biol Med* 1998;218:174–91.
273. Szathmari M, Szucs J, Feher T, et al. Dehydroepiandrosterone sulphate and bone mineral density. *Osteoporos Int* 1994;4:84–8.
274. Praveen EP, Sahoo JP, Kulshreshtha B, et al. Morning cortisol is lower in obese individuals with normal glucose tolerance. *Diabetes Metab Syndr Obes* 2011;4:347–52.
275. Veldhuis JD, Roelfsema F, Iranmanesh A, et al. Basal, pulsatile, entropic (patterned), and spiky (staccato-like) properties of ACTH secretion: Impact of age,

gender, and body mass index. *J Clin Endocrinol Metab* 2009;94:4045–52.

276. Veldhuis JD, Iranmanesh A, Roelfsema F, et al. Tripartite control of dynamic ACTH-cortisol dose responsiveness by age, body mass index, and gender in 111 healthy adults. *J Clin Endocrinol Metab* 2011;96:2874–81.

277. Hatzinger M, Brand S, Herzig N, et al. In healthy young and elderly adults, hypothalamic-pituitary-adrenocortical axis reactivity (HPA AR) varies with increasing pharmacological challenge and with age, but not with gender. *J Psychiatr Res* 2011;45: 1373–80.

278. Parker CR, Jr., Slayden SM, Azziz R, et al. Effects of aging on adrenal function in the human: Responsiveness and sensitivity of adrenal androgens and cortisol to adrenocorticotropin in premenopausal and postmenopausal women. *J Clin Endocrinol Metab* 2000;85:48–54.

279. Laughlin GA, Barrett-Connor E. Sexual dimorphism in the influence of advanced aging on adrenal hormone levels: The Rancho Bernardo Study. *J Clin Endocrinol Metab* 2000;85:3561–8.

280. Pratt JH, Hawthorne JJ, Debono DJ. Reduced urinary aldosterone excretion rates with normal plasma concentrations of aldosterone in the very elderly. *Steroids* 1988;51:163–71.

281. Bauer JH. Age-related changes in the renin-aldosterone system. Physiological effects and clinical implications. *Drugs Aging* 1993;3:238–45.

282. Hegstad R, Brown RD, Jiang NS, et al. Aging and aldosterone. *Am J Med* 1983;74:442–8.

283. Laughlin GA, Barrett-Connor E, Kritz-Silverstein D, et al. Hysterectomy, oophorectomy, and endogenous sex hormone levels in older women: The Rancho Bernardo Study. *J Clin Endocrinol Metab* 2000;85:645–51.

284. Travison TG, O'Donnell AB, Araujo AB, et al. Cortisol levels and measures of body composition in middle-aged and older men. *Clin Endocrinol (Oxf)* 2007;67:71–7.

285. Kern W, Dodt C, Born J, et al. Changes in cortisol and growth hormone secretion during nocturnal sleep in the course of aging. *J Gerontol A Biol Sci Med Sci* 1996;51:M3–9.

286. Ferrari E, Cravello L, Muzzoni B, et al. Age-related changes of the hypothalamic-pituitary-adrenal axis: Pathophysiological correlates. *Eur J Endocrinol* 2001; 144:319–29.

287. Wrosch C, Miller GE, Lupien S, et al. Diurnal cortisol secretion and 2-year changes in older adults' physical symptoms: The moderating roles of negative affect and sleep. *Health Psychol* 2008;27:685–93.

288. Bergendahl M, Iranmanesh A, Mulligan T, et al. Impact of age on cortisol secretory dynamics basally and as driven by nutrient-withdrawal stress. *J Clin Endocrinol Metab* 2000;85:2203–14.

289. Wahbeh H, Kishiyama SS, Zajdel D, et al. Salivary cortisol awakening response in mild Alzheimer disease, caregivers, and noncaregivers. *Alzheimer Dis Assoc Disord* 2008;22:181–3.

290. Kumari M, Badrick E, Chandola T, et al. Measures of social position and cortisol secretion in an aging population: Findings from the Whitehall II study. *Psychosom Med* 2010;72:27–34.

291. Comijs HC, Gerritsen L, Penninx BW, et al. The association between serum cortisol and cognitive decline in older persons. *Am J Geriatr Psychiatry* 2010;18:42–50.

292. Gerritsen L, Geerlings MI, Beekman AT, et al. Early and late life events and salivary cortisol in older persons. *Psychol Med* 2010;40:1569–78.

293. Franz CE, O'Brien RC, Hauger RL, et al. Cross-sectional and 35-year longitudinal assessment of salivary cortisol and cognitive functioning: The Vietnam Era twin study of aging. *Psychoneuroendocrinology* 2011;36:1040–52.

294. Lee BK, Glass TA, McAtee MJ, et al. Associations of salivary cortisol with cognitive function in the Baltimore memory study. *Arch Gen Psychiatry* 2007;64:810–18.

295. Li G, Cherrier MM, Tsuang DW, et al. Salivary cortisol and memory function in human aging. *Neurobiol Aging* 2006;27:1705–14.

296. Evans P, Hucklebridge F, Loveday C, et al. The cortisol awakening response is related to executive function in older age. *Int J Psychophysiol* 2012;84:201–4.

297. Evans PD, Fredhoi C, Loveday C, et al. The diurnal cortisol cycle and cognitive performance in the healthy old. *Int J Psychophysiol* 2011;79:371–7.

298. Greendale GA, Unger JB, Rowe JW, et al. The relation between cortisol excretion and fractures in healthy older people: Results from the MacArthur studies-Mac. *J Am Geriatr Soc* 1999;47:799–803.

299. Reynolds RM, Dennison EM, Walker BR, et al. Cortisol secretion and rate of bone loss in a population-based cohort of elderly men and women. *Calcif Tissue Int* 2005;77:134–8.

300. Hardy R, Cooper MS. Adrenal gland and bone. *Arch Biochem Biophys* 2010;503:137–45.

301. Purnell JQ, Brandon DD, Isabelle LM, et al. Association of 24-hour cortisol production rates, cortisol-binding globulin, and plasma-free cortisol levels with body composition, leptin levels, and aging in adult men and women. *J Clin Endocrinol Metab* 2004;89:281–7.

302. Feldman HA, Longcope C, Derby CA, et al. Age trends in the level of serum testosterone and other hormones in middle-aged men: Longitudinal results from the Massachusetts male aging study. *J Clin Endocrinol Metab* 2002;87:589–98.

303. Muniyappa R, Wong KA, Baldwin HL, et al. Dehydroepiandrosterone secretion in healthy older men and women: Effects of testosterone and growth

hormone administration in older men. *J Clin Endocrinol Metab* 2006;91:4445–52.
304. Tannenbaum C, Barrett-Connor E, Laughlin GA, et al. A longitudinal study of dehydroepiandrosterone sulphate (DHEAS) change in older men and women: The Rancho Bernardo Study. *Eur J Endocrinol* 2004;151:717–25.
305. Muehlenbein MP, Campbell BC, Richards RJ, et al. Dehydroepiandrosterone-sulfate as a biomarker of senescence in male non-human primates. *Exp Gerontol* 2003;38:1077–85.
306. Magri F, Cravello L, Barili L, et al. Stress and dementia: The role of the hypothalamicpituitary-adrenal axis. *Aging Clin Exp Res* 2006;18:167–70.
307. Genazzani AD, Lanzoni C, Genazzani AR. Might DHEA be considered a beneficial replacement therapy in the elderly? *Drugs Aging* 2007;24:173–85.
308. Sorwell KG, Urbanski HF. Dehydroepiandrosterone and age-related cognitive decline. *Age (Dordr)* 2010;32:61–7.
309. Yen SS, Laughlin GA. Aging and the adrenal cortex. *Exp Gerontol* 1998;33:897–910.
310. Ohlsson C, Labrie F, Barrett-Connor E, et al. Low serum levels of dehydroepiandrosterone sulfate predict all-cause and cardiovascular mortality in elderly Swedish men. *J Clin Endocrinol Metab* 2010;95:4406–14.
311. Ponholzer A, Madersbacher S, Rauchenwald M, et al. Vascular risk factors and their association to serum androgen levels in a population-based cohort of 75-year-old men over 5 years: Results of the VITA study. *World J Urol* 2010;28:209–14.
312. Shufelt C, Bretsky P, Almeida CM, et al. DHEA-S levels and cardiovascular disease mortality in postmenopausal women: Results from the National Institutes of Health—National Heart, Lung, and Blood Institute (NHLBI)-sponsored Women's Ischemia Syndrome Evaluation (WISE). *J Clin Endocrinol Metab* 2010;95: 4985–92.
313. Morales AJ, Nolan JJ, Nelson JC, et al. Effects of replacement dose of dehydroepiandrosterone in men and women of advancing age. *J Clin Endocrinol Metab* 1994;78:1360–7.
314. Jankowski CM, Gozansky WS, Van Pelt RE, et al. Oral dehydroepiandrosterone replacement in older adults: Effects on central adiposity, glucose metabolism and blood lipids. *Clin Endocrinol (Oxf)* 2011;75:456–63.
315. Boxer RS, Kleppinger A, Brindisi J, et al. Effects of dehydroepiandrosterone (DHEA) on cardiovascular risk factors in older women with frailty characteristics. *Age Ageing* 2010;39:451–8.
316. Davis SR, Panjari M, Stanczyk FZ. Clinical review: DHEA replacement for postmenopausal women. *J Clin Endocrinol Metab* 2011;96:1642–53.
317. Koutsari C, Ali AH, Nair KS, et al. Fatty acid metabolism in the elderly: Effects of dehydroepiandrosterone and testosterone replacement in hormonally deficient men and women. *J Clin Endocrinol Metab* 2009;94:3414–23.
318. Srinivasan M, Irving BA, Dhatariya K, et al. Effect of dehydroepiandrosterone replacement on lipoprotein profile in hypoadrenal women. *J Clin Endocrinol Metab* 2009;94:761–4.
319. Srinivasan M, Irving BA, Frye RL, et al. Effects on lipoprotein particles of long-term dehydroepiandrosterone in elderly men and women and testosterone in elderly men. *J Clin Endocrinol Metab* 2010;95:1617–25.
320. Baylis D, Bartlett DB, Syddall HE, et al. Immune-endocrine biomarkers as predictors of frailty and mortality: A 10-year longitudinal study in community-dwelling older people. *Age (Dordr)* 2013;35:963–71.
321. Voznesensky M, Walsh S, Dauser D, et al. The association between dehydroepiandosterone and frailty in older men and women. *Age Ageing* 2009;38:401–6.
322. Wolf OT, Neumann O, Hellhammer DH, et al. Effects of a two-week physiological dehydroepiandrosterone substitution on cognitive performance and well-being in healthy elderly women and men. *J Clin Endocrinol Metab* 1997;82:2363–7.
323. Arlt W, Callies F, Koehler I, et al. Dehydroepiandrosterone supplementation in healthy men with an age-related decline of dehydroepiandrosterone secretion. *J Clin Endocrinol Metab* 2001;86:4686–92.
324. Muller M, van den Beld AW, van der Schouw YT, et al. Effects of dehydroepiandrosterone and atamestane supplementation on frailty in elderly men. *J Clin Endocrinol Metab* 2006;91:3988–91.
325. Baulieu EE, Thomas G, Legrain S, et al. Dehydroepiandrosterone (DHEA), DHEA sulfate, and aging: Contribution of the DHEAge Study to a sociobiomedical issue. *Proc Natl Acad Sci U S A* 2000;97:4279–84.
326. von Muhlen D, Laughlin GA, Kritz-Silverstein D, et al. Effect of dehydroepiandrosterone supplementation on bone mineral density, bone markers, and body composition in older adults: The DAWN trial. *Osteoporos Int* 2008;19:699–707.
327. Bhagra S, Nippoldt TB, Nair KS. Dehydroepiandrosterone in adrenal insufficiency and ageing. *Curr Opin Endocrinol Diabetes Obes* 2008;15:239–43.
328. Flynn RW, Macdonald TM, Jung RT, et al. Mortality and vascular outcomes in patients treated for thyroid dysfunction. *J Clin Endocrinol Metab* 2006;91:2159–64.
329. Basaria S, Coviello AD, Travison TG, et al. Adverse events associated with testosterone administration. *N Engl J Med* 2010;363:109–22.

# 24

# Endocrine emergencies

*Simon Aylwin, Ben Whitelaw*

Urgent and emergency presentations of endocrine disorders are relatively uncommon, but they carry a significant mortality, especially if unrecognized. The endocrinologist may solely be responsible for the care of the patient or may be contacted to interpret a complex multisystem presentation, to verify a diagnosis, and to guide management. This chapter covers a range of endocrine emergencies and is divided into five sections: (1) pituitary emergencies, (2) adrenal emergencies, (3) thyroid emergencies, (4) salt and mineral emergencies, and (5) neuroendocrine emergencies. The related topic of diabetes emergencies is not discussed.

## *Pituitary emergencies (see Chapter 1)*

### *Pituitary apoplexy*

Pituitary apoplexy is a rare emergency that occurs due to hemorrhage and/or infarction of the pituitary.[1] It almost always occurs in the context of a preexisting pituitary tumor, but in up to 80% of cases the tumor is not identified before the apoplexy (Figure 24.1).[2] Occasionally, pituitary apoplexy occurs on a background of a normal pituitary gland, classically in the case of acute severe postpartum hemorrhage (Sheehan's syndrome).

A separate condition of subclinical, asymptomatic pituitary hemorrhage is recognized. This condition is normally identified on routine imaging or histopathology and is not normally considered to be part of the clinical presentation of pituitary apoplexy.[1]

About 80% of patients with acute apoplexy will have deficiency of one or more anterior pituitary hormones at presentation.[3] Adrenocorticotropic hormone (ACTH) deficiency leading to secondary hypocortisolemia is the most clinically significant hormone deficiency and is a major source of mortality in this condition.[1] Secondary hypothyroidism affects about 50% of cases.[4] Diabetes insipidus (DI) is a rare consequence, affecting only about 2% overall.[4]

Clinically, the presentation is characterized by sudden onset severe headache that is normally retro-orbital, together with vomiting. Ocular palsy, most commonly third cranial nerve palsy, occurs in about 70% of cases due to compression effects in the cavernous sinus.[5] Acute onset of visual field defects and reduced visual acuity is a common feature. Extravasation of blood to the subarachnoid space can cause meningism and photophobia. The clinical presentation can be acute or subacute. Risk factors for the precipitation of apoplexy include hypertension; anticoagulation, cardiac bypass, trauma, surgery, and pituitary function testing.

#### *Diagnosis and assessment*

The diagnosis should be considered in patients who present with a severe headache, with or without neuro-ophthalmological signs. Apoplexy can mimic subarachnoid hemorrhage, meningitis, and stroke. Computed tomography (CT) scan is often the initial imaging modality used, and this scan will identify abnormalities in 80% of cases but is diagnostic in only

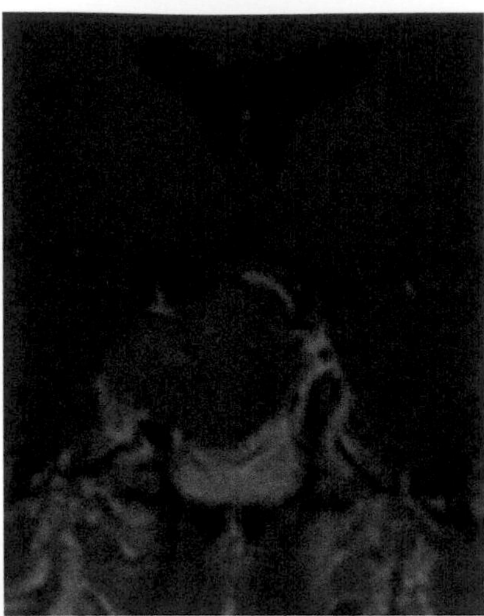

***Figure 24.1***
*Apoplexy.*

| *Pituitary apoplexy score (PAS)* | *Points* |
|---|---|
| **Level of consciousness** | |
| Glasgow coma scale 15 | 0 |
| Glasgow coma scale 8–14 | 2 |
| Glasgow coma scale <8 | 4 |
| **Visual acuity** | |
| Normal 6/6 | 0 |
| Reduced—unilateral | 1 |
| Reduced—bilateral | 2 |
| **Visual field defects** | |
| Normal | 0 |
| Unilateral defect | 1 |
| Bilateral defect | 2 |
| **Ocular palsy** | |
| Absent | 0 |
| Present—unilateral | 1 |
| Present—bilateral | 2 |

*Source:* Rajasekaran S et al., *Clinical Endocrinology*, 74, 9–20, 2011.

***Table 24.1***
*Pituitary apoplexy score (PAS).*

about 20%–30% of cases.[2] Magnetic resonance imaging (MRI) pituitary scan will therefore be required in most cases. Cerebrospinal fluid (CSF) analysis, if performed, may show polymorphs or lymphocytes but is sterile on culture.[6]

Clinical and biochemical assessment of endocrine status must be performed.[1] Because apoplexy normally occurs in the context of a preexisting but unidentified tumor, assessment must include considering whether the tumor was functioning or nonfunctioning. Apoplexy in functioning tumors will often reduce or abolish the excess autonomous hormone secretion. Evaluation will include clinical and biochemical assessment for deficiency of anterior or posterior pituitary function. Assessment of visual acuity, eye movements, and visual fields is essential. Visual fields should be formally assessed, by Goldmann perimetry, as soon as practically possible.

The U.K. apoplexy guidelines[1] propose that four aspects of the presentation are scored giving rise to pituitary apoplexy score (PAS) of 0–10 (Table 24.1).[1] The four areas assessed are level of consciousness, visual acuity, visual fields, and ocular palsy. Higher scores favor earlier surgical intervention.[7]

## Management

### Hormone replacement

In some circumstances, patients are relatively stable, allowing assessment of baseline cortisol status. Otherwise, the initial treatment is with hydrocortisone 100–200 mg i.v. bolus. Followed by 50–100 mg q.d.s. intramuscular hydrocortisone, or a hydrocortisone infusion of 2–4 mg/h. Intermittent intravenous injections of hydrocortisone are less appropriate because much of the hydrocortisone will be rapidly cleared from the circulation. Once the patient is clinically stable, the dose of hydrocortisone should quickly be reduced to 20–30 mg/day in two to three divided doses.

### Surgery

In cases where there is reduced level of consciousness and/or significant visual field deficit, it is widely agreed that neurosurgical decompression is appropriate. This is reflected in such patients having a high PAS.[7] In other cases, the role and timing of neurosurgical intervention are controversial. Some authorities report that, in general, early neurosurgical decompression gives better visual and endocrine outcome[8,9]; other studies suggest there is no difference in outcome.[10]

Management must be by a combined endocrine–neurosurgical team with access to specialist endocrinology and ophthalmological expertise.

**Apoplexy case study**

A 50-year-old man presented with sudden onset severe frontal headache associated with right-sided ptosis complete right ophthalmoplegia. He also reported a 9-month history of weight loss, vomiting, cold intolerance, poor concentration, and loss of libido. The MRI scan shows a sella mass with right parasellar extension into the cavernous sinus.

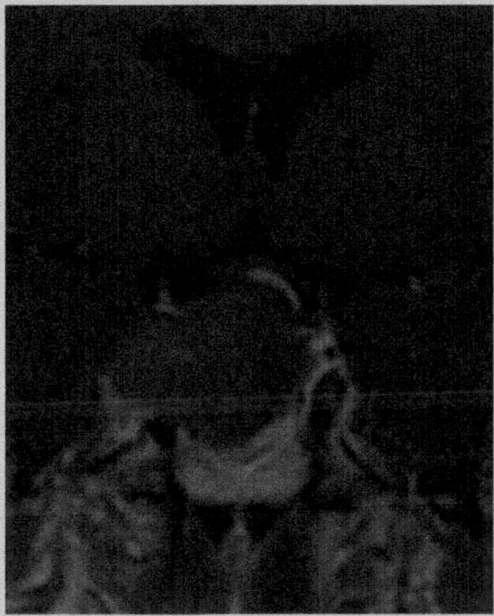

The presentation is typical of pituitary apoplexy in the context of undiagnosed nonfunctioning pituitary adenoma. Hydrocortisone replacement treatment was given and urgent endoscopic transsphenoidal surgery was performed. Postoperatively, the ptosis and ophthalmoplegia resolved completely by 3 months.

## Rapid pituitary tumor growth/ mass effect/impending visual loss

The majority of pituitary tumors are benign and slow growing, with a small proportion exhibiting more aggressive behavior. Tumors may present with mass effect or may demonstrate mass effect as part of tumor progression or recurrence. The most common symptom is a visual field loss due to pressure on the optic chiasm or other parts of the optic tracts or nerves. Invasion of the cavernous sinus is also seen in aggressive tumors, leading to both pain and cranial nerve palsies. Symptoms from hydrocephalus or brain stem compression may be seen in severe cases (Figure 24.2).

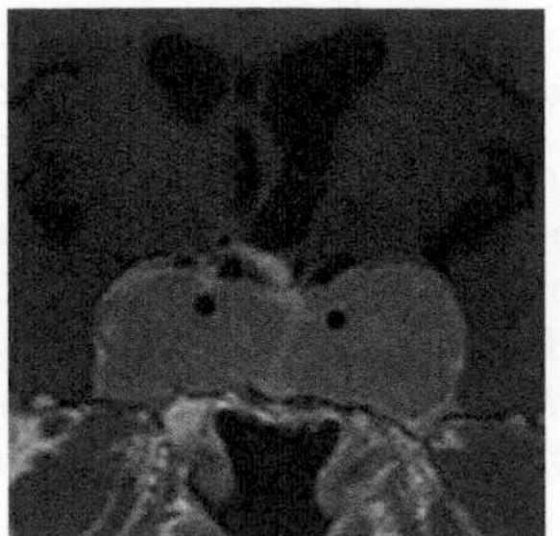

***Figure 24.2***
*Aggressive pituitary tumor.*

### *Diagnosis and assessment*

This presentation is an indication for urgent intervention to achieve tumor control and to maximize the possibility of reversing neurological damage. Urgent measurement of serum prolactin is mandatory to evaluate the possibility of the tumor being a prolactinoma and therefore amenable to shrinkage with dopamine agonist therapy. A baseline of assessment of neurological status together with a clinical and biochemical assessment endocrine function should be performed if possible so that subsequent interventions can be evaluated.

### *Management*

Assuming the lesion is not thought to be a prolactinoma, surgical decompression is the first-line intervention if possible. Surgery will be the quickest method of obtaining tumor decompression and will also provide tumor histology, as this is not already available.

If surgery is not possible, then other modalities singularly or in combination, should be considered. Radiotherapy (fractionated or single fraction) may be used in this situation, but its use may be limited by proximity of the optic nerves or chiasm.

About 70% of pituitary tumors will show tumor shrinkage with the use of temozolomide chemotherapy. This treatment is normally characterized as a salvage therapy, for use when all conventional therapies have failed,[11] but in selected cases it may be appropriate to use temozolomide earlier in the treatment algorithm.[12] There is evidence that temozolomide is most effective in tumors that are depleted of the enzyme $O^6$-methylguanine-DNA methyltransferase (MGMT).

**Tumor mass effect case study**

A 34-year-old man who had previously had surgery and radiotherapy for a resistant prolactinoma presented with worsening headaches and bitemporal visual field loss. Over the next few weeks, he developed blindness in the left eye, painful proptosis, and bilateral cranial nerve VI palsies. MRI showed a 6-cm tumor recurrence with extension into both orbits.

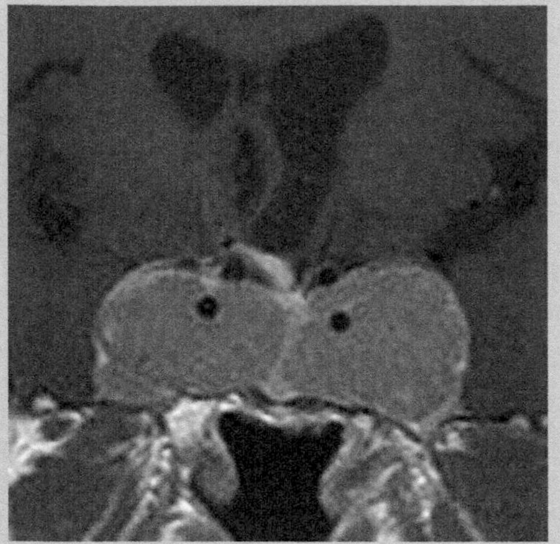

Craniotomy and tumor decompression were unsuccessful. The patient was commenced on temozolomide chemotherapy leading to a dramatic clinical improvement and radiological tumor regression.

# Acute severe Cushing's syndrome

Cushing's syndrome can arise from ACTH or non–ACTH-based pathology. The clinical presentation is a spectrum from mild, subtle, and chronic features to an acute, severe phenotype. In its most severe form, Cushing's syndrome can manifest with severe psychiatric symptoms, including psychosis. Other severe features can include proximal myopathy, accelerated hypertension, resistant hypokalemia, and cardiomyopathy.[13] These patients are significantly immunosuppressed and are at risk of atypical infections such as tuberculosis and *Pneumocystis carinii* pneumonia (PCP). Cushing's syndrome has a significant mortality, estimated as four times that of age-matched controls, and the urgency for treatment is especially high in those cases presenting with severe features.[14]

### *Management*

After the initial investigations have confirmed the diagnosis, life-saving disease control measures will be required, often before the more definitive treatment, such as transsphenoidal surgery or adrenalectomy. Regardless of the underlying cause, the control of acute severe Cushing's can potentially be obtained by either medical treatment or bilateral adrenalectomy.

The commonest regimen for medical blockade is metyrapone, ketoconazole, or both. Metyrapone blocks 11β-hydroxylase, the final step of cortisol synthesis. The usual dose required for blockade is 2–4 g in three or four divided doses. The dose is titrated to achieve a serum cortisol level of 150–300 mmol/L on a day curve. Ketoconazole blocks adrenal cortisol synthesis at multiple points and is normally used at a dose of 200–400 mg three times daily. Etomidate is an intravenous anesthetic agent that can be used for control of severe hypercortisolemia, especially in an intensive care environment. An infusion of 1.2–2.5 mg/h will normally block cortisol synthesis without precipitating general anesthesia. These agents may be used as a "block & replace" regime with glucocorticoids added back in the form of hydrocortisone or dexamethasone.

Mitotane is an adrenolytic drug that also blocks cortisol synthesis. It has an established role in the treatment of adrenocortical cancer.[15] It has a slow onset of action that limits its use in emergency blockade. However, combination use of mitotane with metyrapone and ketoconazole has recently been show to give good results.[16]

Mifepristone is a glucocorticoid receptor antagonist that can be used to block the effects of acute severe Cushing's syndrome. There are reports of it being used effectively when other agents have failed.[17] In Cushing's syndrome, the hypercortisolemia can overwhelm the protective effects of the enzyme 11β-hydroxysteroid dehydrogenase type 2. This leads to mineralocorticoid effects such as severe hypokalemia. Because mifepristone blocks only the glucocorticoid receptor, the mineralocorticoid pathology remains untreated and hypokalemia remains a significant problem with mifepristone treatment.

Bilateral adrenalectomy may be needed to achieve rapid control of severe Cushing's syndrome. This can be done after a period of medical blockade if needed. Postoperatively, the patient will require permanent glucocorticoid and mineralocorticoid replacement.

**Severe Cushing's case study**

A 42-year-old lady presented with progressive proximal muscle weakness, weight gain, and changes in facial appearance over several weeks. On examination, she was profoundly Cushingoid with severe proximal muscle weakness. Investigations showed serum cortisol levels >2000 nmol/L unresponsive to dexamethasone. Serum ACTH levels were 500 pmol/L. Imaging showed a normal pituitary gland and multiple metastatic liver deposits consistent with a neuroendocrine tumor. The patient was commenced on medical blockade therapy with metyrapone and ketoconazole and then proceeded to have bilateral adrenalectomy for control of the cortisol excess.

**Severe hypokalemia in Cushing's syndrome**

A serum potassium of <2.5 mmol/L is regarded as potentially severe. Symptoms include muscle weakness and paralysis, hypotonia, arrhythmias, cramp, and tetany. The electrocardiogram (ECG) may show reduced amplitude T waves and prominent U waves. Hypokalemia in Cushing's syndrome is normally caused by high levels of cortisol saturating the protective effects of 11β-hydroxysteroid dehydrogenase enzyme, allowing cortisol to exert a mineralocorticoid effect.

**Treatment**

Intravenous potassium chloride treatment should be given. The recommended infusion rate is to not exceed 10 mmol/h. Central venous access should be obtained for this because concentrated potassium solutions can cause pain and phlebitis in peripheral veins. In emergency situations, potassium has been given at rates of up to 40 mmol/h.[18] Patients with abnormal ECG due to hypokalemla should have continuous cardiac monitoring during treatment until the abnormalities resolve.

Specific treatments for mineralocorticoid hypokalemia would include mineralocorticoid antagonists such as spironolactone and eplerenone. Severe Cushing's syndrome leading to hypokalemia can be treated, in part, by blocking cortisol synthesis using ketoconazole, metyrapone, or both as described above.

## *Diabetes insipidus (see Chapter 5)*

Hypothalamic DI is a condition characterized by the inappropriate and excess production of dilute urine, due to deficiency of vasopressin. The causes of hypothalamic DI are listed in Table 24.2 along with causes of nephrogenic DI.

### *Diagnosis and assessment*

DI is not normally an endocrine emergency (Figure 24.3). If the patient is alert, has an intact thirst mechanism, and has unrestricted access to fluid, then the situation is not dangerous. When one of these elements is absent, the need to identify the clinical situation and manage it become urgent.

In the acute situation, the diagnosis of uncontrolled DI is based on identifying inappropriately dilute polyuria. For these purposes, polyuria is defined as passing >200 mL/h for two consecutive hours, in a catheterized patient or >800 mL in 4 h for a noncatheterized patient. When this occurs, blood and urine samples should be sent simultaneously for urgent assessment of osmolality. Elevated plasma osmolality (>295 mOsm/kg) with inappropriately low urine osmolality (<600 mOsm/kg) is diagnostic of DI. The exact values used for diagnostic cut off vary.[19–21]

### *Management*

A patient with known or suspected DI is at risk of severe dehydration and hypernatremia if they are kept nil by mouth or if they have a reduced level of consciousness for any reason. In these circumstances, the maintenance of a fluid balance chart is essential to identify if a patient is developing a significant negative fluid balance. Patients who are nil by mouth should have intravenous fluid prescribed. The rate of infusion should be adjusted to maintain a neutral fluid balance. One method is to administer each hour the amount of fluid lost in urine the previous hour.

In addition to maintaining fluid balance, treatment of DI using desmopressin will terminate polyuria. In an inpatient setting, the dose used is normally 0.5–1 μg by subcutaneous injection every 12–24 h. Fluid balance and electrolytes should be regularly reevaluated to avoid over or undertreatment with desmopressin.

| Causes of hypothalamic DI | Causes of nephrogenic DI |
|---|---|
| Inflammatory conditions | Hypercalcemia |
| Lymphocytic hypophysitis, sarcoidosis, Langerhans' cell histiocytosis, tuberculosis | Hypokalemia |
| Trauma and neurosurgery | Hyperglycemia |
| Vascular infarction or sickle cell | Drugs, e.g., lithium, demecolcine |
| Infection—meningitis, encephalitis | Vascular |
| Tumor, e.g., craniopharyngioma, pituitary metastasis | Chronic kidney disease |
| Hypothalamic disease | Genetic/Familial syndromes |
| Genetic—vasopressin gene mutation (AD) DIDMOAD | Postobstructive uropathy |
| DIDMOAD is a genetic cause so should follow on from the line above | |
| Idiopathic | |

AD, autosomal dominant; DIDMOAD, Diabetes insipidus, diabetes mellitus, optic atrophy, and deafness.

***Table 24.2***
*Causes of hypothalamic DI and nephrogenic DI.*

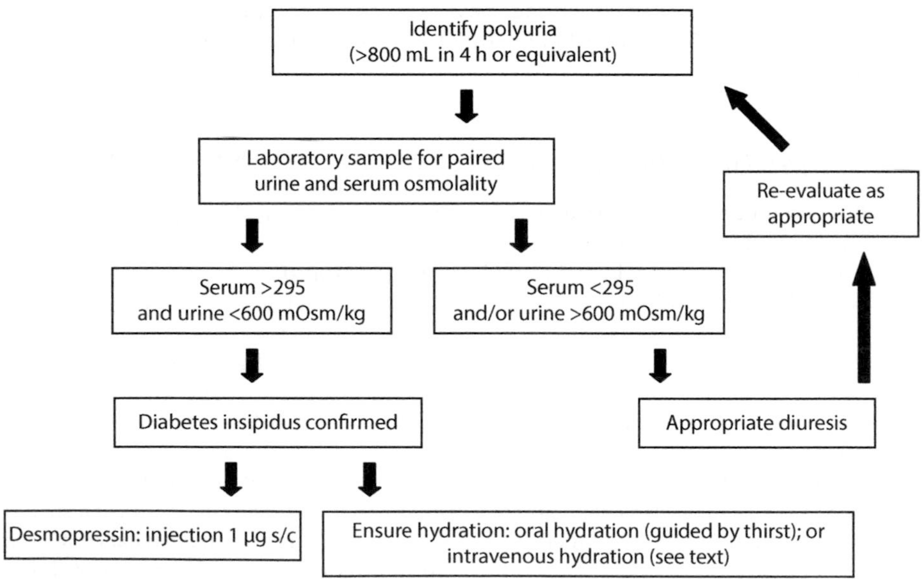


***Figure 24.3***
*Algorithm for inpatient assessment of suspected. Desmopressin.*

**DI case study**

A 35-year-old man with known DI, normally managed with oral desmopressin, was admitted after a road traffic accident. He was taken for urgent surgery to his right leg. He is kept nil by mouth preoperatively, and postoperatively he is drowsy. The orthopedic team gives him intravenous fluid (1 L of 0.9% saline over 8 h). The following day he is very drowsy and confused, blood tests show hypernatremia, and the patient's fluid chart suggests he may have passed 8 L of urine.

Serum sodium 158 mmol/L
Serum osmolality 332 mOsm/kg
Urine osmolality 85 mOsm/kg

This case demonstrates the potentially severe consequences of untreated DI in circumstances where the patient does not have free access to fluids. The management at this point is to give desmopressin 1 μg s.c. and to give Intravenous fluids with monitoring in a high-dependency environment.

# Adrenal emergencies

## Pheochromocytoma crisis[5]

Pheochromocytomas and paragangliomas are chromaffin-derived tumors of the adrenal medulla or the extra-adrenal autonomic nervous system, respectively. They may be functioning, meaning that they secrete adrenaline, noradrenaline, dopamine, or a combination, or they may be nonfunctioning.[22] Pheochromocytomas can present in a variety of ways. The patient may present with symptoms either continuously or paroxysmal. It is becoming increasingly common for pheochromocytoma to be first identified from abdominal imaging done for another purpose. In such cases, retrospective history-taking may identify symptoms attributable to catecholamine excess.[23]

Pheochromocytoma crisis is a rare, life-threatening emergency. The most severe form of presentation is pheochromocytoma multisystem crisis. It is characterized by multiorgan failure, hyperpyrexia, encephalopathy, and hypertension or hypotension.[24] The presentation can mimic sepsis, leading to a delay in diagnosis. The term "adrenergic apoplexy" has been used to describe this presentation. Other manifestations of the pheochromocytoma crisis include cardiovascular and respiratory compromise, such as hypertensive crisis, shock, arrhythmias, acute myocardial infarction, pulmonary edema, and myopathy.[25]

Catecholamine cardiomyopathy is rare but well recognized. The classic presentation is symptoms and signs consistent with myocardial infarction but no evidence of coronary artery stenosis. Echocardiogram demonstrates transient left ventricular apical ballooning. The condition has been called takotsubo cardiomyopathy because it is said that the shape of the heart resembles a Japanese octopus fishing pot called a takotsubo. Inverted takotsubo cardiomyopathy has also been described with basal and midventricular hypokinesia and sparing of the apex.[26,27]

The pathological process underlying all the aspects of the crisis is acute excess catecholamines. In most cases, the precipitant cause is unclear. Potential precipitating factors include surgery and anesthesia some studies have suggested a relation to administration of glucagon[28] and glucocorticoids.[29–31]

### *Diagnosis and assessment*

The diagnosis should be considered in patients with acute unexplained left ventricular failure, lactic acidosis, multisystem failure, or hypertensive crisis. Urine and plasma samples should be obtained for assessment of catecholamines and metabolites (metanephrines). It should be recognized that in the context of acute illness there is no established normal range.

Imaging should be obtained to confirm or exclude the presence of an adrenal or extra-adrenal mass. It should be recognized that incidental adrenal nodules are common, found on approximately *2%–4%* of CT scans, so clinicians should be cautious about overinterpreting the finding of a nodule.[32] Extra-adrenal pheochromocytomas (functioning paragangliomas) can be the source of a catecholamine crisis, and these can be found in a variety of locations; most commonly they are in a paraspinal location arising from the sympathetic chain, but also can be retroperitoneal, mediastinal, cervical, and pelvic.[25]

### *Management*

Supportive management is required, normally in an intensive care environment. Presentations with severe cardiac failure may be complicated by cardiac arrest and may require mechanical treatment of severe left ventricular failure, such as intra-aortic balloon pump therapy[33] or extracorporeal membrane oxygenation therapy.[34,35]

Patients with pheochromocytoma crisis are often significantly hypovolemic, and expansion of the circulating volume, with intravenous fluids, will be required, concurrent with or before commencement of α blockade, to prevent severe hypotension.[36]

Once the diagnosis is suspected, α blockade should be initiated. Phenoxybenzamine, a noncompetitive α-blocker, is the preferred drug. This drug can be given enterally, normally by nasogastric tube, or intravenously. The enteral starting dose is 10 mg three times daily, normally increasing to 60–80 mg/day in three to four divided doses.[33,37] Entral doses up to 250 mg/day have been required.[38] In the context of a crisis, intravenous phenoxybenzamine is given at a dose of 1–2 mg/kg.[39]

Phentolamine is an alternative α-blocker, but it is a short acting and thus less useful to establish stable blockade. It can be used intravenously at a dose of 1 mg/min to correct severe hypertensive crisis due to pheochromocytoma. An infusion of 20–100 mg in 500 mL of dextrose can be used for maintenance. Doxazosin is a competitive α-antagonist and is therefore not a preferred choice because high levels of adrenaline and noradrenaline would overcome the antagonist effect.

In addition to α blockade, intravenous magnesium has been shown to improve hemodynamic status in acute pheochromocytoma crisis.[40] The dose used is 4 g as an intravenous bolus followed by an infusion of 1 g/h.

After adequate α blockade has been established, β-blockers can subsequently be used to control reflex tachycardia or tachyarrhythmia. β-Blockers must not be used before α blockade because the unopposed α adrenergic activity can exacerbated a hypertensive crisis. The combined α- and β-blocker labetalol is not recommended as a single agent because its β-blocker activity exceeds the α activity that can exacerbate hypertensive crisis.[41]

Surgical removal of the pheochromocytoma is the definitive treatment, and this surgery should be arranged urgently once α and β blockade are established.

If surgical cure is not possible, for example, in unresectable or metastatic disease, the most established systemic treatment is MIBG radionucleotide therapy. Alternative targeted therapies such as the multikinase inhibitor sunitinib have also been used.[42]

**_Pheochromocytoma case study_**

A 50-year-old lady presented with collapse and breathlessness. She was found to have severe hypertension, severe left ventricular failure, and acute renal failure. Serum troponin I was elevated (>50 μg/L). She was admitted to intensive care and given supportive management for presumed acute coronary syndrome. Coronary angiogram was normal and further imaging demonstrated left suprarenal mass. The patient reported an 8-year history of palpitations, sweating, acute episodes of pallor, and resistant hypertension.

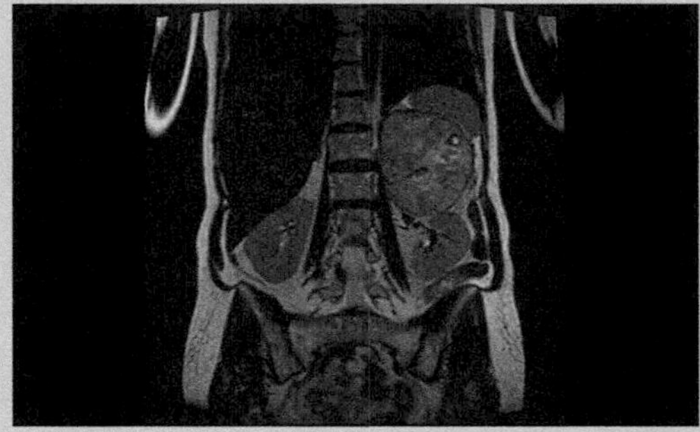

Biochemistry confirmed the diagnosis of pheochromocytoma that was treated surgically after preoperative α and β blockade.

## *Addisonian crisis/acute adrenal insufficiency (see Chapters 13, 20)*

Acute adrenal crisis is a potentially life-threatening complication of adrenal insufficiency.

It most frequently affects patients known to have chronic adrenal insufficiency in the context of a precipitating event such as intercurrent illness. Alternatively, it may be the first presentation of previously undiagnosed adrenal insufficiency.

Adrenal insufficiency may be primary or secondary. The causes of primary adrenal insufficiency include autoimmune adrenalitis, infiltration, infection (particularly tuberculosis), adrenal hemorrhage, and infarction. Secondary causes are due to hypothalamic–pituitary pathology, leading to ACTH deficiency, and consequent glucocorticoid deficiency. In secondary adrenal insufficiency, mineralocorticoid activity is preserved because it is under the control of the renin angiotensin system, rather than ACTH. The prolonged use of exogenous steroids, including inhaled steroids,[43] is a common cause of suppression of the hypothalamic–pituitary–adrenal (HPA) axis and secondary adrenal insufficiency.

The acute presentation is highly variable. Hypotension, shock, and circulatory failure are the classic symptoms in a patient with combined glucocorticoid and mineralocorticoid deficiency.[44] There are many other symptoms that may be present and may precede the crisis, including headache, nausea, vomiting, abdominal pain, weakness, lethargy, and confusion. There are reports of atypical presentations such as cerebral edema[45] and suspected myocardial infarction.[46]

The incidence of adrenal crisis in patients with known adrenal insufficiency is 3%–5% per annum. This incidence is confirmed by a survey of 444 patients with known adrenal insufficiency that reported that 42% had experienced at least one episode of adrenal crisis.[47] The patients in the survey had adrenal insufficiency for a median of 10 years, and a crisis was defined as acute illness requiring hospital admission and intravenous hydrocortisone.

## *Diagnosis and assessment*

Clinical features are often nonspecific and may be atypical. The most important aspect of making the diagnosis is to consider the condition at all. The diagnosis will clearly be easier to suspect in patients with known preexisting pituitary or adrenal pathology. The initial available investigations may demonstrate hyponatremia and hyperkalemia, in primary adrenal failure, that will increase the degree of suspicion.

Other groups of patients who should be considered at risk include patients known to have a personal or family history of autoimmune disorders. Infectious diseases known to cause adrenalitis, such as tuberculosis, cytomegalovirus, and human immunodeficiency virus (HIV), are a risk factor. Medications that either reduce cortisol synthesis, such as ketoconazole, or increase cortisol metabolism, such as rifampicin or phenytoin, also give increased risk of crisis.

Investigation, in the context of acute hypotension and circulatory compromise, needs to be brief, because of the requirement to proceed with treatment. A serum sample should be obtained to measure cortisol. If possible, baseline samples for ACTH, renin, and aldosterone should also be obtained, recognizing that these samples have more stringent requirements for collection and need to be transferred to the laboratory urgently. If the patient is stable, an ACTH stimulation (Synacthen) test can be performed. Often, it is necessary to commence glucocorticoid replacement urgently, in which case it can either be subsequently interrupted or the ACTH stimulation test can be conducted on dexamethasone. Acute adrenal insufficiency is unlikely if either the basal or the 30-min stimulated cortisol samples are >550 nmol/L.[48,49]

|  | *Primary hypoadrenalism* | *Secondary hypoadrenalism* |
|---|---|---|
| Sodium | ↓↓ | ↓ |
| Potassium | ↑ | ↔ |
| pH | ↓ | ↔ |
| Renin | ↑ | ↔ |
| Aldosterone | ↓ | ↔ |
| ACTH | ↑ | ↓ |

***Table 24.3***
***Primary hypoadrenalism as distinguished from secondary hypoadrenalism.***

If hypocortisolemia is identified, primary adrenal disease may be distinguished on the basis of elevated ACTH, low aldosterone, and high renin. Secondary adrenal insufficiency is associated with low ACTH (Table 24.3).

The presentation and investigations may demonstrate associated hypoglycemia and hypercalcemia. Thyroid function may be abnormal for a variety of reasons. Elevated TSH with low free levothyroxine (fT4) is known to occur in untreated hypoadrenalism in the absence of any separate thyroid disorder. The TSH is normally only slightly elevated to <10 U/L and normalizes once the hypoadrenalism has been treated.[50] In addition, primary autoimmune hypothyroidism is associated with autoimmune adrenalitis; and in hypopituitarism, secondary thyroid and adrenal deficiency are often observed together.

## *Management*

### *General measures*

Fluid and electrolyte replacement can begin as soon as there is a clinical need and/or a suspicion of adrenal insufficiency.[50] Normally, treatment would be with intravenous 0.9% saline, guided by clinical assessment of circulatory status. Hypoglycemia should be treated with 10% or 20% glucose infusion (see section: Neuroendocrine emergencies "Severe hypoglycemia").

Precipitating conditions such as infection should be treated after appropriate investigation and cultures have been taken.

*Specific measures*
Hydrocortisone is given intravenously or intramuscular at a dose of 100–200 mg initially. The maintenance dose is normally 100 mg intramuscular four times per day while the patient is acutely unwell, or a hydrocortisone infusion of 2–4 mg/h.[44] Intermittent intravenous injections of hydrocortisone are sometimes used but are in principle less appropriate because much of the hydrocortisone will be rapidly cleared from the circulation. Separate mineralocorticoid replacement is not required while high doses of hydrocortisone are being administered, because the high-dose hydrocortisone has adequate mineralocorticoid activity.

Once the patient is clinically stable, the hydrocortisone can be administered orally, and the dose can quickly be reduced to 20–30 mg/day, in two to three divided doses. A standard regime would be 10 mg on first waking, followed by 5 mg at noon and 5 mg at 4 p.m. Patients who have primary adrenal deficiency will also need fludrocortisone therapy at a dose 50–200 μg, guided by blood pressure, electrolytes, and plasma renin.

# Massive adrenal tumor (see Chapter 10)

Small adrenal nodules are relatively common and radiological series suggest a 5% prevalence, with the overwhelming majority being nonfunctioning adenoma.[51] Adrenal lesions that are massive (>10 cm in size) are more likely to be adrenocortical carcinoma (ACC).[52] Adrenocortical carcinoma may present with the endocrine effects of the tumor, such as features of Cushing's or virilization. In the majority, the tumor is hormone silent, in which case it may be detected incidentally or because of mass effect. A suspected ACC requires urgent preoperative clinical and biochemical endocrine assessment to enable appropriate staging, identification of preoperative tumor markers, and appropriate perioperative hormone management. Interestingly, although up to 50% of ACCs are said to be clinically silent, it has been shown that the urinary steroid profile of these patients has a very high sensitivity for distinguishing an ACC from a nonadrenal tumor.[53]

### Management
Although usually stable, patients with large adrenal masses frequently present with abdominal pain and may require urgent investigation in the hospital. Further management normally includes complete resection of the primary tumor and then the use of adjuvant mitotane chemotherapy.[54]

**Massive adrenal tumor case study**

A 25-year-old man presented with left-sided abdominal pain. Found to have a palpable left upper quadrant mass. CT scan showed a 20-cm left adrenal tumor consistent with ACC, confirmed with preoperative urine and serum biochemical assessment. Staging was completed with axial imaging and fluorodeoxyglucose-positron emission tomography (FDG PET), demonstrating two lung metastases.

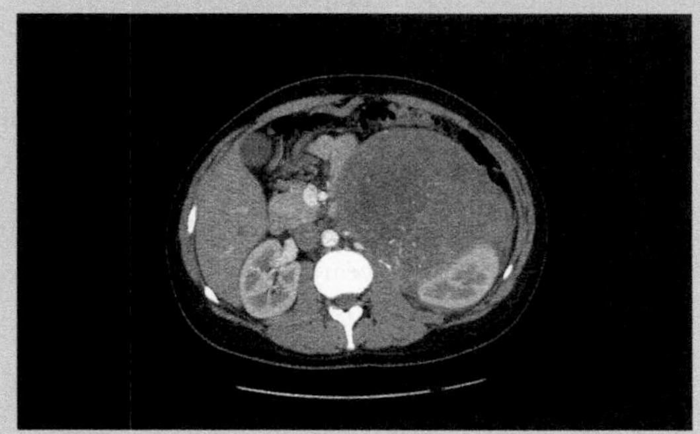

The primary tumor was surgically resected. Subsequently, the two pulmonary metastases were surgically resected in a planned second-stage procedure. The patient was commenced on adjuvant therapy with mitotane and remains well 4 years later, with no evidence of recurrence.

# Thyroid emergencies (see Chapter 13, 14)

## Thyroid storm

Thyroid storm, also known as accelerated hyperthyroidism, is an acute presentation of severe hyperthyroidism. It is now exceptionally uncommon. The mortality is reported as 20%–50%,[55] but there are no data from the modern era. Presentation may be precipitated by surgery, infection, or trauma.

### Diagnosis and assessment
The diagnosis is based on the clinical features. Patients are likely to have tachycardia, pyrexia, delirium, or agitation.

Congestive cardiac failure, hypotension, and cardiovascular collapse can occur. Abdominal pain, vomiting, and diarrhea may be present.

Thyroid storm is the most severe end of a spectrum of hyperthyroidism, but there are no clear or universally accepted criteria to distinguish it from severe hyperthyroidism. A scoring system was proposed in 1993 by Burch and Wartofsky to clarify the diagnostic criteria[55] (Table 24.4).[56] The scoring system evaluates seven different symptoms or physiological parameters (fever, tachycardia, cognitive effects, cardiac failure, atrial fibrillation, gastrointestinal (GI) symptoms, and precipitating factors). The maximum score is 140. A score of more than 45 is highly suggestive of thyroid storm; conversely, a score of less than 25 makes thyroid storm unlikely.

Thyroid function tests will demonstrate primary hyperthyroidism. The levels of T3 and T4 are not significantly higher in patients with thyroid storm compared with patients with uncomplicated hyperthyroidism. The reasons why some experience more severe clinical features are unknown but is thought to be related to enhanced susceptibility to the effects of thyroid hormone, adrenergic effects, or both. Other investigations will be aimed at assessing the severity of the presentation, including chest x-ray and ECG; or identifying an underlying cause, including at technetium thyroid uptake scan, thyroid peroxidase (TPO), and TSH receptor antibodies.

*Burch–Wartofsky score[13]*

| *Criteria* | *Points* | *Criteria* | *Points* |
|---|---|---|---|
| **Fever** | | **Tachycardia** | |
| 37.2–37.7 | 5 | 99–109 | 5 |
| 37.7–38.3 | 10 | 110–119 | 10 |
| 38.3–38.9 | 15 | 120–129 | 15 |
| 38.9–39.4 | 20 | 130–139 | 20 |
| 39.4–40 | 25 | >140 | 25 |
| >40 | 30 | | |
| **Central nervous system (CNS) effects** | | **Congestive cardiac failure** | |
| Absent | 0 | Absent | 0 |
| Mild (agitation) | 10 | Mild (peripheral edema) | 5 |
| Moderate (delirium, psychosis, extreme lethargy) | 20 | Moderate (bibasal crepitations) | 10 |
| | | Severe (pulmonary edema) | 15 |
| Severe (seizures, coma) | 30 | **Atrial fibrillation** | |
| **GI disturbance** | | Absent | 0 |
| Absent | 0 | Present | 10 |
| Moderate (diarrhea, nausea, vomiting, abdominal pain) | 10 | | |
| Severe (unexplained jaundice) | 20 | | |
| **Precipitating event** | | | |
| Absent | 0 | | |
| Present | 10 | | |

*Source:* Sarlis NJ, Gourgiotis L, *Reviews in Endocrine & Metabolic Disorder,* 4, 129–36, 2003.
*Note:* Overall score is obtained by adding the scores from each of the seven criteria (range, 0–140); Score >45—highly suggestive of thyroid storm; score 25–45—suggests impending storm; score <25—unlikely thyroid storm.

***Table 24.4***
*Burch–Wartofsky scoring system for thyroid storm as distinguished from severe hyperthyroidism.*

### Management

Treatment is aimed at stabilizing and supporting the patient and rapidly reducing the levels of active circulating thyroid hormones. Supportive treatment includes monitoring and management of ventilatory and circulatory state in an intensive care environment. Sedation with benzodiazepines may be needed to treat agitation. Active cooling and paracetamol are first-line treatments for pyrexia. Chlorpromazine can be used to treat both agitation and pyrexia. Dantrolene is the treatment for resistant hyperpyrexia.

There are four groups of medications that are likely to be used to reduce circulating thyroid hormones:

β-blockers, antithyroid medication, iodine-containing agents, and glucocorticoids.

#### *β-Blockers*

β-Blockers are routinely used to control adrenergic symptoms of hyperthyroidism, and their use is recommended in accelerated hyperthyroidism. Propranolol is a nonselective β-blocker and is the drug of choice due to both its nonselectivity and also because it can block peripheral conversion of T4 to T3.[57] The recommended oral or nasogastric dose is 40–60 mg four times daily. Higher doses may be required because propranolol is metabolized faster in thyrotoxicosis.[58] The intravenous dose of propranolol is 0.5–1 mg given over 10 min.

Many patients presenting with thyroid storm will have congestive cardiac failure, a core part of the syndrome. β-Blockers are an essential part of the management of thyroid storm, and control of severe tachycardia can improve cardiac function. However, some caution should be used because of the risk of exacerbating cardiac failure and precipitating cardiovascular collapse.[59] Intravenous use of the short-acting β-blocker esmolol is thought to be safer if there is significant congestive cardiac failure. The initial loading dose is 250–500 μg/kg i.v., followed by an infusion of 50–100 μg/kg/min.[60] If β-blockers are contraindicated, then nondihydropyridine calcium channel blockers, such as diltiazem, can be considered, but their effectiveness is disputed.[59,61]

#### *Antithyroid drugs*

Propylthiouracil and carbimazole (and methimazole in the United States) are antithyroid drugs (ATDs) that inhibit the enzyme thyroperoxidase and therefore block synthesis of thyroid hormone. Large doses of ATDs are recommended as part of the treatment of thyroid storm.[56,62] Propylthiouracil is preferred to carbimazole because of its additional ability to block peripheral conversion of T4 to T3. The recommended dose is 200 mg four times daily oral or nasogastric, if the patient cannot swallow.

#### *Iodine and iodine-containing contrast agents*

In the thyrotoxic state, short-term administration of iodine blocks the release of preformed thyroid hormone from the thyroid gland and also inhibits further thyroid hormone synthesis (Wolff–Chaikoff effect). This may seem paradoxical because iodine is an essential substrate of thyroid hormone production, but the effect is well documented. Levels of fT4 can show a 50% fall by day 4 and normalization at day 9.[63]

Iodine-containing contrast agents such as sodium ipodate (Orografin®) are thought to be even more effective than iodine because they both block the release of preformed thyroid hormone and inhibit the peripheral conversion of T4 to T3.[64]

After this initial rapid blockade of thyroid hormone release, the further administration of iodine or ipodate may be ineffective. This effect is described as "escape" from the inhibitory effects of iodine that can potentially lead to enrichment of thyroid iodine stores, and ultimately worsening of the hyperthyroidism.[65] For this reason, it is important that iodine is either used concurrently with other treatments or is used before planned date of surgery, normally after 7–10 days of iodine treatment.

The dosing of iodine and iodine contrast agents can be confusing because there are several preparations, and many texts refer to oral iodine in "drops," a nonstandard unit. The classic preparation is Lugol's iodine, named after French physician Jean Lugol (1786–1851), who originally promoted its use to treat tuberculosis. Lugol's iodine is a solution of elemental iodine and potassium iodide in water. The full-strength solution contains 5% iodine and 10% potassium iodide. The iodine content of the solution means that it is potentially irritant to mucosa and should be used in dilution. A dose of 10 mL of 5% Lugol's is reported to cause gastric erosions.[66] Dosing recommendations vary from 3 drops twice per day[67] to 10 drops every 8 h.[68]

There are 20 drops to a milliliter, making one drop equal to 0.05 mL.

An alternative preparation to Lugol's is saturated solution of potassium iodide (SSKI) that contains 1000 mg of potassium iodide per milliliter of solution. This preparation contains iodide rather than iodine and is not irritating to mucosa. Again the recommended doses vary from 1 to 5 drops, two to four times per day.[68] Five drops of SSKI is estimated to provide 250 mg of iodide. The recommended oral dose of the contrast agent sodium ipodate is 500–1000 mg daily.

### *Steroids/glucocorticoids*

Glucocorticoids inhibit the release of thyroid hormone from the thyroid gland and also inhibit the peripheral conversion of fT4 to fT3. They are therefore useful adjunctive treatments in thyroid storm to aid control of the thyrotoxicosis. Normally, hydrocortisone or dexamethasone is used intravenously or by nasogastric tube.

### *Combined treatment*

Initially, propranolol (40 mg q.d.s.) and propylthiouracil (200 mg q.d.s.) are commenced. At least 1 h after these medications have been commenced, oral iodine can be given (five drops = 0.25 mL; can be given four times per day). The rationale for a slight delay in commencing the iodine is that the effect of iodine on the thyroid is not entirely predictable. There is a theoretical risk that iodine can exacerbate hyperthyroidism, hence the delay in introducing it. Glucocorticoids can be given at any stage.

Aspirin should be avoided if possible because it can increase fT4 and fT3 levels by interfering with protein binding. If conventional treatment is unsuccessful, plasma exchange could be considered because there has been some success reported[69] (Table 24.5).

## *Myxedema coma*

Myxedema coma is a presentation with severe and decompensated hypothyroidism.[70] It is a rare condition, mostly seen in elderly women. The mortality is estimated at up to 50%.[71–73] Clinical features may include hypothermia, bradycardia, hypotension, hypoglycaemia, altered mental state, and circulatory and respiratory failure. Despite the wide use of the term, coma is not required to make the diagnosis, because confusion and other more minor degrees of altered mental state are sufficient. Some studies suggest that the term "myxoedema crisis" should be used in preference to myxedema coma.[67]

### ***Diagnosis and assessment***

The diagnosis should be considered in patients who have unexplained altered mental state, especially if they have hyponatremia, hypoglycemia, or hypothermia (Box 24.1). The essential elements of the condition are clinical and biochemical hypothyroidism, significantly altered mental state, with or without hypothermia.[73,74]

| | Medication | Dose | Rationale |
|---|---|---|---|
| β-Blockers | Propranolol<br>Esmolol i.v. | 40–80 mg oral 6 hourly<br>250–500 μg/kg i.v., then 50–100 μg/kg/min | Controls adrenergic symptoms |
| ATDs | Propylthiouracil (PTU)<br>Carbimazole (CBZ) | 200 mg oral 6 hourly<br>20 mg oral 6 hourly | Inhibit synthesis of thyroid hormone (PTU also blocks peripheral conversion of T4 to T3) |
| Iodine and iodine-containing agents | Lugol's iodine<br>Potassium iodide (SSKI)<br>Sodium ipodate | 0.5 mL (10 drops) 8 hourly<br>1–5 drops 6–12 hourly<br>500–1000 mg daily | Inhibit the release and synthesis of thyroid hormone |
| Glucocorticoids | Dexamethasone | 2 mg 6 hourly | Inhibit the release of thyroid hormone and block peripheral conversion of T4 to T3 |

***Table 24.5***
*Management of thyroid storm.*

**Box 24.1** *Diagnosis of myxedema coma*

**Myxedema coma requires all of the following:**

1. Clinical features of severe hypothyroidism, including at least one of the following: hyponatremia, hypoglycemia, bradycardia, and hypothermia
2. Altered mental state
3. Biochemical evidence of hypothyroidism, either primary or secondary

Most studies demonstrate that older patient have a worse outcome.[72,75] The other factors that predict poor outcome in myxedema coma are lower level of consciousness, as measured by Glasgow coma score (GCS), and greater physiological derangement (e.g., Acute Physiology and Chronic Health Evaluation II score [APACHE II] score).[73] Often, the acute presentation with myxedema coma relates to a precipitating factor, such as infection, myocardial infarction, stroke, CNS depressant medication, or electrolyte imbalance. One series reported that infection was the precipitant in 74% of cases diagnosed.[71]

## Management

There are three aspects to management of myxedema coma. The first aspect is general supportive treatment and includes circulatory and ventilatory support, often requiring intubation and ventilation, and intravenous volume expansion in an intensive care unit. Other aspects of supportive management include intravenous glucose for hypoglycemia and active warming for hypothermia.

The second aspect of management is treatment of any underlying precipitant, such as infection, cardiovascular event, or withdraw a precipitating drug. The third aspect is the urgent replacement of thyroid hormone. The optimal replacement regime is controversial, and there are minimal trial data to guide management. The clinical questions center on whether a loading dose is required before maintenance therapy, whether intravenous preparations are preferable, and finally whether T3 should be used in preference to T4 or whether a combination of T3 and T4 is best.[70]

### *Loading dose of T4*

Some studies recommend a loading dose of T4.[67,76] The rationale is to saturate thyroid hormone stores and to rapidly achieve steady-state hormone replacement. However, it is widely believed that a loading dose is unnecessary and potentially dangerous.[77,78] It is therefore appropriate to proceed straight to maintenance replacement treatment.

### *Intravenous or enteral replacement*

Some studies recommend that thyroid hormone treatment should be given intravenously; others argue that enteral administration is as effective as intravenous administration. The justification for intravenous treatment is that the poor circulatory and hypometabolic state may make enteral absorption unpredictable.[76] In the United Kingdom, intravenous liothyronine (T3) is available but intravenous T4 may be unavailable or difficult to obtain urgently.

### *Maintenance dose: T4, T3, or both*

The options for maintenance treatment are either to give T4 alone, T3 alone, or a combination of T4 and T3. Again, there is controversy surrounding the recommendations. The argument for giving T3 maintenance treatment is that it has greater biological activity and a more rapid onset of action that would, theoretically, lead to more rapid restoration of thyroid action at a cellular level. Conversely, T4 has a lower level of biological activity, and the conversion of T4 to T3 by 5-deiodinase is impaired during acute illness.

The theoretical advantages of giving T3 replacement to treat myxedema coma have not led to any clear evidence of improved outcomes associated with its use. In fact, the administration of higher doses of T3, and/or the presence of higher calculated levels of T3, have been shown to correlate with increased mortality.[72]

Yamamoto et al. report a series of eight patients. The first three were treated with high-dose T3 and all died; the subsequent five cases were treated with low-dose T3 or T4 and all survived. They subsequently reviewed the published literature and concluded that a daily replacement dose of >75 μg T3 or >500 μg T4 is associated with an increased mortality at 1 month.[78]

One accepted maintenance replacement treatment regime is to give T4 50–100 μg/day either oral (by nasogastric tube if required) or intravenous. T4 can be supplemented with T3 at a dose of 5–10 μg every 8 h.[67]

It is recommended that patients presenting with myxedema coma are given a stress dose of hydrocortisone replacement to treat possible coexistent hypocortisolemia. Normally, this dose would be 50–100 mg q.d.s. i.m. hydrocortisone (see section on Addisonian crisis) (Box 24.2).

**Box 24.2** *Acute management of myxedema coma*

1. General supportive treatment
2. Treatment of any underlying precipitant
3. Thyroid hormone replacement (T4 or T3 or both can be given)
4. Hydrocortisone treatment 100 mg 6 hourly i.v.

# Salt and mineral emergencies

## Severe hypercalcemia (see Chapter 11)

Severe hypercalcemia is normally defined on the basis of serum calcium >3.5 mmol/L (>14 mg/dL). If severe symptoms are present together with a serum calcium 3.0–3.5 mmol/L, this condition would also be included.

The emergency presentation is characterized by confusion, vomiting, and dehydration.

### Diagnosis and assessment

The range of possible symptoms is extensive and includes GI, neurological, cardiovascular, and renal systems. Severe cases may present obtunded or comatose with dehydration and acute kidney injury. Severe hypercalcemia leads to a widening of the QRS complexes and widening of the T waves progressing to arrhythmia and, on occasions, cardiac arrest. The commonest causes are malignancy, accounting for 50% of hospital inpatient cases, and primary hyperparathyroidism. Other causes are shown in Box 24.3 and investigations in Box 24.4.

**Box 24.3** *Causes of hypercalcemia*

Hyperparathyroidism—Primary

Tertiary

Malignancy—parathyroid hormone-related protein (PTHrp)-mediated

Bone metastases

Myeloma

Granulomatous conditions, e.g., sarcoidosis

Addison's disease

Hyperthyroidism

Familial hypocalciuric hypercalcemia (calcium-sensing receptor [CaSR] mutation)

Vitamin D toxicity and milk alkali syndrome

Drugs: thiazides, bendroflumethiazide, lithium, vitamin A

Immobilization

Renal failure

Congenital, e.g., William's syndrome

**Box 24.4** *Investigation of hypercalcemia*

Parathyroid hormone (PTH)

Thyroid function tests

9 a.m. cortisol (± ACTH stimulation test)

Serum electrophoresis/immunoglobulins

Serum angiotensin-converting enzyme (ACE)

PTHrp

CXR ± CT chest/abdomen/pelvis

Urinary calcium/creatinine

### Treatment

The initial standard treatment of severe hypercalcemia is intravenous fluid together with bisphosphonates and calcitonin (Table 24.6). Large volumes of normal saline should be given to restore the intravascular circulation. The rate at which fluid can safely be given will vary, but initial rates are 200–300 mL/h, aiming for 3–6 L/day, provided the patient is not edematous. Frusemide can be given if the patient becomes edematous, but it is not routinely recommended because the injudicious use of frusemide will promote dehydration, which worsens hypercalcemia. Frusemide also depletes other electrolytes (potassium and magnesium) that increase the risk of arrhythmia.

Calcitonin can be used as a short-term, rapid-onset agent to lower serum calcium levels. It works by inhibiting both bone resorption and tubular calcium reabsorption. The dose of salmon calcitonin is 4–8 U/kg given intramuscularly every 6–12 h. Onset of action is within 2 h, but there is tachyphylaxis after 2–3 days. Hemodialysis can be used for the treatment of life-threatening hypercalcemic crisis, for example, with

| | Treatment | Dose | Onset | Duration |
|---|---|---|---|---|
| Calcitonin | Salmon calcitonin | 4–8 U/kg i.m. every 6–12 h | 2 h | Tachyphylaxis after 2 days |
| Bisphosphonate | Pamidronate | 60–90 mg i.v. (2 h) | 2 days | 2 weeks |
| | Zoledronic acid | 4 mg i.v. (15 min) | 2 days | 3–4 weeks |

***Table 24.6***
*Initial standard treatment of severe hypercalcemia.*

a serum calcium of >4.5 mmol/L, which is not rapidly responding to initial treatment.

Intravenous bisphosphonates inhibit bone resorption and are an effective treatment for hypercalcemia. Pamidronate (60–90 mg) or zoledronic acid (4 mg) is normally used as an intravenous infusion. The serum calcium begins to fall with 2 days and reaches its maximum effect after 5–7 days. The infusion can be repeated at intervals of 1–4 weeks as required.

Treatment of the underlying cause, such as parathyroidectomy, should be considered. Steroids are effective in the treatment of hypercalcemia caused by vitamin D intoxication, granulomatous disease, and myeloma, but they are not recommended outside of these circumstances. Cinacalcet is a calcium mimetic that can be used to lower serum calcium levels in hyperparathyroidism caused by parathyroid cancer.

## Severe hypocalcemia (see Chapter 11)

Acute hypocalcemia causes neuromuscular excitability. Symptoms, if present, include paraesthesia that classically affects the hands, feet, or lips; carpopedal spasm; tetany; laryngospasm; and seizures. Chvostek's sign (twitching of the facial muscles in response to tapping facial nerve) and Trousseau's sign (carpal spasm in response to occlusion of the blood supply to the upper arm) may be seen. Arrhythmias may occur, and ECG may show a prolonged QT interval. Hypotension due to hypocalcemia-mediated vasodilation may be observed (Box 24.5).

**Box 24.5** *Causes of hypocalcemia*

- Vitamin D deficiency
- Hypoparathyroidism—post neck surgery
  - Autoimmune
  - Infiltrative: hemochromatosis, Wilson's, granulomatous
- Genetic defects—abnormal glandular development, e.g., De George syndrome
  - PTH mutations and CaSR mutations
- Hyperphosphatemia
- Hypomagnesemia—gives rise to PTH resistance
- Drugs: chelating agents, bisphosphonates, cinacalcet, cisplatin, foscarnet
- Pancreatitis
- Rhabdomyolysis
- Sepsis
- Pseudohypoparathyroidism (PTH resistance syndromes)

### Diagnosis and assessment

Acute symptomatic hypocalcemia should be treated as an emergency. The level that acute symptomatic hypocalcemia is likely to be seen is serum calcium <1.9 mmol/L. Approximately 50% of serum calcium is bound to albumin, leaving the remaining 50% in the ionized biologically active form. The albumin binding is affected by pH. Assessment should include measurement of the serum calcium together with the assessment of magnesium, phosphate, renal function, pH, and bicarbonate. Vitamin D and PTH should also be assessed.

### Treatment

Emergency treatment is with intravenous calcium gluconate. The usual dose is 10 mL of 10% (contains 90 mg or 2.25 mmol of elemental calcium) administered over 10 min in 50–100 mL of 5% dextrose.

Stronger solutions of calcium can cause phlebitis. This initial dose can be repeated. A maintenance infusion of (1.7 × patient's weight in kg) mL of 10% calcium gluconate in 1000 mL of glucose or saline can then be infused over 24 h.

Hypomagnesemia inhibits PTH secretion and gives rise to resistant hypocalcemia. Coexisting hypomagnesemia should be treated with an intravenous infusion.

Oral vitamin D preparations should be commenced as part of the longer term treatment for hypocalcemia. Alfacalcidol and calcitriol are the more effective and rapid-onset treatments. The normal doses used are 0.5–2 μg/day. Cholecalciferol (D3) can be used if there is vitamin D deficiency, but it is not recommended in situations when hypoparathyroidism is suspected because activation of D3 by 1α-hydroxylase is PTH-dependent.

## *Severe hyponatremia (see Chapter 11)*

Hyponatremia (serum Na <135 mmol/L) is common amongst inpatients, with some hospitals reporting a prevalence of up to 47%.[79] Mild hyponatremia is often asymptomatic but can be associated with an increased risk of falls especially in the elderly. Severe hyponatremia (Na <120 mmol/L) may give rise to significant symptoms, including headache, confusion, seizures, and coma, due in part to associated cerebral edema. The symptoms are more pronounced and severe if the hyponatremia has developed over a short period, such as over several hours; conversely, even biochemically severe hyponatremia may be well tolerated if it has developed slowly. Severe hyponatremia affects about 1% of hospital inpatients[79] (Table 24.7).

### *Diagnosis and assessment*

Disorders of salt and water metabolism are complex. It is beyond the scope of this chapter to review the topic in full; for details, please see Janicic and Verbalis.[80] Assessment should involve initially checking the plasma osmolality to exclude pseudohyponatremia, caused by excess lipids or paraproteins, or a translocational hyponatremia, due to elevated serum glucose or another osmotic active solute. Once the serum sodium is confirmed as genuinely low, hypocortisolemia and hypothyroidism should be excluded by measuring thyroid function tests and a 9 a.m. cortisol blood test, with subsequent short Synacthen test if necessary. Sodium losing medications especially diuretics and angiotensin-converting enzyme inhibitor (ACEi)/angiotensin receptor blocker (ARB) medications should be considered as potential contributing causes. An assessment should be made of the intravascular volume status. If hypovolemic, then the likely cause of the hyponatremia is sodium loss in excess of concurrent fluid loss, a situation that occurs in the state of cerebral salt wasting.

If the patient is edematous with peripheral fluid overload, then the hyponatremia is likely to relate to congestive cardiac failure, liver disease, or hypoalbuminemia. In these circumstances, the mechanism of the hyponatremia is secondary to the decreased effective circulatory volume.

If euvolemic, the diagnosis may be inappropriate antidiuretic hormone secretion (SIADH). The paired urine and serum osmolality should be assessed to confirm inappropriately elevated urine osmolality.

### *Management*

Treatment will depend on an assessment of the likely underlying cause. If the cause can be quickly determined and treated, other interventions may not be required. Severe hyponatremia will sometimes require urgent treatment to manage the neurological complications of confusion and seizure. The usual treatment in this situation is to give hypertonic saline to bring the sodium to a level >125 mmol/L and then reassess. Hypertonic saline is available as 1.8% or 3% solutions.

| *Hypovolemic* | *Euvolemic* | *Fluid overloaded* |
|---|---|---|
| Renal salt wasting | Hypothyroidism | Cirrhosis |
| Cerebral salt wasting | SIADH | Congestive cardiac failure |
| Addison's | Medication | Hypoalbuminemia |
| Excess GI or skin salt loss | | |

***Table 24.7***
*Causes of hyponatremia.*

Sodium be corrected slowly at a rate of <0.5 mmol/h to reduce the risk of pontine or extrapontine myelinolysis.[81] An expert panel has recommended a correction rate of not more than 10 mmol/L in the first 24 h and 18 mmol/L in the first 48 h.[82]

The infusion rate formula is as follows[83]: [total body water (60% of body weight in kg) × desired correction rate (e.g., 0.5–1.0 mmol/L/h)] × [1000/total mmol of sodium in 1 liter of proposed fluid]. For example, for a 70-kg man, being treated with twice normal saline (1.8%), which has 308 mmol sodium/L): [(60% × 70 kg) × 0.5] × [1000/308] = 68 ml/h.

Tolvaptan is an oral vasopressin antagonist that is selective for the V2 receptor, causing a water diuresis. It can be used in euvolemic or hypervolemic hyponatremia but is contraindicated in hypovolemic hyponatremia.[84]

# Neuroendocrine emergencies

## Carcinoid crisis (see Chapter 8)

Carcinoid crisis is a rare, acute presentation characterized by severe flushing, hypotension, tachycardia, diarrhea, and hyperthermia.[85] It is an extreme version of the carcinoid syndrome that affects some patients with neuroendocrine tumors that secrete serotonin and other biologically active substances. Normally, the liver can inactivate these amines and peptides released into the portal circulation. Carcinoid syndrome is most common in patients who have neuroendocrine tumors of the small intestine and the proximal colon, with significant liver metastasis. It can also occur in ovarian and bronchial carcinoids that secrete mediators directly into the systemic circulation.

Crisis may be precipitated by manipulation of the tumor at surgery, biopsy, anesthesia, arterial embolization procedures, chemotherapy, or infection.[86] Pretreatment with somatostatin analogs reduces the risk of a crisis.[87]

### Diagnosis

The diagnosis is made clinically on the basis of the clinical features, in the context of a known or suspected neuroendocrine tumor. The most discriminating feature is fluctuation in blood pressure with predominance of hypotension. The serum and urinary markers of neuroendocrine tumors (chromogranin and 5-hydroxyindoleacetic acid [5HIAA]) are likely to be elevated. There are no commonly used criteria to confirm a crisis.

### Management

Treatment is with intravenous octreotide infusion 50–100 μg/h.[88] Antihistamine H1 and H2 blockers are also used, together with supportive treatment such as intravenous fluids.[89]

## Severe hypoglycemia

Hypoglycemia is most often observed in the context of treatment for diabetes. Outside of that situation, hypoglycemia is rare and there are a range of causes (Box 24.6).

### Diagnosis and assessment

Clinically, an episode of hypoglycemia will present with characteristic symptoms that include autonomic elements (sweating and shaking) together with neuroglycopenic symptoms (e.g., hunger, poor concentration, confusion). Hypoglycemia must be confirmed by laboratory glucose measurement; bedside fingerprick testing is insufficiently

**Box 24.6** *Causes of hypoglycemia*

**Diabetes treatment-related**

Sepsis and infection (including malaria)

Critical illness and malnutrition

Drug-induced (alcohol, quinine, β-blockers, ACEi, quinolones)

Hypocortisolemia

Hypothyroidism

Renal impairment

Insulinoma

Nesidioblastosis

Nonislet cell tumor (IGF2 mediated)

Factitious

**Box 24.7** *Diagnosis of hypoglycemia*

1. Symptoms of hypoglycemia
2. Low levels of plasma glucose
3. Resolution of the symptoms with treatment/correction of the glucose level

accurate for diagnosis. Robust diagnosis of hypoglycemia, summarized in Box 24.7, is based on demonstrating the three elements proposed by Whipple.[90]

On biochemical testing, the pathological threshold for hypoglycemia is a plasma glucose of <2.2 mmol/L (<40 mg/dL). The majority of patients will require investigation with a controlled fast to identify an episode of hypoglycemia and obtain the necessary biochemistry.

Controlled fast is performed as an inpatient and the patient is allowed only water from the start of the fast. Capillary blood glucose is measured every 2 hours and once readings fall below 3.3mmol/L (60 mg/dL) laboratory glucose samples are taken and processed at each time point. If a blood glucose of below 2.2 mmol/L (40 mg/dL) is confirmed then samples are taken for insulin, pro-insulin and c-peptide (See Table 24.8) The fast may then be terminated and hypoglycaemia treated. A sulphonylurea screen (blood and urine) should also be obtained. The controlled fast can be continued for up to 72 hours. The test is used both to confirm pathological hypoglycemia and to determine whether it is insulin or non-insulin mediated.

### Management

The emergency treatment of hypoglycemia requires administration of glucose. If the patient is conscious, this treatment can often be done by giving oral fast-acting glucose. The recommended amount is 15–20 g of rapidly absorbed carbohydrate. This amount is achieved by giving 100–200 mL of lucozade or fruit juice or five or six glucose tablets.[91]

If the patient is unconscious, treatment is with intravenous glucose; 150 mL of 10% glucose or 75 mL of 20% glucose is a recommended initial dose. The use of 50% glucose solutions is discouraged because it is no more effective and can cause extravasation injuries.[92]

The most severe cases of neuroendocrine hypoglycemia may be due to metastatic insulinoma. These cases may require a continuous glucose infusion. In this situation, glucocorticoids and diazoxide are sometimes used to reduce hypoglycemia burden. Surgical treatment to debulk the tumor can used together with other multimodal therapies. In this context, everolimus, an mammalian target of rapamycin (mTOR) inhibitor, has shown specific effects of ameliorating hypoglycemia in addition to the neuroendocrine tumor chemotherapy effects.[93]

## Severe neuroendocrine diarrhea (VIPoma, gastrinoma)

Diarrhea is a common symptom with a wide differential diagnosis for its cause. Functioning neuroendocrine tumors are a rare cause of diarrhea, accounting for <1% of cases.[94] Carcinoid tumors and pancreatic neuroendocrine tumors (pNETs), including VIPoma, gastrinoma cause this syndrome.

The most severe presentations are likely to be due to vasoactive intestinal polypeptide (VIP)-secreting pNETs. VIP binds to receptors on intestinal epithelial cells (known as cholera receptors) and activates intracellular messengers, giving rise to secretory diarrhea that is often severe and can lead to dehydration, renal failure, electrolyte imbalance, and can be life-threatening.[95] The clinical syndrome is known as watery diarrhea, hypokalemia, achlorhydria (WDHA).

### Management

Initial supportive treatment will involve intravenous fluids and the replacement of depleted electrolytes, especially potassium. Blood samples should be taken for gut hormones and chromogranin A and B. The samples are

| Tests that must be done during an episode of hypoglycemia | Tests that need not be done during hypoglycemia |
|---|---|
| Glucose | Cortisol (9 a.m.) |
| Insulin | IGF-II/IGF-I |
| Proinsulin | Insulin antibodies |
| c-Peptide | Thyroid function test (TFT) |
| β-Hydroxybutyrate | |
| Sulfonylurea screen | |

***Table 24.8***
*Investigation of hypoglycemia.*

taken in a blood bottle containing the enzyme inhibitor aprotinin (Trasylol®). Aprotinin inhibits proteolytic enzymes and prevents their degradation before analysis.

Octreotide injections are a specific treatment for this form of severe diarrhea. Octreotide inhibits the secretion of neuroendocrine peptides such as VIP. The initial dose of octreotide is 50–100 μg s.c. 8 hourly.

If there is a clinical suggestion of gastrinoma, high-dose proton pump inhibitor medication should be used first line to inhibit the production of gastric acid, resolve diarrhea, and reduce the risk of peptic ulceration and perforation.

After stabilization of the patient and control of the diarrhea, multimodal therapy is normally needed to treat the underlying neuroendocrine tumor.

# References


*1. Rajasekaran S, Vanderpump M, Baldeweg S, et al. UK guidelines for the management of pituitary apoplexy. *Clinical Endocrinology*. 2011;74(1):9–20.
2. Sibal L, Ball SG, Connolly V, et al. Pituitary apoplexy: A review of clinical presentation, management and outcome in 45 cases. *Pituitary*. 2004;7(3):157–63.
3. Ayuk J, McGregor EJ, Mitchell RD, et al. Acute management of pituitary apoplexy—surgery or conservative management? *Clinical Endocrinology*. 2004;61(6):747–52.
4. Veldhuis JD, Hammond JM. Endocrine function after spontaneous infarction of the human pituitary: Report, review, and reappraisal. *Endocrine Reviews*. 1980;1(1):100–7.
5. Randeva HS, Schoebel J, Byrne J, et al. Classical pituitary apoplexy: Clinical features, management and outcome. *Clinical Endocrinology*. 1999;51(2):181–8.
6. Valente M, Marroni M, Stagni G, et al. Acute sterile meningitis as a primary manifestation of pituitary apoplexy. *Journal of Endocrinological Investigation*. 2003;26(8):754–7.
7. Reddy NL, Rajasekaran S, Han TS, et al. An objective scoring tool in the management of patients with pituitary apoplexy. *Clinical Endocrinology*. 2011;75(5):723.
8. Bills DC, Meyer FB, Laws ER, Jr., et al. A retrospective analysis of pituitary apoplexy. *Neurosurgery*. 1993;33(4):602–8.
9. Arafah BM, Harrington JF, Madhoun ZT, et al. Improvement of pituitary function after surgical decompression for pituitary tumor apoplexy. *Journal of Clinical Endocrinology and Metabolism*. 1990;71(2):323–8.
10. Gruber A, Clayton J, Kumar S, et al. Pituitary apoplexy: Retrospective review of 30 patients—is surgical intervention always necessary? *British Journal of Neurosurgery*. 2006;20(6):379–85.
11. Casanueva FF, Molitch ME, Schlechte JA, et al. Guidelines of the Pituitary Society for the diagnosis and management of prolactinomas. *Clinical Endocrinology*. 2006;65(2):265–73.
12. Whitelaw BC, Dworakowska D, Thomas NW, et al. Temozolomide in the management of dopamine agonist-resistant prolactinomas. *Clinical Endocrinology*. 2012;76(6):877–86.
13. Yong TY, Li JY. Reversible dilated cardiomyopathy in a patient with Cushing's syndrome. *Congestive Heart Failure*. 2010;16(2):77–9.
14. Arnaldi G, Angeli A, Atkinson AB, et al. Diagnosis and complications of Cushing's syndrome: A consensus statement. *Journal of Clinical Endocrinology and Metabolism*. 2003;88(12):5593–602.
15. Terzolo M, Angeli A, Fassnacht M, et al. Adjuvant mitotane treatment for adrenocortical carcinoma. *New England Journal of Medicine*. 2007;356(23):2372–80.
16. Kamenicky P, Droumaguet C, Salenave S, et al. Mitotane, metyrapone, and ketoconazole combination therapy as an alternative to rescue adrenalectomy for severe ACTH-dependent Cushing's syndrome. *Journal of Clinical Endocrinology and Metabolism*. 2011;96(9): 2796–804.
17. Castinetti F, Fassnacht M, Johanssen S, et al. Merits and pitfalls of mifepristone in Cushing's syndrome. *European Journal of Endocrinology/European Federation of Endocrine Societies*. 2009;160(6):1003–10.
18. Hamill RJ, Robinson LM, Wexler HR, et al. Efficacy and safety of potassium infusion therapy in hypokalemic critically ill patients. *Critical Care Medicine*. 1991;19(5):694–9.
19. Druce MGAB. BARTS ENDOCRINE E-PROTOCOLS PITUITARY FUNCTION. 2009. Available from: http://bartsendocrinology.co.uk/resources/PITUITARY_Barts_protocol_$5Bfinal$5D.pdf.
20. Adams JR, Blevins LS, Jr., Allen GS, et al. Disorders of water metabolism following transsphenoidal pituitary surgery: A single institution's experience. *Pituitary*. 2006;9(2):93–9.
*21. Loh JA, Verbalis JG. Disorders of water and salt metabolism associated with pituitary disease. *Endocrinology and Metabolism Clinics of North America*. 2008;37(1):213–34.
22. Lenders JW, Eisenhofer G, Mannelli M, et al. Phaeochromocytoma. *Lancet*. 2005;366(9486):665–75.
23. Kopetschke R, Slisko M, Kilisli A, et al. Frequent incidental discovery of phaeochromocytoma: Data from a German cohort of 201 phaeochromocytoma. *European Journal of Endocrinology/European Federation of Endocrine Societies*. 2009;161(2):355–61.
24. Newell KA, Prinz RA, Pickleman J, et al. Pheochromocytoma multisystem crisis. A surgical emergency. *Archives of Surgery*. 1988;123(8):956–9.


* Key or Classic references.

25. Brouwers FM, Eisenhofer G, Lenders JW, et al. Emergencies caused by pheochromocytoma, neuroblastoma, or ganglioneuroma. *Endocrinology and Metabolism Clinics of North America*. 2006;35(4):699–724.
26. Kim S, Yu A, Filippone LA, et al. Inverted-Takotsubo pattern cardiomyopathy secondary to pheochromocytoma: A clinical case and literature review. *Clinical Cardiology*. 2010;33(4):200–5.
27. Zielen P, Klisiewicz A, Januszewicz A, et al. Pheochromocytoma-related 'classic' takotsubo cardiomyopathy. *Journal of Human Hypertension*. 2010;24(5):363–6.
28. Hosseinnezhad A, Black RM, Aeddula NR, et al. Glucagon-induced pheochromocytoma crisis. *Endocrine Practice: Official Journal of the American College of Endocrinology and the American Association of Clinical Endocrinologists*. 2011;17(3):e51–4.
29. Yi DW, Kim SY, Shin DH, et al. Pheochromocytoma crisis after a dexamethasone suppression test for adrenal incidentaloma. *Endocrine*. 2010;37(1):213–19.
30. Rashid-Farokhi F, Cheraghvandi A, Masjedi MR. Pheochromocytoma crisis due to glucocorticoid administration: A case report and review of the literature. *Archives of Iranian Medicine*. 2009;12(2):190–4.
31. Rosas AL, Kasperlik-Zaluska AA, Papierska L, et al. Pheochromocytoma crisis induced by glucocorticoids: A report of four cases and review of the literature. *European Journal of Endocrinology/European Federation of Endocrine Societies*. 2008;158(3):423–9.
32. Barzon L, Sonino N, Fallo F, et al. Prevalence and natural history of adrenal incidentalomas. *European Journal of Endocrinology/European Federation of Endocrine Societies*. 2003;149(4):273–85.
33. Carey M, Carter J, Nesbitt I. Phaeochromocytoma crisis presenting under anaesthesia with profound left ventricular failure—successful treatment with intra-aortic balloon pump. *Journal of the Intensive Care Society*. 2010;11(3):192–5.
34. Grinda JM, Bricourt MO, Salvi S, et al. Unusual cardiogenic shock due to pheochromocytoma: Recovery after bridge-to-bridge (extracorporeal life support and DeBakey ventricular assist device) and right surrenalectomy. *Journal of Thoracic and Cardiovascular Surgery*. 2006;131(4):913–14.
35. Chao A, Yeh YC, Yen TS, et al. Phaeochromocytoma crisis—a rare indication for extracorporeal membrane oxygenation. *Anaesthesia*. 2008;63(1):86–8.
36. Schnelle N, Ferris DO, Schirger A. The use of blood volume determination in patients undergoing surgery for pheochromocytoma. *Anesthesia and Analgesia*. 1964;43:641–5.
37. Committee SfEsC. Protocol using oral phenoxybenzamine to prepare patients with catecholamine-secreting phaeochromocytoma and paraganglioma for surgery. 2010 [cited 2012 10/1/12]; Available from: http://www.endocrinology.org/policy/docs/10-10_Protocol_using_oral_phenoxybenzamine.pdf.
38. Bajwa SS, Bajwa SK. Implications and considerations during pheochromocytoma resection: A challenge to the anesthesiologist. *Indian Journal of Endocrinology and Metabolism*. 2011;15(Suppl 4):S337–44.
39. Temple WJ, Voitk AJ, Thomson AE, et al. Phenoxybenzamine blockade in surgery of pheochromocytoma. *Journal of Surgical Research*. 1977;22(1):59–64.
40. James MF, Cronje L. Pheochromocytoma crisis: The use of magnesium sulfate. *Anesthesia and Analgesia*. 2004;99(3):680–6, table of contents.
41. Chung PC, Li AH, Lin CC, et al. Elevated vascular resistance after labetalol during resection of a pheochromocytoma (brief report). *Canadian Journal of Anaesthesia = Journal canadien d'anesthesie*. 2002;49(2):148–50.
42. Grogan RH, Mitmaker EJ, Duh QY. Changing paradigms in the treatment of malignant pheochromocytoma. *Cancer Control: Journal of the Moffitt Cancer Center*. 2011;18(2):104–12.
43. Grossman AB, Tomlinson JW. Position statement of the Society for Endocrinology on the endocrine effects of inhaled corticosteroids in respiratory disease. Society for Endocrinology; 2011; Available from: http://www.endocrinology.org/policy/docs/11-07_Endocrine%20effects%20of%20inhaled%20steroids%20in%20respiratory%20disease.pdf.
*44. Bouillon R. Acute adrenal insufficiency. *Endocrinology and Metabolism Clinics of North America*. 2006;35(4):767–75.
45. Myers KA, Kline GA. Addison disease presenting with acute neurologic deterioration: A rare presentation yields new lessons from old observations in primary adrenal failure. *Endocrine Practice: Official Journal of the American College of Endocrinology and the American Association of Clinical Endocrinologists*. 2010;16(3):433–6.
46. Akpa MR, Odia OJ. Addison's disease presenting as acute chest syndrome: Case report and review of literature. *Nigerian Journal of Medicine: Journal of the National Association of Resident Doctors of Nigeria*. 2006;15(4):451–2.
47. Hahner S, Loeffler M, Bleicken B, et al. Epidemiology of adrenal crisis in chronic adrenal insufficiency: The need for new prevention strategies. *European Journal of Endocrinology/European Federation of Endocrine Societies*. 2010;162(3):597–602.
48. Oelkers W. Adrenal insufficiency. *New England Journal of Medicine*. 1996;335(16):1206–12.
49. Le Roux CW, Meeran K, Alaghband-Zadeh J. Is a 0900-h serum cortisol useful prior to a short synacthen test in outpatient assessment? *Annals of Clinical Biochemistry*. 2002;39(Pt 2):148–50.
50. Arlt W. The approach to the adult with newly diagnosed adrenal insufficiency. *Journal of Clinical Endocrinology and Metabolism*. 2009;94(4):1059–67.
51. Song JH, Chaudhry FS, Mayo-Smith WW. The incidental adrenal mass on CT: Prevalence of adrenal disease in 1,049 consecutive adrenal masses in patients

with no known malignancy. *AJR American Journal of Roentgenology*. 2008;190(5):1163–8.

52. Terzolo M, Ali A, Osella G, et al. Prevalence of adrenal carcinoma among incidentally discovered adrenal masses. A retrospective study from 1989 to 1994. Gruppo Piemontese Incidentalomi Surrenalici. *Archives of Surgery*. 1997;132(8):914–19.
53. Arlt W, Biehl M, Taylor AE, et al. Urine steroid metabolomics as a biomarker tool for detecting malignancy in adrenal tumors. *Journal of Clinical Endocrinology and Metabolism*. 2011;96(12):3775–84.
*54. Fassnacht M, Allolio B. Clinical management of adrenocortical carcinoma. *Best Practice & Research Clinical Endocrinology & Metabolism*. 2009;23(2):273–89.
55. Burch HB, Wartofsky L. Life-threatening thyrotoxicosis. Thyroid storm. *Endocrinology and Metabolism Clinics of North America*. 1993;22(2):263–77.
56. Sarlis NJ, Gourgiotis L. Thyroid emergencies. *Reviews in Endocrine & Metabolic Disorders*. 2003;4(2):129–36.
57. Harrower AD, Fyffe JA, Horn DB, et al. Thyroxine and triiodothyronine levels in hyperthyroid patients during treatment with propranolol. *Clinical Endocrinology*. 1977;7(1):41–4.
58. Klein I, Ojamaa K. Thyrotoxicosis and the heart. *Endocrinology and Metabolism Clinics of North America*. 1998;27(1):51–62.
59. Ngo SY, Chew HC. When the storm passes unnoticed—a case series of thyroid storm. *Resuscitation*. 2007;73(3):485–90.
60. Isley WL, Dahl S, Gibbs H. Use of esmolol in managing a thyrotoxic patient needing emergency surgery. *American Journal of Medicine*. 1990;89(1):122–3.
61. Klein I, Becker DV, Levey GS. Treatment of hyperthyroid disease. *Annals of Internal Medicine*. 1994;121(4):281–8.
62. Nayak B, Burman K. Thyrotoxicosis and thyroid storm. *Endocrinology and Metabolism Clinics of North America*. 2006;35(4):663–86.
63. Wartofsky L, Ransil BJ, Ingbar SH. Inhibition by iodine of the release of thyroxine from the thyroid glands of patients with thyrotoxicosis. *Journal of Clinical Investigation*. 1970;49(1):78–86.
64. Robuschi G, Manfredi A, Salvi M, et al. Effect of sodium ipodate and iodide on free T4 and free T3 concentrations in patients with Graves' disease. *Journal of Endocrinological Investigation*. 1986;9(4):287–91.
65. Martino E, Balzano S, Bartalena L, et al. Therapy of Graves' disease with sodium ipodate is associated with a high recurrence rate of hyperthyroidism. *Journal of Endocrinological Investigation*. 1991;14(10):847–51.
66. Sreedharan A, Rembacken BJ, Rotimi O. Acute toxic gastric mucosal damage induced by Lugol's iodine spray during chromoendoscopy. *Gut*. 2005;54(6):886–7.
67. Wondisford FE, Radovick S. *Clinical Management of Thyroid Disease*. Philidephia: Saunders Elsevier; 2009. 423 p.
68. Ross DS. The medical management of Graves' disease. *Endocrine Practice: Official Journal of the American College of Endocrinology and the American Association of Clinical Endocrinologists*. 1995;1(3):193–9.
69. Muller C, Perrin P, Faller B, et al. Role of plasma exchange in the thyroid storm. *Therapeutic Apheresis and Dialysis: Official Peer-Reviewed Journal of the International Society for Apheresis, the Japanese Society for Apheresis, the Japanese Society for Dialysis Therapy*. 2011;15(6):522–31.
70. Wartofsky L. Myxedema coma. *Endocrinology and Metabolism Clinics of North America*. 2006;35(4):687–98.
71. Dutta P, Bhansali A, Masoodi SR, et al. Predictors of outcome in myxoedema coma: A study from a tertiary care centre. *Critical Care*. 2008;12(1):R1.
72. Hylander B, Rosenqvist U. Treatment of myxoedema coma—factors associated with fatal outcome. *Acta Endocrinologica*. 1985;108(1):65–71.
73. Rodriguez I, Fluiters E, Perez-Mendez LF, et al. Factors associated with mortality of patients with myxoedema coma: Prospective study in 11 cases treated in a single institution. *Journal of Endocrinology*. 2004;180(2):347–50.
74. Mathew V, Misgar RA, Ghosh S, et al. Myxedema coma: A new look into an old crisis. *Journal of Thyroid Research*. 2011;2011:493462.
75. Jordan RM. Myxedema coma. Pathophysiology, therapy, and factors affecting prognosis. *The Medical Clinics of North America*. 1995;79(1):185–94.
76. Holvey DN, Goodner CJ, Nicoloff JT, et al. Treatment of myxedema coma with intravenous thyroxine. *Archives of Internal Medicine*. 1964;113:89–96.
77. Pereira VG, Haron ES, Lima-Neto N, et al. Management of myxedema coma: Report on three successfully treated cases with nasogastric or intravenous administration of triiodothyronine. *Journal of Endocrinological Investigation*. 1982;5(5):331–4.
78. Yamamoto T, Fukuyama J, Fujiyoshi A. Factors associated with mortality of myxedema coma: Report of eight cases and literature survey. *Thyroid: Official Journal of the American Thyroid Association*. 1999;9(12):1167–74.
79. Doshi SM, Shah P, Lei X, et al. Hyponatremia in hospitalized cancer patients and its impact on clinical outcomes. *American Journal of Kidney Diseases: The Official Journal of the National Kidney Foundation*. 2012;59(2):222–8.
80. Janicic N, Verbalis JG. Evaluation and management of hypo-osmolality in hospitalized patients. *Endocrinology and Metabolism Clinics of North America*. 2003;32(2):459–81.
81. Gujjar A, Al-Mamari A, Jacob PC, et al. Extrapontine myelinolysis as presenting manifestation of adrenal

failure: A case report. *Journal of the Neurological Sciences*. 2010;290(1–2):169–71.

*82. Verbalis JG, Goldsmith SR, Greenberg A, et al. Hyponatremia treatment guidelines 2007: Expert panel recommendations. *American Journal of Medicine*. 2007;120(11 Suppl 1):S1–21.

83. Adrogue HJ, Madias NE. Hyponatremia. *New England Journal of Medicine*. 2000;342(21):1581–9.

84. Robertson GL. Vaptans for the treatment of hyponatremia. *Nature Reviews Endocrinology*. 2011;7(3):151–61.

85. Melmed S, Polonsky KS, Larsen PR, et al. *Williams Textbook of Endocrinology*. 12th ed. Philadelphia: Elsevier; 2011. 1897 p.

86. Vaughan DJ, Brunner MD. Anesthesia for patients with carcinoid syndrome. *International Anesthesiology Clinics*. 1997;35(4):129–42.

87. Kinney MA, Warner ME, Nagorney DM, et al. Perianaesthetic risks and outcomes of abdominal surgery for metastatic carcinoid tumours. *British Journal of Anaesthesia*. 2001;87(3):447–52.

88. Kvols LK, Martin JK, Marsh HM, et al. Rapid reversal of carcinoid crisis with a somatostatin analogue. *New England Journal of Medicine*. 1985;313(19):1229–30.

89. Roberts LJ 2nd, Marney SR, Jr., Oates JA. Blockade of the flush associated with metastatic gastric carcinoid by combined histamine H1 and H2 receptor antagonists. Evidence for an important role of H2 receptors in human vasculature. *New England Journal of Medicine*. 1979;300(5):236–8.

90. Whipple AO. Islet cell tumors of the pancreas. *Canadian Medical Association Journal*. 1952;66(4):334–42.

91. Choudhary P, Amiel SA. Hypoglycaemia: Current management and controversies. *Postgraduate Medical Journal*. 2011;87(1026):298–306.

92. Moore C, Woollard M. Dextrose 10% or 50% in the treatment of hypoglycaemia out of hospital? A randomised controlled trial. *Emergency Medicine Journal: EMJ*. 2005;22(7):512–15.

93. Kulke MH, Bergsland EK, Yao JC. Glycemic control in patients with insulinoma treated with everolimus. *New England Journal of Medicine*. 2009;360(2):195–7.

94. Jensen RT. Overview of chronic diarrhea caused by functional neuroendocrine neoplasms. *Seminars in Gastrointestinal Disease*. 1999;10(4):156–72.

95. Sjoqvist U, Permert J, Lofberg R, et al. Life threatening diarrhoea ultimately cured by surgery. *European Journal of Gastroenterology & Hepatology*. 1998;10(11):963–7.

# Appendix

## Pituitary function testing

*William M. Drake, Peter J. Trainer*

### *Introduction*

Pituitary function testing for hypopituitarism is required in two quite distinct clinical situations. The first scenario is in the assessment of a new patient in whom the diagnosis of hypopituitarism has been raised. Patients in this group include those with target organ failure (such as hypogonadism or hypoadrenalism) without appropriate elevation of the relevant pituitary trophic hormone; patients with cranial diabetes insipidus; patients with mechanical symptoms consequent upon a pituitary tumor, such as headache and visual failure; and patients in whom a pituitary lesion is documented incidentally during radiological evaluation of an unrelated symptom. The second clinical situation is in the follow-up of patients in whom evolving endocrinopathy is anticipated. External radiotherapy is the best-studied cause of insidious pituitary failure and can be either pituitary-directed treatment or as scatter from therapy for a central nervous system (CNS) or head and neck tumor. With improved imaging, surgery, and medical therapy, radiotherapy is less frequently required in the management of pituitary or peripituitary tumors while the greatly improved prognosis of many CNS, and "head and neck" tumors means such cancer survivors constitute the greater workload but with the confounding complication challenge that they are rarely under surveillance by an endocrinologist. Traumatic brain injury is increasingly recognized as a cause of late, and frequently unrecognized, pituitary failure, that represents particular challenges because head injury is common and the order of development of hormone deficiencies may vary from that seen in most other conditions (see Chapters 1, 5).

Sarcoidosis, Langhan's cell histiocytosis, and other such inflammatory conditions, where progressive hypothalamo–pituitary destruction may occur, can result in the delayed development of hormone deficiencies. Determining, for each subgroup of patients, the optimal frequency of pituitary function testing is not always easy, and, for example, in irradiated patients requires knowledge of the biologically effective dose delivered to the pituitary and hypothalamus.

Hypopituitarism consequent upon a pituitary adenoma and/or its treatment usually develops in a predictable order with growth hormone (GH) deficiency preceding gonadotropin deficiency and failure of thyroid-stimulating hormone (TSH) and adrenocorticotropic hormone (ACTH) secretion occurring later.

For patients in both groups, pituitary function testing may help identify those patients with hypopituitarism sufficiently severe to threaten their safety; and exclude or provide evidence for hormonal deficiencies as a cause of symptoms such as lethargy and fatigue. A sound knowledge of the physiological basis behind pituitary function tests and their limitations is vital if correct decisions are to be made about patient management. This appendix discusses various tests of pituitary function and their interpretation, with the aim of producing a rational, reliable, and safe strategy for diagnosing hypopituitarism. The clinical features and biochemical diagnosis of the various pituitary syndromes of hypersecretion are discussed elsewhere.

# *Principles of pituitary assessment*

The diagnostic evaluation of pituitary function has several complementary limbs involving laboratory and radiological investigations. In new patients with suspected hypopituitarism, clinical suspicion arises because of symptoms related to target organ failure. Hence, it is first necessary to demonstrate target organ hormonal insufficiency, such as low levels of thyroid hormone or gonadal steroid. Paired testing of both hormones in the pituitary-target organ feedback loop, sometimes in combination with provocative testing, will prove that target organ failure is consequent upon lack of stimulation by the relevant pituitary trophic hormone. Additional tests may occasionally be performed to determine whether the pituitary itself is at fault, or whether pituitary failure is secondary to understimulation by the hypothalamus—a distinction that has no bearing on the need for hormone replacement therapy. Magnetic resonance imaging is required to look for possible causes of hypothalamo-pituitary destruction, and together with careful neuro-ophthalmological assessment, helps determine the mechanical effects of any hypothalamo-pituitary mass lesion. Finally, where the cause of pituitary failure is believed to be a systemic illness (such as sarcoidosis), more specific investigations may be needed.

# *Types of laboratory tests*

## *Basal pituitary function tests*

Basal blood tests are taken with the patient resting, unstressed, and with no physiological or pharmacological manipulation of the pituitary cell–target cell feedback loop. Such investigations are performed between 7 and 9 a.m., when serum cortisol and testosterone levels are highest, thereby maximizing the chances of basal investigations yielding sufficient information to avoid the need for more complex tests. Where appropriate, paired measurement of both limbs of a pituitary hormone–target hormone loop is required for interpretation of the target hormone level: low levels of target hormone in association with low or normal levels of the relevant pituitary trophic hormone indicate understimulation by the pituitary as the cause of target gland failure.

## *Stimulation tests*

If basal investigations do not yield sufficient diagnostic information about suspected pituitary cell hypofunction, then provocative tests are used; these tests are complementary to basal investigations rather than being superior to them. Such tests assess the ability of a given cell type to respond acutely to a stimulus, but they do not necessarily provide information about the adequacy of day-to-day hormone production under basal conditions. Two types of provocative tests are used: tests that stimulate hormone release indirectly (such as the insulin stress [tolerance] and glucagon tests) and direct stimulation tests in which pharmacological doses of synthetically manufactured peptide are injected and the target-cell hormone response is measured. Examples include hypothalamic releasing hormone tests and the short Synacthen test (see below). The virtue of indirect provocation tests is that the integrity of an entire hypothalamo–pituitary-target-cell loop is tested.

Hypothalamic releasing hormone tests, with thyrotropin-releasing hormone (TRH), gonadotropin-releasing hormone (GnRH), and growth hormone–releasing hormone (GHRH), discussed below, have no value in the diagnosis of hypopituitarism and cannot predict future pituitary failure. Occasionally, they may help differentiate hypothalamic from pituitary disease, because a normal response to the injection of hypothalamic releasing hormone implies a hypothalamic defect. The major use of releasing hormone tests has been as a tool to increase our understanding of the neuroregulation of pituitary hormone secretion.

# *Hypothalamo-pituitary adrenal axis testing*

This testing is probably the most controversial component of pituitary function testing, mainly because assessment of the adequacy of the hypothalamo–pituitary–adrenal (HPA) axis has the most far-reaching consequences for patient health. Biochemical assessment of the HPA axis is performed in two distinct clinical settings, with the aim of establishing adequate cortisol production being common to both. In some patients, symptoms such as tiredness, listlessness, and malaise lead to an assessment of ACTH reserve, but a more common clinical scenario is that of a patient known to be at risk of developing secondary adrenal insufficiency, due either to previous treatment with supraphysiological doses of corticosteroids; or after surgery and/or radiotherapy directed at the pituitary. In asymptomatic "at-risk patients," it is necessary to assess the patient's ability to mount a response to physiological stress and hence judge the need for emergency steroid cover. Dynamic tests provide an indication of a given patient's ability to respond to physiological stress, but they do not assess the appropriateness of basal, unstressed cortisol secretion. An inadequate "stress response" necessitates steroid cover for surgery, sepsis, and accidental trauma, but it does not automatically indicate a need for life-long glucocorticoid replacement. The limitations of the assessment of the basal cortisol production rate must be borne in mind and consideration given to patients' symptoms and well-being when instigating life-long glucocorticoid replacement.

## Cortisol production in health

Measurement of the target hormone (cortisol) is common to all tests of the HPA axis. Synthesis and secretion of cortisol is controlled by pituitary-derived ACTH that, in turn, is regulated by hypothalamic corticotrophin-releasing hormone (CRH) and vasopressin. A change in cortisol production rate is the "final common pathway" for the effect of various neural and humoral inputs that modulate the system at both hypothalamic and pituitary levels; hence, the use of serum cortisol levels for the assessment of ACTH reserve. It has the added practical advantage of ease of collection, because ACTH samples require cold centrifugation and flash-freezing, whereas cortisol is measured in serum.

The clinical spectrum of ACTH deficiency varies between hypotension with oliguria and electrolyte abnormalities to a more subtle dysfunction precipitated only by acute physiological stress such as major surgery or sepsis. A study of the cortisol response to major abdominal surgery in normal and corticosteroid-treated individuals showed that the peak serum cortisol was at least 580 nmol/L.[1] This study used a fluorimetric method[2] to measure serum cortisol, a technique that, unlike modern radioimmunoassays (RIAs), also detects cortisone. In the same study,[1] serum cortisol responses to hypoglycemia were shown to correlate well with the peak perisurgical serum cortisol measurement. Controlled iatrogenic hypoglycemia is widely accepted as the "gold standard" by which to judge an individual's ability to mount an adequate cortisol response to physiological stress. The adoption of RIA means that the "cut-off" serum cortisol level adequate for physiological stress should be lowered from 580 to 500 nmol/L, because modern RIAs measure approximately 15% lower than fluorometry.[3] This is supported by studies in normal volunteers,[4] although no comparison with cortisol levels during stress has been undertaken.

It is an important point to note that there is considerable variability in serum cortisol measurements according to the assay methodology used.[5] This makes comparisons of cortisol responses between different laboratories extremely difficult and emphasizes the desirability for each endocrine unit to establish its own local reference range, rather than select rigid cut-off values that will almost certainly have been established using different methodologies.

## Measurement of cortisol

Cortisol is generally measured by RIA, although there is a trend toward adoption of tandem mass spectroscopy. Prednisolone, methylprednisolone, and various cortisol metabolites (see "Metyrapone test") all cross-react in cortisol immunoassays, resulting in misleadingly high values, a problem that is eliminated by mass spectroscopy. Serum cortisol measurement refers to total levels, and it must be appreciated that only 5%–10% of cortisol is free and biologically active, with the remainder bound to albumin and cortisol-binding globulin (CBG). Plasma CBG levels therefore significantly alter measurements of serum cortisol. Similar to sex hormone–binding globulin (SHBG), the rate of hepatic CBG synthesis is increased in pregnancy and by oral estrogen preparations that undergo "first-pass" metabolism by the liver. Accurate assessment of the HPA axis in pregnancy is extremely difficult, and oral estrogens should be discontinued 6 weeks before assessment of the HPA axis.[6] Other circumstances in which CBG and albumin levels may complicate assessment of the HPA axis include nephrotic syndrome and hepatic cirrhosis. GH decreases circulating CBG, such that levels are low in acromegaly and fall with initiation of GH therapy in GH-deficient adults. Genetic variation in CBG concentrations and activity (cortisol affinity) is being described with increasing frequency and, although not associated with a phenotype, can be a cause of diagnostic confusion.[7]

Measurement of serum-free cortisol is complex, controversial, and not routinely available, but salivary cortisol measurement is a potential surrogate for serum free cortisol. Although salivary cortisol is extensively used in the investigation of Cushing's syndrome, there are very few data on its use basally or during stimulation tests in the diagnosis of cortisol deficiency. Furthermore, its adoption is inhibited by the differences assay performance (bias), thus there are no consensus criteria for diagnostic cut-offs.

Appreciation of the physiology of the HPA axis is important to interpretation of serum cortisol. First, cortisol is part of a short (pituitary) and a long (hypothalamic) feedback loop, such that falling cortisol levels stimulate a rise in ACTH and CRH secretion from the pituitary and hypothalamus, respectively, and vice versa. Second, in the absence of a trophic signal, the adrenal gland undergoes reversible atrophy, with secondary failure of cortisol production. Last, the normal, diurnal pattern of ACTH and cortisol secretion is dramatically modified by pathophysiological stimuli such as trauma and sepsis.

## Basal serum cortisol

Is it possible to infer from measurements of basal serum cortisol whether the HPA axis is capable of responding normally to stress in a given individual? Conversely, below which level does a basal cortisol measurement make dynamic testing unnecessary to confirm ACTH deficiency? Endogenous HPA activity is maximal in the early morning, and samples should be drawn between 7 and 9 a.m. In cases of suspected pituitary insufficiency, a basal morning serum cortisol of <100 nmol/L strongly indicates ACTH deficiency, dynamic testing is not necessary, and glucocorticoid replacement should commence immediately, and, in most patients, will be permanent. However, in cases of ACTH deficiency before surgery for a pituitary tumor, recovery of ACTH reserve after surgical decompression may occur, and the axis should be reassessed postoperatively. Published evidence suggests that a basal level of 400 nmol/L or above is sufficient to avoid the need for an IST.[8]

In summary, when basal serum cortisol lies between 100 and 400 nmol/L, stimulation test is indicated, but values outside this range indicate adrenal insufficiency and a normally functioning HPA axis, respectively.

## Emergency assessment of the HPA axis

In acutely sick patients with suspected hypoadrenalism, a morning cortisol and/or a dynamic test of ACTH reserve are impractical, and glucocorticoid support must commence immediately. Circadian variation of ACTH release will be absent, and activity of the HPA axis should be maximal. If adrenal insufficiency is suspected, then random serum cortisol and plasma ACTH measurements will suffice. If, subsequently, the random cortisol level is shown to have been appropriate to the clinical situation (>500 nmol/L) glucocorticoids may be withdrawn. If not, steroid support should continue and dynamic testing must follow resolution of the acute clinical situation. A plasma ACTH will differentiate primary from secondary adrenal insufficiency: a serum cortisol <200 nmol/L with a plasma ACTH >200 pg/mL is diagnostic of primary adrenal failure. An elevated plasma renin activity with an inappropriately low serum aldosterone provides additional evidence of primary adrenal disease.

## Insulin stress (tolerance) test (IST) (Table A1.1)

The IST[9] seeks to simulate physiological "stress" in a controlled, supervised environment by inducing hypoglycemia with intravenous, short-acting insulin. Hypoglycemia is a powerful stress stimulus that, in the intact pituitary and hypothalamus, induces ACTH and GH release and a rise in serum cortisol levels. It therefore assesses the integrity of the entire HPA axis and has traditionally been regarded as the gold standard for this purpose. Its reproducibility amongst healthy volunteers is good[10] but not known amongst patients with pituitary disease. The assumption underlying the use of the test is that an ability to respond to insulin-induced hypoglycemia will translate into an appropriate cortisol rise during acute illness or major surgery (see above).

Although some physicians are uncomfortable with the use of the IST, particularly in children, the morbidity of this investigation in experienced hands in a designated metabolic investigation unit is reassuringly low, provided that the exclusion criteria detailed in Table A1.1 are adhered to.[8] The initial dose of insulin used varies in different centers between 0.1 and 0.15 IU/kg, increasing to 0.3 IU/kg for patients with acromegaly, Cushing's syndrome, or other conditions associated with insulin resistance. It is contraindicated in patients with ischemic heart disease or epilepsy and requires careful supervision.

The immediate counterregulatory response to hypoglycemia is characterized by catecholamine release with consequent hepatic short Synacthen test (SST) glycogenolysis and correction of hypoglycemia. Glucocorticoids are not part of this phenomenon, although the laying down of hepatic glycogen stores does require glucocorticoid. Hence, in patients with long-standing ACTH deficiency and inadequate glycogen stores, recovery from hypoglycemia may be delayed. It is usual practice to administer oral glucose in the form of a sugary drink, together with a meal, at the conclusion of the test.

## Short Synacthen test (Table A1.2)

This investigation was originally introduced as a test for primary adrenal failure[11] and involves the injection of a pharmacological dose (250 μg) of synthetic ACTH, with measurement of the serum cortisol response. The basis of its use in the context of hypopituitarism, as an alternative to the IST, is that chronic underexposure of the adrenal

| *Indications* | *Assessment of ACTH and GH reserve* |
|---|---|
| Contraindications | Ischemic heart disease |
| | Epilepsy/unexplained syncopal episodes |
| | Severe hypoadrenalism (basal serum cortisol <100 nmol/L) |
| | Glycogen storage disease |
| | Untreated hypothyroidism |
| Protocol | Must be performed by experienced metabolic nurse and/or physician |
| | Resting electrocardiogram (ECG) to be certified normal by attendant physician |
| | Ensure emergency intravenous dextrose and dexamethasone available |
| | Patient must be fasting from 2400 hours |
| | Insert intravenous cannula approximately 30 min before commencement of test |
| | Draw sample for basal cortisol |
| | Administer 0.15 IU/kg soluble insulin (e.g., Actrapid®) as a bolus |
| | Document clinical signs of neuroglycopenia. If not present after 45 min, consider repeating same dose of insulin |
| | In cases of severe, prolonged hypoglycemia, syncope or presyncope, termination of the test with intravenous dextrose should be seriously considered. Continue sampling |
| | Draw samples for plasma glucose (fluoride bottle), cortisol, and GH (both serum) at 30, 45, 60, 90, and 120 min |
| | Glucose drink and meal at conclusion of test |
| | NB. Patients with active Cushing's syndrome, acromegaly, and other causes of insulin resistance may be insulin resistant and require 0.3 IU/kg of soluble insulin |
| Interpretation | Plasma glucose <2.2 mmol/L with symptoms and signs of neuroglycopenia necessary for assessment of the adequacy of the stimulus to ACTH/GH release |
| | Serum cortisol should rise >500 nmol/L |
| | Peak GH 3 μg/L or less indicates severe GHD |

***Table A1.1***
*Protocol for the ITT test.*

glands to ACTH will result in a blunted cortisol response to exogenously administered ACTH. The test does not distinguish primary from secondary adrenal insufficiency: clinical assessment (pigmentation) and measurement of basal plasma ACTH are usually sufficient for this distinction. The major argument in favor of the SST is its simplicity, because it requires no specialist staff and takes only an hour to complete. The SST does not assess GH reserve. It is universally accepted that the SST cannot be used for the assessment of ACTH reserve in acute hypopituitarism, such as after pituitary infarction (apoplexy) or immediately postoperatively. It takes at least 2 weeks for the adrenal zona fasciculata to involute after withdrawal of ACTH stimulation, during which time the adrenal cortex will remain responsive to supraphysiological doses of ACTH. In addition, it should be remembered, in the assessment of new patients with suspected hypothalamic–pituitary disease that the duration of ACTH deficiency may be unknown and that, as after pituitary surgery or apoplexy, a falsely reassuring cortisol response may result.

The increment in serum cortisol after Synacthen has been advocated as a measure of the ability of the HPA axis to respond to stress, but it is a poor index of adrenal responsiveness, because there is considerable overlap between normal volunteers and patients with secondary adrenal insufficiency.[12] Furthermore, the cortisol increment is inversely correlated with the basal value; hence, a smaller increment is seen in the early morning when plasma ACTH and serum cortisol levels are at their highest.[13] The peak serum cortisol response after Synacthen shows no diurnal variation and is now the accepted index of adrenal responsiveness.

Serum cortisol levels 30 min after injection of Synacthen and the peak cortisol achieved during an IST

| *Indications* | *Assessment of ACTH and GH deficiency in cases where IST contraindicated* |
|---|---|
| Contraindications | Glycogen storage disease |
| | Severe hypoadrenalism (basal cortisol <100 nmol/L) |
| | Untreated hypothyroidism |
| Protocol | Patient must be fasting from 2400 hours |
| | Insert intravenous cannula approximately 30 minutes before commencement of test |
| | Draw sample for basal cortisol |
| | Administer 1 mg of glucagon s.c. (1.5 mg if >90 kg) |
| | Draw samples for plasma glucose (fluoride bottle), cortisol, and GH (both serum) at 90, 120, 150, 180, 210, and 240 min |
| Interpretation | Plasma glucose should peak at 90 min |
| | Serum cortisol should rise >500 nmol/L |

***Table A1.2***
*Protocol for glucagon stimulation test.*

are clearly correlated, and it is argued by some that the IST can be restricted to patients who fail to reach a given threshold 30 min post-Synacthen cortisol level (usually between 550 and 600 nmol/L), or who require simultaneous assessment of GH reserve. The SST is increasingly being used in preference to the IST.

Despite its increasing use as a test of ACTH reserve, there is no study showing that a normal SST indicates that the HPA axis is capable of responding normally to major illness or stress. Critics of the use of the SST point to reports of patients with pituitary disease with symptoms and signs of adrenal failure, corrected by glucocorticoid replacement, having recently had a reassuringly "normal" SST. This problem cannot be corrected by application of a more "stringent" threshold of serum cortisol as in two such reported patients the peak serum cortisol value was >950 nmol/L 30 min after Synacthen. However, it should be stressed that reports exist of patients who have developed acute adrenal crisis after a "normal" IST. SSTs should be initiated at 9 a.m. or earlier as under such circumstances a low basal (time 0) cortisol should arouse suspicion of hypoadrenalism and reduce the risk of false reassurance based on a good peak serum cortisol.

The SST is very safe and side effects are rare, but catastrophic anaphylaxis has been reported, with a history of atopy being a risk. This side effect is particularly relevant when testing the HPA axis in asthmatics on exogenous glucocorticoid therapy.

## *Low-dose short Synacthen test*

There have been reports of the use of a very low dose of ACTH (typically 1 μg) for the assessment of secondary hypoadrenalism because the conventional dose of 250 μg produces plasma concentrations that are supraphysiological and beyond the top of the ACTH/cortisol dose–response curve. Proponents of the low-dose SST argue that chronically understimulated adrenal glands may mount a satisfactory cortisol response to unphysiological concentrations of ACTH but that only normal glands will respond to 1 μg. Plasma ACTH levels after injection of 1 μg are comparable to those reached during an IST in healthy volunteers.[14] The test is quick (a single sample only is drawn 30 min after injection of ACTH) and may be performed at any time of day.

A study of the cortisol responses to the standard and low-dose ACTH tests and to the IST in patients with suspected or proven pituitary disease[15] showed that, when a serum cortisol of 500 nmol/L was used as a "pass" on the IST, the low-dose short Synacthen test (LDSST) had a sensitivity of 100% and specificity of 80% with an adequate response defined as a serum cortisol >600 nmol/L. In other words, there was no patient in whom a serum cortisol level of >600 nmol/L provided false reassurance about their ability to pass the IST. A serum cortisol level <600 nmol/L after 1 μg ACTH indicated the need for an IST and the study advocates the LDSST as a screening procedure for the investigation of secondary ACTH deficiency, reserving the IST for patients with a borderline response. In a comparison of normal volunteers and patients with pituitary disease, false reassurance was provided in 70% of patients with known secondary adrenal failure by using a 30-min serum cortisol value after injection of 5 or 250 μg of ACTH, whereas the 1-μg LDSST identified all patients with proven ACTH deficiency.[16] This may partly be accounted for by the use of different protocols for ACTH dilution.

Although the LDSST is theoretically an attractive proposition, its widespread adoption is hindered by the absence of a commercial 1-μg preparation of ACTH. Currently, the diagnostic accuracy of the LDSST test is premised upon the reproducibility of 250-fold dilution of a 1-mL vial of Synacthen compounded by the concern about the extent to which ACTH may be adsorbed onto the plastic of syringes or saline bags. Improved standardization and reproducibility of the LDSST are required before its widespread recommendation for the assessment of ACTH deficiency.[17]

## *Glucagon stimulation test (Table A1.3)*

The subcutaneous injection of glucagon, by unknown mechanisms, induces ACTH and GH release, and this response has led to its widespread use as a means of assessing the reserve of these two hormones. Glucagon is a less potent and reliable stimulus of ACTH release than hypoglycemia and false-negative results are common. Its injection makes patients feel unwell with nausea and, occasionally, abdominal pain and vomiting, but serious complications are very rare. The glucagon test has not been as extensively studied as other investigations, and its interpretation relies upon criteria established for the IST. However, it remains a useful method of assessing the HPA and GH axes, particularly when the IST is contraindicated.[18]

## *Metyrapone test*

Metyrapone inhibits 11β-hydroxylase, the final enzyme involved in cortisol synthesis. The fall in cortisol levels that follow administration of metyrapone stimulates ACTH release from the intact pituitary; corticosteroidogenesis increases; and serum levels of cortisol precursors such as 11-deoxycortisol, which lacks glucocorticoid action and does not suppress ACTH secretion, rise. In patients with secondary adrenal insufficiency, a fall in cortisol does not stimulate an increase in ACTH secretion; hence, no rise in 11-deoxycortisol level occurs. A typical protocol entails oral administration of 30 mg/kg metyrapone in the hospital at midnight. Simultaneous cortisol and 11-deoxycortisol levels are taken between 8 and 9 a.m. and oral glucocorticoids are subsequently administered if the index of suspicion of ACTH deficiency is high. An 11-deoxycortisol level of >200 nmol/L indicates normal adrenal function, whereas levels <200 nmol/L strongly suggest secondary adrenal insufficiency.[19] A low 9 a.m. serum cortisol (as evidence of adequate pituitary stimulation) is required for the interpretation of the test. Anticonvulsant therapy such as phenytoin accelerates the metabolism of metyrapone, and an alternative test of the HPA axis should be used in such patients.

A major limitation on the widespread adoption of the metyrapone test has been the challenge of the accurate measurement of 11-deoxycortisol and cortisol, in the presence of elevated 11-deoxycortisol levels. Even in cortisol assays that purport to have minimal cross-reactivity for 11-deoxycortisol, our studies have indicated this is not necessarily to be the case with significant overestimation of circulating cortisol levels.[20] 11-Deoxycortisol assays are not available for most of the commercial multichannel analyzers; therefore, the assay can be expensive and labor-intensive, with delayed results due to sample batching. Mass spectroscopy overcomes the problems of cross-reactivity and allows simultaneous measurement of both steroids in a single analytical run.

| *Indications* | *Assessment primary and secondary adrenal failure* |
|---|---|
| Contraindications | History of atopy |
| Protocol | Nonfasting |
| | Insert intravenous cannula approximately 30 min before commencement of test |
| | Draw sample for basal cortisol |
| | Administer 250 μg of Synacthen intramuscularly |
| | Draw samples for cortisol at 30 and 60 min |
| Interpretation | The 30-min cortisol should rise to at least 550 nmol/L (most useful during longitudinal follow-up of a patient known to be at risk of developing secondary adrenal failure (e.g., after pituitary irradiation) |

***Table A1.3***
*Protocol for short Synacthen test.*

The increasing access to mass spectroscopy may make the metyrapone test, an intrinsically more physiological test, a preferable alternative to the SST, particularly in patients with asthma on glucocorticoid therapy.

## Conclusions

It is inevitable that the debate about the optimum method for the assessment of the HPA axis will continue. Practical issues such as cost and staff availability will, to a large extent, affect local policy but the fundamental clinical issue of patient safety remains the same. Dynamic tests of the integrity of the HPA axis support, rather than substitute for, clinical decisions, and it is important to recognize that the use of sophisticated statistical methods for the comparison of serum cortisol levels in groups of people with or without endocrine disease can never substitute for clinical awareness in the individual patient. Even the IST cannot provide complete reassurance that an individual will not develop secondary adrenal insufficiency during physiological stress. Changes in methodology and regional variation in the assays used for cortisol measurements hinder comparisons between published experiences of HPA testing and make it difficult to recommend the use of a single protocol. Endocrine physicians should educate their patients about the implications of pituitary disease in terms of the stress response, particularly when an evolving endocrine deficit is anticipated, such as after pituitary irradiation. The IST is the single most reliable test of the ability of the HPA axis to respond to stress but should only be performed under close supervision in specialist centers. If there is any doubt about the adequacy of ACTH reserve, it is sensible to err on the side of caution with respect to the provision of emergency steroid cover and to consider a trial of oral glucocorticoid replacement therapy in patients with symptoms suggestive of chronic adrenal insufficiency and an equivocal response to dynamic testing. A suboptimal peak cortisol response to a dynamic test does not equate to a subnormal basal cortisol production rate and should not result in automatic initiation of life-long glucocorticoid replacement therapy.[21]

# Pituitary–thyroid axis

Diagnosing TSH deficiency, and the initiation of replacement therapy, in a timely manner is a major challenge. TSH is rarely undetectable in hypopituitarism but more typically is in the lower part of the reference range and therefore cannot be used in isolation in the diagnosis of secondary hypothyroidism.

Similar to other pituitary cell types, thyrotrophs interact with their target cells by feedback inhibition, although the diurnal and ultradian variations that characterize ACTH and GH release are less marked. Secondary hypothyroidism is strongly suggested by low levels of circulating thyroxine in the presence of a low or low normal TSH, with stimulation tests having no part to play. The difficulty is that to wait until thyroxine levels are below the lower limit of the reference range implies the patient will be symptomatically hypothyroid. In the context of TSH deficiency, the thyroxine level may fall significantly while still remaining in the reference range, and the goal must be to intervene before levels are subnormal. Knowledge of the status of the other pituitary hormones is important as TSH deficiency is one of the last hormones to be affected by any insult to the pituitary. If a patient with pituitary disease is not GH or gonadotropin deficient, then TSH deficiency is improbable. For several decades, there has been little progress in diagnosing TSH deficiency or defining the moment for introducing levothyroxine (T4) replacement therapy, but recently the concept of a TSH concentration corrected for the thyroxine level has been described (the "TSH index"). Preliminary data suggest that TSH index may have a role in identifying patients with TSH deficiency, although further work is required to validate these findings.[22]

The differential diagnosis of TSH deficiency includes illness ("sick euthyroid" syndrome), thyroxine-binding globulin deficiency, supraphysiological doses of glucocorticoids, and drugs such as phenytoin also may produce a similar picture. The interpretation of the results is dependent on the overall clinical context and is assisted by measurement of free T4 and tissue markers of thyroid hormone action such as SHBG.

## TRH testing

TRH testing is of no value in diagnosing secondary hypothyroidism or predicting imminent TSH deficiency. In normal individuals, intravenous injection of TRH produces a rise in TSH, with levels at 20 min being greater than those at 60 min. Patients with hypothalamic disease classically show a delayed response to TRH, with the 60-min value greater than that at 20 min. Patients with pituitary disease typically have an absent TSH response to TRH, although it is recognized that some patients will respond. This is thought to be due to the fact that some pituitary tumors cause functional disconnection of the hypothalamus from the pituitary, thereby simulating a hypothalamic lesion. Renal failure, depression, malnutrition, and extreme illness may all be associated with delayed or absent TRH responses. The TRH test is associated with syncope and carries a small risk of precipitating pituitary apoplexy in patients with pituitary tumors. The TRH test is now very seldom used in the assessment of pituitary function.

## GH axis

Normal GH secretion is pulsatile; in adults, four to six pulses per 24 h punctuate long periods when GH levels in the blood are extremely low. Hence, basal blood samples are unlikely to yield significant diagnostic information, unless it coincides with a GH surge. Measurement of 24-hr spontaneous GH profiles has been used in children but has proved disappointing in adult practice because considerable overlap exists between the integrated growth hormone concentration (IGHC) of normal subjects and those of hypopituitary patients.[23] Sleep and exercise are both associated with GH release, but assessing GH secretion by these methods is prohibitively time-consuming for routine clinical use.

Most, if not all, actions of GH are mediated through insulin-like growth factor (IGF)-I. However, measurement of serum IGF-I is of limited value in the diagnosis of adult-onset growth hormone deficiency (GHD), because 30% of patients with proven severe GHD have a serum IGF-I in the lower part of the age-related normal range,[24] but a serum IGF-I below the age-related reference range in the presence of pituitary disease is strongly indicative of GH deficiency. Proof of GHD by two dynamic tests is the current requirement for the prescription of recombinant human (rh) GH in many countries.

Pharmacological stimulation of GH release is the most practical and reproducible method of assessing GH reserve and the IST (see above) has been the most frequently used test in this regard. Severe GHD is defined as a peak GH response of 3 μg/L or less,[25] although variability (bias) in GH assays between centers must be borne in mind when applying international consensus guidelines to local practice.

Where the IST is contraindicated, alternative provocative tests of GH reserve include the glucagon (Table A1.2) and arginine tests. Arginine stimulates GH release, with a peak occurring between 30 and 120 min after infusion and is frequently used when a second dynamic test of GH reserve is required and the IST is contraindicated. It involves the intravenous infusion of 0.5 g/kg (maximum dose 30 g) in 100 mL of normal saline over 30 min and sampling for 2 hr thereafter. Clonidine testing is of no value for the diagnosis of GHD in adults.

Growth hormone secretagogue testing with GHRH and GHRP has fallen out of favor due to the lack of commercial supplies of the various secretagogues.

## Assessment of the pituitary–gonadal axis

Regular menstruation in a woman implies normal gonadotroph function and measurement of gonadotropins and estradiol add little to the clinical assessment. Ovulation is not necessarily implied by regular menstruation: measurement of luteal phase progesterone levels is required for the assessment of subfertility in a patient with pituitary disease and a regular cycle. Unlike hydrocortisone and thyroxine substitution, social and age-related factors may influence the need to correct any underlying gonadal deficiency in men and women. The benefits of gonadal steroid replacement in terms of avoiding cardiovascular complications and loss of bone mineral density must be set against the temporal relationship of normal physiology. For example, an 80-year-old patient with secondary hypogonadism is likely to feel differently about gonadal steroid replacement therapy than a patient of 30.

Basal measurements of gonadotropin hormones and sex steroid levels are usually sufficient for assessment of the pituitary–gonadal axis. Estradiol and testosterone bind to SHBG: simultaneous measurement of SHBG and gonadal steroid levels is therefore required to assess the "free" (biologically active) levels of these hormones. Testosterone is measured at 9 a.m., because levels show considerable diurnal variation. Estradiol is best measured in the follicular phase of the menstrual cycle, if patients are menstruating. Ovulation is assessed by measurement of progesterone in the luteal phase (days 18–25) of the cycle.

Dynamic tests may help in the differential diagnosis of secondary gonadal failure but do not significantly alter clinical management. Previously, a combination of clomiphene and luteinizing hormone (LH)–releasing hormone (LHRH) tests were believed to provide useful evidence in distinguishing hypothalamic from pituitary causes of secondary gonadal failure. Such information has little clinical value, because modern radiological imaging is usually able to distinguish these two groups of causes. Central hypogonadism may be isolated;

it may occur in the context of a hypothalamo-pituitary tumor or its treatment, or it may be the earliest sign of incipient panhypopituitarism. Isolated gonadotropin deficiency is either congenital (e.g., Kallman's syndrome) where it is associated with delayed/absent pubertal development, or acquired and secondary to systemic illness (e.g., AIDS), excessive exercise (e.g., long-distance runners), opiate use, or psychological disturbance (e.g., anorexia nervosa). In all cases, detailed pituitary function testing and imaging is mandatory.

## *Gonadotropin-releasing hormone testing*

GnRH (LHRH) stimulates LH and follicle-stimulating hormone (FSH) release from the pituitary in a dose-dependent manner between 25 and 100 µg. An absent response is characterized by a failure to rise above three times the within-assay coefficient of variation of the basal values. The GnRH test is not used for the diagnosis of hypogonadism but may assist in establishing its etiology, although with modern imaging techniques is rarely indicated.

In a patient with secondary hypogonadism, a normal response to GnRH implies that hypogonadism is the result of understimulation by the hypothalamus. This may be due to a hypothalamic lesion or disconnection of the pituitary from the hypothalamus by a functional pituitary stalk lesion. Occasionally, the GnRH test also may provide an index of hypothalamic function. GnRH is required for both LH synthesis and release, such that flat or subnormal responses may both be seen in hypothalamic disease with GnRH deficiency.

# *Prolactin*

A clinical syndrome due to prolactin deficiency is not recognized and its measurement serves only as a guide to the etiology of hypopituitarism. Prolactin physiology differs from that of other anterior pituitary hormones in that its secretion is principally under tonic inhibition by release of dopamine from the hypothalamus. Levels do not show significant diurnal variation and so tests other than basal measurements are very rarely required. Physiological stress and various medications that interfere with dopamine action, such as metoclopramide, prochlorperazine, and various antipsychotics, raise serum prolactin. TRH stimulates prolactin release, but it provides no extra information compared with random serum prolactin measurements, on three separate occasions, to minimize the risk of falsely elevated stress-induced hyperprolactinemia.

# *Conclusions*

Accurate assessment of anterior pituitary function requires a sound knowledge of its normal physiology together with careful integration of clinical and biochemical information. Certain aspects of the optimum method of pituitary function testing, notably the assessment of ACTH reserve, are not universally agreed, such that local circumstances and personal preference may dictate the final choice. Physicians are advised to acquaint themselves with their local laboratory reference ranges and not to allow single hormonal measurements to substitute for clinical awareness, particularly where an evolving endocrine deficit is anticipated, such as after pituitary irradiation. The following protocol is proposed as a reliable and safe strategy for the assessment of suspected hypopituitarism.

## *New patients*

Basal investigations, at 7–9 a.m.: (All serum)

- Cortisol
- Free T4, TSH
- Prolactin
- LH, FSH, testosterone/estradiol, SHBG
- IGF-I
- Urine/plasma osmolality

If basal serum cortisol <400 nmol/L and/or GHD suspected, then proceed to IST. If any abnormality in any of the above-mentioned tests, then proceed to pituitary imaging.

## *At-risk patients*

In at-risk patients (e.g., those who have received pituitary radiotherapy), pituitary function tests should be performed regularly to detect asymptomatic hypopituitarism, although there is a paucity of data on the optimum frequency with which this should be done. Our practice is to check basal pituitary function (0700–0900 h) every year, with a dynamic test of ACTH reserve if the basal serum cortisol is <400 nmol/L every 2 years. If patients exhibit the syndrome of GHD, then the dynamic test of choice will be the IST. GHD occurs early after radiotherapy and, once it has been proven, many physicians use sequential SSTs to document the evolution of ACTH deficiency. Again, data in this regard are scarce such that accurate, robust local reference ranges are essential.

# *References*


1. Plumpton FS, Besser GM. The adrenocortical respone to surgery and insulin-induced hypoglycaemia in corticosteroid-treated and normal subjects. *Br J Surg* (1969); 56: 216–19.
2. Mattingley D. A simple fluorimetric method for the estimation of free 11-hydroxycorticoids in human plasma. *J Clin Pathol* (1962); 15: 374–9.
3. Gashell SJ, Collins CJ, Thorne GC, et al. External quality assessment of assays for cortisol in plasma: Use of target data obtained by GC/mass spectrometry. *Clin Chem* (1983); 29: 862–7.
4. Hurel SJ, Thompson CJ, Watson MJ, et al. The short Synacthen and insulin stress tests in the assessment of the hypothalamic–pituitary–adrenal axis. *Clin Endocrinol* (1996); 44: 141–6.
5. Clark PM, Neylon I, Raggatt PR, et al. Defining the normal cortisol response to the short Synacthen test: Implications for the investigation of hypothalamic-pituitary disorders. *Clin Endocrinol* (1998); 49: 287–92.
6. Brien TG. Human corticosteroid binding globulin. *Clin Endocrinol* (1981); 14: 193–212.
7. Lin HY, Underhill C, Lei JH, et al. High frequency of SERPINA6 polymorphisms that reduce plasma corticosteroid-binding globulin activity in Chinese subjects. *J Clin Endocrinol Metab* (2012); 97: E678–86.
8. Jones SL, Trainer PJ, Perry L, et al. An audit of the insulin tolerance test in adult subjects in an acute investigation unit over one year. *Clin Endocrinol* (1995); 42: 101–2.
9. Greenwood FC, Landon J, Stamp TCB. The plasma sugar, free fatty acid, cortisol and growth hormone response to insulin. *J Clin Invest* (1966); 4: 429–36.
10. Vestergara P, Hoeck HC, Jakobsen PE, et al. Reproducibility of growth hormone and cortisol response to the insulin tolerance test and the short ACTH test in normal adults. *Horm Metab Res* (1997); 29: 106–10.
11. Wood JB, Frankland AW, James VHT, et al. A rapid test of adrenocortical function. *Lancet* (1965); 1: 243–5.
12. Speckart PF, Nicolff JT, Bethune JE. Screening for adrenocortical insufficiency with cosyntropin (synthetic ACTH). *Arch Intern Med* (1971); 128: 761–3.
13. May ME, Carey RM. Rapid adrenocorticotropic hormone test in practice. *Am J Med* (1985); 79: 679–84.
14. Lindholm J, Kehlet H. Re-evaluation of the clinical value of the 30 min ACTH test in assessing hypothalamo–pituitary–adrenal function. *Clin Endocrinol* (1987); 26: 53–9.
15. Abdu TAM, Elhadd TA, Neary R, et al. Comparison of the low dose short synacthen test (1 μg), the conventional dose short synacthen test (250 μg), and the insulin tolerance test for assessment of the hypothalamo–pituitary–adrenal axis in patients with pituitary disease. *J Clin Endocrinol Metab* (1998); 84: 838–43.
16. Tjordman K, Jaffe A, Grazas N, et al. The role of low dose (1 μg) adrenocorticotropin test in the evaluation of patients with pituitary diseases. *J Clin Endocrinol Metab* (1995); 80: 1301–5.
17. Streeten DHP. Shortcomings in the low-dose (1 μg) ATH test for the diagnosis of ACTH deficiency states. *J Clin Endocrinol Metab* (1999); 84: 835–7.
18. Littley MD, Gibson S, White A, et al. Comparison of the ACTH and cortisol responses to provocative testing with glucagon and insulin hypoglycaemia in normal subjects. *Clin Endocrinol* (1989); 31: 527–33.
19. Spiger M, Jubiz W, Meidle W, et al. Single-dose metyrapone test. *Arch Intern Med* (1975); 135: 698–700.
20. Monaghan PJ, Owen LJ, Trainer PJ, et al. Comparison of serum cortisol measurement by immunoassay and liquid chromatography–tandem mass spectrometry in patients receiving the 11β-hydroxylase inhibitor metyrapone. *Ann Clin Biochem* (2011); 48: 441–6.
21. Paisley AN, Rowles SV, Brandon D, et al. A subnormal peak cortisol response to stimulation testing does not predict a subnormal cortisol production rate. *J Clin Endocrinol Metab* (2009); 94: 1757–60.
22. Jostel A, Ryder D, Shalet S. The use of thyroid function tests in the diagnosis of hypopituitarism: Definition and evaluation of the TSH index. *Clin Endocrinol* (2009); 71: 529–34.
23. Shalet SM, Toogood A, Rahim A, et al. The diagnosis of GH deficiency in children and adults. *Endocr Rev* (1998); 19: 203–23.
24. Hoffman DM, O'Sullivan AJ, Baxter RC, et al. Diagnosis of growth hormone deficiency in adults. *Lancet* (1994); 343: 1064–8.
25. Anonymous. Consensus guidelines for the diagnosis and treatment of adults with growth hormone deficiency: Summary statement of the Growth Hormone Research Society Workshop on adult growth hormone deficiency. *J Clin Endocrinol Metab* (1998); 83: 379–81.

# Index

Printed and bound by CPI Group (UK) Ltd, Croydon, CR0 4YY
18/10/2024
01776231-0002